BEHAVIORAL NEUROLOGY AND NEUROPSYCHOLOGY

NOTICE

BEHAVIORAL NEUROLOGY AND NEUROPSYCHOLOGY

EDITORS

Todd E. Feinberg, M.D.

Chief
Betty and Morton Yarmon Division of Neurobehavior and Alzheimer's Disease
Associate Attending, Psychiatry and Neurology
Beth Israel Medical Center
New York, New York
Associate Professor, Neurology and Psychiatry
Albert Einstein College of Medicine
Bronx, New York

Martha J. Farah, PH.D.

Professor of Psychology
Department of Psychology
University of Pennsylvania
Philadelphia, Pennsylvania

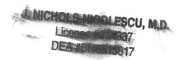

McGraw-Hill
HEALTH PROFESSIONS DIVISION

New York   St. Louis   San Francisco   Auckland   Bogotá
Caracas   Lisbon   London   Madrid   Mexico City   Milan   Montreal
New Delhi   San Juan   Singapore   Sydney   Tokyo   Toronto

McGraw-Hill

*A Division of The **McGraw·Hill** Companies*

BEHAVIORAL NEUROLOGY AND NEUROPSYCHOLOGY

Copyright © 1997 by The McGraw-Hill Companies, Inc. All rights reserved.
Printed in the United States of America. Except as permitted under the
United States copyright Act of 1976, no part of this publication may be
reproduced or distributed in any form or by any means, or stored in a data
base or retrieval system, without the prior written permission of the publisher.

34567890   DOC DOC   98

ISBN 0-07-020361-X

This book was set in Times Roman by Bi-Comp, Inc.
The editors were Joseph A. Hefta and Lester A. Sheinis.
The production supervisor was Richard C. Ruzycka.
The cover designer was Robert Freese.
The indexer was Tony Greenberg, M.D.
R. R. Donnelley & Sons Company was printer and binder.

This book is printed on acid-free paper.

Library of Congress Cataloging-in-Publication Data

Feinberg, Todd E.
    Behavioral neurology and neuropsychology / Todd E. Feinberg,
Martha J. Farah.
       p. cm.
    Includes bibliographical references and index.
    ISBN 0-07-020361-X (alk. paper)
    1. Clinical neuropsychology. 2. Neuropsychiatry. I. Farah,
Martha J.
    [DNLM: 1. Nervous System Diseases. 2. Neuropsychology. WL 140
F299b 1997]
RC341.F36 1997
616.8—dc20
DNLM/DLC
for Library of Congress   95-39574

CONTENTS

v

PART 3   DISORDERS OF PERCEPTION, ATTENTION, AND AWARENESS   237

CONTRIBUTORS

Michael P. Alexander, M.D.
Director, Stroke Rehabilitation program
Braintree Hospital
Braintree, Massachusetts
Department of Neurology
Boston University School of Medicine
Boston, Massachusetts
(Chapter 9)

**Russell M. Bauer, Ph.D., A.B.P.P./
A.B.C.N.**
Associate Professor
Center for Neuropsychological Studies
Departments of Clinical and Health Psychology and
Neurology
University of Florida
Gainesville, Florida
(Chapter 20)

Kathleen Baynes, Ph.D.
Assistant Professor of Neurology
Center for Neuroscience
University of California at Davis
Davis, California
(Chapter 32)

D. Frank Benson, M.D.
Augustus S. Rose Professor of Neurology
Neurology Department
UCLA School of Medicine
Los Angeles, California
(Chapter 30)

Jane Holmes Bernstein, Ph.D.
Assistant Clinical Professor of Psychology
Department of Psychiatry
Harvard Medical School
Director, Neuropsychology Program
Children's Hospital Medical Center
Boston, Massachusetts
(Chapter 59)

F. William Black, Ph.D.
Professor of Psychiatry and Neurology
Director, Neuropsychological Laboratory
Tulane Medical Center
New Orleans, Louisiana
(Chapter 2)

Dana Boatman, Ph.D.
Assistant Professor
Department of Neurology and Cognitive Science
Johns Hopkins Medical Institution
Baltimore, Maryland
(Chapter 53)

François Boller, M.D., Ph.D.
Professor of Neurology
Director of Research
Institut National de la Santé et de la Recherche
Médicale (INSERM)
Paris, France
(Chapter 41)

**John V. Bowler, M.B., B.S., M.D.,
M.R.C.P.(UK)**
Lecturer in Neurology
Academic Unit of Neuroscience
Charing Cross and Westminster Medical School
London, England
(Chapter 46)

Richard J. Caselli, M.D.
Associate Professor of Neurology
Chairman
Division of Behavioral Neurology
Mayo Medical School
Rochester, Minnesota
Department of Neurology
Mayo Clinic
Scottsdale, Arizona
(Chapter 21)

Laird S. Cermak, Ph.D.
Professor of Neurology (Neuropsychology)
Boston University School of Medicine
Director, Memory Disorders Research Center
Department of Veterans Affairs Medical Center
Boston, Massachusetts
(Chapter 48)

H. Branch Coslett, M.D.
Professor of Neurology
Department of Neurology
Temple University School of Medicine
Philadelphia, Pennsylvania
(Chapter 13)

Bruce Crosson, Ph.D.
Associate Professor
Department of Clinical and Health Psychology and
Neurology
Health Science Center
University of Florida
Gainesville, Florida
(Chapter 33)

Jeffrey L. Cummings, M.D.
Professor of Neurology and Psychology
UCLA School of Medicine
Los Angeles, California
(Chapter 40)

Tim Curran, Ph.D.
Assistant Professor of Psychology
Department of Psychology
Case Western Reserve University
Cleveland, Ohio
(Chapter 36)

Antonio R. Damasio, M.D., Ph.D.
M. W. Van Allen Professor and Head of Neurology
University of Iowa College of Medicine
Adjunct Professor
Salk Institute for Biological Studies
La Jolla, California
(Chapter 5)

Hanna Damasio, M.D.
Professor of Neurology
Director of the Human Neuroanatomy and
Neuroimaging Laboratory
University of Iowa College of Medicine
Adjunct Professor
Salk Institute for Biological Studies
La Jolla, California
(Chapter 5)

Martha Bridge Denckla, M.D.
Professor of Neurology, Pediatrics, and Psychiatry
Johns Hopkins University School of Medicine
Director, Developmental Cognitive Neurology
Director, Learning Disabilities Research Center
Kennedy Krieger Institute
Baltimore, Maryland
(Chapter 58)

Maureen Dennis, Ph.D.
Senior Scientist
Department of Psychology and Research Institute
The Hospital for Sick Children
Associate Professor
Department of Surgery, Faculty of Medicine
University of Toronto
Toronto, Ontario, Canada
(Chapter 60)

Ennio De Renzi, M.D.
Professor of Neurology
Chief, Neurological Department
University of Modena
Modena, Italy
(Chapters 18, 23)

Mark D'Esposito, M.D.
Assistant Professor
Department of Neurology
University of Pennsylvania Medical Center
Philadelphia, Pennsylvania
(Chapter 31)

Orrin Devinsky, M.D.
Department of Neurology
NYU Medical Center
Hospital for Joint Diseases
New York, New York
(Chapter 51)

Charles Duyckaerts, M.D., Ph.D.
Professor of Pathology
Laboratoire de Neuropathologie R. Escourolle
Hôpital de la Salpêtrière
Paris, France
(Chapter 41)

Martha J. Farah, Ph.D.
Professor of Psychology
Department of Psychology
University of Pennsylvania
Philadelphia, Pennsylvania
(Chapters 1, 8, 17, 27, 31, 37)

Todd E. Feinberg, M.D.
Chief
Betty and Morton Yarmon Division of
Neurobehavior and Alzheimer's Disease
Associate Attending, Psychiatry and Neurology
Beth Israel Medical Center
New York, New York
Associate Professor, Neurology and Psychiatry
Albert Einstein College of Medicine
Bronx, New York
(Chapters 1, 17, 27, 28, 29)

Ruth B. Fink, M.A., C.C.C.-S.L.P.
Research Associate
Neuropsychology Research Laboratory
Moss Rehabilitation Research Institute
Philadelphia, Pennsylvania
(Chapter 12)

Nancy N. Futrell, M.D.
Associate Professor of Neurology
Associate Professor of Biochemistry and Molecular
Biology
Medical College of Ohio
Department of Neurology
Director, Stroke Division
Toledo, Ohio
(Chapter 49)

Douglas Galasko, M.D.
Associate Professor, Department of Neurosciences
(Neurology)
University of California, San Diego
San Diego, California
(Chapter 43)

Michael S. Gazzaniga, Ph.D.
Director, Center for Neuroscience
Professor of Neurology and Psychology
University of California at Davis
Davis, California
(Chapter 32)

Guido Gainotti, M.D.
Professor, Neurological Rehabilitation
Director, Neuropsychology Service
Universita Cattolica del Sacro Cuove
Facolta di Medicine e Chirurgia
Agostino Gemelli
Intituto di Clinica Mentali
Rome, Italy
(Chapter 55)

Elizabeth L. Glisky, Ph.D.
Associate Professor of Psychology
Department of Psychology
University of Arizona
Tucson, Arizona
(Chapter 39)

Georg Goldenberg, M.D.
Neuropsychological Department
Krankenhaus München Bogenhausen
Munich, Germany
(Chapter 22)

Barry Gordon, M.D., Ph.D.
Associate Professor
Department of Neurology and Cognitive Science
Cognitive Neurology
Johns Hopkins Medical Institution
Baltimore, Maryland
(Chapter 53)

**Neill R. Graff-Radford, M.B.B.Ch.,
M.R.C.P. (UK)**
Professor of Neurology
Mayo Medical School
Rochester, Minnesota
Chair of Neurology
Mayo Clinic Jacksonville
Jacksonville, Florida
(Chapters 34, 50)

Jordon Grafman, Ph.D.
Chief
Cognitive Neuroscience Section
National Institutes of Neurological Disorders and
Stroke
National Institutes of Health
Bethesda, Maryland
(Chapter 15)

Murray Grossman, M.D.
Associate Professor
Department of Neurology
Cognitive Neurology Section
University of Pennsylvania Medical Center
Philadelphia, Pennsylvania
(Chapter 37)

**Vladimir Hachinski, M.D., F.R.C.P. (C),
M.Sc. (D.M.E.), D.Sc. (Med)**
Richard and Beryl Ivey Professor and Chair
Department of Clinical Neurological Sciences
University Hospital
London, Ontario, Canada
(Chapter 46)

John Hart, Jr., M.D.
Assistant Professor
Department of Neurology
Cognitive Neurology
Johns Hopkins Medical Institution
Baltimore, Maryland
(Chapter 53)

Kenneth M. Heilman, M.D.
James E. Rooks, Jr., Professor of Neurology
Department of Neurology
College of Medicine
University of Florida
Gainesville, Florida
(Chapters 16, 24)

Diane M. Jacobs, Ph.D.
Assistant Professor of Neuropsychology
Department of Neurology
Gertrude H. Sergievsky Center
Columbia University College of Physicians and
Surgeons
New York, New York
(Chapter 45)

Daniel I. Kaufer, M.D.
Assistant Professor of Psychiatry and Neurology
University of Pittsburgh Medical Center
Pittsburgh, Pennsylvania
(Chapter 40)

Andrew Kertesz, M.D., F.R.C.P. (C)
Professor
Department of Clinical Neurological Sciences
St. Joseph's Health Centre
University of Western Ontario
London, Ontario, Canada
(Chapter 11)

Daniel Y. Kimberg, Ph.D.
Postdoctoral Fellow
National Institute of Health
Bethesda, Maryland
(Chapter 31)

Marcel Kinsbourne, M.D.
Professor of Psychology
New School for Social Research
New York, New York
Research Professor—Center for Cognitive Studies
Tufts University
Medford, Massachusetts
(Chapters 63, 66)

Robert T. Knight, M.D.
Professor of Neurology
Department of Neurology
Center for Neuroscience
University of California, Davis
Veterans Medical Center
Martinez, California
(Chapter 7)

Kevin S. LaBar, Ph.D.
Postdoctoral Associate
Department of Psychology
Yale University
New Haven, Connecticut
(Chapter 54)

Joseph E. LeDoux, Ph.D.
Professor of Neural Science
Center for Neural Science
New York University
New York, New York
(Chapter 54)

Ronald P. Lesser, M.D.
Professor of Neurology and Neurosurgery
Cognitive Neurology
Johns Hopkins Medical Institution
Baltimore, Maryland
(Chapter 53)

Harvey S. Levin, Ph.D.
Director of Research, Professor
Department of Physical Medicine and Rehabilitation
Baylor College of Medicine
Houston, Texas
(Chapter 38)

Muriel D. Lezak, Ph.D.
Professor, Neurology, Psychiatry, and Neurosurgery
Oregon Health Sciences University
Department of Neurology
Portland, Oregon
(Chapter 3)

David W. Loring, Ph.D.
Professor
Departments of Neurology and Pharmacology/
Toxicology
Medical College of Georgia
Augusta, Georgia
(Chapter 52)

Maureen W. Lovett, Ph.D.
Senior Scientist, Research Institute
The Hospital for Sick Children
Associate Professor
Departments of Paediatrics and Psychology
University of Toronto
Toronto, Ontario, Canada
(Chapter 62)

Richard Mayeux, M.D., M.S.E.
Gertrude E. Sergievsky
Professor of Neurology, Psychiatry, and Public Health
(Epidemiology)
Sergievsky Center
Columbia University
New York, New York
(Chapter 45)

Kimford J. Meador, M.D.
Director, Behavioral Neurology
Professor
Departments of Neurology and Pharmacology/
Toxicology
Medical College of Georgia
Augusta, Georgia
(Chapter 52)

Mario F. Mendez, M.D., Ph.D.
Associate Professor of Neurology
UCLA School of Medicine
Los Angeles, California
(Chapter 44)

M.-Marsel Mesulam, M.D.
Ruth and Evelyn Dunbar Professor of Neurology and
Psychiatry
Department of Neurology and Psychiatry
Northwestern University Medical Center
Chicago, Illinois
(Chapter 4)

Bruce L. Miller, M.D.
Professor of Neurology
UCLA School of Medicine
Reed Neurological Research Institute
Los Angeles, California
(Chapter 30)

Clark H. Millikan, M.D.
Clinical Professor of Neurology
Medical College of Ohio
Toledo, Ohio
(Chapter 49)

Nancy J. Minshew, M.D.
Associate Professor of Neurology and Psychiatry
University of Pittsburgh
Medical Center
Autism and Social Disabilities Clinic
Pittsburgh, Pennsylvania
(Chapter 67)

Robert D. Nebes, Ph.D.
Professor, Department of Psychiatry
University of Pittsburgh Medical School
Pittsburgh, Pennsylvania
(Chapter 42)

Joel Paraiso, M.D.
Amsterdam, New York
(Chapter 51)

Bruce F. Pennington, Ph.D.
Professor
Department of Psychology
University of Denver
Denver, Colorado
(Chapter 65)

Richard W. Price, M.D.
Chief, Neurology Service
San Francisco General Hospital
Professor of Neurology
University of California
San Francisco, California
(Chapter 47)

Robert D. Rafal, M.D.
Professor
Department of Neurology
University of California at Davis
Davis, California
(Chapters 25, 26)

Marcus E. Raichle, M.D.
Co-Director of Radiological Sciences
Professor of Radiology, Neurology, Anatomy:
Neurobiology
Department of Neurology and Radiology
Washington University School of Medicine
St. Louis, Missouri
(Chapter 6)

Timothy Rickard, Ph.D.
Postdoctoral Fellow
Cognitive Neuroscience Section
National Institutes of Neurological Disorders and
Stroke
National Institutes of Health
Bethesda, Maryland
(Chapter 15)

David M. Roane, M.D.
Assistant Professor of Psychiatry
Beth Israel Medical Center
Department of Psychiatry
New York, New York
(Chapter 29)

David P. Roeltgen, M.D.
Neurologist
Williamsport Hospital
Williamsport, Pennsylvania
Adjunct Associate Professor of Neurology
Hahnemann University
Philadelphia, Pennsylvania
(Chapter 14)

Elliott D. Ross, M.D.
Professor and Chairman of Neurology
Department of Neuroscience
University of North Dakota School of Medicine
Director
Clinical Research Program
Neuropsychiatric Research Institute
Chief
Neurology Service
VA Medical Center
Fargo, North Dakota
(Chapter 56)

Leslie J. Gonzalez Rothi, Ph.D.
Associate Professor
Department of Neurology
University of Florida
Speech Pathology Services
VA Medical Center
Gainesville, Florida
(Chapter 16)

Eleanor M. Saffran, Ph.D.
Professor of Communication Sciences and Neurology
Department of Neurology
Temple University School of Medicine
Philadelphia, Pennsylvania
(Chapter 10)

William Samuel, M.D., Ph.D.
Neurology Service
University of California
San Diego, California
(Chapter 43)

Daniel L. Schacter, Ph.D.
Professor of Psychology
Department of Psychology
Harvard University
Cambridge, Massachusetts
(Chapter 36)

Myrna F. Schwartz, Ph.D.
Associate Director
Neuropsychology Research Laboratory
Moss Rehabilitation Research Institute
Philadelphia, Pennsylvania
(Chapter 12)

John J. Sidtis, Ph.D., L.P.
Associate Professor of Neurology
Director, Laboratory of Quantitative Neurology
Department of Neurology
University of Minnesota
Minneapolis, Minnesota
(Chapter 47)

Jonathan M. Silver, M.D.
Associate Professor of Clinical Psychiatry
College of Physicians and Surgeons
Columbia University, Director, Neuropsychiatry
Columbia Presbyterian Medical Center
New York, New York
(Chapter 57)

Yaakov Stern, Ph.D.
Associate Professor of Clinical Neuropsychology
Columbia University
New York, New York
(Chapter 45)

Karin Stromswold, M.D., Ph.D.
Assistant Professor of Psychology and Cognitive Science
Department of Psychology and the Center for Cognitive Science
Rutgers University
New Brunswick, New Jersey
(Chapter 61)

Richard L. Strub, M.D.
Chairman
Department of Neurology
Ochsner Clinic
Clinical Professor of Neurology
Tulane University
New Orleans, Louisiana
(Chapter 2)

Leon J. Thal, M.D.
Professor and Chair
Department of Neurosciences
University of California, San Diego
La Jolla, California
(Chapter 43)

Daniel Tranel, Ph.D.
Professor of Neurology and Psychology
Department of Neurology
University of Iowa Hospital and Clinics
Iowa City, Iowa
(Chapter 19)

Edward Valenstein, M.D.
Professor of Neurology
Department of Neurology
University of Florida
Gainesville, Florida
(Chapter 24)

Mieke Verfaellie, Ph.D.
Associate Professor of Neurology (Neuropsychology)
Boston University School of Medicine
Memory Disorders Research Center
Department of Veterans Affairs
Medical Center
Boston, Massachusetts
(Chapter 48)

Kytja K. S. Voeller, M.D.
Associate Professor of Neurology in Psychiatry
Department of Psychiatry
University of Florida
Gainesville, Florida
(Chapter 64)

Deborah P. Waber, Ph.D.
Associate Professor
Department of Psychiatry
Harvard Medical School
Children's Hospital Medical Center
Boston, Massachusetts
(Chapter 59)

Robert T. Watson, M.D.
Professor
Department of Neurology and Clinical and Health
Psychology
University of Florida
Gainesville, Florida
(Chapters 16, 24)

Stuart C. Yudofsky, M.D.
D.C. and Irene Ellwood Professor and Chairman
Department of Psychiatry
Baylor College of Medicine
Chief of Psychiatry Service
The Methodist Hospital
Houston, Texas
(Chapter 57)

Tricia Zawacki, B.A.
Graduate Student
Center for Neuropsychological Studies
Department of Clinical and Health Psychology
University of Florida
Gainesville, Florida
(Chapter 20)

Stuart Zola, Ph.D.
Research Career Scientist
Veterans Administration Medical Center
Professor in Residence
Departments of Psychiatry and Neurosciences
University of California San Diego School of
Medicine
La Jolla, California
(Chapter 35)

PREFACE

Twelve years ago, a behavioral neurology fellow in Gainesville called a cognitive science postdoc in Cambridge, Massachusetts, to discuss mental imagery in neurologic patients. The conversation lasted well over an hour—or perhaps we should say it lasted twelve years, with the parties on each end of the line moving from Gainesville to New York, and from Cambridge to Pittsburgh to Philadelphia. Throughout this time we have each learned about the other's fields, collaborated on occasional research projects, and significantly bolstered the value of AT&T stock.

It was during one of these long-distance explorations of mind and brain that Dr. Feinberg raised the possibility of a joint book. An editor at McGraw-Hill had approached him with the idea of editing a textbook on behavioral neurology, to complement Adams and Victor's classic *Principles of Neurology*. He was interested, but made a counteroffer—a book that would combine traditional behavioral neurology with current developments in cognitive neuropsychology. McGraw-Hill approved of the idea. So did Dr. Farah, who joined as coeditor.

What motivated us to undertake this project was our sense of how little understanding each of the two fields has of the other's theories, methods, and terminology, despite largely common goals. For example, cognitive neuropsychologists may not be trained in neuroanatomy and may know little about the functional consequences of different etiologies of brain damage. Behavioral neurologists may be unfamiliar with theories of normal

behavior, and as these theories grow more technical (e.g. incorporating concepts from linguistics or computation), they cannot be picked up casually. And of course even within one's own field it is hard to keep up with the last ten years' explosion of new knowledge, for example, in neuroimaging, neuropharmacology, computational modeling, methods of rehabilitation, and theories of memory, frontal function, language, and so on. We intend this book to be used in two ways—as a source of state-of-the-art reviews for researchers and clinicians in their own areas and as an accessible introduction to the major concepts, methods, and findings of these areas for those from the outside.

The success of this project depended almost entirely on the authors who contributed to it. To our delight, almost every one of our first-choice authors agreed to participate. Even better, they delivered excellent manuscripts, sometimes in advance of the deadline. We are especially grateful to them for making the effort to write in a way that can be understood by both specialist and nonspecialist.

Joseph Hefta took over as McGraw-Hill editor for neurology just as the serious work on the book began. He helped keep us organized and dispensed wisdom, moral support, and word-processing tips at the critical times. Lester Sheinis and Heidi Thaens put in long hours in the editing-production phase and were good humored about several last-minute changes and changes to changes. Diana Dyckes-Berke provided invaluable assistance to Dr. Feinberg throughout the project, and Norma Kamen and Michael Hartman provided secretarial support at Beth Israel and Penn, respectively. Paul Bunten of the Oskar Diethelm Library provided research assistance for the first chapter and the cover art. We would also like to acknowledge several funding sources that supported the writing of our chapters—the Alzheimer's Disease Association, the Guggenheim Foundation, the National Institute of Neurological Disease and Stroke, and the National Institute of Mental Health.

Finally, we wish to acknowledge those who contributed to this book in less direct, but no less important, ways. For their collegial support and guidance over many years Todd thanks Ken Heilman, Leslie Gonzalez Rothi, Arnold Winston, Matthew Fink, Thomas Killip, Robert Newman, and Morton Hyman. He thanks Betty and Morton Yarmon for their enormous generosity in supporting the Division of Neurobehavior and Alzheimer's Disease at Beth Israel and making projects like this book possible. Also, for valuable discussions and clinical material he thanks Dr. Joseph Giacino and Dr. John Deluca. Most especially he thanks his parents, Gloria and Mortimer Feinberg, his wife, Marlene, and his children, Rachel and Josh, who make it all worthwhile. Martha thanks her many wonderful colleagues at Penn, Temple, and elsewhere. She also thanks her postdocs, students, and research assistants, past and present, who make neuropsychology perennially interesting and new. Finally, for help and support while this book was being written and edited (which coincided with the start of another major project), she thanks her friends and family, especially "Uncles" David and Bob, "Aunts" Janet, Paddy, and Ginny, "Grannies" Lois and Hermine, real Aunt Najla, cousins Cathy and Suzie, and little Theodora Najla Farah, who helped most of all by sleeping through the night a month before the production deadline.

BEHAVIORAL
NEUROLOGY
AND
NEUROPSYCHOLOGY

Part 1
GENERAL PRINCIPLES

Chapter 1

THE DEVELOPMENT OF MODERN BEHAVIORAL NEUROLOGY AND NEUROPSYCHOLOGY

Todd E. Feinberg
Martha J. Farah

HISTORICAL ROOTS OF BEHAVIORAL NEUROLOGY AND NEUROPSYCHOLOGY

The history of the study of brain function could be said to start with a different organ, the heart. The ancient Egyptians held that the heart and diaphragm were the seats of mental life. They held this belief despite their observations of the behavioral effects of head injury, including descriptions of aphasia dating back as far as 3500 B.C.[1-6] In ancient Greece, we see the first statements of and debate over a cerebrocentric view of the mind. Alcmaeon of Croton,[6] a Greek of the fifth-century B.C. who may have been a pupil of Pythagoras,[2,7] could well be considered the first neurologist or neuropsychologist. On the basis of his clinical and pathologic investigations, he proposed that the brain was the organ responsible for sensation and thought. He also taught that the various sensations each had a particular localization in the brain,[2,3,6,8] thus articulating for the first time a localist view of brain function. Starting in the eighteenth century, localism would become such a controversial hypothesis that it would polarize the field and become the driving motivation for almost 300 years of research.

A century after Alcmaeon, the writings of Hippocrates constitute another major turning point. Hippocrates believed that the brain was responsible for the intellect, senses, knowledge, emotions, and even mental illness.[9] A particularly revolutionary idea, recorded in the Hippocratic tract entitled "On the Sacred Disease," was that epilepsy is a medical condition and not the result of demonic possession.[2] However, even at this point the issue of cerebrocentrism versus cardiocentrism was not yet settled for all time. Plato, a contemporary of Hippocrates, accepted a cerebrocentric view of the mind, but a century later Aristotle rejected it in favor of the more traditional cardiocentric view.[2,3,8] Furthermore, even in the cerebrocentric camp, more than a few details concerning mind-brain relations remained to be worked out. Herophilus of Chalcedon, a follower of Hippocrates in the third century B.C. and a pioneer in the practice of human dissection, believed that the brain's ventricles, particularly the fourth ventricle, were the seat of human intelligence.[3,6,7,10]

The Greek natural philosophers taught an influential "doctrine of the spirits."[7] They proposed that a *spiritus naturalis* originated in the liver and was transported to the heart and lungs. Here it was mixed with air and thereby transformed into the *spiritus vitalis*, which was identified with the essential principle of life. Finally it is transported to the brain where it is converted into the *spiritus animalis,* the essence of the soul and mind. The doctrine of the spirits was to appear in various forms over the centuries and was frequently incorporated into later theories that were based on more objective knowledge of the brain.

One of the great physicians of the classical period was Galen of Pergamus (A.D. 131–201).[2,3] Galen firmly rejected the cardiocentric position of

Aristotle and reaffirmed the position of the brain as the seat of the psyche. His thinking on brain physiology reflected the continuing belief in the spirit doctrine and the importance of the ventricular system in brain functioning. He taught that the *vital spirits,* produced by the left ventricle of the heart, were transferred via the vessels to the brain where, in the *rete mirabile,* they were transformed into *animal spirits.* The *rete mirabile,* previously described by Herophilus, is a vascular network that surrounds the pituitary gland and is prominently present in the ox but absent in humans. This error is testament to the degree to which the ancients relied upon animal dissection for the knowledge of anatomy. After transformation in the *rete mirabile,* the animal spirits could be stored in the ventricles and, when needed, sent through the nerves to the rest of the body for use in action or sensation.[10] While Galen taught that the ventricles were crucial to action and sensation, he also believed that brain tissue itself played a role in mental life.[11]

For the entire period of the middle ages in Europe (approximately the fourth to fourteenth centuries), the ventricles continued to be the focus of theories relating mind and brain.[11] For example, according to fourth-century church fathers, the anterior ventricles were associated with perception (later to be known as the *sensorium commune*), the middle with reason, and the posterior with memory.[10] It has been suggested that this focus on the ventricles accorded better with the dualism of Christian theology, as the hollow cavities could be said to contain the soul without hypothesizing an identity between mind and the physical substrate of brain tissue.[11] Figure 1-1 shows an early illustration of the ventricular system.

During the Renaissance, the ventricular doctrine and the role of the *rete mirabile* began to lose their influence on theories of mind-brain relations.[4,10,12] The seventeenth-century writings of René Descartes mark a transitional phase, in which the interaction between fluid in the ventricles and brain tissue itself was hypothesized to explain intelligent action, as shown in Fig. 1-2. For reflexive action, Descartes proposed a simple loop, in which stimulated nerves caused the release of animal spirits in the ventricles, which, in turn,

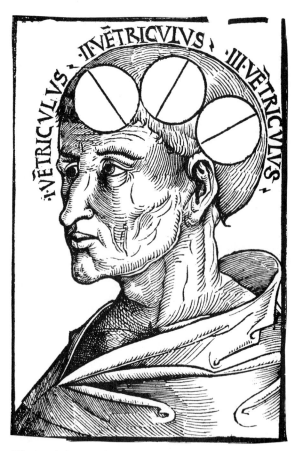

Figure 1-1
The ventricular system according to Albertus Magnus from his Philosophia naturalis *(1506).*[10]

caused efferent nerves and muscles to act. For intelligent human action, this loop was modulated by the soul via its effects on the pineal gland. The pineal gland was chosen in part because it is unpaired and centrally located and also because it is surrounded by cerebrospinal fluid. It was also mistakenly thought to be uniquely human. Of course, the pineal gland was just the vehicle for the mind's influence on the body; Descartes' theory still denied any form of identity between the mind and neural tissue.[4,13–16]

Descartes' theory was formulated at a time when neuroanatomic knowledge was quite primitive. This situation began to change with the work of such figures as Thomas Willis later in the seven-

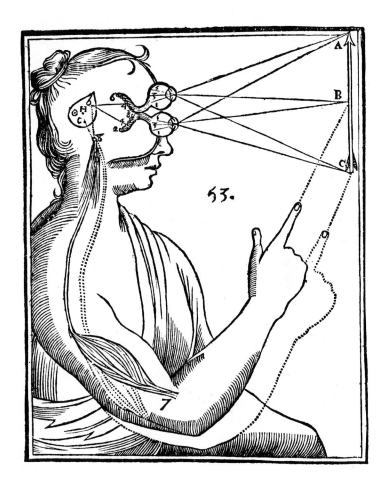

Figure 1-2
Descartes' conception of sensation and action as conceived in his De homine *(1662). Light was transferred from the retina to the ventricles, causing the release of animal spirits. The pineal gland modulated this mechanism for voluntary action.*[3]

teenth century[4,17] and Malpighi Pacchioni and Albrecht von Haller in the eighteenth.[8,18] For example, Von Haller stimulated the nerves of live animals in an effort to discover the pathways for perception and motor action, thus establishing the experimental method in neurophysiology. This work set the stage for the explosion of experimental and clinical research of the nineteenth century, in which the brain organization underlying perception, action, language, and many other cognitive functions was revealed.

Some of the earliest inroads into meaningful localization in the nervous system began not with the brain but the peripheral nervous system. Von Haller had suggested that the same nerves subserved motor and sensory functions.[2] Sir Charles Bell and François Magendie, independently, dis-covered the segregation of sensory functions to the posterior spinal roots and motor functions to the anterior spinal roots, which has come to be known as the Bell-Magendie law. The clear-cut division of function provided by these observations, coupled with a straightforward anatomic basis and its proof by experiment, was both a model for localization of function within the nervous system and a triumph for the experimental method.[2,4,8,18–20]

THE LOCALISM/HOLISM DEBATE OF THE NINETEENTH CENTURY

One of the more notorious figures in the history of behavioral neurology is Franz Josef Gall, shown

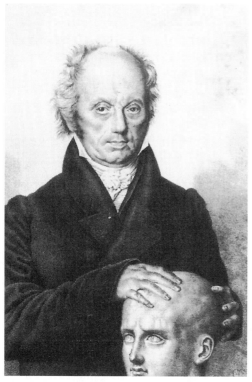

Figure 1-3
Franz Josef Gall (1758–1828).

associated them with particular brain centers that could affect the shape of the skull, as shown in Fig. 1-4. These included memory of things and facts, sense of spatial relations, vanity, God and religion, and love for one's offspring.[23] His theory was based on hundreds of skulls and casts of humans and beasts. For instance, the disposition to murder and cruelty was based on a bump above the ear possessed by carnivorous animals. He located the same feature in sadistic persons whom he had examined personally,[4] skulls of famous criminals, and the busts and paintings of famous murderers.[18] Gall taught and practiced medicine in Vienna from 1781 to around 1802, until Emperor Francis I banned Gall's public lectures because they were materialistic and thus opposed to morality and religion.[18] Gall then took to the road, lecturing across Europe to enthusiastic popular audiences. By the time he settled in Paris in 1807, he

Figure 1-4
An example of a porcelain phrenology bust with demarcations that demonstrate the reflection of the human faculties on the skull. (Photograph courtesy of Joseph A. Hefta.)

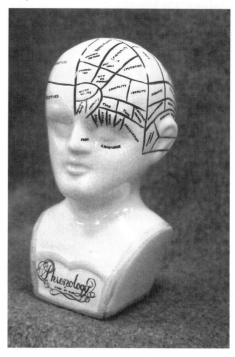

in Fig. 1-3. In the late eighteenth and early nineteenth centuries, he and his collaborator Johann Spurzheim made a number of important contributions to functional neuroanatomy, including proving by dissection the crossing of the pyramids and establishing the distinction between gray and white matter.[21–23] Gall is also credited with one of the earliest descriptions of aphasia linked to a lesion of the frontal lobes.[24] He is most famous, however, for his general theory of cerebral localization, known today as phrenology. At the age of 9, Gall had noted that his schoolmates who excelled at rote memory tasks had quite prominent eyes, *"les yeux à fleur de tête"* (cow's eyes). He reasoned that this was the result of the overdevelopment of the subjacent regions of the brain, and speculated that these regions of the brain might be particularly involved in language functions and especially verbal memory.

Gall identified 27 basic human faculties and

was hugely popular and internationally known. However, phrenology continued to create controversy in scientific circles.

The best-known critic of Gall was Marie-Jean-Pierre Flourens. Flourens mounted a scientific research program to disprove Gall's theory, but it appears to have been motivated at least as much by religious discomfort with the implications of Gall's straightforward mind-brain equivalences as by scientific considerations. Flourens viewed Gall's theory as tantamount to denying the existence of the soul, because it divided the mind and brain into functionally distinct parts and Flourens believed the soul to be unitary.[18,25–27] He carried out extensive lesion experiments on a variety of animal species to demonstrate the equipotentiality of cortex.

Gall's status as a popularizer, and Flourens's empirical attacks, helped to push localism out of the mainstream of contemporary scientific thought in the early nineteenth century. When, in 1825, Jean-Baptiste Bouillaud, shown in Fig. 1-5, presented a large series of clinical cases of loss of

Figure 1-5
Jean-Baptiste Bouillaud (1796–1881).

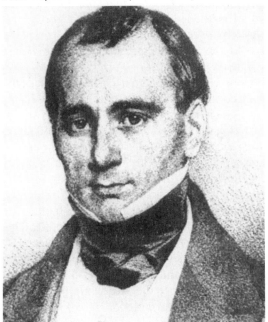

speech following frontal lesions,[21,27,28] his work was largely ignored. This landmark work, in which speech per se was distinguished from nonspeech movements of the mouth and tongue, is still relatively unknown.

Bouillaud was not the only one to suggest a frontal location for language functions. During this period and lasting up to the 1860s, numerous clinical reports of patients with frontal lobe damage and loss of speech were recorded in Europe and America. Indeed, this idea had considerable historical precedence throughout antiquity.[5,29,30] However, intense interest in localization of brain functions, particularly language, was now developing. It was during this time that Marc Dax noted the association between left-hemispheric damage, right hemiplegia, and aphasia, based upon his examination of 40 patients over a 20-year period. This paper was handwritten in 1836 and not published at the time,[31] but copies may have been distributed to friends and colleagues.[4]

It was not until 1861 that the field reconsidered localism with a more open mind. That year the Société d'Anthropologie in Paris held a series of debates between Pierre Gratiolet, arguing in favor of holism or equipotentiality, and Ernest Auburtin, the son-in-law of Bouillaud, arguing in favor of localism.[21,32,33] Auburtin, shown in Fig. 1-6, reported his clinical observations of a patient whose frontal bone was removed following a suicide attempt. He reported that when the blade of a spatula was applied to the "anterior lobes," there was complete cessation of speech without loss of consciousness.[4,21,33] Auburtin went on to describe a patient of Bouillaud's who had a speech disturbance and was near death. Auburtin boldly vowed if this patient lacked a frontal lesion he would renounce his views.[21,32–35]

The 1861 debate is best known not for the presentations of Gratiolet and Auburtin but for the eventual participation of the society's founder and secretary, Paul Broca, shown in Fig. 1-7. Although Broca did not initially take a strong position, his observations of a patient then under his care led him to play a pivotal role in the debate. His patient, Leborgne, suffered from epilepsy, right hemiplegia, and loss of speech, the last for a period of over 20 years. Leborgne had been institutional-

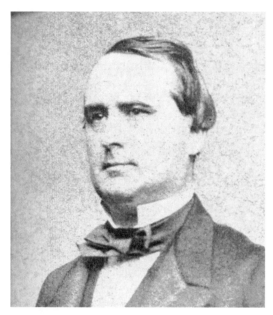

Figure 1-6
Ernest Aubertin (1825–1865).

Figure 1-7
Paul Broca (1824–1880).

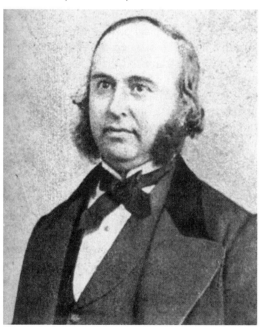

ized for some 31 years and throughout the hospital was known by the name "Tan," as this was his only utterance along with a few obscenities.[3,4] In light of Auburtin's declaration, Broca invited him to examine Tan, which Auburtin did and afterward concluded that indeed the patient met the criteria of his prior challenge. Six days later Leborgne died; the following day, April 18, 1961, Broca presented the brain to the society along with a brief statement but without firm conclusions.[33] Figure 1-8 shows the brain of Leborgne.

Four months later, at a meeting of the Société Anatomique de Paris in August, Broca made a more extensive report. The brain of Leborgne had demonstrated an egg-sized fluid-filled cavity located in the posterior second and third frontal convolutions, with involvement of adjacent structures as well, including the corpus striatum.[36] In this report, Broca claimed that his findings would "support the ideas of M. Bouillaud on the seat of the faculty for language";[33,36] he later suggested a possible localization of speech functions to the second or more probably third frontal convolution. Later the same year, Broca presented another patient with speech disturbance, an 84-year-old laborer whose lesion also involved the left second and third frontal convolutions. The lesion was more circumscribed than that found in Leborgne and strengthened the association of those structures with speech localization.

In the mid-1860s the issue of hemispheric asymmetry entered the debate on localization. The previous cases strongly suggested that speech is localized to the left hemisphere, and an additional series of eight cases published by Broca in 1863 were exclusively left-sided.[4,31,37] In spite of the strong lateralization of lesion locus in these cases, Broca made note of this "remarkable" observation but made no further claims.[31] In this same year and shortly before Broca's paper was presented,[4] Gustave Dax, son of Marc Dax, sent a handwritten copy of his father's manuscript to the Académie de Médecine in Paris. In this document, Marc Dax had previously described his view on the relation between speech and the left hemisphere. The paper was read before the Académie in December 1864 and published in 1865.[38,39] By 1865, Broca

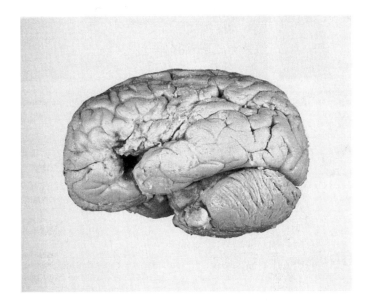

Figure 1-8
Photograph of the brain of Broca's first patient, Leborgne ("Tan"). It is now housed in the Musée Dupuytren.

clearly expressed the opinion that the left hemisphere played a dominant role in speech production.[40,41] As far as the issue of priority of discovery is concerned (a matter of controversy among historians), most writers agree that the Dax paper in its original form in 1836 had no influence on Broca or the scientific community when first written. This paper did, however, make clear the association of language functions and the left hemisphere. While Broca alone clarified the role of the second and third frontal convolutions, he apparently did not take a firm position on the specific role of the left hemisphere until after the Dax paper was read before the Académie de Médecine in Paris in December 1964.[4] It appears that the reemergence of the Dax manuscript and Broca's discovery were nearly simultaneous events.

THE AFTERMATH OF 1861: THE EMERGENCE OF MODERN BEHAVIORAL NEUROLOGY AND NEUROPSYCHOLOGY

The events in Paris in the 1860s constituted a turning point in the history of ideas regarding brain function. The concepts and methods developed in the course of debating the localization of speech were extended to a variety of different higher functions, and experimental work on animals also developed apace. From this period onward, it is impossible to trace a single line of scientific development. Here we simply present a summary of some of the major advances seen in the behavioral neurology and neuropsychology of the late nineteenth and early twentieth centuries.

In the decade following Broca's contributions, two important developments took place in Germany. First, Edward Hitzig and Gustav Fritsch performed a series of experiments in which the cortex of a dog was stimulated while the dog lay on a dressing table in Hitzig's Berlin home.[3,4,42] These experiments established that motor functions are localized to anterior cortex and demonstrated experimentally the somatotopic organization of motor cortex inferred indirectly from previous clinical-anatomic correlations in humans. In their report, the investigators specifically noted that their results refuted the holism of Flourens. Following their work, Sir David Ferrier in England confirmed the findings of Hitzig and Fritsch and improved upon their method of stimulation to discover more detailed structure-function relationships.[18]

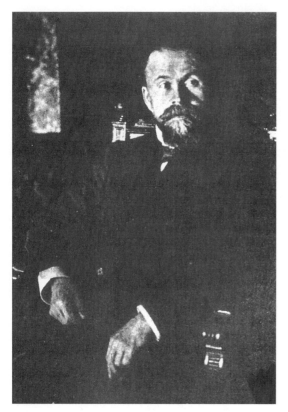

Figure 1-9
Carl Wernicke (1848–1904).

About the same time, the German neurologist Carl Wernicke began to investigate language functions other than speech. Wernicke, shown in Fig. 1-9, documented a form of aphasia different from the nonfluent variety that followed frontal damage. In what he called sensory aphasia, a posterior lesion in the region of the first temporal gyrus caused a disturbance in auditory comprehension, inappropriate word selection in spontaneous speech, and impaired naming and writing. In his landmark monograph *Der aphasische Symptomencomplex,* Wernicke reasoned that Broca's area was the center for the motor representation of speech, and the posterior first temporal gyrus was the center for "sound images." Wernicke also described global aphasia and explained it as a result of destruction of both anterior and posterior language areas. He also made a prediction that a disturbance

of the pathways between these two areas would produce another variety of aphasia he called "conduction aphasia," in which comprehension would be preserved but output would be as impaired as in sensory aphasia.[43–46] Wernicke had, in effect, proposed a model that could explain a number of different aphasic syndromes by lesions to different combination of centers and connections between centers. This type of theorizing came to be known as "associationism," because language use was viewed in terms of associating representations in different brain centers, or as "connectionism," because of the emphasis that view put on the connections between centers, as shown in Fig. 1-10.

The connectionist paradigm was quickly extended to explain other disorders. Ludwig Lichtheim placed pure word deafness in this

Figure 1-10
Wernicke's model of the speech mechanism.[44] The auditory areas (a) project to centers subserving vocal output (b) and areas which contain tactile (c) and visual (d) images.

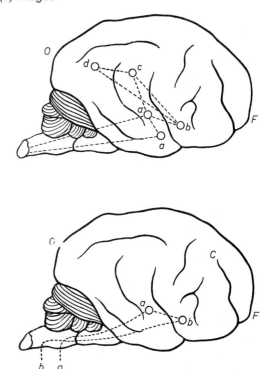

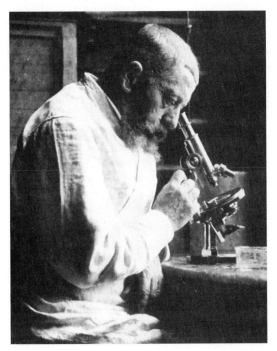

Figure 1-11
Joseph Jules Déjerine (1849–1917).

framework, predicting the critical lesion site as well as noting that, given the connectionist explanation for this syndrome, a disturbance in repetition should accompany conduction aphasia.[46,47] Hugo Liepmann described the apraxias, including ideomotor apraxia,[48] and, with Maas, callosal apraxia,[49] explaining them in terms of connectionist principles. Joseph Jules Déjerine, shown in Fig. 1-11, also used the framework of centers and connections in his explanation of alexia without agraphia.[50]

The nineteenth-century connectionist framework proved to have both parsimony and explanatory power. Rather than hypothesizing a new center for every ability or every observed deficit, after the fashion of Gall, a relatively small number of basic centers (vision, sound images, motor outputs) could be combined through connections to explain a wide variety of higher functions and their deficits. Connectionist explanations of aphasia, apraxia, alexia, and other disorders survived well into the twentieth century; indeed, Norman

Geschwind, one of the most influential behavioral neurologists of our time, championed them throughout his career.[51] Despite the current proliferation of theories and approaches in our field, the theories of Déjerine, Liepmann, Lichtheim, and Wernicke are still held to be correct by many.

Nevertheless, as successful as the connectionist framework was in late nineteenth century in explaining a variety of disorders, skeptics continued to reject the localism implicit in it. One of the most influential of these was the English neurologist John Hughlings Jackson, shown in Fig. 1-12. He viewed the nervous system not as a series of centers connected by pathways but rather as a hierarchically organized and highly interactive whole that could not be understood piecemeal.[32]

Figure 1-12
John Hughlings Jackson (1835–1911).

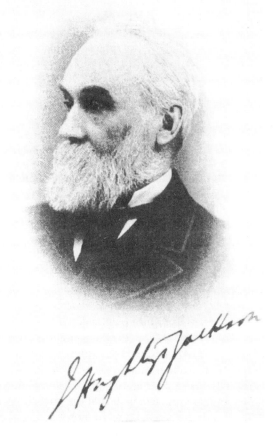

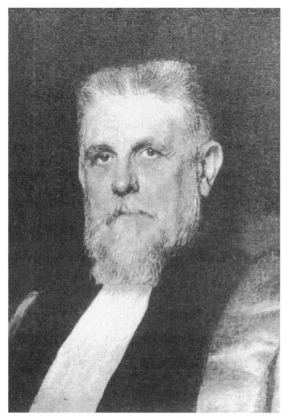

Figure 1-13
Pierre Marie (1853–1940).

When aphasia is viewed this way, a network of specialized centers is superfluous. A movement toward holism continued into the early twentieth century, with Jackson and Marie followed by a number of influential neurologists and psychologists, including Henry Head in England,[32] shown in Fig. 1-14, Kurt Goldstein in Germany,[53–55] shown in Fig. 1-15, and Karl Lashley in the United States.[56–59] This swing of the pendulum back toward holism has been explained by the waning of German influence following World War I[60] and the growing influence of Gestalt psychology.[61]

While these workers emphasized the brain's unity, other researchers had pointed out the difference between brain regions in cellular morphology, cell densities, and lamination and produced the first cytoarchitectonic maps. Oskar and Cécile Vogt[62,63] and Alfred W. Campbell[64,65] produced some of the earliest examples of these architectonic maps, followed by many others, including

Figure 1-14
Henry Head (1861–1940).

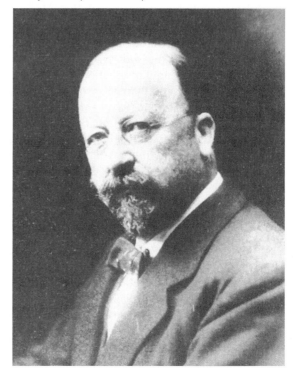

Figure 1-13 shows Pierre Marie, a Parisian student of Broca and Charcot, who also took issue with the connectionist theorizing of the late nineteenth century. His style was direct, to say the least. One of his articles was so offensive to Déjerine that it provoked the latter to challenge Marie to a duel. His article questioning the empirical basis of the early claims concerning speech localization was entitled *"La troisiéme circonvolution frontale gauche ne joue aucun rôle spécial dans la fonction du langage"* ("The third frontal convolution plays no special role at all in the function of language").[52] Marie believed that there was just one basic form of aphasia, a posterior aphasia, which was a type of general intellectual loss not specific to language per se. He held that the speech problems of anterior aphasics were motoric in nature.

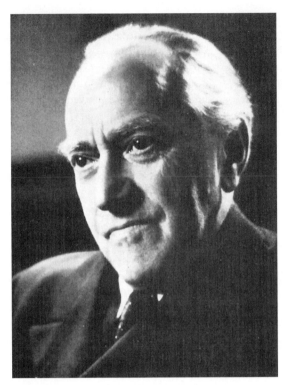

Figure 1-15
Kurt Goldstein (1878–1965).

latter nineteenth century was the description by Wernicke and Korsakoff (shown in Fig. 1-16) of the syndrome that bears their names, including Korsakoff's observations of what he called "pseudo-reminiscence," now known as confabulation.[70,71]

In 1881, Hermann Munk reported that when he ablated the occipital lobes of dogs, they seemed unable to recognize objects despite seeing well enough to navigate the visual environment.[72] Shortly thereafter, Lissauer presented one of the earliest clinical descriptions of visual recognition impairment in a human and suggested the distinction between apperceptive and associative impairment—a clinical dichotomy still in use today.[73] Freud would later introduce the term *agnosia* to describe these conditions.[74] In the decades that followed, the visuospatial functions of the right hemisphere finally attracted the attention of neurologists and neuropsychologists.[75–77] The rela-

Figure 1-16
Sergei S. Korsakoff (1853–1900).

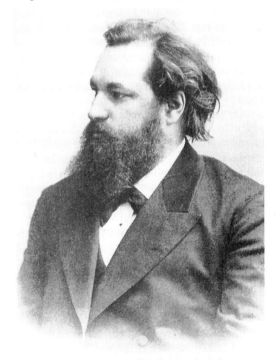

those of Korbinian Brodmann,[66] whose cortical maps of the human brain have had the most widespread application. While these workers did not agree on the number and location of cortical areas (the Vogts counted over 200, Brodmann only 52[4]) it could not be contested that there were clear regional neuroanatomic differences.

The late nineteenth century also saw the beginnings of the modern study of memory and vision. Theodule Ribot introduced the distinction between anterograde and retrograde memory impairments and observed what is now known as "Ribot's law," that the most recently laid down memories were the most vulnerable to brain damage.[67–69] Ribot can also be credited with describing preserved learning in amnesia, thus anticipating the distinction between declarative and nondeclarative forms of memory that has been so intensively investigated in our own recent times. An additional contribution to memory research in the

tively delayed entry of this realm of functioning into the research arena is probably a result of the field's original focus on language and the left hemisphere, reflected in the nineteenth-century terminology of *major* and *minor hemisphere.*

THE RISE OF EXPERIMENTAL NEUROPSYCHOLOGY

Most of the advances described so far in this chapter were made by studying individual patients, or at most a small series of patients with similar disorders. In many instances, particularly before the middle of this century, patients' behavior was studied relatively naturalistically, without planned protocols or quantitative measurements. In the nineteen sixties and seventies, a different approach to the study of brain-behavior relations took hold. Neurologists and neuropsychologists began to design experiments patterned on research methods in experimental psychology.

Typical research designs in experimental psychology involved groups of normal subjects given different experimental treatments (for example, different training or different stimulus materials), and the effects of the treatments were measured in standardized protocols and compared using statistical methods such as analysis of variance. In neuropsychology, the "treatments" were, as a rule, naturally occurring brain lesions. Groups of patients with different lesion sites or behavioral syndromes were tested with standard protocols, yielding quantitative measures of performance, and these performances were compared across patient groups and with non-brain-damaged control groups. Unlike the impairments studied previously in single-case designs, which were so striking that control subjects would generally have been superfluous, experimental neuropsychology often focused on group differences of a rather subtle nature, which required statistical analysis to substantiate.

The most common question addressed by these studies concerned localization of function. Often the localization sought was no more precise than left versus right hemisphere or one quadrant

of the brain (which, in the days before computed tomography, often amounted to left versus right hemisphere with presence or absence of visual field defects and/or hemiplegia). Given the huge amount of research done during this period on language, memory, perception, attention, emotion, praxis, and so-called executive functions, it would be hopeless even to attempt a summary. For those interested in some examples of this approach, we cite here some classic papers from a variety of the active laboratories of the period, addressing the question "Is the right hemisphere specialized for spatial perception of properties such as location,[78–80] orientation,[81,82] and large-scale topography?[83,84]"

The influential research program of the Montreal Neurological Institute also began during this period. In the wake of William Scoville's discovery that the bilateral medial temporal resection he performed on epileptic patient H.M. resulted in permanent and dense amnesia, Brenda Milner and her colleagues investigated this patient and groups of other operated epileptic patients. This enabled them to address questions of functional localization with the anatomic precision of known surgical lesions (e.g., see Refs. 85 and 86 for reviews of research from that period on frontal lobe function and temporal lobe function, respectively). At the same time, another surgical intervention for epilepsy, callosotomy, also spawned a productive and influential research program. Roger Sperry and his students and collaborators were able to address a wide variety of questions about hemispheric specialization by studying the isolated functioning of the human cerebral hemispheres.[87]

In addition to answering questions about localization, the experimental neuropsychology of the sixties and seventies also uncovered aspects of the functional organization of behavior. By examining patterns of association and dissociation among abilities over groups of subjects, researchers tried to determine which abilities depend on the same underlying functional systems and which are functionally independent. For example, the frequent association of aphasia and apraxia had been taken by some to support the notion that aphasia was not language-specific but was just one manifestation of a more pervasive loss of the ability to symbolize or represent ("asymbolia"). A classic group study by Goodglass and Kaplan[88] undermined this position by showing that severity of apraxia and aphasia were uncorrelated in a large sample of left-hemisphere-damaged subjects. A second example of the use of dissociations between groups of patients from this period is the demonstration of the functional distinction, by Newcombe and Russell, within vision between pattern recognition and spatial orientation.[89]

By the end of the seventies, experimental neuropsychology had matured to the point where many perceptual, cognitive, and motor abilities had been associated with particular brain regions, and certain features of the functional organization of these abilities had been delineated. Accordingly, it was at this time that first editions of some of the best-known neuropsychology texts appeared, such as those by Hécaen and Albert,[90] Heilman and Valenstein,[91] Kolb and Whishaw,[92] Springer and Deutsch,[93] and Walsh.[94]

Despite the tremendous progress of this period, experimental neuropsychology remained distinct from and relatively unknown within academic psychology. Particularly in the United States, but also to a large extent in Canada and Europe (the three largest contributors to the world's psychology literature), experimental neuropsychologists tended to work in medical centers rather than university psychology departments and to publish their work in journals separate from mainstream experimental psychology. An important turning point in the histories of both neuropsychology and the psychology of normal human function came when researchers in each area became aware of the other.

THE MARRIAGE OF EXPERIMENTAL NEUROPSYCHOLOGY AND COGNITIVE PSYCHOLOGY

The predominant approach to human experimental psychology in the 1970s was cognitive psychology. The hallmark of this approach was the assumption that all of cognition (broadly construed to include perception and motor control) could be viewed as information processing. Although the effects of damage to an information-processing mechanism might seem to be a good source of clues as to its normal operation, cognitive psychologists of the seventies were generally quite ignorant of contemporary neuropsychology.

The reason that most cognitive psychologists of the 1970s ignored neuropsychology stemmed from an overly narrow conception of information processing, based on the digital computer. A basic tenet of cognitive psychology was the computer analogy for the mind: the mind is to the brain as software is to hardware in a computer. Given that the same computer can run different programs and the same program can be run on different computers, this analogy suggests that hardware and software are independent and that the brain is therefore irrelevant to cognitive psychology. If you want to understand the nature of the program that is the human mind, studying neuropsychology is as pointless as trying to understand how a computer is programmed by looking at the circuit boards.

The problem with the computer analogy is that hardware and software are independent only for very special types of computational systems: those systems that have been engineered, through great effort and ingenuity, to make the hardware and software independent, enabling one computer to run many programs and enabling those programs to be portable to other computers. The brain was "designed" by very different pressures, and there is no reason to believe that, in general, information-processing functions and the physical substrate of those functions will be independent. In fact, as cognitive psychologists finally began to learn about neuropsychology, it became apparent that cognitive functions break down in characteristic and highly informative ways after brain damage. By the early 1980s, cognitive psychology and neuropsychology were finally in communication with one another. Since then, we have seen an explosion of meetings, books, and new journals devoted to so-called cognitive neuropsychology. Perhaps more important, existing cognitive psychology journals have begun to publish neuropsychological studies, and articles in existing neuro-psychology and neurology journals frequently include discussions of the cognitive psychology literature.

Let us take a closer look at the scientific forces that drove this change in disciplinary boundaries. By 1980, both cognitive psychology and neuropsychology had reached stages of development that were, if not exactly impasses, points of diminishing returns for the concepts and methods of their own isolated disciplines. In cognitive psychology, the problem concerned methodologic limitations. By varying stimuli and instructions and measuring responses and response latencies, cognitive psychologists made inferences about the information processing that intervened between stimulus and response. But such inferences were indirect, and in some cases they were incapable of distinguishing between rival theories. In 1978 the cognitive psychologist John Anderson published an influential paper[95] in which he called this the "identifiability" problem and took as his example the debate over whether mental images were more like perceptual representations or linguistic representations. He argued that the field's inability to resolve this issue, despite many years of research, was due to the impossibility of uniquely identifying internal cognitive processes from stimulus-response relations. He suggested that the direct study of brain function could, in principle, make a unique identification possible, but he indicated that such a solution probably lay in the distant future.

That distant future came to pass within the next 10 years, as cognitive psychologists working on a variety of different topics found that the study of neurologic patients provided a powerful new source of evidence for testing their theories. In the case of mental imagery, taken by Anderson to be emblematic of the identifiability problem, the finding that perceptual impairments after brain damage were frequently accompanied by parallel imagery impairments strongly favored the perceptual hypothesis.[96] The study of learning and memory within cognitive psychology was revolutionized by the influx of ideas and findings on preserved learning in amnesia, leading to the hy-pothesis of multiple memory systems.[97-99] In the study of attention, cognitive psychologists had for years focused on the issue of early versus late attentional selection without achieving a resolution, and here too neurologic disorders were crucial in moving the field forward. The phenomena of neglect provided dramatic evidence of selection from spatially formatted perceptual representations, and the variability in neglect's manifestations from case to case helped to establish the possibility of multiple loci for attentional selection as opposed to a single early or late locus. The idea of separate visual feature maps, supported by cases of acquired color, motion, and depth blindness, provided the inspiration for the most novel development in recent cognitive theories of attention—namely, feature integration theory.[100]

What did neuropsychology gain from the rapprochement with cognitive psychology? The main benefits were theoretical rather than methodologic. Traditionally, neuropsychologists studied the localization and functional organization of *abilities,* such as speech, reading, memory, object recognition, and so forth. But few would doubt that each of these abilities depends upon an orchestrated set of *component cognitive processes,* and it seems far more likely that the underlying cognitive components, rather than the task-defined abilities, are what is implemented in localized neural tissue. The theories of cognitive psychology therefore allowed neuropsychologists to pose questions about the localization and functional organization of the components of the cognitive architecture, a level of theoretical analysis that was more likely to yield clear and generalizable findings.

Among patients with reading disorders, for example, some are impaired at reading nonwords (e.g., *plif*) while others are impaired at reading irregular words (e.g., *yacht*). Rather than attempt to localize nonword reading or irregular word reading per se and delineate them as independent abilities, neuropsychologists have been able to use a theory of reading developed in cognitive psychology to interpret these disorders in terms of damage to a whole-word recognition system and a grapheme-to-phoneme translation system, respectively.[101] This interpretation has the advantage of correctly predicting additional features of patient behavior, such as the tendency to misread nonwords as words of overall similar appearance when operating with only the whole-word system.

In recent years the neurology and neuropsychology of every major cognitive system has adopted the theoretical framework of cognitive psychology in a general way, and in some cases specific theories have been incorporated. This is reflected in the content and organization of the present book. For the most intensively studied areas of behavioral neurology and neuropsychology—namely, visual attention, memory, language, frontal lobe function, and Alzheimer disease—integrated pairs of chapters review the clinical and anatomic aspects of the relevant disorders and their cognitive theoretical interpretations. Chapters on other topics will cover both the clinical and theoretical aspects together.

NEW TOOLS FOR THE STUDY OF MIND AND BRAIN

In the past two decades, behavioral neurology and neuropsychology have been transformed not only by the influx of theoretical ideas from cognitive psychology but also by the advent of powerful new methods for studying brain activity during cognition. The first of these methods to find wide use was functional neuroimaging.

Functional Neuroimaging

Following its introduction in the 1970s, positron emission tomography (PET) was quickly embraced by researchers interested in brain-behavior relations. This technique provides images of regional glucose utilization, blood flow, oxygen consumption, or receptor density in the brains of live humans. Resting studies, in which subjects are scanned while resting passively, have provided a window on differences between normal and pathologic brain function in a number of neurologic and psychiatric conditions. With the use of radioactive ligands, abnormalities can be localized to specific neurotransmitter systems as well as specific anatomic regions. Activation studies, in which separate images are collected while normal subjects perform different tasks (typically one or more active tasks and one resting baseline) yielded new insights on the localization of cognitive processes. These localizations were not studied region by region, as necessitated by the lesion technique, but could be apprehended simultaneously in a whole intact brain. Examples of images obtained by PET may be found in Figs. 6-1 and 6-3. Figure 1-17 shows a subject in a PET scanner.

Positron emission tomography was soon joined by other techniques for measuring regional brain activity, each of which has its own strengths and weaknesses. Single photon emission computed tomography (SPECT) was quickly adapted for some of the same applications as PET, providing a less expensive but also less quantifiable and spatially less accurate method for obtaining images of regional cerebral blood flow. With new developments in the measurement and analysis of electromagnetic signals, the relatively old techniques of electroencephalography (EEG) and event-related potentials (ERPs), as well as magnetoencephalography (MEG), joined the ranks of functional imaging techniques allowing some degree of anatomic localization of brain activity, with temporal resolution that is superior to the blood flow and metabolic techniques. Most recently, functional magnetic resonance imaging (fMRI) has provided a particularly attractive package of reasonably good anatomic and temporal resolution, using techniques that are noninvasive and can be implemented with equipment available for clinical purposes in many hospitals.

Much of the early work with functional neuroimaging could be considered a form of "calibration," in that researchers sought to confirm well-established principles of functional neuroanatomy using the new techniques—for example, demonstrating that visual stimulation activates visual cortex. As functional neuroimaging matured, researchers began to address new questions, to which the answers were not already known in advance. An important development in this second wave of research was the introduction of theories and

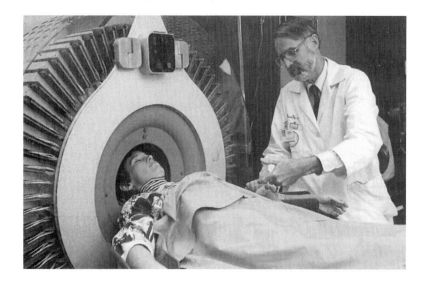

Figure 1-17
A subject about to undergo positron emission tomography. (From Marcus E. Raichle, M.D., Washington University, St. Louis, Missouri, with permission.)

methods from cognitive psychology, which specified the component cognitive processes involved in performing complex tasks and provided a means of isolating them experimentally. In neuroimaging studies of normal subjects, as with the purely behavioral studies of patients, the entities most likely to yield clear and consistent localizations are these component cognitive processes and not the tasks themselves. Starting in the mid-1980s, a collaboration between cognitive psychologist Michael Posner and neurologist Marcus Raichle at Washington University led to a series of pioneering studies in which the neural circuits underlying language, reading, and attention were studied by PET (see Ref. 102 for a review). Since then, researchers at Washington University and a growing number of other centers around the world have adapted neuroimaging techniques to all manner of topics in behavioral neurology and neuropsychology. This progress is reflected in many of the chapters of this book, illustrating the synergism that is possible between behavioral studies with patients and neuroimaging studies with both patients and normal subjects.

Computational Modeling of Higher Brain Function

A second and even more recent methodologic development is computational modeling of higher brain function. Computational models enable us to test hypotheses about the functioning of complex, interactive systems and about the effects of lesions to individual parts of such a system by building, running, and "lesioning" the models.

The roots of the computational approach can be traced back to earlier thinking in both behavioral neurology and cognitive psychology. Within behavioral neurology, the perennial critiques of localizationism can be viewed as an early expression of the need to consider the brain as "more than the sum of its parts" for purposes of understanding cognition. Aleksandr Luria's concept of "functional systems"[103] placed explicit emphasis on the importance of the system or circuit as the correct level of analysis for understanding brain function, and this point has been reemphasized more recently by such writers as Marcel Mesulam,[104] Kenneth Heilman,[105] and Patricia Goldman-Rakic.[106] The most radical reconceptualization of brain function in terms of global system properties as opposed to local centers can be attributed to Marcel Kinsbourne,[107,108] who has argued that local phenomena such as spreading activation or competition between reciprocally connected areas can lead the system as a whole to become "captured" in certain global states of attention, awareness, or asymmetrical hemispheric control of behavior.

Within cognitive psychology, a parallel evolution has taken place, from discrete-stage models of human information processing, in which cognition unfolds through a series of functionally and temporally isolable stages, to models in which information is processed simultaneously and interactively over a network of processors. The latter type of model, similar in spirit to behavioral neurology's system-level theorizing, often takes the form of a running computer simulation in cognitive psychology. Such models have been termed "parallel distributed processing" (PDP) models, calling attention to the parallel or simultaneous nature of processing at multiple loci within the model and the distributed as opposed to localist nature of representation and processing within the model. They have also been called "artificial neural networks," calling attention to the analogy between the units in the network and neurons in the brain. Like neurons, PDP units are highly interconnected; they process information by summing inputs received from other units across excitatory and inhibitory connections and sending outputs to a large number of other units in the same way.

The initial development of such computational models in cognitive psychology was largely due to David Rumelhart, James McClelland, and their collaborators.[109] Figure 1-18 illustrates an early PDP theory of word perception, showing a high degree of interactivity among letter feature, letter, and word representations. In addition to activation flowing from letters to words, it also flows between words (through inhibitory connections, thus helping the most strongly supported word "win out" over other possible words) and from words to letters (through excitatory connections, thus explaining the previously puzzling finding that letters are perceived more clearly in words than in isolation).

By embodying the general ideas of distributedness, parallelism, and interactivity in concrete computer simulations, the specific predictions of hypotheses could be derived and tested. This is valuable because predictions about the effects local lesions in a highly interactive network on the behavior of the network as a whole can be difficult to derive by intuition alone and can sometimes be quite counterintuitive. Pioneering work in the application of PDP models to problems in behav-

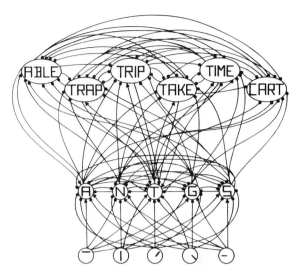

Figure 1-18
An illustration of part of the network of letter feature, letter, and word representations in McClelland and Rumelhart's "parallel distributed processing" (PDP) model of word recognition.

ioral neurology and neuropsychology was done in the realm of acquired disorders of reading by Geoffrey Hinton, David Plaut, and Tim Shallice,[110,111] Karalyn Patterson and colleagues,[112] and Michael Mozer and Marlene Behrmann.[113] Since then, such models have been applied to disorders of perception, attention, memory, frontal lobe function, and language. A comparison of conventional and PDP approaches to neuropsychology can be found in Ref. 114.

CONCLUSIONS

Six years ago the U.S. Congress declared the 1990s the "Decade of the Brain," acknowledging the progress that has been made in understanding brain function and anticipating an acceleration in new insights and discoveries as we approach the close of the century. The chapters that follow show this to have been a good call. When viewed in the context of its development through the centuries, our current understanding of higher brain functions is surely one of humanity's most impressive achievements, all the more valuable because of its application to treating neurologic and psychological disorder. We are proud of the cumulative contributions of past and present colleagues in behavioral neurology and neuropsychology, summarized in the remaining chapters of this book.

REFERENCES

1. Breasted JH: *The Edwin Smith Surgical Papyrus.* Chicago: University of Chicago Press, 1930.

2. McHenry LC Jr: *Garrison's History of Neurology.* Springfield, IL: Charles C Thomas, 1969.

3. Clarke E, O'Malley CE: *The Human Brain and Spinal Cord.* Berkeley, CA: University California Press, 1968.

4. Finger S: *Origins of Neuroscience. A History of Explorations into Brain Function.* New York: Oxford University Press, 1994.

5. Sondhaus E, Finger S: Aphasia and the CNS from Imhotep to Broca. *Neuropsychology* 2:87–110, 1988.

6. Woollam DHM: Concepts of the brain and its functions in classical antiquity, in Poynter FNL (ed): *The Brain and Its Functions.* Oxford, England: Blackwell, 1958, pp 5–18.

7. Bruyn GW: The seat of the soul, in Rose FC, Byrum WF (eds): *Historical Aspects of the Neurosciences.* New York: Raven Press, 1981, pp 55–81.

8. Mazzolini RG: Schemes and models of the thinking machine. In Corsi P (ed): *The Enchanted Loom: Chapters in the History of Neuroscience.* New York: Oxford University Press, 1991, pp 68–143.

9. Hippocrates: The sacred disease, in Adams F (trans): *The Genuine Works of Hippocrates.* New York: William Wood, 1932.

10. Clarke E, Dewhurst K: *An Illustrated History of Brain Function.* Berkeley, CA: University of California Press, 1972.

11. Pagel W: Medieval and Renaissance contributions to knowledge of the brain and its functions, in Poynter FNL (ed): *The Brain and Its Functions.* Oxford, England: Blackwell, 1958, pp 95–114.

12. Bakay L: *An Early History of Craniotomy.* Springfield, IL: Charles C Thomas, 1985.

13. Wozniak RH: *Mind and Body: René Descartes to William James.* National Library of Medicine, Bethesda, MD, and the American Psychological Association, Washington, DC, 1992.

14. Riese W: Descartes' ideas of brain function, in Poynter FNL (ed): *The Brain and Its Functions.* Oxford, England: Blackwell, 1958, pp 115–134.

15. Descartes R: *De homine figuris et latinitate donatus a Florentio Schuyl.* Leyden: Franciscum Moyardum and Petrum Leffen, 1662.

16. Descartes R: *Les passions de l'âme. Paris:* Henry Le Gras, 1649.

17. Willis T: *Cerebri anatome: Cui accessit nervorum descriptio et usus.* London: Martyn and Allestry, 1664.

18. Young RM: *Mind, Brain and Adaptation in the Nineteenth Century.* New York: Oxford University Press, 1990.

19. Bell C: *Idea of a New Anatomy of the Brain: Submitted for the Observations of His Friends.* London: Strahan and Preston, 1811.

20. Magendie F: Expériences sur les fonctions des racines des nerts rachidiens. *J Physiol Exp Pathol* 2:276–279, 1822.

21. Stookey B: A note on the early history of cerebral localization. *Bull NY Acad Med* 30:559–578, 1954.

22. Ackerknecht EH: Contribution of Gall and the phrenologist to knowledge of brain function, in Poynter FNL (ed): *The Brain and Its Functions.* Oxford: Blackwell, 1958, pp 149–153.

23. Pogliano C: Between form and function: A new science of man, in Corsi P (ed): *The Enchanted Loom: Chapters in the History of Neurosciences.* New York: Oxford University Press, 1991, pp 144–203.

24. Brown JW, Chobor KL: Phrenological studies of aphasia before Broca: Broca's aphasia or Gall's aphasia? *Brain Lang* 43:475–486, 1992.

25. Flourens P: *Phrenology Examined* (Charles De Lucena Meigs, trans). Philadelphia: Hogan and Thompson, 1846.

26. Flourens P: *Recherches Expérimentales sur les Propriétés et les Fonctions du Système Nerveux dans les Animaux Vertèbras* (1824), 2d ed. Paris: Baillière, 1842.

27. Harrington A: Beyond phrenology: Localization theory in the modern era, in Corsi P (ed): *The Enchanted Loom. Chapters in the History of Neuroscience.* New York: Oxford University Press, 1991, pp 207–239.

28. Bouillaud JB: *Traité clinique et physiologique de l'encephalite ou inflammation du cerveau.* Paris: Baillière, 1825.

29. Benton AL, Joynt RJ: Early descriptions of aphasia. *Arch Neurol* 3:205–221, 1960.

30. Benton AL, Joynt RJ: Three pioneers in the study of aphasia. *J His Med Sci* 18:381–383, 1963

31. Joynt RJ, Benton AL: The memoir of Marc Dax on aphasia. *Neurology* 14:851–854, 1964.

32. Head H: *Aphasia and Kindred Disorders of Speech.* New York: Macmillan, 1926.

33. Stookey BL: Jean-Baptiste Bouillaud and Ernest Aubertin: Early studies on cerebral localization and the speech center. *JAMA* 184:1024–1029, 1963.

34. Critchley M: The Broca-Dax controversy, in Critchley M (ed): *The Divine Banquet of the Brain and Other Essays.* New York: Raven Press, 1979.

35. Joynt RJ: Centenary of patient "Tan": His contribution to the problem of aphasia. *Arch Intern Med* 108:953–956, 1961.

36. Broca P: Remarques sur le siège de la faculté du langage articulé: Suivies d'une observation d'aphémie. *Bull Soc Anat (Paris)* 6:330–357, 1861.

37. Broca P: Localisation des fonctions cérébrales: Siège du langage articulé. *Bull Soc Anthropol (Paris)* 4:200–203, 1863.

38. Dax M: Lesions de la moitié gauche de l'encéphale coincident avec l'oublie des signes de la pensée. *Gaz hbd Méd Chir (Paris)* 2:259–262, 1865.

39. Dax G: Notes sur la mème sujet. *Gaz hbd Méd Chir (Paris)* 2:262, 1865.

40. Broca P: Sur le siège de la faculté du langage articulé. *Bull Soc Anthropol* 6:337–393, 1865.

41. Berker EA, Berker AH, Smith A: Translation of Broca's 1865 report: Localization of speech in the third left frontal convolution. *Arch Neurol* 43:1065–1072, 1986.

42. Fritsch G, Hitzig E: On the electrical excitability of the cerebrum (1870), in von Bonin G (ed): *Some Papers on the Cerebral Cortex.* Springfield, IL: Charles C Thomas, 1960, pp 73–96.

43. Geschwind N: Wernicke's contribution to the study of aphasia. *Cortex* 3:449–463, 1967.

44. Wernicke C: *Der aphasische Symptomemkomplex: Eine psychologische Studie auf anatomischer Basis.* Breslau: Cohn und Weigert, 1874.

45. Lecours AR, Lhermitte F: From Franz Gall to Pierre Marie, in Lecours AR, Lhermitte F, Bryans B (eds): *Aphasiology.* London: Baillière Tindall, 1983.

46. Geschwind N: Carl Wernicke, the Breslau School and the history of aphasia, in Carterette EC (ed): *Brain Function:* Vol III. *Speech, Language, and Communication.* Berkeley, CA: University of California Press, 1963, pp 1–16.

47. Lichtheim L: On aphasia. *Brain* 7:433–484, 1885.

48. Liepmann H: Das Krankheitsbild der Apraxie ("motorische Asymbolie") auf Grund eines Falles von einseitiger Apraxie. *Monatschr Psychiatr Neurol* 8:15–44, 102–132, 182–197, 1900.

49. Liepmann H, Maas O: Fall von linksseitiger Agraphie und Apraxie bei rechtsseitiger Lähmung. *J Psychol Neurol* 10:214–227, 1907.

50. Déjerine J: Contribution à l'étude anatomopathologique et clinique des différentes variétés de cécité verbale. *CRH Séances Mem Soc Biol* 44:61–90, 1892.

51. Geschwind N: Disconnexion syndromes in animals and man. *Brain* 88:237–294, 585–644, 1965.

52. Brais B: The third left frontal convolution plays no role in language: Pierre Marie and the Paris debate on aphasia (1906–1908). *Neurology* 42:690–695, 1992.

53. Goldstein K: *The Organism.* New York: American Book, 1939.

54. Goldstein K: *Language and Language Disturbances.* New York: Grune & Stratton, 1948.

55. Lecours AR, Cronk C, Sébahoun-Balsamo M: From Pierre Marie to Norman Geschwind, in Lecours AR, Lhermitte F, Bryans B (eds): *Aphasiology.* London: Baillière Tindall, 1983.

56. Franz SI, Lashley KS: The retention of habits by the rat after destruction of the frontal portion of the cerebrum. *Psychobiology* 1:3–18, 1917.

57. Lashley KS, Franz SI: The effects of cerebral destruction upon habit-formation and retention in the albino rat. *Psychobiology* 1:71–139, 1917.

58. Lashley KS: *Brain Mechanisms and Intelligence: A Quantitative Study of Injuries to the Brain.* Chicago: University of Chicago Press, 1929.

59. Lashley KS: In search of the engram. *Symp Soc Exp Biol* 4:454–482, 1950.

60. Geschwind N: The paradoxical position of Kurt Goldstein in the history of aphasia. *Cortex* 1:214–224, 1964.

61. Harrington A: A feeling for the "whole": the holistic reaction in neurology from the fin de siècle to the interwar years, in Teich M, Porter R (eds): *Fin de Siècle and Its Legacy.* Cambridge, England: Cambridge University Press, 1990.

62. Vogt O, Vogt C: Zur anatomischen Gliederung des cortex cerebri. *J Psychol Neurol* 2:160–180, 1903.

63. Haymaker WE: Cecile and Oskar Vogt, on the occasion of her 75th and his 80th birthday. *Neurology* 1:179–204, 1951.

64. Campbell AW: Histological studies on cerebral localization. *Proc R Soc* 72:488–492, 1903.

65. Campbell AW: *Histological Studies on the Localization of Cerebral Function.* Cambridge, England: Cambridge University Press, 1905.

66. Brodmann K: *Vergleichende Lokalisationslehre der Grosshirnrinde in ihren Prinzipien dargestellt auf Grund des Zellenbaues.* Leipzig: Barth, 1909.

67. Levin HS, Peters BH, Hulkonen DA: Early concepts of anterograde and retrograde amnesia. *Cortex* 19:427–440, 1983.

68. Ribot T: *Diseases of Memory.* London: Kegan Paul, Trench, 1882.

69. Squire LR, Slater PC: Anterograde and retrograde memory impairment in chronic amnesia. *Neuropsychologia* 16:313–322, 1978.

70. Victor M, Adams RD, Collins GH: *The Wernicke-Korsakoff Syndrome and Related Neurologic Disorders due to Alcoholism and Malnutrition,* 2d ed. Philadelphia: Davis, 1989.

71. Victor M, Yakovlev PI: SS Korsakoff's psychic disorder in conjunction with peripheral neuritis: A translation of Korsakoff's original article with brief comments on the author and his contribution to clinical medicine. *Neurology* 5:394–406, 1955.

72. Munk H: Über die Functionen der Grosshirnrinde: Gesammelte Mitteilungen aus den Jahren. Berlin: Hirschwald, 1877–1880.

73. Lissauer H: Ein fall von seelenblindheit nebst einem Beitrage zur Theori derselben. *Arch Psychiatr Nervenkrankh* 21:222–270, 1980.

74. Freud S: Zur Auffassung der Aphasien. Leipzig and Vienna: Deuticke, 1891.

75. Paterson A, Zangwill OL: Disorders of visual space perception associated with lesions of the right cerebral hemisphere. *Brain* 40:122–179, 1944.

76. Hécaen H, Ajuriaguerra J, Massonet J: Les troubles visuoconstructives par lésion pariéto-occipitale droite. *Encéphale* 40:122–179, 1951.

77. Benton A: Neuropsychology: Past, present and future, in Boller F, Grafman J (eds): *Handbook of Neuropsychology.* New York: Elsevier, 1988, vol 1, pp 3–27.

78. Hannay HJ, Varney NR, Benton AL: Visual localization in patients with unilateral brain disease. *J Neurol Neurosurg Psychiatry* 39:307–313, 1976.

79. Ratcliff G, Davies-Jones GAB: Defective visual localization in focal brain wounds. *Brain* 95:46–60, 1972.

80. Warrington EK, Rabin P: Perceptual matching in patients with cerebral lesions. *Neuropsychologia* 8:475–487, 1970.

81. De Renzi E, Faglioni P, Scotti G: Judgement of spatial orientation in patients with focal brain damage. *J Neurol Neurosurg Psychiatry* 34:489–495, 1971.

82. Carmon A, Benton AL: Tactile perception of direction and number in patients with unilateral cerebral disease. *Neurology* 19:525–532, 1969.

83. Hécaen H, Tzortzis C, Masure MC: Troubles de l'orientation spatiale dans une épreuve de recherche d'itinéraire lors des lesions corticales unilaterales. *Perception* 1:325–330, 1972.

84. Semmes J, Weinstein S, Ghent L, Teuber HL: Correlates of impaired orientation in personal and extrapersonal space. *Brain* 86:747–772, 1963.

85. Milner B: Some effects of frontal lobectomy in man, in Warren JM, Akert K (eds): *The Frontal Granular Cortex and Behavior.* New York: McGraw-Hill, 1964.

86. Milner B: Memory and the medical temporal regions of the brain, in Pribram KH, Broadbent DE (eds): *Biological Bases of Memory.* New York: Academic Press, 1970.

87. Trevarthen C, Roger W: Sperry's lifework and our tribute, in Trevarthen C (ed): *Brain Circuits and Functions of the Mind: Essays in Honor of Roger W. Sperry.* Cambridge, England: Cambridge University Press, 1990.

88. Goodglass H, Kaplan E: Disturbance of gesture and patomime in aphasia. *Brain* 86:703–720, 1963.

89. Newcombe F, Russell W: Dissociated visual perceptual and spatial deficits in focal lesions of the right hemisphere. *J Neurol Neurosurg Psychiatry* 32:73–81, 1969.

90. Hécaen H, Albert ML: *Human Neuropsychology.* New York: Wiley, 1978.

91. Heilman KM, Valenstein E: *Clinical Neuropsychology.* New York: Oxford University Press, 1979.

92. Kolb B, Whishaw I: *Fundamentals of Human Neuropsychology.* New York: Freeman, 1980.

93. Springer SP, Deutsch G: *Left Brain/Right Brain.* San Franciso: Freeman, 1981.

94. Walsh KW: *Neuropsychology: A Clinical Approach.* New York: Churchill Livingstone, 1978.

95. Anderson JR: Arguments concerning representation for mental imagery. *Psychol Rev* 85:249–277, 1978.

96. Farah MJ: Is visual imagery really visual? Overlooked evidence from neuropsychology. *Psychol Rev* 95:307–317, 1988.

97. Schacter DL: Implicit memory: History and current status. *J Exp Psychol Learn Mem Cog* 13:501–518, 1987.

98. Squire L: *Memory and Brain.* New York: Oxford University Press, 1987.

99. Weiskrantz L: On issues and theories of the human amnesic syndrome, in Weinberger N, McGaugh JL, Lynch G (eds): *Memory Systems of the Brain.* New York: Guilford Press, 1985.

100. Treisman A: Features and objects: The fourteenth Bartlett lecture. *Q J Exp Psychol* 40A:201–237, 1988.

101. Coltheart M: Cognitive neuropsychology and the study of reading, in Marin IP, Marin OSM (eds): *Attention and Performance XI.* London: Erlbaum, 1985.

102. Posner MI, Raichle ME: *Images of Mind.* New York: Scientific American Library, 1994.

103. Luria AR: *The Working Brain.* New York: Basic Books, 1973.

104. Mesulam M-M: A cortical network for directed attention and unilateral neglect. *Ann Neurol* 10:309–325, 1981.

105. Heilman KM, Watson RT, Valenstein E: Hemispatial neglect, in Heilman KM, Valenstein E (eds): *Clinical Neuropsychology.* New York: Oxford University Press, 1979.

106. Goldman-Rakic P: Topography of cognition: Parallel distributed networks in primate association cortex. *Annu Rev Neurosci* 11:137–156, 1988.

107. Kinsbourne M: Lateral interactions in the brain, in Kinsbourne M, Smith WL (eds): *Hemispheric Disconnection and Cerebral Function.* Springfield, IL: Charles C Thomas, 1974.

108. Kinsbourne M: Integrated field theory of consciousness, in Marcel AJ, Bisiach E (eds): *Consciousness in Contemporary Science.* Oxford, England: Clarendon Press, 1988.

109. Rumelhart DE, McClelland JL: *Parallel Distributed Processing: Explorations in the Microstructure of Cognition.* Cambridge, MA: MIT Press, 1986.

110. Hinton GE, Shallice T: Lesioning an attractor network: Investigations of acquired dyslexia. *Psychol Rev* 98:74–95, 1991.

111. Plaut DC, Shallice T: Deep dyslexia: A case study of connectionist neuropsychology. *Cog Neuropsychol* 10:377–500, 1993.

112. Patterson KE, Seidenberg MS, McClelland JL: Connections and disconnections: Acquired dyslexia in a computational model of reading processes, in Morris RGM (ed): *Parallel Distributed Processing: Implications for Psychology and Neuroscience.* London: Oxford University Press, 1990.

113. Mozer MC, Behrmann M: On the interaction of selective attention and lexical knowledge: A connectionist account of neglect dyslexia. *J Cognit Neurosci* 5:89–117, 1990.

114. Farah MJ: Neuropsychological inference with an interactive brain. *Behav Brain Sci* 17:43–104, 1994.

Chapter 2

THE MENTAL STATUS EXAM

Richard L. Strub
F. William Black

The mental status examination employed by behavioral neurologists, neuropsychologists, and neuropsychiatrists was developed to elicit and to some extent quantify the behavioral changes that are found in patients with classic organic brain disease or dysfunction. The types of behavior that have characteristically been sampled are largely cognitive or higher cortical functions, though some noncognitive areas such as the changes in comportment seen in the frontal lobe syndrome are also explored.

The current mental status examination has evolved from the nineteenth-century neurologists' interest in aphasia, agnosia, apraxia, alexia, and other specific cognitive dysfunctions. In this century, psychologists, particularly Binet,[1] began to explore global cognitive function by developing tests of intelligence. These were initially used in school placement but have now become the mainstay of neuropsychological testing. In the 1930s, Bender began her work on the gestalt constructional tests, initially investigating their value in assessing developmental changes and later observing their deterioration in disease. In the last half of this century, neurologists and psychologists have borrowed from each other and developed both sophisticated, quantitative neuropsychology batteries and comprehensive bedside mental status examinations.

The primary goals of any neurologically based mental status examination (MSE) include (1) early detection of organically based behavioral changes, (2) screening to determine the need for a comprehensive neuropsychological assessment, and (3) acquisition of data contributing to the diagnosis of both general neurobehavioral syndromes (e.g., dementia) and specific neurobehavioral disorders (e.g., dementia of the Alzheimer type). The mental status examination (MSE) can be used in acute hospital settings, in post–acute rehabilitation settings, or in the office. As an exam, it should be both comprehensive and relatively quick (i.e., 30 to 60 min).

A number of screening procedures or mental status examinations are currently available for clinical use. Some of these tests were designed to evaluate only one cognitive function, such as language (the Aphasia Screening Test[3]), constructional ability (the Bender Gestalt Test[2]), or intelligence (Shipley-Hartford Scale[4]). Others have been developed to diagnose and document the progression of specific neurobehavioral syndromes, the most common condition being dementia. The Blessed, Tomlinson, Roth Dementia Scale—commonly known as the Blessed[5]—the Dementia Rating Scale,[6] and the Mental Status Questionnaire,[7] are typical examples of this type of instrument, many of which contain a mixture of historical information, questions regarding adaptive behavior, and actual patient examination items. Additional measures have been devised to screen for symptoms and degree of dementia, relying primarily on information provided by the family or caregiver (e.g., Alzheimer Dementia Assessment Scale;[8] Cognitive Behavioral Rating Scales[9]).

Other screening tests evaluate a wider range

of cognitive functions, among these tests, the most widely used is the Mini-Mental State Examination,[10] a test designed as a general screening test for "organicity." Because of the inclusion of many verbal memory items, it has been extensively used to screen for and follow the progression of patients with dementia. This test is "objective" in that each item is numerically scored and total score for the test is derived by summing the item scores. Because the test has been standardized and validated on the basis of the total score, it is sensitive in only the most general way—the identification and the degree of organicity. This and similar tests, such as the Cognitive Capacity Screening Exam[11] and the Dementia Rating Scale, are useful in following overall deterioration. For advanced-stage dementia patients, the Severe Impairment Battery[12] has been developed to assess basic cognitive functioning in individuals who are so demented that they are unable to perform validly on conventional measures. Recently, Trzepacz and Baker[13] have published a comprehensive mental status examination directed primarily for use with psychiatric patients but including some areas of neurobehavioral functioning.

The primary problem with most brief screening measures results from the limited number of test items, and although each of the exams has its advantages as well as drawbacks, no absolute statement can be made regarding the relative merits of any single MSE versus another because very few comparative studies of such procedures have been carried out. The sensitivity of the tests varies, the Strub/Black[14] being more sensitive than the Folstein, for example. However, the specificity of the tests depends greatly upon the question asked. No test can validly separate multi-infarct dementia from Alzheimer disease, but many of the comprehensive tests can diagnose an organic amnesic state such as Korsakoff syndrome. See Berg and coworkers[15] or Lezak[16] for further information regarding the utility and potential problems inherent in these screening procedures.

The bedside or office mental status examination described in this chapter is a reasonably comprehensive and broadly derived diagnostic and descriptive examination that represents a structured inventory of the major clinically relevant cognitive functions most often affected in organic mental syndromes. Although primarily a qualitative examination, an objective screening examination based on this exam for use with dementia patients has been standardized for clinical use and does provide a total score for overall rating purposes.[14]

The examination and the individual tasks within the examination are discussed more in terms of their rationale and the usefulness of the function tested rather than offering a detailed explanation of how the evaluation is performed. Performance on some of the cognitive functions show an age-related deterioration irrespective of the presence of disease; these normal changes of aging are pointed out in each section. The examination is organized in a hierarchical fashion, where the latter items on the test require relatively intact performance on earlier items. For example, valid assessment of verbal memory and verbal abstract reasoning requires competence in the basic language system.

HISTORY

As in any medical or psychological examination, the history obtained from the patient and significant others provides extremely important information pertaining to the patient's current complaints and background. The history taken from family members or close friends is particularly important when patients have cognitive disorders. The history should be systematically organized and must include the following areas of clinical concern: (1) information to establish the patient's premorbid level of functioning; (2) data to establish the presence or absence of behavioral indicators of organic dysfunction (e.g., aphasia, memory problems, or social-behavioral dyscontrol); (3) consideration of preexisting or coexisting emotional or behavioral problems; (4) the patient's general medical condition; (5) social and vocational history, including education, vocation, and hobbies; and (6) family medical history, especially of neurologic and psychiatric disease.

EXAMINATION

Behavioral Observations

The mental status evaluation involves more than the testing of specific cognitive functions. The data needed to diagnose such common behavioral syndromes as delirium (acute confusional states), the frontal lobe syndrome, and the denial/neglect syndromes are gathered through structured history taking and observation.

Acute Confusional State (Delirium)   This is a very common clinical condition that is seen in both outpatient practice and the hospital setting (see Chap. 37). Its etiology is primarily toxic (i.e., medication or alcohol/drugs) or metabolic. Such conditions as sepsis, organ failure, significant electrolyte imbalance, or a combination of medical problems plus medication side effects are the most common causes. In delirium, every cell in the brain has been subjected to the general medical derangement; therefore, all cognitive as well as all noncognitive functions can be affected. There are, however, certain features that can validly separate the changes of delirium from other behavioral syndromes—for instance, dementia. The evaluation involves three elements: history of changes over time, examination of the patient at a specific moment in time, and the search for the cause.

History

1.   Speed of onset—hours to days
2.   Fluctuation—common over the 24-h period
3.   Sleep-wake disturbances

Examination

1.   Level of consciousness—almost always altered
2.   Psychomotor activity level—either increased or decreased
3.   Incoherence/disorganization in speech and activity
4.   Hallucinations

5.   Inappropriate behavior
6.   Misinterpretation of surroundings (illusions and delusions)

Items 4, 5, and 6 may be obtained from the history and not be present on examination.

Frontal Lobe Syndrome   During history-taking and throughout the examination, the examiner must ask for and look for the specific behavior changes associated with frontal lobe dysfunction. The primary changes have to do with comportment, goal direction, impulsivity, ability to anticipate the result of one's actions, and drive. Subtle cognitive changes such as difficulty with set-shifting (perseveration), recent memory problems, and serial ordering are also present. (Chapters 30 and 31 fully discuss the frontal lobe syndrome.) With routine mental status testing, the most important thing the examiner can do is to ask other people who have known the patient for many years if the patient has experienced behavior changes typical of frontal lobe disease. For example: "Is the patient now apathetic, euphoric, impulsive, irritable, or doing things that are inappropriate and out of character?" A clear change in behavior is significant. One subtest on the mental status examination that is frequently abnormal in frontal lobe disease is the verbal fluency test (described below), in which the patient must rapidly scan stored memory and come up with a verbal list of items (e.g., animals or words beginning with a single letter).

Neglect   Another behavior function that can be evaluated on patient observation is hemineglect (see Chaps. 24 and 25). In its most dramatic form, the patient may totally neglect one or both sides of the body (e.g., a man might shave only one side of his face) as well as extrapersonal space. In most cases there is only neglect of extrapersonal space; for example, people to one side are ignored or food on one side of the tray is untouched. The neglect can be further elicited on drawing tests, where a flower may have petals on one side or a clock will have all numbers on one side. These patients will also tend to suppress or extinguish stimuli on one side when presented with bilaterally simultaneous stimulations. This extinction can be unimodal (tactile or visual only) or polymodal.

Level of Consciousness and Attention

The term *consciousness* as used medically refers to alertness and the capacity of the patient to react to the environment, both external and internal. Assessment of a patient's level of consciousness is very important, because disease and dysfunction of the brain will frequently affect it. Not only is a change in the level of consciousness often an important behavioral sign of brain dysfunction but impaired consciousness can certainly adversely affect performance of subsequent cognitive tests, especially recent memory/new learning. Although there is a spectrum of levels of consciousness from hyperalert to comatose (see Table 2-1), the levels that are most important in the mental status examination are hyperalert through obtunded.

A second basic and related brain function that requires assessment during mental status testing is attention. Attention (selective attention) implies a capacity to focus on a single stimulus without distraction from extraneous external or internal stimuli. *Vigilance* or *concentration* refers to sustained attention. Conversely, distractibility

and inattention are the symptoms of disordered attention mechanisms. Although many methods of testing attention and vigilance have been devised,[15–17] we have found the procedures outlined below to be both time-efficient and clinically useful.

Observation Information gained during the history taking (from both patient and family members) and careful observation of the patient's behavior can provide important clues to the patient's ability to attend. Attention may be objectively evaluated using a clinical rating system (poor = 0, excellent = 4), or merely qualitatively recorded as a detailed clinical observation.

Digit Repetition Test Digit span has been used as a measure of attention and a component of general intellectual functioning in virtually all standard intelligence tests. Considerable research has demonstrated its utility as a means of quantifying attention or freedom from distractibility. Performance on digit span forward appears to be reasonably specific for auditory attention, while digits backward can be adversely affected by a variety of factors other than basic attention, so the test should not be used for this purpose.[18] The average adult with normal attention should repeat a minimum of seven to nine digits accurately, while fewer than five digits accurately repeated suggests impaired attention.

"A" Test for Vigilance The patient is presented with a verbally administered series of random letters, among which the stimulus letter "A" appears with greater than random frequency. The patient is instructed to indicate whenever he or she recognizes the stimulus letter. The patient's performance is scored for errors of omission, commission, and perseveration. Errors are virtually never made on this test by normals, more than two omission errors being indicative of inattention and two commission errors suggesting impulsivity. More than one inadvertent instance of perseveration is pathologic.

Although various serial subtraction and addition tasks have traditionally been included in

Table 2-1
Levels of consciousness

Hyperalert	Anxiety, mania, or metabolic/toxic excitement from medicines, etc.
Alert	Fully awake and aware of surroundings
Lethargic/somnolent	Not fully alert, tends to drift off to sleep if not stimulated
Obtunded	Requires stimulation to arouse and confused when aroused
Stuporous	Requires vigorous stimulation to arouse; minimal purposeful interaction
Comatose	Unresponsive

many psychiatric and neurologic mental status examinations (e.g., "serial 7s"), most research conducted on such procedures has demonstrated their limited clinical utility. The primary limiting factors for these measures are the confounding influence of intelligence, education, and variable familiarity with tasks of this type.[19]

Both consciousness and attention can be affected by brain dysfunction; the brain dysfunction can be primarily emotional, as in anxiety states, mood disorders or panic disorder, or it may be organic, as in brain tumor, toxic/metabolic delirium, attention deficit disorder, and so on. Since both an alteration in level in consciousness and abnormalities in the ability to sustain attention can prejudice performance on cognitive testing, the examiner must be very cautious in interpreting results obtained in patients who are not fully alert and attentive.

Language

Disruption in language function is a common symptom in brain disease. Structural lesions, especially ischemic stroke in the language-dominant hemisphere, produce the most dramatic and well-known language syndromes (i.e., aphasia—see Chap. 8); however, the generalized cerebral disorders, such as delirium and dementia, also produce changes in language function. Because much of the mental status examination relies upon relatively intact language proficiency, language testing is performed early in the examination. The important features of a true language disturbance (aphasia) are problems in word choice—either trouble with word-finding or poor word choice (e.g., paraphasia, where an improper word is substituted for the correct one); abnormal syntax (e.g., the telegraphic style of Broca's aphasia); or reduced comprehension (e.g., the classic lack of comprehension of Wernicke's aphasia). Since language syndromes differ in left-handed patients with focal lesions, it is important to know the patient's handedness history when the examination findings are being interpreted.

Testing should include (1) assessment of spontaneous running speech for errors in syntax and word choice, (2) verbal fluency testing (e.g., animal names, words beginning with a specific letter produced in 1 min), (3) evaluation of comprehension, (4) repetition testing, (5) naming of objects (common objects (e.g., pen) followed by less common ones (e.g., watch crystal)), and (6) written language—both reading and writing. Testing of comprehension, repetition, naming, and written language should begin with easy or restricted tasks and then go on to tasks that are increasingly difficult and linguistically complex.

Language function changes little with advancing age; the one exception is verbal fluency. The patient under age 70, for example, can produce between 17 and 24 animal names in 1 min, whereas the 70- to 80-year-old produces between 14 and 20 and those over 80 produce from 10 to 20. In dementia and frontal lobe disease, there is a distinct decrease in verbal fluency early in the disease process. Naming errors of low-frequency words (e.g., watch stem, tines of a fork) is also an early sign in dementia.

Memory

The ability to store information and retrieve it at a later time is the basic mental function underlying all learning. It is also a function that is often adversely affected by brain disease and therefore of great interest to clinicians and researchers alike (see Chaps. 33 to 36).

For example, in dementia of the Alzheimer type, deficient memory function is often the initial presenting symptom, while in other conditions (amnesic syndromes)—notably Korsakoff syndrome, posterior cerebral artery strokes, and closed head injury with temporal involvement—memory dysfunction is the primary cognitive defect. Given the sensitivity of the various memory processes to any aberrations in mental function, factors other than organic brain dysfunction, including depression, anxiety, and other primary psychogenic disturbances, can also produce observable problems in memory function. Accordingly, memory dysfunction can be considered to be a highly sensitive mental status finding, although in isolation it is not always specific to a particular neurobehavioral syndrome.

Learning ability varies between individuals and is to some degree related to intelligence, though not a specific element in IQ testing. Memory is also subtly affected in advancing age. Older (age 60 and above) individuals process information more slowly and retains less after a single exposure than younger people. This age-related change is not dramatic but sufficiently great that it must be appreciated during bedside testing (see Table 2-2).

Three principal types of memory are usually evaluated. The first is immediate memory, which involves repeating a short series of items such as numbers immediately after they are given (e.g., digit span testing). In this task, the memory trace is held only long enough for immediate repetition. The second type is recent or short-term memory; this requires that the memory trace be stored and then retrieved after an interval during which the individual is deliberately distracted. This interval can be 10 s, as in certain experimental paradigms, or 5 min, as in clinical mental status testing. The term in common usage also implies retaining personal or historical information over several days or weeks. Third and finally, the term *remote memory* refers to the retrieval of memories stored many years previously, such as the names of school friends, famous people, or historical events.

The basic limbic hippocampal system is the neuroanatomic substrate that facilitates information storage and retrieval. The cortex is the most probable repository of information, but limbic damage prevents the patient from freely accessing it and, to a great degree, from storing new information. This system facilitates memory in all sensory spheres, so damage will affect verbal, visual, and tactile as well as motor memory storage. In order to test recent memory (new learning) in a patient with aphasia, for example, it is important to test visual memory rather than trying to assess the functional integrity of memory by sorting though aphasic responses on verbal memory testing. In testing memory in suspected or established dementia patients, especially Alzheimer dementia, significant emphasis should be placed on new learning tasks, for they have the highest diagnostic sensitivity of all items in the examination.

Testing of recent memory should include several items: orientation, recent news and personal history, and specific new learning tasks both verbal and visual. Orientation to time, place, and person is an excellent indication of how well the patient remembers ongoing events. The elements most frequently missed are the exact date and day of the week. Normal individuals rarely make significant errors in this area; however, it is fairly common not to know the exact date or day of the week.[21] The error is much smaller in college-educated ($\pm$ 1 day) persons than in those who did not go beyond high school ($\pm$ 2 days).

Table 2-2
Recent memory performance

	Normal individuals—age in years					Alzheimer disease patients—stage			
	40–49	*50–59*	*60–69*	*70–79*	*80–89*	*I*	*II*	*III*	*IV*
Four words									
5 min	3.1	2.9	2.0	1.8	2.1	1.6	0.4	0	0
10 min	3.7	3.5	3.0	2.6	2.7	1.9	0.7	0.1	0
30 min	3.7	4.0	3.5	3.1	2.9	1.8	0.6	0.1	0
Story (max = 26 bits of information)	10.1	11.1	9.7	8.2	7.6	5.5	2.8	0.6	0
Five objects	4.6	4.7	4.2	3.9	3.8	2.3	1.1	0.2	0

Patients with early dementia will often be fully oriented; therefore, this is not as sensitive an item as is asking the patient to remember specific new items such as four unrelated words (e.g., *brown, tulip, eyedropper,* and *honesty*) or, a logical memory paragraph (story). If a patient is not fully oriented, then the orientation test can be used as a new learning item. For visual memory testing, the easiest tasks is to have the patient watch you hide five items in the office then attempt to name and locate them after 5 min. Table 2-2 shows the age-related performance with mean and standard deviation for normal and Alzheimer patients (age-pooled). Several important observations can be made from these data: (1) there is a subtle decrease in the ability to learn new things starting in the sixth decade; (2) there is significant difference in performance on the "five hidden objects" test but not on the four-word test between the elderly normal and very early Alzheimer patients; (3) normal older individuals learn across trials (selective reminding) in the four-word test. To avoid making a diagnosis of dementia in a normal elderly patient, the above points must be appreciated.

Constructional Ability

Constructional ability (constructional praxis) refers to the ability to reproduce (draw or construct) printed designs or two- and three-dimensional shapes (e.g., picture puzzles or block designs) from a stimulus or in response to verbal command (see Chap. 19). A variety of tests of this nonverbal cognitive function have traditionally been included in neuropsychological screening exams. We have found paper-and-pencil test items to be valid, reliable, time efficient, and easily transportable in screening patients for constructional impairment. Constructional tasks are good tests to identify nonverbal cortical (and to some extent subcortical) dysfunction. Abnormalities are most often seen in parietal lobe (right > left) disease but can be demonstrated in patients with damage in any area of the brain.

Reproduction Drawings The following two- and three-dimensional items have proved to val-

Figure 2-1
Examples of the 4-point scoring system for Drawings to Command.

idly and reliably differentiate normals (including low-IQ normals) from brain-damaged patients: (1) vertical diamond, (2) two-dimensional cross, (3) three-dimensional box, (4) three-dimensional pipe (smoking implement), and (5) intersecting triangles (triangle within a triangle) (Fig. 2-1). Formal scoring, using a rating system ranging from 0 (poor or impaired reproduction) to 3 (excellent performance) helps to quantify the patient's performance. A score of 0 on any single design is very highly suggestive of neurologic dysfunction (100 percent probability in one study), while a rating of 1 resulted in a probability of 80 percent.[22]

Drawings to Command The patient is requested to draw the following three simple items to verbal command: (1) clock with numbers and

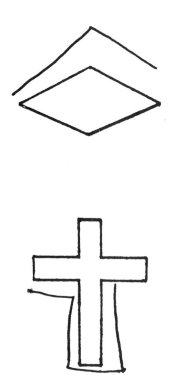

Figure 2-2
Examples of commonly seen "closing in" errors.

hands (hands set at a specific time, such as 2:30), (2) daisy in a flowerpot, and (3) three-dimensional house (Fig. 2-2). In addition to the formal scoring system, instances of perseveration, rotation, closing in, and an interesting tendency to write the name of the object rather than draw the picture are considered strongly indicative of organic pathology. The latter finding is most commonly seen in cases of moderate to advanced dementia or other significant diffuse cortical abnormality. Demented individuals can often draw the clock with all numbers correctly placed but will confuse hand placement and make significant errors. Reproduction and command drawings are remarkably stable throughout life.

In general use with organic patients, we have found drawings to command to be more sensitive to the presence of constructional disorders than reproduction drawings, probably because of the relatively more complex and abstract nature of the task, its integrative nature (auditory input–

motoric output), and the necessity of relying on stored memories for successful performance.

Other Higher Cortical Functions

Higher-order integrative motor and sensory functions and their concomitant dysfunction have been of great interest to neurologists since the mid-nineteenth century. Testing of specific integrative motor function (praxis/apraxia) and sensory perception (gnosis/agnosia) is often carried out during the routine neurologic examination but is equally appropriate to a comprehensive mental status examination.

Praxis or complex integrative motor functions is tested using three types of challenges: (1) asking the patient to perform a specific task (e.g., "Show me how to flip a coin"); (2) having the patient copy the examiner in carrying out the task; and (3) giving the patient the actual object to manipulate. Each aspect of testing involves slightly different neuropsychological processing and can be affected in different ways, depending upon the lesion's location and extent. Errors such as turning the hand over and back or bouncing the coin up and down in the open hand would be considered apraxic.

Praxis testing should include involvement of the buccofacial musculature (e.g., "Blow out a match") as well as limbs and the whole body (e.g., "Show me how you bow" or "Hit a baseball").

Testing using complex multistep commands (e.g., folding a letter, placing it in an envelope, sealing it, then addressing and stamping it) evaluates another type of praxis called ideational praxis. Further discussion of the theory and implications of praxis are covered in Chap. 15.

Gnosis or agnosia testing is performed by presenting an object to the patient in single or multiple sensory modalities (visual, auditory, and tactile). Patients with damage or dysfunction in the association cortices of the specific sense modality will display errors in perception and therefore identification. The resulting agnosia can be modality-specific, such as visual or tactile agnosia (see Chaps. 16 and 23), or multimodal (i.e., object agnosia). Specific agnosias for color (see Chap. 18) and face recognition (prosopagnosia; see Chap. 17) can also be tested using color chips and a gallery of famous faces. Finger gnosis is another specialized function where patients are asked to either verbally identify or display knowledge of the relative positions on the hand of the various fingers (e.g., touch one finger on the patient and ask him or her to point to the same finger on the opposite hand of the examiner).

Right-left orientation is another function that tests the patient's knowledge of body schema that can be tested using verbal labels (e.g., "point to my left ear with your right hand") or by nonverbal means where the examiner touches the patient and asks that the patient touch the same side of the examiner. Testing of these higher functions requires varying degrees of language proficiency, so interpretation of errors made by patients with aphasia must be made with great caution.

Abstract Tasks: Measures of Higher Cognitive Functioning

Abstract tasks, which are typically referred to as among the higher cognitive functions, involve the highest levels of human cognitive functioning that can be readily assessed using standard clinical means. Such abilities involve the application of more basic cognitive functions to the solution of new and changing problems. The manipulation of previous learned knowledge, abstract reasoning, planning and problem solving, and complex arithmetic calculations are examples of such functions. As they represent the highest levels of intellectual development, abstract tasks are frequently disrupted by brain dysfunction of any etiology. Each of these higher cognitive abilities is, however, closely related to basic intelligence, educational exposure and learning, and social experience. The following items have been selected to assess a spectrum of relevant higher cognitive functions.

Proverb Interpretation   Tests of proverb interpretation have commonly been employed as measures of the adequacy of conceptual reasoning. The ability to interpret proverbs accurately (e.g., "Rome wasn't built in a day") requires an adequate fund of general information as well as the ability to retrieve this information from memory

storage, to apply it to novel situations, and to reason in the abstract. Each proverb is scored based on the basis of the degree of abstraction expressed in the patient's response. Gorham[23] and Delis and coworkers[24] have published lists of proverbs and scoring methods that are readily adaptable to mental status testing. A concrete interpretation (e.g., "Rome is a big city; it couldn't be built in a day") of a proverb is suggestive of neurobehavioral dysfunction in all but the mentally retarded, educationally limited, or schizophrenic patient. Performance on proverb interpretation is relatively stable across ages and is reasonably preserved in earliest stage Alzheimer dementia.

Similarities   Verbal similarities is a task of conceptual reasoning that requires the patient to explain the essential similarity between two seemingly different objects or situations (e.g., a car and an airplane). The test assesses the analysis of relationships, the formation of verbal concepts, and logical reasoning. Full credit is given for any abstract similarity (i.e., modes of transportation), a half credit for responses that indicate specific properties of both items (i.e., "Both have motors") in the pair and that constitute a relevant similarity, and no credits are given for responses reflecting properties of only one item of the pair (i.e., "It drives on the road"), generalizations not pertinent to the pair, obviously incorrect responses, and failure to give any response. Performance by normal subjects remains reasonably consistent from age 40 to 89 in our experience, although a number of studies have reported a substantial decline in the seventies and eighties.[16] Our sample of stage I dementia patients performed at a level comparable with that of age peers, with considerable decline in the quality of performance by patients progressing beyond this level.[14]

Deficits in abstract reasoning are most commonly found in patients with diffuse brain dysfunctions regardless of etiology. While such deficits are sensitive to disruption of the brain's integrative functioning in general, they are not well correlated with focal brain lesions of any specific locus. Obviously, a focal lesion that produces a cognitive deficit in one of the basic abilities required to carry out abstract reasoning (e.g., left hemisphere parietal-temporal lesions resulting in an aphasic disorder) will affect the associated higher cognitive function secondarily. Frontal lobe lesions tend not to affect basic cognitive processes adversely but are likely to interfere seriously with social awareness and judgment.

Calculations Arithmetic calculation is taught in grade school the world over; therefore it is a basic cognitive skill that has been acquired by most people, even those of modest educational background. Basic arithmetic involves several separate neuropsychological functions (see Chap. 14): rote memory; the basic arithmetic processes of addition, subtraction, multiplication, division, borrowing, and carrying; and the ability to do written calculations, arranging numbers appropriately on the page. Brain disease, both focal and general, will affect these processes and produce errors in calculation (acalculia—see Chap. 14). Educational level and history of proficiency in arithmetic must be taken into account, for both will definitely affect performance.

Testing always begins with easy examples then proceeds to more complicated items. Verbal as well as written items are useful, but watching the patient solve the written problems is the most instructive in terms of identifying errors. Watching the patient with suspected dementia work through a problem is more valuable than seeing if the final answer is correct. When the patient takes a long time or seems uncertain about the process, using trial and error, the examiner can suspect that a problem exists even though the answer is correct. Calculation testing is useful in the elderly population because there is no age-related decrease in proficiency (Fig. 2-3).

Insight and Judgment Insight and judgment are important aspects of behavior; they are often affected by brain disease, both focal, as in frontal lobe lesions, or general, as in dementia and delirium. Both behaviors are different but very much interrelated. Insight is quite literally the capacity to "see into" or understand either oneself or a situation. Judgment is the more complex mental process of forming an opinion or making a decision

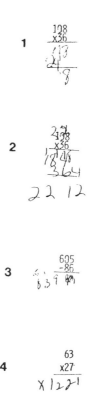

Figure 2-3
Typical errors by mildly moderately demented patients.

by discerning the facts of an issue and then comparing the possible choices against specific established social, cultural, or moral criteria. Judgment usually implies both the decision and the action. One can know what to do but may not exercise good or appropriate judgment in face of an actual situation.

Can these complex functions be accurately tested in a routine examination? To a certain extent the answer is yes; certainly insight is easy to evaluate by asking the patient if he or she is aware of having a problem, such as memory loss. The more difficult function to assess is judgment, which varies so widely in the normal population that determining a patient's judgment in isolation in the office is difficult. With brain disease, however, the question is whether there has been a change in judgment. This question can often be accurately answered by a family member or other observer, and we would encourage all examiners to rely heavily on (hearsay) reports of others in this regard rather than asking abstract questions. Many neuropsychological batteries have specific questions such as "If you found a wallet with money in it, what would you do?" These questions call for complex moral as well as practical judgments; they may be answered appropriately without reflecting the patient's actual behavior.

Other types of questions—such as, "If you locked yourself out of your house, how would you get back in?"—require more of a practical planning or decision-making ability without involving the additional factors of societal values or norms. This type of question poses a problem in abstract reasoning, which certainly can be assessed in the office.

SUMMARY

Data Summary

Upon completion of the examination, the examiner must summarize the findings and separate normal from abnormal performance on the various subtests.

Behavioral Diagnosis

The historical and examination data are now analyzed and organized into patterns of behavioral deficits that define one of the general behavioral syndromes. For example, a patient with a slowly progressive disease that is characterized by apathy, memory problems, and other cognitive deficits without change in level of consciousness presents the syndrome of dementia. The identification of the specific neurobehavioral syndrome—such as dementia, delirium, amnesic state, focal behavioral syndrome (e.g., aphasia, parietal lobe syndrome)—is clinically important because further medical evaluation and management are different for each syndrome.

Clinical Diagnosis

The final step in the diagnostic process is to establish a specific disease diagnosis—for example, de-

mentia of the Alzheimer type or delirium due to sepsis. At some times, the final diagnosis can be made on clinical grounds alone; at others, corroborating laboratory evaluation is necessary.

In conclusion, it is the mental status examination that is the most important diagnostic tool of the behavioral neurologist/neuropsychiatrist/neuropsychologist. The data from this examination permit the clinician to identify organic disease, diagnose the basic behavioral syndromes, and sometimes make a specific neurologic diagnosis. The form used for the Strubb-Black mental status examination is shown in Fig. 2-4.

Figure 2-4
The form used for the Strub-Black mental status examination.

Mental Status Examination Recording Form

PATIENT INFORMATION

Patient name: Date:
Address: Case #:

Phone: Hospital #:
Date of birth: Place of birth:
Age: Sex:
Education:
    Highest level: Age at completion:
    Failures or honors:
Handedness:
    Patient: Family:
Occupation:
Medical diagnosis:
    Onset and nature:

Hemiplegia:
    (Circle)   None   Recovered   Right   Left

Hemianopia:
    (Circle)   None   Recovered   Right   Left

Neurosurgical information:

Electroencephalograph (EEG) focus:

MRI, CT scan, brain scan, angiogram, and so forth:

(Starred items are essential and should be used with all patients.)
*I. Behavioral Observations

  *A. History of behavior change, memory difficulties, bizarre behavior, change in work habits, and the like:

*B. Physical Appearance:

*C. Emotional Status (e.g., confusion, depression, anxiety, lability):

D. Frontal Lobe Test Results (see related cortical functions):

*E. Denial or Neglect:

*II. Level of Consciousness

    *A. Rate: Alert_____ Lethargic_____ Stupor_____ Coma_____

    *B. Describe stimulus necessary to arouse patient, and record patient's response:

*III. Attention

    *A. Observation of patient during examination:
    *B. Digit repetition: Repeat digits at a rate of one per second.

ITEM	CHECK IF CORRECT
3-7	_____
2-4-9	_____
8-5-2-7	_____
2-9-6-8-3	_____
5-7-1-9-4-6	_____
8-1-5-9-3-6-2	_____
3-9-8-2-5-1-4-7	_____
7-2-8-5-4-6-7-3-9	_____

    C. Vigilance: Repeat letters at a rate of one per second. Tell patient to indicate by tapping the table whenever he or she hears the letter "A."

    L T P E A O A I C T D A L A A
    A N I A B F S A M R Z E O A D
    P A K L A U C J T O E A B A A
    Z Y F M U S A H E V A A R A T

    1. Errors of omission: _____

    2. Errors of commission: _____

    D. Unilateral inattention:

*IV. Language

    *A. Spontaneous speech:

        *1. Describe, including fluency, articulation, and presence of paraphasias:

        2. Verbal fluency: Total words: _____

                          Total animals: _____

    *B. Comprehension:

        *1. Patient's response to pointing commands:
        Ask patient to point to one, two, three, then four room objects or body parts in sequence. Record adequacy of performance.

        *2. Patient's response to yes-no questions:
        (e.g., "Is it raining today?" or "Is Grant still president?")

*C. Repetition:

Tell the patient to repeat each of the following:

ITEM	CHECK IF CORRECT
1. Ball	_____
2. Help	_____
3. Airplane	_____
4. Hospital	_____
5. Mississippi River	_____
6. The little boy went home.	_____
7. We all went over there together.	_____
8. The old car wouldn't start on Tuesday morning.	_____
9. The short fat boy dropped the china vase.	_____
10. Each fight readied the boxer for the championship bout.	_____

*D. Naming and Word Finding:

Tell the patient to name the following simple colors and objects:

ITEM	CHECK IF CORRECT
1. Colors	
a. Red	_____
b. Blue	_____
c. Yellow	_____
d. Pink	_____
e. Purple	_____
2. Body parts	
a. Eye	_____
b. Leg	_____
c. Teeth	_____
d. Thumb	_____
e. Knuckles	_____
3. Clothing and room objects	
a. Door	_____
b. Watch	_____
c. Shoe	_____
d. Shirt	_____
e. Ceiling	_____
4. Parts of objects	
a. Watch stem (winder)	_____
b. Coat lapel	_____
c. Watch crystal	_____
d. Sole of shoe	_____
e. Buckle of belt	_____

E. Reading:

Describe level of adequacy (words, sentences, paragraphs) and note types of errors:

F. Writing:

Describe level of adequacy and note types of errors:

G. Spelling:

Describe performance to dictation and note errors:

Figure 2-4 *(Continued)*

*V. Memory: Most of the following memory tasks evaluate verbal memory. In patients with language disturbance (aphasia), the visual memory tests must be used.

   *A. Immediate Recall (short-term memory):
      Refer to Digit Repetition in Section III.

   *B. Orientation:

	CHECK IF CORRECT
*1. Person	
a. Name	_____
b. Age	_____
c. Birth date	_____
*2. Place	
a. Location (at present)	_____
b. City location	_____
c. Home address	_____
*3. Time	
a. Date	_____
b. Day of the week	_____
c. Time of day	_____
d. Season of the year	_____
e. Duration of time with examiner	_____

*C. Remote Memory:

	CHECK IF CORRECT OR ADEQUATE
*1. Personal Information	
a. Where were you born?	_____
b. School information	_____
c. Vocational history	_____
d. Family information	_____
*2. Historic Facts	
a. Four US presidents during your lifetime	_____
b. Last war	_____

*D. New-Learning Ability:
Tell the patient, "I am going to tell you four words, which I want you to remember." Have the patient repeat the four words after they are initially presented and then say that you will ask him or her to remember the words later. Continue with the examination, and at intervals of 5, 10, and 30 minutes, ask the patient to recall the words. Use categoric ("one word is a color") or phonemic ("one word begins with B") cues if he or she is unable to recall the word spontaneously on any trial. Record the type and amount of cuing necessary. Two alternate sets of words are provided.

1. Four Unrelated Words	5 min	10 min	30 min
a. Brown (Fun)	___	___	___
b. Honesty (Loyalty)	___	___	___
c. Tulip (Carrot)	___	___	___
d. Eyedropper (Ankle)	___	___	___

Describe type of cues used if necessary:

Figure 2-4 *(Continued)*

2. Verbal Story for Immediate Recall:
Tell the patient, "I am going to read you a short story, which I want you to remember. Listen closely to what I read because I will ask you to tell me the story when I finish." Read the story slowly and carefully, but without pausing at the slash marks. After completing the paragraph, tell the patient to retell the story as accurately as possible. Record the number of correct memories (information within the slashes) and describe confabulation if it is present.

It was July / and the Rogers / had packed up / their four children / in the station wagon / and were off / on vacation.

They were taking / their yearly trip / to the beach / at Gulf Shores.

This year / they were making / a special / one-day stop / at the Aquarium / in New Orleans.

After a long day's drive / they arrived / at the motel / only to discover / that in their excitement / they had left / the twins / and their suitcases / in the front yard.

  a. Number of correct memories: _____
  b. Describe confabulation if present:

3. Visual Memory (hidden objects):
Tell the patient that you are going to hide some objects around the office, desk, or bed and that you want him or her to remember where they are. Hide four or five common objects (e.g., keys, pen, reflex hammer) in various areas in the patient's sight. After a delay of several minutes, ask the patient to find the objects. Ask patient to name those items he or she is unable to find.

  a. Number of hidden objects found: _____
  b. Number of hidden objects named but not found: _____
  c. Number of locations indicated but objects not named: _____

*4. Visual Memory (visual design reproduction):
(see stimulus cards)

ITEM	SCORE
a. Design 1	_____
b. Design 2	_____
c. Design 3	_____
d. Design 4	_____
Total score: _____	

5. Paired Associated Learning:
Tell the patient that you are going to read a list of words two at a time. The patient will be expected to remember the words that go together (e.g., big—little). When he or she is clear as to the directions, read the first list of words at the rate of one pair per second. After reading the first list, test for recall by presenting the first recall list. Give the first word of a pair and ask for the word that went with it. Correct incorrect responses and proceed to the next pair. After the first recall has been completed, allow a 10-second delay and continue with the second presentation and recall lists.

PRESENTATION LISTS

1	2
a. Weather—Bag	a. House—Income
b. High—Low	b. Weather—Bag
c. House—Income	c. Book—Page
d. Book—Page	d. High—Low

RECALL LISTS

1	2
a. House _____	a. High _____
b. High _____	b. House _____
c. Weather _____	c. Book _____
d. Book _____	d. Weather _____

1. Number of easy paired associates recalled: _____
2. Number of difficult paired associates recalled: _____

*VI. Constructional Ability

*A. Reproduction drawings:
Ask the patient to copy the following drawings in the space provided.

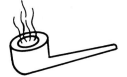

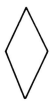

ITEM	SCORE
1. Vertical diamond	_____
2. Two-dimensional cross	_____
3. Three-dimensional cube	_____
4. Three-dimensional pipe	_____
5. Triangle within a triangle	_____
Total score: _____	

*B. Drawings to Command:
Tell the patient to draw the following pictures in the space provided.

Clock with all numbers

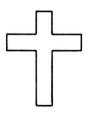

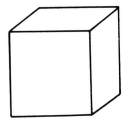

Daisy in flowerpot

Figure 2-4 *(Continued)*

House in perspective

ITEM	SCORE
1. Clock	_____
2. Daisy in flowerpot	_____
3. House in perspective	_____

Total score: _____

C. Block Designs:
       (See stimulus cards)

ITEM	SCORE
1. Design 1	_____
2. Design 2	_____
3. Design 3	_____
4. Design 4	_____

Total score: _____

Describe types of errors:

*VII. Higher Cognitive Functions

A. Fund of Information:

ITEM	CHECK IF CORRECT
1. How many weeks are in a year?	_____
2. Why do people have lungs?	_____
3. Name four US Presidents since 1940.	_____
4. Where is Denmark?	_____
5. How far is it from New York to Los Angeles?	_____
6. Why are light colored clothes cooler in the summer than dark colored clothes?	_____
7. What is the capital of Spain?	_____
8. What causes rust?	_____
9. Who wrote the Odyssey?	_____
10. What is the Acropolis?	_____

Total score: _____

*B. Calculations:
Describe the patient's adequacy in performance and types of errors made on the following types of calculations:

1. Verbal rote examples:

    a. Addition   (4 + 6)
    b. Subtraction   (8 − 5)
    c. Multiplication   (2 × 8)
    d. Division   (56 ÷ 8)

2. Verbal complex examples:

    a. Addition   (14 + 17)
    b. Subtraction   (43 − 38)
    c. Multiplication   (21 × 5)
    d. Division   (128 ÷ 8)

*3. Written complex examples:

    a. Addition   108
                                    + 79

    b. Subtraction   605
                                    − 86

    c. Multiplication   108
                                    × 36

    d. Division   43)559

*C. Proverb Interpretation:
Tell the patient to explain the following sayings. Record the answers.

ITEM	SCORE
1. Don't cry over spilled milk.	_____
2. Rome wasn't built in a day.	_____
3. A drowning man will clutch at a straw.	_____
4. A golden hammer breaks an iron door.	_____
5. The hot coal burns; the cold one blackens.	_____

Total score: _____
Total concrete responses: _____

*D. Similarities

ITEM	SCORE
1. Turnip..........................Cauliflower	_____
2. Car...................................Airplane	_____
3. Desk................................Bookcase	_____
4. Poem ....Novel	_____
5. Horse ....Apple	_____

Total score: _____
Total concrete responses: _____

E. Conceptual Series Completion:

ITEM	CHECK IF CORRECT
1. A B C D ____	_____
2. 1 4 7 10 ____ ____	_____
3. AZ BY CX D ____	_____
4. tote to snow on spun up stab ____ ____	_____
5. elephant 87654321 plan 5732 lap ____ ____ ____	_____

Total score: _____

Figure 2-4   *(Continued)*

VIII. Related Cortical Functions

A. Ideomotor Apraxia:
Describe the adequacy of the patient's performance in carrying out motor acts to command using buccofacial, limb, and whole body commands. Indicate if imitation or use of the real object was necessary to facilitate performance.

ITEM	SCORE
1. Blow out a match.	_____
2. Drink through a straw.	_____
3. Lick crumbs off your lips.	_____
4. Comb your hair.	_____
5. Flip a coin.	_____

B. Ideational Apraxia:
Describe the adequacy of the patient's performance on the following complex motor tasks:

1. Letter-envelope-stamp
2. Candle-holder-match
3. Toothpaste-toothbrush

C. Right-Left Disorientation:

ITEM	CHECK IF CORRECT
1. Identification on self	
a. Show me your right foot	_____
b. Show me your left hand	_____
2. Crossed commands on self	
a. With your right hand touch your left shoulder.	_____
b. With your left hand touch your right ear.	_____
3. Identification on examiner	
a. Point to my left knee.	_____
b. Point to my right elbow.	_____
4. Crossed commands on examiner	
a. With your right hand point to my left eye.	_____
b. With your left hand point to my left foot.	_____

Describe nature and degree of errors made:

D. Finger Agnosia:
Describe the adequacy of the patient's nonverbal and verbal performance.

E. Gerstmann's Syndrome:
Describe the nature and degree of impairment in the following areas if present in the patient:

1. Finger agnosia:	_____
2. Right-left disorientation:	_____
3. Dysgraphia:	_____
4. Dyscalculia:	_____

F. Visual Agnosia:
Describe any deficits in visual identification of objects, naming of objects whose use can be demonstrated, color naming, and facial recognition:

G. Astereognosis:
Describe deficits:

Left hand _____
Right hand _____

H. Geographic Disorientation:
1. Describe evidence of disorientation obtained from history:

2. Map localization:
Describe patient's ability to localize well-known cities on a map:

3. Orientation of self in hospital:
Describe patient's ability to orient self within the hospital environment:

*I. Denial and Neglect:
If present, describe patient's response.

	YES	NO
1. Does patient frankly deny his illness?	____	____
2. Is there evidence of unilateral neglect? (e.g., shaving one side of face, dressing one arm, and so on)	____	____
3. Is there evidence of unilateral neglect on drawings? (e.g., absence of numbers on one side of clock or absence of one side of picture)	____	____

J. Frontal Lobe Tests:
1. Drawings:
Tell the patient to copy and continue the following sequence. Record evidence of perseveration or loss of sequence.

2. Alternating hand sequences:
This is a motor alternation task that uses both hands. Initially, the patient places both hands on the desk, one in a fist and one with the fingers extended palm down. Tell the patient to alternate the position of the two hands rapidly (simultaneously extending the fingers of one hand while making a fist with the other). Record if the patient is unable to maintain the alternating sequence.

SUMMARY OF FINDINGS

1. Describe major areas of impairment:

2. Tentative neurobehavioral diagnosis:

3. Tentative localization:

4. Tentative clinical diagnosis:

5. Proposed management plans:

Figure 2-4   *(Continued)*

<u>**MENTAL STATUS EXAMINATION FOR DEMENTIA**</u>

PATIENT INFORMATION

NAME: DATE:

HOSPITAL OR FILE NUMBER:

AGE: SEX: DIAGNOSIS:

1. VERBAL FLUENCY

    Animals per 60 seconds   Total animals: _____

2. COMPREHENSION   Check if correct:

    a. Point to the ceiling.   _____

    b. Point to your nose and window.   _____

    c. Point to your foot, door, and ceiling.   _____

    d. Point to window, leg, door, and thumb.   _____

3. NAMING AND WORD FINDING

    Parts of objects: Watch stem (winder)   _____

                           Coat lapel   _____

                           Watch crystal   _____

                           Sole of shoe   _____

                           Buckle of belt   _____

4. ORIENTATION

    a. Date   _____

    b. Month   _____

    c. Year   _____

    d. Day of week   _____

5. NEW LEARNING ABILITY

    Four unrelated words: 5 min   10 min

    a. Brown (Fun)   _____   _____

    b. Honesty (Loyalty)   _____   _____

    c. Tulip (Carrot)   _____   _____

    d. Eyedropper (Ankle)   _____   _____

6. VERBAL STORY FOR IMMEDIATE RECALL

    It was July/ and the Rogers/ had packed up/ their four children/ in the
    station wagon/ and were off/ on vacation.

    They were taking/ their yearly trip/ to the beach/ at Gulf Shores.

    This year/ they were making/ a special/ one-day stop/ at The Aquarium/ in
    New Orleans.

    After a long day's drive/ they arrived/ at the motel/ only to discover/ that in
    their excitement/ they had left/ the twins/ and their suitcases/ in the front
    yard.

                           Number of correct memories: _____

7. VISUAL MEMORY (HIDDEN OBJECTS)

    Object   Found

    a. Coin   _____
    b. Pen   _____
    c. Comb   _____
    d. Key   _____
    e. Fork   _____

8. PAIRED ASSOCIATE LEARNING

1	2
a. Weather-Bag	a. House-Income
b. High-Low	b. Weather-Bag
c. House-Income	c. Book-Page
d. Book-Page	d. High-Low

1	2
a. House _____	a. High _____
b. High _____	a. House _____
c. Weather _____	c. Book _____
d. Book _____	d. Weather _____

9. CONSTRUCTIONAL ABILITY

                                                    Score _____

    Daisy in flower pot   Score _____

    House in perspective   Score _____

10. WRITTEN COMPLEX
    CALCULATIONS

    a. Addition   108
                        + 79

    b. Subtraction   605
                        − 86

    c. Multiplication   108
                        × 36

    d. Division   43)559   Number correct _____

Figure 2-4 *(Continued)*

11. PROVERB INTERPRETATION

   a. Don't cry over spilled milk.   Score

_____ _____

   b. Rome wasn't built in a day.

_____ _____

   c. A drowning man will clutch at a straw.

_____ _____

   d. A golden hammer breaks an iron door.

_____ _____

   e. The hot coal burns, the cold one blackens.

_____ _____

12. SIMILARITIES

     a. Turnip......................................Cauliflower _____
     b. Car...Airplane _____
     c. Desk...Bookcase _____
     d. Poem .... Novel _____
     e. Horse ....Apple _____

Figure 2-4   *(Continued)*

REFERENCES

1. Binet A, Simon TH: Le developpement de l'intelligence chez les enfants. *Annee Psychol* 14:1–94, 1908.
2. Bender L: *A Visual Motor Gestalt Test and Its Clinical Use.* Research Monograph, No. 3. New York: American Orthopsychiatric Association, 1938.
3. Halstead WC, Wepman JM: The Halstead-Wepman Aphasia Screening Test. *J Speech Hear Disord* 14:9–15, 1959.
4. Zachary RA: *Shipley Institute of Living Scale: Revised Manual.* Los Angeles: Western Psychological Services, 1986.
5. Blessed G, Tomlinson BE, Roth M: The association between quantitative measures of dementia and senile changes in the cerebral grey matter of elderly subjects. *Br J Psychiatry* 114:797–811, 1968.
6. Mattis S: *Dementia Rating Scale (DRS).* Odessa, FL: Psychological Assessment Resources, 1988.
7. Kahn RL, Miller NE: Assessment of altered brain function in the aged, in Storandt M, Seigler I, Ellis M (eds): *The Clinical Psychology of Aging.* New York: Plenum Press, 1978.
8. Rosen WG, Mohs RC, Davis KL: A new rating scale for Alzheimer's disease. *Am J Psychiatry* 141:1356–1364, 1984.
9. Williams JM: *Cognitive Behavior Rating Scale.* Odessa, FL: Psychological Assessment Resources, 1991.
10. Folstein MF, Folstein SE, McHugh PR: Mini-mental state. *J Psychiatr Res* 12:189–198, 1975.
11. Jacobs JW, Bernhard MR, Delgado A, Strain JJ: Screening for organic mental syndromes in the medically ill. *Ann Intern Med* 86:40–46, 1977.
12. Saxton J, McGonigle-Gibson KL, Swihart AA, et al: Assessment of the severely impaired patient: Description and validation of a new neuropsychological test battery: Psychological assessment. *J Consult Clin Psychol* 2:298–303, 1990.
13. Trzepacz PT, Baker RW: *The Psychiatric Mental Status Examination.* New York: Oxford University Press, 1993.
14. Strub RL, Black FW: *The Mental Status Examination in Neurology,* 3d ed. Philadelphia: Davis, 1993.
15. Berg R, Franzen M, Wedding D: *Screening for Brain Impairment,* 2d ed. New York: Springer, 1994.
16. Lezak MD: *Neuropsychological Assessment,* 3d ed. New York: Oxford University Press, 1995.
17. Spreen O, Strauss E: *A Compendium of Neuropsychological Tests.* New York: Oxford University Press, 1991.
18. Black FW: Digit repetition in brain-damaged adults: Clinical and theoretical implications. *J Clin Psychol* 42:770–782, 1986.
19. Shum DHK, McFarland KA, Bain JD: Construct validity of eight tests of attention: Comparisons of normal and closed head injured samples. *Clin Neuropsychol* 4:151–162, 1990.
20. Signoret J-L: Memory and amnesias, in Mesulum M-M (ed): *Principles of Behavioral Neurology.* Philadelphia: Davis, 1985, pp 169–192.
21. Natelson BH, Haupt EJ, Fleischer EJ, Grey L: Temporal orientation and education: A direct relationship in normal people. *Arch Neurol* 36:444–446, 1979.
22. Strub RL, Black FW, Leventhal B: The clinical utility of reproduction drawing tests with low IQ patients. *J Clin Psychiatry* 40:386–388, 1979.
23. Gorham DR: *Clinical Manual for the Proverbs Test.* Missoula, MT: Psychological Test Specialists, 1956.
24. Delis DC, Kramer J, Kaplan E: *California Proverb Test.* Lexington, MA: Boston Neuropsychological Foundation (undated).

Chapter 3

PRINCIPLES OF NEUROPSYCHOLOGICAL ASSESSMENT

Muriel D. Lezak

EVOLUTION AND APPLICATIONS OF NEUROPSYCHOLOGICAL ASSESSMENT

The rapid development of neuropsychological assessment procedures during the last two decades reflects the growing appreciation of its value for neurodiagnostic issues, for the care and treatment of neurologically impaired patients, and for patients needing cognitive and behavioral rehabilitation. Neuropsychological assessment also contributes significantly to the neurologic sciences, psychiatry, and clinical psychology, both in basic science research and in practical clinical knowledge. In practice, a neuropsychological evaluation may serve one or more purposes. For example, the same information used for diagnostic studies or in a research program may provide a patient's caregivers with the descriptive data on which they can build an individualized rehabilitation program. In other cases, data acquired for research or diagnosis may provide the necessary information for determining the behavioral impact of a cerebral lesion.[1]

The first systematic applications of neuropsychological assessment dealt with diagnosis, for before the days of sophisticated neuroimaging, the identification and—where possible—localization of a cerebral lesion was neuropsychology's most important function.[2–4] As neuropsychologists became more knowledgeable and adept, they not only became more skilled at localizing lesions on the basis of neuropsychological data but also were able to develop criteria for predicting the nature of the lesion—whether it involved damaged or absent tissue, whether the damage was due to a slow or a rapid process.[5–8]

Recent developments in neuroradiologic techniques have greatly reduced the contributions of neuropsychological assessment to diagnosis and lesion localization.[9–11] Nevertheless, the neuropsychological examination continues to provide critical information in the differential diagnosis of the dementias,[12,13] in differentiating depression from dementia in elderly patients,[14–17] as well as in identifying behavioral problems that may presage a developing cerebral disorder.[18,19] Years after a person has sustained a traumatic brain injury[20–22] or been exposed to toxic substances,[23,24] neuropsychological deficits may be the only residual evidence indicating the presence of cerebral damage.

Today, neuropsychological assessment is most often called upon to furnish the detailed behavioral descriptions necessary for intelligent patient care, rational treatment, and appropriate rehabilitation training and vocational/educational placement. For example, to be effective, the goals of rehabilitation as well as the procedures must be based on pertinent and detailed neurobehavioral data.[25–28] The evaluation of medical treatments or neurosurgery also requires appropriate and precise neuropsychological evaluations.[29–32] Repeated neuropsychological examinations help to predict the degree and quality of improvement in acute conditions (e.g., stroke, head trauma) or of decline in deteriorating conditions (e.g., dementias, multiple sclerosis).[33–36]

Descriptive neuropsychological data can provide the information needed for patients or their caregivers to make practical decisions necessitated by the patient's neurologic disorder. These decisions may concern the patient's legal status or financial options; whether the patient returns to work or when return to work is feasible; or such domestic issues as whether the patient needs help with household chores or is ready to return home from a care facility.

Contributions of neuropsychological assessment to research in the clinical neurosciences have proven invaluable. These include treatment evaluation, development of criteria for classifying neuropsychological functions, behavioral descriptions of neurologic disorders, and the growing understanding of the functional organization of the nervous system.

Moreover, the findings of neuropsychological evaluations have proven invaluable in the legal domain. More and more, lawyers as well as judges appreciate the importance of cerebral dysfunction in contributing to criminal behavior, mental incompetence, or impaired ability to resume a normal life after an accident, toxic exposure, or other noxious event has resulted in brain damage.

THE NEUROPSYCHOLOGICAL COMPONENTS OF BEHAVIOR

Traditional western epistemology has provided a three-dimensional schema for conceptualizing the psychological components of behavior. Within this framework, the intellect—that is, the cognitive functions—is differentiated from two other, equally important categories of nonintellectual behavior: motivation and the emotions and the executive functions, which include capacities for initiating and carrying out self-directed, goal-directed activities effectively. This conceptual organization has facilitated the identification and classification of behavioral phenomena. It has also received empirical support in that neuropsychological research has shown that these concepts correspond to the major cerebral structural systems.[9,37–39]

Cognitive Functions

Information processing is the province of the cognitive functions. *Perceptual functions* select, organize, and classify stimuli received by the organism. *Memory* functions encode and store this information that *thinking* can reorganize and deal with conceptually or that may determine a *response* in the form of a verbal or motoric activity. For most persons, each of the two cerebral hemispheres is specialized for processing and storing information that in its presentation is either linear (typically the left hemisphere) or configurational (typically the right hemisphere). Moreover, the hemispheres are organized bilaterally to provide for specific processing and storage of information in each perceptual modality as well as in their various combinations.[40] This multidimensional organization of the brain provides for highly specialized information processing for the many subsystems of perception and memory.[41–44]

Several different and independent capacities contribute to the conceptual functions and to different kinds of responses.[1,8,45,46] The variety of mental functions and their relative independence from one another becomes apparent when comparing the many different kinds of cognitive deficits. For example, a patient who can no longer make conceptual classifications may still be able to perform fairly complex arithmetic operations; many aphasic patients are able to make known their intentions and feelings by means of facial expressions, gestures, and posture. Thus the neuropsychological evaluation must include the examination of many distinctly different cognitive functions.

Well before the relationship between specific mental activities and brain structures was known, the cognitive functions had been identified and measured with considerable accuracy.[47–49] It was only after the Second World War that the mental functioning of brain-damaged patients was studied in a systematic manner or that large-scale studies looking for correlations between cerebral and behavioral functions were undertaken.[38,50,51] These studies provided the first scientifically grounded bases and methodologies for the behavioral evaluation of cerebral functioning.

Noncognitive Functions

It is much more difficult to characterize and measure emotional behavior and executive functions than cognitive functions. Since many cerebral disorders can alter emotional behavior, often in a quite characteristic manner,[1,52–54] we need reliable and accurate techniques to identify and quantify specific aspects of emotional behavior. However, the fact that many emotional responses are both multidetermined and multidimensional makes it difficult if not impossible to delineate precisely the differences between the effects of a lesion, of personality predispositions, and of situational reactions, particularly since most often the patient's emotional behavior results from interactions between these factors. Thus, in comparison with the cognitive functions, both the understanding and assessment of the emotional alterations accompanying cerebral damage are less well developed.

The executive functions comprise capacities for volitional activity (initiation, self-awareness), planning, carrying out activities effectively, and self-regulation.[38,55] The executive functions are integral to all independently undertaken goal-directed activities. Some of the executive function disorders are now known to be associated with specific focal lesions, mostly involving well-defined areas of the frontal lobes.[1,37,56,57] Yet despite good practical understanding of the executive functions, it has been difficult to develop satisfactory methods for demonstrating and quantifying them. The structured nature of most examinations rarely gives the patient the opportunity to exercise any independent judgment or activity—that is, to make use of the executive functions. Moreover, executive behavior or its absence typically becomes evident in the qualitative aspects of the patient's test performances, such as abilities to identify and correct errors, to develop an effective

solution strategy, or even to recognize that erasure crumbs should be swept from the page. Complicating the problem of measuring the executive functions is the tendency for the most common and obvious cognitive deficits to mask them. Too often examiners who do not understand the behavioral disorders that can accompany brain damage tend to misinterpret serious executive disorders, such as apathy or impulsivity, as emotional problems or personality aberrations.

THE ASSESSMENT OF NEUROPSYCHOLOGICAL DEFICIT

Cognitive Defects and Cognitive Deficits

Given that psychology's involvement in the identification and measurement of cognitive functions dates back more than a century,[58] it is not surprising that the neuropsychological examination has focused on these functions especially. The evaluation of cognitive disorders concerns their severity, how they affect the patient's behavior generally, the interrelations between specific defects and deficits, as well as the correlations between specific aspects of cognitive dysfunction and underlying neuropathology.

Cognitive dysfunction can appear in the form of measurable *deficits* in skills, knowledge, or intellectual capacities, or it can appear as specific *defects*. Pathognomonic phenomena such as the patient's inattention to what occurs on the left of his or her midline, or characteristic behavioral symptoms, such as the telegraphic speech of patients with Broca's aphasia, are examples of cognitive defects. Many of these defects tend to be obvious to any observer; most of them will be identified in a careful neurologic examination. A neuropsychological examination providing a systematic review of functions may bring to light subtle defects that would not be apparent to a naive observer.

Cognitive deficits appear in the relative weakening or diminution of skills or knowledge. Fine-grained examinations are not necessary for identifying the presence of these deficits when they are obvious, as when the patient cannot tell what happened more than 5 min ago. However, in many cases, cognitive impairment may not become evident without an adequate neuropsychological examination. For example, a retired elderly person may no longer need to use highly refined visuospatial skills and thus may not appreciate that they have been compromised by a stroke. Also, many patients tend to avoid activities involving the affected functions and thus do not complain about losing these skills or understandings. Neuropsychological assessment may also be the best means of documenting mildly diminished cognitive capacities when they are of sufficient magnitude to affect the patient's functioning but not severe enough to be obvious. This is a not uncommon occurrence for persons whose mathematical abilities had been of *high average* or *superior* caliber but who, after sustaining brain damage, may be able to solve arithmetic problems at only an *average* level. In such cases, isolated deficits do not provide diagnostic information, and the patient's complaints about mental troubles may be misinterpreted until the examiner takes account of the patient's history (e.g., a software engineer; a physician) to make an objective comparison between premorbid functioning and the patient's present relatively lower level of mathematical competence.

Identifying Deficit

Finding an Appropriate Comparison Standard   The premorbid level of patients' cognitive abilities provides a comparison standard that allows the examiner to determine whether they have been impaired to a significant degree. The identification of cognitive impairment is easiest when there is concrete evidence of premorbid competencies, such as school or army test scores, course grades, and so on. However, such information is often not available, forcing the examiner to turn to other sources to make a reasonable estimate. While some examiners have used population means as comparision standards for this purpose, this practice is not only inappropriate but can be grossly misleading, since a quarter of the population perform at levels above the *average* range and a quarter fall below it.

Another method for estimating premorbid ability levels is based on the highest test scores or historical indicators of mental competence.[1] Underlying this practice are the assumptions that *by and large, people who perform well in one area perform well in others, and vice versa;* that *cognitive potential can be either realized or reduced by external influences but that it is not possible to function at a higher level than biological capacity will permit; that marked discrepancies between the levels at which a person performs different cognitive functions or skills probably reflect disease, developmental anomalies, cultural training biases or deficiencies, emotional disturbances, or some other condition that has interfered with the full expression of that person's ability potential;* and that *for cognitively impaired persons, the least depressed abilities are the best remaining behavioral representatives of the original cognitive potential.* Moreover, since, *within the limits of chance variations, a person's ability to perform a task is at least as high as the level of performance of that task,* the patient's best performances, whether they be in the neuropsychological examination or taken from historical data, are probably the best indicators of premorbid ability. Since chance variations do occur, the wise examiner who has access to test performances only will not rely on a single high score but look for a cluster of highest scores on which this estimate can be based.

Some examiners use demographic data,[59,60] residual ability to read phonetically irregular words,[61–63] or a combination of these.[64] However, these methods have not proven satisfactory, overpredicting high scores and underpredicting low ones,[65,66] thus estimating only from one-half[67] to two-thirds[66] of cases correctly.

Measurement of Deficit   The presence of a cognitive impairment is most readily demonstrated when related functions show a deficit relative to other kinds of cognitive functions. For example, when scores on tests involving visuospatial organization run significantly lower than performance levels on tests of language and verbal reasoning, a neuropsychological deficit may be hypothesized. Studies involving patients with different kinds of deficits and those suffering from the many known cerebral disorders have documented many distinctive deficit patterns that aid in diagnosing and understanding the patients' disorders and cerebral functioning.[1,12,13,68] These known deficit patterns also help the knowledgeable clinician to distinguish organically based conditions from diminished cognitive functioning due to different sociocultural experiences or to poor education.[69-71]

TESTS IN NEUROPSYCHOLOGICAL ASSESSMENT

Test Contributions to the Neuropsychological Examination

The data of the neuropsychological examination consist of observations by the examiner and reports by others—such as those from caregivers or spouses, data about the patient's psychosocial and medical history, and findings from psychometric tests and other psychological examination techniques. Observation of the patient's behavior during the examination provides important information about the patient's emotional status, social skills, and both cognitive and executive functioning. The patient's history and medical reports provide the context for developing hypotheses to guide the direction of the examination and for interpreting its data.

Tests can serve several purposes. They can be used to establish a comparison standard—that is, for estimating premorbid ability. They may elicit behavioral indications of a cerebral disorder. They are indispensable for making precise comparisons between test performances on different functions or at different times (e.g., for evaluating treatments, following a patient's course). Tests may also elicit behavioral abnormalities that require special attention in a rehabilitation program, in readaptation to living at home, and so on.

Many of the tests used by neuropsychologists have their origins in the tests of mental abilities, academic performance, and various aptitudes that have been used for educational placement and guidance since the early 1900s.[72,73] A well-devel-

oped psychometric technology provides the theoretical and statistical foundations for the tests and measurements used in neuropsychology. For example, the Wechsler Intelligence Scales (WIS)[3,74] owe much of their popularity to these technological accomplishments.

Other popular neuropsychological tests and examination techniques have come from quite different sources: Porteus's *Mazes*[75] and Raven's *Progressive Matrices*[76] were responses to the desire for culture-free measures of mental ability. The original purpose of the Bender-Gestalt Test[77] was to examine the perceptual development of children. Industry's need for efficient selection of employees led to a number of interesting tests, such as the *MacQuarrie Test for Mechanical Ability*[78] and the *Purdue Pegboard Test.*[79] Neuropsychologists have also developed tests, typically to examine specific neuropsychological functions.[68,80]

Test Selection

Hundreds of tests are available for examining different aspects of the many cognitive functions; they vary in presentation format, complexity of the tasks involved, scoring criteria, and adequacy of standardization. Moreover, each year dozens of new tests appear in the literature and in test catalogues. By selecting appropriately from this profusion of tests, innovative examiners acquire the means to identify most of the organically-based cognitive disorders and, often, to describe them with considerable precision. However, in order to establish the parameters of a patient's cognitive status and the severity of dysfunction, it is also necessary to have baseline data from a broad-range assessment that considers both those functions known or suspected to be impaired and those that have been relatively spared by the patient's organic condition.

Because of the need for baseline data, many examiners always use the same general-purpose battery, which will both measure a number of specific functions and provide a fairly global evaluation. Some of these batteries are available commercially, such as the *Halstead-Reitan Battery;*[81,82] others are assembled by the individual examiner.[1,50] Another advantage of using a test battery is that repeated experience with a specific set of tests enhances the examiner's ability to use and interpret them. Two important technical advantages of formalized batteries are their provision of standardized assessment procedures and their reproducibility for comparisons between examinations and for research. Their chief disadvantage is that none are fully appropriate for any particular patient, resulting in both overtesting and undertesting in every case. Additionally, examiners who rely on a formalized battery are less likely to explore their patients' unique strengths and deficits and less likely to have the tools or experience to make such explorations.

Most neuropsychologists compromise between a completely individualized examination and a set battery approach.[1,83] The usual practice consists of choosing a core set of tests that will provide a general review of cognitive functions. Based on the findings obtained from this standardized and wide-ranging assessment, the examiner can identify problem areas that need further individualized exploration. Ideally, this exploration can be conducted with well-established tests, but the examiner may select tests that are less well known or well standardized when they are most appropriate for the specific issues presented by the patient.

INTERPRETING NEUROPSYCHOLOGICAL TEST DATA

Application and Limitations of Test Scores

Test scores are essentially abstractions from observations. A score obtained from a standardized test is a mathematical calculation representing a performance level that has been evaluated relative to the performance of a normative group on a well-defined task. The score serves as an objective reference point on a linear scale of values. Objective tests benefit from uniformity in their items, in administration procedures, in the standardizations that determine their scores, and in their normative populations. Standard scores are powerful tools, for, by using them, statistically sound comparisons can be made between an individual's performance on different tests, between different tests examining the same or similar abilities, between different persons taking the same tests, or between groups from different cultures or with different educational backgrounds.

These characteristics of standardized test scores make them particularly useful in the neuropsychological evaluation. Because of their objective nature, they can become comparison standards when evaluating deficits in an individual's test performance. However, test scores are not appropriate comparison standards for persons who have suffered global deterioration or who have a psychosocial or cultural background that may compromise their cognitive development.

By comparing a patient's test scores with one another, the examiner can identify both cognitive strengths and cognitive weaknesses. Moreover, particular cerebral disorders tend to affect cognitive functioning differently, producing score patterns characteristic of many of these disorders. For example, early in the course of Alzheimer disease, scores on the *Block Design* and *Digit Symbol* tests of the WIS battery tend to drop significantly, as do scores on most memory tests, while many verbal abilities as well as immediate verbal memory span remain unchanged or close to premorbid levels.[84,85] In contrast, patients with early symptoms of another dementing disorder, progressive supranuclear palsy, tend to do everything extremely slowly,[86] so that, even when most cognitive functions are still fairly well preserved and these patients' memory performance is still intact, they may appear impaired if not properly examined.[87,88]

Nevertheless, because they are abstractions from observations, test scores offer only an artificially attenuated description of the test performance. Test scores taken in isolation from other scores and from the history and observations of the patient can easily be misinterpreted. When scores are reported without any information about the qualitative aspects of the patient's test performance, it is not possible to know, for example, whether they are valid representations of the patient's ability, whether they were based on a too restrictive test format so that a full knowledge of the patient's strengths or deficits could not become apparent, or whether improper administrative procedures affected the patient's performance.

This problem of test score limitations is well illustrated by the *Arithmetic* test in the WIS battery.[74] Since the administration instructions require the subject to solve, mentally and within time limits, problems that the examiner reads once, patients whose auditory-verbal span is reduced, who have difficulty performing complex mental operations without visual supports, or whose mental processing is abnormally slow will receive low scores regardless of their level of mathematical competence. Unless the examiner allows these patients to work out the problems on paper and/or acknowledges the validity of slow but accurate responses, these patients' actual arithmetic ability will not become apparent to the examiner, and the nature and practical implications of their actual deficits will not be documented or appreciated.

For valid test interpretation, an appropriate reference group must be used to evaluate the patient's scores. Even though age is the most important variable affecting cognitive functioning,[89–91] a number of popular tests still lack adequate age norms. When age norms are not used, in most instances an older person's test scores are compared with a younger normative group, resulting in artificially lowered scores that can be misinterpreted as indicating some kind of abnormality.[92] Education is also a powerful variable for cognitive functioning. The effects of education on tests of verbal and academic abilities are obvious. Less obvious have been its significant contributions to scores on tests of nonverbal and nonacademic mental abilities[69,93–95] and memory abilities.[96–98]

Moreover, the way in which patients respond to the requirements of the examination reveals important information about the practical ramifications of their impairments as well as about the presence and nature of these impairments. For example, observations on whether a patient introduces strategies when solving problems or initiates, self-monitors, and self-regulates activities appropriately if at all, or how well a patient follows directions and can maintain an instructional set become invaluable information when evaluating for rehabilitation potential or for educational or vocational planning. This kind of information may also contribute to a better understanding of the nature of the patient's lesion or lesions.[1,21,99,100]

Methods of Interpreting Test Data

Three methods have proven value in neuropsychological assessment. Since each of these methods is most suitable for different problems or different tests, all three can contribute to the interpretation of the findings of a single examination.

Cutting Scores Some tests were developed to detect organic brain damage or a particular cerebral dysfunction. These tests are based on observations that patients who have sustained certain specific injuries often show characteristic cognitive aberrations rarely seen in normal subjects. For example, most people can locate the middle of a horizontal line fairly accurately, but patients with left-sided visuospatial inattention tend to mark the middle at a point situated somewhat to the right of the line's center.[101] For diagnostic purposes, the cutting score aids in discriminating between persons who show such pathological characteristics to a significant degree and those who do not. Although not all patients who have the condition of interest will perform below the cutting score (*false-negative* cases), very few—typically less than 5 percent—normal subjects will perform at abnormal levels (*false-positive* cases) when age especially[102] but also education[69,103] are taken into account. Thus cutting scores indicate only the probability that brain damage—or a particular kind of cerebral dysfunction—is present or absent. Moreover, no diagnostic decisions can rest on the score obtained for any single test, regardless of how far below the designated level of abnormality;

nor does the cutting score provide much information about the nature of the abnormality that a low score reflects.

Double Dissociation   This procedure requires performance on at least three—preferably more—tests to identify the critical neuropsychological disorder underlying poor performances on complex tasks.[8,104] Most cognitive tests call upon two or more different functions. For example, the task of copying a complex design requires at least visuoperceptual accuracy, visuospatial analyzing and synthesizing abilities, visuomotor integrity, and fine hand coordination: failure in any one of these areas would result in a poorly constructed copy. Thus, in the individual case, only one of these functions may be impaired. In order to determine which this is, the examiner can compare performances on different tests which each measure just one or two of the several functions in question. Thus, to identify the source of a problem in copying a complex design, the examiner would give the patient a visuomotor task—such as one calling for symbol substitutions, which has virtually no visuospatial components; a visual recognition test, which has neither visuospatial nor motor components; and a task involving visuospatial analysis and synthesis, which also has no motor component. Failure on one or two of these tests when the other or others are performed adequately will indicate which functions necessary for drawing from a copy are impaired and which preserved. By means of this kind of procedure, the functions making the critical contribution to the impaired performance may best be identified.

Pattern Analysis   This approach takes into account the scores from all of the tests.[1,8,83,97] The examiner compares the pattern of cognitive strengths and weaknesses with the deficit patterns characteristic of particular disorders or lesion sites or evaluates the score pattern to determine whether it makes neuropsychological or neurologic sense. Competent pattern analysis requires a neuropsychologically sophisticated examiner.

Integrated Interpretation

In evaluating test performance, most neuropsychologists consider the patient's background, personality, and current situation along with the medical history. They also pay attention to neuropsychologically relevant behavioral characteristics, such as idiosyncrasies of speech, inappropriate emotional responses, carelessness or overcautiousness, distractibility, perseveration, and confabulation, characteristics that can often convey as much or more information about the patient as the test data. While recognizing that formal testing procedures constitute the basis of most neuropsychological evaluations, a valid and meaningful interpretation of test findings requires the integration of all available data. The neuropsychological examination is not a psychometric exercise but rather an opportunity for understanding the patient's behavioral functioning in the broadest sense, as appropriate for the needs and circumstances that led to the examination.

REFERENCES

1. Lezak MD: *Neuropsychological assessment,* 3d ed. New York: Oxford University Press, 1995.
2. Teuber HL: Neuropsychology, in Harrower MR (ed): Recent advances in diagnostic psychological testing. Springfield, IL: Charles C. Thomas, 1948, pp 30–52.
3. Reitan RM: Problems and prospects in studying the psychological correlates of brain lesions. *Cortex* 2:127–154, 1966.
4. Yates AJ: The validity of some psychological tests of brain damage. *Psychol Bull* 51:359–379, 1954.
5. Anderson SW, Damasio AR, Tranel D: Neuropsychological impairments with lesions caused by tumor or stroke. *Arch Neurol* 47:397–405, 1990.
6. Crosson B: *Subcortical Functions in Language and Memory: A Working Model.* New York: Guilford, 1992.
7. Jones-Gotman M. Localization of lesions by neuropsychological testing. *Epilepsia* 32(suppl 5):S41–S52, 1991.
8. Walsh KW: *Neuropsychology,* 2d ed. Edinburgh: Churchill Livingstone, 1987.
9. Kertesz A (ed): *Localization and Neuroimaging in*

Neuropsychology. New York: Academic Press, 1994.

10. Thatcher RW, Hallett M, Zeffiro T, et al (eds): *Functional Neuroimaging.* New York: Academic Press, 1994.

11. Theodore WH (ed): *Clinical Neuroimaging.* New York: Liss, 1988.

12. Derix MMA: *Neuropsychological Differentiation of Dementia Syndromes.* Berwyn PA: Swets & Zeitlinger, 1994.

13. Parks RW, Zec RF, Wilson RS (eds): *Neuropsychology of Alzheimer's Disease and Other Dementias.* New York: Oxford University Press, 1993.

14. Caine ED: The neuropsychology of depression: The pseudo-dementia syndrome, in Grant I, Adams KM (eds): *Neuropsychological Assessment of Neuropsychiatric Disorders.* New York: Oxford University Press, 1986, pp 221–243.

15. Godwin-Austin R, Bendall J: *The Neurology of the Elderly.* New York: Springer-Verlag, 1990.

16. Kaszniak AW, Sadeh M, Stern LZ: Differentiating depression from organic brain syndromes in older age, in Chaisson-Stewart GM (ed): *Depression in the Elderly: An Interdisciplinary Approach.* New York: Wiley, 1985, pp 161–189.

17. Marcopulos BA: Pseudodementia, dementia, and depression: Test differentiation, in Hunt T, Lindley CJ (eds): *Testing Older Adults: A Reference Guide for Geropsychological Assessments.* Austin, TX: Pro-ed, 1989.

18. Strauss, ME, Brandt J: Attempt at preclinical identifiation of Huntington's disease using the WAIS. *J Clin Exp Neuropsychol* 8:210–218, 1986

19. Zec RF: Neuropsychological functioning in Alzheimer's disease, in Park RF, Zec RF, Wilson RL (eds): *Neuropsychology of Alzheimer's Disease and Other Dementias.* New York: Oxford University Press, 1993, pp 3–80.

20. Levin HS, Mattis S, Ruff RM, et al: Neurobehavioral outcome of minor head injury. *J Neurosurg* 66:234–243, 1987.

21. Lezak MD (ed): *Assessment of the Behavioral Consequences of Head Trauma.* New York: Liss, 1989.

22. Stuss DT, Ely P, Hugenholtz H, et al: Subtle neuropsychological deficits in patients with good recovery after closed head injury. *Neurosurgery* 17:41–47, 1985.

23. Morrow LA: Cuing attention: Disruptions following organic solvent exposure. *Neuropsychology* 8:471–476, 1994.

24. White RF, Feldman RG, Proctor SP: Neurobehavioral effects of toxic exposures, in White RF (ed): *Clinical Syndromes in Adult Neuropsychology: The Practitioner's Handbook.* New York: Elsevier, 1992.

25. Diller L, Gordon WA: Interventions for cognitive deficits in brain-injured adults. *J Consult Clin Psychol* 49:822–834, 1981.

26. Kreutzer JS, Wehman PH: *Cognitive Rehabilitation for Persons with Traumatic Brain Injury.* Baltimore, MD: Brookes, 1991.

27. Sohlberg MM, Mateer CA: *Introduction to Cognitive Rehabilitation.* New York: Guilford, 1989.

28. Wilson BA: *Rehabilitation of Memory.* New York: Guilford, 1987.

29. Smith A: Changes in Porteus Maze scores of brain-operated schizophrenics after an eight-year interval. *J Ment Sci* 106:967–978, 1960.

30. Meador KJ, Loring DW, Allen ME, et al: Comparative cognitive effects of carbamazepine and phenytoin in healthy adults. *Neurology* 41:1537–1540, 1991.

31. Meyers CA, Abbruzzese JL: Cognitive functioning in cancer patients: Effect of previous treatment. *Neurology* 42:434–436, 1992.

32. Parker JC, Granberg BW, Nichols WK, et al: Mental status outcomes following carotid endarterectomy: A six-month analysis. *J Clin Neuropsychol* 5:345–353, 1983.

33. Peck EA, Mitchell JB: Normative data for 5338 head injury patients across seven time periods after injury (abstr). *J Clin Exp Neuropsychol* 12:34, 1990.

34. Morris JC, McKeel DW, Storandt M, et al: Very mild Alzheimer's disease: Informant based clinical, psychometric, and pathologic distinction from normal aging. *Neurology* 41:469–478, 1991.

35. Parente FJ, Anderson J: Use of the Wechsler Memory Scale for predicting success in cognitive rehabilitation. *Cogn Rehabil* 2:12–15, 1984.

36. Filley CM, Heaton RK, Thompson LL, et al: Effects of disease course on neuropsychological functioning, in Rao SM (ed): *Neurobehavioral Aspects of Multiple Sclerosis.* New York: Oxford University Press, 1990, pp 136–145.

37. Filley CM: *Neurobehavioral Anatomy.* Niwot, CO: University of Colorado Press, 1995.

38. Luria AR: *Higher Cortical Functions in Man.* Haigh B, trans. New York, Basic Books, 1973.

39. Shepherd GM (ed): *The Synaptic Organization of the Brain.* New York: Oxford University Press, 1990.

40. Goldberg E: Higher cortical functions in humans:

The gradiental approach, in Goldberg E (ed): *Contemporary Neuropsychology and the Legacy of Luria.* Hillsdale, NJ: Erlbaum, 1990, pp 229–276.

41. Benton, AL, Tranel D: Visuoperceptual, visuospatial, and visuoconstructive disorders, in Heilmann KM, Valenstein E (eds): *Clinical Neuropsychology,* 3d ed. New York: Oxford University Press, 1993.

42. Coslett HB, Saffran EM: Disorders of higher visual processing: Theoretical and clinical perspectives, in Margolin DI (ed): *Cognitive Neuropsychology in Clinical Practice.* New York: Oxford University Press, 1992.

43. Damasio AR, Damasio H, Tranel D: Impairments of visual recognition as clues to the processes of memory, in Edelman GM, Gall WE, Cowan WM (eds): *Signal and Sense: Local and Global Order in Perceptual Maps.* New York: Wiley, 1990.

44. Mayes AR: *Human Organic Memory Disorders.* New York: Cambridge University Press, 1988.

45. Andreassi JL: *Psychophysiology: Human behavior and physiological response,* 3d ed. Hillsdale, NJ: Erlbaum, 1995.

46. Heilman KM, Valenstein E, eds: *Clinical Neuropsychology,* 3d ed. New York: Oxford University Press, 1993.

47. Binet A, Simon T: Le developpement de l'intelligence chez les enfants. *Année Psychol* 14:1–94, 1908.

48. Guilford JP: *A Revised Structure of Intellect.* Reports from the Psychological Laboratory of the University of Southern California, No. 19. Los Angeles: University of Southern California, 1957.

49. Thurstone LL. *Primary Mental Abilities.* Chicago: University of Chicago Press, 1938.

50. Newcombe F: *Missile Wounds of the Brain.* London: Oxford University Press, 1969.

51. Teuber H-L. Effects of brain wounds implicating right or left hemisphere in man: Discussion, in Mountcastle VB (ed): *Interhemispheric Relations and Cerebral Dominance.* Baltimore: Johns Hopkins Press, 1962.

52. Lishman WA. *Organic Psychiatry,* 2d ed. Oxford: Blackwell, 1987.

53. Pincus JH, Tucker GJ: *Behavioral Neurology,* 3d ed. New York: Oxford University Press, 1985.

54. Heilman KM, Bowers D, Valenstein E: Emotional disorders associated with neurological diseases, in Heilman KM, Valenstein E (eds): *Clinical Neuropsychology,* 3d ed. New York: Oxford University Press, 1993, pp 461–498.

55. Lezak MD: The problem of assessing executive functions. *Int J Psychol* 17:281–297, 1982.

56. Fuster JM: *The Prefrontal Cortex,* 2d ed. New York: Raven Press, 1989.

57. Stuss DT, Benson DF: *The Frontal Lobes.* New York: Raven Press, 1986.

58. Spearman CE: "General intelligence" objectively determined and measured. *Am J Psychol* 15:72–101, 1904.

59. Barona A, Reynolds CR, Chastain R: A demographically based index of premorbid intelligence for the WAIS-R. *J Consult Clin Psychol* 52:885–887, 1984.

60. Wilson RS, Rosenbaum G, Brown G: The problem of premorbid intelligence in neuropsychological assessment. *J Clin Neuropsychol* 1:49–54, 1979.

61. Nelson HE: *The National Adult Reading Test (NART): Test Manual.* Windsor, Berks, UK: NFER-Nelson, 1982.

62. Crawford JR, Parker DM, Besson JAO: Estimation of premorbid intelligence in organic conditions. *Br J Psychiatry* 153:178–181, 1988.

63. Spreen O, Strauss E: *A Compendium of Neuropsychological Tests.* New York: Oxford University Press, 1991.

64. Crawford JR, Steward LE, Garthwaite PH, et al: The relationship between demographic variables and NART performance in normal subjects. *Br J Clin Psychol* 27:181–182, 1988.

65. Goldstein FC, Gary HE, Levin HS: Assessment of the accuracy of regression equations proposed for estimating premorbid intellectual functioning on the Wechsler Adult Intelligence Scale. *Clin Neuropsychol* 8:405–412, 1986.

66. Karzmark P, Heaton RK, Grant I, Matthews CG. Use of demographic variables to predict full scale IQ: A replication and extension. *J Clin Exp Neuropsychol* 7:412–420, 1985.

67. Silverstein AB: Accuracy of estimates of premorbid intelligence based on demographic variables. *J Clin Psychol* 43:493–495, 1987.

68. McCarthy RA, Warrington EK: *Cognitive Neuropsychology: A Clinical Introduction.* San Diego, CA: Academic Press, 1990.

69. Anger WK: Assessment of neurotoxicity in humans, in Tilson H, Mitchell C (eds): *Neurotoxicology.* New York: Raven Press, 1992, pp 363–386.

70. Dershowitz A, Frankel Y: Jewish culture and the WISC and WAIS test patterns. *J Consult Clin Psychol* 43:126–134, 1975.

71. Vernon PE: *Intelligence: Heredity and Environment.* San Francisco: Freeman, 1979.

72. Anastasi A: *Psychological Testing,* 6th ed. New York: Macmillan, 1988.

73. Cronbach LJ: *Essentials of Psychological Testing,* 4th ed. New York: Harper & Row, 1984.

74. Wechsler D: *WAIS-R Manual.* New York: Psychological Corporation, 1981.

75. Porteus SD: *The Maze Test and Clinical Psychology.* Palo Alto, CA: Pacific Books, 1959.

76. Raven JC: *Raven's Progressive Matrices: Examination Kit.* Los Angeles: Western Psychological Services, no date.

77. Bender L: *A Visual Motor Gestalt Test and Its Clinical Use.* New York: American Orthopsychiatric Association, 1938.

78. MacQuarrie TW: *MacQuarrie Test for Mechanical Ability.* Monterey, CA: CTB/McGraw-Hill, 1925, 1953.

79. Purdue Research Foundation. *Examiner's Manual for the Purdue Pegboard.* Chicago: Science Research Associates, 1948.

80. Benton AL, Hansher K deS, Varney NR, Spreen O: *Contributions to Neuropsychological Assessment.* New York: Oxford University Press, 1983.

81. Boll TJ: The Halstead-Reitan neuropsychology battery, in Filskov SB, Boll TJ (eds): *Handbook of Clinical Neuropsychology.* New York: Wiley-Interscience, 1981, pp 577–615.

82. Reitan, RM, Wolfson D: *The Halstead-Reitan Neuropsychological Test Battery: Theory and Clinical Interpretation.* Tucson, AZ: Neuropsychology Press, 1993.

83. Milberg WP, Hebben N, Kaplan E: The Boston process approach to neuropsychological assessment, in Grant I, Adams KM (eds): *Neuropsychological Assessment of Neuropsychiatric Disorders.* New York: Oxford University Press, 1986.

84. Huff FJ, Becker JT, Belle SH, et al: Cognitive deficits and clinical diagnosis of Alzheimer's disease. *Neurology* 38:786–790, 1988.

85. Storandt M, Botwinick J, Danziger WL: Longitudinal changes: Patients with mild SDAT and matched healthy controls, in Poon LW (ed): *Handbook for Clinical Memory Assessment of Older Adults.* Washington, DC: American Psychological Association, 1986.

86. Grafman J, Litvan I, Gomez C, Chase TN: Frontal lobe function in progressive supranuclear palsy. *Arch Neurol* 47:553–561, 1990.

87. Albert MS, Moss MB, Milberg W: Memory testing to improve the differential diagnosis of Alzheimer's disease, in Igbal K, Wisniewski HM, Winblad B (eds): *Alzheimer's Disease and Related Disorders.* New York: Liss, 1989.

88. Rey GJ, Pirozzolo FJ, Levy J, Jankovic J: Cognitive impairments associated with progressive supranuclear palsy (abstr). *J Clin Exp Neuropsychol* 10:31, 1988.

89. Schaie KW: The course of adult intellectual development. *Am Psychol* 49:304–313, 1994.

90. Storandt M: Longitudinal studies of aging and age-associated dementias, in Boller F, Grafman J (eds): *Handbook of Neuropsychology.* Amsterdam: Elsevier, 1990, vol 4, pp 349–364.

91. Howieson DB, Holm LA, Kaye JA, et al: Neurologic function in the optimally healthy oldest old: Clinical neuropsychological evaluation. *Neurology* 43:1882–1886, 1993.

92. Bornstein RA: Classification rates obtained with "standard" cut-off scores on selected neuropsychological measures. *J Clin Exp Neuropsychol* 8:413–420, 1986.

93. Bornstein RA, Suga LJ: Educational level and neuropsychological performance in healthy elderly subjects. *Dev Neuropsychol* 4:17–22, 1988.

94. Heaton RK, Grant I, Matthews CG: Differences in neuropsychological test performances associated with age, education, and sex, in Grant I, Adams KM (eds): *Neuropsychological Assessment of Psychiatric Disorders.* New York: Oxford University Press, 1986, pp 100–120.

95. Kaufman AS, Reynolds CR, McLean JE: Age and WAIS-R intelligence in a national sample of adults in the 20- to 74-year age range: A cross-sectional analysis with educational level. *Intelligence* 13:235–253, 1989.

96. Stanton BA, Jenkins CD, Savageau JA, et al: Age and educational differences on the Trail Making Test and Wechsler Memory Scales. *Percept Motor Skills* 58:311–318, 1984.

97. Rey A: *L'examen clinique en psychologie.* Paris: Presses Universitaires de France, 1964.

98. Wechsler D: *Wechsler Memory Scale—Revised Manual.* San Antonio, TX: Psychological Corporation, 1987.

99. Bigler ED: Neuropathology of traumatic brain injury, in Bigler ED (ed): *Traumatic Brain Injury.* Austin, TX: Pro-ed, 1990.

100. Stuss DT, Eskes GA, Foster JK: Experimental neuropsychological studies of frontal lobe functions, in Boller F, Grafman J (eds): *Handbook*

of Neuropsychology. Amsterdam: Elsevier, 1994, vol 9.

101. Schenkenberg T, Bradford DC, Ajax ET: Line bisection and visual neglect in patients with neurologic impairment. *Neurology* 30:509–517, 1980.
102. Bornstein RA, Paniak C, O'Brien W: Preliminary data on classification of normal and brain-damaged elderly subjects. *Clinical Neuropsychol* 1:315–323, 1987.
103. Stern Y, Andrews H, Pittman J, et al: Diagnosis of dementia in a heterogeneous population: Development of a neuropsychological paradigm-based diagnosis of dementia and quantified correction for the effects of education. *Arch Neurol* 40:8–14, 1992.
104. Milner B, Teuber H-L: Alteration of perception and memory in man: Reflections on methods, in Weiskrantz L (ed): *Analysis of Behavior Change.* New York: Harper & Row, 1968, chap 11.

Chapter 4

ANATOMIC PRINCIPLES IN BEHAVIORAL NEUROLOGY AND NEUROPSYCHOLOGY

M.-Marsel Mesulam

The student of human neuroanatomy faces many challenges. There is no universal agreement on terminology, no distinct boundaries that completely separate one region from another, and, in most instances, no one-to-one correspondence among lobar designations, traditional topographic landmarks, cytoarchitectonic boundaries, and behavioral specializations. One part of the brain can have more than one descriptive name and cytoarchitectonic (striate cortex), functional (primary visual cortex), and topographic (calcarine cortex) terms can be used interchangeably to designate the same area.

Cytoarchitectonic maps, especially that of Brodmann,[1] have introduced a useful and widely used approach to the parcellation of the cerebral hemispheres. Brodmann delineated individual architectonic areas on the basis of microscopic criteria. In contemporary usage, however, a statement such as "activation was seen in area 9" almost invariably means that the investigator estimated the area of activation to be in a part of the hemisphere analogous to the part that Brodmann designated area 9. This usage can lead to potential inaccuracies, since the topographic fit between the imaged brain slice and Brodmann's hand-drawn brain may not be exact and there may be interindividual differences in the distribution of cytoarchitectonic areas. Brodmann's map is also quite unclear about cytoarchitectonic designations for sulcal banks, which contain a very significant proportion of the cerebral cortex.

There is no immediate solution to these difficulties, but it is important to be aware of their existence. In this chapter, descriptive neuroanatomic designations are used whenever possible. For example, with regard to primary auditory cortex, the term *Heschl's gyrus*, which refers to an easily identifiable topographic landmark, is preferred to a cytoarchitectonic designation such as *area 41-42*, which is based on microscopic critera. When used, cytoarchitectonic designations follow the nomenclature of Brodmann. Since the anatomic information in this chapter is highly condensed, the reader may want to consult more comprehensive treatments of this subject by Brodmann (now available in English translation[1]), Duvernoy,[2] Nieuwenhuys and coworkers,[3] Pandya and Yeterian,[4] and Mesulam.[5]

Neurons of the central nervous system are engaged in three major operations: (1) reception and registration of sensory stimuli from outside and from within (input); (2) planning and execution of complex motor acts (output); and (3) intermediary processing interposed between input and output. Thought, language, memory, self-awareness and even many aspects of mood and affect constitute different manifestations of intermediary processing. The neural substrates for these intermediary processes are located principally within the limbic system and cortical association areas. From a behavioral point of view, therefore, the cerebral hemispheres can be divided into four major components: primary sensory cortex, primary motor cortex, association cortex, and limbic-paralimbic cortex (Table 4-1). It is the latter two com-

Table 4-1

Types of cortical areas and their corresponding Brodmann numbers

Primary Sensory and Motor Cortex

Primary visual (area 17)

Primary auditory (areas 41, 42)

Primary somatosensory (areas 1, 2, 3 but mostly area 3b)

Primary motor (area 4 and caudal part of area 6)

Association Cortex

Unimodal visual (areas 18, 19, 20, 21, ? 37)

Unimodal auditory (area 22)

Unimodal somatosensory (area 5, rostral area 7)

Unimodal motor (rostral area 6, caudal area 8, area 44)

Heteromodal prefrontal (areas 9, 10, 11, 45, 46, 47, ? rostral area 8, rostral area 12, rostral area 32)

Heteromodal parietotemporal (areas 39, 40, caudal area 7, banks of superior temporal sulcus, ? area 36)

Limbic System (cortical components)

Corticoid formations (amygdala, substantia innominata, septal nuclei)

Allocortex (hippocampus, pyriform olfactory cortex)

Paralimbic cortex [insula (areas 14, 15), temporopolar cortex (area 38), caudal orbitofrontal cortex (caudal areas 11, 12, 13), cingulate complex (areas 23, 24, 33, 31, 26, 29) parolfactory region (area 25, caudal area 32), parahippocampal cortex (areas 28, 34, 35, 30)]

---

ponents, those associated with intermediary processing, that are most relevant to behavioral neurology and neuropsychology and which will receive the most emphasis in this chapter.

CORTICAL TYPES

Regions of the cerebral cortex display a variety of architectures. The simplest type of cortex is located in the basal forebrain. Components of the basal forebrain such as the septal nuclei, the substantia innominata, and the amygdaloid complex are situated directly on the ventral and medial surface of the hemispheres and are thus considered part of the cortical mantle. These structures contain the simplest and most undifferentiated type of cortex. The organization of the constituent neurons is rudimentary and no consistent lamination or dendritic orientation can be discerned. These three components of the basal forebrain could be designated as having a "corticoid," or cortexlike, structure. Corticoid areas (especially the amygdala) have architectonic features that are in part cortical and in part nuclear.[5]

The next stage of cortical differentiation is known as allocortex. This type of cortex contains one or two principal bands of neurons arranged into moderately differentiated layers. The two allocortical formations of the brain are (1) the hippocampal formation, which also carries the designation of archicortex, and (2) the piriform or primary olfactory cortex, which is also known as paleocortex. Corticoid and allocortical formations collectively make up the limbic zone of cortex.

The next level of structural complexity is encountered in the paralimbic zone of the cerebral cortex (Fig. 4-1). These areas are intercalated between allocortex and isocortex so as to provide a gradual transition from one to the other. Allocortical cell layers often extend into the periallocortical component of paralimbic areas. Several gradual changes in the direction of increased complexity and differentiation occur from the allocortical toward the isocortical side of paralimbic regions. These changes include (1) progressively greater accumulation of small granular neurons in layer IV and then in layer II, (2) sublamination and columnization of layer III, (3) differentiation of layer V from layer VI and of layer VI from the underlying white matter, and (4) an increase of intracortical myelin, especially along the outer layer of Baillarger (layer IV).

There are five major paralimbic formations in the primate brain: (1) the caudal orbitofrontal cortex; (2) the insula; (3) the temporal pole; (4) the parahippocampal gyrus (includes the entorhinal, prorhinal, perirhinal, presubicular, and parasubicular areas); and (5) the cingulate complex (includes the retrosplenial, cingulate, and parolfactory areas). These five paralimbic regions form an

Figure 4-1

Distribution of functional zones in relation to Brodmann's map of the human brain. The boundaries are not intended to be precise. Much of this information is based on experimental evidence obtained from laboratory animals and must be confirmed in the human brain. The primary sensory and motor zone is shown in blue, the unimodal zone in yellow, the heteromodal zone in magenta, the paralimbic zone in green, and the limbic zone in white. Abbreviations: AA = auditory association cortex; AG = angular gyrus; A1 = primary auditory cortex; CG = cingulate cortex; F = fusiform gyrus; INS = insula; IPL = inferior parietal lobule; IT = inferior temporal gyrus; MA = motor association cortex; MPO = medial parietooccipital area; MT = middle temporal gyrus; M1 = primary motor area; OF = orbitofrontal region; PC = prefrontal cortex; PH = parahippocampal region; PO = parolfactory area; PS = peristriate cortex; RS = retrosplenial area; SA = somatosensory association cortex; SG = supramarginal gyrus; SPL = superior parietal lobule; ST = superior temporal gyrus; S1 = primary somatosensory area; TP = temporopolar cortex; VA = visual association cortex; V1 = primary visual cortex. (From Mesulam,[5] with permission.)

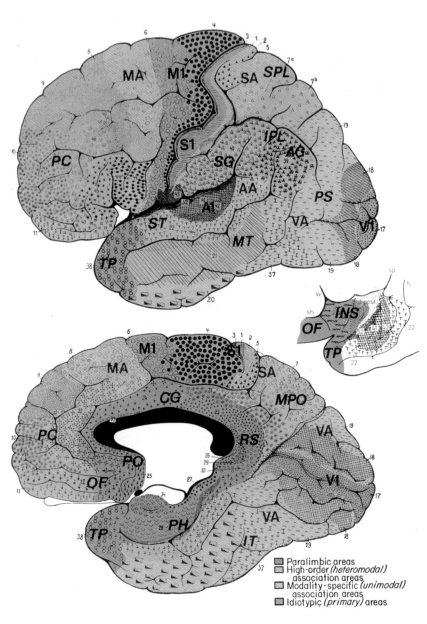

uninterrupted girdle surrounding the medial and basal aspects of the cerebral hemispheres.[6]

The greatest extent of the cortical surface in the human brain consists of six-layered homotypical isocortex, also known as association cortex. Association isocortex can be subdivided into two major types: modality-specific (unimodal) isocortex and high-order (heteromodal) isocortex. Unimodal association isocortex is defined by three essential characteristics: (1) the constituent neurons are almost exclusively responsive to stimulation in only a single sensory modality; (2) the predominant cortical inputs are provided by the primary sensory cortex or by other unimodal regions in that same modality; (3) damage yields modality-specific deficits confined to tasks guided by cues in that modality.

The unimodal areas for the three major sensory modalities have been determined experimentally in the brain of the macaque monkey. Such experiments have shown that the superior temporal gyrus is the unimodal auditory association area, that the superior parietal lobule provides the somatosensory unimodal association area, and that the peristriate, midtemporal, and inferotemporal regions provide the unimodal association regions in the visual modality.[5]

The heteromodal component of isocortex is identified by the following characteristics: (1) neuronal responses are not confined to any single sensory modality, (2) the cortical inputs originate from unimodal areas in more than one modality and/or from other heteromodal areas, and (3) damage to this type of cortex leads to deficits that transcend any single modality. Some neurons in heteromodal association areas respond to stimulation in more than one modality, indicating the presence of direct multimodal convergence. More commonly, however, there is an admixture of neurons with different preferred modalities. Defined in this fashion, heteromodal cortex includes the types of regions that have been designated as high-order association cortex, polymodal cortex, multimodal cortex, polysensory areas, and supramodal cortex.[5]

There are essentially two and perhaps three major heteromodal fields in the brain of the monkey. One is in the prefrontal region, including the anterior orbitofrontal surface and the dorsolateral frontal convexity. The second heteromodal field includes the inferior parietal lobule and extends into the banks of the superior temporal sulcus and perhaps into parts of the midtemporal gyrus. There may be a third heteromodal region in the posterior part of the ventral temporal lobe.

There are some relatively subtle architectonic differences between unimodal and heteromodal areas. In general, the unimodal areas have a more differentiated organization, especially with respect to sublamination in layers III and V, columnarization in layer III, and more extensive granularization in layer IV and especially layer II. On these architectonic grounds, it would appear that heteromodal cortex is closer in structure to paralimbic cortex and that it provides a stage in the hierarchy of architectonic differentiation intercalated between paralimbic and unimodal areas.

The koniocortex of primary sensory areas and the macropyramidal cortex of the primary motor region constitute unique and highly specialized regions that can be designated as having an idiotypic architecture. There are two divergent opinions about these primary areas. One is to consider them as the most basic and elementary components of cortex; the other is to see these areas as the most advanced and highly differentiated components of the cortical mantle. I favor the latter point of view. The location of idiotypic regions is well known: the primary visual area covers the occipital pole and the banks of the calcarine fissure, the primary auditory cortex covers Heschl's gyrus on the supratemporal plane, the primary somatosensory cortex covers the postcentral gyrus, and the primary motor area is located in the precentral gyrus.

A GENERAL PLAN OF ORGANIZATION FOR PATTERNS OF BEHAVIORAL SPECIALIZATION AND NEURAL CONNECTIVITY IN CORTEX

The preceding discussion shows that the hemispheric surface can be subdivided into five zones (limbic, paralimbic, unimodal, heteromodal, and idiotypic) which collectively provide a spectrum of cytoarchitectonic differentiation ranging from the simplest to the most differentiated (Fig. 4-1).

All types of cortical areas, including association isocortex, receive direct hypothalamic projections.[7] For the great majority of cortical regions, this hypothalamic input is quite minor. The only exception is provided by the limbic structures. Thus, the septal nuclei, basal nucleus of the substantia innominata, amygdaloid complex, piriform cortex, and hippocampus stand out by the presence of substantial hypothalamic connections. Another major source of connections for limbic structures originates in the paralimbic zone. For example, the amygdala receives an extensive cortical input from the insula; the hippocampus from the entorhinal sector of the parahippocampal region; and the piriform cortex as well as the nucleus basalis from insular, temporopolar, and orbitofrontal paralimbic areas. Paralimbic areas have extensive monosynaptic connections with limbic and heteromodal areas; heteromodal areas with paralimbic and unimodal areas; unimodal areas with primary and heteromodal areas. Primary areas derive their major cortical connections from unimodal areas and major subcortical connections from the relevant thalamic relay nuclei.[5]

These patterns are relative rather than absolute. For example, the amygdala is also known to receive direct input from association isocortex, but this does not appear to be as substantial as the connections of this limbic structure with the hypothalamus and with paralimbic regions. In some cases, however, there are more rigid distinctions. The primary areas in the more advanced primates, for example, do not seem to receive any limbic or paralimbic cortical input. This may ensure that the initial processing of sensory information is not influenced by drive and mood. Perhaps this is why emotional state does not alter the shape of an object or the pitch of a sound. The adaptive value of this arrangement is evident. In other mammalian species such as the rat, however, this separation may be less complete, since direct connectivity between primary and paralimbic areas has been reported.[8]

Many cortical areas have connections with other constituents of the same functional zone.

These are extremely well developed within the limbic, paralimbic, and heteromodal zones. For example, of all the cortical neurons that directly projected to a subsector of prefrontal heteromodal cortex, 26 percent were located within unimodal areas, 13 percent in paralimbic regions, and 61 percent in other heteromodal cortex.[9] Furthermore, the insula as well as the cingulate cortex have interconnections with virtually each of the other paralimbic regions of the brain. Although unimodal regions may receive extensive input from other unimodal areas in the same modality, there is essentially no interconnectivity between areas belonging to different modalities. In a similar vein, except for the intimate interconnections between the primary somatosensory and motor areas, there are no neural projections among primary areas belonging to separate modalities. It appears, therefore, that there is a premium on channel width within the limbic, paralimbic, and heteromodal zones, whereas the emphasis is on fidelity within the unimodal and primary zones.

As noted above, the corticoid and allocortical areas, collectively designated as "limbic" structures, are the parts of the cerebral cortex that have the closest association with the hypothalamus. Through neural and also hormonal mechanisms, the hypothalamus is in a position to coordinate electrolyte balance, blood glucose levels, basal temperature, metabolic rate, autonomic tone, sexual phase, circadian oscillations, and even immunoregulation. The hypothalamus is essentially the head ganglion of the internal milieu and also a major coordinating structure for drives and instincts that promote the survival of the self and of the species. In keeping with these functions of the hypothalamus, areas in the limbic zone of the cerebral cortex assume an important role in the regulation of behaviors such as memory and learning, the modulation of drive, the emotional coloring of experience, and the higher control of hormonal balance and autonomic tone. These specializations of limbic structures are related to the maintenance of the internal milieu (homeostasis) as well as to the associated operations necessary for the preservation of the self and the species.[5]

At the other pole of the cytoarchitectonic

spectrum lie the most highly specialized primary sensory and motor areas. These are the parts of cortex that are most closely related to the extrapersonal space, since sensory input from the environment has its first cortical relay in primary koniocortical areas and motor cortex coordinates actions that lead to the manipulation of the extrapersonal world.

Intercalated between these two extremes, the zones of association and paralimbic cortex provide neural bridges that link the internal milieu to the extrapersonal environment. The heteromodal and unimodal areas are predominantly involved in perceptual elaboration and motor planning, whereas the paralimbic zone is involved predominantly in directing drive and emotion to the appropriate extrapersonal and intrapsychic targets. Collectively, the unimodal, heteromodal, and paralimbic areas enable the needs of the individual to be discharged according to relevant opportunities and limitations that exist in the environment.

Within the group of isocortical association areas, the unimodal association cortices provide the principal neuronal machinery for the modality-specific elaboration and encoding of sensory input. Unimodal areas can be divided into *upstream* and *downstream* components. Upstream components receive their major modality-specific information directly from the corresponding primary area, whereas the downstream areas receive their major modality-specific input from the corresponding upstream unimodal areas. In the visual modality, for example, the peristriate region (areas 18 and 19), constitutes an upstream unimodal association area, whereas inferotemporal cortex (areas 20 and 21) constitutes a downstream unimodal association area.

Heteromodal cortex receives convergent input from multiple unimodal areas, especially downstream unimodal areas, whereas paralimbic cortex acts as a relay between sensory association cortices and the limbic zone of the cerebral cortex.[4] Heteromodal and paralimbic formations support two major types of neural processing: (1) the associative linkage of unimodal sensory information into distributed templates that encode multimodal knowledge and (2) the integration of this information with drive and emotion. In contrast to the idiotypic and unimodal belts, which are characterized by relatively more "dedicated" and homogeneous neural mechanisms confined to single modalities of information processing, the heteromodal and paralimbic areas support a more "generalized" type of processing, with heterogeneous input-output relationships, so that no uniform behavioral specialization can be assigned to individual components of the paralimbic and heteromodal zones.

SUBCORTICAL STRUCTURES: STRIATUM AND THALAMUS

The striatum can be divided into three components: the caudate, the putamen, and the olfactory tubercle-nucleus accumbens complex. Each striatal component receives cortical input but none projects back to the cortex. The caudate and putamen, which are also collectively designated as the dorsal striatum, receive cortical input predominantly from association cortex and primary idiotypic areas. The dopaminergic input to these striatal components originates in the pars compacta of the substantia nigra. The cortical input to the olfactory tubercle-nucleus accumbens complex originates in limbic and paralimbic parts of the brain. The nucleus accumbens, for example, receives convergent input from the amygdala and the hippocampus. On the basis of this connectivity pattern, the nucleus accumbens-olfactory tubercle complex can be designated as the limbic striatum.[10] The dopaminergic innervation of the limbic striatum originates in the ventral tegmental area of Tsai, which is just medial to the substantia nigra, and dopamine turnover is higher in the limbic striatum than in the neostriatum.[11]

All parts of cortex project to the striatum. These corticostriatal projections obey a complex topographic arrangement. One feature of this arrangement is that the input from each cortical area forms multiple patches of axonal terminals within the striatum. Yeterian and Van Hoesen[12] made the interesting suggestion that terminal patches from separate cortical areas are more likely to show partial overlap if the relevant cortical areas are interconnected with each other. This implies that there may be some replication of corticocortical interaction patterns within the striatum.

The caudate may have a lesser role than the putamen in motor control. For example, motor cortex projects to the putamen but not to the caudate.[13] The head of the caudate receives most of its input from dorsolateral prefrontal cortex. It is therefore interesting to note that lesions in the head of the caudate yield deficits that are essentially identical to those that emerge upon ablating prefrontal cortex.[14] This raises the possibility that each striatal region may have behavioral specializations similar to those of the cortical area, from which it receives its major cortical input.

Lesions in the head of the caudate and in the putamen have been associated with aphasia and also with unilateral neglect. However, in almost all such cases the adjacent white matter is also involved, so that it is not possible to determine whether these deficits reflect damage to the striatum or to the adjacent fibers, which interconnect cortical areas related to language and attention. We have seen one ambidextrous patient with multi-infarct dementia who also had a substantial infarction in the head of the left caudate. This patient had no motor deficit, aphasia, or amnesia. His mental state deficits were characterized by a severe lack of judgment, insight, and planning. This patient raises the possibility that damage to the head of the caudate may give rise to mental changes similar to those seen in conjunction with prefrontal cortex lesions.[5]

The globus pallidus of the primate has four easily identifiable components: (1) the outer (lateral) segment, (2) the inner (medial) segment, (3) the ventral pallidum, and (4) the pars reticulata of the substantia nigra. The globus pallidus receives projections from the striatum and projects to the thalamus. The globus pallidus is thus an essential link in the striatopallidothalamocortical loops, which are thought to have important organizing roles in a number of complex behavioral domains.

There is essentially no disagreement about the crucial role of the globus pallidus in motor control. In humans, lesions of the globus pallidus are frequently associated with severe extrapyramidal disturbances. However, the relationship of the globus pallidus to movement may be quite complex and appears to involve substantial sensorimotor integration. For example, local cooling in the area of the globus pallidus in monkeys yields a severe and reversible breakdown of a learned flexion-extension movement, but only when the animal is blindfolded. In the presence of visual input, the deficit is no longer observed.[15]

The medial zone of the inner pallidal segment and also the ventral pallidum have close associations with limbic structures. For example, in contrast to the more dorsal parts of the pallidum, which receive their striatal input from the caudate and putamen, the ventral pallidum receives its major striatal projections from the nucleus accumbens. Furthermore, a substantial number of ventral pallidal neurons respond to amygdaloid stimulation.[16]

In the monkey, the core of the internal pallidal segment projects to the motor thalamus. However, a medial crescent of this pallidal segment projects predominantly to the lateral habenula, which is generally considered as a structure closely related to the limbic regions of the brain.[17] In keeping with this anatomic pattern, some types of pallidal lesions interfere with behaviors generally associated with limbic mechanisms. For example, MacLean[18] showed that damage to the medial globus pallidus of monkeys severely disrupts species-specific sexual display patterns. Thus, the ventral pallidum and the medial portion of the inner pallidal segment could be considered as having preferential limbic affiliations.

The pars reticulata of the substantia nigra is a caudal extension of the globus pallidus. There is evidence suggesting that this portion of the pallidal complex may participate in the programming of saccadic eye movements in response to actual or remembered targets.[19]

One function of the thalamus is to relay subcortical lemniscal inputs to cortical areas. Almost all thalamic nuclei have well-developed reciprocal connections with cortex. The one exception is the reticular nucleus, which receives subcortical and cortical input but does not project back to cortex.[20]

There is very little interconnectivity among individual thalamic nuclei, so that there is very little interaction at the thalamic level among the different types of information that are being relayed to cortex. The one exception is provided by the reticular and intralaminar nuclei, which have extensive connections with other thalamic nuclei.

The large number of thalamic nuclei can be subdivided into several functional groups on the basis of their preferred cortical and subcortical projections.[5] The primary relay nuclei are the easiest to identify (Fig. 4-2). The caudal part of the ventroposterior lateral nucleus (VPL_c) and the principal division of the ventroposterior medial

Figure 4-2

Schematic diagram of the four major groups of thalamic nuclei. Abbreviations: AD = anterior dorsal; AM = anterior medial; AV = anterior ventral; LD = laterodorsal; LGN = lateral geniculate; LP = lateroposterior; MD = medialis dorsalis; MGN = medial geniculate; Pi = inferior pulvinar; Pl = lateral pulvinar; Pm = medial pulvinar; Po = oral pulvinar; VA = ventral anterior; VL = ventral lateral; VPL = ventroposterior lateral; VPM = ventroposterior medial. (From Mesulam,[5] with permission).

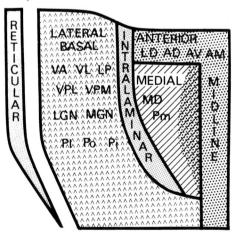

RETICULAR ACTIVATING

MODALITY SPECIFIC

HETEROMODAL + PARALIMBIC

LIMBIC + PARALIMBIC

nucleus (VPM) receive fibers from the medial lemniscus and quintothalamic tract and constitute the somatosensory relay nuclei of the thalamus. The lateral geniculate nucleus (LGN) and the part of the medial geniculate nucleus (MGN) that receives the brachium of the inferior colliculus are the primary relay nuclei for the visual and auditory modalities, respectively. Damage to the VPL_c or to the LGN gives rise to hemihypesthesia and hemianopia, respectively. Since inputs from both ears reach the MGN in each hemisphere, unilateral damage to this thalamic nucleus does not lead to deafness in the contralateral ear. In fact, unilateral MGN lesions may be extremely difficult to detect clinically. The major thalamic input into primary motor cortex (M1) comes from the caudal ventrolateral nucleus (VL_c) and the oral ventroposterior lateral nucleus (VPL_o). The behavioral effects of lesions in these nuclei are poorly understood.

A second group of thalamic nuclei project predominantly to unimodal association areas (see Ref. 5 for a review of the evidence). In the rhesus monkey, the major thalamic projections to the somatosensory association cortex of the superior parietal lobule (area 5) come from the lateroposterior nucleus (LP) and perhaps also from the oral subdivision of the pulvinar nucleus (P_o). In the visual modality, the nuclei that provide the major projection to visual unimodal association areas include the inferior (P_i) and lateral (P_l) subdivisions of the pulvinar nucleus. In the auditory modality, the unimodal association region receives its major thalamic input from the anterior MGN and probably also from a ventral rim of the medial pulvinar. Thus, the MGN is the source of thalamic projections not only to A1 but also to the auditory association cortex. The motor association cortex receives its major thalamic input from the oral ventrolateral nucleus (VL_o) and from parts of the ventral anterior nucleus (VA).

A third group of thalamic nuclei have no specific modality affiliations and project predominantly to heteromodal and limbic cortex. The lateral part of the medial dorsal nucleus (MD) is the major thalamic nucleus for the prefrontal heteromodal fields, whereas the medial pulvinar nucleus (P_m) and parts of the adjacent lateral posterior nucleus (LP) are the major nuclei for the heteromodal fields in the inferior parietal lobule and within the banks of the superior temporal sulcus.

The close interaction between cortical heteromodal and paralimbic zones is also reflected in the arrangement of thalamic connectivity patterns. Thus, the MD and P_m nuclei, which are the major nuclei for heteromodal cortical areas, also have extensive paralimbic connections. For example, the medial part of MD (including the magnocellular MD_{mc} component) is the major thalamic nucleus for the orbitofrontal paralimbic region, while the P_m has reciprocal projections with all components of the paralimbic belt and is probably the major nucleus for the temporopolar paralimbic area. The MD and P_m also have direct limbic connections. Thus, the medial and magnocellular parts of MD have connections with the amygdala, piriform cortex, and septal region. Furthermore, the P_m has also been shown to have reciprocal projections with the amygdaloid complex (see Ref. 5 for a review of the evidence).

Another group of dorsally and medially placed nuclei are collectively known as the nuclei of the "anterior tubercle." These nuclei include the anterior thalamic nucleus [including its dorsal (AD), ventral (AV), and medial (AM) components] and the laterodorsal nucleus (LD). They provide the major thalamic connections for the posterior cingulate cortex, the retrosplenial area, and some of the parahippocampal paralimbic areas. The anterior thalamic nucleus receives the mammillothalamic tract and is therefore an important component of the Papez circuit.

A number of nuclei that are situated close to the thalamic midline are collectively known as midline nuclei. These include the paratenial, paraventricular, subfascicular, central, and reuniens nuclei. These nuclei have extensive connections with paralimbic areas (e.g., temporal pole and anterior cingulate gyrus) and also with the hippocampal formation.

The effects of lesions in these nuclei are consistent with their patterns of cortical connectivity. For example, in the rhesus monkey, bilateral MD lesions reproduce deficits in spatial delayed alternation similar to those associated with prefrontal ablations.[21] On the other hand, more medial MD lesions, which also involve adjacent midline nuclei, lead to deficits in visual object recognition similar to those obtained after medial temporal ablations.[22] In some patients, even unilateral lesions in the more medial parts of the MD and in the anterior tubercle nuclei have been associated with severe amnestic conditions.[23] In Wernicke encephalopathy, involvement of the MD and P_m is thought to play a major role in the genesis of the amnestic state.[24] Lesions of the right pulvinar nucleus, including its medial component, have been described in conjunction with contralateral neglect for the left extrapersonal space.[25] Electrical stimulation of the left medial pulvinar has been reported to induce transient anomia.[26] These behavioral relations are consistent with the connections of the P_m with the parietotemporal parts of heteromodal cortex and with limbic-paralimbic structures.

A fourth group of thalamic nuclei are closely affiliated with the ascending reticular activating system. The reticular nucleus of the thalamus as well as the intralaminar nuclei (e.g., the limitans, paracentralis, centralis lateralis, centromedian, and parafascicularis) have strong associations with the ascending reticular activating pathways. In contrast to other thalamic nuclei, which have somewhat restricted projection zones, the intralaminar nuclei have more widespread connections and are also known as "diffuse projection nuclei."

THE ASCENDING RETICULAR ACTIVATING SYSTEM

The cerebral cortex has three sources of afferent neural projections: cortical, thalamic, and extrathalamic. The existence of corticocortical and thalamocortical projections had been established by classic neuroanatomic methodology. During the past 20 years, the advent of more powerful methods based on axonally transported tracers has helped to uncover a third set of subcortical but extrathalamic afferents with origins in the ventral tegmental area (dopaminergic), raphe nuclei (serotonergic), nucleus locus ceruleus (noradrenergic), hypothalamus (mostly histaminergic), and basal forebrain (cholinergic and GABAergic). These extrathalamic afferents exert a modulatory influence upon cortical activity and constitute important components of what is currently emerging as the modern concept of the ascending reticular activating system.[27]

Moruzzi and Magoun[28] had introduced the concept of a brainstem reticular activating system that acted to desynchronize the cortical electroencephalogram via a relay in the thalamus. Subsequent work revealed that a most important component in this system consists of a cholinergic reticulothalamic pathway that facilitates the activation of corticopetal relay neurons in the thalamus.[29–33] It is becoming quite clear that the original concept of the ascending reticular activating system (ARAS) needs to be expanded to include at least three interconnected sources of ascending projections, one in the brainstem, a second in the basal forebrain, and a third in the thalamus.

The brainstem contingent of the ascending activating pathways displays considerable complexity. In addition to ascending cholinergic projections from the laterodorsal tegmental and pedunculopontine nuclei, there are also dopaminergic projections from the substantia nigra–ventral tegmental area, serotonergic projections from the raphe nuclei, noradrenergic projections from the nucleus locus ceruleus, and excitatory amino acid projections from the rostral reticular formation.[27,34] The ascending monoaminergic projections are predominantly directed to the cerebral cortex (without a thalamic relay), whereas the ascending cholinergic and excitatory amino acid projections are directed predominantly to the thalamus. Although all thalamic nuclei receive cholinergic projections from the brainstem, the reticular and intralaminar nuclei are traditionally considered to have the most intimate relation to the ARAS.

The nucleus basalis of the substantia innominata provides the source of a very substantial cholinergic projection directed to the entire cerebral cortex and the amygdala. These projections have complex effects upon cortical neurons but generally tend to act as excitatory neuromodulators that increase the impact of behaviorally relevant sensory events upon cortical neurons.[35] The ascending corticopetal cholinergic projection originating from the nucleus basalis is a crucial telencephalic component of the ARAS.

The cerebral cortex is not only the target of ascending projections from the brainstem, basal forebrain, and thalamus but also the source of descending feedback projections to several components of the ARAS. Almost all parts of the cerebral cortex project to the reticular nucleus and therefore influence its inhibitory effect upon other thalamic nuclei.[20] The projection from the cerebral cortex to the reticular nucleus of the thalamus is mostly excitatory, whereas the projections to this thalamic nucleus from the brainstem cholinergic nuclei are inhibitory. The reticular nucleus is thus in a position to gate thalamocortical transmission in a way that reflects the integrated influence of the brainstem and cerebral cortex.

Although the basal forebrain projects to the entire cerebral cortex, it receives feedback projections from a very limited set of cortical areas, namely those that belong to the limbic and paralimbic zones of the cerebral cortex.[36] This asymmetry is a feature of all the other extrathalamic ascending pathways of the ARAS: they project widely to the cerebral cortex but receive very few reciprocal connections from the cerebral cortex.[37] These pathways of the ARAS collectively provide the physiologic matrix for modulating a wide range of cortical functions related to arousal and attention.

NEURAL NETWORKS

The anatomic substrate of individual cognitive domains takes the form of large-scale neurocognitive networks that contain interconnected cortical and subcortical nodes.[34] Each major node of such a network belongs to multiple intersecting networks. Consequently, the same cognitive domain may be disrupted after damage to several different regions of the brain, and damage confined to a single region may yield more than one type of cognitive deficit.

At least four large-scale neurocognitive networks can be identified in the human brain: the left hemisphere language network, the right hemisphere attentional network, the limbic system, and the frontal network.[34] The major cortical nodes of the language network are located in Broca's area (areas 44 and 45) and Wernicke's area (posterior part of area 22 and parts of areas 39 and 40) of the left hemisphere. These two nodes are interconnected with several perisylvian cortical areas and with specific regions of the thalamus and striatum. Damage to components of this network leads to distinct aphasic disturbances whose clinical features reflect the specializations of the primary lesion site. The three major cortical nodes of the attentional network are located in the frontal cortex, posterior parietal cortex, and cingulate gyrus of the right hemisphere. Damage to cortical or subcortical components of this network leads to the various manifestations of the spatial neglect syndrome. The limbic system includes the limbic and paralimbic cortical areas, limbic striatum, limbic nuclei of the thalamus, and hypothalamus. Damage to components of this network leads to deficits of retentive memory, emotion, motivation, and affiliative behaviors. The frontal network includes the heteromodal and paralimbic cortices of the frontal lobes, the head of the caudate nucleus, and the mediodorsal nucleus of the thalamus. Damage to components of this network leads to complex deficits of the attentional matrix, personality, and comportment.

Experimental investigation of interconnections between major cortical nodes of individual networks shows that pairs of such areas are interconnected not only with each other but also with an additional set of identical cortical areas.[38] This architecture of connectivity is compatible with parallel and distributed processing. In resolving a cognitive problem, a set of cortical areas interconnected in this fashion can execute an extremely rapid survey of a vast informational landscape until the entire system settles into a best fit with respect to the multiple goals and constraints engendered by the problem.[34] This computational architecture is quite compatible with cognitive tasks such as deciding which words best express a thought or how to reconstruct a specific complex

memory. There are no single "correct" solutions to such tasks but an entire family of possibilities, each leading to a different compromise within the relevant matrix of goals and constraints.

Anatomic experiments have shown that members of an interconnected pair of cortical areas in a network are likely to send interdigitating and partially overlapping projections to the striatum.[12] The striatum receives cortical input but does not project back to cortex and could act as an "efference synchronizer" for the set of cortical areas in a large-scale network.[34] Cortical areas have extensive corticocortical connections, so that each member of the association cortex is likely to belong to multiple intersecting networks. Thalamic subnuclei, however, have almost no interconnections among each other and may thus play an important role in setting coactivation boundaries for individual networks.[34] Cortical components, together with corresponding regions of the thalamus, striatum, and reticular pathways, make up large-scale distributed networks that provide the immediate anatomic substrates of individual cognitive domains.

Several computational models can be proposed for understanding how the central nervous system converts simple sensory input into knowledge and experience. One possibility is to postulate the existence of a hierarchical synaptic chain for the transfer of information from primary sensory areas first to upstream unimodal areas, then to downstream unimodal areas, and finally to multimodal areas where knowledge is encoded in convergent form. This convergent encoding model faces several serious objections.[39] An alternative selectively distributed processing model proposes that the most veridical building blocks of experience are encoded at the level of unimodal rather than heteromodal association cortex.[39,40] According to this model, heteromodal, paralimbic, and limbic areas of the cerebral cortex provide transmodal nodes for binding this modality-specific information into coherent but distributed (nonconvergent) multidimensional knowledge. Lesions that interrupt the flow of information within unimodal areas or from unimodal to transmodal areas result in disconnection syndromes such as pure alexia, pure word deafness, and prosopagnosia.[41]

Depending on their location, connectivity, and affiliations with specific large-scale networks, individual transmodal zones provide critical nodes for coordinating complex mental phenomena in the realms of memory encoding, retrieval, object recognition, language comprehension, and spatial awareness. The cerebral substrate for cognition is thus both distributed and regionally specialized but neither modular nor diffuse. This model, based predominantly on the anatomic organization of the cerebral cortex, lends itself to a variety of experimental approaches for probing the complex relationship between cerebral structure and cognitive phenomena.

REFERENCES

1. Brodmann K: *Localisation in the Cerebral Cortex.* London: Smith-Gordon, 1994.
2. Duvernoy H: *The Human Brain.* Vienna: Springer-Verlag, 1991.
3. Nieuwenhuys R, Voogd J, van Huijzen C: *The Human Central Nervous System.* Berlin: Springer-Verlag, 1988.
4. Pandya DN, Yeterian EH: Architecture and connections of cortical association areas, in Peters A, Jones EG (eds): *Cerebral Cortex.* New York: Plenum Press, 1985, vol 4, pp 3–61.
5. Mesulam M-M: Patterns in behavioral neuroanatomy: Association areas, the limbic system, and hemispheric specialization, in Mesulam M-M (ed): *Principles of Behavioral Neurology.* Philadelphia: Davis, 1985, pp 1–70.
6. Mesulam M-M, Mufson EJ: Insula of the old world monkey: I. Architectonics in the insulo-orbito-temporal component of the paralimbic brain. *J Comp Neurol* 212:1–22, 1982.
7. Mesulam M-M, Mufson EJ, Levey AI, Wainer BH: Cholinergic innervation of cortex by the basal forebrain: Cytochemistry and cortical connections of the septal area, diagonal band nuclei, nucleus basalis (substantia innominata), and hypothalamus in the rhesus monkey. *J Comp Neurol* 214:170–197, 1983.
8. Vogt BA, Miller MW: Cortical connections between rat cingulate cortex and visual motor and postsubicular cortices. *J Comp Neurol* 216:192–210, 1983.
9. Barbas H, Mesulam M-M: Organization of afferent input to subdivisions of area 8 in the rhesus monkey. *J Comp Neurol* 200:407–431, 1981.
10. Heimer L, Wilson RD: The subcortical projections of the allocortex: Similarities in the neural associations of the hippocampus, the piriform cortex and the neocortex, in Santini M (ed): *Golgi Centennial Symposium: Proceedings.* New York: Raven Press, 1975, pp 177–193.
11. Walsh FX, Thomas TJ, Langlais PJ, Bird ED: Dopamine and homovanillic acid concentrations in striatal and limbic regions of the human brain. *Ann Neurol* 12:52–55, 1982.
12. Yeterian EH, Van Hoesen GW: Cortico-striate projections in the rhesus monkey: The organization of certain cortico-caudate connections. *Brain Res* 139:43–63, 1978.
13. Künzle H: Bilateral projections from precentral motor cortex to the putamen and other parts of the basal ganglia: An autoradiographic study in *Macaca fascicularis. Brain Res* 88:195–209, 1975.
14. Iversen SD: Behavior after neostriatal lesions in animals, in Divac I, Oberg RGE (eds): *The Neostriatum.* Oxford: Pergamon Press, 1979.
15. Horel J, Meyer-Lohmann J, Brooks VB: Basal ganglia cooling disables learned arm movements of monkeys in the absence of visual guidance. *Science* 195:584–586, 1977.
16. Yim CY, Mogenson GJ: Response of ventral pallidal neurons to amygdala stimulation and its modulation by dopamine projections to nucleus accumbens. *J Neurophysiol* 50:148–161, 1983.
17. Parent A, de Bellefeuille L: Organization of efferent projections from the internal segment of the globus pallidus in primate as revealed by fluorescence retrograde labeling method. *Brain Res* 245:201–213, 1982.
18. MacLean PD: Effects of lesions of globus pallidus on species-specific display behavior of squirrel monkey. *Brain Res* 149:175–196, 1978.
19. Hikosaka O, Wurtz RH: Visual and oculomotor functions of monkey substantia nigra pars reticulata: III. Memory-contingent visual and saccade responses. *J Neurophysiol* 49:1268–1284, 1983.
20. Jones EG: Some aspects of the organization of the thalamic reticular complex. *J Comp Neurol* 162:285–308, 1975.
21. Isseroff A, Rosvold HE, Galkin TW, Goldman-Rakic PS: Spatial memory impairments following damage to the mediodorsal nucleus of the thalamus in rhesus monkeys. *Brain Res* 232:97–113, 1982.

22. Aggleton JP, Mishkin M: Visual recognition impairment following medial thalamic lesions in monkeys. *Neuropsychology* 21:189–197, 1983.

23. Michel D, Laurent B, Foyatier N, et al: Étude de la mémoire et du langage dans une observation tomodensitométrique d'infarctus thalamique paramedian gauche. *Rev Neurol (Paris)* 138:533–550, 1982.

24. Signoret J-L: Memory and amnesias, in Mesulam M-M (ed): *Principles of Behavioral Neurology.* Philadelphia: Davis, 1985, pp 169–192.

25. Cambier J, Elghozi D, Strube E: Lésion du thalamus droit avec syndrome de l'hémisphère mineur: Discussion du concept de négligence thalamique. *Rev Neurol (Paris)* 136:105–116, 1980.

26. Ojemann GA, Fedio P, VanBuren JM: Anomia from pulvinar and subcortical parietal stimulation. *Brain* 91:99–116, 1968.

27. Mesulam M-M: Cholinergic pathways and the ascending reticular activating system of the human brain. *Ann NY Acad Sci* 757:169–179, 1995.

28. Moruzzi G, Magoun HW: Brain stem reticular formation and activation of the EEG. *Electroencephalogr Clin Neurophysiol* 1:459–473, 1949.

29. Dingledine R, Kelly JS: The brainstem stimulation and acetylcholine-invoked inhibition of neurons in the feline nucleus reticularis thalami. *J Physiol* 271:135–154, 1977.

30. Hoover DB, Jacobowitz DM: Neurochemical and histochemical studies of the effect of a lesion of the nucleus cuneiformis on the cholinergic innervation of discrete areas of the rat brain. *Brain Res* 70:113–122, 1970.

31. Hoover DB, Baisden RH: Localization of putative cholinergic neurons innervating the anteroventral thalamus. *Brain Res Bull* 5:519–524, 1980.

32. McCance I, Phillis JW, Westerman RA: Acetylcholine-sensitivity of thalamic neurons: Its relationship to synaptic transmission. *Br J Pharmacol* 32:635–651, 1986.

33. Phillis JW, Tebecis AK, York DH: A study of cholinoceptive cells in the lateral geniculate nucleus. *J Physiol* 192:695–713, 1967.

34. Mesulam M-M: Large-scale neurocognitive networks and distributed processing for attention, language, and memory. *Ann Neurol* 28:597–613, 1990.

35. Mesulam M-M: Structure and function of cholinergic pathways in the cerebral cortex, limbic system, basal ganglia, and thalamus of the human brain, in Bloom FE, Kupfer DJ (eds): *Psychopharmacology: The Fourth Generation of Progress.* New York: Raven Press, 1994, pp 135–146.

36. Mesulam M-M, Mufson EJ: Neural inputs into the nucleus basalis of the substantia innominata (Ch4) in the rhesus monkey. *Brain* 107:253–274, 1984.

37. Mesulam M-M: Asymmetry of neural feedback in the organization of behavioral states. *Science* 237:537–538, 1987.

38. Morecraft RJ, Geula C, Mesulam M-M: Architecture of connectivity within a cingulo-fronto-parietal neurocognitive network for directed attention. *Arch Neurol* 50:279–284, 1993.

39. Mesulam M-M: Neurocognitive networks and selectively distributed processing. *Rev Neurol (Paris)* 150:564–569, 1994.

40. Seeck M, Schomer D, Mainwaring N, et al: Selectively distributed processing of visual object recognition in the temporal and frontal lobes of the human brain. *Ann Neurol* 37:538–545, 1995.

41. Geschwind N. Disconnection syndromes in animals and man. *Brain* 88:237–294, 1965.

Chapter 5

THE LESION METHOD IN BEHAVIORAL NEUROLOGY AND NEUROPSYCHOLOGY

Hanna Damasio and Antonio R. Damasio

The lesion method aims at establishing a correlation between a circumscribed region of brain damage, a lesion and a pattern of alteration in some aspect of an experimentally controlled cognitive or behavioral performance. The brain-damaged region is conceptualized as part of a large-scale network of cortical and subcortical sites that operate in concert, by virtue of their interlocking connectivity, to produce a particular function. Given a theoretical framework for how such networks are constituted and carry out that particular function, a lesion is thus a *probe* to test a specific hypothesis. A lesion probe allows the investigator to decide whether damage to a component of the putative network, responsible for function X, alters the network behavior according to the predictions made for it. In other words, given a theory about the operations of a normal brain, lesions are a means to support or falsify the theory.

The subjects for the lesion method may be humans or animals. The lesions may have been produced by neurologic disease alone or incurred in the process of treating it (e.g., a surgical procedure). They may be small or large and may be studied in vivo or at postmortem. The indispensable requirements are that lesions be stable, well demarcated, and referable to a neuroanatomic unit. In this chapter we focus on human lesions, produced by neurologic disease or surgical ablation, and studied in vivo with modern neuroimaging techniques.

The lesion approach provided the first method in what was to become neuroscience. In the very least, it dates to Morgagni's demonstration of an association between unilateral brain disease and contralateral sensory and motor disabilities. Bouillaud's and Broca's finding of a correlation between speech and focal damage to the frontal lobe are reasonable signposts to mark the modern era of lesion studies.

In the latter decades of the nineteenth century, the lesion method led to pathbreaking discoveries. But although most of the findings have stood the test of time and gained wide acceptance, the theories that were associated with them did not. The pioneering neurologists conceived of the existence of brain centers capable of performing complex psychological functions with relative independence. What little interaction there was among those few and noncontiguous centers was achieved by unidirectional pathways. These concepts were subject to deserved criticism, the best known of which came from Sigmund Freud and Hughlings Jackson. As the theoretical account lost influence, the lesion method, which was closely interwoven with the theory, lost favor as a means of valid scientific inquiry.

The lesion method began to regain some prominence in the 1960s, perhaps as a reaction to the impasses of "equipotential" antilocalizationism and "black-box" behaviorism. The revival was spearheaded by Geschwind's reflections on the work of Wernicke, Lichtheim, Liepmann, and Déjerine and by the work of notable neuropsychologists, among whom were A. R. Luria, Henri Hécaen, Brenda Milner, Arthur Benton, Hans-

69

Lukas Teuber, and Oliver Zangwill. The full value of the lesion method, however, only began to be appreciated after the development of new neuroimaging technologies—computed tomography (CT), which had its inception in 1973, and magnetic resonance imaging (MRI), which emerged a decade later.

It has gradually become evident that the lesion method should be separated from the theoretical accounts historically connected with it. As with any other approach, this method has limitations and misapplications. Nonetheless, it is one entity, with its virtues and pitfalls, and the theoretical constructs that make use of it represent another. Nothing prevents practitioners of the lesion method from proposing the richest and most dynamic accounts of brain function.

In short, the classically discovered links between certain brain regions of the cerebral cortex and signs of neuropsychological dysfunction have been validated, remain a staple of clinical neurology, and allow for relatively accurate predictions of *localization of damage* from neurologic signs. That is, more often than not, the presence of certain neuropsychological defects indicates to the clinical expert that there is dysfunction in a specific brain area. These valid links, however, should not be taken to mean that the functions disturbed by the lesion were inscribed in the tissue that the lesion destroyed. The complex psychological functions, which usually constitute the target of neuropsychological studies in humans, are not localizable at that level.

The neural architectures revealed by neuroanatomy and neurophysiology and the cognitive architectures revealed by experimental neuropsychology suggest that single-center functions, single-purpose pathways, and unidirectional cascades of information process are unrealistic. Moreover, the residual performance that follows focal brain insults, and the ensuing patterns of recovery, suggest that knowledge must be widely distributed, at multiple neural levels, and complex psychological functions must emerge from the cooperation of multiple components of integrated networks.

Two key developments made human lesion studies rewarding again. First, lesion studies in nonhuman primates brought major advances to the understanding of the neural basis of vision and memory, as demonstrated, among others, by Mishkin and colleagues. Second, the advent of CT and MRI began to permit human lesion studies in vivo. It is apparent now that the lesion method is indispensable to cognitive neuroscience, especially when it comes to human studies. The *new* lesion method is not concerned with "localizing functions," nor is it a contest for "localizing lesions." It is a means to test, at systems level, hypotheses regarding *both* neural structure *and* cognitive processes. What investigators from Déjerine to Geschwind gleaned from single cases can now be replicated systematically in a suitable group of subjects. Hypotheses old and new, including some advanced by the pioneer neuropsychologists, can be tested experimentally.

Beyond their intrinsic value, the results from the new lesion method in humans provide a welcome complement to results from neuroanatomic and neurophysiologic experiments in animals. Lesion work in humans has revealed characteristics of neural systems that could not have been investigated in experimental animals. The example of linguistic processes is the most obvious. Lesion results have also been the source of hypotheses that were further investigated in animals and in humans. Ungerleider and Mishkin's study of ventral and dorsal visual pathways in nonhuman primates[1] was inspired by Newcombe's work in humans.[2] Conversely, Ungerleider and Mishkin's work was followed up in humans, and the inferotemporal system has now been anatomically and functionally fractionated.[3–5] Moreover, the lesion method offers the possibility of conducting indepth experiments on some cognitive operations whose temporal characteristics are not suitable for other approaches (for instance, experiments requiring the monitoring of psychophysiologic variables).

We also see the lesion method as joining forces with two other approaches to the investigation of human brain function: electrophysiologic studies and functional imaging. The first includes the use of event-related potentials, the study of cognitive and behavioral changes induced by electrical stimulation of exposed cerebral cortex, and the direct recording of activity from cerebral cortex. The second involves the imaging of brain activity inferred from the differential emission of radio signals. It encompasses positron emission tomography (PET), single photon emission computed tomography (SPECT), and functional magnetic resonance imaging (fMRI). The combination of results from the lesion method with those from the other approaches will strengthen our conceptualization of the human brain and bring to light discrepancies that require new theorizing and experimentation. Many well-established facts from the lesion method remain the benchmark against which some results of the new dynamic methods must be measured. Moreover, the actual combination of procedures is likely to generate more powerful tools. This will become reality, for instance, with the performance of PET and fMRI studies in patients with focal lesions causing specific cognitive disorders.

The lesion method does have its limitations. Not every anatomic region of the human nervous system can be properly sampled by natural lesions, and the size of the lesions provides a natural limit to the structures the method can probe with confidence. And yet, in its modern incarnation, the approach provides data currently unavailable through other means.

Only a concerted set of approaches from the molecular to the systems levels, in both humans and experimental animals, can eventually provide answers to the questions currently posed in cognitive neuroscience. The lesion method is a key partner in systems-level studies.

THE MODERN PRACTICE OF THE LESION METHOD IN HUMANS

There are at least five prerequisites for the modern practice of the lesion method: first, the availability of fine-grained structural imaging of the living human brain; second, the availability of a reliable method for the anatomic study of lesion probes; third, access to a large pool of subjects with lesions in varied brain sites, so that hypotheses regarding the operation of different systems can be experimentally tested in comparable target subjects and in appropriate controls; fourth, the availability of reliable techniques for various cognitive measurements; and fifth, the guidance of testable hypotheses concerning the neural basis of specific cognitive processes at systems level. In the following pages, we discuss some of these requisites.

Neuroanatomy from Neuroimaging

For many years, we have conceptualized the systematic neuroimaging studies pursued in our laboratory as a means to practice *human neuroanatomy from imaging data,* i.e., a means for detection and description of a lesion and consideration of its placement in the context of the anatomic systems to which it belongs. This purpose, which requires detailed knowledge of human neuroanatomy, is distinguishable from the traditional role of neuroimaging in *clinical neurologic diagnosis,* i.e., the detection of structural alterations and the prediction of its possible neuropathologic basis. The original tool for these studies was the template technique,[6] but we have since developed a new technique for individualized lesion analysis based on the three-dimensional (3D) reconstruction of the human brain from high-resolution MRI.[7] This new technique is known as BRAINVOX. It permits us to identify reliably, in vivo, every major gyrus and sulcus of the human brain; to slice and reslice the human brain in whatever incidence is necessary for anatomic analysis; and to define and measure volumes or surfaces of interest in single cases and across groups. The technique dispenses with charting onto brain templates and permits instead a customized definition of each subject. We will comment on this technique first and complete this section with a review of the template technique.

BRAINVOX

BRAINVOX is a 3D volumetric imaging and analysis system. The software was originally developed to facilitate the 3D display and mapping of acquired human brain lesions using a volume-rendering approach, but it has grown to support a wide range of advanced multimodality neuroanatomic visualization and analysis techniques. Although BRAINVOX was designed for the analysis of high-resolution volumetric MRI, it can be used with CT and PET.

BRAINVOX consists of several interconnected software components: (1) a slice/contour–based tracing module, (2) a multivolume 3D rendering system, (3) a set of general-purpose volume-manipulation tools, (4) a basic volume–data-handling system, (5) a palette editor, and (6) a volumetric object-measurement system.

BRAINVOX allows for explicit definition of volumes bounded by tracings that can be separated from the full MRI volume. The software allows users to define many such volumes simultaneously, slice by slice, taking advantage of common borders, edge tracking, and flexible trace-editing tools. Volume and intersection volume statistics can be computed for all objects defined in this manner. Histograms of volumes and individual slices can be computed.

Lesion Analysis with BRAINVOX

Using the 3D reconstructed brain to determine which anatomic sectors of each hemisphere are damaged obviates the need to adjust the angle in which the MRI sections are obtained to the angle of available template systems. The accuracy of interpretation no longer depends on the "reading" of a template with the transferred lesion but rather on the direct reading from the identified landmarks in the unique brain in question.

The new technique permits a direct identification of gyri and sulci, comparable to what can be achieved at the autopsy table in a postmortem brain after the meninges have been removed. The technique permits the accurate marking of such structures in coronal axial or parasagittal slices, with the advantage that the extension of lesions into the depths of sulci can also be determined (Fig. 5-1, Plate 1).

Other advantages of the new technique are as follows. First, the identification of anatomic structures is based on each individual brain rather than on an idealized "average" brain. The standard landmarks of each area of interest can be localized in the brain of each individual subject rather than on a template. Although templates use anatomic constants, they cannot account for individual variation and thus introduce an error of measurement, albeit small in some cases. Second, because each area of interest has been customized for each subject, it is possible to determine with

Figure 5-1

Three-dimensional reconstruction (obtained from 124 contiguous thin coronal MRI slices) of the brain of a subject with an infarct in the left frontal lobe. Acutely, the subject had a nonfluent aphasia and mild paresis of the right face and arm. At the time of the MRI (1 year later), both language deficit and paresis had improved.

Several sulci were identified and color-coded on the 3D reconstructed brain: central sulcus (red), precentral sulcus (green), inferior frontal sulcus (yellow), superior frontal sulcus (brown), and sylvian fissure (magenta).

Inspection of the left lateral and top views of the brain shows that the area of infarct is centered on the precentral sulcus, which is clearly visible only in the top view. The most anterior sector of the precentral gyrus is damaged, as well as the posterior sector of the middle frontal and inferior frontal gyrus.

The brain volume was also resectioned in axial (ax), coronal (co), and parasagittal (ps) slices (as shown in the three rows of brain slices in the lower segment of the image). Whenever any of the slices intersected a color-coded sulcus, the color automatically appeared on the slice, thus permitting an accurate identification of sulci and of gyri. Resectioning allowed us to inspect the lesion in depth and show that it extended all the way to the insula, which is compromised in its most superior sector (best seen in slice ps-3).

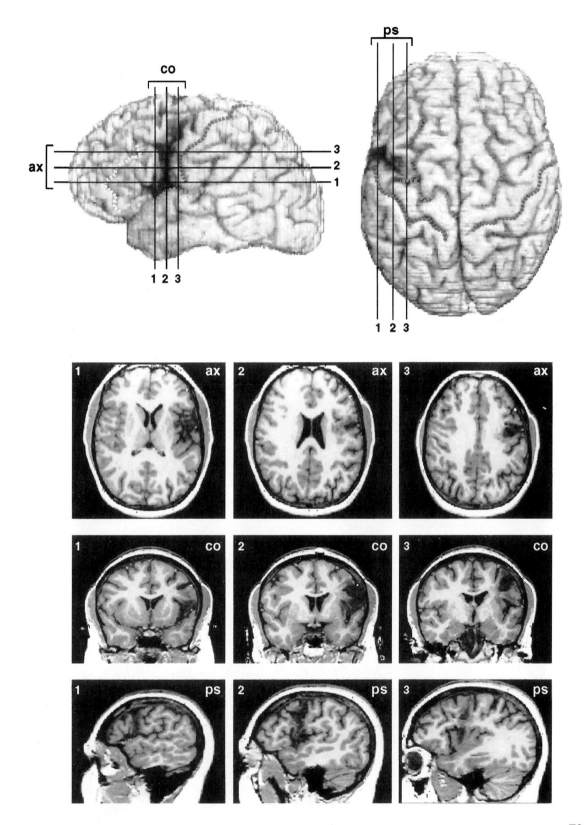

73

considerable rigor the proportion of a given area that has been destroyed by a lesion as well as the proportion of subjacent white matter that has been involved by the lesion (Fig. 5-2, Plate 2). Again, error is reduced.

This new technique requires a T_1-weighted MRI scan with contiguous thin slices (1.5 mm). For best results, the scan should be performed in the chronic stage. Regular MRI scans obtained for diagnostic purposes with thicker slices, interslice

Figure 5-2

Three-dimensional reconstruction of a human brain with a lesion in the left frontal lobe. The questions addressed here concerned the size of the lesion and the percentage of volume it occupied in the whole brain, in the left frontal lobe (LFL), and in some subdivisions of the frontal lobe: the pars triangularis (pars triang.) and the pars opercularis (pars operc.), the posterior half of the middle frontal gyrus (post. MFG), and the precentral gyrus in its inferior (inf. preCG) and middle thirds (mid. preCG). The limits of all of these regions of interest (ROI) were marked on the 3D reconstructed brain. On all coronal slices, the several ROIs are individually traced, as is the contour of the lesion. Six coronal slices are shown as an example. The different ROIs are color- and texture-coded. The automatically calculated absolute volumes and the percentage of damage in each of them are recorded on the top right-hand corner.

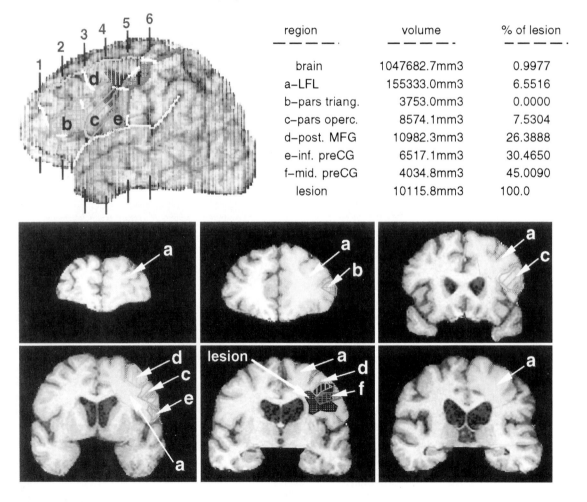

region	volume	% of lesion
brain	1047682.7mm3	0.9977
a–LFL	155333.0mm3	6.5516
b–pars triang.	3753.0mm3	0.0000
c–pars operc.	8574.1mm3	7.5304
d–post. MFG	10982.3mm3	26.3888
e–inf. preCG	6517.1mm3	30.4650
f–mid. preCG	4034.8mm3	45.0090
lesion	10115.8mm3	100.0

gaps, and other pulse specifications are not adequate for reconstruction. Furthermore, application of this elaborate procedure to acute lesions would be a waste of effort.

The Template Technique

Whenever MRI or CT scans are obtained with regular parameters (thick slices, and, in the case of MRI, interslice gaps), anatomic analyses must rely on the template technique.

The template technique relies on film transparencies of MRI or CT. For research purposes, it is advisable to have a technician collect all the films for a given case, mask the subject identification in all of them, and substitute a numerical entry code on the basis of which imaging data can be stored. This step ensures that the investigator performing the anatomic study is blind to the neurologic and neuropsychological data available for the same subject.

As with the previous technique, detailed knowledge of human neuroanatomy is indispensable. Needless to say, the investigator must be conversant with the imaging techniques themselves. The template technique relies on the availability of brain templates of the normal brain such as those published by us in 1989 and 1995. The key steps are as follows:

1.   Determine the angle of incidence in which CT or MRI were obtained. This can be achieved on the basis of a pilot scan or by inspection of the lower axial slices in which the relative positions of structures in the three main cranial fossae can be observed.

2.   On the basis of the above determination, select the set of templates that best fits the subject's films.

3.   Chart the lesion on the templates at every level at which it occurs, using an *X/Y* plotting strategy.

4.   Superimpose over the template an appropriate "in register" transparency that contains anatomic cells representing neural "areas of interest" in both gray and white matter structures. Each of those cells is limited by a linear boundary and

has a letter and number code on the basis of which it can be anatomically identified.

5.   Assign the area of damage charted in the template to the cells that encompass the abnormal images.

6.   Assign the estimation of the amount of involvement within target cells. We usually code this 0 when there is less than 25 percent involvement of the total, 1 if the involvement is between 25 and 75 percent; and 2 if more than 75 percent of the total area is damaged. This step can be achieved in two ways: (a) using a transparent square grid and counting the number of units involved by the lesion at each level, then calculating the percentage in relation to the total number of units encompassed by each area of interest (which is the sum of units occupied by the region at each template level); or (b) transferring the template system into computer software, tracing the lesion's limits as marked on the template with a digitizer, and then using automated determination of the percentage of area involved.

The number of cuts in the scan and in the correctly chosen set of templates may not coincide for two reasons: varied thickness of cuts and variations in individual brain size. Therefore, the investigator must search for the most appropriate scan/template matches, on a cut-by-cut basis, using all available anatomic constants—for example, ventricular system and prominent sulci. Fortunately, current MRI resolution provides such a wealth of landmarks that finding appropriate correspondences is no longer a daunting task. Correspondences are a necessary complement to the *X/Y* plotting approach. The results of *X/Y* plotting should be counterchecked by inspection of identifiable landmarks, since "blind" plotting may produce an inaccurate chart. This is why we do not advocate the use of fully automated lesion analysis with the template technique.

The major source of error in the template technique is the choice of the wrong template set. The key to the correct choice of templates is the inspection of *all* available brain cuts, especially the lower ones, which contain crucial landmarks for the determination of the incidence of a particular scan. In practical terms, it is necessary to compare the proportion of frontal lobe, temporal lobe, and posterior fossa structures shown in the scan with those seen in the various template sets and to select the best match. It is not possible to find the right match based on the inspection of high cuts alone, because in high-lying cuts, the cues from anatomic constraints such as the ventricular system or bony landmarks are lost.

Improved Template Technique

The availability of BRAINVOX and of 3D reconstructed normal brains has allowed us to improve the template technique. It is now possible to create "customized templates" for any set of CT or MRI slices. Instead of using published templates, a 3D reconstructed normal brain can be resliced so as to match the incidence of cut and the level of slices in the CT or MR images to be analyzed (Fig. 5-3, Plate 3). The key steps are as follows:

1.   All major sulci are identified and colorcoded in the 3D reconstructed normal brain.

2.   The normal brain is resliced on the computer screen so as to match the slice orientation and thickness of the 2D images of the brain to be analyzed, creating an equal number of brain slices (the "customized template set"). The color codes generated in (1) are automatically transferred onto the single brain slices.

3.   On each matched pair of normal/abnormal brain slices, the lesion is transferred in much the same manner as described for the basic template technique.

4.   The result is a 3D transfer of the lesion, which can then be "read off" the normal 3D reconstructed brain.

Analysis of Groups of Subjects

Whenever a study involves a large number of subjects, it may be advantageous to create maps of lesion overlap. For this purpose we have developed a technique that permits the determination of the region of maximal overlap in terms of brain surface ("Map-2," a 2D map), or in volumetric terms ("Map-3," a 3D map). Each of these techniques entails the transfer of all individual lesions onto a normal reference brain.

For Map-2, the steps are as follows:

1.   For each case, each view of the 3D brain showing the lesion is matched with the corresponding view of the normal reference brain, in terms of spatial coordinates.

2.   The surface contour of the lesion is transferred from the subject's brain and fitted onto the normal reference brain, taking into account its relation to sulcal and gyral landmarks.

3.   The lesions are then superimposed to form a surface map. A region of maximal lesion overlap is determined on the basis of the superimpositions and assigned a numerical weight based on the number of contributing lesions.

To obtain a Map-3, we transfer and fit the limits of all the target lesions onto the normal reference brain reconstructed in 3D (by transferring the contour of each lesion as seen in each slice into the corresponding slices of the reference brain in the way described above). The sum total of lesion contours for each case constitutes a 3D object. Given the collection of such objects, we then determine the intersection of their volumes in whatever plane we prefer. This allows us to determine overlap in both cortical "surface" and white matter "depth." We refer to the area of maximal overlap as the "center of volume."

Identifying Lesions with Computed Tomography and Magnetic Resonance Imaging

The identification of neuropathologic changes using CT depends on the detection, within a given brain region, of an x-ray absorption that departs from the norm. The presence of cerebral infarction, edema, or tumor at a specified anatomic location alters the standard x-ray absorption for that region and produces an abnormal image.

In the case of MRI, the identification of neuropathologic changes depends on the production of a locally different rate of hydrogen proton spinning, within the affected brain region, after the brain is exposed to a magnetic field. In other

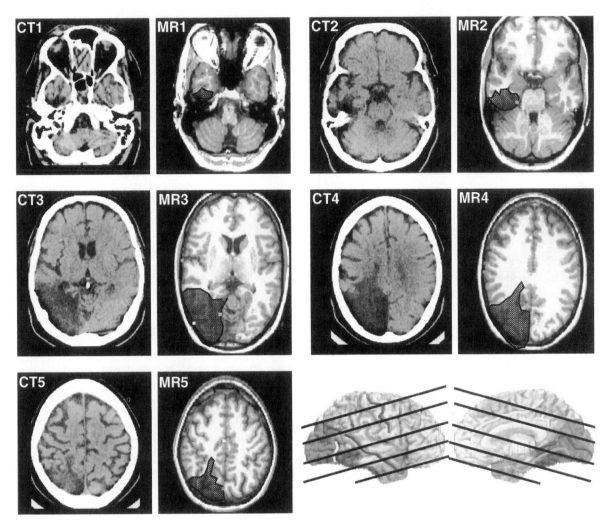

Figure 5-3

Demonstration of the improved template method. Brain CT (CT 1-5) of a subject who could not undergo an MRI study. A normal 3D reconstructed brain was resliced so as to match the orientation and level of the CT slices (MR 1-5). The lesion seen on the CT slices was transferred onto each matched MR slice, taking into account all identifiable sulci and gyri. Once the sulci were color-coded on the 3D reconstruction, the lesion could be read off each individual slice. The object defined by the transferred traces could be fused with the normal brain to visualize the lesion's surface extent (right lower corner).

words, after the brain is subjected to a magnetic field, with varied magnetic pulse sequence parameters, the presence of a pathologic brain region due to edema, infarction, or tumor will determine hydrogen proton spinning rates within the area that are different from what normally would be

expected for the given anatomic structure subjected to the same magnetic pulse sequence. Lesion-detection sensitivity with either method varies according to the specific procedure, the nature of the pathology, the stage at which the imaging measurement is made in relation to the onset of the pathologic process, and the quality of the equipment and proficiency of the technique.

The potential for false negatives or false positives is considerable, their magnitude depending on the factors listed above. For example, CT is often negative in the first 24 h following an infarct but is usually positive in the days after. However, in the second and third weeks after an infarct, because the infarcted tissue absorbs x-rays at the same rate as normal tissue, the CT may become negative again if not performed after the injection of a contrast-enhancing substance. Contrast seeps out of damaged vessels in the damaged region and increases the density of the area.

Neuroanatomic Resolution

The limits of resolution in the lesion method are set by the state of the technology. Current-generation CT and MRI scanners detect lesions as small as 1 mm on the plane of section. From the perspective of microstructure, these seemingly astounding resolutions are actually modest, since such small areas contain so many neurons and connections. Nonetheless, from the perspective of cytoarchitecture or of cortical regions defined neurophysiologically, this resolution is quite respectable. In short, current imaging technology visualizes neural structure at a level that permits the neuroanatomic definition of most lesions resulting from acquired neurologic disease or neurosurgical ablations.

Neither CT nor MRI can detect discrete cellular pathology except when a fairly large cortical region or subcortical nucleus is affected over a sizable surface or volume that turns out to be, in the aggregate, larger than the lower limit of resolution discussed above. This is why, in the early stages of degenerative dementia of either the Alzheimer or Pick types, when neuropsychological assessment already reveals marked cerebral dysfunction, CT and MRI studies may be so deceptively normal. At the same stage, however, dynamic neuroimaging using emission tomography procedures, of either the SPECT or PET types, may show changes in cerebral blood flow or metabolism.

Decreased radio signal in posterior temporal

and temporoparietal regions is quite characteristic of Alzheimer's dementia.[8–11] This is probably the consequence of both local pathologic changes and local physiologic changes brought about by anterior temporal lesions.

In moderate to advanced stages of Alzheimer's disease, CT and MRI often show fairly widespread cerebral atrophy or ventricular enlargement. In addition, MRI studies may also show a reduction in the volume of medial temporal structures, the result of accumulated damage in entorhinal and perirhinal cortices, and subsequent degeneration in hippocampus.[12,13]

In Pick's disease, autopsy studies have shown repeatedly that the characteristic pathology is especially evident in the frontal and anterior temporal cortices,[14] and in moderate to advanced cases, anatomic analysis of CT or MRI of patients with progressive dementia does reveal severe atrophy localized to those regions.[15]

The Choice of Neuropathologic Specimens

The choice of pathologic specimen is a major technical consideration in the lesion method, given that the neuropathologic characteristics of infarctions, intraparenchymal hemorrhages, or varied types of tumor are entirely different.

Nonhemorrhagic infarctions provide the best specimens for neuroanatomic investigation and correlation with neuropsychological findings, because cerebral infarctions actually destroy brain parenchyma. The infarcted area is eventually replaced by scar tissue and by cerebrospinal fluid, and CT or MRI in the chronic state provide a clear demarcation of the infarct. In CT, the damage is depicted as an area of decreased density, seen as a darker area in the gray scale that accompanies the images. In MRI, infarctions show as a dark area in T_1-weighted images and a white bright signal region in T_2-weighted images.

Herpes simplex encephalitis provides comparable anatomic detail. In adults, the virus has an affinity for a limited set of brain structures, mostly within the limbic system, and it destroys those areas rather completely by a mechanism that includes vascular collapse. In the chronic state, both CT and MRI produce extremely accurate images of the involved territories.

In most other varieties of neuropathologic process, the precise anatomic definition of lesions is less accurate and the functional impact of the lesion itself is less well defined. For instance, earlier in their growth, *gliomas* infiltrate brain tissue by dislocating local populations of neurons but may not destroy them immediately. Moreover, the region of low or high density seen on the CT or MRI of such tumors corresponds not just to the tumor tissue but also to edema surrounding it and to brain tissue that may still be functionally competent. In other words, in such cases it may be impossible to decide that the brain parenchyma is destroyed or that the area is functionally inoperative, or, for that matter, that an area without apparent abnormality is free of tumor. For these reasons, we do not believe that patients with glial tumors are a first choice for the lesion method. This point is made clear in a study by Anderson and coworkers,[16] who compared the neuropsychological profile of patients with confirmed gliomas to that of patients with strokes in the same regions.

Where subjects with glial tumors pose problems for the lesion method, those in whom *meningiomas* have been excised and who have had a circumscribed ablation of brain tissue are actually ideal cases. The images from such cases are entirely appropriate to establish a link between the anatomic site of the ablation and the neuropsychological profile obtained *after* the ablation has taken place.

Patients who have had ablations for seizure treatment also afford a good opportunity for behavioral and anatomic studies. In those cases, MRI obtained with T_1-weighted images can help delineate the extent of brain tissue removal with extraordinary precision, although some caution is recommended in the interpretation of neuropsychological data obtained in such patients. Some patients who undergo surgical removal of brain tissue for the treatment of uncontrollable seizures may have developmental brain defects. Those whose seizures began early in life are likely to have had some degree of compensatory brain reor-

ganization before surgery. Frequent and long-standing seizural discharges may also produce changes elsewhere in the brain. The participation of such patients in lesion studies must be evaluated on an individual basis.

The inclusion in lesion method studies of subjects with *metastatic disease, intracerebral hemorrhages,* or *severe head injury* must also be decided on an individual basis, lest it contaminate otherwise valid results. For instance, data from patients with a single brain metastasis, removed surgically, and studied in the stable, postoperative state, concomitantly with a good-quality CT or MRI, are quite acceptable.

Intracerebral hemorrhages affect the brain by two different mechanisms. They destroy neural tissue, as nonhemorrhagic infarctions do, and they cause a space-occupying blood collection that displaces neurons, as tumors do. During the acute phase of a hemorrhage, neither CT nor MRI provides an accurate picture of the abnormality, because within the area of abnormal signal some neurons are truly destroyed, whereas others are simply displaced. The amount and location of tissue destruction can be estimated only after the resolution of the hematoma.

In conclusion, the specimen of choice for the purpose of establishing correlates between dysfunction and site of brain destruction are cases of nonhemorrhagic infarction and herpes encephalitis. Surgical ablations performed for the treatment of meningiomas also provide excellent material. Other material should be used on an individual basis, after careful assessment of the dynamics of lesion development.

Timing of Imaging

The timing of CT and MRI data collection is of the essence, especially in relation to subjects with stroke. Both CT and MRI may fail to show *any* abnormality when they are obtained immediately after the occurrence of a stroke. With modern-generation CT and MRI scanners, most images will be positive after 24 h. This is certainly not the case with older scanners, however. It is important to keep in mind that many CT (or even MRI) studies obtained less than 24 h after the onset of a stroke may be negative, especially when a patient with an acute stroke happens to have a CT or MRI that shows a well-demarcated area of low density with sharp margins. Such an image, early after stroke, should suggest a previous infarct, probably unrelated to the new set of symptoms.

Positive CT images obtained in the first week post onset usually show areas of abnormality that are far larger than the region of actual structural damage because of confounding phenomena—for example, edema. This commonly occurs and means that the results of observations and experiments conducted at later epochs should not be correlated with the anatomic analysis performed in the acute images.

When CT is obtained in the second or third week after a stroke's onset without intravenous infusion of a contrast-enhancing substance, the images are negative in a good number of cases. The image can change even after a previous CT obtained earlier showed a large area of decreased density. During this period, the damaged area can show the same density as the normal tissue. On the other hand, in contrast-enhanced CT images, those normal-looking areas will appear as areas of increased density (primarily due to seepage of contrast substance through the walls of newly formed vessels in the affected region). In the chronic stage, which we define as 3 months post onset and beyond, most CT studies of infarction are unequivocally positive. Even then, however, when strokes are small and located close to a major sulcus or to the wall of a ventricle, the chronic CT may mislead the observer, resembling images of focal "atrophy" with sulcal enlargement or images of ventricular dilatation. When no previous images are available for comparison with those obtained in the chronic stage, the correct interpretation and the establishment of an adequate behavioral/anatomic correlation may not be possible.

Similar problems befall MRI with images obtained with only one pulse sequence. T_1-weighted images obtained with an inversion recovery (IR) pulse sequence provide maximal anatomic detail. With this pulse sequence, however, infarctions appear as dark areas, in precisely the same range of grays used to depict the ventricular system or any region filled with cerebrospinal fluid, such as the cerebral sulci and fissures. When infarcts are small and close to one of these structures, they may not be readily distinguishable. Images obtained with different pulse sequences on MRI (proton density or T_2-weighted) show the damaged area as a region of intense bright signal, more easily distinguishable from the bright signals generated by white and even gray matter.

A meaningful relation between an anatomic image and a particular neuropsychological pattern require reasonable temporal closeness between the epochs at which the image and the neuropsychological data were obtained. Because, during the acute period, edema and brain distortion often occur, it is not easy to define precisely the location and amount of destroyed tissue. The pairing of such images with observations made in the chronic state may lead to error. Likewise for the inverse situation—that is, pairing the results of acute neuropsychological observations obtained in the acute state with the anatomy gleaned during the chronic stage. The most reliable anatomic and neuropsychological data are obviously those obtained in the chronic stage.

Other Considerations

A traditional limitation of the lesion method in humans has been the excessive reliance on single cases. Many of the important observations made in the past were uncontrolled and went unreplicated, the significance of the results being thus diminished. Notable exceptions—for instance, Milner's collection of epileptic patients with surgical ablations in temporal and frontal lobe, Newcombe's head injury project, or Gazzaniga's group of epileptics with split brain interventions—simply confirm the rule. In our laboratory, we have obviated this limitation by creating a continuously renewed population of patients with lesions in varied neural systems who would be willing to participate in neuropsychological experiments. The goal was to conduct multiple single-subject studies in target patients and in controls with an approach as rigorous as the one used in the traditional experimental setting and to make it possible to design and carry out experiments in which certain hypotheses regarding anatomy and function could be probed comprehensively, using many individual data sets.

It goes without saying that, given optimal neuroanatomic analysis, the lesion method will be only as successful as the quality of the cognitive tasks used in the experiments and the quality of the theoretical framework and hypotheses being tested. The rapidly evolving fields of cognitive science and experimental neuropsychology have provided investigators with many useful tasks applicable to most aspects of cognition and behavior likely to be studied with the lesion method. There are also many relevant theoretical developments concerning the conceptualization of both the cognitive and neural architectures in humans. The traditional divisions between behaviorist and cognitivist views seem to have been largely overcome by theoretical positions that combine the best of both (see, for examples, Refs. 17 to 19). The conceptualization of neural structures and of their operations, insofar as mental processes and behaviors are concerned, has also changed radically, as indicated at the beginning of this chapter. Neural signaling is seen as both massively parallel and massively sequential, and, no less importantly, massively recurrent. The prevalence of feedforward and feedback loops disposed along as well as across neural streams has been duly noted, and so has the convergent/divergent nature of those neuron streams. The dependence on timing mechanisms for the normal operations of these networks is well accepted.[20-24]

REFERENCES

1. Ungerleider LG, Mishkin M: Two cortical visual systems, in Ingle DJ, Mansfield RJW, Goodale MA (eds): *The Analysis of Visual Behavior.* Cambridge, MA: MIT Press, 1982.
2. Newcombe F, Russell WR: Dissociate visual, perceptual and spatial deficits in focal lesions of the right hemisphere. *J Neurol Neurosurg Psychiatry* 332:73–81, 1969.
3. Damasio A, Tranel D, Damasio H: Face agnosia and the neural substrates of memory. *Annu Rev Neurosci* 13:89–109, 1990.
4. Damasio AR, Damasio H, Tranel D, Brandt JP: Neural regionalization of knowledge access: Preliminary evidence. *Symposia on Quantitative Biology* 55:1039–1047, 1990.
5. Tranel D, Damasio H, Damasio AR, Brandt JP: Separate concepts are retrieved from separate neural systems: Neuroanatomical and neuropsychological double dissociations (abstr). *Soc Neurosci* 21:1497, 1995.
6. Damasio H, Damasio A: *Lesion Analysis in Neuropsychology.* New York, Oxford University Press, 1989; Japanese edition, Tokyo: Igaku-Shoin, 1992.
7. Damasio H: *Human Brain Anatomy in Computerized Images.* New York: Oxford University Press, 1995.
8. Chase TN, Foster NL, Fedio P, et al: Regional cortical dysfunction in Alzheimer's disease as determined by positron emission tomography. *Ann Neurol* 15(suppl):S170–S174, 1984.
9. Foster NL, Chase TN, Mansi L, et al: Cortical abnormalities in Alzheimer's disease. *Ann Neurol* 16:649–654, 1984.
10. Friedland RP, Budinger TF, Ganz E, et al: Regional cerebral metabolic alterations in dementia of the Alzheimer type: Positron emission tomography with (18F) Fluorodeaxyglucose. *J Comp Assist Tomogr* 7:590–598, 1983.
11. Rezai K, Damasio H, Graff-Radford N, et al: Regional cerebral blood flow abnormalities in Alzheimer's disease. *J Nucl Med* 26(5):105, 1985.
12. Hyman BT, Damasio AR, Van Hoesen GW, Barnes CL: Cell specific pathology isolates the hippocampal formation in Alzheimer's disease. *Science* 225:1168–1170, 1984.
13. Van Hoesen, Damasio A: Neural correlates of the cognitive impairment in Alzheimer's disease, in Plum F (ed): *The Handbook of Physiology.* Bethesda, MD: American Physiological Society, 1987, pp 871–898.
14. Escourelle R, Poirier J: *Manual of Basic Neuropathology.* Philadelphia: Saunders, 1978.
15. Graff-Radford NR, Damasio AR, Hyman BT, et al: Progressive aphasia in a patient with Pick's disease: A neuropsychological, radiologic and anatomic study. *Neurology* 40:620–626, 1990.
16. Anderson SW, Damasio H, Tranel D: The use of tumor and stroke patients in neuropsychological re-

search: A methodological critique. *J Clin Exp Neuropsychol* 10:32, 1988.

17. Kosslyn SM: *Image and Brain: The Resolution of the Imagery Debate.* Cambridge, MA: Bradford Books/ MIT Press, 1994.

18. Damasio AR: *Descartes' Error: Emotion, Reason and the Human Brain.* New York: Grosset/Putnam, 1994.

19. Churchland PS, Sejnowski JF: *The Computational Brain: Models and Methods on the Frontiers of Computational Neuroscience.* Cambridge, MA: Bradford Books/MIT Press, 1992.

20. Damasio AR: The brain binds entities and events by multiregional activation from convergence zones. *Neural Comput* 1:123–132, 1989.

21. Damasio AR, Damasio H: Cortical systems for retrieval of concrete knowledge: The convergence zone framework, in Koch C (ed): *Large-Scale Neuronal Theories of the Brain.* Cambridge, MA: MIT Press, 1994, pp 61–74.

22. Crick F: *The Astonishing Hypothesis: The Scientific Search for the Soul.* New York: Scribner's, 1994.

23. Edelman G: *Neural Darwinism.* New York: Basic Books, 1987.

24. Rockland KS (ed): Special issue: Local cortical circuits. *Cerebral Cortex* 3:361–498, 1993.

Chapter 6

FUNCTIONAL IMAGING IN BEHAVIORAL NEUROLOGY AND NEUROPSYCHOLOGY

Marcus E. Raichle

Early discussions of the "mind-brain problem" treated the brain largely as a "black box." Then, in 1861, French surgeon and anthropologist Pierre Paul Broca described a clear relationship between a patient's difficulty speaking and an injury to a specific part of the patient's brain due to a stroke. Since this seminal observation, a vast body of scientific literature has accumulated implicating various parts of the human brain in specific aspects of human behavior, including language. The remarkable level of sophistication to which this work has risen is detailed in the preceding chapter by Drs. Antonio and Hanna Damasio.

The features of brain organization arising from the study of patients with brain injury nevertheless raise some questions of interpretation. The size and location of brain injury varies greatly from patient to patient, making a precise correlation between damage to a particular area of the brain and the function normally served by that area sometimes difficult to determine. Furthermore, each patient may be assumed to have some features of brain organization that are unique to him or her. Finally, it remains uncertain whether one can simply attribute a lost or disrupted function to a particular area of injury. Because of the interconnected nature of areas of the brain, injury in one area is likely to have effects on other areas that cannot necessarily be predicted from the location and size of the injury itself. Thus, as valuable as our insights concerning the organization of the human brain have been, from the study of patients with stroke and other types of brain injury, it has

remained an open question exactly how this information relates to the normal organization of the human brain.

Only recently have scientists interested in this question had the opportunity to explore it analytically—to peer inside the black box as it functions normally. This ability stems from the developments in imaging technology over the past 20 years, most notably positron emission tomography (PET) and magnetic resonance imaging (MRI). These techniques can now capture precisely localized physiologic changes in the normal human brain associated with behaviorally induced changes in neuronal activity.[1,2]

It is important to point out that the underlying assumptions of current brain-mapping studies with PET and functional MRI (fMRI) are not a modern version of phrenology. The phrenologists of the past century posited that single areas of the brain, often identified by bumps on the skull, uniquely represented specific thought processes and emotions. In contrast, modern thinking posits that single areas of the brain each contribute quite simple mental operations that form the elementary components of the observable behaviors. Observable behaviors and thought processes emerge through the cooperative interactions of many such areas. So, just as diverse instruments of a large orchestra are played in a coordinated fashion to produce a symphony, a group of diverse brain areas, each performing quite elementary and unique mental operations, work together in a coordinated fashion to produce human behavior. The prerequisite for such analyses is the conviction that complex behaviors can be broken down into sets of constituent mental operations.

HISTORY OF FUNCTIONAL BRAIN IMAGING

The modern era of medical imaging began in the early 1970s, when the world was introduced to a remarkable technique called x-ray computed tomography, now known as x-ray CT or just CT. South African physicist Allan M. Cormack and British engineer Sir Godfrey Hounsfield independently developed its principles. Hounsfield constructed the first CT instrument in England. Both investigators received the Nobel prize in 1979 for their contributions.

Computed tomography takes advantage of the fact that different tissues absorb varying amounts of x-ray energy. The denser the tissue, the more it absorbs. A highly focused beam of x-rays traversing the body will exit at a reduced energy level depending on the tissues and organs through which it passes. A beam of x-rays passed through the body at many different angles through a plane collects sufficient information to reconstruct a picture of that body section. It was crucial to the development of CT that clever computing and mathematical techniques emerged for processing the vast amount of information necessary to create the images themselves. Without the availability of sophisticated computers, the task would have been impossible to accomplish.

Computed tomography had two consequences. First, it changed the practice of medicine forever, because it was much superior to standard x-rays. For the first time, physicians could safely and effectively view living human tissue such as the brain with no discomfort or risk to the patient. Standard x-rays revealed only bone and some surrounding soft tissue. Second, CT immediately stimulated scientists and engineers to consider alternative ways of creating images of the body's interior using similar mathematical and computer strategies for image construction. These efforts went beyond the picture of human anatomy provided by CT to focus on function.

One of the first groups to be intrigued by the possibilities opened by CT consisted of experts in tissue autoradiography, a method used for many years in animal studies to investigate organ metabolism, biochemistry, and blood flow. In tissue autoradiography, a radioactively labeled compound is injected into a vein. After the compound has accumulated in the organ under investigation, the animal is sacrificed and the organ (e.g., the brain) removed for study. The organ is then carefully sectioned, and the individual slices are laid on a piece of film sensitive to radioactivity. Much as the film in a camera records a scene as it was originally viewed, this x-ray film records the distribution of radioactively labeled compound in each slice of tissue.

When the x-ray film is developed, scientists have a picture of the distribution of radioactivity within the organ and hence can deduce the organ's specific functions. The type of information is determined by the radioactive compound injected. A radioactively labeled form of glucose, for example, measures brain metabolism, because glucose is the primary source of energy for the cells of the brain. Central to functional brain imaging with PET is the measurement of brain blood flow, which is accomplished by the injection of radioactively labeled water.

Investigators adept at tissue autoradiography were fascinated when CT was introduced. They suddenly realized that if they could reconstruct the anatomy of an organ by passing an x-ray beam through it, as CT did, they could also safely reconstruct the distribution of a previously administered radioisotope. One had simply to measure the emission of radioactivity from the body section. This realization was the birth of autoradiography of living human subjects.

One crucial element in the evolution of human autoradiography was the choice of radioisotope. Workers in the field selected a class of radioisotopes that emit positrons, which resemble electrons except that they carry a positive charge. A positron produced within the tissue almost immediately combines with a nearby electron. The positron and electron annihilate one another in this interaction, emitting two high-energy gamma rays in the process. Since the gamma rays travel in nearly opposite directions, radiation detection devices arrayed in a circle around the organ of interest can detect the pairs of gamma rays and, with the aid of computers, locate their origin with remarkable precision. The crucial role of positrons in human autoradiography gave rise to the name positron emission tomography (PET).

More recently, another imaging technique has emerged and taken its place alongside PET in revealing the function of the human brain. This technique, MRI, derives from the potent laboratory technique known as nuclear magnetic resonance (NMR), which was designed to explore detailed chemical features of molecules. It garnered a Nobel prize for its developers, Felix Bloch of Stanford University and Edward Purcell of Harvard University, in 1972. The method depends on the fact that many atoms behave as little compass needles in the presence of a magnetic field. By skillfully manipulating the magnetic field, scientists can align the atoms. Applying radio-wave pulses to the sample under these conditions briefly perturbs the atoms from their aligned state in a precise manner. As a result, they emit detectable radio signals unique to the number and state of the particular atoms in the sample. Careful adjustments of the magnetic field and the radio-wave pulses yield particular information about the sample under study.

Nuclear magnetic resonance moved from the laboratory to the clinic when Paul C. Lauterbur of the University of Illinois found that NMR can form images by detecting protons. Protons are useful because they are abundant in the human body, being found primarily in water and fat. Using mathematical techniques again borrowed initially from x-ray CT but later modified extensively, images of the anatomy of organs of the living human body were produced that far surpassed in detail those produced by CT. Because the term *nuclear* made the procedure sound dangerous to some, NMR soon became known as magnetic resonance imaging. The current excitement over both PET and functional MRI (fMRI) for the imaging of normal brain function stems from the ability of these techniques to detect signals related to

changes in neuronal activity through changes in local brain blood flow. Below, we turn briefly to the nature of these changes in blood flow and their relationship to changes in neuronal activity.

MEASURING BRAIN FUNCTION WITH IMAGING

Measurements of blood flow to local areas of the brain are at the heart of assessing brain function with either PET or fMRI.[2] The idea that blood flow is intimately related to brain function is a surprisingly old one. English physiologists Charles S. Roy and Charles S. Sherrington formally presented the idea in a publication in 1890 (for a detailed review of this history, see Refs. 2 and 3). They suggested that an "automatic mechanism" regulated the blood supply to the brain. The amount of blood depended on local variations in activity. Although subsequent experiments have amply confirmed the existence of such an automatic mechanism, no one is yet entirely certain about its exact nature. It obviously remains a challenging area for research.

Positron emission tomography measures blood flow in the human brain by adapting an autoradiographic technique for laboratory animals developed in the late 1940s by Seymour S. Kety of the National Institute of Mental Health and his colleagues (for a detailed review, see Ref. 3). Positron emission tomography relies on radioactively labeled water, specifically hydrogen combined with oxygen-15, a radioactive isotope of oxygen. The labeled water, which emits copious numbers of positrons as it decays, is administered into a vein in the arm. In less than a minute thereafter, the radioactivity accumulates in the brain, forming an image of blood flow.

Functional MRI measures a complex function of blood flow related to the fact that when blood flow increases during normal brain function, the amount of oxygen consumed by the brain does not.[3a] Under these circumstances, more oxygen is present locally in the tissue because the blood flow (i.e., supply) has increased but the demand for oxygen has not. Since the amount of oxygen in the tissue affects its magnetic properties, a fact first noted in 1935 by Linus Pauling,[4] fMRI can detect a change, which is often referred to as the "BOLD" or blood oxygen level–dependent effect.[5-7] An actual measurement of blood flow equivalent to that measured by PET with oxygen-15–labeled water has proven difficult with fMRI primarily because of the short "half-life" (i.e., the T_1 relaxation time) of the water protons in the fMRI experiment (i.e., the T_1 relaxation time of the water proton in brain tissue is approximately 1 s, whereas the half-life of oxygen-15–labeled water is 123 s, which is ideal for the measurement of blood flow in the human brain).

IMAGING STRATEGY

A distinct strategy for the functional mapping of neuronal activity has emerged during the past 15 years. Initially developed for PET, it has been extended, with modifications which will be discussed a bit further on, to fMRI.

This approach extends an idea first introduced to psychology in 1868 by Dutch physiologist Franciscus C. Donders. Donders proposed a general method to measure thought processes based on a simple logic. He subtracted the time needed to respond to a light (say, by pressing a key) from the time needed to respond to a particular color of light. He found that discriminating color required about 50 ms. In this way, Donders isolated and measured a mental process for the first time by subtracting a *control state* (i.e., responding to light) from a *task state* of interest (i.e., discriminating the color of the light).

The current functional imaging strategy is designed to accomplish a similar subtraction, but adding information about the areas of the brain that distinguish the task state from the control state. In particular, images of blood flow, or blood flow–related changes in the case of fMRI (i.e., the BOLD signal; see above), taken in a control state are subtracted from those obtained when the brain is engaged in the task. Scientists carefully choose the control state and the task state so as to isolate

as well as possible a limited number of mental operations when subtracting the two states. Subtracting blood flow–dependent measurements made in the control state from those made in the task state should isolate those parts of the brain uniquely responsible for the performance of the task.

To obtain reliable data, scientists take the average of responses across many individual subjects (usually the case with PET) or of many experimental trials in the same person (usually the case with fMRI). Averaging enables researchers to detect changes in blood flow associated with mental activity that would otherwise easily be confused with spurious shifts resulting from statistical noise in the resulting images. The averaging of results across individuals has another important feature in that it gives us the opportunity to learn what features of brain organization we share. Knowledge of such common principles of brain organization is an essential basis for an understanding of the unique and universal capacity of humans for language, for example. The image subtraction and averaging strategy used for PET is illustrated in Fig. 6-1. A typical imaging paradigm used for fMRI is illustrated in Fig. 6-2.

The remainder of this review focuses on studies of language, largely from the author's own laboratory, for several reasons: (1) the work nicely illustrates the implementation of the strategies described above; (2) the work reflects substantial input from both cognitive scientists and neuroscientists; (3) results are promising in relation to cognitive theories of brain function, and (4) important lessons have been learned about how best to conduct functional imaging research and what conclusions to draw from the results of these studies. The following discussion is not intended as a review of functional imaging studies of language but, rather, as a review of functional brain imaging strategies as employed in laboratories throughout the world, using our studies of language for illustrative purposes only. For those interested in a more in-depth review of human cognition and functional brain imaging, a recently published book is recommended.[2]

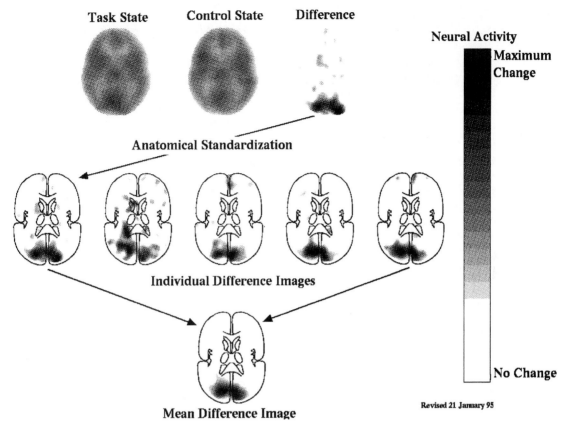

Figure 6-1

Image subtraction and image averaging are crucial steps in the development of PET images of brain function. In the top row are two PET blood-flow images in a normal human subject, one labeled Task State *and the other labeled* Control State. *These images represent horizontal slices throughout the center of the brain. In each image, the front of the brain is on top and the left side is to the reader's left. Areas that are darker have higher blood flow than those that are lighter. During the task state, the subject passively viewed a flashing annular checkerboard (i.e., a potent visual stimulus) while holding visual fixation on a small dot in the middle of the screen. During the control state, the subject simply maintained fixation. The difference in blood flow between the two states is shown in the difference image on the right. Once such a difference image is obtained, computer techniques are used to fit it to a standard brain so that comparisons can be made with other individuals (second row of difference images). From these individual difference images an averaged or mean difference image (bottom image) is made. Because the changes in blood flow are small, individual difference images tend to be somewhat variable due to the presence of statistical noise in the images and individual differences among the subjects. Therefore, averaging is necessary in order to determine the presence of significant changes that reflect changes common to a sample of all individuals. In such a process, noise is suppressed whereas consistent signals are enhanced. All of the remaining images in this chapter (with the exception of the fMRI images in Fig. 6-2) are mean difference images formed in the above manner.*

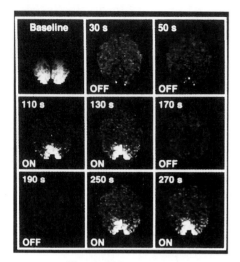
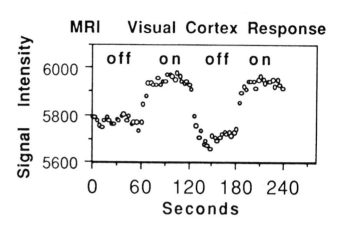

Figure 6-2

Data obtained by fMRI during visual stimulation in a single normal subject. The baseline image was acquired during darkness (upper left) *and was subtracted from the subsequent images obtained during darkness* (labeled OFF) *and during visual stimulation* (labeled ON). *A total of 80 images was obtained at the rate of one every 3.5 s. These images are oriented so that the front of the brain is on top and the visual cortices are on the bottom. Note the increase in signal intensity during visual stimulation. The graph on the right plots this signal intensity as a function of time and the presence or absence of a visual stimulus. (From Kwong et al.,[7] with permission.)*

STUDY OF LANGUAGE: AN EXAMPLE

The manner in which language skills are acquired and organized in the human brain has been the subject of intense investigation for more than a century. As recounted in Chap. 1, the Paris debate of 1861 spurred a number of investigators to examine the effects of focal brain lesions on the ability to speak, and, later, the ability to comprehend language. From these beginnings has emerged a concept of language organization in the human brain which, in broad outline, posits the following: information flows from visual and auditory reception areas to areas at the junction between the left temporal and parietal lobes for comprehension and then on to frontal areas for verbal response selection and speech production. As pointed out above, almost all of this information was gleaned from patients with brain damage. Could this organization represent the actual organization in the normal brain?

In the mid-1980s, the author and his colleagues Steven E. Petersen, Michael I. Posner, Peter T. Fox, and Mark A. Mintun began a series of experiments[8–11] designed to answer this question. We elected to begin our work with an analysis of the manner in which the normal human brain processes single words from perception to speaking. We designed our initial experiments in an hierarchical manner in which several levels of information processing of increasing complexity were employed. This design is in keeping with the experimental model discussed above. In these experiments, words were presented to the subjects either on a television monitor or through earphones. The presentation to follow focuses on those aspects of the study involving the *visual presentation* of words.

Opening the Eyes

Regardless of the task to be performed by our subjects, they were always asked to fix their gaze on a small fixation point in the middle of a television monitor. This was done to prevent the unwanted activation of brain areas concerned with saccadic eye movements from complicating our analysis. When one compares this simple act of opening one's eyes and fixing on a small dot in the middle of a television monitor with lying quietly with one's eyes closed (Fig. 6-3, top row), it is readily apparent that there is a significant increase in brain activity in the back of the brain in those areas known to respond to visual stimuli. It is important to realize that subsequent changes build upon this already present activity produced simply by opening the eyes and fixing the gaze.

Words as Passive Visual Stimuli

Putting common English nouns on the television monitor at the rate of one per second while subjects continued to fix their gaze on the fixation point produced a marked increase in the extent and complexity of brain activity in the visual areas of the brain, as shown in Fig. 6-3 (second row). The subjects were not instructed to process the words in any way, simply to fix their gaze on the fixation point. These results suggested that words had special properties as visual stimuli that had powerful effects on the visual system of the human brain. The question was what those properties might be. Clearly, further analysis of words as visual stimuli was needed.

In studying words as visual stimuli, we considered at least four properties as important contributors to the response we observed. First, words must be viewed as complex collections of *visual features*. They consist of varying numbers of units made up of connected lines with varying spatial orientations. Second these units of connected lines are not a random arrangement of lines but come from a unique set of 26 units representing the *letters* of the English alphabet. Third, the letters in words are not randomly distributed but are arranged in combinations of vowels and consonants according to the *rules* of the English language. These rules reflect the ways in which English letters can be put together to make words (orthography) and, to some extent, the ways in which the

letters are pronounced. Finally, words convey *meaning*.

It is reasonable to suppose that the responses we observed in the human visual system to the passive presentation of words represented a combination of responses to any or all of these features of words. We wished to begin the process of connecting, in the best possible way, active areas to specific features of words. To dissect the overall responses into their component parts, we needed to determine the component operations involved in reading a word. We believed at the outset that these operations related to visual features, letters and letter combinations, but not to the word meaning, which we did not expect to be processed in the visual system of the brain.

We devised four different visual stimuli,[10] shown in Table 6-1, that systematically varied the different features of the words. We then observed the effects of these different stimuli on the visual system of the brain as recorded by a PET scan. The four stimuli consisted of false fonts, consonant letter strings, pseudowords, and words; each represented one of the four suggested features of interest to us. The computer-generated false fonts incorporated all of the visual features of words but none of the other features. Consonant letter strings added the letter code but obviously could not be pronounced according to English rules of pronunciation. Pseudowords contained both consonants and vowels and could be pronounced because they had been arranged according to English rules of pronunciation. For most individuals, pseudowords do not convey meaning (an occasional individual will recognize a Hungarian word or the name of a neighbor inadvertently included among the pseudowords). Finally, words contain all of the aforementioned features plus meaning.

A group of normal individuals was instructed to observe the stimuli passively. By scanning the subjects as they were shown false fonts, consonant letter strings, pseudowords, or words, it was possible to distinguish among responses to the visual features, letters, orthographic regularity, and meaning. If the activation to words was attributable to the visual features of the stimulus and nothing else, then all stimuli should produce the

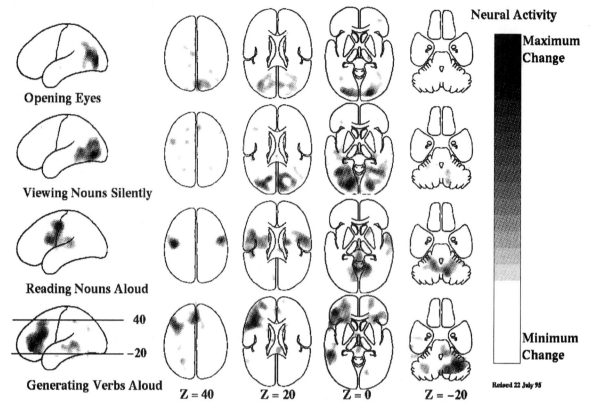

Neural Activity

Maximum Change

Minimum Change

Opening Eyes

Viewing Nouns Silently

Reading Nouns Aloud

40

−20

Generating Verbs Aloud

Z = 40   Z = 20   Z = 0   Z = −20

Revised 22 July 95

Figure 6-3

Four different task states are represented in these mean difference PET images from a group of normal subjects performing a hierarchically designed series of language tasks. Each row represents the mean difference between images of the designated task state and those of a control state. The images on the left represent projections of the changes as seen on the lateral surface of the brain with the front of the brain to the reader's left. The horizontal lines through the bottom left image denote the orientation of the horizontal slices throughout the same data as seen to the right of this first image. These horizontal images are oriented with the front of the brain on top and the left side to the reader's left. The markings Z = 40 and so on indicate millimeters above or below a horizontal plane through the brain at Z = 0. The row labeled Opening Eyes *indicates those areas of the brain with increased activity when subjects maintained fixation on a small dot of light in the middle of an otherwise blank television monitor, as compared with lying quietly with eyes closed. The row labeled* Viewing Nouns Silently *indicates those areas of the brain with increased activity when subjects passively viewed common English nouns as they appeared on the television monitor as compared to simply maintaining fixation on a small dot of light (row 1). The row labeled* Reading Nouns Aloud *indicates those areas of the brain with increased activity when subjects read aloud the nouns as they appeared on the screen. The control state was passively viewing the same nouns (row 2). Finally, the row labeled* Generating Verbs Aloud *indicates those areas of the brain with increased activity when subjects said aloud an appropriate verb for each noun as it appeared on the television monitor. The control state was reading the nouns aloud (row 3). Taken together, these difference images, arranged in a hierarchical fashion, are designed to demonstrate the spatially distributed nature of the processing going on in the normal human brain during a simple language task. By designing and presenting the experiment in this way, it is possible to take the first steps toward an understanding of the neural circuitry underlying various aspects of human language and the particular role played by individual areas within these circuits.*

COLOR PLATES

1 *Three-dimensional recon-struction (obtained from 124 contiguous thin coronal MRI slices) of the brain of a subject with an infarct in the left frontal lobe. Acutely, the subject had a nonfluent aphasia and mild paresis of the right face and arm. At the time of the MRI (1 year later), both language deficit and paresis had improved.*

Several sulci were identified and color-coded on the 3D reconstructed brain: central sulcus (red), precentral sulcus (green), inferior frontal sulcus (yellow), superior frontal sulcus (brown), and sylvian fissure (magenta).

Inspection of the left lateral and top views of the brain shows that the area of infarct is centered on the precentral sulcus, which is clearly visible only in the top view. The most anterior sector of the precen-tral gyrus is damaged, as well as the posterior sector of the middle frontal and inferior frontal gyrus.

The brain volume was also resectioned in axial (ax), coro-nal (co), and parasagittal (ps) slices (as shown in the three rows of brain slices in the lower segment of the image). Whenever any of the slices intersected a color-coded sulcus, the color automatically appeared on the slice, thus permitting an accurate identifi-cation of sulci and of gyri. Resectioning allowed us to inspect the lesion in depth and show that it extended all the way to the insula, which is compromised in its most superior sector (best seen in slice ps-3).

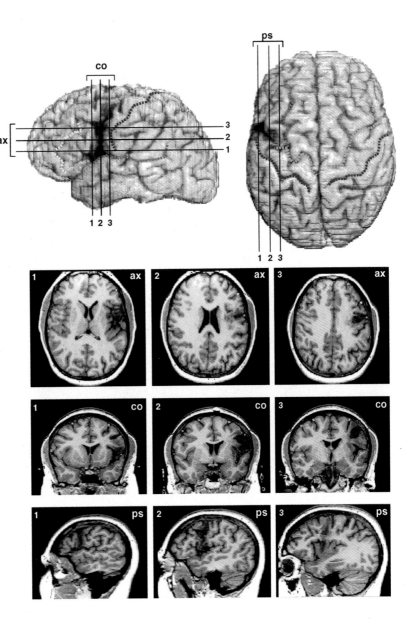

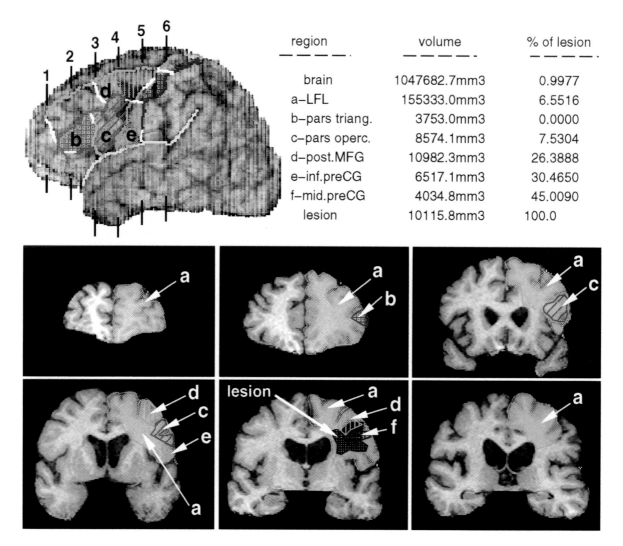

region	volume	% of lesion
brain	1047682.7mm3	0.9977
a–LFL	155333.0mm3	6.5516
b–pars triang.	3753.0mm3	0.0000
c–pars operc.	8574.1mm3	7.5304
d–post.MFG	10982.3mm3	26.3888
e–inf.preCG	6517.1mm3	30.4650
f–mid.preCG	4034.8mm3	45.0090
lesion	10115.8mm3	100.0

2 *Three-dimensional reconstruction of a human brain with a lesion in the left frontal lobe. The questions addressed here concerned the size of the lesion and the percentage of volume it occupied in the whole brain, in the left frontal lobe (LFL), and in some subdivisions of the frontal lobe: the pars triangularis (pars triang.) and the pars opercularis (pars operc.), the posterior half of the middle frontal gyrus (post. MFG), and the precentral gyrus in its inferior (int. preCG) and middle thirds (mid. preCG). The limits of all of these regions of interest (ROI) were marked on the 3D reconstructed brain. On all coronal slices, the several ROIs are individually traced, as is the contour of the lesion. Six coronal slices are shown as an example. The different ROIs are color- and texture-coded. The automatically calculated absolute volumes and the percentage of damage in each of them are recorded on the top right-hand corner.*

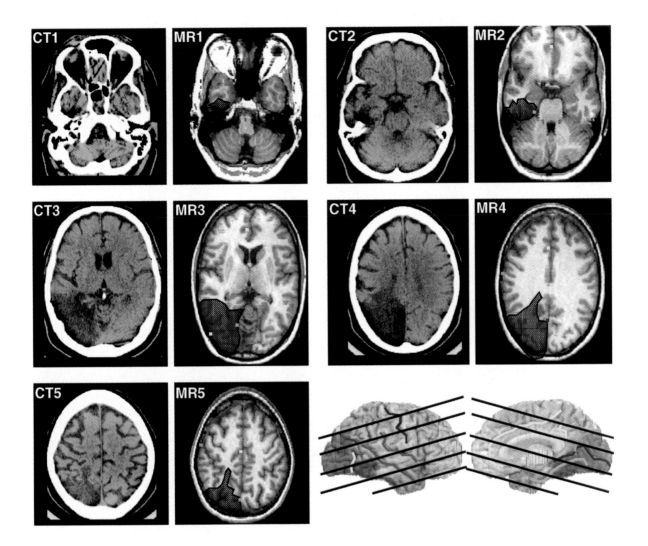

3 *Demonstration of the improved template method. Brain CT (CT 1-5) of a subject who could not undergo an MRI study. A normal 3D reconstructed brain was resliced so as to match the orientation and level of the CT slices (MR 1-5). The lesion seen on the CT slices was transferred onto each matched MR slice, taking into account all identifiable sulci and gyri. Once the sulci were color-coded on the 3D reconstruction, the lesion could be read off each individual slice. The object defined by the transferred traces could be fused with the normal brain to visualize the lesion's surface extent* (right lower corner).

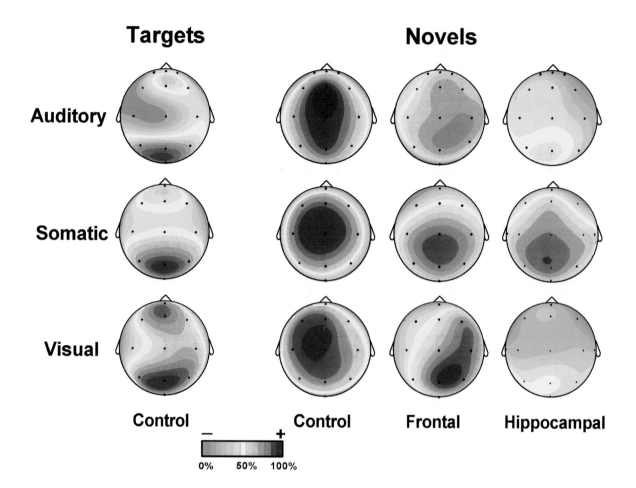

Targets **Novels**

Auditory

Somatic

Visual

Control   Control   Frontal   Hippocampal

−   +

0%   50%   100%

4 *This figure shows the scalp voltage topographies for target and novel stimuli in controls. Note the marked increase in prefrontal activity to the novel stimuli in all sensory modalities. The effects of prefrontal or hippocampal lesions on the brain novelty response are shown on the right. Unilateral prefrontal damage results in multimodal decrease in the novelty response. Unilateral hippocampal damage results in severe bilateral reductions in the novelty response, maximal at prefrontal sites. These findings implicate a prefrontal-hippocampal network in the detection of perturbations in the environment (see text for details).*

5 *Three-dimensional reconstruction (using Brainvox[20]) of a T$_1$-weighted magnetic resonance imaging in a typical patient with hemiachromatopsia, pure alexia, and category-specific visual object agnosia (animals impaired; tools/utensils normal). The lesion is centered in the left occipitotemporal region and involves parts of the lingual and fusiform gyri.*

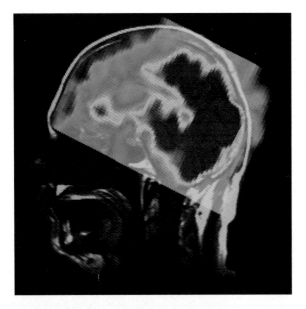

6 This is a xenon-133–corrected-HMPAO SPECT coregistered upon a T_2-weighted MRI scan from a patient with frontotemporal dementia. There is profound frontal hypoperfusion.

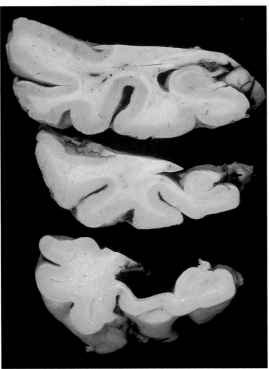

7 Atrophy of the hippocampus: The upper section comes from a control without neurologic symptoms. The hippocampus has a normal volume. The two other sections come from patients with Alzheimer disease at various stages. Maximal atrophy is seen in the lowest section.

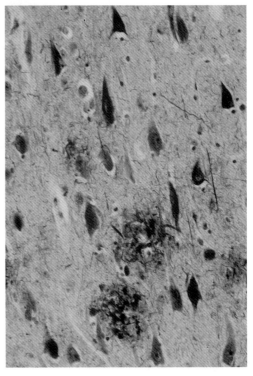

8 The two main lesions of Alzheimer disease: (1) neurofibrillary tangles are located in the neuronal cell body and appear in black; (2) senile plaques are seen as spheres made of entangled neurites. Bielschowsky silver impregnation counterstained by cresyl violet. Staining performed by Dr. Joachim Kauss. Initial magnification: x750.

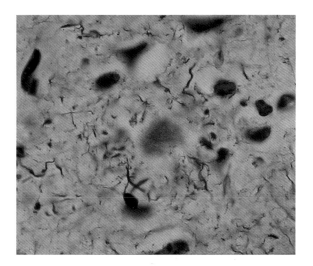

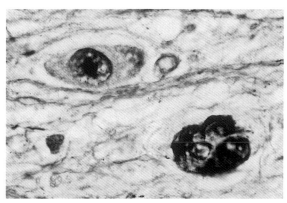

9 *Senile plaques. The plaque in the center of the picture is a composite lesion. Its center, stained gray, consists of amorphous extracellular material mainly composed of Aß peptide. Other stains, such as Congo red, would show its "amyloid" nature. Around the amyloid center, a crown of degenerating neurites is clearly seen. The nuclei that are in contact with the plaque belong, for the most part, to microglial cells. Initial magnification: x1200.*

10 *Neurofibrillary tangles. This high-power view of the nucleus basalis of Meynert shows two neurons; the cytoplasm of the normal neuron appears light brown. The second neuron contains a neurofibrillary tangle consisting of deep black fibrils surrounding and partly overlapping the nucleus. Bodian silver impregnation. Initial magnification: x2500.*

Plates 11 and 12 are located on the following page.

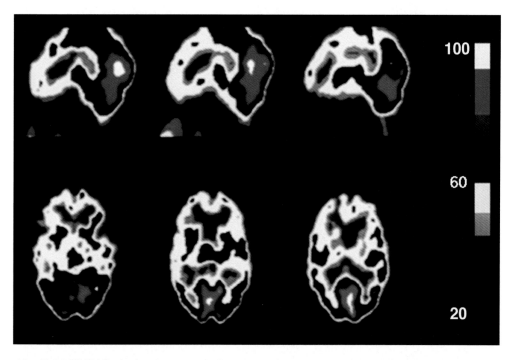

13 *Tc99-HMPAO single-photon emission tomography scans (gray scale) of a patient with Pick disease, demonstrating frontal and anterior temporal hypometabolism (lighter anterior regions).*

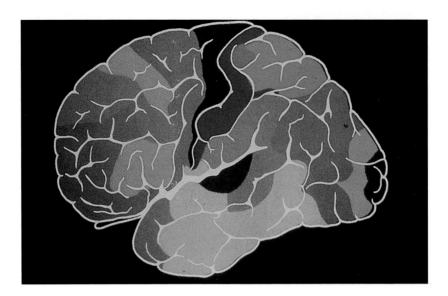

11 *Comparison of the distribution of neurofibrillary tangles (NFT) with the functional organization of the cortical areas. Distribution of the cortical neurofibrillary tangles. The density of lesions is indicated by the following color scale: dark blue (no lesion); light blue, green, yellow, and orange (maximal density of lesions). (From Arnold et al.,[107] with permission.)*

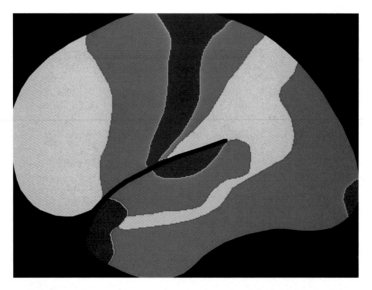

12 *Comparison of the distribution of neurofibrillary tangles (NFT) with the functional organization of the cortical areas. Schematic cytoarchitectonic map showing primary cortex (blue), unimodal association areas (green), multimodal association areas (yellow), and paralimbic cortex (red). There is a clear overlap between the density of NFT and the hierarchy of connections from primary (low density) to multimodal association and paralimbic cortex (high density).*

Table 6-1

Example of the four types of visual stimuli

Words	Pseudowords	Letter strings	False fonts
ANT	GEEL	VSFFHT	ᴙᴂᴈ
RAZOR	IOB	TBBL	ᴊᴂᴊᴂ
DUST	RELD	TSTFS	ᴚᴆᴣᴂ
FURNACE	BLERCE	JBTT	ⱶᴦᴈᴨ
MOTHER	CHELDINABE	STB	ᴂᴙᴂᴊᴮ
FARM	ALDOBER	FFPW	ᴚᴧᴆᴂ

same response. If the activation was attributable to the letters, then the activation should be produced only by letter strings, pseudowords, and words. If the activation was attributable to the orthographic regularity of words regardless of their meaning, then the results produced with words and pseudowords should be identical. Finally, if activation to words was attributable to the meaning of words, even during passive presentation, then words would produce a unique response. Thus, using the methods of cognitive science, we were able to break down the passive perception of words into a group of component mental operations and to set the stage for an imaging experiment designed to determine where in the brain these mental operations were implemented.

The results,[10] shown in Fig. 6-4, were of considerable interest. All four groups of stimuli produced responses in visual areas of the brain as compared with looking at a fixation point. The areas reacted to the complex visual features of the stimuli regardless of whether they consisted of groups of false fonts or letters. However, only pseudowords and words produced the dramatic responses originally observed with words alone. The heightened responses unique to words and pseudowords occurred along the inner surfaces of the left hemisphere of the brain, as shown in Fig. 6-4.

Two levels of analysis appear to be occurring in the visual system as we passively view words. At one level, the brain analyzes the visual features of the stimuli regardless of their relationships to letters and words. These visual features appear to be processed in multiple areas of the visual system on both sides of the brain. Responses to the false fonts that contain only meaningless features are particularly strong on the right side of the brain (not well illustrated in Fig. 6-4 because of the selection of slices).

At a second level, the brain analyzes the visual word form. It seems clear that visual stimuli incorporating the pronunciation rules of the English language uniquely activate a group of areas in the visual system of fluent readers of English. This coordinated response among a group of areas clustered in one part of the visual system must be acquired as we learn to read, and its existence is probably critical to the facility with which skilled readers handle words.

Reading Words Aloud

Following the hierarchical design of the original experiment, the subjects were next asked to read aloud the words (i.e., common English nouns) as they appeared on the television monitor in front of them. For most individuals fluent in their native languague, this is an easy task to perform. One might easily envision that such a task could be performed effortlessly while, at the same time, another, unrelated task was being performed. The point is that such a task requires little of our conscious attention.

Not surprisingly for those knowledgeable about the location of the motor areas of the brain,

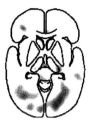 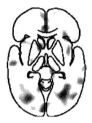 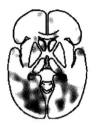 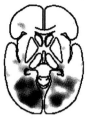

False Font   **Letter Strings**   **Pseudowords**   **Words**

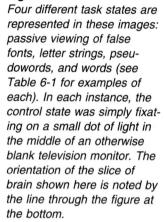

Figure 6-4
Four different task states are represented in these images: passive viewing of false fonts, letter strings, pseudowords, and words (see Table 6-1 for examples of each). In each instance, the control state was simply fixating on a small dot of light in the middle of an otherwise blank television monitor. The orientation of the slice of brain shown here is noted by the line through the figure at the bottom.

these areas were activated when individuals spoke the words they read on the television monitor. As shown in Fig. 6-3 (third row), these areas included the primary motor cortices in both cerebral hemisphere (Fig. 6-3, third row, Z = 40). In addition, other motor areas buried more deeply within the cerebral hemispheres (Fig. 6-3, third row, Z = 20) were also activated, including the cerebellum (Fig. 6-3, third row, Z = −20). At this point it should be noted that the act of speaking words, seen in its simplest form during reading aloud single words, did not produce activity in the classic areas of the left cerebral hemisphere known as Broca's and Wernicke's areas. This was probably one of the first surprises to emerge from the studies of language in normal people made with modern imaging techniques. The classic theories of language organization based on more than a century of research on patients with brain injury would have predicted clear-cut activity in these areas.

Although not mentioned above, listening to words does produce activity in posterior left temporal cortex at the temporoparietal junction in the region classically thought of as Wernicke's area. Furthermore, this area remains active when normal individuals repeat aloud the words they hear. However, it is important to the standard theory

of language organization that this area was not activated when the same individuals read aloud the words that were presented visually. Clearly, Wernicke's area as classically defined from studies of brain-injured patients is not active in an obligatory fashion when we speak. Critics of this new view are quick to point out that the new imaging techniques, such as PET and fMRI, might simply not have been sensitive enough to pick up a change in Wernicke's area when people read aloud. Were it not for the findings in the next stage of the experiment (generating verbs aloud for visually presented nouns) this would have been a difficult criticism to refute.

Generating Verbs Aloud

Generating a verb aloud for a noun presented visually (e.g., see *car*, say *drive*) may seem an unnecessarily complex next step in the hierarchical design of this experiment (linguists have been particularly critical!). After all, it involves a number of complex mental operations such as determining the meaning of the presented word (semantics) and the relation between the meaning of the word and the choice of an appropriate verb (syntax). Additionally, it is a very powerful episodic memory encoding task as well as a semantic retrieval task. Concerns about such issues obscure a most important difference between this task and reading or repeating words aloud. This difference lies in the requirement that the subjects devote considerable conscious attention to the task and, among other things, suppress the tendency to speak the word they see and to substitute an appropriate verb. Furthermore, this must be done rapidly, because in our experiments nouns were being presented at the rate of 40 to 60 per minute. It was very clear to us that subjects found this task difficult when they first attempted it. They often fell behind and occasionally skipped nouns.

The changes we observed in the brain (Fig. 6-3, bottom row) clearly indicated that this task of generating verbs for visually presented nouns placed a significant additional burden on the processing resources of the brain. In addition to areas previously activated, new areas within the left frontal (Fig. 6-3, bottom row, Z = 40, 20, and 0) and temporal (Fig. 6-3, bottom row, Z = 0) lobes were activated along with an area along the midline in front (Fig. 6-3, bottom row, Z = 40). Areas qualifying as Broca's and Wernicke's areas were clearly active, along with the surprising additional involvement of the right cerebellum (Fig. 6-3, bottom row, Z = −20). Recall that some of the cerebellum was active during reading aloud (Fig. 6-3, third row, Z = −20), but this additional activation in the right cerebellar hemisphere during verb generation represented a distinctly separate area. Whatever else might have been predicted about the neural substrate of this task, the right cerebellar hemisphere was not on anyone's mind prior to obtaining the results.

The fact that some areas of the motor system active during word reading (see Fig. 6-3, third row, Z = 20) were actually inactive during verb generation was an additional surprise. (Because of the nature of the color scale used in Fig. 6-3, where only positive differences between the task state and the control state can be shown, this inactivation cannot be illustrated. Suffice it to say that these areas, very active during reading aloud, were mysteriously inactive during verb generation.) This particular result (i.e., some areas being added while other areas were dropped) hinted at the possibility that the task of verb generation actually required *different* brain circuits rather than simply additional brain circuits for speech production. Our thinking in this regard was dramatically affected by an entirely serendipitous event.

While an additional group of subjects were being studied on the verb-generation task, a single subject was actually given practice on the task to ensure that he could do it with less difficulty and greater accuracy (never before had subjects practiced the verb-generation task prior to performing it in the PET scanner). Little did we suspect the effect this would have on our results. We immediately noticed that practice not only improved performance but also resulted in the failure to activate any of the areas seen in our previous study of verb-generation task (see Fig. 6-3, bottom row). In this individual, practice on the verb-generation task appeared to allow the brain to perform the task with the same circuits used for simple word reading aloud (for reference, see Fig. 6-3, row 3). If true, this was, indeed, a surprising finding. Therefore we set about studying the effect of practice on the brain circuits used for speech production.

Practice Effects

The first task was to examine in greater detail the actual effect of practice on the verb-generation task itself. What we learned[11] was that when normal subjects practiced generating verbs for the same list of 40 common English nouns, their reaction times became significantly shorter over a period of about 10 min. During this time, they were able to go through the same word list 10 times, each time being encouraged by the examiner to be as quick as possible in responding. Another remarkable feature of the learning process was the fact that as they became practiced, they became quite stereotyped in their responses. While each of the words on the list could be associated with several verbs, practice led to the repeated selection of just one verb. In a sense, an automated stimulus-response pattern of behavior had been established. If, after learning had occurred, a new word list was substituted, their behavior returned to the unpracticed state (i.e., significantly slower and unstereotyped). It should also be noted that regardless of the amount of practice or whether the subjects were speaking verbs or nouns, the actual time needed to say the word did not change. What did change was the time necessary to begin the response and the nature of the response (i.e., stereotyped versus not stereotyped). Armed with this more complete information concerning the behavioral effects of practice, we were in a position to evaluate the effect of practice on the brain circuits in a new imaging experiment.

In the new imaging experiment,[11] we studied normal subjects performing the verb-generation task to visually presented nouns, naively and after 10 min of practice. The control task was simply reading aloud the same words as they were presented on the television monitor. Consistent with our earlier experiments, the naive generation of verbs for visually presented nouns showed again the same brain areas involved, a reassuring finding, which supported our confidence in the imaging method. The changes with practice were dramatic. The areas in the frontal and temporal cortex in the left hemisphere and the right side of the cerebellum needed to accomplish the verb-generation task in the naive state (top row, Fig. 6-5) were completely replaced by areas deep within the brain hemispheres after a few minutes' practice (bottom row, Fig. 6-5). These latter areas were actually used as well for the far simpler task of reading nouns aloud. In addition, areas in left occipital cortex seen active during the passive visual presentation of words (see Fig. 6-3, second row, $Z = 0$) and unchanged during reading nouns aloud (see Fig. 6-3, third row, $Z = 0$) and naively generating verbs for visually presented nouns (see Fig. 6-3, fourth row, $Z = 0$) significantly increased their activity after practice on the verb-generation task (Fig. 6-6).

These results strongly support the hypothesis that we actually utilize different brain circuits when performing a task like verb generation for the first time than after practice when we have perfected or automated the task. Why should such an arrangement of brain circuitry be necessary? Why two circuits? Why not just do a better job of utilizing existing brain circuits as we learn? The answer may not be simply that the brain needs two circuits, one for the nonconscious performance of highly automated tasks and the other for the performance of novel, nonautomated tasks. It may, instead, be related to our need to strike a balance between the efficiency conferred by automation of much of our behavior and the occasional need to modify our programmed behavior in accordance with unexpected contingencies in our environment. Only further research will allow us to clarify such issues. What is clear is that functional brain imaging adds a remarkable new dimension to our thinking about how language and other cognitive activities are implemented in the normal human brain.

Practical Implications

In our initial study of lexical processing,[8] we introduced the concept of hierarchical subtractions to modern functional imaging as a means of isolating the functional anatomy of specific mental operations (see Fig. 6-3). The logic of the subtraction analysis was that the passive presentation of nouns minus no presentation (i.e., fixation point only) would isolate areas involved in passive sensory processing (row 2, Fig. 6-3); reading aloud visually presented nouns minus the passive presentation of nouns would isolate areas involved in articulatory output and motor programming (row 3, Fig. 6-3); and the verb-generation task minus reading nouns aloud would isolate areas involved in high-level processes such as semantic analysis (row 4, Fig. 6-3).

In its simplest form, the type of hierarchical subtraction method used for the design of this study (see Fig. 6-3) involved accepting the assumption that processing done by previously added areas does not change with the addition or deletion of new areas (i.e., each area is functionally isolated). Also assumed in this approach is that the subject does not change strategies with the addition of another task, nor do the task combinations interact with each other.[12–14]

The limitations of the "additive" method were first discussed in terms of reaction-time studies of human performance.[12–14] For studies of this

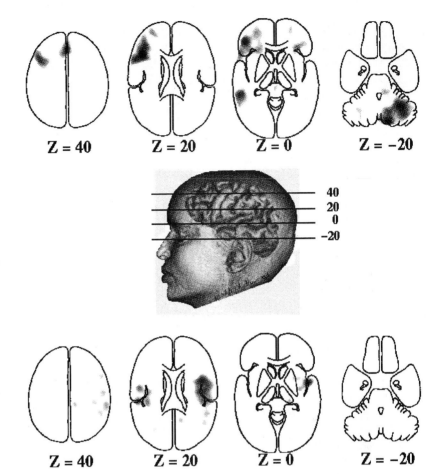

Figure 6-5
A single task state is represented in the images in this figure. In this task, subjects were asked to generate verbs aloud for visually presented common English nouns. The control state for these subtraction images was simply reading aloud the same visually presented nouns. The top row of images shows those areas of the brain used in the performance of this task when it is first undertaken. A brief period of practice markedly improves performance on this difficult task and dramatically alters the areas of the brain uniquely utilized for the task (bottom). Additional practice-induced changes are shown in Fig. 6-6.

type, the validity of the underlying assumptions cannot be directly tested and, as a result, controversy has occasionally arisen about their interpretation. For functional imaging studies, however, empirical testing is theoretically possible. The locations of areas added at different stages in a task hierarchy can be identified, and the magnitude of their activity at each level in the imaging sequence can be monitored. If a brain area is not functionally isolated, then the magnitude of its activity will be modulated by the addition of new tasks. In fact, our study of the effect of practice on the verb-generation task had its genesis in part because of the discovery that generation aloud of a verb appropriate to a visually presented noun (compared to reading the same noun aloud) modulated

areas activated by the reading aloud of the noun. Furthermore, these imaging results (see Figs. 6-5 and 6-6) clearly indicate that the actual areas supporting a task and their relationship with other areas can change dramatically as a result of practice. Such observations underscore the utility of combining the hierarchical subtraction method of psychology with modern functional imaging techniques such as PET and fMRI to further our understanding of the functional anatomy of the normal human brain. They should also impart a note of caution in placing neurobiological interpretations on behavioral data in the absence of direct information about how a process is actually implemented in the brain.

Because of the potential for rapid change in

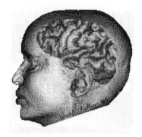 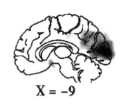

X = −9

Figure 6-6

The task state represented in Fig. 6-5 is again represented in this figure. In this task, subjects were asked to generate verbs aloud for visually presented common English nouns. The control state for these subtraction images was simply reading the same visually presented nouns aloud. The difference image to the right, which represents a sagittal slice of the brain 9 mm to the left of the midline, demonstrates the marked increase in blood flow in the medial occipital cortices occurring as the result of practice on the verb-generation task.

the use of brain circuitry resulting from the practice of an unfamiliar task, interpretation of repeated or time-intensive within-subject functional imaging measurements must be made with care. It would appear that 15 minutes of practice on an unfamiliar task such as the verb-generation task is sufficient to significantly alter the brain circuitry underlying the task. At what time these changes in brain circuitry actually occurred within this 15-min time period remains to be determined. That they may have occurred much earlier than 15 min remains a distinct possibility.

With regard to the actual imaging measurement duration and the effect of practice, the selection of an imaging measurement strategy will also be critical. In the study of the effect of practice on the verb-generation task, functional imaging was performed with PET and measurements of blood flow. The measurement of blood flow was selected because of its simplicity and also because of the short measurement time. The total measurement time for blood flow with PET is 40 s. This is to be contrasted with measurement of glucose metabolism, an equally good marker of neuronal activity,[3] which requires 30 to 45 min to com-

plete.[15,16] Clearly studies of the verb-generation task would have yielded very different results had such a lengthy measurement strategy been selected. The advent of fMRI with even more rapid measurements of functional change with the human brain than anything achievable with PET (see Fig. 6-2) portends an even more precise description of the events surrounding the shift in brain circuitry with practice.

THE TEMPORAL DIMENSION

While functional imaging studies with PET provide remarkable insights into the functional brain *anatomy* of neuronal circuits underlying various cognitive activities in the normal human brain, they do not provide any information on the temporal sequence of information processing within these circuits. Conceptually, one might think of a network of brain areas (see Fig. 6-3) as a group of individuals in the middle of a conference call. The temporal information sought would be equivalent to knowing who was speaking when and who was in charge. Such information is critical in understanding how specific brain areas are coordinated as a network to produce observable human behavior.

Viewing the temporally varying changes in brain activity revealed by fMRI (see Fig. 6-2) has raised the possibility that fMRI, with its speed of data acquisition approaching a few tens of milliseconds, might provide both the anatomy and the timing of information processing within functional brain circuits in the human brain. The stumbling block, however, is the speed of neuronal activity compared with the rate of change of the fMRI signal. Signals from one part of the brain can travel to another in as little as a few milliseconds. Unfortunately, changes in blood flow and blood oxygenation (which is dependent on changes in blood flow) often require several seconds to occur after the onset of a change in neuronal activity. In all likelihood, the only methods that respond quickly enough are the electrical recording techniques such as electroencephalography (EEG) and magnetoencephalography (MEG), which are reviewed in detail in Chap. 7.

One might reasonably ask why these techniques have not been used to provide the types of maps now forthcoming from PET and fMRI. The limitations are spatial resolution and sensitivity. Even though great strides have been made, particularly with MEG, accurate localization of the source of brain activity remains difficult with electrical recording devices used in isolation. Furthermore, the resolution becomes poorer the deeper into the brain information is sought.

Neither PET nor fMRI suffers from this difficulty. They can both sample all parts of the brain with equal spatial resolution and sensitivity. Recently several successful attempts have been made to combine the spatial information from functional imaging studies with the temporal information from electrical studies.[17,18] One such attempt brought together investigators from our laboratory and the University of Oregon to study the temporal dynamics of the naive verb-generation task.[18] Event-related potentials (ERPs) were recorded during both verb generation and reading nouns aloud. Difference ERPs were then computed. From this study, it became clear that information processing unique to naive verb generation began in midline frontal cortices between 180 and 200 ms after the noun was presented. This was followed by a spread of activity laterally to the left prefrontal cortex between 220 and 240 ms. Only later did activity arise in the left posterior temporal cortex, peaking between 620 and 640 ms after stimulus onset (Fig. 6-7). These data, admittedly preliminary, provide important information about the role of specific areas of the brain in the information processing requirements underlying the verb-generation task. For example, the activation in posterior temporal cortex (see Fig. 6-3, fourth row, Z = 0, and Fig. 6-7) in the vicinity of the classic Wernicke's area is rather late to be involved in many rapid semantic tasks that produce reaction times much faster than 600 ms. The later Wernicke's area activation may relate more to the integration of word meanings to obtain the overall meaning of phrases, sentences, or other units more complex than words. Regardless of

their final interpretation, *combined data* of this type are likely to constrain our models of information processing in the human brain and certainly represent an important future direction in functional brain imaging.

RELATIONSHIP TO LESION STUDIES

Functional brain imaging studies in normal humans add a new dimension to the lesion-based studies of behavioral neurology and neuropsychology. Two examples will serve to illustrate this new relationship. In our studies of the processing of single words, which have been used primarily to illustrate the strategy and some of the new findings from functional brain imaging, a new role for the cerebellum was unexpectedly identified. The role of the cerebellum was expected when subjects read aloud words from a television monitor (see Fig. 6-3, third row, Z = −20), as would be the case for any overt motor activity. The presence of robust activity in the right cerebellar hemisphere during verb generation (see Fig. 6-3, fourth row, Z = −20) after subtraction of the activity associated with speaking a word (see Fig. 6-3, third row, Z = −20) was, indeed, a surprise. Although others had speculated about a role for the cerebellum in nonmotoric, cognitive activity,[19] direct evidence for this assertion in normal human subjects was lacking. The PET findings left little doubt about an important role, but the exact nature of the contribution of the cerebellum could not be determined from the imaging results in normals.

At this point we turned to the study of patients with lesions of the cerebellum.[20] Specifically, we wanted to know the performance of individuals who had lesions confined to the right cerebellar hemisphere. Such an individual was located and studied extensively over a period of 2 years.[20] Beginning with the task that produced the right cerebellar PET activation (see Fig. 6-3), we studied this 49-year-old right-handed male (RC1) with right cerebellar damage on a variety of tasks involving complex nonmotor processing. Whereas RC1's performance on standard tests of memory, intelligence, "frontal function," and language skills was

Figure 6-7

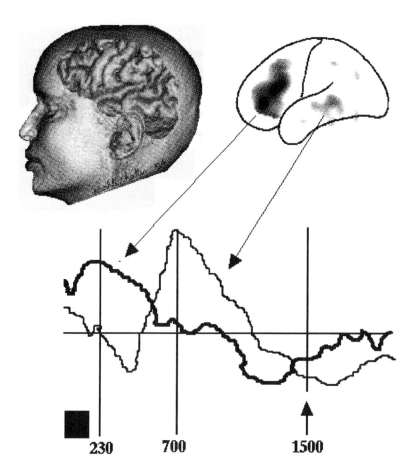

The PET difference image in this figure presents the increase in blood flow occurring in left frontal and temporal cortices during the naive performance of the verb-generation task (see Figs. 6-3 and 6-6 for additional information) along with selected event-related potential (ERP) difference (i.e., verb generation aloud minus reading nouns aloud) waveforms obtained for the same task. The arrows connect the PET blood-flow responses with difference ERP waveforms recorded at the nearest overlying electrode (heavy line = F7; light line = T5). The short horizontal bar below ERP waveforms indicates the visual presentation of the word and the vertical arrow indicates the response cue. Note that activity in frontal cortex precedes that in temporal cortex by over 400 ms. The numbers below the vertical lines represents times in milliseconds after presentation of the word. More complete descriptions of these ERP data are presented in Ref. 18.

excellent, he had profound deficits in two areas: (1) practice-related learning and (2) detection of errors. Considered in relation to cerebellar contributions to motor tasks, the results suggested to us that some functions performed by the cerebellum may be generalized beyond a purely motor domain. Clearly this was an important advance in our understanding of human cerebellar function and its role in human cognition made possible by new knowledge from functional brain imaging of normals coupled with focused studies in patients with lesions.

Our experience with this patient, RC1, suggests to us a paradigm shift in which information about the organization of the normal human brain, obtained from modern functional imaging studies, uniquely guides the bedside evaluation of patients with specific lesions. RC1's very specific cognitive deficits were not apparent to him (remarkably, even during specific testing, he seemed almost completely unaware of his cognitive performance deficits). Likewise, his physicians were pleased to note that his classic cerebellar symptoms and signs of imbalance and incoordination had completely resolved. New knowledge of right cerebellar activation in normals and the specific class of tasks necessary to elicit this activation were critical to the evaluation of RC1 and future patients.

Experience with a second patient[21] reveals another aspect of the role played by functional imaging studies in the evaluation of patients with specific lesions. This patient (LF1) had a lesion of the left frontal cortex secondary to a stroke. Such lesions are known to produce speech-production impairments (nonfluent aphasia). These impairments vary from patient to patient and performance on certain speech-production tasks can be relatively preserved in some patients. It was, therefore, not entirely surprising to find that LF1 had a small island of preserved function. The task on which he performed entirely normally was word-stem completion. In this task, subjects are shown the first three letters of a word and asked to respond with the first word that comes to mind (e.g., see *str*, say *street*). Functional brain imaging in normals has shown that performance of this task activates a discrete area of left frontal cortex in Brodmann area 44.[22] This area had been completely destroyed in LF1.

A possible explanation for preservation of function under these circumstances is that areas outside left prefrontal cortex are used to compensate for the injured brain. We tested this hypothesis in LF1 by having him perform the word-stem completion task, which he was able to do normally despite the lesion in his left frontal cortex, while being scanned with PET. Remarkably, he activated an homologous region in the right frontal cortex. These findings are consistent with the hypothesis that preserved function can be the result of compensatory changes in the circuitry supporting the task performance. Building upon this experience, it should be possible to better understand the manner in which the human nervous system compensates for injury. Also, this experience should inject a note of caution in the behavioral interpretation of a lesion in the absence of a clear understanding of the function or functions performed by the lesioned area in the normal brain.

SUMMING UP

Modern functional brain imaging with PET and fMRI, complemented by ERPs, will play an important role in our understanding of the functional organization of the normal human brain. These new tools, guided by the principles of cognitive science, now permit us to dissect the basic mental operations underlying our behavior and to relate them to specific circuitry within the normal human brain. A glance back at Fig. 6-3 reveals that, as we undertake even relatively simple cognitive tasks, extensive areas of the brain are recruited to assist in the performance of these tasks. Although we can begin making statements about the roles of such groups of areas or circuits, it remains for further studies to determine the more basic mental operations to be assigned to the individual brain areas within a given circuit. The studies of words presented in this chapter give some indication of the manner in which such an analysis might proceed. This information—coupled with studies of patients with brain injury and guided anew by information from normals as well as more basic studies in laboratory animals using a variety of sophisticated techniques—bodes well for our future understanding of human brain function. Armed with such information, we will be in a much better position to appreciate the basis of human behavior.

REFERENCES

1. Posner MI, Petersen SE, Fox PT, Raichle ME: Localization of cognitive operations in the human brain. *Science* 240:1627–1631, 1988.
2. Posner MI, Raichle ME: *Images of Mind.* New York: Freeman, 1994.
3. Raichle ME: Circulatory and metabolic correlates of brain function in normal humans, in *Handbook of Physiology, The Nervous System. Higher Functions of the Brain.* Bethesda, MD: American Physiological Society, 1987, vol V, pp 643–674.
3a. Fox PT, Raichle ME, Minton MA, Deuce C: Nonoxidative glucose consumption during focal physiologic neural activity. *Science* 241:462–464, 1988.
4. Pauling L, Coryell CD: The magnetic properties

and structure of hemoglobin, oxyhemoglobin and carbonmonoxyhemoglobin. *Proc Natl Acad Sci USA* 22:210–216, 1936.

5. Ogawa S, Lee TM, Tank DW: Brain magnetic resonance imaging with contrast dependent on blood oxygenation. *Proc Natl Acad Sci USA* 87:9868–9872, 1990.

6. Ogawa S, Tank DW, Menon R, et al: Intrinsic signal changes accompanying sensory stimulation: Functional brain mapping with magnetic resonance imaging. *Proc Natl Acad Sci USA* 89:5951–5955, 1992.

7. Kwong KK, Belliveau JW, Chesler DA, et al: Dynamic magnetic resonance imaging of human brain activity during primary sensory stimulation. *Proc Natl Acad Sci USA* 89:5675–5679, 1992.

8. Petersen SE, Fox PT, Posner MI, et al: Positron emission tomographic studies of the cortical anatomy of single word processing. *Nature* 331:585–589, 1988.

9. Petersen SE, Fox PT, Posner MI, et al: Positron emission tomographic studies of the processing of single words. *J Cogn Neurosci* 1:153–170, 1989.

10. Petersen SE, Fox PT, Synder AZ, Raichle ME: Activation of extra striate and frontal cortical areas by visual words and word-like stimuli. *Science* 249:1041–1044, 1990.

11. Raichle ME, Fiez JA, Videen TO, et al: Practice-related changes in human brain functional anatomy during non-motor learning. *Cereb Cortex* 4:8–26, 1994.

12. Kulpe OO: The analysis of compound reactions, in Bradford-Tichener E (ed): *Outlines of Psychology.* New York: Macmillan, 1909, pp 410–422.

13. Donders FC: On the speed of mental processes (reprint). *Acta Psychol* 30:412–431, 1969.

14. Sternberg S: The discovery of processing stages: Extensions of Donders' method. *Acta Psychol* 30:276–315, 1969.

15. Sokoloff L, Reivich M, Kennedy C, et al: The [14C]deoxyglucose method for the measurement of local cerebral glucose utilization: Theory, procedure and normal values in the conscious and anesthetized albino rat. *J Neurochem* 28:987–917, 1977.

16. Reivich M, Alavi A, Wolf A, et al: Glucose metabolic rate kinetic model parameters determination in humans: The lumped constants and rate constants for [18F]fluorodeoxyglucose and [11C]deoxyglucose. *J Cereb Blood Flow Metab* 5:179–192, 1985.

17. Heinze HJ, Mangun GR, Burchert W, et al: Combined spatial and temporal imaging of brain activity during visual selective attention in humans. *Nature* 372:543–546, 1994.

18. Snyder AZ, Abdullaev YG, Posner MI, Raichle ME: Scalp electrical potentials reflect regional cerebral blood flow responses during processing of written words. *Proc Natl Acad Sci USA* 92:1689–1693, 1995.

19. Leiner HC, Leiner AL, Dow RS: Does the cerebellum contribute to mental skills? *Behav Neurosci* 100:443–454, 1986.

20. Fiez JA, Petersen SE, Cheney MK, Raichle ME: Impaired non-motor learning and error detection associated with cerebellar damage. *Brain* 115:155–178, 1992.

21. Buckner RL, Corbetta M, Schatz J, et al: Preserved speech abilities and compensation following prefrontal damage. *Proc Natl Acad Sci USA,* 1996.

22. Buckner RL, Petersen SE, Ojemann JG, et al: Functional anatomical studies of explicit and implicit memory retrieval tasks. *J Neurosci* 15:12–29, 1995.

Chapter 7

ELECTROPHYSIOLOGIC METHODS IN BEHAVIORAL NEUROLOGY AND NEUROPSYCHOLOGY

Robert T. Knight

Electrophysiologic recording techniques are widely employed to study cognitive processing in normal and clinical populations.[1-3] Frequency analysis of the ongoing electroencephalogram (EEG) and extraction of evoked potentials embedded in the ongoing EEG can be used to provide information on tonic and phasic changes in brain activity during cognitive processing. Analysis of EEG frequencies is particularly valuable for the study of alterations in regional neural activity in a time domain extending from one to several seconds. The temporal window measured by EEG frequency analysis techniques approximates that accessed by blood-flow-based physiologic techniques described in Chap. 6, such as positron emission tomography (PET) or functional magnetic resonance imaging (fMRI). Recent efforts to record EEG and fMRI simultaneously represent a particularly exciting approach to linking neuronal and regional blood flow changes during mental activity. Evoked potential methods can extract stimulus- or cognition-related neural activity from the ongoing EEG in the millisecond-to-second range, providing a method for real-time assessment of changes in neural activity during cognitive processing. Metabolic techniques such as PET and fMRI currently provide better spatial resolution of cognitive activity, but their temporal resolution is limited to the second or minute range, depending on the individual method. Thus, converging data from evoked potential, PET, and fMRI will likely provide the strongest insights into the neural regions and mechanisms involved in mental activity. This review focuses predominantly on the use of evoked potentials in behavioral neurology. Several excellent sources are available for extensive discussions of the role of EEG frequency analysis methods in the study of cognition.[4]

GENERAL ISSUES

Neural activity in axonal pathways and inhibitory (IPSPs) and excitatory (EPSPs) postsynaptic potentials on the soma and dendrites of active neurons contribute to scalp recorded field potentials, with the brunt of scalp EEG activity due to summed IPSPs and EPSPs. A major limitation of scalp electrical and magnetic recording is uncertainty about the precise brain locations of the signal sources. Rapid accumulation of data from research utilizing intracranial recording, mathematical dipole modeling, lesion populations, and animal models is providing information on the intracranial sources and pharmacologic systems underlying both sensory and cognitive brain potentials (see Swick and associates[5] for review). These efforts are markedly enhancing the spatial localizing power of scalp recording techniques.

Evoked potentials are classified as either exogenous (sensory) or endogenous (cognitive). The latency and amplitude of exogenous responses are determined predominantly by stimulus parameters such as intensity and rate. Examples of exogenous responses include the brainstem auditory evoked response (BAEP), the pattern shift P100 visual evoked potential (VEP), and primary so-matosensory evoked potentials (SEP). Since these responses are largely resistant to cognitive influences, they are widely employed in a variety of neurologic conditions to measure neural activity in sensory pathways. In contrast, endogenous potentials are sensitive to the cognitive parameters of the task. The degree of attention [P300 (P for positive, 300 for latency in milliseconds)], effort [CNV (contingent negative variation)], movement preparation (movement-related potentials; MRPs), and linguistic analysis [N400 (N for negative, 400 for latency in milliseconds)] are examples of cognitive factors determining the amplitude, latency, and scalp distribution of different types of endogenous brain potentials (see Knight,[6] Picton,[7] Hillyard and Picton,[1] for reviews). Since endogenous potentials are generated in response to some cognitive event, they are also referred to as event-related potentials (ERPs) in the literature.

TECHNICAL CONSIDERATIONS

The local intracranial geometry of intracranial neural sources places an important constraint on scalp or extracranial EEG or magnetoencephalography (MEG) recording. Neural sources must have an open-field configuration to generate dipole sources recordable at a distance.[8] Simply put, an open-field geometry occurs when neurons assume a local organized cellular structure wherein neurons are oriented in the same direction. Examples of open-field geometry would include the laminar structure of the cortex or the hippocampus where electromagnetic fields of synchronously active neurons are aligned and sum to produce a dipole field recordable at the scalp. A closed-field geometry occurs when a neuronal structure lacks a clear local cellular anatomic substructure such as the intralaminar thalamic nuclei. In this situation, neurons may fire synchronously but the local extracellular fields are not well aligned and will cancel out locally and not generate a summed dipole field recordable at a distance. This constraint of open- versus closed-field geometry is shown schematically in Fig. 7-1. On the left are two neurons that are aligned in the same direction in an open-field

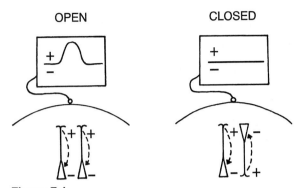

Figure 7-1

Schematic of an idealized open- and closed-field neuronal configuration. In the open-field situation, extracellular fields sum and can be recorded at a distance. In the closed-field condition, the extracellular fields of the two synchronously active neurons cancel and no evoked field is recorded at a distance.

configuration. If these neurons fire synchronously, their extracellular fields will sum and this activity can be recorded by volume conduction at a distant site such as the scalp. On the right are the same two neurons firing synchronously but aligned 180° out of phase in a closed-field configuration. In this situation their extracellular fields would cancel out and no electrical field would be recorded at a distance. A single unit recording electrode would record equivalent activity in both the open- and closed-field condition, and metabolic techniques would also record comparable activity in each situation.

The distance of an active neuronal source from the recording site has a major influence on the strength of the signal recorded at the scalp since electric and magnetic fields drop in amplitude as an inverse power function of the distance of the active neuronal elements from a recording site. Intracranial neuronal generators can be classified as near- or far-field sources. An example of a near-field source would be the primary SEP generated in the depths and crown of the postcentral gyrus. Since this neuronal source is on the surface of the hemisphere, the scalp field will be large and focally distributed in parietal scalp electrodes situated over the postcentral gyrus (see Fig. 7-2). A classic far-field source would be the brainstem

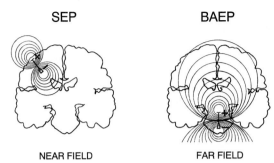

SEP   BAEP

NEAR FIELD   FAR FIELD

Figure 7-2
On the left is the near field of the primary SEP. The evoked field changes rapidly over small distances on the scalp. On the right is an example of the far-field response of the BAEP. Note that the field is broadly distributed over the scalp, since the neural source is deep in the brainstem. See text for details. (Modified from Knight,[30] with permission.)

auditory evoked potential (BAEP). The BAEP is generated by sequential activity of auditory structures located in the brainstem extending from the eighth nerve to the inferior colliculus. The dipole field of these generators is broadly distributed over the scalp and small in amplitude due to its distance from the scalp (see Fig. 7-2). Because of this biophysical constraint, the brunt of electrical activity recorded at scalp sites arises in near-field generators in neocortical regions.

Evoked potentials range in amplitude from 0.5 μV for the exogenous BAEP to 10 to 20 μV for longer-latency endogenous potentials such as the P300, N400, and CNV. These evoked signals are buried in the ongoing EEG, which typically varies from 10 to 200 μV. In order to extract these signals from the ongoing EEG, the evoked response to a discrete sensory stimulus or cognitive manipulation must be averaged over multiple trials. Since the background EEG can be approximated as random noise, the sum of repetitive EEG epochs will tend to average to zero. Conversely, the evoked response, which is time-locked to a specific stimulus or response, will summate and emerge from the background EEG. The signal-to-noise ratio, which can be viewed as a measure of the ability to confidently identify the evoked signal in the background EEG "noise," is proportional

to the square root of the number of stimulus repetitions. In general, smaller signals require many more trials before a reliable potential is seen. The effects of signal averaging for the small, far-field, exogenous BAEP is shown in Fig. 7-3. Note that no signal is apparent in the evoked potential average of the first 16 trials. A clear but noisy signal is seen after 144 trials, and by 1024 trials, a clean

Figure 7-3
The signal averaging of the BAEP. Note that a clear signal is not observable for at least 144 trials, since the BAEP is small (<0.5 μV) and buried in the background EEG activity.

BAEP AVERAGING

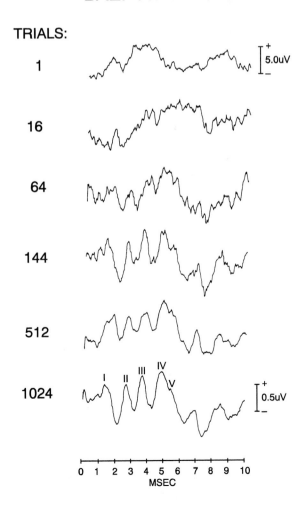

TRIALS:

1

16

64

144

512

1024

0 1 2 3 4 5 6 7 8 9 10
MSEC

signal shows the principal five components of the BAEP. A different pattern is seen in Fig. 7-4, which shows the averaging of a P300 response to unexpected novel sounds over 1 to 36 trials in two subjects. Since the P300 to these unexpected sounds is in the range of 10 to 30 μV for a single stimulus, it rapidly emerges from the background EEG noise after a few trials. Indeed, in subject 1, it can be seen in a single trial, and it is clear by four trials in subject 2. Note that the EEG continues to flatten out with repetitive trials, which can be most easily seen in the prestimulus epoch. Several techniques have been developed to extract single trials from the ongoing EEG during cognitive tasks that generate large responses (see Gevins and Remond[9] for extensive reviews of signal processing techniques).

Figure 7-4
The signal averaging of novelty P3a responses in two subjects. Since the P3a amplitude is large (>10 μV), the signal is well seen in only a few trials.

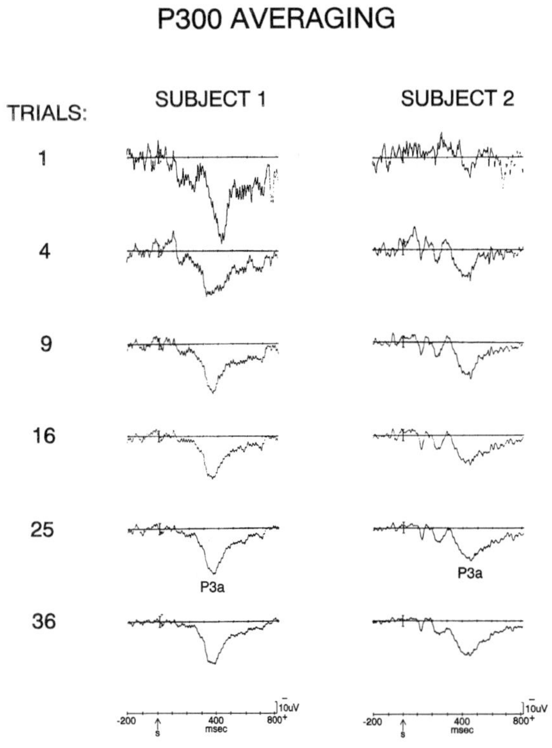

P300 AVERAGING

APPLICATION OF EVOKED POTENTIAL TECHNIQUES TO BEHAVIORAL NEUROLOGY

Evoked potentials have been applied to the study of several behavioral problems, including dementia, frontal lobe dysfunction, and aphasia. Recent advances in three-dimensional (3-D) lesion construction and contributions from the field of neuropsychology[10] have been coupled with evoked potential recording in an effort to delineate the anatomic and physiologic underpinnings of neurobehavioral syndromes (see Fig. 7-5 for examples of 3-D lesion reconstructions). The application of evoked potential techniques to the analysis of attention capacity with a particular emphasis on human prefrontal cortex will be reviewed in an effort to show how combined approaches can contribute to our understanding of cognitive mechanisms in humans.

Dorsolateral prefrontal cortex is crucial for the control of sustained and phasic attention to environmental events.[11] Attention and orienting ability have been studied using sensory and cognitive evoked potential recording techniques in neurologic patients with damage centered in Brodmann's areas 9 and 46 and in patients with posterior cortical and mesial temporal damage. Electrophysiologic and behavioral data from these patients have indicated that problems with inhibitory control of sensory inputs, deficits in sustained attention, and abnormalities in the detection of novel events are central to prefrontal disease.

The role of prefrontal cortex in the regulation of sustained and phasic attention is crucial for maintenance of working memory. The term *working memory* refers to the on-line ability to manipulate information generated by either external sensory events or internal mental activity. The concept of working memory encompasses a range of cognitive activities.[12,13] A trivial example would be the rehearsal of a new phone number while waiting to dial. A more complex example would be conscious comparison of an observed event to a previous experience or a potential future outcome. Dorsolateral prefrontal cortex, including areas 9 and 46 in humans and the corresponding sulcus

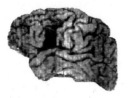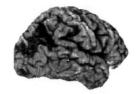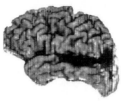

Figure 7-5
Three-dimensional in vivo MRI reconstructions of three stroke patients with lesions in Broca's area, the right parietal lobe, and the left superior temporal plane. These reconstructions were obtained with the Brain Vox software.[142]

principalis region in monkeys, functions as a central executive to control the distributed neocortical networks engaged during working memory.[2,14–17] At intervals of less than 5 s working memory is largely independent of access to the long-term store and relies predominantly on distributed neocortical networks.[18] Thus, working memory is largely intact in patients with diencephalic or hippocampal amnesia.

SENSORY GATING AND EVOKED POTENTIALS

Inability to inhibit internal representations of previous responses that are now incorrect may underlie the poor performance of prefrontal subjects on the Wisconsin Card Sorting Task and on the Stroop Phenomenon.[19] The attention deficits of a patient with a prefrontal lesion and the behavioral phenomena of perseveration in advanced prefrontal disease have also been linked to problems with inhibitory control of posterior sensory and perceptual mechanisms.[20,21] Physiologic data indicates that this lack of inhibitory control may extend to early sensory processing in primary cortical regions.

Neural inhibition by prefrontal regions has been reported in a variety of mammalian preparations. A net inhibitory output to both subcortical[21a] and cortical regions has been documented.[21b] Cryogenic blockade of a prefrontal-thalamic gating system in cats results in enhancement of amplitudes of primary sensory cortex evoked responses.[22,22a] This prefrontal-thalamic inhibitory system provides a potential mechanism for intermodality suppression of irrelevant inputs at an early stage of sensory processing.

Support for a similar mechanism in humans has been obtained from the observation of patients with prefrontal damage due to stroke. Task-irrelevant auditory and somatosensory stimuli were delivered to patients with damage to dorsolateral prefrontal cortex and to patients with comparably sized lesions in the temporoparietal junction or the lateral parietal cortex. Evoked responses from primary auditory[23] and somatosensory[24–26] cortices were recorded in these patients and in age-matched controls (see Fig. 7-6). The stimuli consisted of either monaural clicks or brief electric shocks to the median nerve, eliciting a small opponens pollicis twitch.

Lesions of the posterior association cortex invading either the primary auditory or somatosensory cortex reduced early latency (20 to 40 ms) evoked responses generated in these regions. Lesions in posterior association cortex, sparing primary sensory regions, had no effects on the amplitudes or latencies of the primary cortical evoked responses; such patients served as a brain-lesioned control group. Prefrontal damage resulted in disinhibition of both the primary auditory and somatosensory evoked responses generated from 20 to 40 ms poststimulation.[27,28] Spinal cord and brainstem potentials were unaffected by prefrontal damage, indicating that amplitude enhancement of primary cortical responses was due to abnormalities in either prefrontal-thalamic or direct prefrontal-sen-

Frontal Gating

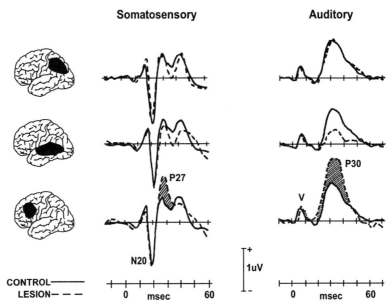

Figure 7-6

Primary cortical auditory and somatosensory evoked potentials are shown for controls (solid line) *and patients* (dashed line) *with focal damage in the lateral parietal cortex (top, n = 8), temporal-parietal junction (middle, n = 13), or dorsolateral prefrontal cortex (bottom, n = 13). Reconstructions of the center of damage in each patient group are shown on the left. Somatosensory evoked responses were recorded from area 3b (N20) and areas 1 and 2 on the crown of the postcentral gyrus (P26). Stimuli were square-wave pulses of 0.15 ms duration delivered to the median nerve at the wrist. Stimulus intensity was set at 10 percent above opponens twitch threshold, and stimuli were delivered at a rate of 3/s. Damage in posterior cortical regions sparing primary somatosensory cortex had no effect on the N20 or earlier spinal cord potentials. Prefrontal damage resulted in a selective increase in the amplitude of the P26 response (hatched area). Auditory stimuli were clicks delivered at a rate of 13/s at intensity levels of 50 dB HL. Unilateral damage in the temporoparietal junction extending into primary auditory cortex reduces P30 responses. Lateral parietal damage sparing primary auditory has no effect on P30 responses. Dorsolateral prefrontal damage results in normal inferior collicular potentials (wave V) but an enhanced P30 primary cortical response (hatched area). The shaded area in each modality indicates the area of evoked potential amplitude enhancement.*

sory cortical mechanisms. Chronic disinhibition of sensory inputs may contribute to many of the behavioral sequelae of prefrontal damage. For instance, decision confidence is decremented by a noisy internal milieu, and the orienting response would be habituated.[29,30]

FOCUSED ATTENTION, SUSTAINED ATTENTION, AND THE CONTINGENT NEGATIVE VARIATION

Selective attention to a sensory channel such as an ear, a portion of the visual field, or a finger increases the amplitude of evoked potentials generated to all stimuli delivered to that region.[31] This amplitude enhancement onsets by 25 ms after stimulation in the auditory modality, indicating that neurologically intact humans are able to exert attention effects on sensory inputs to primary cortical regions.[32,33] Early-onset selective attention effects have also been reported in the visual and somatosensory modalities,[34,35] supporting an early sensory filtering mechanism in humans.[36–38] In the visual modality, attention may not modulate primary sensory activity in calcarine cortex but instead acts on subsequent stages of processing in visual association cortex.[39]

Auditory selective attention capacity has been examined in patients with unilateral damage localized to left or right dorsolateral prefrontal cortex. Lesions were due to infarction of the precentral branch of the middle cerebral artery and centered in areas 9 and 46. In dichotic selective attention tasks, normal subjects generate an enhanced negativity to all stimuli in an attended channel with onset from 25 to 50 ms after delivery of an attended auditory stimulus. Control subjects generated comparable selective attention effects for both left- and right-ear stimulation. Left prefrontal patients generate reduced attention effects in both ears. Patients with right prefrontal damage show electrophysiologic and behavioral evidence of a dense hemi-inattention to left-ear stimuli.[40] The prefrontal patients' evoked potential deficits parallel the human hemineglect syndrome, which is more common after right prefrontal or temporoparietal lesions.[41–44] Posterior association cortex lesions in the temporoparietal junction have comparable attention deficits for left- and right-sided lesions, indicating that these areas are not asymmetrically organized for auditory selective attention.[45] This suggests that some aspects of hemineglect subsequent to temporoparietal damage may be due to remote effects of disconnection from asymmetrically organized prefrontal regions.

Attention capacity improves at short versus long interstimulus intervals in patients with prefrontal lesions. This could be interpreted to support either a temporal bridging or a distractibility deficit in the patients. Prefrontal cortex is proposed to be critical for bridging temporal disconti-

nuities,[46] and deficits should be more apparent at longer interstimulus intervals. However, at longer interstimulus intervals, prefrontal subjects are also more likely to encounter distracting intervening and irrelevant stimuli. Distractibility is a prominent behavioral feature of animals and humans with prefrontal lesions.[47–49] Indeed, the classic delayed response deficit in animals with prefrontal lesions may be due to distractibility in the delay interval.[50,51]

The evoked potential experiments in patients with prefrontal lesions provided some evidence supporting the distractibility hypothesis. In normal subjects, delivery of an irrelevant stimulus in the nonattended ear during a dichotic experiment has no effect on attention effects to a subsequent stimulus in the attended channel. However, presentation of an irrelevant stimulus reduces attention to a subsequent stimulus in patients with prefrontal lesions. This effect is particularly pronounced in the ear contralateral to a prefrontal lesion at long interstimulus intervals. Since attention performance is improved in these patients if no irrelevant stimuli are present, the results favor distractibility as the major cause of the attention deficits.[52] Recent behavioral experiments have also documented an important role for prefrontal cortex in inhibiting response to irrelevant sensory information in delay tasks ranging from 2 to 12 s. Of interest are observations that patients with mesial temporal damage show gating deficits similar to the those of frontal patients with frontal lesions at delays over 8 s. This suggests that at long delays (>8 s) limbic circuits need to be engaged to hold information in auditory working memory.[53]

The CNV is a negative-polarity brain potential maximal over frontal-central scalp sites generated during a delay period initiated by a warning stimulus. The CNV is terminated by a behavioral response that is contingent on information delivered in the warning stimulus.[54] The behavioral structure of tasks that generate a CNV shares attributes with paradigms associated with working memory in monkeys and humans.[55–57a] The CNV potentials are focally reduced by discrete prefrontal damage supporting a generator of the CNV in prefrontal cortex[58,59] (see Fig. 7-7). These data provide a further link between prefrontal regions

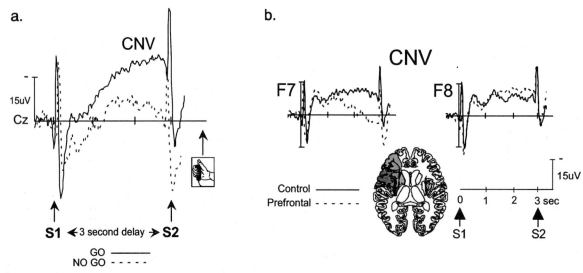

Figure 7-7

This figure shows the results of classic auditory contingent negative variation (CNV) experiment in patients with focal prefrontal (PFCx) damage. On the left (A) are the results of a CNV task in normals. A warning stimulus (S1) triggers either a GO or NO/GO trial which is terminated by the imperative S2 stimulus. GO trials generate a large DC shift maximal over frontocentral scalp sites, referred to as the CNV. Damage to the PFCx results in severe attenuation in the CNV over lesioned cortex (B), reductions observed throughout the lesioned hemisphere (see Rosahl and Knight[59] for details). On the bottom right are the group-averaged lesion reconstructions in 10 patients with prefrontal damage. Posterior lesions focally reduce the CNV over lesioned cortex but do not result in widespread hemispheric declines. These data provide evidence of PFCx involvement in sustaining distributed neural activity during delay periods.

and sustained attention and working memory capacity.

PHASIC ATTENTION, P300, AND CORTICAL-HIPPOCAMPAL CIRCUITS

The P300 component is a scalp-recorded brain potential that can be used to study phasic attention mechanisms in humans. The P300 component of the human ERP was first reported in 1965[60,61] and since that time has been the subject of extensive cognitive research in both normal and clinical populations. This prominent scalp response has been described in a range of mammalian species, including rats[62,63] (see Fig. 7-8), cats,[64–66] and monkeys.[67–70] The ubiquitous occurrence across species indicates that the P300 phenomenon may represent activity of a basic neural system involved in the early detection and encoding of sensory stimuli.

Theories centered on attention and memory processing have been proposed to account for the cognitive basis of the P300, although no clear consensus has emerged.[71,72] Much of this disagreement in the previous literature is due to the fact that the P300 is not a unitary brain potential arising from a discrete brain region or cognitive process, as had been initially proposed. Instead, scalp positivities generated during cognitive processing in the 300- to 700-ms poststimulus delivery reflect serial and parallel activation of multiple neocorti-

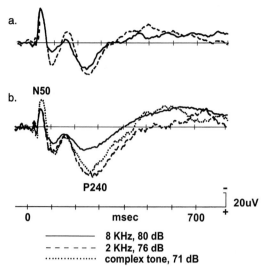

a.

b. N50

P240

20uV

0　　　　　　　 msec　　　　 700

——————— 8 KHz, 80 dB
– – – – – 2 KHz, 76 dB
················ complex tone, 71 dB

Figure 7-8

*Experiments were performed to examine whether a
novelty P3a potential could be recorded in the unre-
strained rat. Stimuli were pure tones (8 kHz, 80 dB; 2
kHz, 76 dB; and complex tones, 71 dB). The complex
tones were recordings of rat vocalizations. In one condition, only the two pure tones were presented, each
50 percent of the time. Comparable waveforms were
obtained (A). In another condition, 8 kHz tone occurred
on 80 percent of the trials. Two kHz pure tones and
the rat vocalizations were delivered randomly on 10
percent of the trials. These infrequent stimuli generated
an enhanced positive potential at 240 ms which may
represent the rodent homologue of the human P3a (B).
(From Yamaguchi et al.,[63] with permission.)*

cal and limbic regions. For instance, long-latency
positive scalp potentials differing in both scalp topography and latency have been linked to both
voluntary and involuntary attention in addition to
different aspects of memory processing. Support
for these conclusions derives from scalp topographical studies in normals,[73–79] intracranial recording in epileptic patients,[80–86] and lesion studies
in neurologic patients.[30,87–91]

　　Subcomponents of the P300 phenomenon
have been proposed to measure engagement of
early attention and working memory mechanisms
in humans. Voluntary detection of a task-relevant
stimulus in either the visual, auditory, or somato-

sensory modality generates a prominent P300
response maximal over posterior scalp regions
(P3b). The P3b has been proposed to underlie a
range of cognitive processes. One proposal is that
the P3b is generated during closure of a perceptual
task.[71,84] According to this theory, the P3b represents inhibition of a discrete epoch of stimulus
processing. A P3b is generated by inhibition of
regional negativity in activated neocortex or mesial temporal sites associated with the termination
of voluntary processing of an expected stimulus.[92,93] This theory has the strength of being directly testable in animal P300 models, although
no such data are available at present. Another
prominent theory supported by extensive cognitive psychophysiologic research is that the P3b
indexes updating of information in working memory.[72] Other proposals, such as those linking P3b
and template matching, may be subsumed under
the concept of context updating in working memory.[94] The modality specificity of the P3b has also
been extensively studied. Scalp topography studies
in normals[95–97] and temporal lobectomy patients[98]
and magnetoencephalographic studies in normals[99,100] report that modality-specific activity contributes to scalp P3b potentials.

　　Delivery of an unexpected and novel stimulus generates an earlier-latency P300 response
(P3a), which is recorded over widespread anterior
and posterior scalp sites. The P3a potential has a
more frontocentral scalp distribution than the P3b
in all sensory modalities and has been proposed
to be a central marker of the orienting response.[29,30,74,75] A longer-latency posterior posi-
tivity generated during recognition memory tasks
(~600 ms) predicts subsequent memory for the
eliciting stimulus and appears to be distinct from
the P3b based on scalp topography, intracranial
recording, and lesion studies.[81,101–105] Ruchkin and
colleagues have provided evidence that longer-
latency scalp positivities index activity in phonological and visuospatial systems of working
memory.[76–78]

　　Intracranial recording supports the view that
multiple regions are activated during the temporal
window for recording scalp P3b and P3a potentials. A great deal of excitement was generated

by reports of large endogenous potentials in the hippocampal region during tasks that produced scalp P3b responses.[106] Subsequent studies reporting intact parietal P3bs in patients with mesial temporal damage due to hypoxia,[107] anterior temporal lobectomy,[87] herpes simplex encephalitis,[108,109] tumor,[104] and hippocampal infarction[2,110,111] indicate that although the hippocampus is clearly activated by stimuli that generate scalp P3b potentials, it is unlikely that the brunt of the scalp P3b recorded at midline and posterior scalp sites is due to volume conducted field potentials from hippocampal regions. An extensive study involving scalp and intracranial recording pre- and postoperatively in epileptic patients undergoing anterior temporal lobectomy revealed that P3b responses were intact at midline sites after mesial temporal removal.[80] This finding—coupled with latency data from the same study reporting that hippocampal P3-like activity peaked from 30 to 50 ms after the scalp P3b—further indicated that hippocampal structures could not be the prime generator of scalp P3b activity. It should be noted that anterior temporal lobectomies,[80] bilateral mesial temporal lesions due to herpes simplex encephalitis,[108] and unilateral posterior hippocampal infarctions[110] result in significant P300 reductions at far lateral temporal and frontal sites. This suggests that mesial temporal structures may either be generating field potentials that propagate to the surface at these sites or are providing modulatory input necessary for P300 generation in these regions. In addition to the well-described hippocampal potentials, intracranial recording has also reported P3b potentials in several cortical sites, including superior temporal sulcus, inferior parietal lobe, and possibly superior parietal lobe.[84–86,112]

Intracranial recordings in the visual, auditory, and somatosensory modalities have shown that multiple neocortical and limbic regions are activated during tasks that generate scalp novelty-dependent P3a potentials.[84–86,112,113] Intracranial P3a activity has been recorded in widespread areas of frontal and posterior association cortex in addition to cingulate and mesial temporal regions.

These intracranial novelty-related P3a potentials have been proposed to measure neural activity in a distributed multimodal corticolimbic orienting system. Similar theories have been suggested for the scalp P3a response.[30,73,74] Of interest are recent data showing the galvanic skin response (GSR), a peripheral marker of the orienting response, is also reduced by damage to the prefrontal and posterior association cortex.[114]

Further support for the existence of multiple P300 generators has been provided by lesion data recorded from neurologic patients with focal damage in either dorsolateral prefrontal cortex, temporoparietal junction, lateral parietal cortex, or hippocampal regions. Discrete damage in the temporoparietal junction results in severe reduction of P3a and P3b activity at posterior scalp sites in both the auditory[27,88] and somatosensory[89,115] but not the visual modality[91] (see Fig. 7-9). Verleger and colleagues recently confirmed that the auditory P3b was markedly reduced by temporoparietal damage and also noted that the visual P3b was not as much reduced as the auditory response in their patients.[116] These data provide additional evidence that modality-specific regions contribute to the scalp P3b.

The human temporoparietal junction may correlate anatomically to multimodal area cSTP[117] and auditory association area Tpt in monkeys. These regions, located in the posterior superior temporal sulcus of the monkey, have bidirectional connections to area TH in the parahippocampal gyrus and have been implicated in learning and memory in animals and humans.[118] The P3b reductions in the patients with temporoparietal lesions are accompanied by attention and memory deficits.[45,110] Temporoparietal lesions in monkeys also result in auditory memory deficits.[119] These studies suggest that the posterior scalp P3b component marks activity in posterior association cortex generated during engagement of early attention and memory processes. This posterior neocortical system may interact with hippocampal regions during encoding of sensory inputs.[120] For instance, hippocampal field potentials are generated about 50 ms after the posterior scalp P3b,[80] indicating that the

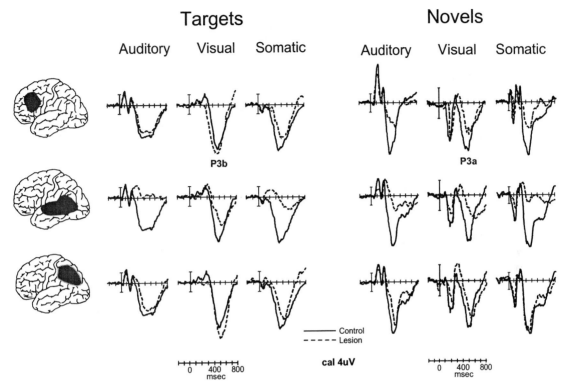

Figure 7-9

Summary of the target P3b and novelty P3a effects in controls and three patient groups with focal cortical damage. The center of the damage in each group is shown on the left. The waveforms from selected electrodes with maximal response amplitude (Pz for targets, Fz for novels) are shown for both target and novel stimuli in the auditory, visual, and somatosensory modalities in patients and controls. Prefrontal and lateral parietal lesions had no significant effect on the latency or amplitude of the target P3b generated in this simple detection task in the auditory, somatosensory, or visual modalities, implying that substantial regions of dorsolateral, prefrontal, and parietal association cortex are not critical for the parietal maximal P3b. Conversely, focal infarction in the temporal-parietal junction resulted in marked P3b reductions in the auditory and somatosensory modalities and partial reductions in the visual modality. On the right are the results of the novelty experiments. Lateral parietal damage again had no significant effect on the P3 to novel stimuli and served as a brain lesioned control. Both prefrontal and temporoparietal damage resulted in multimodal reductions of the novelty P3a.

scalp P3b may index readout of cortical information to limbic regions.

Prefrontal damage results in differential effects on scalp P3a and P3b responses. The parietal maximal P3b generated to expected and correctly detected stimuli in simple sensory discrimination tasks is unaffected by prefrontal damage. However, parietal P3b reductions after prefrontal damage are observed in more complex tasks.[121] P3a responses generated over prefrontal scalp sites to unexpected novel stimuli are reduced by prefrontal lesions, with reductions observed throughout

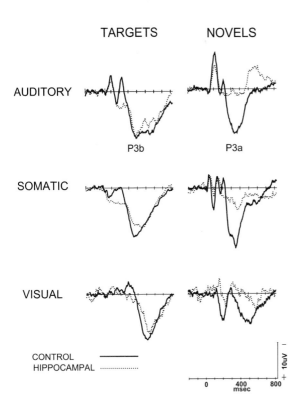

Figure 7-10

Group-averaged event-related potential (ERP) data from controls and patients with hippocampal lesions (n = 7) for auditory, visual, and somatosensory target and novel stimuli. Subjects were seated in a sound-attenuated booth and instructed to press a button upon detection of a designated target stimulus during each experiment. Auditory stimuli consisted of blocks of repetitive standard 1000-Hz monaural tone bursts (60 dB HL; 50 ms duration, 1 s ISI). Tone bursts of 1500 Hz occurred randomly on 10 percent of the trials and served as targets. Unexpected novel tones consisting of complex computer-generated sounds, and environmental noises such as bells or barks were randomly delivered on 10 percent of the trials. A similar paradigm was employed in the visual modality. Visual stimuli consisted of repetitive presentation of triangles. On 10 percent of the trials, inverted triangles served as target stimuli. On an additional 10 percent of trials, random line drawings or pictures of irrelevant stimuli served as novel events. Somatosensory stimuli consisted of repetitive taps to the index finger, with targets being random taps to the ring finger that occurred on 10 percent of the trials. Novel stimuli consisted of brief random shocks to the median nerve on 6 percent of the trials. The ERPs shown are from the electrode where maximal response were recorded (Pz for targets; Fz for novels). The novelty P3a is markedly reduced at prefrontal sites in all three modalities, and the target P3b is spared.

the lesioned hemisphere. These data support distributed interaction between prefrontal and posterior regions during both voluntary and involuntary attention and working memory.[41,122] Comparable P3a decrements have been observed in the auditory,[30,123] visual,[91] and somatosensory modalities in humans with prefrontal damage[89] (see Fig. 7-10). Reductions appear to be more severe after right prefrontal damage.[90] These findings support a prefrontal source for the frontal scalp component of the novelty P300 and converge with both clinical observations and animal experimentation supporting a critical role of prefrontal structures in the detection of novel stimuli.[124,125] The results of the selective attention and novelty detection experiments provide converging evidence of a right pre-

frontal dominance in both sustained and phasic attention in humans.[2]

Unilateral damage centered in the posterior hippocampal region has no effect on parietal P3b activity generated to auditory, visual, and somatosensory stimuli but reduces frontocentral P3 activity to both target and novel stimuli in all modalities. Reductions are most prominent over frontal regions and for novel stimuli[111,125] (see Fig. 7-11, Plate 4). These reductions are comparable in amplitude to those observed after focal prefrontal damage. However, unilateral hippocampal damage reduces P300 potentials over both prefrontal cortices, whereas prefrontal damage results in predominantly unilateral reductions over the lesioned hemisphere. These observations support involve-

Figure 7-11

This figure shows the scalp voltage topographies for target and novel stimuli in controls. Note the marked increase in prefrontal activity to the novel stimuli in all sensory modalities. The effects of prefrontal or hippocampal lesions on the brain novelty response are shown on the right. Unilateral prefrontal damage results in multimodal decreases in the novelty response. Unilateral hippocampal damage results in severe bilateral reductions in the novelty response, maximal at prefrontal sites. These findings implicate a prefrontal-hippocampal network in the detection of perturbations in the environment (see text for details).

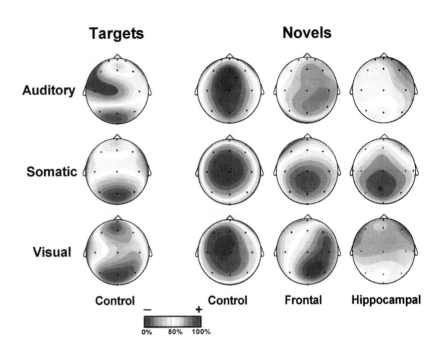

ment of a prefrontal-hippocampal system in the detection of deviancies in the ongoing sensory stream and indicate that the hippocampal formation has bilateral facilatory input to prefrontal cortex.

Reciprocal pathways coursing through the caudomedial lobule of the mesial temporal lobe provide a potential anatomic substrate for prefrontal-hippocampal interactions during sensory and mnemonic processing.[56] Studies with PET have also documented frontal hypometabolism in patients with medial temporal amnesia.[126] Prefrontal-hippocampal interactions may contribute to classic memory phenomena such as the von Restorff effect, where novel or out of context stimuli are better remembered.[127-129]

These results, in conjunction with the data from intracranial and lesion studies, provide further evidence that the P300 phenomenon is not a unitary phenomenon but represents distributed neural activity in corticolimbic regions engaged during both voluntary and involuntary response to discrete en-

vironmental events. Although this view is more complicated than initial proposals of a unitary nature of P300 activity, it strengthens the potential utility of scalp ERP recording, since it provides a means for the measurement of neural activity in distributed brain regions in the time domain of cognitive processing.

N400 AND LANGUAGE PROCESSING

Another cognitive evoked potential extensively studied in language processing tasks is the N400, a negative potential peaking at about 400 ms post-stimulus (see Ref. 130 for review). The N400 was first described by Kutas and Hillyard[131] as being elicited by violations of semantic expectancies at the end of sentences ("She takes her coffee with cream and *dog*" rather than ". . . cream and *sugar*"). The N400 amplitude is modulated by the extent to which a word is related to its prior context. General theories of N400 have addressed whether or not this component reflects retrieval of information from long-term memory.[130-132] Another contentious point is whether the N400 is entirely linguistic in nature or instead reflects semantic processing in a more generic sense. Nonverbal stimuli such as faces,[133] pictures,[18,134,135] and environmental noises[94] have also been reported to elicit N400-type components, although deviant endings to melodies did not.[82,136] It is conceivable that multiple intracranial regions contribute to the scalp N400 with different subcomponents related to various aspects of cognitive processing, as has been suggested for P300 phenomena. Indeed, a recent report suggests there are at least four subcomponents that contribute to the N400 that differ in latency and scalp topography.[137]

Intracranial recordings in the anterior medial temporal lobe (MTL) have revealed potentials resembling the scalp N400 in verbal recognition memory, lexical decision, semantic priming, and picture-naming tasks.[138-140] MTL-N460 amplitudes have been reported to be largest in the left MTL following new words, while an MTL-P620 potential was largest to repeated words and was reduced in a passive condition. Puce and colleagues[81] found similar MTL potentials to both verbal stimuli and abstract "nonverbalizable" patterns during recognition memory. Following the presentation of auditory word pairs, elderly controls and Broca's aphasics demonstrated semantic and associative priming effects manifested by a decreased N400 to related targets versus unrelated targets, while Wernicke's aphasics failed to show priming effects.[141] Additionally, N400 amplitudes were reduced in Wernicke's aphasics with lesions encompassing the temporoparietal junction. Conversely, N400 amplitudes were reported to be normal in Broca patients with frontal lesions. These data suggest that a posterior cortical-mesial-temporal network is engaged during N400 generation.

ACKNOWLEDGMENTS

Special thanks to Clay C. Clayworth for technical assistance in all phases of the work. Supported by NINDS Javits Award NS21135, PO NS17778 from the NINDS, and the Veterans Administration Medical Research Service.

REFERENCES

1. Hillyard SA, Picton TW: Electrophysiology of cognition, in Plum F (ed): *Handbook of Physiology: the Nervous System.* Baltimore: American Physiological Society, 1987, pp 519–584.
2. Knight RT: Attention regulation and human prefrontal cortex, in Thierry AM, Glowinski J, Goldman-Rakic P, Christen Y (eds): *Motor and Cognitive Functions of the Prefrontal Cortex: Research and Perspectives in Neurosciences.* Berlin, Heidelberg: Springer-Verlag, 1994, pp 160–173.
3. Egan MF, Duncan CC, Suddath RL, et al: Event-related potential abnormalities correlate with structural brain alterations and clinical features in patients with chronic schizophrenia. *Schizophr Res* 11:259–271, 1994.
4. Lopes da Silva FH, Storm van Leewen W, Remond A: Clinical applications of computer analysis of EEG and other neurophysiological signals, in *Handbook of Electroencephalography and Clinical Neurophysiology.* Philadelphia: Elsevier, 1987, vol 2.
5. Swick D, Kutas M, Neville HJ: Localizing the neural generators of event-related brain potentials, in Kertesz A (ed): *Localization in Neuroimaging in Neuropsychology.* New York: Academic Press, 1994, pp 73–121.
6. Knight RT: Electrophysiology in behavioral neurology, in Mesulam M-M (ed): *Principles of Behavioral Neurology.* Philadelphia: Davis, 1985, pp 327–346.
7. Picton TW: Human event-related potentials, in *Handbook of Electroencephalography and Clinical Neurophysiology.* Philadelphia: Elsevier, 1987, vol 3.
8. Klee M, Rall W: Computed potentials of cortically arranged populations of neurons. *J Neurophysiol* 40:647–666, 1977.
9. Gevins AS, Remond A: Methods of analysis of brain electrical and magnetic signals, in *Handbook of Electroencephalography and Clinical Neurophysiology.* New York, Elsevier, 1987, vol 1.
10. Robertson LC, Knight RT, Rafal R, Shimamura AP: Cognitive neuropsychology is more than single case studies. *J Exp Psychol* 19:710–717, 1993.
11. Stuss DT, Benson DF: *The Frontal Lobes.* New York: Raven Press, 1986.

12. Baddeley A: Working memory. *Science* 255:556–560, 1992.

13. Baddeley A: Working memory: The interface between memory and cognition. *J Cogn Neurosci* 4:281–288, 1992.

14. Goldman-Rakic PS: Circuitry of primate prefrontal cortex and regulation of behavior by representational memory, in Plum F (ed): *Handbook of Physiology: The Nervous System.* Baltimore: American Physiological Society, 1987, pp 373–417.

15. Petrides M, Alivisatos B, Meyer E, Evans AC: Functional activation of the human prefrontal cortex during the performance of verbal working memory tasks. *Proc Natl Acad Sci USA* 90:878–882, 1993.

16. Petrides M, Alivasatos B, Meyer E, Evans EC: Dissociation of human mid-dorsolateral from posterior dorsolateral frontal cortex in memory processing. *Proc Natl Acad Sci USA* 90:873–877, 1993.

17. Jonides J, Smith EE, Koeppe RA, et al: Spatial working memory in humans as revealed by PET. *Nature* 363:623–625, 1993.

18. Nielsen-Bohlman LC, Knight RT: Rapid memory mechanisms in man. *NeuroReport* 5:1517–1521, 1994.

19. Shimamura AP: Memory and the frontal lobe, in Gazzaniga M (ed): *The Cognitive Neurosciences.* Cambridge, MA: MIT Press, 1994, pp 803–813.

20. Lhermitte F: Human autonomy and the frontal lobes: Part II. Patient behavior in complex and social situations: The "environmental dependency syndrome." *Ann Neurol* 19:335–343, 1986.

21. Lhermitte F, Pillon B, Serdaru M: Human anatomy and the frontal lobes: Part I. Imitation and utilization behavior: A neuropsychological study of 75 patients. *Ann Neurol* 19:326–334, 1986.

21a. Edinger HM, Siegel A, Troiano R: Effect of stimulation of prefrontal cortex and amygdala on diencephalic neurons. *Brain Res* 97:17–31, 1975.

21b. Alexander GE, Newman JD, Symmes D: Convergence of prefrontal and acoustic inputs upon neurons in the superior temporal gyrus of the awake squirrel monkey. *Brain Res* 116:334–338, 1976.

22. Skinner JE, Yingling CD: Central gating mechanisms that regulate event-related potentials and behavior, in Desmedt JE (ed): *Progress in Clinical Neurophysiology* Basel: Karger, 1977, vol 1, pp 30–69.

22a. Yingling CD, Skinner JE: Gating of thalamic input to cerebral cortex by nucleus reticularis thalami, in Desmedt JE (ed): *Progress in Clinical Neurophysiology.* Basel: Karger, 1977, vol I, pp 70–96.

23. Kraus N, Ozdamar O, Stein L: Auditory middle latency responses (MLRs) in patients with cortical lesions. *Electroencephalogr Clin Neurophysiol* 54:275–287, 1982.

24. Leuders H, Leser RP, Harn J, et al: Cortical somatosensory evoked potentials in response to hand stimulation. *J Neurosurg* 58:885–894, 1983.

25. Sutherling WW, Crandall PH, Darcey TM, et al: The magnetic and electric fields agree with intracranial localizations of somatosensory cortex. *Neurology* 38:1705–1714, 1988.

26. Wood CC, Spencer DD, Allison T, et al: Localization of human sensorimotor cortex during surgery by cortical surface recording of somatosensory evoked potentials. *J Neurosurg* 68:99–111, 1988.

27. Knight RT, Scabini D, Woods DL: Prefrontal cortex gating of auditory transmission in humans. *Brain Res* 504:338–342, 1989.

28. Yamaguchi S, Knight RT: Gating of somatosensory inputs by human prefrontal cortex. *Brain Res* 521:281–288, 1990.

29. Sokolov EN: Higher nervous functions: The orienting reflex. *Annu Rev Physiol* 25:545–580, 1963.

30. Knight RT: Decreased response to novel stimuli after prefrontal lesions in man. *Electroencephalogr Clin Neurophysiol* 59:9–20, 1984.

31. Hillyard SA, Hink RF, Schwent UL, Picton TW: Electrical signs of selective attention in the human brain. *Science* 182:177–180, 1973.

32. McCallum WC, Curry SH, Cooper R, et al: Brain event–related potentials as indicators of early selective processes in auditory target localization. *Psychophysiology* 20:1–17, 1983.

33. Woldorff MG, Hillyard SA: Modulation of early auditory processing during selective listening to rapidly presented tones. *Electroencephalogr Clin Neurophysiol* 79:170–191, 1991.

34. Desmedt JE, Hut NT, Bourguet M: The cognitive P40, N60, and P100 components of somatosensory evoked potentials and the earliest signs of sensory processing in man. *Electroencephalogr Clin Neurophysiol* 56:272–282, 1983.

35. Woods DL: The physiological basis of selective attention: Implications of event-related potential studies, in Rohrbaugh JW, Parasuraman R, Johnson R Jr (eds): *Event-Related Brain Potentials.* New York: Oxford University Press, 1990, pp 178–210.

36. Broadbent DE: *Perception and Communication.* London: Pergamon Press, 1958.

37. Treisman AM: Contextual cues in selective listening. *Q J Exp Psychol* 12:242–248, 1960.

38. Kahneman D, Treisman A: Changing views of attention and automaticity, in Parasuraman R, Davies R (eds): *Varieties of Attention.* San Diego, CA: Academic Press, 1984, pp 29–61.

39. Gonzalez CMG, Clark VP, Fan S, et al: Sources of attention-sensitive visual event-related potentials. *Brain Topogr* 7:41–51, 1994.

40. Knight RT, Hillyard SA, Woods DL, Neville HJ: The effects of frontal cortex lesions on event-related potentials during auditory selective attention. *Electroencephalogr Clin Neurophysiol* 52: 571–582, 1981.

41. Mesulam MM: A cortical network for directed attention and unilateral neglect. *Ann Neurol* 10:309–325, 1981.

42. Kertesz A, Dobrolowski S: Right-hemisphere deficits: Lesion size and location. *J Clin Neurophysiol* 3:283–299, 1981.

43. Hier DB, Mondlock J, Caplan LR: Recovery of behavioral abnormalities after right hemisphere stroke. *Neurology* 33:345–350, 1983.

44. Stein S, Volpe BT: Classic "parietal" neglect syndrome after subcortical right frontal lobe infarction. *Neurology* 33:797–799.

45. Woods DL, Knight RT, Scabini D: Anatomical substrates of auditory selective attention: Behavioral and electrophysiological effects of temporal and parietal lesions. *Cogn Brain Res* 1:227–240, 1993.

46. Fuster JM: *The Prefrontal Cortex.* New York: Raven Press, 1980.

47. Bartus RT, Levere TE: Frontal decortication in rhesus monkeys: A test of the interference hypothesis. *Brain Res* 119:233–248, 1977.

48. Milner B: Some cognitive effects of frontal lesions in man. *Philos Trans R Soc Lond* 298:211–226, 1982.

49. Zattore RJ, Samson S: Role of the right temporal neocortex in retention of pitch in auditory short-term memory. *Brain* 114:2403–2407, 1991.

50. Jacobsen CF: Functions of frontal association areas in primates. *Arch Neurol Psychiatry* 33:568–569, 1935.

51. Brutkowski S: Functions of prefrontal cortex in animals. *Physiol Rev* 45:721–746, 1965.

52. Woods DL, Knight RT: Electrophysiological evidence of increased distractibility after dorsolateral prefrontal lesions. *Neurology* 36:212–216, 1986.

53. Chao L, Knight RT: Human prefrontal lesions increase distractibility to irrelevant sensory inputs. *NeuroReport* 6:1605–1610, 1995.

54. Walter WG, Cooper R, Aldridge V, et al: Contingent negative variation: An electrical sign of sensorimotor association and expectancy in the human brain. *Nature* 203:380–384, 1964.

55. Goldman-Rakic PS: Cellular and circuit basis of working memory in prefrontal cortex of nonhuman primates. *Progr Brain Res* 85:325–336, 1990.

56. Goldman-Rakic PS, Selemon LD, Schwartz ML: Dual pathways connecting the dorsolateral prefrontal cortex with the hippocampal formation and parahippocampal cortex in the rhesus monkey. *Neuroscience* 12:719–743, 1984.

57. Funahashi S, Bruce CJ, Goldman-Rakic PS: Dorsolateral prefrontal lesions and oculomotor delayed-response performance: Evidence for mnemonic "scotomas." *J Neurosci* 13:1479–1497, 1993.

57a. Goldman-Rakic PS, Bates JF, Chefee MV: The prefrontal cortex and internally generated motor acts. *Curr Opin Neurobiol* 2:830–835, 1992.

58. Chao LL, Knight RT: Age related prefrontal changes during auditory memory. *Soc Neurosci* 20:1003, 1994.

59. Rosahl S, Knight RT: Prefrontal cortex contribution to the contingent negative variation. *Cereb Cortex* 5:123–134, 1995.

60. Sutton S, Baren M, Zubin J, John ER: Evoked potentials correlates of stimulus uncertainty. *Science* 150:1187–1188, 1965.

61. Desmedt JE, Debecker J, Manil J: Mise en evidence d'un signe electrique cerebral associe a la detection par le sujet d'un stimulus sensoriel tactile. *Bull Acad R Med Belgique* 5:887–936, 1965.

62. Ehlers CL, Wall TL, Chapin RI: Long latency event-related potentials in rats: Effects of dopaminergic and serotonergic depletions. *Pharmacol Biochem Behav* 38:789–793, 1991.

63. Yamaguchi S, Globus H, Knight RT: P3-like potentials in rats. *Electroencephalogr Clin Neurophysiol* 88:151–154, 1993.

64. Wilder MB, Farley GR, Starr A: Endogenous late positive component of the evoked potential in cats corresponding to P300 in humans. *Science* 211:605–607, 1981.

65. O'Connor T, Starr A: Intracranial potentials correlated with an event-related potential, P300, in the cat. *Science* 339:27–28, 1985.

66. Katayama Y, Tsukiyama T, Tsubokawa T: Thalamic negativity associated with the endogenous positive component of cerebral evoked potentials

(P300): Recording using discriminative aversive conditioning in humans and cats. *Brain Res Bull* 14:223–226, 1985.

67. Arthur DL, Starr A: Task-relevant late positive component of the auditory event-related potential in monkeys resembles P300 in humans. *Science* 223:186–188, 1984.

68. Neville HJ, Foote SL: Auditory event-related potentials in the squirrel monkey: Parallels to human late wave responses. *Brain Res* 298:107–116, 1984.

69. Paller KA, Zola-Morgan S, Squire LR, Hillyard SA: P3-like brain wave in normal monkeys and in monkeys with medial temporal lesions. *Behav Neurosci* 102:714–725, 1988.

70. Pineda JA, Foote SL, Neville HJ: Effects of locus coeruleus lesions on auditory, long-latency, event-related potentials in monkeys. *J Neurosci* 9:81–93, 1989.

71. Verleger R: Event-related potentials and cognition: A critique of the context updating hypothesis and an alternative interpretation of P3. *Behav Brain Sci* 11:343–356, 1988.

72. Donchin E, Coles MGH: Is the P300 component a manifestation of context updating? *Behav Brain Sci* 11:357–427, 1988.

73. Squires N, Squires K, Hillyard SA: Two varieties of long-latency positive waves evoked by unpredictable auditory stimuli in man. *Electroencephalogr Clin Neurophysiol* 38:387–401, 1975.

74. Courchesne E, Hillyard SA, Galambos R: Stimulus novelty, task relevance, and the visual evoked potential in man. *Electroencephalogr Clin Neurophysiol* 39:131–143, 1975.

75. Yamaguchi S, Knight RT: P300 generation by novel somatosensory stimuli. *Electroencephalogr Clin Neurophysiol* 78:50–55, 1991.

76. Ruchkin DS, Johnson R Jr, Canoune H, Ritter W: Short-term memory storage and retention: An event-related brain potential study. *Electroencephalogr Clin Neurophysiol* 76:419–439, 1990.

77. Ruchkin DS, Johnson R Jr, Canoune HL, et al: Multiple sources of P3b associated with different types of information. *Psychophysiology* 27:157–176, 1990.

78. Ruchkin DS, Johnson R Jr, Grafman J, et al: Distinctions and similarities among working memory processes: An event-related potential study. *Cogn Brain Res* 1:53–66, 1992.

79. Bruyant P, Garcia-Larrea L, Mauguiere F: Target side and scalp topography of the somatosensory P300. *Electroencephalogr Clin Neurophysiol* 88:468–477, 1993.

80. McCarthy G, Wood CC, Williamson PD, Spencer DD: Task-dependent field potentials in human hippocampal formation. *J Neurosci* 9:4253–4260, 1989.

81. Puce A, Andrewes DG, Berkovic SF, Bladin PF: Visual recognition memory: Neurophysiological evidence for the role of temporal white matter in man. *Brain* 114:1647–1666, 1991.

82. Paller KA, McCarthy G, Roessler E, et al: Potentials evoked in human and monkey medial temporal lobe during auditory and visual oddball paradigms. *Electroencephalogr Clin Neurophysiol* 84:269–279, 1992.

83. Paller KA, McCarthy G, Wood CC: Event-related potentials elicited by deviant endings to melodies. *Psychophysiology* 29:202–206, 1992.

84. Halgren E, Baudena P, Clarke JM, et al: Intracerebral potentials to rare target and distractor auditory and visual stimuli: I. Superior temporal plane and parietal lobe. *Electroencephalogr Clin Neurophysiol* 94:191–220, 1995.

85. Halgren E, Baudena P, Clarke JM, et al: Intracerebral potentials to rare target and distractor stimuli: II. Medial, lateral and posterior temporal lobe. *Electroencephalogr Clin Neurophysiol* 94:229–250, 1995.

86. Baudena P, Halgren E, Heit G, Clarke JM: Intracerebral potentials to rare target and distractor auditory and visual stimuli: III. Frontal cortex. *Electroencephalogr Clin Neurophysiol* 94:251–264, 1995.

87. Johnson R Jr: Scalp-recorded P300 activity in patients following unilateral temporal lobectomy. *Brain* 111:1517–1529, 1988.

88. Knight RT, Scabini D, Woods DL, Clayworth CC: Contribution of the temporal-parietal junction to the auditory P3. *Brain Res* 502:109–116, 1989.

89. Yamaguchi S, Knight RT: Anterior and posterior association cortex contributions to the somatosensory P300. *J Neurosci* 11:2039–2054, 1991.

90. Scabini D: Contribution of anterior and posterior association cortices to the human P300 cognitive event related potential. PhD dissertation. University of California, Davis: University Microfilms International, 1992.

91. Knight RT: Distributed cortical network for visual stimulus detection. *J Cogn Neurosci*. In press.

92. Heit G, Smith ME, Halgren E: Neuronal activity

in the human medial temporal lobe during recognition memory. *Brain* 113:1093–1112, 1990.

93. Schupp HT, Lutzenberger W, Rau H, Birbaumer N: Positive shifts of event-related potentials: A state of cortical disfacilitation as reflected by the startle reflex probe. *Electroencephalogr Clin Neurophysiol* 90:135–144, 1994.

94. Chao L, Nielsen-Bohlman L, Knight RT: Auditory event-related potentials dissociate early and late memory processes. *Electroencephalogr Clin Neurophysiol* 96:157–168, 1995.

95. Barrett G, Neshige R, Shibasaki H: Human auditory and somato-sensory event-related potentials: Effects of response condition and age. *Electroencephalogr Clin Neurophysiol* 66:409–419, 1987.

96. Johnson R Jr: Developmental evidence for modality-dependent P300 generators: A normative study. *Psychophysiology* 26:651–667, 1989.

97. Naumann E, Huber C, Maier S, et al: The scalp topography of P300 in the visual and auditory modalities: A comparison of three normalization methods and the control of statistical type II error. *Electroencephalogr Clin Neurophysiol* 83:254–264, 1992.

98. Johnson R Jr: Auditory and visual P300s in temporal lobectomy patients: Evidence for modality-dependent P300 generators. *Psychophysiology* 26:633–650, 1989.

99. Rogers RL, Baumann SB, Papanicolaou AC, et al: Localization of the P3 sources using magneto-encephalography and magnetic resonance imaging. *Electroencephalogr Clin Neurophysiol* 79:308–321, 1991.

100. Rogers RL, Papanicolaou AC, Baumann SB, Eisenberg HM: Late magnetic fields and positive evoked potentials following infrequent and unpredictable omissions of visual stimuli. *Electroencephalogr Clin Neurophysiol* 83:146–152, 1992.

101. Fabiani M, Karis D, Donchin E: P300 and recall in an incidental learning paradigm. *Psychophysiology* 23:298–300, 1986.

102. Neville HJ, Kutas M, Chesney G, Schmidt A: Event-related potentials during encoding and recognition memory of congruous and incongruous words. *J Memory Lang* 25:75–92, 1986.

103. Paller KA, Kutas M, Mayes AR: Neural correlates of encoding in an incidental learning paradigm. *Electroencephalogr Clin Neurophysiol* 55:417–426, 1987.

104. Rugg MD, Pickles CP, Potter DD, Roberts RC: Normal P300 following extensive damage to the left medial temporal lobe. *J Neurol Neurosurg Psychiatry* 54:217–222, 1991.

105. Rugg MD, Roberts RC, Potter DD, et al: Event-related potentials to recognition memory: Effects of unilateral temporal lobectomy and temporal lobe epilepsy. *Brain* 114: 2313–2332, 1991.

106. Halgren E, Squires NK, Wilson CL, et al: Endogenous potentials generated in the human hippocampal formation and amygdala by infrequent events. *Science* 210:803–805, 1980.

107. Polich J, Squires LR: P300 from amnesic patients with bilateral hippocampal lesions. *Electroencephalogr Clin Neurophysiol* 86:408–417, 1993.

108. Onofrj M, Fulgente T, Malatesta G, et al: P3 recordings in patients with bilateral temporal lobe lesions. *Neurology* 42:1762–1767, 1992.

109. O'Donnell BF, Cohen RC, Hokama H, et al: Electrical source analysis of auditory ERPs in medial temporal lobe amnestic syndrome. *Electroencephalogr Clin Neurophysiol* 87:394–402, 1993.

110. Knight RT: Evoked potential studies of attention capacity in human frontal lobe lesions, in Levin H, Eisenberg H, Benton F (eds): *Frontal Lobe Function and Dysfunction,* New York: Oxford University Press, 1991, pp 139–153.

111. Knight RT: Effects of hippocampal lesions on the human P300 (abstr). *Soc Neuroscience* 17:657, 1991.

112. Smith ME, Halgren E, Sokolik ME, et al: The intra-cranial topography of the P3 event-related potential elicited during auditory oddball. *Electroencephalogr Clin Neurophysiol* 76:235–248, 1990.

113. Scabini D, McCarthy G: Hippocampal responses to novel somatosensory stimuli (abstr). *Soc Neurosci* 19:564, 1993.

114. Tranel D, Damasio H: Neuroanatomical correlates of electrodermal skin conductance responses. *Psychophysiology* 31:427–438, 1994.

115. Yamaguchi S, Knight RT: Effects of temporal-parietal lesions on the somatosensory P3 to lower limb stimulation. *Electroencephalogr Clin Neurophysiol* 84:139–148, 1992.

116. Verleger R, Heide W, Butt C, Kompf D: Reduction of P3b potentials in patients with temporo-parietal lesions. *Cogn Brain Res* 2:103–116, 1994.

117. Hikosaka K, Iwai E, Saito H, Tanaka K: Polyresponse properties of neurons in the anterior bank of the caudal superior temporal sulcus of the macaque monkey. *J Neurophysiol* 60:1615–1637, 1988.

118. Amaral DG, Inausti R, Cowan WM: Evidence for a direct projection from the superior temporal gyrus to the entorhinal cortex in the monkey. *Brain Res* 275:263–277, 1983.

119. Colombo M, D'Amato MR, Rodman HR, Gross CG: Auditory association cortex lesions impair auditory short-term memory in monkeys. *Science* 247:3336–338, 1990.

120. Eichenbaum H, Otto T, Cohen N: Two functional components of the hippocampal memory system. *Behav Brain Sci* 17:449–518, 1994.

121. Swick D, Knight RT: Effects of frontal cortex lesions on ERPs and repetition priming in a lexical decision task (abstr). *Soc Neurosci* 19:791, 1993.

122. Friedman HR, Goldman-Rakic PS: Coactivation of prefrontal and inferior parietal cortex in working memory tasks revealed by 2DG functional mapping in the rhesus monkey. *Neuroscience* 14:2775–2788, 1994.

123. Scabini D, Knight RT: Frontal lobe contributions to the human P3a. *Soc Neurosci* 15:477, 1989.

124. Kimble DP, Bagshaw MH, Pribram KH: The GSR of monkeys during orienting and habituation after selective partial ablations of the cingulate and frontal cortex. *Neuropsychology* 3:121–128, 1965.

125. Knight RT, Grabowecky M: Escape from linear time: Prefrontal cortex and conscious experience, in Gazzaniga M (ed): *The Cognitive Neurosciences.* Cambridge, MA: MIT Press, 1994, pp 1357–1371.

126. Perani D, Bressi S, Cappa SF, et al: Evidence of multiple memory systems in the human brain: A 18F FDG PET metabolic study. *Brain* 116:903–919, 1993.

127. Karis D, Fabiani M, Donchin E: "P300" and memory: Individual differences in the Von Restorff effect. *Cogn Psychol* 16:177–216, 1984.

128. Fabiani M, Gratton G, Chiarenzo GA, Donchin E: A psychophysiological investigation of the von Restorff paradigm in children. *J Psychophysiol* 4:15–24, 1990.

129. Metcalfe J: Novelty monitoring, metacognition, and control in a composite holographic associative recall model: Implications for Korsakoff amnesia. *Psychol Rev* 100:3–22, 1993.

130. Kutas M, Van Petten C: Event-related brain potential studies of language, in Ackles PK, Jennings JR, Coles MGH (eds): *Advances in Psychophysiology.* Greenwich, CT: JAI Press, 1988, vol 3.

131. Kutas M, Hillyard SA: Reading senseless sentences: Brain potentials reflect semantic incongruity. *Science* 207:203–205, 1980.

132. Noldy-Cullum NE, Stelmack RM: Recognition memory for pictures and words: The effect of incidental and intentional learning on N400, in Johnson R Jr, Rohrbaugh JW, Parasuraman R (eds): *Current Trends in Event-Related Potential Research.* Amsterdam: Elsevier, 1987, EEG suppl. 40:350–354.

133. Barrett SE, Rugg MD, Perrett DI: Event-related potentials and the matching of familiar and unfamiliar faces. *Neuropsychology* 26:105–117, 1988.

134. Friedman D: Cognitive event-related potential components during continuous recognition memory for pictures. *Psychophysiology* 27:136–148, 1990.

135. Nigam A, Hoffman JE, Simons RF: N400 to semantically anomalous pictures and words. *J Cogn Neurosci* 4:15–22, 1992.

136. Besson M, Macar F: An event-related potential analysis of incongruity in music and other nonlinguistic contexts. *Psychophysiology* 24:14–25, 1987.

137. Nobre AC, McCarthy G: Language-related ERPs: Scalp distributions and modulation by word type and semantic priming. *J Cogn Neurosci* 6:233–255, 1994.

138. Smith ME, Stapleton JM, Halgren E: Human medial temporal lobe potentials evoked in memory and language tasks. *Electroencephalogr Clin Neurophysiol* 63:145–159, 1986.

139. McCarthy G, Nobre AC, Bentin S, Spencer DD: Language-related field potentials in the anterior-medial temporal lobe: I. Intracranial distribution and neural generators. *J Neurosci* 15:1080–1089, 1995.

140. Nobre AC, McCarthy G: Language-related field potentials in the anterior-medial temporal lobe: II. Effects of word type and semantic priming. *J Neurosci* 15:1090–1098, 1995.

141. Hagoort P, Brown CM, Swaab T: Lexical-semantic event-related potential effects in left hemisphere patients with aphasia and right hemisphere patients without aphasia. *Brain.* In press.

142. Damasio H, Frank R: Three-dimensional in vivo mapping of brain lesions in humans. *Arch Neurol* 40:138–142, 1992.

Chapter 8

COMPUTATIONAL MODELING IN BEHAVIORAL NEUROLOGY AND NEUROPSYCHOLOGY

Martha J. Farah

COGNITION AS COMPUTATION

If the insights of cognitive psychology had to be boiled down to a single statement, a good candidate would be "cognition is computation." Starting with the work of Allen Newell and Herbert Simon in the sixties,[1] psychologists have been able to explain a wide range of human behavior in terms of information encoded from the environment, information stored in memory, and mechanisms for combining these two sources of information to select appropriate actions.

Viewing cognition as computation freed the field of psychology from the constraints of Skinnerian behaviorism, in which all psychological explanation was confined to directly observable entities such as stimulus and response. According to behaviorism, to hypothesize about the internal mental states intervening between stimulus and response was unscientific, nonexplanatory, and downright mystical. The information processing of computers provided a concrete demonstration that the states intervening between stimulus and response could also be within the domain of objective science. Hypothesizing about the knowledge that caused a person to act one way rather than another is no more mystical than hypothesizing about the stored data in a computer that caused it to give one output rather than another. The computational view of the mind made it possible to have a *psychological* level of explanation—dealing with entities such as memory, knowledge, inference, and decision—that could be understood as a function of perfectly nonmystical *physical* mechanisms.

There are many different ways that physical mechanisms can process information. The best known, and in many ways the most powerful, is the way computers work. Symbolically coded information is retrieved from a particular physical memory location, operated upon in a physically distinct central processing unit according to stored instructions, and then reentered into memory. Most of the early theories of cognitive psychology assumed this type of computational architecture. More recently, a very different computational architecture has been explored by computer scientists, psychologists, and neuroscientists, which has more in common with brains than with office computers. This is the parallel distributed processing (PDP) architecture. Because PDP is similar in many ways to neural information processing, PDP models have increasingly come to be used in neuropsychology.

Computation has played two roles in cognitive psychology and neuropsychology. In some cases theories are simply expressed in terms of the concepts of computation: the informational content and format of representations, the parallel or serial nature of searches, and the like. In other cases, researchers implement their theories as running computer simulations. With the advent of the PDP architecture, computer simulation is increasingly used. One reason for this is that the behavior of PDP systems is not always obvious or predictable by intuition alone.

PARALLEL DISTRIBUTED PROCESSING

Parallel distributed processing systems consist of a large number of highly interconnected neuronlike units. These units are connected to one another by weighted connections that determine how much activation from one unit flows to another. There is no central controller governing the behavior of the network. Rather, each part of the network functions locally and in parallel with the other parts, hence the first P in PDP. Representations consist of the pattern of activation distributed over a population of units, and long-term memory knowledge is encoded in the pattern of connection strengths distributed among a population of units, hence the D. Alternative terms for PDP include *connectionism* (not to be confused with the center-and-pathway approach of Wernicke and his followers, which has also been called connectionism), *brain-style computation,* and *artificial neural networks.* For more than the brief overview offered here, the reader is directed to Rumelhart and McClelland's classic two-volume book on PDP[2] or more recent books by Anderson[3] (for a technical introduction) or Bechtel and Abrahamsen[4] (for a conceptual and philosophical introduction).

There are many types of PDP networks with different computational properties. Among the features that determine network type are the activation rule, connectivity, and the learning rule. The activation rule governs how the activation values of units are updated given a certain input activation. Units' activations can be discrete or continuous, and activations may be increased in direct proportion to the sum of the inputs (a *linear activation function*) or as a nonlinear function of the inputs (generally a sigma-shaped function). The activation rule has a variety of consequences for network behavior, some of which are not immediately obvious. For example, as noted below, purely linear networks will not be able to learn certain kinds of associations.

A major distinguishing feature is connectivity, which can be unidirectional, in which case the network is called *feedforward,* or bidirectional, in which case it is called *interactive.* Feedforward networks may consist simply of a set of input units and a set of output units. A pattern associator can be made from such a network if the weights between the first- and second-layer units are set so that each of a set of patterns of activation over the units in the first layer evokes an associated pattern over the units in the second layer. Some feedforward networks have an additional set of so-called *hidden units* interposed between the input and output units. With nonlinear systems, the additional set of units is useful in transforming the input patterns of activation to the desired output patterns; indeed, certain types of problems (such as associating input patterns 00 and 11 with one output and 01 and 10 with another, the "XOR" problem) can be solved only with hidden units. In *recurrent networks,* later layers loop back to earlier layers. In interactive networks, some or all connections are bidirectional. In recurrent and interactive networks, "downstream" units can influence "upstream" units; more than one processing step is therefore needed to arrive at their final activation state. These networks are said to "settle into" a stable state after the addition of an input pattern of activation.

Learning in neural networks consists of adjusting the weights between units so that, given a set of input activation patterns, in each case the network ends up in the desired activation state. For example, for a network to learn that a certain name goes with a certain face, the weights among units in the network are adjusted so that presentation of either the face pattern in the units representing faces or the name pattern in the units representing names causes the corresponding other pattern to become activated.

There is a wide variety of learning algorithms, and the choice depends in part on the type of network and the task to be learned. A learning rule proposed many decades ago by the neuroscientist Donald Hebb[5] forms the basis for many current learning algorithms. The gist of the *Hebb rule* is: Neurons that fire together wire together. In other words, when there is a positive correlation in the activity of two units, strengthen their connection so that future activation of one will be even more likely to activate the other. This form of the rule enables *unsupervised learning*—that is, learning without a teacher to direct what is learned. Networks that use unsupervised learning are called *self-organizing,* as they develop their own representations of regularities in their input—for example, developing edge representations from center-surround-like inputs[6] or semantic representations from patterns of word co-occurrence[7] (see Ref. 8 for additional information on self-organizing systems).

The Hebb rule can also be used to learn to associate patterns, but only if the input patterns are orthogonal, a rather stringent requirement. When the object is to learn to associate or complete patterns, then *supervised* learning is normally used. The *delta rule* is an example of a supervised learning rule that can be viewed as a variant of the Hebb rule. Both learning rules change weights proportionate with a comparison between activation values; in the case of supervised learning, the comparison is between desired activation value and actual activation value, an error measure. Networks with hidden units demand yet a further modification of the learning rule, as the weights to be changed do not directly link the input with the output units from which the error measure is derived. The *generalized delta rule,* or *backpropagation,* is often used in this case. With this rule, the error in the output units is propagated back to alter the weights of the (nonadjacent) input units.

Further discussion of learning rules is beyond the scope of this chapter, except to note that learning in PDP models is often not intended to simulate real learning. Rather, it is frequently used as a tool for setting the weights in a network so that the network can simulate some aspect of cognition in its mature end state. Backpropagation is sometimes criticized for being physiologically implausible. This may or may not be a valid criticism, depending on the goal of the simulation. For example, if one were interested in studying the effects of damage to the face-recognition system, one would need a model of face recognition that embodied a set of associations between facial appearance and other knowledge about people, on which one could inflict damage. As it is virtually impossible to "hand wire" networks of more than a few units, learning rules would be used to build in these associations. However, they would not be simulating in the way in which people learn face recognition. For this reason it might be less confusing to refer to learning algorithms for neural networks as weight-setting algorithms unless the learning process is explicitly being modeled.

How Realistic Are PDP Models?

Of course, there are cases when real human learning is the subject of the model, and then we are right to inquire whether or in what sense the model's learning is similar to human learning. More generally, it is important to consider whether PDP is a reasonable model for human brain function.

Parallel distributed processing models differ from real neural networks, including the human brain, in numerous ways: Even the biggest PDP networks are tiny compared to the brain; PDP models have just one kind of unit, compared to a variety of types of neurons; and just one kind of activation (which can act excitatorily or inhibitorily), rather than a multitude of different neurotransmitters; and so on. Yet these differences are not necessarily cause to reject the PDP approach. No model is identical in all respects to the system being modeled; models possess theory-relevant and theory-irrelevant attributes. Furthermore, science must often simplify nature in order to understand it. Parallel distributed processing models should be viewed as simplifications of the brain, possessing enough theory-relevant attributes of the brain to be informative on many questions but clearly leaving out or even contradicting many known aspects of brain function.

Among the theory-relevant aspects of PDP models are the use of distributed representations, the large number of inputs to and outputs from each unit, the modifiable connections between units, and the existence of both inhibitory and excitatory connections, summation rules, bounded activations, and thresholds. Parallel distributed processing models allow us to find out what aspects of behavior, normal and pathologic, can be explained by this set of theory-relevant attributes. Of course, some behavior may be explainable only with the incorporation of other features of neuro-anatomy and neurophysiology not currently used in PDP models. This seems quite likely, and the discovery of such instances will be extremely informative with respect to the functional significance of these features of our biology. However, note that this problem does not apply to cases in which the current models perform well. In such cases, the only danger associated with nonrealism is that the model's success might depend on a theory-irrelevant simplification. For example, scale is generally treated as theory-irrelevant, but it is possible that certain mechanisms will work only for small networks or small amounts of knowledge. We must be on the lookout for such cases but also recognize that it is unlikely that the success of most models will happen to depend critically on their unrealistic features.

Spatial Analogies for Understanding the Behavior of PDP Networks

Spatial analogies are useful for visualizing certain aspects of network dynamics, including the way in which the network's patterns of activation change under the influence of an input and the way in which the ensemble of weights changes during learning. The activation state of the network at any point in time can be represented as a point in a high-dimensional space called *activation space*. The dimensions of this space represent the level of activation of each unit in the network, assuming a fixed set of weights. In addition to the dimensions representing the activation levels of the units, there is one additional dimension, representing the overall "fit" between the current activation pattern and the weights.

When units that are both active have a large positive weight between them, so that they reinforce each other's activation, this is an example of a good fit. If both units are active and the weight between them is negative (i.e., inhibitory), the fit will be poor. This measure of fit is called "energy," with low energy representing a better fit. The energy value associated with each pattern of activation defines a surface in activation space.

When an input pattern is presented to the network, the corresponding initial position in activation space is defined by the activation levels on the input units, along with resting-level values for the dimensions representing the other units in the network. The weights in the rest of the network will not fit well with uniform resting-level activation values over their portion of the network. Thus, the initial point in activation space will be in a region of high energy. As activation propagates through the network, the pattern of activation changes and the point representing this pattern moves along the energy surface in activation space. The movement will be generally downward, as the network lowers its energy, much as a ball rolls down a hill to lower its potential energy. To see why this would happen in terms of network dynamics rather than by analogy with rolling balls, consider the examples given earlier of high- and low-energy activation states. For example, active units connected by negative weights (a poor-fit, high-energy pattern) will tend to change their activations until one is active and the other is not (a good-fit, low-energy pattern).

The energy minima toward which the network tends are termed *attractors*. Attractors are useful in network computation not only for associating patterns and completing partial patterns but also for their ability to "clean up" a noisy input by transforming a pattern similar to a known pattern into that known pattern (i.e., a pattern just uphill from an attractor will roll down into the attractor).

The shape of the energy landscape is determined by the network's weights. In an untrained network, the landscape will be generally flat with random hills and valleys. When the network has learned a certain association, its weights will create an energy landscape in activation space in which the point corresponding to the input pattern and the attractor point corresponding to the complete associated pattern are connected by a smoothly and steeply sloping path that causes the one state to "roll" down into the other.

The weights that determine the attractor structure of activation space can themselves be used to define a space, and this space is useful for visualizing the process of learning. In *weight space*, each of the weights in a network corresponds to one dimension of a space, so that we can represent the sum total of the network's knowledge as a point in this high-dimensional space. If one additional dimension is now added to the space, representing the performance of the network at associating names and faces (an error measure of some sort), then there will be a surface defined by each combination of weights and their associated error measure. Learning consists of moving along this surface in weight space, changing weight values, until a sufficiently low point has been reached.

APPLICATIONS OF COMPUTATIONAL MODELING TO BEHAVIORAL NEUROLOGY AND NEUROPSYCHOLOGY

For most of the history of behavioral neurology and neuropsychology, the lesion method has been our primary source of insights into human brain organization. Yet the interpretation of lesion effects is not always as transparent as one would like. As early as the nineteenth century, authors such as John Hughlings-Jackson[9] cautioned that the brain is a distributed and highly interactive system, such that local damage to one part can unleash new modes of functioning in the remaining parts of the system. As a result, one cannot assume that a patient's behavior following brain damage is the direct result of a simple subtraction of one or more components of the mind, with those that remain functioning normally. More likely, it results from a combination of the subtraction of some components and changes in the functioning of other components that had previously been influenced by the missing components.

Parallel distributed processing provides a conceptual framework, and concrete tools, for reasoning about the effects of local lesions in distributed, interactive systems.[10] It has already proven helpful in understanding a number of different neuropsychological disorders. Each of the examples reviewed here constitutes a reinterpretation of a well-known disorder, with qualitatively different implications for the normal organization of the

brain and the functional locus of damage within that organization.

Deep Dyslexia: Interpreting Error Types

Patients with deep dyslexia (see Chap. 13) make two very different types of reading errors, which have been interpreted as indicating that two functionally distinct lesions are needed to account for these errors. Deep dyslexics make semantic errors, that is, errors that bear a semantic similarity to the correct word, such as reading *cat* as "dog." They also make visual errors—that is, errors that bear a visual (graphemic) similarity to the correct word, such as reading *cat* as "cot." The fact that both semantic and visual errors are common in deep dyslexia has been taken to imply that deep dyslexics have multiple lesions, with one affecting the visual system and another affecting semantic knowledge. However, a consideration of the effects of single lesions in a network with attractor states suggests that a single lesion is sufficient to account for these patients' errors. Furthermore, it suggests that mixtures of error types will be the rule rather than the exception when the system that has been damaged normally functions to transform the stimulus representation from one form that has one set of similarity relations (e.g., visual, in which *cot* and *cat* are similar) to another form with different similarity relations (e.g., semantic, in which *cot* and *bed* are similar).

Hinton and Shallice[11] trained the recurrent network shown in Fig. 8-1 to produce semantic representations of a set of words, given their printed orthography as input. The grapheme-to-"sememe" (their term for elements of semantic representation) mapping is carried out with the aid of hidden units, and the sememes are interconnected among themselves and connected to a final layer of semantic representation that connects, recurrently, back to the sememes. This pattern of connectivity in the semantic layers creates attractor states for the network. The input to the semantic layers need not be perfectly on target for the semantics of a particular word; as long as it is sufficiently similar to the correct semantics, which is an attractor state, it will be pulled in (i.e., as

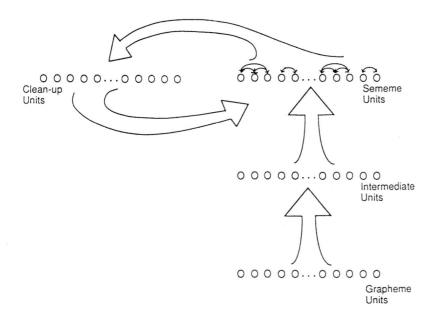

Clean-up
Units

Sememe
Units

Intermediate
Units

Grapheme
Units

Figure 8-1
Hinton and Shallice's[11] *PDP model of reading, in which visual graphemic representations are associated with semantic representations. Single lesions in this model produce a mixture of visual and semantic errors. (From Hinton and Shallice,*[11] *with permission.)*

long as it falls in a region of activation space that slopes downward to the correct activation pattern, it will be transformed into that pattern). Damage to the network from the removal of units or connections distorts the shape of activation space. Figure 8-2 illustrates the normal attractor structure of a region of activation space containing *cot, cat,* and *bed* and the altered structure following damage to semantics. Whereas before damage, "cat" fell into the *cat* basin of attraction, after damage, the edges of the basins have shifted and "cat" falls into the *cot* basin of attraction. Thus, one need not hypothesize damage to visual representations to account for the visual errors in deep dyslexia.

Plaut and Shallice[12] have demonstrated the generality of Hinton and Shallice's account by replicating their simulation results with a variety of different networks, with different patterns of connectivity, and with different training procedures. As long as there are attractors that serve to transform input patterns whose similarity relations are based on visual appearance into semantic representations whose similarity relations are based on meaning, the landscape of the activation space will be organized by both visual and semantic similarity, and distortions of that landscape due to net-

work damage will result in both visual and semantic errors.

Neglect Dyslexia: Localizing the Functional Lesion

Patients with left visual neglect omit or misidentify letters on the left side of letter strings. When the letter string is a word, this pattern of performance is termed *neglect dyslexia* (see Chap. 13). Surprisingly, neglect dyslexics are more likely to report the initial letters of a word than of a nonword letter string, even when the initial letters of the word cannot simply be guessed on the basis of the end of the word.[13] This seems to imply that the breakdown in the processing of neglected stimuli comes at a late stage, after word recognition, for how else could lexical status (word versus nonword) affect performance?

The concept of attractors is helpful here, too, in localizing the functional lesion in neglect dyslexia at a stage prior to visual pattern recognition. Mozer and Behrmann[14] simulated neglect dyslexia by damaging the attentional mechanism in a computational model of printed word recognition so that attention is distributed asymmetrically over

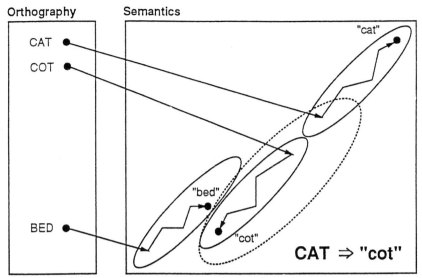

Figure 8-2
Part of the activation space of the Hinton and Shallice model, as represented by Plaut and Shallice,[12] showing attractors for three words. After damage to semantic units, the basins of attraction shift from those shown in solid lines to those shown in dotted lines, resulting in visual errors. (From Plaut and Shallice,[12] with permission.)

letter strings. In their model, attention *precedes* word recognition. In fact, it gates the flow of information out of early visual feature maps. Neglect therefore results in full information from the right side of a letter string but only partial information from the left being transmitted to word representations.

According to this model, the errors that occur with nonword letter strings result from partial visual information about the letter features on the left side of the string, which is not sufficient to identify precisely which letters are present. In contrast, the same partial information about the initial letters of a word, with good-quality information about the remaining letters of a word, will result in an activation pattern that is similar to the activation pattern for that word. Because known words are attractors, the network will settle into the pattern of the word, complete with initial letters. In this way, it is possible to explain why neglect dyslexics read words better than nonwords without giving up the hypothesis that neglect is a disorder

of visual perception, affecting stimulus processing prior to the word recognition stage.

Computational models make predictions that can be tested empirically. According to this model of neglect dyslexia, if the asymmetry of attention is too extreme, no information about the initial letters will get through to word representations and the resulting activation state will not fall within the basin of attraction for the word. Behrmann and colleagues tested this prediction with a patient who had severe neglect.[15] As predicted, he did not show better perception of the initial letters of words than of nonwords. Furthermore, when his attention was drawn to the left and the attentional asymmetry thereby was made less extreme, he then showed the usual difference between word and nonword letter strings. Conversely, a patient who normally showed this difference between words and nonwords was stopped from doing so by attentional manipulations that increased his attentional asymmetry.

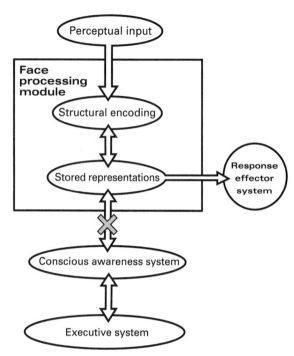

Figure 8-3

A model proposed by De Haan, Bauer, and Greve[16] to account for covert face recognition in prosopagnosia. There is a separate mechanism hypothesized for conscious awareness, distinct from the mechanisms of face recognition, and covert recognition is explained by a lesion at location 1, disconnecting the two parts of the model. (From De Haan et al.,[16] with permission.)

Covert Face Recognition: Dissociation without Separate Systems

Prosopagnosia is an impairment of face recognition that can occur relatively independently of impairments in object recognition (see Chap. 18). A number of recent findings seem to suggest that the underlying impairment, in at least some patients, is not in face recognition per se but in awareness of recognition (see Chap. 27). This would seem to imply that recognition and awareness depend on dissociable and distinct brain systems, as shown in Fig. 8-3.[16] My colleagues and I built a computer simulation that is able to account for covert recognition in three very different tasks.[17] The network

is shown in Fig. 8-4 and consists of face recognition units, semantic knowledge units, and name units (embodying knowledge of people's facial appearance, general information about them, and their names, respectively). Hidden units were interposed between these layers to assist the network in learning to associate faces and names by way of semantic information. There is no part of the network that is dedicated to awareness.

The first finding to be simulated was that some prosopagnosics can learn to associate facial photographs with names faster when the pairings are true (e.g., Harrison Ford's face with Harrison

Figure 8-4

A model proposed by Farah, Vecera, and O'Reilly[17] to account for covert face recognition in prosopagnosia. The dissociation between overt and covert face recognition emerges when the face-recognition system is damaged. (From Farah et al.,[17] with permission.)

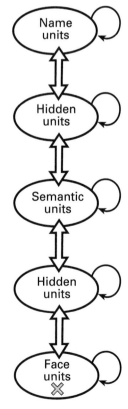

Ford's name) than when they are false (e.g., Harrison Ford's face with Michael Douglas's name).[18] This result was initially taken to imply that these patients were recognizing the faces normally and that the breakdown in processing lay downstream from vision, as shown in Fig. 8-3. However, when some of the face units were eliminated from our model, thus simulating a lesion in the visual system, the network also relearned old face-name pairings faster than new ones. Why should this be? Recall that learning can be viewed as a process of moving through weight space. After damage, the network is in a high-error region of weight space for both old face-name pairings and new ones, and for this reason the network cannot overtly associate any faces with any names. However, that region of weight space is closer to a low-error region for the old pairings than for the new ones, because the residual weights (connecting intact units) have the correct values for the old pairings, and the learning process is therefore shorter.

A second finding, that previously familiar faces are perceived more quickly in the context of a same/different matching task, has also been interpreted as evidence for intact visual face processing.[18] However, after lesions to the face units in our model, the remaining face units settled into a stable state faster for previously familiar face patterns. This can be understood in terms of the distortion of the network's attractor structure after damage. The original structure was designed to take familiar face patterns as input and settle quickly to a stable state. After damage, these patterns will still find themselves on downward-sloping parts of the energy landscape more often than novel patterns, even if the energy minima into which they roll have changed.

Finally, in a task that requires classifying a printed name as belonging to an actor or a politician, a face from the opposite occupational category shown in the background slows the responses of both normal subjects and a prosopagnosic, again implying that the face is recognized despite prosopagnosia.[18] In simulating this finding, face units were removed until the network's overt performance at classifying faces according to occupation

was as poor as the patient's. At this level of damage, wrong-category faces slowed performance in the name-classification task. This can be understood in terms of the distributed nature of representation in neural networks, which allows for partial representation of information when some but not all units representing a face have been eliminated. The partial information generally raises the activation of the appropriate downstream occupation units, thus biasing their responses to the printed names, but it is not generally able to raise their activations above threshold to allow an explicit response to faces.

REFERENCES

1. Newell A, Simon HA: *Human Problem Solving.* Englewood Cliffs, NJ: Prentice Hall, 1972.
2. Rumelhart DE, McClelland JL: *Parallel Distributed Processing: Explorations in the Microstructure of Cognition.* Cambridge, MA: MIT Press, 1986.
3. Anderson JA: *An Introduction to Neural Networks.* Cambridge, MA: MIT Press, 1995.
4. Bechtel W, Abrahamsen A: *Connectionism and the Mind.* Cambridge, MA: Blackwell, 1991.
5. Hebb DO: *The Organization of Behavior.* New York: Wiley, 1949.
6. Linsker R: From basic network principles to neural architecture: Emergence of orientation-selective cells. *Proc Natl Acad Sci USA* 83:8390–8394, 1986.
7. Ritter H: Self-organizing maps for internal representations. *Psychol Res* 52:128–136, 1990.
8. Kohonen T: *Self-Organizing Maps.* New York: Springer-Verlag, 1995.
9. Jackson JH: On the anatomical and physiological localization of movements in the brain. *Lancet* 1:84–85, 162–164, 232–234, 1873.
10. Farah MJ: Neuropsychological inference with an interactive brain. *Behav Brain Sci* 17:90–104, 1994.
11. Hinton GE, Shallice T: Lesioning an attractor network: Investigations of acquired dyslexia. *Psychol Rev* 98:96–121, 1991.
12. Plaut DC, Shallice T: Deep dyslexia: A case study of connectionist neuropsychology. *Cog Neuropsychol* 10:377–500, 1993.
13. Sieroff E, Pollatsek A, Posner MI: Recognition of

visual letter strings following injury to the posterior visual spatial attention system. *Cog Neuropsychol* 5:427–449, 1988.

14. Mozer MC, Behrmann M: On the interaction of selective attention and lexical knowledge: A connectionist account of neglect dyslexia. *J Cog Neurosci* 2:96–123, 1990.

15. Behrmann M, Moscovitch M, Black S, Mozer M: Perceptual and conceptual mechanisms in neglect dyslexia: Two contrasting case studies. *Brain* 113:1163–1183, 1990.

16. De Haan EHF, Bauer RM, Greve KW: Behavioral and physiological evidence for covert recognition in a prosopagnosic patient. *Cortex* 28:77–95, 1992.

17. Farah MJ, O'Reilly RC, Vecera SP: Dissociated overt and covert recognition as a emergent property of lesioned attractor networks. *Psychol Rev* 100:751–788, 1993.

18. De Haan EHF, Young AW, Newcombe F: Face recognition without awareness. *Cog Neuropsychol* 4:385–415, 1987.

Part 2

APHASIA AND OTHER DOMINANT HEMISPHERE SYNDROMES

Chapter 9

APHASIA: CLINICAL AND ANATOMIC ASPECTS

Michael P. Alexander

The clinical study of aphasia began in 1861 with the observations of Paul Broca.[1] Within 40 or 50 years, all of the basic clinical phenomena reviewed here had been described and many of the major flashpoints of clinical and theoretical disagreement had been identified. In the past 20 years, fresh interest has come to clinical aphasia research from two directions: modern neuroimaging and cognitive neurosciences. Together, they have additionally provided tools to carry out aphasia-related language experiments in normals. Furthermore, old questions such as cerebral laterality, the influence of handedness, the effects of gender and bilingualism on aphasia, and the mechanisms of recovery have been reexplored. Much of this chapter—which reviews the basic clinical features of aphasia—could have been written 20, 50, or even 100 years ago. In 1995, it is possible to consider this material with greater appreciation of the variability found in the basic syndromes, of their anatomic complexities, of the natural history of recovery, and (although here only briefly) of the cognitive and linguistic deficits that fundamentally underlie the classic syndromes. The chapters on neuroimaging and on cognitive analysis of aphasia should be read along with this chapter.

CLINICAL SYNDROMES

The description of syndromes of aphasia arose out of much the same motivation as the identification of other clinical neurologic syndromes: the need

to identify clinically useful associations between specific clusters of signs and the likely anatomy of the lesion producing them. The most clinically transparent signs of aphasia have generally been taken to be independent signs of brain damage. Thus, syndromes have been constructed out of reduced language output as well as impaired comprehension, repetition, and naming. Disorders of written language have been divided into additional syndromes only as reading and writing have been impaired beyond spoken language impairments. Using three independent signs will generate eight syndromes, assuming naming to be impaired in all aphasics.

Although these syndromes have reasonable clinical validity, there are numerous limitations to this type of syndrome construction. First, the syndromes depend on a sign being normal or not, much as a hemiparesis is present or absent; but the complexity of impairments in comprehension and language production are less amenable to simple dichotomous judgments. Thus, distinctions come to depend on the statistical properties and structural assumptions of the test. Second, there is no certainty that signs all have the same pathophysiologic mechanism in all patients. For comprehension at the sentence level, in particular, there may be several independent pathways to impairment.[2] Third, the syndromes are not stable even when the anatomy is. A patient with a temporoparietal stroke may have an initial Wernicke's aphasia, but, over weeks, language improves to reach the clinical diagnosis of conduction aphasia.[3] Does one conclude that the behavioral-anatomic correlations are with Wernicke's or conduction aphasia? Can one be certain that there are two distinct syndromes if they blur into each other? Should one conclude that only the early-phase correlations hold, that all correlations have built in corollaries about recovery, or that both are true? Fourth, most syndromes are polytypic—that is, they are defined by several criteria.[4] What do we conclude if only some of the criteria are met? Would this be a less severe syndrome? A subsyndrome? A different syndrome altogether?

Despite these limitations, the classic syndromes do have utility. They serve as a type of shorthand for clinical communications. If told that a patient has transcortical motor aphasia 2 weeks after a stroke, one would know approximately what to expect of language examinations, what the range of possible brain lesions would be, what the prognosis should be, and what some reasonable treatments might be. If inclined, one would even know what interesting cognitive neuroscience issues the patient might illuminate.

Broca's Aphasia

In Broca's aphasia, language output is nonfluent—that is, it is reduced in phrase length and grammatical complexity. This reduction can range from no recognizable output or repeated meaningless utterances to short, truncated phrases using only the most meaning-laden words (substantives). There is usually considerable hesitation and delay in production. Speech quality is impaired. Articulation is poor (dysarthria). Melodic line is disrupted (dysprosody), partly due to dysarthria but often more than just secondary to it. Volume is usually reduced at first (hypophonia). With time, speech takes on hyperkinetic (dystonic and spastic) qualities. Language comprehension is adequate although rarely normal. Response to word-recognition tasks, simple commands, and routine conversation is generally good. Response to multistep commands and complex syntactical requests is generally poor. Repetition is poor, although often better than speech. Relational words (functors—articles, conjunctions, modifiers, etc.)

may be produced in repetition, but they are exceedingly uncommon in spontaneous speech. Written language parallels spoken, although some patients, while never regaining useful speech, develop writing that is telegraphic. Oral reading is usually agrammatic; so-called deep dyslexia (see Chap. 13) may emerge with this.[5] Naming is usually poor, but it may be surprisingly good in chronic patients. All types of errors can occur, although semantic errors are most typical for substantive words.[6] Objects are frequently named better than are actions.[7]

Broca's aphasia is commonly accompanied by right hemiparesis, buccofacial apraxia, and ideomotor apraxia of the left arm (or both arms in the nonparetic case). Right-sided sensory loss and right visual field impairments (extinction and/or lower-quadrant deficit) are less frequent. Depression, frequently major, develops in approximately 40 percent of patients with Broca's aphasia.[8]

Many patients have fractional syndromes of Broca's aphasia. Because all of these fractional disorders are still taxonomically closer to Broca's aphasia than to any of the other seven classic diagnoses, many aphasia systems will classify them all as Broca's aphasia.[9] In analyzing reports of Broca's aphasia, it is crucial to understand the taxonomic rules of the report's assessment tool. If all fractional cases are considered Broca's aphasia, the clinicoanatomic correlations will seem imprecise. This is an example of the difficulty inherent in building syndromes with polytypic qualities. Analysis of the clinicoanatomic relationships within these fractional cases may be much more informative than lumping them all together on the basis of some overlap with the full syndrome.

Chronic Broca's Aphasia

This syndrome, as described above, often emerges out of global aphasia.[10] Damage can vary in extent; there does not seem to be a necessary and sufficient lesion profile. The most common pattern is extensive dorsolateral frontal, opercular, rolandic, and anterolateral parietal cortical damage plus lateral striatal and extensive paraventricular white

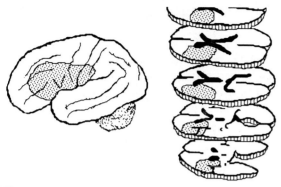

Figure 9-1
Typical lesion associated with severe chronic Broca's aphasia.

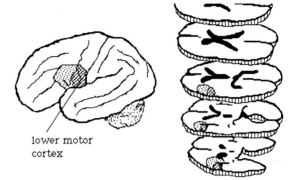

lower motor cortex

Figure 9-2
Lesion distributions of incomplete forms of Broca's aphasia. The entire lesion would produce "acute" Broca's aphasia. The anterior component involved alone (stippled area) would typically evolve toward transcortical motor aphasia. The posterior component involved alone would typically evolve toward aphemia. In either case, the residual aphasia would be mild.

matter damage (Fig. 9-1).[11] Particularly critical to chronic Broca's aphasia is the subcortical extension of the lesion.[12] Long-lasting mutism can be seen after anterior deep lesions, undercutting supplementary motor area and cingulate-caudate projections.[13] Deep anterior periventricular white matter lesions disrupt dorsolateral frontal-caudate systems involved in ready access to complex output procedures.[14] They may also disrupt ascending anterior thalamic-frontal projections. Anterior supraventricular deep white matter lesions disrupt callosal frontal projections. Large periventricular and subcortical white matter lesions can disrupt all of the long parietotemporal to frontal projection pathways. All the distant corticocortical systems will be disrupted. A combination of these systems' disruptions seems to be the structural basis of persistent Broca's aphasia even with subcortical lesions only.

Acute Broca's Aphasia

Infarctions or trauma that produce acute Broca's aphasia often involve the frontal operculum, lower motor cortex, lateral striatum, and subcortical white matter (Fig. 9-2).[9,15] These patients recover over weeks to months, with variable mixtures of initiation delay, syntactic simplification, paraphasias, speech impairment, and usually with impaired repetition.

"Broca's Area" Lesion

Damage to the frontal operculum (areas 44 and 46) produces an acute aphasic disorder roughly compatible with Broca's aphasia (Fig. 9-2), but there is quite rapid improvement usually to transcortical motor aphasia or even just mild anomic aphasia.[9,15] Damage to the dorsolateral frontal cortex (areas 44, 46, 6, and 9) produces classic transcortical motor aphasia[13] (discussed in detail below). Damage to the subcortical frontal white matter or even to the dorsolateral caudate nuclei may produce the same deficit.[14] These observations suggest the existence of a "frontal-caudate" regional network required for construction of complex output procedures of language—syntax and narrative discourse at a minimum. Damage to this system is part of classic Broca's aphasia.

Lower Motor Cortex Lesion

Damage to the lower 50 percent of the prerolandic gyrus can acutely produce a deficit pattern roughly compatible with mild Broca's aphasia, but there is rapid recovery to a much more limited disorder of speech—predominantly of articulation and prosody—sometimes called aphemia (Fig. 9-2).[16] Damage to the subcortical outflow of lower motor cortex can produce the same speech deficit, suggesting the existence of a local (rolandic) network for articulation and some aspects of prosody that project to the brainstem. This, too, is part of classic Broca's aphasia.

A rare variant of this restricted damage to motor systems of speech production is the foreign-accent syndrome.[17] A small number of cases have been described, usually emerging out of mild Broca's aphasia. In these patients, the predominant deficit is in speech prosody, but the quality of the prosodic deficit sounds to the listener like a foreign accent, not pathologic prosody. The reported lesions have all been in some component of the motor system for speech, either lower motor cortex[16] or putamen or deep connections between lower motor cortex and basal ganglia.[18,19] The precise speech impairment has not been consistent, and the foreign accent syndrome probably represents a heterogeneous group with partial damage to the motor speech apparatus.

For all of these variants and fractional syndromes of Broca's aphasia, some improvement can be expected. The severe cases that often emerge from global aphasia typically have better recovery of comprehension than of speech; this recovery that may continue over a very long time.[3,20] Minimal recovery of spoken or written output from essentially none to classic telegraphic output is usually accompanied by lesion extent throughout the deep frontal white matter from the middle periventricular region to the region anterior and superior to the frontal horn.[12] The outcome of the milder cases is partly determined by lesion size,[9] but for these smaller lesions, precise lesion site seems to best account for evolution into the various fractional systems.[10,15,16] In both severe and milder cases, some patients may recover by reorganizing cerebral functions to allow some right-brain control of speech. Evidence for this comes from patients with serial frontal lesions[21] and from temporary inactivation of the right brain (Wada test) after left-brain stroke has produced severe nonfluent aphasia.[22]

Wernicke's Aphasia

In this disorder, language output is fluent—that is, normal in mean phrase length, generally sentence-length, and using all grammatical elements available in the language. Content may be extremely paraphasic[6] or empty. Paraphasic speech conforms to the general rules of the language but contains substitutions at the phonemic level (phonemic paraphasias such as "smoon" for spoon), the word level (semantic paraphasias such as "cup" for spoon), or entirely novel but phonologically legal words (neologisms such as "snopel"). Empty speech may consist of either vague circumlocutions or single words (thing, one, unit, it, going, etc.). Lengthy, complex, phonologically rich output with varied neologisms is jargonaphasia. Although statements may be of sentence length, grammar may become quite imprecise, usually because of semantic ambiguity; this is paragrammatism.[23] Speech is normal. Language comprehension is poor at the levels of word recognition, simple commands, and simple conversation. Repetition is very poor. Written language is comparable to spoken. Naming is very poor. Errors are paraphasias, circumlocutions, and nonresponses.

Apraxia to command is common, but when the patient is given a model to imitate, performance can be extremely variable, from persistently severe apraxia to normal performance.[24] Deficits in the right visual field are common. In the acute phase, patients may be anosognosic; but with awareness of deficits, agitation and suspiciousness may emerge.

Fractional syndromes of Wernicke's aphasia are less common but can occur. Some patients have relatively better auditory comprehension (and usually repetition); others have relatively better reading comprehension. Severe limb apraxia (both ideomotor, even with imitation of gestures, and ideational) is sometimes seen.

The minimal lesion producing Wernicke's aphasia is damage to the superior temporal gyrus back to the end of the sylvian fissure (Fig. 9-3).[11] If damage includes additional adjacent structures, either the deep temporal white matter or the supramarginal gyrus or both, problems will be more

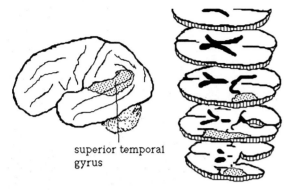

Figure 9-3
Typical lesion producing Wernicke's aphasia. Persistence and severity would depend on lesion extent (see text).

superior temporal gyrus

persistent.[25–27] If damage includes middle and interior temporal gyri, initial deficits will be more severe, anomia will be more persistent, and reading comprehension will be poor even if auditory comprehension improves. Patients with lesions restricted to the superior temporal gyrus may have predominantly auditory comprehension difficulties with relatively little anomia and much less reading impairment. The differential effects of lesion placement in the posterior temporal lobe certainly reflect variable damage to converging regional networks for several language processing systems. The auditory language system may be more specifically temporal, thus the relatively greater impairment of auditory comprehension. Visual language processing surely emerges out of the more posterior temporooccipitoparietal association cortex.[28] Cross-modal lexical and semantic knowledge emerges out of a broad range of regions in the posterior association cortex, but available evidence highlights the inferior temporal and middle temporal/angular gyrus transition as the particularly key regions for word retrieval.[29]

Severe and persistent Wernicke's aphasia seems to require damage to all of these regions or to their deep functional connections. The mechanisms of recovery are not completely known. As noted above, the brain regions involved in lexical-semantic function are broadly distributed in posterior association cortex. Size of lesion in these re-

gions, extent of involvement of the superior temporal gyrus,[25,27] and extent of coincident damage to supramarginal and angular gyri[26] have all been implicated as factors in recovery of comprehension. Studies with positron emission tomography (PET) have demonstrated a variety of effects related to recovery. Heiss and colleagues, studying subacute recovery in a mixed group of aphasic syndromes, demonstrated that recovery of comprehension was proportional to recovery of resting blood flow in the surviving left hemisphere, particularly the temporoparietal junction.[30] Weiller and coworkers demonstrated that recovery in Wernicke's aphasia is closely related to a shift in PET activation to semantic tasks from left temporal in normals to right temporal in Wernicke's aphasics who recover.[31] The precise meaning of these related studies is not known, but they all converge on the importance of posterior association cortex, either left or, if it is too damaged, right for recovery of comprehension.

Pure word deafness is sometimes considered a separate syndrome reflecting exclusive impairment to the auditory language processing system.[32] Most patients are only relatively "pure," emerging out of Wernicke's aphasia with relatively better recovery of reading comprehension for anatomically specific reasons proposed above. Some patients have had only small left temporal lesions;[32] others have had bilateral temporal lesions.[33] Depending upon the relative size and location of the bilateral lesions, these patients may be effectively deaf[37] (cortical deafness: bilateral Heschl gyrus lesions) or have agnosia for the meaning of all sounds (machinery, animals, musical instruments, etc.) even though they hear them (auditory environmental agnosia: large right lesion, whatever the left lesion[34]). Also, depending on specific lesion sites, language output can be variably abnormal, although to be "pure," it should be normal. In this case, the implication is that underlying knowledge of word phonology is preserved because spontaneous production is normal. Depending on lesion site, "relatively pure" cases may have considerable phonemic paraphasia or anomia.

The mechanism of pure word deafness is presumably damage to a system that converts the acoustic signal into a phonologically meaningful stimulus.[33] This is necessary but not sufficient for comprehension; for example, normals can repeat sentences in languages phonologically similar to their native one without understanding anything. There must still be merger of the processed acoustic signal with a semantic system. In some patients with Wernicke's aphasia, the phonological process seems very impaired; in others, the mapping to semantics and in yet others both are impaired.

Conduction Aphasia

In conduction aphasia, language output is fluent. Content is paraphasic, usually predominantly phonemic.[6] There may be frequent hesitations and attempts to correct ongoing phonemic errors (so-called *conduit d'approche*). Speech is normal. Language comprehension is good except for auditory span. Repetition is poor, not always worse than spontaneous output but dominated by phonemic paraphasias on substantive words, particularly phonologically complex target words ("happy hippopotamus") or words embedded in phonologically complex sentences ("Dogs chase but rarely catch clever cats"). Written language is extremely variable in this syndrome. Writing is rarely better than speech, but it can be much more impaired. Oral reading is usually comparable to speech but can be better or worse. Reading comprehension is usually comparable to auditory but can be worse. Patients with the agraphia with alexia syndrome usually have conduction aphasia. Naming is also extremely variable, from extremely poor to nearly normal. Errors are paraphasias (phonemic especially).

Limb ideomotor apraxia is common initially but clears in most patients.[24] Right-sided sensory loss or visual field impairment (extinction and/or lower quadrant deficit) are common.

Most patients with conduction aphasia have prominently reduced auditory verbal short-term memory (STM), tested as digit-span, word-span, or sentence-length effect in repetition. There is, however, little specificity of the STM problem, as many patients with perisylvian aphasias have a similar problem. The STM deficit also has little

relevance to the language production problem, as similar output occurs in spontaneous output, oral reading and naming, as well as repetition. There is converging evidence that the inferior parietal lobule, particularly the supramarginal gyrus, is critical for all aspects of phonologic processing. Thus, lesions there have been blamed for pure STM deficits,[35] phonologic agraphia,[36,37] and phonologic alexia, all of which commonly emerge from conduction aphasia.

The necessary and sufficient lesion to produce conduction aphasia is damage to supramarginal gyrus[38] (Fig. 9-4). The classic correlation was with the arcuate fasciculus, putatively connecting temporal lobe to frontal lobe.[39] Lesions in subcortical parietal white matter disrupt this fasciculus and may represent the classic correlation.[40] Lesions in white matter deep to sensory cortex or in the subinsular extreme capsule as well as supramarginal cortex lesions may also produce conduction aphasia.[41] These observations suggest that temporoparietal short association pathways (i.e., a regional network) may support the phonologic output structure of speech. This network is required for phonologic accuracy in spontaneous output, repetition, oral reading, and naming. If disturbed phonologic structure of output is the hallmark of conduction aphasia, this would be the criterion structural basis.

Some patients have very extensive parietal

Figure 9-4

Typical lesion producing conduction aphasia. Smaller lesions within this region may also produce similar aphasia (see text).

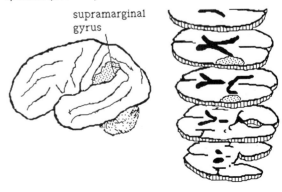

supramarginal gyrus

lesions with more severe anomia, agraphia, and limb ideomotor apraxia. Partial involvement of the superior temporal gyrus can produce initial Wernicke's aphasia that evolves into conduction aphasia with *very* paraphasic output and severe anomia. Again, the overlap of syndromes should be evident. Patients whose perisylvian arterial architecture just happens to catch the superior temporal lobe in a predominantly parietal stroke will have elements of pure word deafness (decreased auditory comprehension) with conduction aphasia (phonemic paraphasias, anomia, and agraphia). That combination would be indistinguishable from Wernicke's aphasia; in fact, it probably *is* Wernicke's aphasia except that recovery of comprehension would be "surprisingly" good.

Most patients with acute conduction aphasia have good recovery over a few weeks, although residual writing impairments, mild anomia, and occasional phonemic errors can be observed.[3] For the more severe cases with marked anomia and very paraphasic output, recovery is less complete. The combination of significant phonologic and semantic deficits despite good comprehension can be very long-lasting. Over time, patients become less neologistic and more empty and circumlocutory, even if the basic deficits do not improve.[42]

Global Aphasia

In many ways global aphasia is the easiest syndrome to define. By definition, patients have significant impairments in all aspects of language. Language output is severely limited—there is no more than "yes," "no," and a recurring stereotypic utterance ("da, da," "no way, no way," etc.). In some global aphasics (and Broca aphasics) the recurring utterance may be repeated rapidly in a richly inflected manner that suggests fluent output if only it could be comprehended.[43] This is not jargonaphasia; it has none of the phonological richness or preservation of grammatical infrastructure of jargonaphasia. The mechanism of this richly inflected stereotype is unknown, and it has no known prognostic significance.

Comprehension is very impaired. The Boston Diagnostic Aphasia Examination (BDAE) definition allows comprehension up to the 30th percentile for an aphasic population.[44] This is compatible with considerable single-word comprehension. The language comprehension tasks most likely to be preserved in global aphasia are pointing to a named location on a map,[45] pointing to personally highly familiar names from multiple choice or acknowledging them when they are presented auditorily, and a small subset of commands ("take off your glasses," "close your eyes," "stand up").[24] Some global aphasics can do those tasks but little else. There is no repetition, naming, or writing.

Buccofacial and limb apraxia, to command and imitation, are nearly universal.[24] Right hemiplegia, hemisensory loss, and visual field impairments are all common but not invariable.

The most typical lesion involves or substantially undercuts the entire perisylvian region.[11] At least, this would require a combination of the Broca's and Wernicke's aphasia lesions, but much clinical variability is seen. Some patients with Broca's aphasia lesions present as global aphasics without evident temporal lesions.[46,47] Conversely, some patients with very extensive posterior lesions that extend into subrolandic white matter present with global aphasia without *any* definite frontal or even anterior periventricular lesion.[9] The mechanism of severe comprehension loss without a temporal lesion in a substantial fraction of global aphasics, is not known. The same effect is not seen without coincident frontal lesions—that is, even enormous cortical and subcortical parietal lesions alone do not cause such deficits in comprehension. The coincident frontal lesion may produce additional cognitive problems—such as inattention, underactivation, unconcern, poor problem solving (particularly relevant when the Token Test is the defining tool of comprehension), or perseveration—that interact with more modest phonologic/semantic deficits to produce more profound functional comprehension deficits. Alexander and associates have suggested that a sufficiently great lesion of the deep temporal white matter might undercut connections to the temporal lobe.[48] Naeser and colleagues found these deep temporal lesions to be associated with poor comprehension in many global aphasics.[25] There was good recovery of comprehension in cases with deep temporal lesions but intact temporal cortex. Heisse and co-workers have demonstrated a very high correlation between reduced temporoparietal blood flow in resting PET and poor comprehension, whatever the anatomic limits of the infarction.[30] Vignolo and associates[46] and DeRenzi and colleagues,[47] who have provided the most meticulous description of global aphasia without temporal lesions, have not found that temporal white matter lesions easily account for the deficits in comprehension.

Some patients with global aphasia have no hemiparesis. As a group, they are likely to have only a large frontal lesion or separate frontal and temporal lesions.[49] The purely frontal lesions are again presumably causing a quasicomprehension deficit due to inattention, activation, perseveration, and so on. These patients are also likely to have a better prognosis, but absence of hemiparesis is not a guarantee of a good outcome, as the absence of hemiparesis only means that a small portion of paraventricular white matter has been spared.[50]

When caused by infarction, global aphasia has a poor prognosis. Smaller lesions (some without hemiparesis) will improve quickly. After infarction, patients still meeting taxonomic criteria for global aphasia at 1 month postonset have a very low probability of improving substantially.[3] Large hemorrhages may be associated with more late recovery, but by 2 months without improvement, the prognosis remains grim. Many patients show gradually improving comprehension over weeks and months and eventually reach taxonomic criteria for severe Broca's aphasia.

Transcortical Motor Aphasia

In this syndrome, language output is commonly viewed as nonfluent because there is substantial initiation block, reduction in average phrase length, and simplification of grammatical form.[13] Many patients with transcortical motor aphasia (TCMA) are initially mute and may remain mute or nearly so for days or weeks. Note that, if they are mute, repetition is obviously absent and, by strict taxonomic criteria, such patients would initially be called Broca's aphasics. Frank agrammatism is uncommon; responses are simply terse and delayed. Echolalia in various forms is frequently observed. Completely uninhibited echolalia is unusual, but fragmentary echoing, particularly of commands, may be observed. Incorporation echolalia is more common. The patient incorporates a portion of a question into the initial portion of his response. Speech quality is normal in the classic case. Repetition is, by definition, normal or at least vastly superior to spontaneous output. Recitation of even very complex overlearned material (e.g., the Lord's Prayer) may be flawless. Language comprehension is supposed to be normal, but, as observed above, the large frontal lesions most often associated with TCMA may produce substantial impairment of comprehension. Writing is usually similar to spoken output, but patients rarely write to dictation as well as they repeat. Reading comprehension parallels auditory. Oral reading may be quite normal if initial prompts are provided. Naming is quite variable; errors are nonresponses, semantic paraphasias, or perseverations.[6]

Transcortical motor aphasia may have any range of associated motor deficits, depending upon lesion site. The classic case has no motor deficit. Hemiparesis accompanies many cases of subcortical TCMA.[14] Inverted hemiparesis (leg worse than arm) and a contralateral grasp reflex accompany medial frontal TCMA.[13] Sensory loss and visual field deficits are not usually seen except in subcortical cases. Buccofacial apraxia may be seen, but limb ideomotor apraxia is less common.[24]

The classic patient has a large dorsolateral frontal lesion, typically extending into the deep frontal white matter (Fig. 9-5).[13] Identical cases have been reported with just a white matter lesion abutting the frontal horn of the lateral ventricle.[48] Very similar cases involve the capsulostriatal region, particularly the dorsolateral caudate and adjacent paraventricular white matter (Fig. 9-6).[14] The similarity of the aphasia associated with these disparate lesions is paralleled by the nearly identical reduction in blood flow seen on resting PET or single proton emission computed tomography (SPECT) in dorsolateral frontal cortex, whatever

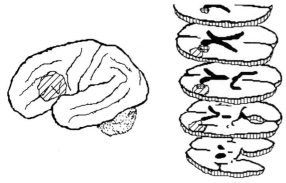

Figure 9-5

Typical lesions producing transcortical motor aphasia. Note overlap with Broca's area lesions (Fig. 9-2).

the lesion site.[51,52,57] The more posteriorly the lesion extends along the paraventricular white matter, the likelier the presence of dysarthria (see discussion of aphemia, above) and hemiparesis. Damage to the medial frontal lobe, particularly the supplementary motor area, produces TCMA-like disturbance.[53] Mutism may be more prolonged. When patients begin to speak, they rarely show any frankly aphasic qualities. They simply do not speak much.

Analysis of cortical and subcortical cases

Figure 9-6

Large lenticulostriate lesion, which is often associated with transcortical motor aphasia, frequently accompanied by speech disturbance and hemiparesis. Smaller lesion (cross-hatched area) may produce mild transcortical motor aphasia without motor deficits.

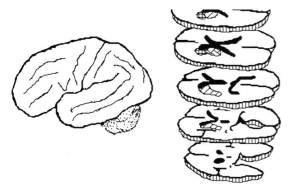

with TCMA suggests that one fundamental deficit is in generative language tasks.[14,54] The patients seem to have very limited capacity to generate complex syntax. They may reuse the syntax in a question they are asked (incorporation echolalia). They may produce short responses, even short sentences, quite well. When asked an open-ended question, however, they do not have timely access to the range of syntax needed to answer.[54,55] Bedside generative tasks—word-list generation, storytelling, or producing sentences using provided main verbs—will be impaired out of proportion to other language tasks. Patients with large dorsolateral frontal lesions may have little or no aphasia on standard tests but still be unable to tell a story or recite a narrative in normal fashion.

A second fundamental deficit in TCMA is reduction in activation to speak (or to write). Analysis of lesion site effects, particularly the profound mutism that occurs with medial frontal damage, suggests that reduced activation is due to loss of ascending dopaminergic pathways. The medial frontal regions are primary targets of the nonnigral dopaminergic system.[56] Bilateral damage to this system anywhere from the upper midbrain to the frontal cortex results in akinetic mutism,[57] evolving into less flagrant forms often called abulia.[58] Transcortical motor aphasia may represent a subsyndrome of akinetic mutism with more rapid clearing of mutism and less global akinesia because the lesion is only unilateral. The improvement in fluency and speech rate after administration of direct dopamine agonists supports this proposition.[59,60] Improvement with bromocriptine is almost uniquely seen in TCMA.

Transcortical Sensory Aphasia

In transcortical sensory aphasia (TCSA), language output is fluent. Content is very empty, with semantic paraphasia predominating. All patients make abundant use of one-word circumlocutions and nonspecific filler words, such as *one, things, does,* etc. Phonemic paraphasias and neologistic jargon are less common, so that output is more accurately described as extended English jargon. Content is also often perseverative. Speech quality is normal. Repetition is, by definition, normal. Language comprehension is impaired. In particular, single-word comprehension may be quite poor. When accompanied by accurate repetition of the test words and even their incorporation in sentences, ("A watch? I should know that. Is one of these a watch?"), the behavior has been called alienation of word meaning.[61] There may be category-specific comprehension impairments with particularly good performance at following commanded actions and very poor performance at pointing to named targets. Many patients will accept incorrect names or quibble over accuracy. ("You could call it a watch, but I don't think it is one.") Naming is poor, and again some category-specificity may be observed. Some patients are worse at naming animals, insects, and other animate objects than tools and other inanimate objects.[62] There is no important discrepancy between naming performance to different sensory modalities. Many patients respond quickly to phonemic cues but will then reject or be uncertain about the correct response. This behavior has been called a two-way naming impairment.[63] Written output may be similar to spoken, but patients usually do not write extensively and are very perseverative. Reading aloud and reading comprehension are both abnormal. In many patients reading comprehension is even worse than auditory comprehension.

Transcortical sensory aphasia has been described after lesions in middle and inferior temporal gyri (Fig. 9-7).[61] The temporal lesion may produce a right visual field defect if white matter extent reaches the geniculocalcarine pathways. Many cases of TCSA have unexpected lesion sites involving the entire perisylvian cortex, a lesion much likelier to produce global aphasia.[64] The mechanism for this is unknown, although some variant on bilateral language representation is usually recruited. Some cases with temporal lesions may also involve the inferior temporooccipital region—for instance, after posterior cerebral artery infarction. These patients will certainly have very impaired reading.[28] Many have associative agnosia.[65] Not only can they not name an object or point to a named object but they cannot indicate

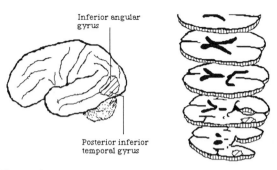

Figure 9-7
Typical lesion producing transcortical sensory aphasia. Lesions more medial and inferior, usually posterior cerebral artery infarctions, may produce similar aphasia (see text).

its use or sort it into a correct functional category (i.e., put a pencil with chalk rather than with a knife). Thus, the deficit is not restricted to *lexical* semantic knowledge but involves actual semantic knowledge. This may be modality-specific, with visually presented tasks more impaired,[65] or it may affect all modalities equally.[66]

Transcortical sensory aphasia is almost monotypic in that it is fundamentally a disorder of semantic processing. Nevertheless, different aspects of semantic knowledge and access to semantic knowledge may be impaired in different cases. The inability of patients with TCSA to associate a name with an object is the result of a semantic disorder at the interface between language and semantic memory. When semantic memory is more globally affected, patients are unable to demonstrate recognition of objects by nonverbal means as well (see Chap. 37). This is most commonly seen in degenerative diseases with a predilection for temporal cortex, such as Alzheimer Disease, Pick Disease, and so-called Semantic Dementia.[29,62,67–69]

Anomic Aphasia

Anomic aphasia is a much less homogeneous grouping than any of the other classic syndromes. By definition, language is fluent, comprehension good, and repetition good. The only deficit in spoken language is in word retrieval. Paraphasias are infrequent. Word-finding problems usually produce filler words[6] or circumlocutions. Other impairments vary with lesion site.

Anomic aphasia is the residual state of many aphasic disorders after time for improvement.[21] As a primary diagnosis, anomic aphasia usually accompanies lesions in the same regions as TCMA or TCSA.[10,11]

As noted, most patients with TCMA are or at least become basically fluent but with terse, unelaborated utterances. When it is accompanied by word-finding deficits, this condition would qualify as anomic aphasia. Anomic aphasia is also the mildest form of TCSA, representing a deficit only in lexical retrieval from semantic stores. Thus, when anomic aphasia is caused by a dorsolateral frontal lesion, there are no accompanying neurologic signs. When it is caused by a deep frontal-striatal lesion, there may be dysarthria, hemiparesis, and buccofacial apraxia, depending upon lesion extent. When it is caused by a posterior association cortex lesion, there may be a visual field deficit and alexia, depending upon lesion extent. When anomic aphasia is the residual of partly recovered conduction or Broca's aphasia, the accompanying signs are as expected for those disorders.

Mixed Transcortical Aphasia

In mixed transcortical aphasia (MTA), language output is nonfluent. Comprehension is impaired. Naming is poor. Repetition is preserved. Echolalia and fragmentary sentence starters ("I don't . . . ," "Not with the . . .") are common. Speech quality is normal. Writing and reading are similarly reduced.

In the patient whose case report defined this syndrome, MTA was due to bilateral hypoxic neuronal loss in the arterial border zones,[70] but ischemic damage in the left border zones could presumably cause the same disorder. The implication is that MTA requires a combination of the lesions of TCMA and TCSA, with perisylvian structures allowing repetition preserved. Most cases are actually due to large frontal lesions in the region of

TCMA lesions. The comprehension defect is probably due to a mixture of frontal impairments, exactly as described for restricted frontal lesions and global aphasia. Comprehension improves, and patients evolve toward TCMA. Associated lesions are as described for TCMA.

Large anterior thalamic lesions also produce MTA.[71–73] Most cases have involved the anterior, ventrolateral, and dorsomedian nuclei at a minimum.[71,72] Damage to those three nuclei effectively deprives the frontal lobe of thalamic input and modulation. Patients are often mute initially. When they speak, the reduction in narrative and terseness of structure are similar to those of TCMA. The impairment in comprehension may be due to the speculative "frontal" mechanisms. The associated signs depend upon lesion extent out of the thalamus. Recovery of language is usually good.

CROSSED APHASIA AND APHASIA IN LEFT-HANDERS

The foregoing review is valid for most right-handers with lesions of the left hemisphere. For the 10 percent of the population that is left-handed and for the approximately 2 to 5 percent of the right-handed population that becomes aphasic after a right-brain lesion (crossed aphasia), some modifications of the clinical rules are required. For left-handers, the phenomenology of aphasia is complicated by the very issue of left-handedness. More than right-handers, all left-handers are not created equal; they vary greatly in degree and nature of hemispheric specialization for language. For both populations the phenomenology is further complicated by irregularities in lateral dominance for other typically lateralized functions, such as praxis and some aspects of visuospatial function. Only a brief summary of these issues is possible here.

Crossed Aphasia

The incidence of crossed aphasia has been reported as anywhere from 1 to 13 percent.[74–76] The stroke population[74] is least contaminated by possible bilateral lesions, but in all populations methodological limitations (defining handedness and aphasia testing strategies) leave the actual incidence uncertain. A reasonable estimate is 2 to 5 percent.

Patients with crossed aphasia fall into two broad categories. About 70 percent have a standard aphasia syndrome associated with, at least approximately, the lesion site expected in the left hemisphere.[77] All types of aphasia profiles can occur with the expected lesions (albeit in the right hemisphere). The other 30 percent have striking anomalies in the aphasia-lesion relationship.[77] In this group, unexpectedly mild aphasia syndromes occur despite large lesions that would typically cause a more severe aphasia. Conduction aphasia or phonologic agraphia have been seen despite large perisylvian lesions.[77,78] In other patients with large perisylvian lesions, transcortical sensory aphasia or anomic aphasia has been described.[64,87] Alexander and Annett have suggested that these anomalous cases point to possible discrepant lateralizations of phonologic and semantic functions.[79] Patients with crossed aphasia may have a better capacity for recovery.

Lateralization of praxis and visuospatial functions in crossed aphasia has not been as definitely addressed as the language functions. Castro-Caldos and coworkers claim that these functions show anomalous lateralization less frequently than language, asserting that praxis remains in the left hemisphere contralateral to the preferred right hand and that visuospatial functions remain in the right hemisphere.[74] Others have disputed this, arguing from case reports that all functions show a high rate of anomalous lateralization.[80] Alexander and coworkers have reviewed the case reports of anomalous visuospatial lateralization to the left hemisphere in right-handers.[81] They have proposed that there is a subset of right-handers who have chance lateralization of all functions. These authors, among others, have even proposed that a genetic basis for the inheritance of handedness and laterality of cognitive functions such as the right shift theory of Annett[77,79] can

account for the rates of all anomalies. The biological basis of crossed aphasia, however, remains unknown.

Aphasia in Left-Handers

Left-handers make up 10 percent of the population, but they are a much more heterogeneous group than right-handers. If a strict criterion for left-handedness is used, most of the left-handed population becomes relabeled as being mixed-handed.[76] Thus, some authorities simply refer to non-right-handers. The rate of cerebral lateralization of left-handers depends to some extent on the criteria used to define the group. Large studies of left-handed aphasics have been reasonably consistent, however, in finding that about 70 percent have left-brain lesions and 30 percent have right-brain lesions.[82] Hécaen has computed that approximately 15 percent probably would be aphasic after a lesion of either hemisphere; that is, they have bilateral language representation. Whether aphasic after left or right brain lesions, the proportion of cases with anomalous aphasia-lesion relationships is higher than in right-handers.[83] It has been claimed that left-handers have better recovery than right-handers,[82] but, as with crossed aphasia, this question is muddied by the higher proportion of mild aphasics.[83] It is also unclear if better recovery means bilateral language capacity so all functions have higher potential for recovery or divergent lateralization of functions so that some are left uninvolved by any lateralized lesion.[75,79,84] Both factors are probably operative, but in different patients.

Lateralization of praxis and visuospatial function shows anomalies at a rate similar to those of crossed aphasia. Every possible arrangement of impaired and preserved functions has been reported after left or right lesions.[94] Since the biological basis of neither handedness nor the lateralization of cognitive functions has been established, it remains an open question how these anomalies occur in left-handers as well as right-handers.

EFFECT OF ETIOLOGY

Infarctions

Almost all of the foregoing is based on the literature accumulated from strokes. Infarcts have numerous advantages for clinicoanatomic correlations. They are sudden in onset, and there is therefore no accommodation and compensation prior to clinical presentation. Boundaries between damaged and nondamaged brain are fairly precise, so correlations are clearer. Nevertheless, the vascular system cannot provide every topographic variation of brain injury; therefore much of what has come to us as classic syndromes could easily be partially artifactual correlations produced by the limited independence of lesions sites from infarctions.

There are some aphasic syndromes that are commonly believed to be caused by emboli because the distribution of infarction seems most plausibly to be in the territory of a branch of the middle cerebral artery. The fractional Broca's aphasias, conduction aphasia, and Wernicke's aphasia all seem likely to have an embolic basis when due to infarction. Global aphasia and Broca's aphasia require more extensive damage in the territory of the middle cerebral artery. There is, however, no basis for presuming an infarction mechanism simply on the basis of these aphasia types.

Hemorrhages

All of the rules established for infarctions apply for hemorrhages if the hemorrhage happens to be in the same brain topography as an infarction pattern. Patients with hemorrhages may be much more impaired initially because of physiologic deficits not primarily related to aphasia—mass effects, intraventricular blood, and so on. Hemorrhages are not constrained by vascular patterns, so entirely novel arrangements of lesions can be seen. This may be exemplified most clearly with lesions of the lenticulostriate region. Infarctions tend to be partially or completely limited to the middle cerebral artery perforators, but hemorrhages can dissect out of that limited region. Much of the variability reported after lenticulostriate lesions[85] may be due to idiosyncratic extensions of hemorrhages.[86]

Trauma

Focal contusions can occur anywhere, depending upon the direction of the blow, skull fragments, and so forth. When the contusion is in a perisylvian region, the resulting aphasia will usually follow the rules established by infarctions. Conduction and Wernicke's aphasias may be seen with predominantly superficial lesions and so may be quite typical. Cortical contusions rarely cause injury deep enough to damage all of the required deep structures (see above) and thus to produce nonfluent aphasia. There is a strong tendency for traumatic contusions to arise from basal structures due to inertial effects. Focal contusions of the inferior temporal lobe will cause anomic aphasia. If the lesions are large and extend into lateral temporal lobe or hemorrhage dissects up into the deep temporal white matter, patients may present with Wernicke's aphasia or TCSA. Trauma can also cause large epidural or subdural hematomas that do not directly affect language zones. They cause cerebral herniation with entrapment of the posterior cerebral artery, causing occipitotemporal infarctions with alexia and anomia. This herniation-caused infarction can be superimposed on direct temporal contusion, resulting in a very severe fluent aphasia.

Tumors

The lesson for aphasia is no different than that for any cognitive function. In general, large tumors produce relatively much less cognitive impairment than an infarction of the same size would produce, but tumors produce symptoms qualitatively appropriate for the region involved. Tumors tend to infiltrate and gradually disrupt function, allowing substantial compensation as the disorder progresses. The conformity with patterns established by infarctions will be correlated largely with the malignancy and speed of growth of the tumor.

Herpes Simplex Encephalitis

Although rare, herpes simplex encephalitis (HSE) has a predilection for the medial temporal lobes, basal-medial frontal lobes, and insular cortices. Survivors of HSE frequently have severe amnesia.[62,87] Patients with extensive left-sided HSE lesions, including the inferotemporal lobe, commonly show category-specific semantic deficits.[62,87]

Dementia

The most common dementing illnesses—DAT and multi-infarct dementia (MID)—both cause language impairments. Dementia of the Alzheimer type typically presents with memory and language disturbances.[68] The language problem begins as anomia and is often misidentified by families as memory impairment. With time, the language disorder evolves toward TCSA, and the patients' semantic memory erodes.[88] The structure of this erosion is fairly predictable. Highly typical semantic associations survive longer than the semantic associations and attributes of low typicality.[88] For instance, the patients may still recognize the words and concepts behind "cat," but not the words and then even the concepts of "leopard," "fang," or "litter." It has been proposed that this slow erosion of semantic knowledge—first words and then concepts—is the fundamental cognitive deficit of DAT.[89] Its presumed pathologic basis is the loss of neurons in posterior association cortex.

If one of the infarcts is in the language zone, MID may cause aphasia directly. The more typical pathology of MID is, however, numerous small infarcts in subcortical regions. These lesions may produce a variety of motor speech impairments such as articulatory problems, hypophonia, dysprosody, and rate disturbances. A recognizable aphasic syndrome does not occur, but patients may show cognitive deficits similar to those seen with frontal lobe lesions, including disturbances in all aspects of generative language: reduced word-list generation, terse or unelaborate utterances, and poor narrative ability. It has been suggested that a single small infarct in the genu of the left internal capsule is sufficient to disconnect frontal-thalamic circuitry and produce these deficits.[90]

A rarer form of degenerative dementia, primary progressive aphasia, is virtually restricted to language deficits.[91] The most common form is progressive loss of semantics and has therefore also been called semantic dementia[92] (see Chap. 37). The presentation is usually similar to the language impairments of DAT—anomia initially progressing to TCSA and finally to loss of semantic concepts and knowledge. Unlike DAT, other cognitive functions remain intact in these cases. Pathology is restricted to the anterior inferior temporal lobes, and the histopathology is usually Pick disease.[69,92,93] Nonfluent forms of primary progressive aphasia have also been described;[94] however, the pathology has not always been established.

REFERENCES

1. Broca P: Perte de la parole. Ramollissement chronique et destruction partielle du lobe antérieur gauche du cerveau. *Bull Soc Anthropol* 2:235, 1861.
2. Goodglass H: *Understanding Aphasia.* San Diego, CA: Academic Press, 1983, pp 247–250.
3. Kertesz A, McCabe P: Recovery patterns and prognosis in aphasia. *Brain* 100:1–18, 1977.
4. Caramazza A: The logic of neuropsychological research and the problem of patient classification in aphasia. *Brain Lang* 21:9–20, 1984.
5. Marshall JC, Newcombe F: Patterns of paralexia. *J Psycholing Res* 2:175–199, 1973.
6. Ardila A, Rosselli M: Language deviations in aphasia: A frequency analysis. *Brain Lang* 44:165–180, 1993.
7. Kohn SE: Verb finding in aphasia. *Cortex* 25:57–69, 1989.
8. Robinson RG, Kubos KL, Starr LB, et al: Mood disorders in stroke patients: Importance of location of lesion. *Brain* 107:81–93, 1984.
9. Mazzocchi F, Vignolo LA: Localisation of lesions in aphasia: Clinical-CT scan correlations in stroke patients. *Cortex* 15:627–654, 1979.
10. Mohr JP, Pessin MS, Finkelstein S, et al: Broca's aphasia: Pathologic and clinical. *Neurology* 28:311–324, 1978.
11. Naeser MA, Hayward RW: Lesion location in aphasia with cranial computed tomography and the Bos-

ton Diagnostic Aphasia Exam. *Neurology* 28:545–551, 1978.

12. Naeser MA, Palumbo CL, Helm-Estabrooks N, et al: Severe nonfluency in aphasia: Role of the medial subcallosal fasciculus and other white matter pathways in recovery of spontaneous speech. *Brain* 112:1–38, 1989.

13. Freedman M, Alexander MP, Naeser MA: Anatomic basis of transcortical motor aphasia. *Neurology* 34:409–417, 1984.

14. Mega MS, Alexander MP: Subcortical aphasia: The core profile of capsulostriatal infarction. *Neurology* 44:1824–1829, 1994.

15. Alexander MP, Naeser MA, Palumbo C: Broca's area aphasia. *Neurology* 40:353–362, 1990.

16. Schiff HB, Alexander MP, Naeser MA, Galaburda AM: Aphemia: Clinical-anatomic correlations. *Arch Neurol* 40:720–727, 1983.

17. Monrad-Krohn GH: Dysprosody or altered "melody of language." *Brain* 70:405–415, 1947.

18. Blumstein SE, Alexander MP, Ryalls JH: The nature of the foreign accent syndrome: A case study. *Brain Lang* 31:215–244, 1987.

19. Graff-Radford NR, Cooper WE, Colsher PL, Damasio AR: An unlearned foreign "accent" in a patient with aphasia. *Brain Lang* 28:86–94, 1986.

20. Prin RS, Snow E, Wagenaar E: Recovery from aphasia: Spontaneous speech versus language comprehension. *Brain Lang* 6:192–211, 1978.

21. Basso A, Gardelli M, Grassi MP, Mariotti M: The role of the right hemisphere in recovery from aphasia: Two case studies. *Cortex* 25:555–556, 1989.

22. Kinsbourne M: The minor hemisphere as a source of aphasic speech. *Trans Am Neurol Assoc* 96:141–145, 1971.

23. Goodglass H: *Understanding Aphasia.* San Diego, CA: Academic Press, 1983, pp 107–109.

24. Alexander MP, Baker E, Naeser MA, et al: Neuropsychological and neuroanatomical dimensions of ideomotor apraxia. *Brain* 118:87–107, 1992.

25. Naeser MA, Helm-Estabrooks N, Haas G, et al: Relationship between lesion extent in Wernicke's area on computed tomographic scan and predicting recovery of comprehension in Wernicke's aphasia. *Arch Neurol* 44:73–82, 1987.

26. Kertesz A, Lau WK, Polk M: The structural determinants of recovery in Wernicke's aphasia. *Brain Lang* 44:153–164, 1993.

27. Selnes OA, Knopman DS, Niccum N, et al: Computed tomographic scan correlates of auditory com-

prehension deficits in aphasia: A prospective recovery study. *Ann Neurol* 13:558–566, 1983.

28. Henderson VW, Friedman RB, Teng EL, Weiner JM: Left hemisphere pathways in reading: Inference from pure alexia without hemianopia. *Neurology* 35:962–968, 1985.

29. Damasio A: Synchronous activation in multiple cortical regions: A mechanism for recall. *Semin Neurosci* 2:287–296, 1990.

30. Heiss W, Kessler J, Karbe H, et al: Cerebral glucose metabolism as a predictor of recovery from aphasia in ischemic stroke. *Arch Neurol* 50:958–964, 1993.

31. Weiller C, Isensee C, Rijintjes M, et al: Recovery from Wernicke's aphasia: A positron emission tomography study. *Ann Neurol* 37:723–732, 1995.

32. Takahashi N, Kawamura M, Shinotou H, et al: Pure word deafness due to left hemisphere damage. *Cortex* 28:295–303, 1992.

33. Auerbach SH, Allard T, Naeser MA, et al: Pure word deafness: Analysis of a case with bilateral lesions and a defect at the prephonemic level. *Brain* 105:271–300, 1982.

34. Fujii T, Fukatsu R, Watabe S, et al: Auditory sound agnosia without aphasia following a right temporal lobe lesion. *Cortex* 26:263–268, 1990.

35. Paulesu E, Frith CD, Frackowiack RSJ: The neural correlates of the verbal component of working memory. *Nature* 362:342–345, 1993.

36. Roeltgen DP, Sevush S, Heilman KM: Phonological agraphia: Writing by the lexical semantic route. *Neurology* 33:755–765, 1983.

37. Alexander MP, Friedman RB, Loverso F, Fischer RF: Lesion localization in phonological agraphia. *Brain Lang* 43:83–95, 1992.

38. Palumbo CL, Alexander MP, Naeser MA: CT scan lesion sites associated with conduction aphasia in Se K (ed): *Conduction Aphasia.* Hillsdale NJ: Erlbaum, 1992, pp 51–75.

39. Benson DF, Sheremata WA, Bouchard R, et al: Conduction aphasia: A clinicopathological study. *Arch Neurol* 28:339–346, 1973.

40. Mendez MF, Benson DF: Atypical conduction aphasia: A disconnection syndrome. *Arch Neurol* 42:886–891, 1985.

41. Damasio H, Damasio AR: The anatomical basis of conduction aphasia. *Brain* 103:337–350, 1980.

42. Kertesz A, Benson DF: Neologistic jargon: A clinicopathological study. *Cortex* 6:362–386, 1970.

43. Poeck K, de Bleser R, von Keyserlingk DG: Neurolinguistic status and localization of lesions in aphasic

patients with exclusively consonant vowel recurring utterances. *Brain* 107:199–217, 1984.

44. Goodglass H, Kaplan E: *The Assessment of Aphasia and Related Disorders.* Philadelphia: Lea & Febiger, 1983, p 97.

45. Wapner W, Gardner H: A note on patterns of comprehension and recovery in global aphasia. *J Speech Hearing Res* 29:765–771, 1979.

46. Vignolo LA, Boccardi E, Caverni L: Unexpected CT-scan finding in global aphasia. *Cortex* 22:55–69, 1986.

47. DeRenzi E, Colombo A, Scarpa M: The aphasic isolate. *Brain* 114:1719–1730, 1991.

48. Alexander MP, Naeser MA, Palumbo CL: Correlations of subcortical CT lesion sites and aphasia profiles. *Brain* 110:961–991, 1987.

49. Tranel D, Biller J, Damasio H, et al: Global aphasia without hemiparesis. *Arch Neurol* 44:304–308, 1987.

50. Legatt AD, Rubin AJ, Kaplan LR, et al: Global aphasia without hemiparesis. *Neurology* 37:201–205, 1987.

51. Alexander MP: Speech and language deficits after subcortical lesions of the left hemisphere: a clinical, CT, and PET study, in Vallar G, Cappa SF, Wallesch C-W (eds): *Neuropsychological Disorders Associated with Subcortical Lesions.* Oxford, England: Oxford Science Publications, 1991, pp 454–477.

52. Démonet JF, Puel M: "Subcortical" aphasia: Some proposed pathophysiological mechanisms and their rCBF correlates revealed by *SPECT. J Neuroling* 6:319–344, 1991.

53. Rubens AB: Transcortical motor aphasia. *Studies Neuroling* 1:293–306, 1976.

54. Luria AR, Tsvetkova LS: Towards the mechanism of "dynamic aphasia." *Acta Neurol Psychiatr Belg* 67:1045–1067, 1967.

55. Costello A de L, Warrington EK: Dynamic aphasia. *Cortex* 25:103–114, 1989.

56. Lindvall O, Bjorklund A, Moore RY, Stenevi U: Mesencephalic dopamine neurons projecting to neocortex. *Brain Res* 81:325–331, 1974.

57. Alexander MP: Disturbances in language initiation: Mutism and its lesser forms, in Joseph AR, Young RR (eds): *Movement Disorders in Neurology and Psychiatry.* Boston: Blackwell, 1992, pp 389–396.

58. Fisher CM: Abulia minor vs. agitated behavior. *Clin Neurosurg* 31:9–31, 1985.

59. Albert ML, Bachman DL, Morgan A, Helm-Estabrooks N: Pharmacotherapy for aphasia. *Neurology* 38:877–879, 1988.

60. Saba L, Leiguarda R, Starkstein SE: An open-label trial of bromcriptine in nonfluent aphasia. *Neurology* 42:1637–1638, 1992.

61. Alexander MP, Hiltbronner B, Fischer R: The distributed anatomy of transcortical sensory aphasia. *Arch Neurol* 46:885–892, 1989.

62. Warrington EK, Shallice T: Category-specific semantic impairment. *Brain* 107:829–854, 1984.

63. Benson DF: Neurologic correlates of anomia, in Whitaker H, Whitaker HA (eds): *Studies in Neurolinguistics.* New York: Academic Press, 1979, pp 293–328.

64. Berthier ML, Starkstein SE, Leiguarda R, et al: Transcortical aphasia. *Brain* 114:1409–1427, 1991.

65. Feinberg TE, Dyckes-Berke D, Miner CR, Roane DM: Knowledge, implicit knowledge and metaknowledge in visual agnosia and pure alexia. *Brain* 118:789–800, 1995.

66. Feinberg TE, Rothi LJG, Heilman KM: Multimodal agnosia after unilateral left hemisphere lesion. *Neurology* 36:864–867, 1986.

67. Riddoch MJ, Humphreys GW, Coltheart M, Funnell E: Semantic systems or system? Neuropsychological evidence re-examined. *Cogn Neuropsychol* 5:3–25, 1988.

68. Price BH, Gurvit H, Weintraub S, et al: Neuropsychological patterns and language deficits in 20 consecutive cases of autopsy-confirmed Alzheimer's disease. *Arch Neurol* 50:931–937, 1993.

69. Graff-Radford NR, Damasio AR, Hyman BT, et al: Progressive aphasia in a patient with Pick's disease. *Neurology* 40:620–626, 1990.

70. Geschwind N, Quadfasel FA, Segarra JM: Isolation of the speech area. *Neuropsychologia* 6:327–340, 1968.

71. McFarling D, Rothi LJ, Heilman KM: Transcortical aphasia from ischemic infarcts of the thalamus. *J Neurol Neurosurg Psychiatry* 45:107–112, 1982.

72. Graff-Radford NR, Damasio H, Yamada T, et al: Nonhemorrhagic thalamic infarction. *Brain* 108:485–516, 1985.

73. Cappa SF, Vignolo L: "Transcortical" features of aphasia following left thalamic hemorrhage. *Cortex* 19:227–241, 1979.

74. Castro-Caldas A, Confraria A, Poppe P: Nonverbal disturbances in crossed aphasia. *Aphasiology* 1:403–413, 1987.

75. Bryden MP, Hécaen H, DeAgostini M: Patterns of cerebral organization. *Brain Lang* 20:249–262, 1983.

76. Annett M: *Left, Right, Hand and Brain: The Right Shift Theory.* Hillsdale, NJ: Erlbaum, 1985.

77. Alexander MP, Fischette MR, Fischer RS: Crossed aphasia can be mirror image or anomalous. *Brain* 112:953–973, 1989.

78. Basso A, Capitani E, Laiacona M, Zanobio ME: Crossed aphasia: One or more syndromes? *Cortex* 1:25–45, 1985.

79. Alexander MP, Annett M: Crossed aphasia and related anomalies of cerebral organization: Case reports and a genetic hypothesis. *Brain Lang.* In press.

80. Trojano L, Balbi P, Russo G, Elefante R: Patterns of recovery in verbal and nonverbal function in a case of crossed aphasia. *Brain Lang* 46:637–661, 1994.

81. Fischer RS, Alexander MP, Gabriel C, et al: Reversed lateralization of cognitive functions in right handers. *Brain* 114:245–261, 1991.

82. Hécaen H, DeAgostini M, Monzon-Montes A: Cerebral organization in lefthanders. *Brain Lang* 12:261–284, 1981.

83. Basso A, Farabola M, Grassi MP, et al: Aphasia in left-handers. *Brain Lang* 38:233–252, 1990.

84. Naeser MA, Borod JC: Aphasia in lefthanders. *Neurology* 36:471–488, 1986.

85. Puel M, Démonet JF, Cardebat I, et al: Aphasies sous-corticales: Étude neurolinguistigue avec scanner x de 25 cas. *Rev Neurol* 140:695–710, 1984.

86. D'Esposito M, Alexander MP: Subcortical aphasia: Distinct profiles following left putaminal hemorrhages. *Neurology* 45:33–37, 1995.

87. DeRenzi E, Lucchelli F: Are semantic systems separately represented in the brain? The case of living category impairment. *Cortex* 30:3–25, 1994.

88. Smith S, Faust M, Beeman M, et al: A property level analysis of lexical semantic representation in Alzheimer's disease. *Brain Lang* 49:263–279, 1995.

89. Hodges JR, Salmon DP, Butters N: Semantic memory impairment in Alzheimer's disease: Failure of access or degraded knowledge? *Neuropsychologia* 30:301–314, 1992.

90. Tatemichi TK, Desmond DW, Prohovnik I, et al: Confusion and memory loss from capsular genu infarction: A thalamocortical disconnection syndrome? *Neurology* 42:1966–1979, 1992.

91. Weintraub S, Rubin NP, Mesulam MM: Primary progressive aphasia: Longitudinal course, neuropsychological profile and language features. *Arch Neurol* 47:1329–1335, 1990.

92. Hodges JR, Patterson K, Oxbury S, Funnell E: Semantic dementia. *Brain* 115:1783–1806, 1992.

93. Kertesz A, Hudson L, MacKenzie IRA, Munoz DG: The pathology and nosology of primary progressive aphasia. *Neurology* 44:2065–2072, 1994.

94. Mesulam MM: Slowly progressive aphasia without generalized dementia. *Ann Neurol* 11:592–598, 1982.

Chapter 10

APHASIA: COGNITIVE NEUROPSYCHOLOGICAL ASPECTS

Eleanor M. Saffran

As is evident from the preceding chapter, much was known about aphasia prior to the emergence of cognitive neuropsychology in the 1970s. Symptoms had been described, diagnostic and treatment protocols developed, anatomic correlates established, and models proposed that interpreted aphasic phenomena within an anatomic theory based on aphasic data (see Ref. 1 for a review). The cognitive neuropsychological approach represents a shift from clinical and anatomic concerns to an emphasis on functional architecture. One assumption that underlies this approach is that language breakdown patterns reflect the natural divisions of the language system and hence that the disorders reveal its componential structure. This school of neuropsychological research is closely tied to developments in cognitive psychology and psycholinguistics. Normative models guide the investigation of pathologic phenomena, which, in turn, provide fertile ground for testing and extending theories of language function.

The concern with functional architecture has implications not only for the types of questions that are addressed by aphasia research but also for methodology. Earlier investigators had relied extensively on the classic aphasia syndrome categories (e.g., Broca's aphasia, Wernicke's aphasia) as the basis for identifying and grouping subjects. While useful as behavioral descriptors and pointers to lesion site, the syndrome designations allow a considerable amount of variability.[2,3] Moreover, these fairly gross breakdown patterns did not map very neatly onto the models of normal

language processing that psycholinguists were developing. The investigative focus therefore moved from what might be regarded as "typical" aphasic manifestations*—for example, the combination of receptive and expressive symptoms that define Wernicke's aphasia—to deficits that were (1) of a more circumscribed nature and (2) had some clear relationship to models of language processing.† An early statement of the assumptions underlying the approach was provided by Marin and colleagues:[4]

> . . . the behavior of the patient with organic brain disease largely reflects capacities which existed in the premorbid state. We should therefore be able to make some inferences about the organization of normal language function from patterns of functional preservation and impairment: if process X is intact where process Y is severely compromised or absent, and especially if the converse is found in other patients, there is reason to believe

*Although any experienced clinician would agree that many patients are not easily assigned to the classic syndrome categories.

†This is not to imply that the cognitive neuropsychology approach is without clinical relevance. The assumption is that analyses of disorders in terms of loci of disruption within processing models should provide the basis for developing treatment programs tailored to the underlying disturbance (e.g., Chap. 12 in Ref. 105).

that X and Y reflect different underlying mechanisms in the normal state. At the very least, the resulting matrix of intact and impaired functions should yield a taxonomy of functional subsystems. It may not tell us how these subsystems interact—but it should identify and describe what distinct capacities are available (e.g., it might, to take a hypothetical instance, describe a semantic process that is distinct from a syntactic process). The method is, of course, limited by the functional topology of the brain. Because functions may overlap in their anatomical substrates, we cannot state with assurance that every functional system which could be observed will be observed. But positive evidence that functions are organized independently should be significant for a theory of the language process [pp. 869–870].

It follows from this emphasis on dissociations that, for investigative purposes, greater value is placed on the purity of the impairment than on its frequency of occurrence in the aphasic population. Since circumscribed deficits are relatively rare, studies of single patients are not only admissible but, in the view of some investigators (e.g., Ref. 5), constitute the only valid source of neuropsychological data for the purpose of testing models of cognitive function (see Chap. 10 in Ref. 6 for discussion). Many cognitive neuropsychologists do not subscribe to this position, and group studies that involve sets of patients identified as having a particular cognitive impairment (e.g., "asyntactic" comprehension; see below) are not uncommon. Moreover, although the case study approach clearly departs from the random sampling from a population that is standard for behavioral research, the data are nevertheless cumulative. Delineation of an impairment in a single case report often leads to the identification of other patients with similar impairments and ultimately to compilations of data from a number of cases whose deficits appear quite similar (e.g., Refs. 7 and 8).

The cognitive neuropsychological approach is clearly well suited to the investigation of cognitive systems with modular architectures, that is,

systems with components that are discrete and isolable, both functionally and anatomically (cf. Ref. 9). In a system so constituted, the effects of damage to a single component should be quite local; other components should continue to function much as they did before the damage was incurred (see Ref. 6 for discussion). According to this view, the behavioral deficit should directly reflect the nature of the underlying impairment; Caramazza[1] refers to this as the "transparency" assumption. We will return to this point again at the end of the chapter, after reviewing the major contributions of cognitive neuropsychology to the study of aphasia.*

COMPONENTS OF LANGUAGE PROCESSING

Most psycholinguists would agree that a model of language processing should include the components identified in Fig. 10-1. The model distinguishes among three types of information—semantic, syntactic, and phonologic; it does not, however, specify the extent to which these forms of information are processed independently, a matter that is still much debated (see, for example, Refs. 10 to 12). The model includes procedures for recognizing and producing spoken words and for recovering and generating syntactic structures; the extent to which components are shared by the comprehension and production streams is another open question (e.g., Refs. 13 and 14). Language breakdown patterns are germane to both of these issues.

Assuming that the model is correct and that the processes and components identified in Fig. 10-1 can be disrupted independently, it should be possible to find patients with deficits that reflect breakdown at particular loci in the model. We will examine evidence for such disorders in the sections that follow.

---

*Although the approach was first applied in the study of acquired dyslexia (e.g., Ref. 7), reading disorders are the subject of another chapter in this volume (Chap. 12) and are not discussed here.

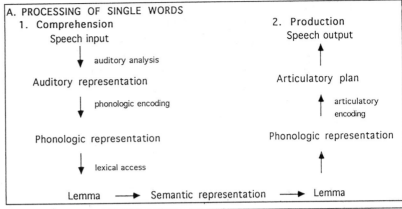

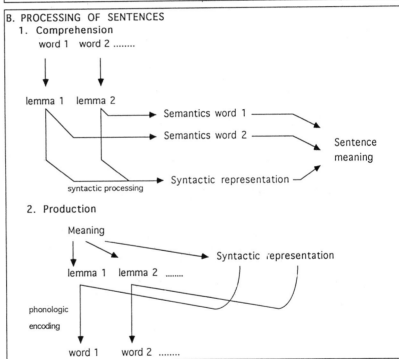

Figure 10-1

Stages in language processing. A. Processing of single words. The lemma refers to a processing level at which the word is specified with respect to meaning and grammatical class but not encoded phonologically. B. Processing of sentences.

DISORDERS OF LANGUAGE PROCESSING

Processing of Single Words: Comprehension

Impairments in the comprehension of spoken words are common in aphasia, and it is evident from Fig. 10-1 that there are a number of ways in which comprehension might fail: faulty phonologic processing prior to lexical access; loss of or impaired access to the phonologic forms of words; and/or loss of or impaired access to word meanings. Disorders of the first type can be ruled out by tests of phoneme perception and the second by lexical decision tasks in which the patient is asked to determine whether a string of phonemes is or is not a word. If a semantic deficit is present, it should be manifest not only on tests of auditory word comprehension but on written word comprehension and production tasks as well. This follows from the widely held assumption that comprehension and production, in both oral and written modalities, rely on a common conceptual base (cf. Ref. 14).

Phonologic Processing The task for the perceiver of spoken language is to recover meaningful units (words) from the complex and variable sound patterns produced by the human vocal tract. Phonemes, such as *d*, *ow*, and *t*, which are the basic building blocks of words, consist of several distinct frequency bands (formants) that may differ in their relative onset times as well as undergo transient shifts in frequency. These acoustic properties can vary depending on the context in which the phoneme occurs; compare the *d* sound in "ride" with the *d* sound in "rider." A further complication is that the boundaries between words are not systematically marked by gaps in the acoustic stimulus, as they are in written text. Thus the processing of speech input is a complicated matter, which, it has been argued, requires specialized mechanisms that are distinct from those used to process other types of acoustic stimuli (e.g., Ref. 15).

The fact that the processing of speech sounds can be selectively disrupted by brain damage supports this view. Disorders that meet this description are labeled "pure word deafness." They are the product of small lesions, usually embolic in nature, that affect the superior temporal lobe on the left, or, in other cases, bilaterally. In its pure form, the disorder is relatively rare. In most cases the lesion is more extensive, resulting in the set of symptoms associated with Wernicke's aphasia, which may include features of word deafness (e.g., Ref. 16).

The hallmark of pure word deafness is that the patient has great difficulty comprehending and repeating what he or she hears but can read and speak virtually normally. The audiometric exam is essentially normal, and nonspeech sounds are interpreted without difficulty. Some patients have shown suppression of right-ear input under dichotic listening conditions, suggesting that auditory

input is being processed in the right hemisphere[17,18] (but see Ref. 19). Auditory comprehension improves significantly when lipreading is allowed (e.g., Ref. 19), speech is slowed down (e.g., Ref. 17), and/or contextual constraints are provided. For example, Saffran and coworkers[18] described a patient whose ability to repeat words was better with semantically constrained than random word lists. These observations suggest that the auditory information available for word identification is in some way inadequate or degraded. Studies in which speech perception has been carefully examined have demonstrated deficits in the discrimination and identification of phonemes (e.g., Refs. 18 to 20). Vowels, made up of steady-state formants, tend to be better preserved than consonants, in which there are transient frequency shifts (e.g., Ref. 20). The processing of nonspeech sounds has not been examined as systematically. Although word-deaf patients are generally able to identify environmental stimuli such as the sounds of animals and musical instruments, they have seldom been called upon to make fine-grained judgments outside the speech domain, involving, for example, the temporal and waveform parameters that are manipulated in speech perception tasks. In the few studies that have included such investigations, deficits in the resolution of repetitive click stimuli have been identified.[17,19,21] This finding points to an impairment in auditory processes that are essential to phoneme perception but are not necessarily specific to speech. Auerbach and coworkers[19] have suggested that there may, in fact, be two forms of word deafness, one reflecting impairment of prephonetic auditory processing and the other specific to phonetic operations. This proposal requires further investigation.

Lexical Processing Lexical access entails matching of the acoustic input to an entry in lexical memory that represents the word's phonologic form. Loss or degradation of lexical phonology is a possible cause of comprehension failure. Deciding whether a speech sound is a word or not (auditory lexical decision) should be impaired under these conditions, but it should still be possible to repeat words, treating them as one would normally treat nonwords. Lexical decision and comprehension of written words should be preserved. Deficits in word comprehension, with relatively preserved repetition, have been described under the label "word-meaning deafness."[22–24] These patients are reported to have no comparable difficulty with written words and may resort to writing down spoken words in order to understand them. However, data on lexical decision have not been provided, and evidence for the critical phenomenon—failure to comprehend spoken words that can be understood in written form—is limited to a small number of examples.

The model outlined in Fig. 10-1 also suggests the possibility of preserved access to phonologic form with failure of access to word meaning. Franklin and associates[25] have recently reported a case that meets this description, at least for abstract words. This patient performed well on phonologic processing and auditory lexical decision tasks but was impaired in the auditory—but not written—comprehension of abstract words. He also had difficulty repeating abstract words as well as nonwords. Word meaning was clearly a significant factor in his repetition performance, as further indicated by a tendency to produce semantic errors in repeating single words. This pattern of repetition performance is termed "deep dysphasia" (for case reports, see Refs. 26 to 28). As will be seen below, this is but one of several disorders in which particular types of words are disproportionately affected.

Semantic Processing Deficits that involve the loss of word meaning are frequently reported, although often in the context of other impairments (e.g., as in Wernicke's aphasia). Relatively pure cases have been described under the label "transcortical sensory aphasia," a disorder in which repetition is spared relative to comprehension and spontaneous production (e.g., Refs. 29 and 30). Semantic disturbances are also found in cases of herpes encephalitis (e.g., Refs. 31 and 32) and, in progressive form ("semantic dementia"), in association with degenerative brain disease (e.g., 33 and 34); these disorders involve damage to middle and inferior temporal lobe structures that lie out-

side the perisylvian zone usually associated with language function (see Chap. 37).

In some cases, the deficit is remarkably selective, affecting some categories of words more than others. The pattern that has been most frequently reported is a disproportionate loss of knowledge of biological kinds, such as animals, fruits, and vegetables; knowledge of artifacts, such as tools and furniture, is at least relatively preserved (see Ref. 35 for review). The semantic deficit is manifest on naming tasks as well as on a variety of measures of word comprehension. This "category-specific" disorder has most often been described in cases of herpes encephalitis but has also been found in one case of semantic dementia (e.g., Ref. 36). There have been attempts to account for this pattern in terms of confounding factors such as the greater visual complexity and lesser familiarity of animals relative to objects such as tools (e.g., Refs. 37 and 38), but the category differences have been shown to persist even when these factors are well controlled (e.g., Ref. 39). Moreover, the opposite pattern—better performance on living things—has been demonstrated in patients with frontoparietal lesions (see Ref. 35 for review). One possible account of this double dissociation is that biological kinds and artifacts depend in different degrees on different types of semantic information (e.g., Refs. 31 and 40). For example, animals are distinguished largely on the basis of perceptual characteristics such as shape and color (compare *lion* and *tiger,* for example), while artifacts are defined primarily by their function (namely, the diverse objects that qualify as radios).

These considerations are compatible with the view that semantic memory is distributed across subsystems specialized for different types of knowledge (but see Ref. 41). Figure 10-2, from Allport,[42] illustrates such a model: the shape of a telephone is stored in one subsystem, its sound in another, its function (not shown) in still another. Although represented in different subsystems, the properties of an object are linked in memory by virtue of the fact that they consistently occur together. When some features of an object (e.g., its shape) are accessed, properties that reside in other

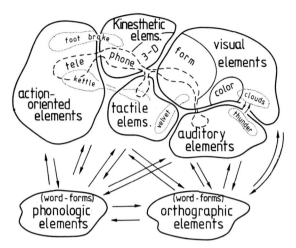

Figure 10-2
Schematic of a distributed model of conceptual representation. (From Allport,[42] with permission.)

subsystems (e.g., function) are automatically activated, instantiating the distributed activation pattern that corresponds to full knowledge of the object.

Semantic breakdown also occurs along the abstractness/concreteness dimension. Normal subjects show an advantage for concrete words (e.g., Ref. 43), and it would not be surprising if brain damage magnified this effect. This is, in fact, the result that is most frequently reported. For example, repetition of abstract words is disproportionately impaired in deep dysphasia (e.g., Refs. 26 to 28), a pattern that also holds for oral reading in deep dyslexia (cf. Ref. 7). It is unlikely, however, that this effect simply reflects the greater difficulty of abstract words, as there are patients who show the reverse pattern, performing better on abstract than concrete words (e.g., Refs. 36, 44, and 45). There is some evidence that abstract word superiority is associated with differential impairment within the class of concrete words, specifically, worse performance on words denoting living things than those denoting artifacts.[32,36] This would suggest that both patterns reflect disproportionate loss of perceptual components of meaning, which are irrelevant

to abstract words and more salient for some categories of concrete words than others.

Processing of Single Words: Production

Psycholinguists conceive of production as a multistage process that begins with a concept and ends with movement of the articulators (e.g., Refs. 11, 46, and 47). Here we will concern ourselves only with the processes exemplified in Fig. 10-1, which involve selection of a lexical entry (lemma) that corresponds to the concept to be communicated, followed by access to the phonologic form of the word. We will not review the evidence that supports the two-stage retrieval process here (see Refs. 11, 46, and 47), but consideration of the tip-of-the-tongue phenomenon—knowing that one knows a word without being able to encode it phonologically—suggests that there is a stage of lexicalization that precedes access to phonology. The second stage, phonologic encoding, is a complex process involving retrieval of a set of phonemes, arranging them in the correct serial order, and specifying their stress pattern (e.g., Ref. 11).

Although there is general agreement that word retrieval is a two-step process, the nature of the relationship between the two stages is controversial. Some theorists maintain that lemma selection precedes and is entirely uninfluenced by phonologic encoding (e.g., Ref. 11). Others view lexical retrieval as an interactive process, involving feedback from phonology as well as activation in the forward direction, with the result that phonology can affect lemma selection (e.g., Refs. 10 and 48). Observations that favor the latter account include the fact that mixed errors that bear both a semantic and a phonologic relationship to the target word (e.g., carrot → cabbage) are more frequent than would be expected by chance (e.g., Refs. 49 and 50). This finding suggests that phonologic feedback interacts with feedforward activation from semantics to promote the selection of alternatives that bear both a semantic and a phonologic relationship to the target.

Models of word production are based to a

large extent on normal speech error patterns (e.g., Refs. 46 and 47). It should be possible to account for aphasic speech errors within the same theoretical framework. The errors produced by normal speakers include word substitutions that are semantically (e.g., fork → spoon), or phonologically related to the target (e.g., index → insect) as well as the mixed errors referred to above. Semantic errors are common in aphasics, and, although the literature suggests that phonologically related word substitutions are rare (cf. Ref. 51), there are some patients who do produce high rates of these "formal paraphasias."[52,53] Perhaps the major difference between aphasic and normal speech errors (aside from the increase in overall rate of error production) is the frequency with which aphasics generate errors that are not words; these are referred to as phonemic paraphasias, or neologisms. Some of these errors bear a clear phonologic relationship to the target (e.g., scout → scut); others, sometimes referred to as abstruse neologisms (e.g., Ref. 54), do not.

Although patients generally produce both semantic and phonologic errors, there are cases in which one type of error dominates. For example, Caramazza and Hillis[55] describe a patient who produced only semantic errors, while Caplan and coworkers[56] report a case in which errors were exclusively phonologic. In general, the error patterns of aphasics are consistent with the two-stage model, with indications that semantic and phonologic processes can, on occasion, be disrupted independently.

Recently, there have been efforts to bring aphasic data to bear on the question of independent stage versus interactive models of lexical retrieval. As noted earlier, the interactive model predicts that mixed (semantic + phonologic) errors should exceed levels expected by chance; this prediction should hold for aphasics as well as for normals. Martin and coworkers[57] examined a corpus of errors elicited from aphasics in a picture-naming task and found that it does. Martin and her colleagues[53] were also able to simulate error patterns of a patient who produced a high rate of form-based word substitutions by altering parameter settings on an implemented version of an interactive computational model.[10]

Grammatical class is another important variable in lexical retrieval. It is not unusual to find patients who show significant differences in their ability to retrieve nouns versus verbs (e.g., Refs. 58 and 59). Case studies include those of McCarthy and Warrington[60] of a patient with a selective disturbance in verb production and comprehension and Zingeser and Berndt,[61] whose patient showed preservation of action naming relative to object naming. Different lesion sites have been implicated in these selective impairments—specifically, a frontal locus for verbs and a temporal locus for nouns (e.g., Ref. 62). But the functional basis for these grammatical class effects is not entirely clear. As grammatical class reflects a conceptual distinction, one might expect this factor to be operative early in word retrieval; indeed, the lemma is assumed to specify grammatical class (e.g., Ref. 11). However, Caramazza and Hillis[63] have argued that phonologic output from the lexicon is also organized with respect to grammatical class. This proposal follows from their study of two patients who showed selective deficits for verbs in a single modality—oral production in one case and written production in the other. They interpret these patterns to reflect selective impairment for verbs at the level of orthographic or phonologic encoding.

Sentence-Level Processing: Comprehension

As inspection of the sentences below will indicate, the meaning of a sentence is not solely a function of its lexical content. Failure to comprehend such sentences—interpreting sentence 1 to indicate that the cat was the chaser or that the dog was black—is not uncommon in aphasics, even when they understand all of the individual words. In an influential study, Caramazza and Zurif[64] demonstrated such an impairment in Broca's aphasics. Although their subjects had no difficulty understanding sentences like sentence 2, they performed at chance on sentences like sentence 1.

1. The cat that the dog chased was black.
2. The apple that the boy ate was red.

The difference between the two sentences, which have the same syntactic structure, is that the second one is semantically constrained (apples can't eat boys) while the first is not. In order to interpret sentence 1 correctly, it is necessary to recover the syntax of the sentence and to use this information to assign the nouns to the thematic roles specified by the verb (i.e., dog to the role of agent, or chaser, and cat to the role of theme, or the entity being chased). Caramazza and Zurif's experiment showed that the aphasics had difficulty utilizing syntactic information for this purpose, although they were clearly able to make use of semantic constraints. These authors showed, further, that performance was a function of syntactic complexity: although the patients did relatively well on simple active declarative sentences, their performance broke down on more complex structures, such as passives and object relatives (sentence 1, for example). Caramazza and Zurif interpreted this result to indicate that the patients were using heuristics such as "assign the preverbal noun the agent role and the postverbal noun the role of theme." Reliance on heuristics, together with semantic constraints, would account for the fact that sentence comprehension appears relatively preserved in Broca's aphasics.

Difficulty in sentence production—the pattern known as "agrammatism"—is also part of the symptom complex in Broca's aphasia. The fact that syntactic impairments in comprehension and production occurred in the same patients* gave rise to the hypothesis that the co-occurring deficits were due to a central syntactic deficit, character-

---

*The comprehension deficit is not, however, unique to Broca's aphasics. It is also demonstrated by conduction aphasics (e.g., Refs. 64 and 106), who, like Broca's, have little or no difficulty in comprehending single words. In fact, most aphasics tend to perform worse on semantically reversible sentences (e.g., The boy kissed the girl.); the critical point is that some patients are selectively impaired, performing virtually without error on nonreversible sentences.

ized as a loss of grammatical knowledge (e.g., Ref. 65). Another influential view was that both disturbances reflect impairment to the closed class vocabulary, consisting of elements such as prepositions and tense markers, which convey syntactic information (e.g., Ref. 66). Both hypotheses were subsequently challenged by two sources of evidence: reports of cases in which production was agrammatic but comprehension was intact (e.g., Ref. 67) and the demonstration that agrammatic Broca's aphasics with the "asyntactic" comprehension pattern described by Caramazza and Zurif[64] were able to detect grammatical violations such as those in sentences 3a and 3b.[68,69]

3a. How many did you see birds in the park?
3b. John was finally kissed Louise

These results, subsequently replicated in other laboratories (e.g., Refs. 70 and 71), present difficulty for both accounts of the agrammatic impairment. The ability to detect such violations requires knowledge of the grammar as well as sensitivity to the absence or presence and identity of the grammatical morphemes on which most of them depend.

What, then, is the basis for the "asyntactic" comprehension pattern? Linebarger and coworkers[68] suggested two possible accounts. The first of these is the limited capacity hypothesis. The patients have limited processing resources that will not suffice for parsing and interpretive operations; if they parse, they cannot interpret, and vice versa. Schwartz and coworkers[72] tested this hypothesis in a study in which patients judged the plausibility of sentences such as sentences 4a and 4b. The "padding" in sentence 6a should increase the difficulty of parsing relative to sentence 4b; on the limited capacity hypotheses, one might therefore expect worse performance on the padded sentences.

4a. The chicken killed the farmer.
4b. In the early part of the day, the chicken drank some water and then killed and ate the farmer.
4c. The farmer was killed by the chicken.

The results showed, however, that the effect of padding was negligible for the "asyntactic" comprehenders (though not for other aphasics); in contrast, the effect of the syntactic manipulation in sentence 4c, which involves movement of the nouns from their canonical (preverbal agent, postverbal theme) positions, was seriously detrimental. The second account is the mapping hypothesis. The patients are able to parse sentences but cannot carry out additional operations on the structures computed by the parser, such as mapping from a syntactic representation to thematic roles.

Interpretation of the "asyntactic" comprehension pattern remains controversial. The mapping and limited capacity hypotheses are still debated, as are other interpretations motivated by recent developments in linguistic theory (see Ref. 69 for discussion). The mapping hypothesis has led to the development of treatment programs directed at the mapping operation (see Refs. 73 and 74 and Chap. 12, this volume), which have produced gains in some chronic aphasics. The capacity limitation hypothesis has received support from studies conducted with normal subjects; it turns out that a variety of manipulations that might be expected to tax processing capacity (e.g., rapid serial visual presentation of the words in a sentence; divided attention; elimination of grammatical morphemes) result in comprehension patterns that mirror those of the aphasics (e.g., Refs. 75 to 77). However, this evidence in itself is not compelling. Assuming that it is the recovery of syntactic information and/or the mapping from syntactic to semantic structures that are most vulnerable under these conditions, one would expect other factors that contribute to sentence interpretation to be more influential; these include a tendency to assign the preverbal noun the role of agent, which it often is in English sentences (e.g., Ref. 78). Other proposals have come from linguists, who have attempted to interpret the asyntactic comprehension pattern in terms of constructs in linguistic theory (see Ref. 69 and other papers in that volume). To a large extent, these accounts emphasize the difficulty that these aphasics have in comprehending sentences with moved arguments; these structures are marked with "traces" (indicated by t)

linked to the argument that has been moved, as in sentence 5:

5. The farmer was killed t by the chicken.

It is assumed that the necessity to link the moved argument (the farmer, in sentence 5) to the trace complicates sentence processing for the aphasics. Often ignored by proponents of these views, however, is the fact that "asyntactic" patients frequently have difficulty with sentences that (at least according to most theories) lack traces, such as the simple active declarative[79,80] and locative[79,81] sentences exemplified by sentences 6a and 6b.

6a. The boy follows the girl.
6b. The paper is on the book.

Thus, while the basic phenomena are well established, there is as yet no generally accepted interpretation of the "asyntactic" comprehension pattern.

Short-Term Memory and Sentence Processing

Other studies of aphasics have focused on the role of short-term memory (STM) in sentence processing. Although most aphasics show some degree of short-term verbal memory impairment (see Ref. 82 for review), there are cases in which STM capacity, as measured by digit and word span, is markedly deficient in the context of relatively preserved language abilities (e.g., Refs. 83 and 84). The STM deficit appears to reflect impairment of a phonologic component of STM (e.g., Ref. 8). Most STM patients have difficulty with sentence comprehension, demonstrating the performance pattern characteristic of agrammatic aphasics that was described above (e.g., Ref. 85). It has proved difficult, however, to specify the relationship between these two impairments. One complicating factor is that the two are not perfectly correlated; there are instances in which reduced memory span is not accompanied by impairment in comprehension (e.g., Refs. 86 and 87). Studies of normal sentence processing indicate, moreover, that syntactic and semantic encoding occur on line (e.g., Ref. 88), so that there would seem to be no need to maintain the input in phonologic form. But while phonologic memory may not be necessary for first-pass encoding operations, it may serve as a backup store that allows the listener to revise interpretations in light of information that comes later in the sentence (for discussion, see Refs. 89 and 90).

Sentence-Level Processing: Production

A schema for sentence production is outlined in Fig. 10-1. Although not explicitly represented in the diagram, most psycholinguists assume that sentence production involves retrieval of a syntactic frame that stipulates word order (e.g., determiner-noun-auxiliary-verb. . .) and serves as a template into which phonologically specified words are later inserted (e.g., Refs. 47 and 48). While there are other aphasics who are impaired in some aspects of sentence production (e.g., Ref. 91), it is the deficits of agrammatical Broca's aphasics that have drawn most attention. The production of such patients is characterized by the limited use of syntactic structures and the omission of grammatical morphemes, such as tense markers (e.g., *-ed*), determiners (e.g., *the*), and prepositions (e.g., *to*).* It seems likely that frame retrieval is seriously impaired in such patients, reflecting a reduction in the inventory of syntactic structures, their inaccessibility, or both (e.g., Ref. 92). The fact that patients occasionally produce utterances that are more complex than those constituting the bulk of their corpora suggests that inaccessibility of these structures is at least part of the problem (e.g., Ref. 93). In light of evidence from normals that use promotes further use,[94,95] it seems likely that a tendency to rely on a limited set of structures will render other structures progressively less accessible. There is some evidence that frame retrieval can be disrupted independently of access to grammatical morphology[67,96] and that bound (i.e., inflectional) and freestanding grammatical morphemes can be selectively affected.[97,98]

---

*Omission is common in English, which is not highly inflected. In other languages, such as Hebrew, substitution of grammatical morphemes is the dominant error pattern (e.g., Ref. 107).

NEW DIRECTIONS

Cognitive neuropsychology adopted the box-and-arrow information processing models that were favored by cognitive psychologists in the 1970s. The boxes stood for modules whose internal operations were largely unknown; the arrows symbolized the flow of information between them. More recently, cognitive theorists have turned to computer-implemented (neural network or "connectionist") models that specify more precisely how information is represented and processed (see Chap. 8). The models are networks of units that represent information; the informational significance of the units is either specified by the modeler (in "localist" models; e.g., Ref. 48) or acquired during learning trials (in parallel distributed processing, or PDP, models; e.g., Refs. 40 and 99). In the latter, inner layers of units are initially connected randomly to input and output layers in which units are specified for content. Thus, for example, models that learn to read aloud have input units that stand for individual letters or groups of letters and output units that stand for specific phonemes or groups of phonemes. Explorations of effects of "lesioning" these models (for example, by randomly eliminating units or altering the strength of connections between units) have revealed some interesting properties that have implications for fundamental assumptions in cognitive neuropsychology.

One major result of the simulation studies is that symptoms are not necessarily a direct reflection of the type of representation that is lesioned. For example, Shallice and colleagues[99,100] have developed a connectionist model of reading in which learning procedures are used to train graphemic units to activate units of meaning ("sememes" such as "brown," "has legs," etc.) which ultimately activate phoneme units. In other words, the model learns to pronounce written words by looking up their meanings. Lesioning this model can result in semantic errors (e.g., reading *night* as *sleep*) of the sort that are produced by patients with deep dyslexia (see Chapter 12, this volume). These errors were generally thought to reflect impairment at the semantic level (e.g., Ref. 101). The simulations on this model demonstrate, however, that semantic errors can be generated by lesions elsewhere in the network. A related point is made by data from a study by Farah and McClelland,[40] who lesioned a semantic network to simulate the disorders involving living and nonliving things. The model included two semantic subsystems, one representing functional properties and the other visual properties, which predominated for living things. As a result of the connectivity patterns within the network, damage to the visual subsystem rendered the functional properties of living things inaccessible. The "symptoms" therefore reflected perturbations that extended well beyond the subsystem targeted by the lesion. The implication of these findings is that the relationship between symptom and deficit may not be as direct as it is often taken to be (cf. Ref. 102).

Other simulation studies demonstrate that performance patterns that appear selective can be generated by "lesions" that are widespread. Employing a localist model of word retrieval,[10] which allows activation to feed back from phonemes to lemma to semantic units as well as to proceed in the forward direction, our group has shown that shifts in the dominant error types can be produced by altering different parameters of the model.[53,103] The two parameters are connection strength, which affects the ease with which activation flows (in both directions) from one level to another, and decay rate, which affects the persistence of activation within representational levels. Different error patterns result from connection weight and decay rate "lesions," both applied uniformly throughout the lexical system. A decrease in connection strength reduces the flow of activation to target-related units, resulting in an increase in nonword errors. Decay rate "lesions" have a different effect on the distribution of activation, shifting error production in the direction of semantic and formal substitutions. Lest it be thought that this is merely a formal exercise, manipulation of these two parameters closely simulated the individual error patterns of almost all (20/23) of the fluent aphasics that we tested.

How seriously should we take these demonstrations of nonlocal effects of lesions, and do they in any way invalidate the 20-year research program in cognitive neuropsychology? Computational modeling in the language domain is relatively new, and it is too soon to determine how useful this approach will prove to be. However, recent psycholinguistic studies indicate that normal language processing is characterized by a good deal of interaction among processing components (e.g., Refs. 10, 95, and 104). Interactive processing architectures complicate the task of inferring the locus of the deficit from a patient's performance. As Farah[102] has observed, the relationship between symptom and impaired process is no longer transparent; semantic errors, for example, need not necessarily reflect perturbation of a semantic process. But while it will be necessary to interpret new data more cautiously, and, perhaps, to reexamine earlier conclusions, the effort to tie phenomena of language breakdown to models of normal language function remains useful and valid. Neuropsychological data extend the database and testing ground for normative models, and the models, in turn, provide a coherent framework for the investigation and interpretation of clinical phenomena.*

ACKNOWLEDGMENT

Preparation of this chapter was supported by grant DC00191 from the National Institutes of Health.

REFERENCES

1. Goodglass H, Geschwind N: Language disorders (aphasia), in Carterette EC, Friedman MP (eds): *Handbook of Perception.* New York: Academic Press, 1976.
2. Caramazza A: The logic of neuropsychological re-

---

*One impediment to the clinical application of cognitive neuropsychological approaches to language disorders has been the dearth of appropriate diagnostic instruments. However, new tests that are intended to provide a psycholinguistic analysis of aphasic deficits are becoming available (e.g., Refs. 89 and 108).

search and the problem of patient classification in aphasia. *Brain Lang* 21:9–20, 1984.

3. Schwartz MF: What the classical aphasia categories can't do for us and why. *Cogn Neuropsychol* 21:3–8, 1984.

4. Marin OSM, Saffran EM, Schwartz MF: Dissociations of language in aphasia: Implications for normal function. *Ann NY Acad Sci* 280:868–884, 1976.

5. Caramazza A: On drawing inferences about the structure of normal cognitive systems from the analysis of patterns of impaired performance: The case for single-patient studies. *Brain Cogn* 5:41–66, 1986.

6. Shallice T: From neuropsychology to mental structure. Cambridge, England: Cambridge University Press, 1988.

7. Coltheart M, Patterson KE, Marshall JC (eds): *Deep Dyslexia.* London: Routledge, 1980.

8. Vallar G, Shallice T (eds): *Neuropsychological Deficits in Short-Term Memory.* Cambridge, England: Cambridge University Press, 1990.

9. Fodor JA: *The Modularity of Mind.* Cambridge, MA: MIT Press, 1983.

10. Dell GS, O'Seaghdha PG: Mediated and convergent lexical priming in language production: A comment on Levelt et al. *Psychol Rev* 98:604–614, 1991.

11. Levelt WJM. Accessing words in speech production: Stages, processes and representations. *Cognition* 42:1–21, 1992.

12. Mitchell DC: Sentence parsing, in Gernsbacher MA (ed): *Handbook of Psycholinguistics.* San Diego, CA: Academic Press, 1994.

13. Allport DA: Speech production and comprehension: One lexicon or two? in Prinz W, Sanders AF (eds): *Cognition and Motor Processes.* Berlin: Springer-Verlag, 1984.

14. Monsell S: On the relation between lexical input and output pathways for speech, in Allport A, MacKay D, Prinz W, Sheerer E (eds): *Language Perception and Production.* London: Academic Press, 1987.

15. Liberman AM, Studdert-Kennedy M: Phonetic perception, in Held R, Lebowitz H, Teuber H-L (eds): *The Handbook of Sensory Physiology: Perception.* Heidelberg: Springer-Verlag, 1978, vol 8, pp. 143–178.

16. Caramazza A, Berndt RS, Basili AG: The selective impairment of phonological processing: A case study. *Brain Lang* 18:128–174, 1983.

17. Albert ML, Bear D: Time to understand: A case study of word deafness with reference to the role of time in auditory comprehension. *Brain* 97:373–384, 1974.

18. Saffran EM, Marin OSM, Yeni-Komshian G: An analysis of speech perception in word deafness. *Brain Lang* 3:209–228, 1976.

19. Auerbach SH, Allard T, Naeser M, et al: Pure word deafness: Analysis of a case with bilateral lesions and defect at the prephonemic level. *Brain* 105:271–300, 1982.

20. Denes G, Semenza C: Auditory modality-specific anomie: Evidence from a case of pure word deafness. *Cortex* 14:41–49, 1975.

21. Tanaka Y, Yamadori A, Mori E: Pure word deafness following bilateral lesions. *Brain* 110:381–403, 1987.

22. Bramwell B: Illustrative cases of aphasia (case 11). *Lancet* 1:1256–1259, 1897. Reprinted with an introduction by A W Ellis in *Cogn Neuropsychol* 1:245–258, 1984.

23. Kohn SE, Friedman RB: Word-meaning deafness: A phonological semantic dissociation. *Cogn Neuropsychol* 3:291–308, 1986.

24. Schacter DL, McGlynn SM, Milberg WP, Church BA: Spared priming despite impaired comprehension: Implicit memory in a case of word-meaning deafness. *Neuropsychology* 7:107–118, 1993.

25. Franklin S, Howard D, Patterson K: Abstract word meaning deafness. *Cogn Neuropsychol* 11:1–34, 1994.

26. Howard D, Franklin S: *Missing the Meaning? A Cognitive Neuropsychological Study of Processing of Words by an Aphasic Patient.* Cambridge, MA: MIT Press, 1988.

27. Katz R, Goodglass H: Deep dysphasia: An analysis of a rare form of repetition disorder. *Brain Lang* 39:153–185, 1990.

28. Martin N, Saffran EM: A computational account of deep dysphasia: Evidence from a single case study. *Brain Lang* 43:240–274, 1992.

29. Berndt RS, Basili A, Caramazza A: Dissociation of functions in a case of transcortical sensory aphasia. *Cogn Neuropsychol* 4:79–101, 1987.

30. Martin N, Saffran EM: Factors underlying repetition and short-term memory in transcortical sensory aphasia. *Brain Lang* 37:440–479, 1990.

31. Warrington EK, Shallice T: Category specific semantic impairments. *Brain* 107:829–854, 1984.

32. Sirigu A, Duhamel J-R, Poncet M: The role of sensorimotor experience in object recognition. *Brain* 114:2555–2573, 1991.

33. Snowden JS, Goulding PJ, Neary D: Semantic dementia: A form of circumscribed cerebral atrophy. *Behav Neurol* 2:167–182, 1989.

34. Hodges JR, Patterson K, Oxbury S, Funnell E: Semantic dementia: Progressive fluent aphasia, with temporal lobe atrophy. *Brain* 115:1783–1806, 1992.

35. Saffran EM, Schwartz MF: Of cabbages and things: Semantic memory from a neuropsychological perspective—A tutorial review, in Umilta C, Moscovitch M (eds): *Attention and Performance: XV. Conscious and Nonconscious Processes.* Cambridge, MA: MIT Press, 1994.

36. Breedin SD, Saffran EM, Coslett HB: Reversal of the concreteness effect in a patient with semantic dementia. *Cogn Neuropsychol* 11:617–660, 1994.

37. Funnell E, Sheridan J: Categories of knowledge? Unfamiliar aspects of living and non-living things. *Cogn Neuropsychol* 9:135–154, 1992.

38. Stewart F, Parkin AJ, Hunkin NM: Naming impairments following recovery from herpes simplex encephalitis: Category specific? *Q J Exp Psychol* 44A:261–284, 1992.

39. Farah MJ, McMullen PA, Meyer MM: Can recognition of living things be selectively impaired? *Neuropsychologia* 29:185–193, 1991.

40. Farah MJ, McClelland JL: A computational model of semantic memory impairment: Modality specificity and emergent category. *J Exp Psychol (Gen)* 120:339–357, 1991.

41. Caramazza A, Hillis AE, Rapp B, Romani C: The multiple semantics hypothesis: Multiple confusion? *Cogn Neuropsychol* 7:161–189, 1990.

42. Allport DA: Distributed memory, modular subsystems and dysphasia, in Newman SK, Epstein R (eds.), *Current Perspectives in Dysphasia.* Edinburgh: Churchill Livingstone, 1985, pp 32–60.

43. Paivio A: Dual coding theory: Retrospect and current status. *Can J Psychol* 45:255–258, 1991.

44. Warrington EK: The selective impairment of semantic memory. *Q J Exp Psychol* 27:635–657, 1975.

45. Cipolotti L, Warrington EK: Semantic memory and reading abilities: A case report. *J Int Neuropsychol Soc* 1:104–110, 1995.

46. Fromkin VA: The non-anomalous nature of anomalous utterances. *Language* 47:27–52, 1971.

47. Garrett MF: Levels of processing in sentence production, in Butterworth B (ed): *Language Production.* New York: Academic Press, 1980, vol 1.

48. Dell GS: A spreading activation theory of retrieval in language production. *Psychol Rev* 93:283–321, 1986.

49. Dell GS, Reich PA: Stages in sentence production: An analysis of speech error data. *J Verb Learn Verb Behav* 20:611–629, 1981.

50. Martin N, Weisberg R, Saffran EM: Variables influencing the occurrence of naming errors: Implications for models of lexical retrieval. *J Mem Lang* 28:462–485, 1989.

51. Ellis AW: The production of spoken words, in Ellis AW (ed): *Progress in the Psychology of Language.* Vol 2. London: Erlbaum, 1985.

52. Blanken G: Formal paraphasias: A single case study. *Brain Lang* 38:534–554, 1990.

53. Martin N, Dell GS, Saffran EM, Schwartz MF: Origins of paraphasias in deep dysphasia: Testing the consequences of a decay impairment to an interactive spreading activation model of lexical retrieval. *Brain Lang* 47:609–660, 1994.

54. Schwartz MF, Saffran EM, Bloch DE, Dell GS: Disordered speech production in aphasic and normal speakers. *Brain Lang* 47:52–88, 1994.

55. Caramazza A, Hillis AE: Where do semantic errors come from? *Cortex* 26:95–122, 1990.

56. Caplan D, Vanier M, Baker C: A case study of reproduction conduction aphasia: I. Word production. *Cogn Neuropsychol* 3:99–128, 1986.

57. Martin N, Gagnon DA, Schwartz MF, et al: Phonological facilitation of semantic errors in normal and aphasic speakers. *Lang Cogn Process.* In press.

58. Miceh G, Silveri MC, Romani C, Caramazza A: On the basis for the agrammatic's difficulty in producing main verbs. *Cortex* 20:207–220, 1984.

59. Kohn SE, Lorch MP, Pearson DM: Verb finding in aphasia. *Cortex* 25:57–69, 1989.

60. McCarthy R, Warrington EK: Category specificity in an agrammatic patient: The relative impairment of verb retrieval and comprehension. *Neuropsychologia* 23:709–727, 1985.

61. Zingeser LB, Berndt RS: Retrieval of nouns and verbs in agrammatism and anomia. *Brain Lang* 39:14–32, 1990.

62. Daniele A, Giustolisi L, Silveri MC, et al: Evidence for a possible neuroanatomical basis for lexical processing of nouns and verbs. *Neuropsychologia* 32:1325–1341, 1994.

63. Caramazza A, Hillis AE: Lexical organization of nouns and verbs in the brain. *Nature* 349:788–790, 1991.

64. Caramazza A, Zurif EB: Dissociations of algorithmic and heuristic processes in language compre-

hension: Evidence from aphasia. *Brain Lang* 3:572–582, 1976.

65. Caramazza A, Berndt RS: Semantic and syntactic processes in aphasia: A review of the literature. *Psychol Bull* 85:898–918, 1978.

66. Bradley DC, Garrett MF, Zurif EB: Syntactic deficits in Broca's aphasia, in Caplan D (ed): *Biological Studies of Mental Processes.* Cambridge, MA: MIT Press, 1980.

67. Miceli G, Mazzuchi A, Menn L, Goodglass H: Contrasting cases of Italian agrammatic aphasia without comprehension disorder. *Brain Lang* 19:65–97, 1983.

68. Linebarger MC, Schwartz MF, Saffran EM: Sensitivity to grammatical structure in so-called agrammatic aphasics. *Cognition* 13:641–662, 1983.

69. Linebarger MC: Agrammatism as evidence about grammar. *Brain Lang* 50:52–91, 1995.

70. Berndt RS, Salasoo A, Mitchum CC, Blumstein S: The role of intonation cues in aphasic patients' performance of the grammaticality judgment task. *Brain Lang* 34:65–97, 1988.

71. Shankweiler D, Crain S, Gorrell P, Tuller B: Reception of language in Broca's aphasia. *Lang Cogn Process* 4:1–33, 1989.

72. Schwartz MF, Linebarger M, Saffran EM, Pate DS: Syntactic transparency and sentence interpretation in aphasia. *Lang Cogn Process* 2:85–113, 1987.

73. Byng S: Sentence comprehension deficit: Theoretical analysis and remediation. *Cogn Neuropsychol* 5:629–676, 1988.

74. Schwartz MF, Saffran EM, Fink RB, et al: Mapping therapy: A treatment program for agrammatism. *Aphasiology* 8:19–54, 1994.

75. Miyake A, Carpenter PA, Just MA: A capacity approach to syntactic comprehension disorders: Making normal adults perform like aphasics. *Cogn Neuropsychol* 11:671–717, 1994.

76. Blackwell A, Bates E: Inducing agrammatic profiles in normals: Evidence for the selective vulnerability of morphology under cognitive resource limitation. *J Cogn Neurosci* 7:228–257, 1995.

77. Pulvermüller F: Agrammatism: Behavioral description and neurobiological explanation. *J Cogn Neurosci* 7:165–181, 1995.

78. Bever TG: The cognitive basis for linguistic structures, in Hayes JR (ed): *Cognition and the Development of Language.* New York: Wiley, 1970.

79. Schwartz MF, Saffran EM, Marin OSM: The word order problem in agrammatism: 1. Comprehension. *Brain Lang* 10:263–288, 1980.

80. Berndt RS, Mitchum CC, Haendiges AN: Comprehension of reversible sentences in "agrammatism." *Cognition.* In press.

81. Kolk H, Van Grunsven MJE: Agrammatism as a variable phenomenon. *Cogn Neuropsychol* 2:347–384, 1985.

82. Saffran EM: Short-term memory impairment and language processing, in Caramazza A (ed): *Advances in Cognitive Neuropsychology and Neurolinguistics.* Hillsdale, NJ: Erlbaum, 1990.

83. Saffran EM, Marin OSM: Immediate memory for word lists and sentences in a patient with deficient auditory short term memory. *Brain Lang* 2:420–433, 1975.

84. Vallar G, Baddeley AD: Phonological short-term store, phonological processing and sentence comprehension: A neuropsychological case study. *Cogn Neuropsychol* 1:121–142, 1984.

85. Saffran EM, Martin N: Short-term memory impairment and sentence processing, in Vallar G, Shallice T (eds): *Neuropsychological Impairments of Short Term Memory.* Cambridge, England: Cambridge University Press, 1990.

86. Butterworth B, Campbell R, Howard D: The uses of short-term memory: A case study. *Q J Exp Psychol* 38:705–737, 1986.

87. Martin RC: Articulatory and phonological deficits in short-term memory and their relation to syntactic processing. *Brain Lang* 32:159–192, 1987.

88. Marslen-Wilson W, Tyler LK: The temporal structure of spoken language understanding. *Cognition* 8:1–71, 1980.

89. Caplan D: *Language: Structure, Processing and Disorders.* Cambridge, MA: MIT Press, 1992.

90. Gathercole SE, Baddeley AD: *Working Memory and Language.* Hillsdale, NJ: Erlbaum, 1993.

91. Butterworth B, Howard D: Paragrammatisms. *Cognition* 26:1–38, 1987.

92. LaPointe S, Dell GS: A synthesis of some recent work on sentence production, in Tanenhaus MK, Carlson G (eds): *Linguistic Structure in Language Processing.* Dordrecht: Kluwer, 1988.

93. Menn L, Obler LK (eds): *Agrammatic Aphasia: A Cross-Language Narrative Sourcebook.* Philadelphia: John Benjamins, 1990.

94. Bock JK: Syntactic persistence in language production. *Cogn Psychol* 18:355–387, 1986.

95. Bock JK: Structure in language: Creating form in talk. *Amer Psychol* 45:1221–1236, 1990.

96. Saffran EM, Schwartz MF, Marin OSM: Evidence from aphasia: Isolating the components of a pro-

duction model, in Butterworth B (ed): *Language Production.* London: Academic Press, 1980, pp 221–240.

97. Nespoulous J-L, Dordain M, Perron C, et al: Agrammatism in sentence production without comprehension deficits: Reduced variability of syntactic structures and/or of grammatical morphemes? A case study. *Brain Lang* 33:273–295, 1988.

98. Saffran EM, Berndt RS, Schwartz MF: A scheme for the quantitative analysis of agrammatic production. *Brain Lang* 37:440–479, 1989.

99. Plaut D, Shallice T: Deep dyslexia: A case study of connectionist neuropsychology. *Cogn Neuropsychol* 10:377–500, 1993.

100. Hinton GE, Shallice T: Lesioning an attractor network: Investigations of acquired dyslexia. *Psychol Rev* 98:74–95, 1991.

101. Shallice T, Warrington EK: Single and multiple component central dyslexic syndromes, in Coltheart M, Patterson KE, Marshall JC (eds): *Deep Dyslexia.* London: Routledge, 1980, pp 119–145.

102. Farah MJ: Neuropsychological inference with an interactive brain: A critique of the "locality assumption." *Behav Brain Sci* 17:43–104, 1994.

103. Dell GS, Schwartz MF, Martin N, et al: Lesioning a connectionist model of lexical retrieval to simulate naming errors in aphasia. Presented at conference on Neural Modeling of Cognitive and Brain Disorders; June 9, 1995; College Park, MD.

104. MacDonald MC, Pearlmutter NJ, Seidenberg MS: Lexical nature of syntactic ambiguity resolution. *Psychol Rev* 101:676–703, 1994.

105. Howard D, Hatfield FM: Aphasia therapy: Historical and contemporary issues. Hillsdale, NJ: Erlbaum, 1987.

106. Heilman KM, Scholes RJ: The nature of comprehension errors in Broca's, conduction, and Wernicke's aphasics. *Cortex* 12:258–265, 1976.

107. Grodzinsky Y: The syntactic characterization of agrammatism. *Cognition* 16:99–120, 1984.

108. Kay J, Lesser R, Coltheart M: *Psycholinguistic Assessment of Language Processing in Aphasia (PALPA).* London: Erlbaum, 1992.

Chapter 11

RECOVERY OF APHASIA

Andrew Kertesz

Recovery of cognition after brain damage is a complex phenomenon with great theoretical and practical significance. Recovery from aphasia is an important model because language function has been extensively studied and quantitated. Loss of language is particularly disabling to a patient, and rehabilitation of language function is a major issue after stroke and trauma. Approximately 25 percent of stroke patients have significant aphasia.[1] Clinicians have recognized that aphasic syndromes are dynamic and that recovery takes place to a considerable extent after stroke and to an even greater extent after trauma. Wernicke[2] postulated much of the recovery from aphasic symptoms is affected by *right hemispheric compensation;* subsequently, Henschen[3] restated this principle, which was named *Henschen's principle.* Von Monakow[4] formulated his *diaschisis* theory on observations with aphasics and on the analogy of spinal shock, which was well established by physiologists. He even said: *"The temporary nature is one of the most important characteristics of aphasia."* Diaschisis is an active process by which acute brain damage deprives the surrounding or functionally connected areas from a trophic influence initially causing a more severe deficit than would be expected from the loss of affected area alone. The deprived areas recover by acquiring reinnervation from the original source or a neuron or become active after adapting to the state of partial denervation. The concept of diaschisis has been developed pharmacologically and physiologically using various modern neuroscience techniques, particularly cerebral blood flow (CBF) and metabolic studies.[5]

Animal experiments and clinical observations suggested that "silent" areas or structures, not usually involved in the functions that were lost due to a specific structure damaged, take over the function or account for the compensation. This was called *vicariation* or *vicarious functioning* by Fritsch and Hitzig,[6] who observed the recovery of hemiplegia in dogs after removing the motor cortex, and by Munk, who documented the recovery of visual loss in animals. The concept implied a built-in redundancy in the central nervous system (CNS), which is a difficult premise to accept. It is more parsimonious biologically to assume, however, that all compensatory structures have some role, even though partial, in the function in question prior to brain damage. The CNS is considered as a dynamically organized network capable of substitution and change of function rather than as permanently determined distinct centers. Functional plasticity is quite extensive and reorganization of cerebral networks is evident from converging sources. Nevertheless, there is a finite amount of cortex subserving certain functions, so that, when damaged in humans, permanent deficits result.

The considerable neuroplasticity allowing recovery is a subject of great interest in recent biological and anatomic research. Reorganization may take place by functionally connected tissue substituting for some of the functions lost by altering complex polysynaptic connections and physiologic mechanisms.[7] This form of recovery in humans is probably subject to retraining and pharmacotherapy. Particularly in the early stages of recovery, a substantial imbalance of neurotransmitters may occur, not only in damaged tissue but also in the surrounding or functionally connected areas that have suddenly become denervated.[8] Much of the pharmacotherapy of stroke has concentrated on reperfusion, or neuroprotection, at early stages of the injury. Replacing neurotransmitters may provide a form of pharmacotherapy that goes beyond neuroprotection in the very brief time window following a stroke. Denervation hypersensitivity to remaining albeit diminished excitatory transmitters and the reversal of inhibitory chemical neurotransmitters may also contribute to recovery. Axonal sprouting, regrowth, and collateral sprouting are important processes of repair following brain damage and have been observed centrally as well as in the peripheral nervous system. Recently, the area of brain tissue grafting and transplantation has been developed to promote local physiologic, pharmacologic, and structural repair. Despite the demonstration of axonal regrowth in central autografts[9] and in cerebral tissue transplantation, particularly for Parkinson disease,[10] it is likely that recovery from lesions of any substantive size in the brain takes place not as a result of axonal regrowth but mainly as a result of functional reorganization. This implies strengthening of certain connections based on biochemical changes, such as long-term potentiation, and even microstructural alterations, such as increasing the number of dendritic spines.

Functional analysis of deficits and their relationship to clinical brain lesions provides much of the information about the reorganization of brain function in humans. The complexity and variability of cognitive impairment renders longitudinal measurement and analysis of deficits difficult. The reproducibility of observations is influenced by many biological and psychological factors. The main areas investigated are language, visuospatial cognition, praxis, attention, and memory. The complexity of deficit analysis in cognition and in aphasia has been increasingly recognized and quantitation has been achieved by several advances in methodology. Aphasia tests for a language-disordered population have become better standardized and more specific, and the methods of follow-up and statistical evaluation of change have become more sophisticated.[11–15] Advances in cognitive psychology and linguistics have also contributed to deficit analysis[16] (see Chaps. 1 and 10). Development in neuroimaging, as in computed tomography (CT) and magnetic resonance imaging (MRI), allow us to localize and quantitate lesions in patients who can be concomitantly examined in detail with neuropsychological tests or psychophysiological experiments (see Chap. 5). More recently, functional activation of cerebral metabolism and blood flow with positron emission tomography (PET) and functional MRI (fMRI) are contributing to issues of recovery and compensation of function (see Chap. 6). Prognostic factors, such as initial severity, time from onset, etiology, age, handedness, aphasia type, lesion size and location, and the effect of therapy have been extensively investigated.

FACTORS IN RECOVERY

Initial Severity

The extent of initial language deficit is one of the most important prognostic factors in recovery. Early investigators considered initial severity to have highly predictive value.[17–23] Final outcome is clearly better in patients who are less severely affected on the initial examination. The severity of deficit at onset has a different effect on recovery rates, because mildly affected aphasics do not have much room for recovery (a "ceiling effect") and severely affected aphasics often have a long way to go. This explains why some studies claim that those with global aphasia recover the most.[24] The difference between outcome measures and recovery rates is discussed further in the section dealing with lesion size. A recent study indicated a 6-month post-onset examination may be a better predictor of 24-month outcome than an initial examination.[25] Some of this may be attributable to the relatively low number of individuals who participated in the regression analysis and also the variability of severity that was obtained at 1 month, by which time some individuals often show considerable recovery. Several investigators explored the possibility that individual language behaviors may be predictive for eventual recovery. Some suggested that the initial level of auditory comprehension is an important prognostic factor.[26–29] Gestural or praxis scores were also found to be predictive, but these are associated substantially with auditory comprehension, with high correlation between the subscores.[13,30] Treated patients tend to be selected from the less severe groups and to bias outcome results.[31,32] The failure to control for initial severity renders some studies of treatment unreliable. There are various methods of controlling for initial severity, such as analysis of covariance or the change expressed as a ratio or percentage of initial severity. Each of these statistical methods has some limitations on either end of the severity scale.

Time from Onset

Time from onset of the assessment is also an important variable. When patients are entered into studies at various stages in their recovery curve, comparison becomes very difficult. In our studies, we begin our evaluation within the acute period, between 10 to 45 days after a stroke.[23] Since most of our patients were examined at exactly 14 days post onset, this provides a rather homogeneous population. Only the more severely affected patients, who could not be examined at that time because of intercurrent medical illness or obtundation, were kept until the upper limit of the acute period. On subsequent follow-up examinations, a considerable amount of attrition of patients can be expected for various reasons. Therefore, studies examining patients' performance may be difficult to interpret if the comparison is between segments of various recovery slopes unless the number of patients at each intersect are statistically accounted for.

Most recovery occurs in the first 2 to 3 months. Recovery curves show an exponential decrease in the 3- to 6-month interval, a 6- to 12-

month interval reaching a plateau after 1 year.[23,24] However, studies have shown some further recovery after 1 year, even though some of these were only a few patients who improved with treatment. These studies claim that treatment produces further recovery in periods where spontaneous recovery is not expected.[32,33] A recent study suggests that severe aphasics improve most in the second 6 months of recovery.[25]

Etiology

Different etiologies produce different types of damage and compensatory mechanisms. Some intracerebral hemorrhages, especially from a subarachnoid bleed, recover rather quickly.[34,35] The difference between infarcts and hemorrhage is unclear. There are some anecdotal reports of hemorrhages recovering to a greater extent than ischemic infarcts.[25] It appears that the size and the location of the hemorrhage have to be compared with the size and location and dry infarcts before such a conclusion can be reached, even though some of the initially large hemorrhages occupying a substantial volume in the brain often become absorbed and only leave a slitlike lesion in the subcortical tissues. There is some pathologic evidence showing that hemorrhages tend to displace tissues rather than to destroy them, in certain parts of the hemorrhage at any rate. Major hemorrhages, on the other hand, are quite destructive, and the patients are less likely to survive because of the intraventricular extension or edema.

Traumatic aphasia, for instance, recovers well unless it is related to penetrating head injury.[34,36] Persisting dysarthria is common in severe trauma, and this often disrupts communication to such a degree that the extent of posttraumatic aphasia is difficult to determine. Penetrating head injury affects a different age group, and there is a variability in the speed and path of the missiles and the associated concussion. Therefore, posttraumatic aphasia is biologically different from the vascular type. There are many similarities nonetheless, indicating that the recurring patterns of aphasic types are not necessarily related to the distribution of vascular lesions. A recent study by

Ludlow and coworkers,[36] for instance, on Vietnam veterans, showed that the lesions that produce a persisting asyntactic or Broca's aphasia are large, involving the subcortical structures and the parietal area in addition to Broca's area. This study on penetrating missile injuries reached very much the same conclusions that have been obtained in studying stroke recovery.

Multiple lesions confound the pattern of recovery. Several small lesions produce an accumulating deficit, the sum of which is less than the deficit caused by a single large lesion. This has been observed clinically by Dax[37] in the description of recovery from motor aphasia. The added lesion effect[38] has been studied physiologically in animals and is a model to explain why slowly growing tumors cause so much less deficit than the functional loss of a sudden large lesion. Accumulating lesions avoid the diaschisis effect of a single large lesion. There is often a critical stage when the amount of deficit becomes irreversible.

There is a prevalent view among speech and rehabilitation specialists showing that younger patients recover better, but the issue of age as a factor in recovery is more complex than it appears on the surface. Age is a major variable in recovery if one takes into consideration the superior recovery rates of immature individuals. This is called the *Kennard principle,* after a series of experiments in animals indicating much better recovery in the young.[39] Childhood aphasia is also said to recover better when compared with that of adults. When a child sustains brain damage, the plasticity of the brain probably allows for almost complete compensation by the homologous hemisphere, whether it is related to a hemispherectomy in a young child[40] or childhood aphasia due to other etiologies.[41] In addition to the plasticity, however, one should also consider that children have different etiologies, such as infection and trauma, causing a different aphasia from that of strokes.[42] There is also the problem of older patients having multiple vascular lesions or degenerative diseases, in addition to their aphasic stroke, influencing recovery. Weisenburg and McBride,[43] for instance, studied only patients under 60 so as to avoid complicating the picture by "senile changes." When certain studies combine all aphasics in a clinic, including posttraumatic or encephalitic patients, the issue of etiology is confounding.[44] Most investigators find that when they control for etiology and take a relatively homogeneous stroke population, age has little or no influence.[23,31,45–50]

Sex

Sex differences in recovery have been postulated, but only a few studies support better recovery in females that would suggest more distributed bilateral interhemispheric organization of speech functions.[51,52] We have not found any sex differences in our studies of recovery[30] and neither have other studies.[53] Another study found better recovery for males than for females on a multivariate analysis of factors in recovery.[54]

FUNCTIONS, SYMPTOMS, OR SYNDROMES

In order to study recovery of any function, one must define and measure the function in question. Clinicians tend to study symptoms, syndromes (clusters of symptoms that are coherent), and concurrent symptoms that are usually reproduced by a certain etiology. Psycholinguists argue for testing functions based on theoretical concepts. Many of these concepts are defined in terms of computer science or artificial intelligence, and may have little if any relationship to a real psychological or even less to a physiologic function.[55] Computational models that incorporate the parallelism and interactivity of cerebral functions are just beginning to be developed (see Chap. 8). Reduction of a complex behavior to its components is also fraught with the hazard of losing the meaning and biological significance of the behavior to the organism.

From the point of view of localization, more complex behaviors are likely to have widespread input and will be affected by lesions in many areas. Indirect measures of function—such as electroencephalography (EEG), event-related averaged potentials, or the distribution of neurotransmitters—also support the diffuse and interactive nature of cerebral activity. Cerebral blood flow studies[56] and recent evidence from PET and MRI studies of functional activation indicate a considerable cortical spread of activation during linguistic processes.[57,58] Physiologic and computational considerations suggest that mental processes operate in parallel and not in a series of temporally separated stages.[59,60] Seemingly elementary yet cognitively complex linguistic processes, such as naming, are impaired from multiple lesion sites, providing converging evidence for widely distributed localization.[61] On the other hand, syndromes are more likely to correlate with localizable lesions. The syndrome approach is clinically productive and more valid for rehabilitation, because it consists of a set of coherent symptoms reliably associated with certain lesion size and location. Clinicians generally attempt to deal with syndromes, as they represent the total deficit picture in the patient, although they may undertake symptom analysis that goes beyond the syndromes. Isolated or pure psychological phenomena, representing single modules of function, are difficult to define and even more difficult to localize, yet this route is often chosen by experimental psychologists. Often one function is emphasized only to establish a theoretical point, and other symptoms are ignored. Drawing the line between a symptom and a cluster of related functions may be impossible.

The taxonomy issue is a crucial one in many aspects of recovery. Some discrepancies are simply related to the same terminology applied to different behaviors, such as the different definition of transcortical motor aphasia. Sometimes the opposite also occurs and similar behaviors are grouped differently; therefore, the conclusions are contradictory. An example of this is the use of the term *jargon* for the stereotypies of global aphasia instead of restricting it to fluent Wernicke's aphasia. These disagreements may come about because a phenomenon is poorly defined and described only qualitatively. Even when standardized tests are used, classifications differ, because the criteria for each syndrome or deficit are different.[62] Despite some of these differences, as long as the behavioral criteria are clearly defined on the basis of standardized measurements, various groups can be compared with reasonable efficiency, and correlation with lesion sites has been successful and convincingly consistent for many syndromes of higher cerebral function.[13,63,64]

Articulated language output is an example of complex cognitive function subserved by a network in the central nervous system. Speech output differs substantially whether it is (1) in response to questions (responsive speech), (2) an extemporaneous expression of ideas, (3) descriptive speech, or (4) repetition. Spoken language incorporates many subfunctions, which have been categorized by linguists as articulation, fluency, prosody, phonologic processing, lexical retrieval, syntax, pragmatics, and so on. Nevertheless, all or most of the functional components tend to be involved to some extent in the clinical syndrome of Broca's aphasia, which can be reliably defined by standardized test scores[13] or by careful clinical description. The more standardized the description, the more reliable the localization. Many identifiable, even dissociable phenomena, such as agrammatism or dysprosody, contribute to the syndrome, but they do not have a consistent localization by themselves.

LESION SIZE AND LOCATION

Lesion size and location are interrelated and complex factors in aphasia recovery. Clinicians have relied on autopsy correlations, but modern neuroimaging has provided an opportunity to study lesion characteristics in vivo. We found, in our first study of lesion size measured on CT and recovery from aphasia, that the larger the lesion, the poorer the outcome; in other words, outcome correlated negatively with lesion size.[61] This has been known to clinicians since Hughlings Jackson suggested, in principle, the "mass effect".[65] Experimental psychologists, through animal lesions, have placed the importance of lesion size or mass effect above lesion location. Recovery rates also showed, with one exception, a trend of negative correlation with lesion size in our study.[61] The recovery rate of comprehension was found to be correlated positively with lesion size. This can best be understood if we look at another study of ours in which the best recovered modality was found to be comprehension.[27] Patients with large lesions having global or severe Broca's aphasia often show greater improvement in comprehension. Patients with smaller lesions, such as anomic aphasics, already have good comprehension; therefore they have less room for recovery (a ceiling effect). The large lesions with more recovery and small lesions with little change give rise to a consistently positive correlation unless the initial severity is covaried, as in our subsequent studies.[30]

Structural limitation of recovery allows compensation to take place only in certain areas, such as the adjacent cortex, contralateral homologous cortex, or hierarchically connected structures such as the subcortical ganglia.[65,66] The issue of a primary, noncompensable cortex for language function similar to the primary motor or visual cortex has become an important question for research. The existence of such a primary language cortex is supported by the large number of permanently aphasic patients and the anatomic and physiologic evidence for networks for language output and comprehension. The clinical characteristics of such networks can be summarized as follows: (1) a single, complex function is supported by multiple sites, therefore lesions from multiple sites can produce a similar deficit; (2) each area may belong to several overlapping networks, therefore a lesion in a single area often produces multiple deficits; and (3) severe and lasting deficit of function occurs when all or most structural components of a network are involved.

NONFLUENT APHASIA AND RECOVERY

Broca's aphasia has been associated with lesions from several structures outside Broca's area. These lesions often extend beyond the "foot" of the inferior frontal convolution,[61,67] involving the rolandic operculum,[68,69] anterior insula, subcortical (capsulostriatal) area,[70,71] and the periventricular or centrum semiovale region.[72] Involvement of only Broca's area is usually followed by good recovery.[67] Such lesions often produce a transient motor aphasia (also called "cortical motor aphasia," "aphemia," "pure motor aphasia," or "verbal apraxia"). *Pure motor aphasia,* or verbal apraxia, has been associated with anterior subcortical, as well as opercular, inferior rolandic, and insular cortical lesions.[71,73] Recovered Broca's aphasics often regain their fluency and syntax, but articulatory and prosodic aspects of language may remain affected and the clinical condition widely known as verbal apraxia continues.[13]

Large lesions that include not only Broca's area (posterior third of F3 and the frontal operculum) but also the inferior parietal and often the subcortical regions[30,61,67] cause persisting *Broca's aphasia.* In previous studies, impaired fluency has been associated with lesions extending to the rolandic cortical region and underlying white matter.[30,74,75] The involvement of the central white matter is also important for the fluency deficit in the head-injured population[36,76] and in stroke.[71] The centrum semiovale or periventricular white matter, which is involved in persistent cases of global or Broca's aphasia, often includes the pyramidal tract, thalamocortical somatosensory projections, striatocortical connections, callosal radiations,[71] subcallosal fasciculus,[77] thalamocortical projections forming the dorsomedial and ventrolateral nuclei,[78] and occipitofrontal fasciculus.[79]

We evaluated lesion location in Broca's aphasics who were divided at the median for poor and good recovery. In both groups, certain structures showed significant involvement (more than 50 percent). These were the inferior frontal gyrus, especially the pars opercularis and triangularis, and the insula. The difference between patients with persisting Broca's aphasia and those who show good recovery was most prominent in the involvement of the precentral, postcentral, and supramarginal gyri in the cases of poor recovery. The subcortical regions showed significant differences in the involvement of the putamen and the caudate, which was twice as frequent in the persistent cases.[30]

Lesion size and lesion location in the recovery of nonfluent aphasia in stroke was further studied in our laboratory. The target population consisted of all the consecutively examined nonfluent aphasics in whom localization with CT or MRI was available. In a 10-year period, 71 right-handed stroke patients with single lesions, ages 30 to 80, with nonfluent aphasia were followed from the acute examination period between 10 and 45 days poststroke to 12 months poststroke with a standardized comprehensive aphasia test, the Western Aphasia Battery (WAB).[14] Nonfluent aphasia was defined as having a fluency score of 4.0/10 or less as well as a repetition score of 6.9/10 or less on the WAB. Broca's aphasia was further differentiated from global aphasia as having a comprehension score of 4.0/10 or above on the WAB. The lesion areas were digitized using an area-from-contour algorithm.[80] Regions of Interest (ROI) check-listing was carried out to determine the location of the lesions. The ROIs were chosen for their physiologic importance and anatomic distinctiveness and were defined according to the CT atlas of Matsui and Hirano[81] and a new set of templates for MRI based on a cadaver study with gadolinium-filled markers.[82]

Outcome measures had a high negative correlation with lesion size throughout. Naming was an interesting exception, possibly indicating a ceiling effect combined with the relative persistence of a moderate naming deficit in many recovered nonfluent aphasics. All of these patients were treated with a variable amount of language therapy, some of them for the duration of the study, while others participated in a formal study of language therapy.[83]

The most common pattern by which a vascular lesion could produce Broca's aphasia involved the frontal opercular and central cortex and the anterior insula with or without significant subcortical involvement. With the exception of one who had central cortical, insular, and subcortical involvement, these patients recovered quite well. One patient with only an anterior insular lesion, which undercut the underlying white matter for Broca's area, showed a moderate amount of recovery. Another patient with central and insular le-

sions as well as one patient with central and subcortical lesions showed poor recovery. This suggests a certain amount of variability in how the components of the network are affected, producing different degrees of recovery.

Global aphasia is defined by the loss of speech output and comprehension as well, usually associated with destruction of both the anterior and posterior language areas.[61,84,85] However, in patients who are initially global aphasics, the Wernicke's area may be spared.[13,86] These patients tend to recover toward Broca's aphasia. Even Broca's area cortex may not be destroyed, although it is usually disconnected from the rest of the language cortex by white matter involvement.[71,74] Occasionally white matter lesions alone may produce persistent global aphasia.[61,71] Some studies have indicated that subcortical lesions associated with nonfluent aphasia tend to recover,[85] although there are exceptions to this depending on the size and number of structures involved. There are also case reports of patients with initial global aphasia without hemiplegia who recover dramatically when they have lesions affecting the posterior frontal and posterior temporal regions but sparing the central structures.[87,88] We have also seen such a case; the double lesions and the sparing of central cortex is illustrated in Figure 11-1.

The classification of severely nonfluent aphasics influences the results of recovery studies. For instance, in the Boston Diagnostic Aphasia Examination (BDAE),[11] a large group of what others would classify as severe Broca's aphasics may be labeled, at times, as "mixed anterior aphasics." In the classification system of Aachen Aphasia Test (AAT),[15] many global aphasics would be reclassified as Broca's aphasics in other clinics. Some of these problems in taxonomy have been studied systematically in the comparison of aphasia batteries and how their scoring systems affect classification.[62] Global and Broca's aphasias, as defined by our taxonomy and methods of measurements, have similar spontaneous language characteristics. In our previous taxonomic studies,[89] these were the two closest groups in the nearest-neighbor-network analysis. The major difference between

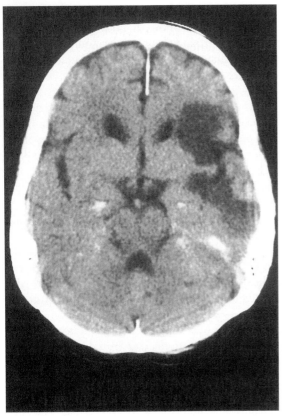

Figure 11-1

This CT scan indicates a double lesion. The anterior portion includes inferior frontal cortical and subcortical regions undercutting Broca's area and the posterior portion, a patchy temporal lesion undercutting Wernicke's area. The sparing of the central regions is noteworthy and accounts for an excellent recovery from the initial global aphasia without hemiplegia.

the two groups is in the extent of comprehension deficit. Since comprehension often recovers well, there are a great number of patients who change from global to Broca's aphasia during recovery (*Syndromenwandeln*).[90]

In our study, detailed analysis of the smallest lesions (less than 60 cm³) that produce initial global aphasia indicated that the involvement of the centrum semiovale and some involvement of the anterior subcortical basal ganglia, mainly the striatum, produced poor recovery. In two patients where only the centrum semiovale was involved, moderate recovery was seen. Half of global aphasics had both Broca's (defined as the posterior third of the inferior frontal convolution) and Wernicke's (defined as the posterior superior temporal gyrus and the posterior temporal operculum) areas involved, but one-third of globals were spared Wernicke's area and a few were spared Broca's area. These patients had the Broca's area completely undercut, but the cortex was not directly involved.

Transcortical motor aphasia is characterized by poor spontaneous speech but good repetition and comprehension. There is a variable naming deficit and the writing output is also poor. The localization of lesions is characteristically in the mesial frontal region or the supplementary motor area in the dominant hemisphere.[91–95] The importance of this region on the left was recognized by Penfield and Roberts,[96] who renamed it the *supplementary speech area* because of the frequent speech arrest that was found during stimulation of this region. Cytoarchitecturally, the supplementary motor cortex appears to represent a paralimbic extension of the limbic cortex.[97] This suggests a link between the limbic system and initiation of the motor mechanisms of speech. The lack of speech initiation is often considered to be a part of a general hypokinetic syndrome associated with frontal lobe lesions. The term *adynamic aphasia* has also been used to describe this behavior, since Arnold Pick and Kleist. Recovery is usually excellent and these patients are seen only in acute units as a rule.

Motor and premotor phonemic assembly and articulatory output mechanisms are elaborated by an extensive yet definable cortical/subcortical network. Partial damage to one or two components of the network is followed by good recovery. However, if all cortical and subcortical components of the network are impaired, the deficit is more severe and recovery is much less likely. There is converging evidence that the articulatory network for fluency involves the white matter connecting tracts between the components of the network, and lesion in the white matter alone can impair fluency in a persistent fashion.

RECOVERY FROM FLUENT APHASIA WITH COMPREHENSION DEFICIT

Language comprehension is a complex process that involves the analysis of the acoustic and phonologic properties of input as well as the recognition of syntactic and lexical elements.[98] This rapid parallel processing of input and matching it to linguistic precepts is a dominantly left hemispheric function, although the right hemisphere has been shown to recognize words and syntax to a certain degree.[99–100] The auditory association cortex of the superior temporal gyrus region and the planum temporale located behind the Heschl gyrus (Wernicke's area) performs the analysis and decoding of complex verbal stimuli. Wernicke has postulated that the auditory association area plays a monitoring role in language output (presaging modern concepts of feedback and parallel processing) and that its damage results in paraphasic, faulty speech. When the patient complains of not understanding speech but hearing, reading, and speech output remain undisturbed, the diagnostic label of *pure word deafness* is used. Although the condition is not always "pure," good recovery is the rule. *Auditory agnosia* for nonverbal sounds and amusia are often associated, although these symptoms may be seen with right-sided lesions without the verbal component. In *cortical deafness,* which is the result of bilateral temporal lesions, the patient appears clinically deaf with preserved primary hearing, but central auditory processes are impaired and the deficit is often more persisting. The recovery of comprehension seems to be mediated by areas inferior and anterior to the posterior superior temporal gyrus.[101] However, in this study, global and Broca's aphasics were mixed with fluent aphasics.

Neologistic jargon output is distinctive and is associated with lesions of both the superior temporal and inferior parietal regions.[102] *Wernicke's aphasia* with semantic jargon is correlated with lesions that are somewhat smaller, inferior, and more temporal than those in neologisms or phonemic paraphasia.[103] Other CT studies have indicated that patients with semantic substitutions have lesions posterior to those with phonemic parapha-sia.[104] A CT study of Wernicke's aphasia suggests that the extent of involvement of the superior temporal gyrus differentiates groups with good or poor comprehension outcome.[105] These authors also found the temporal isthmus lesions significant for persisting deficit.

Our studies of lesion location and size in recovery from Wernicke's aphasia suggest that ipsilateral connected structures, especially in the inferior parietal lobule, are the most likely to substitute after damage. The supramarginal and angular gyrus appear as the most likely compensating structures.[28] The evolution of Wernicke's aphasia is either in the direction from neologistic jargon to conduction aphasia or to "pure word deafness," and from both of these intermediate stages to anomic aphasia.[13] The importance of temporobasal regions in recovery from several types of aphasia has been shown during periods of treatment.[106] The authors of this study postulated a disconnection between the hippocampal formation and perisylvian language areas that hinders explicit learning of contemporary strategies.

Patients with *transcortical sensory aphasia* who have semantic jargon usually have far more posterior lesions, usually in the watershed area between the middle cerebral and posterior cerebral circulation.[107] These patients are distinguished by preserved repetition. Sometimes the term *semantic aphasia* is applied to patients with similar behavior. Recovery is usually rapid unless the syndrome evolves from a more severe lesion initially producing Wernicke's aphasia. Mixed transcortical aphasia has features of both the motor and sensory symptoms and tends to have a poor prognosis, with nonfluency persisting and not all comprehension returning, depending on the etiology. It occurs relatively uncommonly and the recovery patterns have not been described extensively. In our laboratory, we had two persisting cases, one with stroke and another with posttraumatic syndrome.

Word finding or word access—the retrieval of lexical items (often tested by naming)—is a fundamental process in language, and *anomia* is a feature of most aphasic syndromes. The study of lexical access and semantic processing is a major scientific and clinical topic. Recent advances in this field include the study of modality-specific fields (verbal versus visual) and the category specificity of recognition and retrieval of lexical items. Lexical retrieval is thought to be dependent on a widely distributed cortical network. Lesion studies and functional activation have suggested the role of left temporoparietal and temporooccipital cortex, and functional activation has added the left frontal lobe as having a role in semantic processing.[108] Considering the complex nature of semantic association, narrowly restricted localization of this function is not likely. This is already evidenced from the wide distribution of lesions that result in anomia or anomic aphasia. Patients who have only anomic aphasia de novo usually recover well. Mild word-finding and naming difficulty are very common in acute stroke and can be seen transiently with subcortical, anterior cortical, and posterior cortical lesions and rapid recovery is the rule even before they are transferred to rehabilitation. However, lesion size correlates with the severity of anomic aphasia.[13,109]

RIGHT HEMISPHERE SUBSTITUTION FOR LANGUAGE

Jackson[110] considered the right hemisphere capable of automatic utterances and as responsible for the residual output in severe aphasia. The principle of contralateral homologous cortical substitution was based on patients with large left-hemispheric lesions yet relatively good recovery, where there was very little left hemisphere remaining to take over. More recently CT studies made the same point.[111,112] In addition, in some patients who became aphasic with a single left-hemispheric stroke but recovered, a second, right-hemispheric stroke produced another language deficit.[113–115] These cases, however, may have represented bilateral language organization to begin with, rather than a commonly operating mechanism of functional transfer to the contralateral hemispheres.

    The idea of compensation through right-hemispheric function even after partial left hemispheric damage was also supported by studies of

sodium amytal given to aphasics who had recovered.[116,117] These studies indicated that even though the aphasic disturbance occurred from a left-hemispheric lesion, it was the right-hemispheric injection that increased the language disturbance, implying that the right hemisphere compensated for the previous deficit produced by the left-sided lesion. More recent studies of CBF by PET also suggested right-hemispheric compensation.[118,119] All of these studies, however, demonstrated ipsilateral increase in function as well and acknowledged that it was difficult to separate ipsilateral from contralateral compensation.

FUNCTIONAL AND ANATOMIC ASYMMETRIES

Only a portion of the variation in recovery can be explained by the extent and location of lesions and the rest have been postulated to relate to differences in language laterality, handedness, and anatomic asymmetries. Left-handedness is considered by many, mainly on a theoretical basis, to represent more bilaterally distributed language organization; Subirana's,[120] Luria's,[121] Gloning and coworkers,[122] Hécaen and Sauget's,[123] and Geschwind's[124] suggestions that left-handers and right-handers with a family history of left-handedness recover better from aphasia because of more bilateral language distribution is based on anecdotal evidence. However, subsequent studies could not firm this assumption.[30,125] There was no evidence for atypical patterns of recovery in a group of 19 left-handed aphasic patients.[125] Patients with familial left-handedness did not recover better than those without such a history. Recent studies of anatomic asymmetry on CT, inspired by the demonstration of a commonly larger planum temporale on the left by Geschwind and Levitsky,[126] have correlated better outcome with atypical or less asymmetry.[127] This is also based on the idea that this pattern may be associated with more right-hemispheric language. We have studied the factor of anatomic asymmetry on CT—as measured by occipital width, frontal width, and protuberance (petalia)—and could not confirm that atypical asymmetry played a role in recovery in any of the aphasic groups.[30] It could be that anatomic asymmetries relate more to handedness variables than language distribution, as suggested by some of our studies in normals;[128] therefore we are not seeing an effect on language recovery.

METABOLIC AND FUNCTIONAL STUDIES

Cerebral blood flow (CBF), single photon emission tomography (SPECT), and positron emission tomography (PET) studies of cerebral metabolism provide added functional information to structural or lesion studies of recovery. Recent studies of CBF with xenon 133 have also revealed a right-hemispheric hypometabolism in aphasic strokes, the extent of which has correlated with recovery to a modest degree.[129] Positron emission tomography studies of cerebral metabolism have shown a great deal of hypometabolism surrounding but also remote from cerebral infarcts, thus suggesting that not only surrounding areas but also homologous areas in the contralateral hemisphere play a role in compensation.[118,119] Weiller and colleagues,[119] with a PET 0^{15} activity study, found that both ipsilateral frontal areas and right perisylvian regions are activated in recovered Wernicke's aphasia. However, one CBF study showed no significant contralateral change while clinical recovery occurred in severe aphasics.[130] Patients who improved more showed more blood flow in the left hemisphere. This appears to be the consequence of the size of the lesion, which correlates with the CBF changes. Another CBF study showed better than 60 percent hemispheric flow in patients with good recovery.[131] A PET study also indicated the importance of ipsilateral hemispheric glucose metabolism in recovery from aphasia.[132] We had experience with four aphasics whose distant hypometabolism in the ipsilateral cortex persisted outside their CT lesion, despite significant recovery.[133] Similar results were obtained by Metter and co-workers.[118] Other studies have suggested improved CBF at distant (contralateral) hypometabolic sites with time.[5] The relationship of persisting or improving hypometabolism to recovery remains controversial.

More recent functional activation confirms the importance of the posterior temporal area in auditory perception of language and the central and premotor cortex in articulation, in addition to some newly emphasized components to the language network, such as the mesial frontal and lateral frontal areas in word retrieval and semantic association.[108] The anterior cingulate gyrus appeared to be part of an anterior attentional system, indicated by its activation while monitoring lists of words for semantic category. Some of the continuing work with PET and 0^{15} and recent efforts on MRI functional activation promise to shed further light on these issues.[58,119,134]

CONCLUSION

The size and location of lesions, time from onset, etiology, and initial severity are complex, interdependent factors in the recovery of language loss. Other biological factors—such as age, education, handedness, and sex—play a less significant role when an adult stroke population is followed. Lesion size is undoubtedly a significant factor in the extent of recovery. An exception to the negative correlation between language recovery and lesion size is comprehension. In some patients, even with large lesions, the amount of comprehension recovery is considerable, while patients with small lesions demonstrate a relatively small degree of recovery. One of the unresolved issues remains whether ipsilateral connected adjacent or distant, even contralateral, cortex plays a major role in compensation. The answer is probably both, but our studies of lesion location and recovery in Broca's and Wernicke's aphasia suggest that ipsilateral connected structures play the major role in restoration of function after damage. These are structures that are likely to be used normally in the language network, although for somewhat different functions at different times. The functional participation by these structures implies neuroplasticity rather than a built-in redundancy when recovery from damage occurs. The cytoarchitectonic similarity and anatomic contiguity make some structures prime candidates for substitution. This structural network is capable of a considerable degree of compensation, producing various clinical patterns of deficit, but its substantial destruction results in permanent loss in the majority of individuals. Exceptions to this rule are best explained by contralateral substitution. Functional activation and cortical stimulation provide convergent evidence of such language networks.

REFERENCES

1. Leske MC: Prevalance estimates of communicative disorders in the U.S.: Language, hearing, and vestibular disorders. *ASHA* 23:229–237, 1981.
2. Wernicke C: Die neueren Arbeiten über Aphasie. *Fortschr Med* 4:371–377, 1886.
3. Henschen SE: *Klinische und anatomische Beitrage zur Pathologie des Gehirns.* Stockholm, Nordiska Bokhandel, vols 5–7, 1920–1922.
4. von Monakow C: *Die Lokalisation im Grosshirn und der Abbau der Funktionen durch corticale Herde.* Wiesbaden, Bergmann, 1914.
5. Feeney DM, Baron JC: Diaschisis. *Stroke* 17:817–830, 1986.
6. Fritsch GT, Hitzig E: Über die elektrische Erregbarkeit des Grosshirns. *Archiv Anat Physiol* 300–332, 1870.
7. Merzenich MM, Kaas JH, Wall J, et al: Topographic reorganisation of somatosensory cortical areas 3b and 1 in adult monkeys following restricted deafferentation. *Neuroscience* 8:33–55, 1983.
8. Pappius HM: Brain injury: New insights into neurotransmitter and receptor mechanisms. *Neurochem Res* 16:941–949, 1991.
9. Aguayo AJ, David S, Bray G: Influences of the glial environment on the elongation of axons after injury: Transplantation studies in adult rodents. *J Exp Biol* 95:231–240, 1981.
10. Bjorklund A, Stenevi U: Intracerebral neural implants: Neural replacement and reconstruction of damaged circuitries. *Annu Rev Neurosci* 7:279–308, 1984.
11. Goodglass H, Kaplan E: *Assessment of Aphasia and Related Disorders.* Philadelphia, Lea & Febiger, 1972.
12. Goodglass H, Kaplan E: *Boston Naming Test.* Philadelphia, Lea & Febiger, 1983.
13. Kertesz A: *Aphasia and Associated Disorders: Taxonomy, Localization and Recovery.* New York, Grune & Stratton, 1979.
14. Kertesz A: *The Western Aphasia Battery.* New York, Grune & Stratton, 1982.
15. Huber W, Poeck K, Weniger D, Willmes K: *Aachener-Aphasie Test.* Göttingen, Hogrefe, 1983.
16. McCarthy RA, Warrington EK: *Cognitive Neuropsychology.* San Diego, CA, Academic Press, 1990.
17. Godfrey CM, Douglass E: The recovery process in aphasia. *Can Med Assoc J* 80:618–824, 1959.
18. Schuell A, Jenkins JJ, Pabon J: *Aphasia in Adults.* New York, Harper & Row, 1964.
19. Sands E, Sarno MT, Shankweiler D: Long-term assessment of language function in aphasia due to stroke. *Arch Phys Med Rehabil* 50:202–222, 1969.
20. Sarno MT, Silverman M, Sands E: Speech therapy and language recovery in severe aphasia. *J Speech Hear Res* 13:607–623, 1970.
21. Sarno MT, Silverman M, Levita E: Psychosocial factors and recovery in geriatric patients with severe aphasia. *J Am Geriatr Soc* 18:405–409, 1970.
22. Gloning K, Trappl R, Heiss WD, Quatember R: Prognosis and speech therapy in aphasia in neurolinguistics, in Lebrun Y, Hoops R (eds): *Recovery in Aphasics.* Amsterdam, Swets & Zeitlinger, 1976, vol 4, pp 57–62.
23. Kertesz A, McCabe P: Recovery patterns and prognosis in aphasia. *Brain* 100:1–18, 1977.
24. Sarno MT, Levita E: Recovery in treated aphasia in the first year post stroke. *Stroke* 10:663–670, 1979.
25. Nicholas ML, Helm-Estabrooks N, Ward-Lonergan J, Morgan AR: Evolution of severe aphasia in the first two years post onset. *Arch Phys Med Rehabil* 74:830–836, 1993.
26. Keenan JS, Brassell EG: A study of factors related to prognosis for individual aphasic patients. *J Speech Hear Disord* 39:257–269, 1974.
27. Lomas J, Kertesz A: Patterns of spontaneous recovery in aphasic groups: A study of adult stroke patients. *Brain Lang* 5:388–401, 1978.
28. Kertesz A, Lau WK, Polk M: The structural determinants of recovery in Wernicke's aphasia. *Brain Lang* 44:153–164, 1993.
29. Porch BE, Collins M, Wertz RT, Friden TP: Statistical prediction of change in aphasia. *J Speech Hear Res* 23:312–321, 1980.
30. Kertesz A: What do we learn from recovery from aphasia? in Waxman SG (ed): *Advances of Neurol-*

ogy. *Functional Recovery in Neurological Disease.* New York, Raven Press, 1988, vol 47, pp 277–292.

31. Basso A, Capitani E, Vignolo LA: Influence of rehabilitation on language skills in aphasic patients. *Arch Neurol* 36:190–196, 1979.

32. Poeck K, Huber W, Willmes K: Outcome of intensive language treatment in aphasia. *J Speech Hear Disord* 54:471–479, 1989.

33. Broida H: Language therapy effects in long term aphasia. *Arch Phys Med Rehabil* 58:248–253, 1977.

34. Kertesz A, McCabe P: Recovery patterns and prognosis in aphasia. *Brain* 100:1–18, 1977.

35. Legatt AD, Rubin MJ, Kaplan LR, et al: Global aphasia without hemiparesis: Multiple etiologies. *Neurology* 37:201–205, 1987.

36. Ludlow C, Rosenberg J, Fair C, et al: Brain lesions associated with nonfluent aphasia fifteen years following penetrating head injury. *Brain* 109:55–80, 1986.

37. Dax M: Lesions de la moitie gauche de l'encephale coincidant avec l'oubli des signes de la pensee (lu a Montpellier en 1836). *Gaz Hebd Med Chir* 2:259–262, 1865.

38. Ades HW, Raab DH: Recovery of motor function after two-stage extirpation of area 4 in monkeys. *J Neurophysiol* 9:55–60, 1946.

39. Kennard MA: Age and other factors in motor recovery from precentral lesions in monkeys. *Am J Physiol* 115:138–146, 1936.

40. Basser LS: Hemiplegia of early onset and the faculty of speech with special reference to the effects of hemispherectomy. *Brain* 85:427–460, 1962.

41. Martins IP, Ferro JM: Recovery of acquired aphasia in children. *Aphasiology* 6:431–438, 1992.

42. Woods BT, Teuber HL: Changing patterns of childhood aphasia. *Ann Neurol* 3:273–280, 1978.

43. Weisenburg T, McBride K: *Aphasia: A Clinical and Psychological Study*, 2d ed. New York, Hafner, 1964.

44. Holland AL, Bartlett C: Some differential effects of age on stroke-produced aphasia, in Ulatowska HK (ed): *The Aging Brain: Communication in the Elderly.* San Diego, CA, College Hill, 1985, pp 141–155.

45. Culton G: Reaction to age as a factor in chronic aphasia in stroke patients. *J Speech Hear Disord* 36:563–564, 1971.

46. Kenin M, Swisher L: A study of pattern of recovery in aphasia. *Cortex* 8:56–68, 1972.

47. Sarno MT, Levita E: Some observations on the nature of recovery in global aphasia after stroke. *Brain Lang* 12:1–12, 1981.

48. Messerli P, Tissot A, Rodriquez J: Recovery from aphasia: Some factors of prognosis, in Lebrun Y, Hoops R (eds): *Recovery in Aphasics.* Amsterdam, Swets & Zeitlinger, 1976, pp 124–135.

49. Taylor-Sarno M: Preliminary findings in a study of age, linguistic evolution and quality of life in recovery from aphasia. *Scand J Rehab Med Suppl* 26:43–59, 1992.

50. Lendrem W, Lincoln NB: Spontaneous recovery of language abilities in stroke patients between 4 and 34 weeks poststroke. *J Neurol Neurosurg Psychiatry* 48:743–748, 1985.

51. Basso A, Capitani E, Moraschini S: Sex differences in recovery from aphasia. *Cortex* 18:469–475, 1982.

52. Pizzamiglio L, Mammucari A, Razzano C: Evidence for sex differences in brain organization in recovery in aphasia. *Brain Lang* 25:213–223, 1985.

53. Ferro JM: The influence of infarct location on recovery from global aphasia. *Aphasiology* 6:415–430, 1992.

54. Holland AL, Greenhouse JB, Fromm D, Swindell CS: Predictors of language restriction following stroke: A multivariate analysis. *J Speech Hear Res* 32:232–238, 1989.

55. Crick F: The recent excitement about neural networks. *Nature* 337:129–132, 1989.

56. Ingvar DH, Schwartz MS: Blood flow patterns induced in the dominant hemisphere by speech and reading. *Brain* 97:273–288, 1974.

57. Raichle ME, Herscovitch P, Mintun AM, et al: Dynamic measurements of local blood flow and metabolism in the study of higher cortical function in humans with positron emission tomography. *Neurology* 14:48–49, 1984.

58. Binder JR, Rao SM: Human brain mapping with functional magnetic resonance imaging, in Kertesz A (ed): *Localization and Neuroimaging in Neuropsychology.* San Diego, CA, Academic Press, 1994, pp 185–212.

59. McClelland JL, Rumelhart DE: Parallel distributed processing: *Explorations in the Microstructure of Cognition:* Vol 2. *Psychological and biological models.* London, MIT Press, 1986.

60. Farah MJ: Neuropsychological inference with an interactive brain. *Behav Brain Sci* 17:43–104, 1994.

61. Kertesz A, Harlock W, Coates R: Computer tomo-

graphic localization, lesion size and prognosis in aphasia. *Brain Lang* 8:34–50, 1979.

62. Ferro JM, Kertesz A: Comparative classification of aphasic disorders. *J Clin Exp Neuropsychol* 9:365–375, 1987.

63. Damasio H, Damasio AR: *Lesion Analysis in Neuropsychology*. New York, Oxford University Press, 1982.

64. Kertesz A: *Localization and Neuroimaging in Neuropsychology*. San Diego, CA, Academic Press, 1994.

65. Lashley KS: Factors limiting recovery after central nervous lesions. *J Nerv Ment Dis* 88:733–755, 1938.

66. Bucy PC: The relation of the premotor cortex to motor activity. *J Nerv Mental Dis* 79:621–630, 1934.

67. Mohr JP: Broca's area and Broca's aphasia, in Whitaker H, Whitaker HA (eds): *Studies in Neurolinguistics*. New York, Academic Press, 1976, vol 1, pp 201–235.

68. Levine DN, Sweet E: Localization of lesions in Broca's motor aphasia, in Kertesz A (ed): *Localization in Neuropsychology*. New York: Academic Press, 1983, pp 185–208.

69. Lecours AR, Lhermitte F: The "pure form" of the phonetic disintegration syndrome (pure anarthria): Anatomo-clinical report of a historical case. *Brain Lang* 3:88–113, 1976.

70. Naeser MA, Alexander MP, Helm-Estabrooks N, et al: Aphasia with predominantly subcortical lesion sites: Description of three capsular/putaminal aphasia syndromes. *Arch Neurol* 39:2–14, 1982.

71. Kirk A, Kertesz A: Cortical and subcortical aphasias compared. *Aphasiology* 8:65–82, 1994.

72. Naeser MA, Palumbo CL, Helm-Estabrooks N, et al: Severe nonfluency in aphasia: Role of the medial subcallosal fasciculus and other white matter pathways in recovery of spontaneous speech. *Brain* 112:1–38, 1989.

73. Schiff HB, Alexander MP, Naeser MA, Galaburda AM: Aphemia—Clinical-anatomic correlations. *Arch Neurol* 40:720–727, 1983.

74. Mayendorf, von Niessl E: *Vom Lokalisationsproblem der artikulierten Sprache*. Leipzig, Barth, 1930.

75. Knopman DS, Selnes OA, Niccum N, Rubens AB: A longitudinal study of speech fluency in aphasia: CT scan correlates of recovery and persistent nonfluency, *Neurology* 33:1170–1178, 1983.

76. Russell W, Espir M: *Traumatic Aphasia: A Study of Aphasia in War Wounds of the Brain*. London, Oxford University Press, 1961.

77. Muratoff W: Secundare Degenerationen nach Durchschneidung des Balkens. *Neurologisches Centralblatt* 12:714–729, 1893.

78. Yakovlev PI, Locke S: Limbic nuclei of thalamus and connections of limbic cortex. *Arch Neurol* 5:364–400, 1961.

79. Déjerine J, Déjerine-Klumpke A: *Anatomie des Centres Nerveux*. Paris, Ruef et Cie, 1895.

80. Albinger G: *Sigma-Scan. Version 3.90.* Corte Madera, CA, Jandel Scientific, 1988.

81. Matsui T, Hirano A: *An Atlas of the Human Brain for Computerized Tomography*. New York, Igaku-Shoin, 1978.

82. Na D, Kertesz A: The methodology in MRI localization. *Neurology* 44(suppl 2):A134, 1994.

83. Shewan CM, Kertesz A: Effects of speech and language treatment on recovery aphasia. *Brain Lang* 23:272–299, 1984.

84. Kertesz A, Lesk D, McCabe P: Isotope localization of infarcts in aphasia. *Arch Neurol* 34:590–601, 1977.

85. Ferro JM: The influence of infarct location on recovery from global aphasia. *Aphasiology* 6:415–430, 1992.

86. Mazzochi F, Vignolo LA: Localization of lesions in aphasia: Clinical-CT correlations in stroke patients. *Cortex* 15:627–654, 1979.

87. Van Horn G, Hawes A: Global aphasia without hemiparesis: A sign of embolic encephalopathy. *Neurology* 32:403–406, 1982.

88. Ferro JM: Global aphasia without hemiparesis. *Neurology* 33:1106, 1983.

89. Kertesz A, Phipps J: Numerical taxonomy of aphasia. *Brain Lang* 4:1–10, 1977.

90. Leischner A: Aptitude of aphasics for language treatment, in Lebrun Y, Hoops R (eds): *Recovery in Aphasics*. Swets & Zeitlinger Amsterdam, 1976, pp 112–124.

91. Goldstein K: *Language and Language Disturbances*. New York, Grune & Stratton, 1948.

92. Kornyey E: Aphasie transcorticale et echolalie: Le probleme de l'initiative de la parole. *Rev Neurol* 131:347–363, 1975.

93. Rubens AB: Aphasia with infarction in the territory of the anterior cerebral artery. *Cortex* 11:239–250, 1975.

94. Chusid J, de Gutierrez-Mahoney C, Margules-Lavergne M: Speech disturbances in association with parasagittal frontal lesions. *J Neurosurg* 11:193–204, 1954.

95. Arseni C, Botez MI: Speech disturbances caused by tumors of the supplementary motor area. *Acta Psychiatr Scand* 36:279–299, 1961.

96. Penfield W, Roberts L: *Speech and Brain Mechanisms.* Princeton, NJ, Princeton University Press, 1959.

97. Sanides F: Functional architecture of motor and sensory cortices in primates in the light of a new concept of neocortex evolution, in Noback CR, Montagna W (eds): *The Primate Brain.* New York, Appleton, 1970.

98. Liebermann AM, Cooper FS, Shankweiler DR, Staddert-Kennedy M: Perception of the speech code. *Psychol Rev* 74:431–461, 1967.

99. Zaidel E: Auditory vocabulary of the right hemisphere following brain bisection or hemidecortication. *Cortex* 12:191–211, 1976.

100. Moscovitch M: Right hemisphere language. *Top Lang Disord* 1:41–61, 1981.

101. Selnes OA, Knopman DS, Niccum N, et al: Computed tomographic scan correlates of auditory comprehension deficits in aphasia: A prospective recovery study. *Ann Neurol* 13:558–566, 1983.

102. Kertesz A, Benson DF: Neologistic jargon— A clinicopathological study. *Cortex* 6:362–386, 1970.

103. Kertesz A: Localization of lesions in Wernicke's aphasia, in Kertesz A (ed): *Localization in Neuropsychology.* New York, Academic Press, 1983, pp 209–230.

104. Cappa SF, Cavallotti G, Vignolo LA: Phonemic and lexical errors in fluent aphasia: Correlation with lesion site. *Neuropsychologia* 19:171–179, 1981.

105. Naeser MA, Helm-Estabrooks N, Haas G, et al: Relationship between lesion extent in Wernicke's area on computed tomographic scan and predicting recovery of comprehension in Wernicke's aphasia. *Arch Neurol* 44:73–82, 1987.

106. Goldenberg G, Spatt J: Influence and site of cerebral lesions on spontaneous recovery of aphasia and on success of language therapy. *Brain Lang* 47:684–698, 1994.

107. Kertesz A, Sheppard A, MacKenzie RA: Localization in transcortical sensory aphasia. *Arch Neurol* 39:475–478, 1982.

108. Petersen S, Fox PT, Snyder AZ, Raichle ME: Activation of extrastriate and frontal cortical areas by visual words and word-like stimuli. *Science* 249:1041–1044, 1990.

109. Naeser M, Palumbo CL: Neuroimaging and language recovery in stroke. *J Clin Neurophysiol* 11:150–174, 1994.

110. Jackson JH: On the anatomical and physiological localization of movements in the brain. *Lancet* 1:232–234, 1873.

111. Cummings JL, Benson DF, Walsh MJ, Levine JL: Left-to-right transfer of language dominance: A case study. *Neurology* 29:1547–1550, 1979.

112. Landis T, Cummings JL, Benson DF: Passage of language dominance to the right hemisphere: Interpretation of delayed recovery after global aphasia. *Rev Med Suisse Romande* 100:171–177, 1980.

113. Nielsen JM: *Agnosia, Apraxia, and Aphasia.* New York, Hoeber, 1946.

114. Levine DM, Mohr JP: Language after bilateral cerebral infarctions: Role of the minor hemisphere. *Neurology* 29:927–938, 1979.

115. Cambier J, Elghozi D, Signoret JL, Henin D: Contribution of the right hemisphere to language in aphasic patients: Disappearance of this language after a right-sided lesion. *Rev Neurol* 139:55–63, 1983.

116. Kinsbourne M: The minor cerebral hemisphere as a source of aphasic speech. *Arch Neurol* 25:302–306, 1971.

117. Czopf J: Role of the non-dominant hemisphere in the restitution of speech in aphasia. *Arch Psychiatr Nervenkr* 216:162–171, 1972.

118. Metter EJ, Jackson CA, Kempler D, Hanson WR: Temporoparietal cortex and the recovery of language comprehension in aphasia. *Aphasiology* 6:349–358, 1992.

119. Weiller C, Isensee C, Rijntjes M, et al: Recovery from Wernicke's aphasia: A positron emission tomographic study. *Ann Neurol* 37:723–732, 1995.

120. Subirana A: The prognosis in aphasia in relation to cerebral dominance and handedness. *Brain* 81:415–425, 1958.

121. Luria AR: *Traumatic Aphasia: Its Syndromes, Psychology and Treatment.* Paris, Mouton, 1947.

122. Gloning I, Gloning K, Haub G, Quartember R: Comparison of verbal behavior in right-handed and nonright-handed patients with anatomically verified lesion of one hemisphere. *Cortex* 5:43–52, 1969.

123. Hécaen H, Sauget J: Cerebral dominance in left-handed subjects. *Cortex* 7:19–48, 1971.

124. Geschwind N: Late changes in the nervous system: An overview in plasticity and recovery of function in the central nervous system, in Stein D, Rosen J, Butters N (eds): *Plasticity and Recovery of Function in the Central Nervous System.* New York, Academic Press, 1974, pp 467–508.

125. Borod JC, Carper JM, Naeser M: Long-term lan-

guage recovery in left-handed aphasic patients. *Aphasiology* 4:561–572, 1990.

126. Geschwind N, Levitsky W: Human brain, left-right asymmetries in temporal speech regions. *Science* 161:186–187, 1968.

127. Pieniadz JM, Naeser MA, Koff E, Levine HL: CT scan cerebral hemispheric asymmetry measurements in stroke cases with global aphasia: Atypical asymmetries associated with improved recovery. *Cortex* 19:371–391, 1983.

128. Kertesz A, Polk M, Black SE, Howell J: Anatomical asymmetries and functional laterality. *Brain* 115:589–605, 1992.

129. Knopman DS, Rubens AB, Selnes OR, et al: Mechanisms of recovery from aphasia: Evidence from serial xenon 133 cerebral blood flow studies. *Ann Neurol* 15:530–535, 1984.

130. Demeurisse G, Verhas M, Capon A, Paternot J: Lack of evolution of the cerebral blood flow during clinical recovery of stroke. *Stroke* 14:77–81, 1983.

131. Nagata K, Yunoki K, Kabe S, et al: Regional cerebral blood flow correlates of aphasia outcome in cerebral hemorrhage and cerebral infarction. *Stroke* 17:417–423, 1986.

132. Heiss WD, Kessler J, Karbe H, et al: Cerebral glucose metabolism as a predictor of recovery from aphasia in ischemic stroke. *Arch Neurol* 50:958–964, 1993.

133. Black SE, Garnett ES, Nicholson RL, et al: NMR and PET findings in a crossed dextral aphasic (abstr). *Ann Neurol* 16:155, 1984.

134. Chertkow H, Bub D: Functional activation and cognition: The 0^{15} PET subtraction method, in Kertesz A (ed): *Localization and Neuroimaging in Neuropsychology*. San Diego, CA, Academic Press, 1994, pp 152–184.

Chapter 12

REHABILITATION OF APHASIA

Myrna F. Schwartz
Ruth B. Fink

It is widely accepted that the goal of aphasia rehabilitation is to maximize functional communication skills. There is less agreement on the optimal route to that goal. Speech-language pathologists are exposed to a broad range of approaches and are expected to make informed decisions about the best treatment for an individual patient based on a number of factors (e.g., etiology, severity, type of aphasia, and so on). They are trained to view aphasia as a complex cognitive/linguistic/communication disorder requiring intervention that addresses the social as well as the linguistic needs of the client.[1,2] And they work with patients in a variety of settings (acute care hospitals, rehabilitation units, home care, outpatient facilities) throughout the phases of recovery.

Differences aside, speech-language pathologists typically perform three basic functions: assessment, treatment, and outcome evaluation. The initial assessment is critical for establishing the diagnosis of aphasia and differentiating it from other neuropathologies such as dementia and dysarthria, communicating with other professionals and the patient's family, setting goals, and developing a treatment plan. Following a program of treatment, an outcome evaluation is performed to determine how well the goals have been met. Each of these three functions (assessment, treatment, and outcome evaluation) is carried out at several levels of analysis.

LEVELS OF ANALYSIS: IMPAIRMENT, DISABILITY, AND HANDICAP

The World Health Organization[3] has proposed a useful framework that distinguishes three levels at which functional consequences of a chronic condition such as aphasia may be described and explained: *impairment, disability,* and *handicap.*

"*Impairment* is any loss or abnormality of psychological, physiological, or anatomical structure or function" (p. 47).[3] The classic taxonomy of aphasia (Broca's aphasia, Wernicke's aphasia, conduction aphasia, anomic aphasia) rests on a mix of anatomic-psychological impairment symptoms [e.g., disruption of auditory-phonologic images caused by lesions in the left posterior temporal gyrus (Wernicke's area)]. The contemporary cognitive neuropsychological approach, which we focus on in later sections, derives its impairment categories from cognitive and psycholinguistic theories of the normal language system.

"*Disability* is any restriction or lack (resulting from an impairment) of ability to perform an activity in the manner or within the range considered normal for a human being" (p. 143).[3] While the characterization of impairments is theory-dependent, *disabilities* refers to categories of behavior that have strong face validity (e.g., producing and understanding speech, reading, writing). When speech pathologists characterize an aphasic disturbance, they generally do so in terms of its impact on skills like these, that is, in *disability* terms. On the other hand, such characterizations often make reference to the units affected (e.g., word, phrase, sentence), in which case it becomes difficult to distinguish them from impairment-level characterizations. In general, however, disabilities are observable (at the level of the person), while impairments are inferred from performance on diagnostic tests.*

Handicap refers to the impact of a disability on an individual's capacity to function in society. When communication is compromised by a speech/language disability (e.g., nonfluent speech) such that the individual can no longer function effectively in his or her role as parent, spouse, lawyer, or whatever, a handicap is present. The degree of handicap depends upon factors both within and external to the individual. These include the severity of the disability; the intactness of other avenues of communication, like writing or gesturing; the readiness of others to shoulder the burden of communication; and the ability to use—and to afford—alternate communication systems like computers or communication boards.

THE TRADITIONAL LANGUAGE-ORIENTED SCHOOL OF APHASIA THERAPY

In aphasia rehabilitation, any one of these three levels may be targeted for assessment, treatment, and outcome evaluation. The impairment-disability-handicap (IDH) matrix shown in Fig. 12-1 represents the various possibilities,[4] and the shaded cells locate the endeavor we term the *traditional language-oriented school*. The majority of clinicians in the United States would probably identify themselves with this school, which is eclectic in its approach to assessment and treatment. Assess-

ment draws upon standardized instruments that measure loss at both the disability and impairment levels (e.g., Boston Diagnostic Aphasia Examination,[5] Western Aphasia Battery,[6] Minnesota Test for Differential Diagnosis of Aphasia[7]). The assessment serves as a guide to treatment, which might target several impairments concurrently or bypass the impairment level altogether in favor of direct retraining or stimulation of the compromised language skill. Both the target of treatment and the treatment techniques are tailored to needs of the individual patient. The clinician may choose from several approaches. For example, the "stimulation" approach advocated by Schuell and colleagues[8] uses intensive auditory or multimodality input to elicit language production through a variety of means (e.g., repetition, phonemic cueing, reading) and in a variety of contexts (linguistic and situational). Helm-Estabrooks developed a variant of this technique to facilitate sentence production. Helm's Elicited Language Program for Syntax Stimulation (HELPSS)[9] uses a combined delayed repetition/story elicitation procedure to stimulate production of specific syntactic structures (e.g., yes-no questions; passive voice constructions) in aphasics with grammatical disturbances. The rationale behind the stimulation approach is that aphasia represents reduced access or efficiency. An alternative view is that specific aspects of the language system are lost or disrupted. This view is represented in Shewan and Bandur's "Language-Oriented Therapy,"[10] a comprehensive, psycholinguistically based treatment program that aims to strengthen the impaired function(s) using training methods derived from behavioral learning theory. The common thread among these different approaches is the focus on restoration of language skills as the route to improved functional communication.

The same language-oriented assessments used to evaluate the patient's initial status are generally used as well to measure the gains made in treatment. But this alone does not constitute outcome evaluation. Also required is an assessment of the extent to which the *functional goals* projected for the patient at the outset have been met.

Medicare guidelines[11] specifically require

---

*Frattali and colleagues[15] offer a slightly different interpretation: "*Disability* is a restriction or lack of ability in performance of daily tasks. It is the functional consequence of an impairment. Ex. = difficulty dressing, toileting, communication."

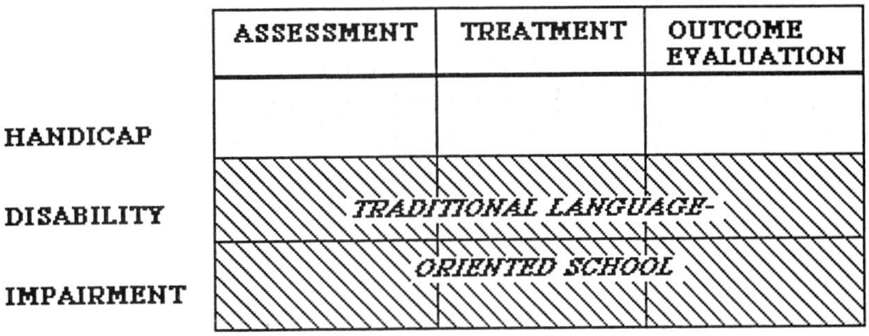

Figure 12-1
The impairment-disability-handicap (IDH) matrix. Assessment, treatment, and outcome evaluation can be directed at any of the three levels. The traditional, language-oriented school of aphasia rehabilitation focuses primarily on the impairment and disability levels.

	ASSESSMENT	TREATMENT	OUTCOME EVALUATION
HANDICAP			
DISABILITY	*TRADITIONAL LANGUAGE-*		
IMPAIRMENT	*ORIENTED SCHOOL*		

that a plan of treatment state functional goals and estimated rehabilitation potential:

Functional goals must be written by the speech and language pathologist to reflect the level of communicative independence the patient is expected to achieve, outside of the therapeutic environment. The long term functional goals must reflect the final level the patient is expected to achieve, be realistic, and have a positive effect on the quality of the patient's everyday functions.

To assess whether functional goals have been met, clinicians often rely on anecdotal reports from patients and family members. While formal assessments of functional communication are available (e.g., Functional Communication Profile,[12] Communicative Abilities in Daily Living,[13] Communicative Effectiveness Index[14]), many clinicians find that they lack the requisite sensitivity or are too cumbersome to administer.[15] A new generation of functional assessments is being developed to better meet the needs of the clinic (e.g., Amsterdam-Nijmegen Everyday Language Test,[16] ASHA's Functional Communication Scales for Adults[17]).

That language-oriented therapy succeeds in enhancing the language skills of treated patients is demonstrated in a number of large-scale group studies (e.g., Refs. 18 to 22), as well as smaller, more focused studies (e.g., Refs. 23 to 27). There is less evidence that these gains translate into reduced handicap and enhanced quality of life. In-

deed, the general view is that language gains evident in the clinic do not generalize well to less constrained tasks or settings.[28] This is one problem with the traditional, language-oriented school of aphasia therapy. A second is its weak theoretical base. Two newer schools have arisen in response to these perceived weaknesses: the functional, or pragmatic, school and the cognitive neuropsychological school.

THE FUNCTIONAL/PRAGMATIC SCHOOL OF APHASIA THERAPY

If linguistic gains made in the clinic do not automatically translate into improved functional communication, then perhaps functional carryover should be programmed in as an integral part of the rehabilitation process. For adherents of the functional/pragmatic school, this means gearing therapy toward the enhancement of *communication*, nonverbal as well as verbal, in functional settings and/or with functional materials. Functional approaches typically capitalize on the patients' strengths and seek to train patients to use compensatory strategies when communicating. Functional approaches may also use behavioral methodology to achieve changes in pragmatic skills, as Doyle and coworkers[29] demonstrated in a study aimed at teaching Broca's aphasics how to make requests. The point of pragmatic treatments is to focus on communication skills that can be used in everyday life. The most widely known pragmatic approach is Promoting Aphasics Communicative Effective-

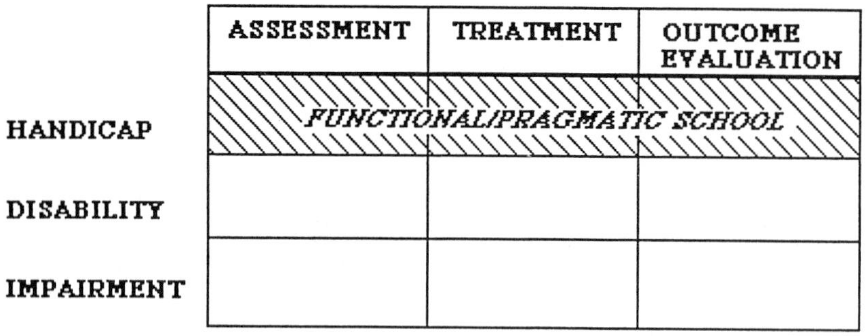

	ASSESSMENT	TREATMENT	OUTCOME EVALUATION
HANDICAP	*FUNCTIONAL/PRAGMATIC SCHOOL*		
DISABILITY			
IMPAIRMENT			

Figure 12-2
The functional/pragmatic school of aphasia rehabilitation focuses primarily on the level of handicap.

ness (PACE),[30] which fosters the communication of new information [the patient conveys a message unknown to the therapist, who must then figure it out using whatever combination of strategies (verbal, written, gestural, graphic) achieves success]. Another pragmatic approach, Conversational Coaching,[31] develops compensatory strategies in treatment sessions simulating conversations that might take place outside the clinic and that include conversations with unfamiliar listeners to further extend generalization. Ultimately, the patient and his or her relatives are trained to use these strategies to communicate with maximum effectiveness.

In its pure form (depicted in Fig. 12-2), the functional/pragmatic philosophy replaces the traditional emphasis on language impairment and disability, with an emphasis on minimizing handicap through enhanced communication. In actuality, however, even its strongest proponents advocate that pragmatic techniques be used in combination with language-based approaches.[31–33]

THE COGNITIVE NEUROPSYCHOLOGY SCHOOL

Practitioners of cognitive neuropsychology (CN) apply information-processing models of normal cognition to the analysis of disorders of higher cortical function, including language. Until recently, CN's major contribution to rehabilitation was the development of model-driven assessments for describing impairments. With increasing fre-

quency, though, cognitive neuropsychologists are involving themselves in treatment. Speech-language pathologists have also begun to apply cognitive models in the clinic. The basic idea is to pursue a more "rational" approach to treatment, in which the goals of the treatment program are informed by theory-based assessment of the patient's language capabilities.*,[34–36]

Cognitive neuropsychological assessments identify and measure impairments. It is not surprising, therefore, that impairments are also the focus of CN treatments and outcome evaluations. This restricted focus is in no way a necessary consequence of using cognitive theory to guide treatment, however. As noted by Caramazza,[37] the outcome of a cognitive assessment does not constrain the choice of therapeutic strategy; having characterized the patient's deficit at the level of impairment, one is perfectly free to target the level of disability or handicap as the focus of treatment and/or outcome. Nevertheless, the bias in CN treatment research, if not in clinical practice, has been to target the impairment level as the focus for assessment, treatment, and outcome assessment (Fig. 12-3).

---

*A recent special issue of the *Journal of Neuropsychological Rehabilitation* (vol 5, March 1995) focuses on the CN approach to aphasia rehabilitation. Additional discussion of the strengths and weaknesses of this approach is available in *Aphasia Treatment: Current Approaches and Research Opportunities*. NIDCD Monograph. Vol 2. NIH Publication No. 93-3424. Bethesda, MD, National Institutes of Health, 1992.

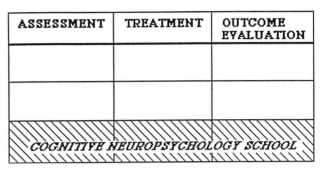

	ASSESSMENT	TREATMENT	OUTCOME EVALUATION
HANDICAP			
DISABILITY			
IMPAIRMENT	*COGNITIVE NEUROPSYCHOLOGY SCHOOL*		

Figure 12-3
The cognitive neuropsychology school of aphasia rehabilitation focuses primarily on the impairment level.

Cognitive Neuropsychological Analysis Applied to Disorders of Word Retrieval (Anomia)

Cognitive neuropsychological assessment begins where traditional assessment ends. For example, having identified a primary disorder of word retrieval, the CN-oriented clinician attempts to locate the deficit within the "functional architecture" of the language production system. The basic assumption is that one must probe for the explanation of a surface symptom like anomia, and that two patients with the same surface symptom may have very different underlying deficits. Probing for underlying deficits proceeds with reference to an information-processing model, using tests and procedures specifically developed with the model in mind.

Figure 12-4 presents a schematic version of a model that has been very influential in the analysis of word-retrieval deficits and, in particular, deficits in picture naming.[38–40] The model subdivides word retrieval into two temporally distinct stages, each of which accomplishes a transcoding, or "mapping," from one type of representation to another. The first stage takes place within the "semantic lexicon"; here, the semantic code that defines the word's meaning is mapped into a phonologic address that provides key information about the word's pronunciation—for example, the initial sound in the word, the number of syllables it contains, and its stress pattern. The second stage takes place within the "phonologic lexicon." Here, the phonologic address for each known word is

mapped onto an ordered string of phonemes specifying the full pronunciation, albeit still in a form more abstract than what the articulatory-motor system can take as input. The transcoding from a phonemic to an articulatory-motor representation occurs at a subsequent step of word production. Disruption of this last step results in verbal "apraxia" of the sort we see in nonfluent (Broca's) aphasia. The types of word-retrieval disorders that are of concern to us here are those that arise earlier in the process, at the first or second word-retrieval stage.

Various diagnostic tests are used to locate a

Figure 12-4
Schematic version of the two-stage model of word retrieval.

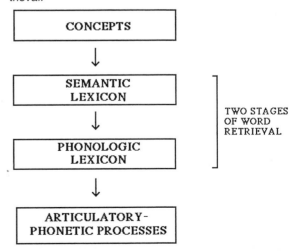

picture-naming deficit at one or the other of these stages (or both). Briefly, when we find that a patient's comprehension of pictures is unimpaired but he or she nevertheless makes semantic errors in naming (e.g., *horse* for *cow*), we immediately think of a problem in the semantic lexicon. If the patient makes semantic errors in comprehension as well as production, it is likely that the meaning representations in the semantic lexicon are degraded.[41] A patient studied by Howard and Orchard-Lisle[42] could not generate any names unless cued with the first phoneme of the target; when this patient was cued with the first phoneme of a semantically related word (e.g., shown a lion and cued with the sound *t*), she showed a reliable tendency to produce the semantic substitution (*tiger*) and to accept that as the correct response. The implication of this "miscuing" effect is that degradation of semantic lexical entries resulted in the subthreshold activation of multiple entries in the semantic lexicon and hence multiple phonologic addresses. Phonemic cues raised the activation value of corresponding addresses to threshold level; when the cue corresponded to the target, the correct name was produced; when it corresponded to a semantic coordinate, a semantic error was produced.

Many anomic patients can be cued phonemically to the correct target but do not show miscuing. Such patients are frequently able to provide partial information about the names they are unable to retrieve (e.g., that it is a long word or short word), and their errors, when they make them, bear a phonologic rather than a semantic relation to the target.[43] These are indications that the problem arises in the retrieval of the full phonologic form at the level of the phonologic lexicon.

Implications for Treatment of Word-Retrieval Deficits

The previous section illustrates the type of evidence that is used to locate a naming deficit within a functional model of the intact system. Reasoning about the treatment implications of such an analysis might proceed as follows: Patients whose deficits are centered in the semantic lexicon—i.e., in

the semantic specification of words or the phonologic addressing mechanism—should benefit from interventions that encourage semantic processing of pictures in conjunction with phonologic processing of their names. A standard way of accomplishing this is to have the patient match pictures to written words, at least some of which bear a semantic relationship to the target name. The semantic component of such tasks should be less important for patients whose deficits are centered in the phonologic lexicon. These patients should benefit as much from purely phonologic techniques, such as repeating the target name or making a rhyme judgment.

Such predictions have rarely been tested directly (but see Refs. 44a and 44b). Instead, the short- and long-term effects of semantic and phonologic facilitation techniques have been compared in undifferentiated groups of subjects with naming deficits,[45,46] with some evidence favoring the semantic techniques. Other studies have used the model-driven analysis to suggest the type of intervention called for (semantic versus phonologic) in single cases or small homogeneous groups, but without examining whether the alternative approach would have been more or less successful. Examples of these model-driven studies can be found in Refs. 44 and 47 through 52. Together, these studies provide conclusive evidence that anomia is amenable to treatment by a variety of semantic and phonologic facilitation techniques, that the benefits are generally limited to treated items, and that these benefits are maintained long after treatment ceases—as much as 1 year in the follow-up study reported in Pring and colleagues.[51]

Cognitive Neuropsychological Analysis Applied to Agrammatism

The term *agrammatism* refers to the simplification and fractionation of morphosyntactic structure in the speech of nonfluent, Broca's aphasics (see Table 12-1). The traditional, language-oriented approach to treating agrammatism uses combinations of stimulation, repetition, and shaping techniques to facilitate production of affected

Table 12-1

Examples of G.R.'s picture description performance at three points in time[a]

TARGET	**THE BOY IS SLEEPING IN THE BED.**
PRE M	Sleep . . . boy . . . bed . . .
POST M	The man is sleeping.
POST V	The boy is sleeping.
TARGET	**THE GIRL IS GIVING FLOWERS TO THE TEACHER**
PRE M	Girl and woman . . . flowers . . .
POST M	The . . . girls is washing . . . daisies.
POST V	The girl is . . . giving the papsies [poppies] to the teacher.
TARGET	**THE ROCK IS FALLING ON THE BOY.**
PRE M	Rock . . .
POST M	The . . . the rock is small big . . . big . . .
POST V	The rock is . . . putting on the man.
TARGET	**THE BOY IS GIVING A VALENTINE TO THE GIRL.**
PRE M	Boy is . . . valentine . . . and . . . girl . . .
POST M	The man . . . valentine's day . . .
POST V	1. The boy is giving the girl to the no . . .
	2. The boy is holding the card to the girl . . . valentine.
	3. The boy is holding the valentine of the girl.
TARGET	**THE TRUCK IS TOWING THE CAR.**
PRE M	One grutch [truck] and one car . . .
POST M	The truck is . . . the car . . .
POST V	The truck is towing the car.
TARGET	**THE BOY IS WATCHING TELEVISION.**
PRE M	Television and man . . .
POST M	The man is TV opening the TV.
POST V	The boy is . . . putting on the TV.
TARGET	**THE BALL IS HITTING THE BOY IN THE HEAD.**
PRE M	Baseball hit . . .
POST M	The baseball is . . . ah no . . .
POST V	The . . . ball is striking the . . . boy.

Source: From Fink et al,[68] with permission.

[a] Pre-mapping therapy (Pre M), 1/20/90; post-mapping therapy (Post M), 5/11/90; post-verb studies (Post V), 12/7/90.

structures. The CN approach aims deeper, at the underlying cause(s) of the impaired production.

Psycholinguist Merrill Garrett[39,53] has produced an account of sentence planning in normal speakers that has been very influential in the CN analyses of agrammatism. The model is illustrated in Fig. 12-5. The first stage involves formulation of the "functional argument structure" (alternatively, predicate- or verb-argument structure), which encodes the who-is-doing-what-to-whom in-

formation in the sentence. The "positional representation" encodes the surface form of the sentence, including the left-to-right order of the content words and grammatical morphemes. Mapping from the functional to positional level is accomplished by means of "planning frames."

Different symptoms of agrammatism arise at different locations in the model. Problems in selecting or pronouncing grammatical morphemes are thought to arise at or after the creation of the

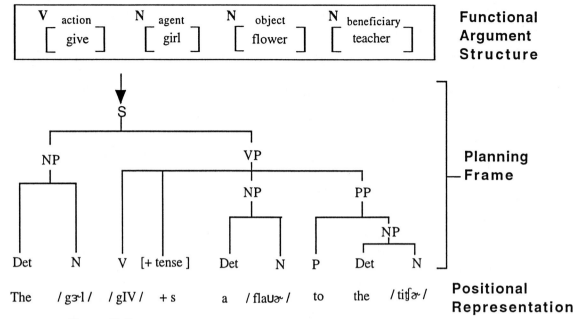

Figure 12-5

Schematic interpretation of Garrett's model of sentence production, applied to the sentence "The girl gives a flower to the teacher." The functional level contains content words only, and these are represented in the abstract format of the semantic lexicon. At the positional level, content words are represented in a phonologic format while grammatical morphemes are represented more abstractly. Abbreviations: S = sentence; NP = noun phrase; VP = verb phrase; PP = prepositional phrase; Det = determiner; N = noun; V = verb; P = preposition.

positional level. Problems in retrieving verbs and their associated argument structures arise earlier, at the functional level, or in the mapping from the functional to the positional level. Schwartz and colleagues[54,55] have also identified faulty mapping between functional and positional representations as the basis for the syntactic comprehension disorder that often accompanies agrammatic speech.

The notion that a deficit in functional-positional level mapping is responsible for production and comprehension impairments in agrammatic aphasics has motivated a number of treatment studies aimed at remediating the mapping deficit.[56–61] These "mapping treatments" represent a radical departure from traditional treatments for agrammatism. We illustrate the mapping-based approach with a 1986 case study by speech pathologist E. Jones.[57]

Jones's patient (B.B.) was a severely nonfluent agrammatic aphasic patient who remained essentially at a single-word level 6 years post onset of a left cerebrovascular accident despite many years of speech therapy. B.B.'s attempts at connected speech contained almost no verbs, but he was able to produce verbs on an action naming test. Asked to describe pictures of simple transitive events, he had difficulty communicating the correct verb-argument structure. Even when supplied with the verb, he continued to have difficulty, for example, leaving out the subject (agent) or reversing the order of agent and object. Referring to the Garrett model, Jones interpreted these findings as evidence of a problem in the early stages of sentence planning—that is, prior to the positional level.

In comprehension testing, B.B. was found to

make errors in comprehending reversible sentences, ordering printed noun and verb constituents to convey the meaning of a picture, and rearranging printed phrases into sentences. Together with the production data, the findings are indicative of a deficit in mapping between sentence form (positional level) and sentence meaning (functional level).

To address this mapping deficit, Jones developed a highly structured treatment program using written sentences. B.B. was first trained to identify the verb in simple sentences, then to identify the arguments of the verb in response to probe questions: "Who (or what) is doing the action? To whom? Where?" After 3 months of this purely receptive treatment, B.B. demonstrated improved sentence comprehension for both written and spoken sentences. Moreover, his production improved as well, as indexed by increased use of correctly inflected verb phrases and increased use of prepositions, particles, and determiners. This improvement in production was noted in the home setting as well as on formal testing.

Jones's report was one of the first in a series of mapping therapy studies (see Refs. 56 and 58 through 61). Most of these studies involved chronic aphasic subjects who underwent detailed, model-driven assessments that yielded evidence consistent with a mapping deficit (e.g., impaired access to verbs and failure to comprehend semantically reversible sentences). In each case a program was designed to remediate the mapping deficit. The specifics of the programs differed, but the general strategy, employed by all but Ref. 59, was to focus the patient's attention on the verb (or preposition in the case of locative sentences like "The pencil is *in* the sink") and the roles it assigns to other constituents in the sentence. In most of the studies, production was not trained directly. Nevertheless, there were posttreatment gains in production, particularly those aspects of production that reflect functional-level processes (i.e., production of verbs; number of arguments produced; reduction in word-order errors).

That a treatment program involving no production training can nonetheless improve production is a striking finding. One possible explanation

is that mapping therapy re-educates patients in mapping rules,[56] which can then be applied across tasks. However, since mapping rules are at least partly verb-specific, one would expect limited generalization to untrained verbs, which is contrary to the findings of Jones's and other mapping therapy studies (e.g., Ref. 56, case 1; also Ref. 61). A more plausible explanation is that the knowledge needed to map correctly is present prior to training but not fully utilized. By drawing the patient's attention to the verb and the meaning it confers on sentence constituents, mapping therapy may shift or facilitate the allocation of processing resources to these aspects of sentence processing. Future studies should help resolve these issues. In any case, it is worth underscoring that the extent of the generalization to untrained materials and tasks that has been reported in some mapping therapy studies is substantially greater than what has been found with more traditional approaches that seek to train production directly.

COGNITIVE NEUROPSYCHOLOGY AND APHASIA REHABILITATION: AN EVALUATION

While the CN approach has much to offer the rehabilitation enterprise, it is not a panacea. Cognitive models are of great value in specifying the locus of impairment in a particular patient, as well as the residual areas of strength, but it still falls to the clinician to use her or his judgment and experience to arrive at the optimal program of treatment—that is, whether to attempt to remediate the impaired process(es), and if so, how. Rehabilitationists are being challenged to develop theories of how the damaged brain relearns and reorganizes itself,[62,63] and it is not clear whether and how cognitive models can contribute to this process (but see Ref. 64 for an encouraging step in this direction).

The length of CN assessments and the need to tailor such assessments to individual patients make them poorly suited to the exigencies of the clinic. The development of model-driven language assessments that are standardized and normed (e.g., Psycholinguistic Assessment of Language Processing in Aphasia, or PALPA),[65] is a great help in this regard. Even so, the CN approach is probably not appropriate for all individuals with aphasia. Pinpointing the functional locus of a deficit rests on a fair degree of selectivity: the more global the deficit, the more problematic the endeavor.

The focus on treating impairments and evaluating success at the impairment level conflicts with the clinical mandate to maximize functional communication. On the other hand, there is no reason why CN interventions could not be used as part of a more comprehensive treatment program that aims to achieve maximal carryover to real-world settings.[66] Recently, our group has outlined an approach that uses CN-motivated treatments as the building blocks or "modules" of a comprehensive treatment program.[67]

THE MODULAR TREATMENTS APPROACH

In preceding sections we have enumerated a set of impairment symptoms that derive from contemporary models of spoken language production. At the level of the lexicon, there are symptoms bearing on the representation and retrieval of meaning and of phonology. At the sentence level, there are symptoms having to do with the verb and its argument structure, the mapping between this and surface syntax, and the retrieval and/or phonologic realization of grammatical morphemes. In other domains, too—spoken language comprehension, written language production, and comprehension—CN studies have elucidated a relatively small set of impairment symptoms that accounts for much of the variability in how disabilities in these domains are expressed.

Most aphasic patients display multiple impairments in more than one domain. The particular combination of impairment symptoms determines the patient's clinical classification. But most impairment symptoms are not restricted to a single clinical classification. For example, the lexical-semantic impairment that compromises word re-

trieval is found in patients with Broca's, Wernicke's, and anomic aphasia.

The goal of a CN assessment is to determine which impairment symptoms are present in the patient and which are amenable to treatment. For many patients, treatment will then aim to strengthen the impaired processes, one at a time or concurrently. To assist the therapist in this enterprise, our group advocates the development of semistandardized treatment "modules," each of which targets a different impairment symptom. Such treatments should be designed to serve as broad a segment of the aphasia population as evinces the target symptom. This can be accomplished by graduating the demands of the treatment task and using multimodality treatment materials whenever possible. In Schwartz, Fink, and Saffran,[67] we illustrate the requirements of treatment modules with experimental and clinical protocols already in use.

The basic idea behind this modular approach is that model-driven treatments that target specific impairments may produce narrow gains, but when they are cumulated over several treatment programs, the effect can be substantial. Consider the case of G.R., a severely agrammatic patient who was 7 years post onset when he joined our mapping therapy study.[61] Comparison of his sentence production before and after mapping therapy revealed nontrivial gains: the percentage of words in sentences increased from 52 to 88; and the percentage of syntactically well-formed sentences increased from 30 to 44. He continued to experience difficulty retrieving verbs, however: the number of verbs produced was 10 before training and 11 after training (maximum 18). We therefore followed mapping therapy with a verb-treatment program designed to facilitate verb retrieval in the context of sentence production.[68] In this study, we compared the effects of two facilitation techniques: a repetition priming technique and a direct production technique that employs cueing and modeling in the context of mapping-type probe questions. The second technique proved more effective in facilitating acquisition of a small set of training verbs and carryover to untrained verbs.

At the end of the verb-treatment study, the number of verbs in G.R.'s picture description attempts increased from 11 to 18, and the number of appropriate verbs increased from 9 to 14. Examples of his picture description attempts at each stage of the treatment program are shown in Table 12-1. Although this was not designed as a test of the modular treatment approach, the results demonstrate the cumulative effects of treatments targeted at specific impairment symptoms.

CONCLUSION

The IDH matrix represents the various levels on which the functional activities of aphasia rehabilitation—assessment, treatment, and outcome evaluation—take place. The different schools of aphasia rehabilitation assign particular emphasis to one or another level, but in reality they are not as distinct from one another as Figs. 12-1 to 12-3 suggest. Cognitive neuropsychology is really a branch of the language-oriented school that advocates using cognitive and psycholinguistic theory to direct rehabilitation activities. And as language-oriented therapists turn their attention to the upper-right-hand cell of the IDH matrix, which insurance providers are increasingly requiring them to do, they are likely to draw on the theoretical and practical tools of the functional/pragmatic school.

What should be clear from even this brief discussion is that the future of aphasia rehabilitation will be shaped by interactions among clinicians and researchers with diverse perspectives and expertise. And there is much that we have not touched upon: Research in neural plasticity is changing the way we think about the brain's capacity for recovery and reorganization after damage; neural models that learn, and that relearn after "lesioning," provide a testing ground for theories of cognitive rehabilitation; and new advances in psychopharmacology and computer technology offer new avenues for treatment. Translating these promising trends into improved care for the individual with aphasia requires opportunities for clinicians, cognitive scientists, and neuroscientists to interact with one another, as well as funding mechanisms to support and sustain such interdisciplinary collaborations.

ACKNOWLEDGMENTS

Preparation of this manuscript was supported by NIH grant #1R01 DC01825. Jessica Myers and Jennifer Bender provided valuable assistance.

REFERENCES

1. Chapey R: An introduction to language intervention strategies in adult aphasia, in Chapey R (ed): *Language Intervention Strategies in Adult Aphasia,* 2d ed. Baltimore, MD: Williams & Wilkins, 1986, pp 2–11.
2. Wepman J: Aphasia therapy: Some "relative" comments and some purely personal prejudices, in Sarno M (ed): *Aphasia-Selected Readings.* New York: Appleton-Century-Crofts, 1972.
3. World Health Organization: *International Classification of Impairments, Disabilities, and Handicaps: A Manual of Classification Relating to the Consequences of Diseases.* Geneva: World Health Organization, 1980.
4. Schwartz MF, Whyte J: *Methodical Issues in Aphasia Treatment Research: The Big Picture.* NIDCD Monograph. Vol 2. Bethesda, MD: NIH Publication No. 93-3424:17–23, 1992.
5. Goodglass H, Kaplan E: *Assessment of Aphasia and Related Disorders.* Philadelphia: Lea & Febiger, 1983.
6. Kertesz A: *Western Aphasia Test Battery.* New York: The Psychological Corporation, 1982.
7. Schuell H: *Minnesota Test for Differential Diagnosis of Aphasia.* Minneapolis: University of Minnesota Press, 1965.
8. Schuell H, Jenkins JJ, Jimenez-Pabon E: *Aphasia in Adults: Diagnosis, Prognosis, and Treatment.* New York: Harper & Row, 1964.
9. Helm-Estabrooks NA: *Helm Elicited Language Program for Syntax Stimulation (HELPSS).* Austin, TX: Exceptional Resources, 1981.
10. Shewan C, Bandur D: *Treatment of Aphasia: A Language-Oriented Approach.* Boston: College-Hill Press, 1986.

11. *Medicare Intermediary Manual, Billing Procedures for Part B Outpatient Speech and Language Services,* 3905.3. Washington, DC: Government Printing Office.

12. Sarno MT: *Functional Communication Profile.* New York: Institute of Rehabilitation Medicine, 1969.

13. Holland AL: *Communicative Abilities in Daily Living: Manual.* Baltimore, MD: University Park Press, 1980.

14. Lomas J, Pickard L, Bester S, et al: The communicative effectiveness index: Development and psychometric evaluation of a functional communication measure for adult aphasia. *J Speech Hear Disord* 54:113–124, 1989.

15. Frattali C, Thompson CK, Wohl CB: Trends in functional assessment. *American Speech-Language Hearing Association Newsletter.* 4:4–9, 1994.

16. Blomart L, Kean ML, Koster CH, Schokker J: Amsterdam-Nijmegen Everyday Language Test: Construction, reliability and validity. *Aphasiology* 8:381–407, 1994.

17. Frattali C, Thompson C, Holland A, et al: The FACS of life: ASHA FACS: A functional outcome measure for adults. *ASHA* 37:40–46, 1995.

18. Basso A, Capitani E, Vignolo LA: Influence of rehabilitation on language skills in aphasic patients: A controlled study. *Arch Neurol* 36:190–196, 1979.

19. Poeck K, Huber W, Williams K: Outcome of intensive language treatment in aphasia. *J Speech Hear Disord* 54:471–479, 1989.

20. Shewan CM, Kertesz A: Effects of speech and language treatment on recovery of aphasia. *Brain Lang* 23:272–299, 1984.

21. Wertz RT, Collins MJ, Weiss D, et al: Veterans administration cooperative study on aphasia: A comparison of individual and group treatment. *J Speech Hear Res* 24:580–594, 1981.

22. Wertz RT, Weiss DG, Aten JL, et al: Comparison of clinic, home, and deferred language treatment for aphasia. *Arch Neurol* 43:653–658, 1986.

23. Doyle PJ, Bourgeois MJ: The effect of syntax training on adequacy of communication in Broca's aphasia: A social validation study, in Brookshire RH (ed): *Clinical Aphasiology.* Vol 16. Minneapolis, MN: BRK Publishers, 1986, pp 123–132.

24. Doyle PJ, Goldstein H, Bourgeois M: Experimental analysis of syntax training in Broca's aphasia: A generalization and social validation study. *J Speech Hear Disord* 52:143–156, 1987.

25. Fink RB, Schwartz MF, Rochon E, et al: Syntax stimulation revisited: An analysis of generalization treatment effects. Presented at Clinical Aphasiology Conference, June 1995, Sunriver, OR.

26. Helm-Estabrooks NA, Ramsberger G: Treatment of agrammatism in long-term Broca's aphasia. *Br J Disord Commun* 21:39–45, 1986.

27. Thompson CK, McReynolds LV: Wh-interrogative production in agrammatic aphasia: An experimental analysis of auditory-visual stimulation and direct-production treatment. *J Speech Hear Res* 29:193–206, 1986.

28. Thompson CK: Generalization research in aphasia: A review of the literature, in Prescott T (ed): *Clinical Aphasiology.* Vol 18. Boston: College-Hill Press, 1989, pp 195–222.

29. Doyle P, Goldstein H, Bourgeois M, Nakles K: Facilitating generalized requesting behavior in Broca's aphasia: A generalization and social validation study. *J Speech Hear Disord* 22:157–170, 1989.

30. Davis GA, Wilcox MJ: *Adult Aphasia Rehabilitation: Applied Pragmatics.* San Diego, CA: College Hill, 1985.

31. Holland AL: Pragmatic aspects of intervention in aphasia. *J Neuroling* 6:197–211, 1991.

32. Davis A: Pragmatics and treatment, in Chapey R (ed): *Language Intervention Strategies in Adult Aphasia,* 2d ed. Baltimore, MD: Williams & Wilkins, 1986, pp 251–265.

33. Springer L, Glindemann R, Huber W, Williams K: How efficacious is PACE-therapy when "language systematic training" is incorporated? *Aphasiology* 5:391–399, 1991.

34. Coltheart M: Editorial. *Cogn Neuropsychol* 1:1–8, 1984.

35. Mitchum CC, Berndt RS: Aphasia rehabilitation: An approach to diagnosis and treatment of disorders of language production, in Eisenbert MG (ed): *Advances in Clinical Rehabilitation.* New York: Springer, 1989.

36. Seron X, Deloche G: Introduction, in Seron X, Deloche G (eds): *Cognitive Approaches in Neuropsychological Rehabilitation.* Hillsdale, NJ: Erlbaum, 1989, pp 1–16.

37. Caramazza A: Cognitive neuropsychology and rehabilitation: An unfulfilled promise? in Seron X, Deloche G (eds): *Cognitive Approaches in Neuropsychological Rehabilitation.* Hillsdale, NJ: Erlbaum, 1989, pp 383–398.

38. Butterworth B: Lexical access in speech production, in Marslen-Wilson W (ed): *Lexical Representation and Process.* Cambridge, MA: MIT Press, 1989, pp 108–135.

39. Garrett MF: Production of speech: Observations from normal and pathological language use, in Ellis A (ed): *Normality and Pathology in Cognitive Functions.* London: Academic Press, 1982.

40. Levelt WJM: *Speaking: From Intention to Articulation.* Cambridge, MA: MIT Press, 1989.

41. Hillis A, Rapp B, Romani C, Caramazza A: *Selective Impairments of Semantics in Lexical Processing: Reports of the Cognitive Neuropsychology Laboratory.* Baltimore, MD: Johns Hopkins University, 1989.

42. Howard D, Orchard-Lisle V: On the origin of semantic errors in naming: Evidence from the case of a global aphasic. *Cogn Neuropsychol* 1:163–190, 1984.

43. Kay J, Ellis A: A cognitive neuropsychological case study of anomia. *Brain* 110:613–629, 1987.

44a. LeDorze G, Pitts C: A case study evaluation of the effects of different techniques for the treatment of anomia. *Neuropsychol Rehabil* 5:51–65, 1995.

44b. Nettleson J, Lesser R: Therapy for naming difficulties in aphasia: Application of a cognitive neuropsychological model. *J Neuroling* 6:139–154, 1991.

45. Howard D, Patterson K, Franklin S, et al: The facilitation of picture naming in aphasia. *Cogn Neuropsychol* 2:48–80, 1985.

46. Howard D, Patterson K, Franklin S, et al: Treatment of word retrieval deficits in aphasia: A comparison of two therapy methods. *Brain* 108:817–829, 1985.

47. Hillis AE: Efficacy and generalization of treatment for aphasic naming errors. *Arch Phys Med Rehabil* 70:632–636, 1989.

48. Greenwald ML, Raymer AM, Richardson ME, Rothi LJG: Contrasting treatments for severe impairments of picture naming. *Neuropsychol Rehab* 5:17–49, 1995.

49. Marshall J, Pound C, White-Thomson M, Pring T: The use of picture/word matching tasks to assist word retrieval in aphasic patients. *Aphasiology* 4:167–184, 1990.

50. Miceli G, Amitrano A, Capasso R, Caramazza A: The remediation of anomia resulting from output lexical damage: Analysis of two cases. *Report* 94-8, 1994.

51. Pring T, White-Thomson M, Pound C, et al: Short report: Picture/word matching tasks and word retrieval: Some follow-up data and second thoughts. *Aphasiology* 4:479–483, 1990.

52. Raymer AM, Thompson CK, Jacobs B, LeGrand HR: Phonological treatment of naming deficits in aphasia: Model-based generalization analysis. *Aphasiology* 7:27–53, 1993.

53. Garrett MF: Levels of processing in sentence production, in Butterworth B (ed): *Language Production.* Vol 1. New York: Academic Press, 1980, pp 177–220.

54. Linebarger M, Schwartz MF, Saffran EM: Sensitivity to grammatical structure in so-called agrammatic aphasics. *Cognition* 13:361–392, 1983.

55. Schwartz MF, Linebarger MC, Saffran EM: The status of the syntactic deficit theory of agrammatism, in Kean MC (ed): *Agrammatism.* New York: Academic Press, 1985.

56. Byng S: Sentence processing deficits: Theory and therapy. *Cogn Neuropsychol* 5:629–676, 1988.

57. Jones EV: Building the foundations for sentence production in a non-fluent aphasic. *Br J Disord Commun* 21:63–82, 1986.

58. LeDorze G, Jacob A, Coderre L: Aphasia rehabilitation with a case of agrammatism: A partial replication. *Aphasiology* 5:63–85, 1991.

59. Mitchum CC, Haendiges AN, Berndt RS: A new approach to treatment of sentence comprehension impairment in aphasia. Presented at the Academy of Aphasia, 1992, Toronto.

60. Nickels L, Byng S, Black M: Sentence processing deficits: A replication of therapy. *Br J Disord Commun* 26:175–199, 1991.

61. Schwartz MF, Saffran EM, Fink RB, et al: Mapping therapy: A treatment program for agrammatism. *Aphasiology* 8:19–54, 1994.

62. Byng S: A theory of the deficit: A prerequisite for a theory of therapy? *Clin Aphasiol* 22:265–273, 1994.

63. Holland AL: Cognitive neuropsychological theory and treatment for aphasia: Exploring the strengths and limitations. *Clin Aphasiol* 22:275–282, 1994.

64. Plaut DC: Relearning after damage in connectionist networks: Toward a theory of rehabilitation. *Brain Lang* (special issue on cognitive approaches to rehabilitation and recovery in aphasia). In press.

65. Kay J, Lesser R, Coltheart M: Psycholinguistic assessment of language processing in aphasia. East Sussex, England: Erlbaum, 1992.

66. Lesser R, Algar L: Towards combining the cognitive neuropsychological and the pragmatic in aphasia therapy. *Neuropsychol Rehabil* 5:67–92, 1995.

67. Schwartz MF, Fink RB, Saffran E: The modular treatment of agrammatism. *Neuropsychol Rehabil* 5:93–127, 1995.

68. Fink RB, Martin N, Schwartz MF, et al: Facilitation of verb retrieval skills in aphasia: A comparison of two approaches. *Clin Aphasiol* 21:263–275, 1993.

Chapter 13

ACQUIRED DYSLEXIA

H. Branch Coslett

The study of acquired dyslexia or disorders of reading dates at least to the contributions of Déjerine, who, in 1891 and 1892, described two patients with quite different patterns of reading impairment. Déjerine's first patient[1] developed an impairment in reading and writing subsequent to an infarction involving the left parietal lobe. Déjerine termed this disorder "alexia with agraphia" and attributed the disturbance to a disruption of the "optical image for words," which he thought to be supported by the left angular gyrus. In an account that in some respects presages contemporary psychological accounts, Déjerine concluded that reading and writing required the activation of these "optical images" and that the loss of the images resulted in an inability to recognize or write familiar words.

Déjerine's second patient[2] was quite different. This patient was unable to read aloud or for comprehension but could write, a disorder that Déjerine designated "alexia without agraphia" (also known as agnosic alexia and pure alexia). The patient had a right homonymous hemianopia from a left occipital lesion, which included the fibers carrying visual information from the right to the left hemisphere. Déjerine explained alexia without agraphia in terms of a "disconnection" between visual information confined to the right hemisphere and the left angular gyrus, which he assumed to be critical for the recognition of words.

After the seminal contributions of Déjerine, the study of acquired dyslexia languished for decades, during which the relatively few investigations that were reported focused primarily on the anatomic underpinnings of the disorders. The study of acquired dyslexia was revitalized, however, by the elegant and detailed investigation by Marshall and Newcombe,[3] demonstrating that by virtue of a careful investigation of the pattern of reading deficits exhibited by dyslexic subjects, distinctly different and reproducible types of reading deficits could be elucidated. These investigators described a patient (GR) who read approximately 50 percent of concrete nouns but was severely impaired in the reading of abstract nouns and all other parts of speech. The most striking aspect of GR's performance, however, was his tendency to produce errors that appeared to be semantically related to the target word (e.g., *speak* read as "talk"). Marshall and Newcombe[3] designated this disorder "deep dyslexia." These investigators also described two patients whose primary deficit appeared to be an inability to derive the pronunciation of irregularly spelled words, such as "yacht." This disorder was designated "surface dyslexia."

On the basis of these data, Marshall and Newcombe[3] concluded that the meaning of written words could be accessed by two separate and distinct procedures. The first was a lexical (whole-word) procedure whereby familiar words activated the appropriate stored representation (or visual word form), which, in turn, activated meaning; reading in deep dyslexia was assumed to involve this procedure, labeled A in Fig. 13-1.

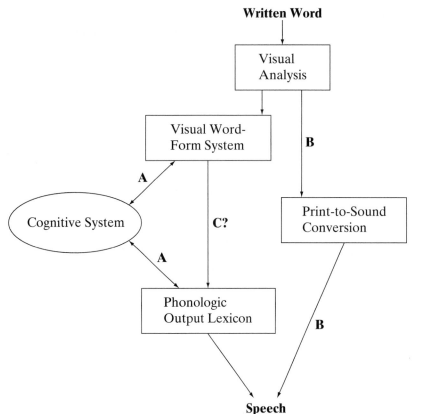

Figure 13-1
A diagram of an information-processing model of reading incorporating three procedures for oral reading.

The second procedure was assumed to be a phonologically based process in which "grapheme-to-phoneme" (hereafter termed "print-to-sound") correspondences were employed to derive the appropriate phonology (that is, "sound out" the word); the reading of surface dyslexics was assumed to be mediated by this nonlexical procedure, labeled B in Fig. 13-1. Although a number of Marshall and Newcombe's specific hypotheses have been criticized, their argument that reading may be mediated by two distinct procedures has received considerable empirical support. Indeed, although it has occasionally been questioned,[4,5] the dual-route model of reading has provided the conceptual framework that has motivated most subsequent study of acquired dyslexias and animates the present discussion.

In this chapter we briefly summarize the clinical features and conceptual basis of the major types of acquired dyslexia. Additionally, the possible role of the right hemisphere in reading is briefly discussed. Finally, recent efforts to develop computational models of normal reading and acquired dyslexia are briefly described.

PERIPHERAL DYSLEXIAS

A useful starting point in the discussion of the dyslexias is the distinction offered by Shallice and Warrington[6] between "peripheral" and "central" dyslexias. The former are conditions characterized by a deficit in the processing of visual aspects of the stimulus that interfere with the matching of a familiar word to its stored orthographic representation or "visual word form."[6] Central dyslexias, in contrast, are attributable to an impairment of the "deeper" or "higher" reading functions by which visual word forms mediate access to meaning or speech production mechanisms. The major types of peripheral dyslexia are briefly described below.

Alexia without Agraphia (Pure Alexia)

The classic syndrome of alexia without agraphia or pure alexia is perhaps the prototypical peripheral dyslexia. As noted above, the traditional account[2,7] of this disorder attributes the syndrome to a "disconnection" of visual information, which is restricted to the right hemisphere, from the left-hemispheric word-recognition system.

Though these patients do not appear to be able to read in the sense of fast, automatic word recognition, many are able to use a compensatory strategy that involves naming the letters of the word in serial fashion; they read, in effect, letter by letter. Using the slow and inefficient letter-by-letter procedure, pure alexics typically exhibit significant effects of word length, requiring more time to read long as compared to short words. In contrast to the central dyslexias, performance is typically not influenced by linguistic factors such as parts of speech (e.g., noun versus functor), the extent to which the referent of the word is concrete (e.g., "table") or abstract (e.g., "destiny"), or whether the word is orthographically regular (that is, can be "sounded out").

A number of alternative accounts of the processing deficit in pure alexia have been proposed. Thus, some investigators have proposed that the impairment is attributable to a limitation in the transmission of letter identity information to the visual word system (e.g., Ref. 8), an inability to directly encode visual letters as abstract orthographic types,[9,10] or an inability to encode multiple visual shapes of any sort in rapid succession.[11,12] Other investigators have argued that the disorder is attributable to a disruption of the visual word-form system itself.[13,14]

Although most reports of pure alexia have emphasized the profound nature of the reading deficit, often stating that patients were utterly incapable of reading without recourse to a letter-by-letter strategy,[7,8] a number of investigators have reported data demonstrating that at least some pure alexic patients are able to comprehend words that they are unable to explicitly identify.[15–17] This capacity has been attributed by some investigators (e.g., Ref. 17) to the operation of a reading procedure based in the right hemisphere.

The anatomic basis of pure alexia has been extensively investigated. Although on rare occasions associated with lesions that "undercut" or disconnect the posterior perisylvian cortex on the left,[18] the disorder is typically associated with a lesion in the posterior portion of the dominant hemisphere, which compromises visual pathways in the dominant hemisphere as well white matter tracts (such as the splenium of the corpus callosum or forceps major) critical for the interhemispheric transmission of visual information.[19,20]

Neglect Dyslexia

Neglect dyslexia, which is most commonly encountered in patients with left-sided neglect, is characterized by a failure to explicitly identify the initial portion of a letter string. Interestingly, the performance of patients with neglect dyslexia is often influenced by the nature of the letter string; thus, patients with this disorder may fail to report the initial letters in nonwords (e.g., the "ti-" in a nonword such as "tiggle") but read real words (e.g., "giggle") correctly (Ref. 21; see also Refs. 22 and 23). The fact that performance is affected by the lexical status of the stimulus has been taken to suggest that neglect dyslexia is not attributable to a failure to register letter information but reflects an attentional impairment at a higher level of representation.

Although neglect dyslexia is generally seen in the context of the neglect syndrome (see Chaps. 24 and 25), it has occasionally been observed in isolation or even in the context of neglect of the opposite side of space.[24]

Attentional Dyslexia

Perhaps the least studied of the acquired dyslexias, attentional dyslexia is characterized by the relative preservation of single-word reading in the context of a gross disruption of reading when words are presented in text or in the presence of other words or letters.[25-28] Patients with this disorder may also exhibit difficulties identifying letters within words, even though the words themselves are read correctly[25] and be impaired in identifying words flanked by extraneous letters (e.g., "lboat"). We[28] have recently investigated a patient with attentional dyslexia secondary to autopsy-proven Alzheimer disease who produced frequent "blend" errors in which letters from one word of a two-word display intruded into the other word (e.g., "take lime" read as "tame"). Although several accounts for this disorder have been proposed, the disorder has been attributed by several investigators to an impairment in visual attention or a loss of location information. As visual attention may be critical to mapping the location of visually presented objects, these accounts are not clearly distinguishable.

CENTRAL DYSLEXIAS

In this section we briefly describe the clinical features and conceptual basis of the major types of central dyslexia including "deep," "phonologic," and "surface" dyslexia. Additionally, the phenomenon of "reading without meaning" is discussed.

Deep Dyslexia

Deep dyslexia, the most extensively investigated central dyslexia (see, for example, Coltheart and colleagues[29]) is in many respects the most compelling. The allure of deep dyslexia is due in large part to the intrinsically interesting hallmark of the syndrome, *semantic errors*. When shown the word *castle*, a deep dyslexic may respond "knight"; similarly, these interesting patients may read *bird* as "canary." At least for some deep dyslexics, it is clear that these errors are not circumlocutions and that the patients are not even aware that they have erred.

While semantic errors are typically regarded as essential for the diagnosis of deep dyslexia, the frequency with which deep dyslexics produce them is quite variable; for some patients, semantic errors may represent the most frequent error type, whereas for others they constitute a small proportion of reading errors. These patients also produce a variety of other types of reading errors, including "visual" errors in which the response bears a clear visual similarity to the target (e.g., *skate* read as "scale") and "morphologic" errors, in which a prefix or suffix is added, deleted, or substituted (e.g., *scolded* read as "scolds"; *governor* read as "government").

Additional hallmarks of the syndrome include a greater success in reading words of high as compared to low imageability. Thus, words such as *table*, *chair*, *ceiling*, and *buttercup*, the referents of which are concrete or imageable, are read more successfully by deep dyslexics than words such as *fate*, *destiny*, *wish*, and *universal*, the referents of which are abstract.

Also characteristic of the syndrome is part-of-speech effect, such that nouns are read more reliably than modifiers (adjectives and adverbs), which are, in turn, read more accurately than verbs. Deep dyslexics manifest particular difficulty in the reading of functors (a class of words that includes pronouns, prepositions, conjunctions, and interrorogatives such as *that*, *which*, *they*, *because*, *under*, etc.). The striking nature of the part-of-speech effect is illustrated by the patient reported by Saffran and Marin[30] who correctly read the word *chrysanthemum* but was unable to read the word *the*! Many errors to functors involve the substitution of a different functor (*that* read as *which*) rather than the production of words of a different class, such as nouns or verbs.

As functors are, in general, less imageable than nouns, verbs, or adjectives, some investigators have claimed that the apparent effect of part of speech is in reality a manifestation of the pervasive imageability effect described above.[31] We have reported a patient,[32] however, whose performance suggests that the part-of-speech effect is not simply a reflection of a more general deficit in the processing of low-imageability words, as the difference remained after functors and content words were matched for imageability.

Finally, all deep dyslexics exhibit a substantial impairment in the reading of nonwords; when confronted with letter strings such as *flig* or *churt*, deep dyslexics are typically unable to employ print-to-sound correspondences to derive phonology; nonwords frequently elicit "lexicalization" errors (e.g., *flig* read as "flag"), perhaps reflecting a reliance on lexical reading in the absence of access to reliable print-to-sound correspondences.

How can deep dyslexia be accommodated by the model of reading depicted in Fig. 13-1? Several alternative explanations have been proposed. Most investigators agree that multiple processing deficits must be hypothesized to account for the full range of symptoms found in deep dyslexia. First, the strikingly impaired performance in reading nonwords and other tasks assessing phonologic function suggest that the print-to-sound conversion procedure is disrupted. Second, the presence of semantic errors and the effects of imageability (a variable usually thought to influence processing at the level of semantics) has been interpreted by many investigators as evidence that these patients also suffer from a semantic impairment; it should be noted in this context, however, that some deep dyslexic patients perform well on tests of comprehension with words they are unable to read aloud. Semantic errors in these patients have been attributed to a deficit in or access to representations in the output phonologic lexicon (Ref. 33; see also Ref. 6). Last, the production of visual errors has been interpreted by some to suggest that these patients suffer from an impairment in the visual word-form system. Other investigators (e.g., Coltheart;[34] Saffran and coworkers[35]) have argued that deep dyslexics' reading is mediated by a system not normally used in reading—that is, the right hemisphere. We will return to the issue of reading with the right hemisphere below.

Although deep dyslexia has occasionally been associated with posterior lesions, this disorder is typically encountered in association with large perisylvian lesions extending into the frontal lobe. As might be expected given the lesion data, deep dyslexia is usually associated with global or

Broca's aphasia but may rarely be encountered in patients with fluent aphasia.

Phonologic Dyslexia: Reading without Print-to-Sound Conversion

First described in 1979 by Derouesne and Beauvois,[36] phonologic dyslexia is, perhaps, the "purest" of the central dyslexias in that the syndrome appears to be attributable to a selective deficit in the procedure mediating the translation from print to sound. Thus, although in many respects less arresting than deep dyslexia, phonologic dyslexia is of considerable theoretical import. It is of interest to note that the existence of this syndrome was *predicted* by dual-route accounts of reading similar to that proposed by Marshall and Newcombe[3] and subsequently identified when dyslexic patients were assessed with theoretically motivated tasks.

Phonologic dyslexia is a relatively mild disorder in which reading of real words may be only slightly impaired. Many patients with this disorder, for example, correctly read 85 to 95 percent of real words (e.g., Refs. 32, 36, 37). Some patients with this disorder read all different types of words with equal facility,[37–39] whereas other patients are relatively impaired in the reading of functors.[40,41] Unlike patients with surface dyslexia, described below, the regularity of print-to-sound correspondences is not relevant to the performance of phonologic dyslexics; thus, these patients typically pronounce orthographically irregular words such as *colonel* and words with standard print-to-sound correspondences such as *administer* with equal facility. Most errors in response to real words appear to have a visual basis, often involving the substitution of visually similar real words (e.g., *topple* read as "table").

The striking and theoretically relevant aspect of the performance of phonologic dyslexics is a substantial impairment in the oral reading of nonword letter strings. A number of investigators have described patients with this disorder, for example, who read more than 90 percent of real words of all types yet correctly pronounce only about 10 percent of nonwords.[32,36] Most errors in nonword reading involve the substitution of a visually similar real word (e.g., *phope* read as "phone") or the incorrect application of print-to-sound correspondences (e.g., *stime* read as "stim," rhyming with "him").

Within the context of the reading model depicted in Fig. 13-1, the account for this disorder is relatively straightforward. The patients' good performance with real words suggests that the processes involved in normal "lexical" reading—that is, visual analysis, the visual word-form system, semantics, and the phonologic output lexicon—are at least relatively preserved. The impairment in nonword reading suggests that the print-to-sound translation procedure is disrupted.

A final point of interest is that a number of phonologic dyslexics exhibit substantial deficits in processing morphologically complex words—that is, words with prefixes and suffixes.[37,41] The explanation for this association is not clear.

Phonologic dyslexia has been observed in association with lesions in a number of sites in the dominant perisylvian cortex and, on occasion, with lesions of the right hemisphere (e.g., Ref. 41). Damage to the superior temporal lobe and angular and supramarginal gyri in particular is found in most but not all patients with this disorder. Although quantitative data are lacking, the lesions associated with phonologic dyslexia appear to be smaller on average than those associated with deep dyslexia.

Just as there is variability with respect to the lesion site associated with phonologic dyslexia, there is variability with respect to the type and severity of aphasia observed in these patients. A phonologic dyslexic reported by Derouesne and Beauvois,[36] for example, did not exhibit a significant aphasia, whereas Funnell's patient WB[37] appears to have had a severe nonfluent aphasia.

Surface Dyslexia

Surface dyslexia is a disorder characterized by the inability to read words with "irregular" or exceptional print-to-sound correspondences. Patients with surface dyslexia are thus unable to read aloud words such as *colonel*, *yacht*, *island*, *have*, and *bor-*

ough, the pronunciation of which cannot be derived by phonologic or "sounding out" strategies. In contrast, these patients read words containing regular correspondences (e.g., *state*, *hand*, *mint*, *abdominal*) as well as nonwords (e.g., *blape*) quite well.

As noted above, normal subjects may read familiar words by matching the letter string to a stored representation of the word and retrieving the pronunciation by means of a mechanism linked to semantics (or, as discussed below, by means of a nonsemantic "direct" route). As this procedure involves the activation of stored representations, the pronunciation of the word is not computed by rules but is retrieved; consequently, the regularity of print-to-sound correspondences would not be expected to play a major role in performance.

In the context of a dual route model of reading, the sensitivity to the regularity of the print-to-sound correspondences provides prima facie evidence that the impairment in surface dyslexia is in the mechanism(s) mediating lexical reading. Similarly, the preserved ability to read regular words and nonwords provides compelling support for the claim that the procedures by which pronunciations are computed by the application of print-to-sound correspondences are at least relatively preserved.

Noting that there is substantial variability in the performance of surface dyslexics with respect to leading latencies as well as accuracy, Shallice and McCarthy[43] suggested that the syndrome of surface dyslexia be fractionated. Type 1 surface dyslexia, they suggested, is characterized by effortless and accurate reading of nonwords and regular words with poor performance with irregular words only. Type 2 surface dyslexia, in contrast, is characterized by slow, effortful reading; although these patients read irregular words less well than regular words and nonwords, they make errors with all types of stimuli. More recently, Shallice[44] suggested that at least for patients with type 2 surface dyslexia, the syndrome may reflect an attempt to compensate for damage to early stages of the reading process.

Other investigators have suggested that the syndrome may be fractionated even more. Thus, for example, surface dyslexia may be associated with disruption of the visual word-form system,[3] with a disruption of semantics (in conjunction with a deficit in the "direct" route),[45,46] or with a lesion involving the phonologic output lexicon.[47] Indeed, Coltheart and Funnell[48] proposed that within the context of a multiroute model of reading, surface dyslexia might be associated with as many as seven distinct types of impairment.

Finally, if as suggested above, patients with surface dyslexia are unable to access semantics by means of a direct lexical procedure, one might ask how these patients derive word meaning. At least for some surface dyslexics, access to a word's meaning appears to occur only after the phonologic form of the word has been derived. Thus, when presented the word *listen*, a patient described by Marshall and Newcombe[3] responded "Liston" and added "that's the boxer."

The anatomic correlate of surface dyslexia has not been well established. Indeed, in recent years the syndrome has been reported most frequently in the context of dementia.[46,49–54] Accordingly, surface dyslexia in demented patients is sometimes termed "semantic dyslexia." Many of these patients have exhibited brain atrophy most prominent in the temporal lobes (e.g., Refs. 50 and 53).

Reading without Meaning

In 1980, Schwartz and coworkers[45] reported a patient (WLP) who exhibited a profound loss of semantics in the context of dementia. Her performance was of particular interest because, unlike patients with surface dyslexia, she correctly read aloud both regular and irregular words that she was unable to comprehend. Thus, for example, when asked to sort written words into their appropriate semantic categories, she correctly classified only 7 of 20 animal names; critically, WLP correctly read aloud 18 of these animal names, including such orthographically ambiguous or irregular words such as *hyena* and *leopard*. The same basic phenomenon—that is, the ability to read aloud regular and irregular words that the patient does not understand—has subsequently been reported

by a number of investigators (see Refs. 55 and 56).

The pattern of performance exhibited by WLP and similar patients is of considerable theoretical interest. Recall that to this point, two procedures have been described by which written words may be pronounced. The first (labeled A in Fig. 13-1) involves the activation of an entry in the visual word-form system, access to semantic information, and ultimately activation of an entry in the phonologic output lexicon. The second (B in Fig. 13-1) involves the nonlexical print-to-sound translation process. Reading without semantics is of interest precisely because it cannot readily be accommodated by such an account. The fact that these patients do not comprehend the words they correctly pronounce indicates that their oral reading is not mediated by the semantically based reading procedure. Additionally, the fact that these patients can read irregular words suggests that they are not relying on a sublexical print-to-sound conversion procedure.

How, then, do these patients read aloud? Several explanations have been proposed. One response was to suggest that oral reading may be mediated by a third mechanism or route (e.g., Ref. 57). This mechanism was assumed to be lexically based, involving the activation of an entry in the visual word-form system and the "direct" activation of an entry in the phonologic output lexicon (C in Fig. 13-1); note that this procedure differs from the lexical procedure described above in that there is no intervening activation of semantic information. Based on the analysis of a phonologic dyslexic's performance across a variety of reading, writing, and repetition tasks, we[32] have reported data providing additional support for the existence of a lexical but nonsemantic reading procedure. An alternative hypothesis was proposed by Shallice and colleagues (Refs. 44 and 46; see also Ref. 58). These investigators attempted to explain reading without semantics within the context of a dual-route model by proposing that the phonologic reading procedure employs not only grapheme-to-phoneme correspondences but also correspondences based on larger units including syllables and even morphemes. Thus, on this account, WLP and similar patient are assumed to compute the pronunciation of irregular words they cannot understand by relying on the multiple levels of print-to-sound correspondences available in the phonologic system. Finally, Hillis and Caramazza[59] have suggested that the apparent ability to read without meaning is attributable to the fact that, while the patient is impaired, the semantic and phonologic reading procedures provide partial information that constrains the subject's responses. Thus, on this account, neither the semantic nor phonologic procedure is assumed to be capable of generating the correct response, but the combination of partial phonologic and incomplete semantic information is often sufficient to identify the stimulus.

READING AND THE RIGHT HEMISPHERE

One important and controversial issue regarding reading concerns the putative reading capacity of the right hemisphere. For many years investigators argued that the right hemisphere was "word blind."[2,6,7] In recent years, however, several lines of evidence have suggested that the right hemisphere may possess the capacity to read. One seemingly incontrovertible line of evidence comes from the performance of a patient who underwent a left hemispherectomy at age 15 for treatment of seizures caused by Rasmussen's encephalitis;[60] after the hemispherectomy, the patient was able to read approximately 30 percent of single words and exhibited an effect of part of speech; she was also utterly unable to use a print-to-sound conversion process. Thus, in many respects this patient's performance was similar to that of a person with deep dyslexia, a pattern of reading impairment that has been hypothesized to reflect the performance of the right hemisphere.[34,35]

The performance of some split-brain patients is also consistent with the claim that the right hemisphere is literate. These patients may, for example, be able to match printed words presented to the right hemisphere with an appro-

priate object.[61,62] Interestingly, the patients are apparently unable to derive sound from the words presented to the right hemisphere; thus, they are unable to determine if a word presented to the right hemisphere rhymes with an auditorially presented word.

Another line of evidence supporting the claim that the right hemisphere is literate comes from evaluation of the reading of patients with pure alexia and optic aphasia.[17,63] We reported data, for example, from four patients with pure alexia who performed well above chance on a number of lexical decision and semantic categorization tasks with briefly presented words that they could not explicitly identify. Three of the patients who regained the ability to identify rapidly presented words explicitly exhibited a pattern of performance consistent with the right-hemisphere reading hypothesis. These patients read nouns better than functors and words of high (e.g., *chair*) better than words of low (e.g., *destiny*) imageability. Additionally, both patients for whom data were available demonstrated a deficit in the reading of suffixed (e.g., *flowed*) as opposed to pseudo-suffixed (e.g., *flower*) words. These data are consistent with a version of the right-hemisphere reading hypothesis postulating that the right-hemisphere lexical-semantic system primarily represents high imageability nouns. On this account, functors, affixed words, and low imageability words are not adequately represented in the right hemisphere.

Finally, we reported data from an investigation with a patient with pure alexia in which transcranial magnetic stimulation (TMS) was employed to directly test the hypothesis that the right hemisphere mediates the reading of at least some patients with acquired dyslexia.[64] We reasoned that if the right hemisphere provides the neural substrate for reading, the transient, localized disruption of cortical processing caused by TMS of the right hemisphere would interfere with reading. An extensively investigated patient with pure alexia who exhibited the reading pattern described above was asked to read aloud briefly presented words, half of which were presented in association with TMS. Consistent with the hypothesis that his reading was mediated by the right hemisphere, stimulation of the right hemisphere interfered with oral reading, whereas left-hemisphere stimulation had no significant effect.

Although a consensus has not yet been achieved, there is mounting evidence that, at least for some people, the right hemisphere is not word-blind but may support the reading of some types of words. The full extent of this reading capacity and whether it is relevant to normal reading, however, remains unclear.

COMPUTATIONAL MODELS OF THE DYSLEXIAS

To this point, the discussion of acquired reading disorders has been motivated by a widely though not universally (see Refs. 4 and 5) accepted multiroute information processing model of reading. In recent years, however, computer-implemented parallel distributed processing (PDP) models of cognitive processing have made important contributions in many domains of cognitive science, including reading (see Chaps. 8 and 10). These models, which differ from traditional information processing models in that they offer (and in fact require) greater specification of the manner in which information is represented and processed, have called into question the necessity of hypothesizing two routes to account for the syndromes reviewed here. Although a detailed discussion of these models is beyond the scope of this chapter, several PDP accounts of reading are briefly summarized below.

Seidenberg and McClelland[65] have reported a PDP model of single-word reading in which the procedure for computing pronunciation directly from orthography (that is, without semantic mediation) is assumed to be mediated by a single network in which orthographic patterns are linked to phonologic representations by means of an intermediate "hidden layer."[65] In contrast to the information processing accounts described above, this model does not postulate a discrete "lexical" or word-representation procedure or distinct lexical and sublexical procedures for the computation of phonology. Of particular relevance in the present context is the fact that investigators have attempted to simulate the performance of dyslexic patients by modifying or "lesioning" this PDP model. Patterson and colleagues,[66] for example, have attempted to model the performance of surface dyslexics by eliminating a proportion of the connections or units at different "lesion" sites. Although the simulations do not appear to capture all of the characteristic features of the performance of surface dyslexics, the lesioned models generate data that are in many interesting and important respects similar to those of patients. More recently, Plaut and Shallice[67] have reported a series of simulations of different PDP architectures in an attempt to model the performance of patients with deep dyslexia.

Several investigators have developed explicit PDP models of single-word reading that incorporate several distinct procedures by which output phonology can be generated. Reggia and coworkers,[68] for example, reported a PDP model that incorporates both lexical and nonlexical procedures for the computation of phonology. This model, which employs a competitive distribution of activation to govern interaction between competing concepts, simulates many aspects of normal reading performance; "lesioning" of the model produces patterns of performance consistent in many respects with the syndromes of phonologic and surface dyslexia. Finally, Coltheart and coworkers[69] have developed a dual-route computational model of visual word recognition and reading aloud that accommodates many of the patterns of performance typical of normal reading. As with the model developed by Reggia and associates,[68] selective disruptions of the model have been demonstrated to simulate surface and phonologic dyslexia.

REFERENCES

1. Déjerine J: Sur en case de cecite verbal avec agraphie, suivi d'autopsie. *C R Seances Soc Biol* 3:197–201, 1891.
2. Déjerine J: Contribution a l'etude anatomo-patho-

logique et clinique des differentes varietes de cecite verbale. *C R Seances Soc Biol* 4:61–90, 1892.

3. Marshall JC, Newcombe F: Patterns of paralexia: A psycholinguistic approach. *J Psycholing Res* 2:175–199, 1973.

4. Marcel AJ: Surface dyslexia and beginning reading: A revised hypothesis of the pronunciation of print and its impairments, in Coltheart M, Patterson KE, Marshall JC (eds): *Deep Dyslexia.* London: Routledge, 1980.

5. Van Orden GC, Pennington BF, Stone GO: Word identification in reading and the promise of subsymbolic psycholinguistics. *Psychol Rev* 97:488–522, 1990.

6. Shallice T, Warrington EK: Single and multiple component central dyslexic syndromes, in Coltheart M, Patterson K, Marshall JC (eds): *Deep Dyslexia.* London: Routledge, 1980.

7. Geschwind N: Disconnection syndromes in animals and man. *Brain* 88:237–294, 585–644, 1965.

8. Patterson K, Kay J: Letter-by-letter reading: Psychological descriptions of a neurological syndrome. *Q J Exp Psychol* 34A:411–441, 1982.

9. Arguin M, Bub DN: Pure Alexia: Attempted rehabilitation and its implications for interpretation of the deficit. *Brain Lang* 47:233–268, 1994.

10. Arguin M, Bub DN: Single-character processing in a case of pure alexia. *Neuropsychologia* 31:435–458, 1993.

11. Kinsbourne M, Warrington EK: A disorder of simultaneous form perception. *Brain* 85:461–486, 1962.

12. Farah MJ, Wallace MA: Pure alexia as a visual impairment: A reconsideration. *Cog Neuropsychol* 8:313–334, 1991.

13. Warrington EK, Shallice T: Word-form dyslexia. *Brain* 103:99–112, 1980.

14. Warrington EK, Langdon D: Spelling dyslexia: A deficit of the visual word-form. *J Neurol Neurosurg Psychiatry* 57:211–216, 1994.

15. Landis T, Regard M, Serrat A: Iconic reading in a case of alexia without agraphia caused by a brain tumor: A tachistoscopic study. *Brain Lang* 11:45–53, 1980.

16. Shallice T, Saffran EM: Lexical processing in the absence of explicit word identification: Evidence from a letter-by-letter reader. *Cog Neuropsychol* 3:429–458, 1986.

17. Coslett HB, Saffran EM: Evidence for preserved reading in pure alexia. *Brain* 112:327–329, 1989.

18. Greenblatt SH: Subangular alexia without agraphia or hemianopia. *Brain Lang* 3:229–245, 1976.

19. Binder JR, Mohr JP: The topography of callosal reading pathways: A case-control analysis. *Brain* 115:1807–1826, 1992.

20. Damasio AR, Damasio H: The anatomic basis of pure alexia. *Neurology* 33:1573–1583, 1983.

21. Sieroff E, Pollatsek A, Posner MI: Recognition of visual letter strings following injury to the posterior visual spatial attention system. *Cog Neuropsychol* 5:427–449, 1988.

22. Behrman M, Moscovitch M, Black SE, Mozer M: Perceptual and conceptual mechanisms in neglect dyslexia. *Brain* 113:1163–1183, 1990.

23. Berti A, Frassinetti F, Umilta C: Nonconscious reading? Evidence from neglect dyslexia. *Cortex* 30:181–197, 1994.

24. Costello AD, Warrington EK: The dissociation of visual neglect and neglect dyslexia. *J Neurol Neurosurg Psychiatry* 50:110–116, 1987.

25. Shallice T, Warrington EK: The possible role of selective attention in acquired dyslexia. *Neuropsychologia* 15:31–41, 1977.

26. Price CJ, Humphreys GW: Attentional dyslexia: The effects of co-occurring deficits. *Cog Neuropsychol* 6:569–592, 1993.

27. Warrington EK, Cipolotti L, McNeil J: Attentional dyslexia: A single case study. *Neuropsychologia* 31:871–886, 1993.

28. Saffran EM, Coslett HB: "Attentional dyslexia" in Alzheimer's disease: A case study. *Cog Neuropsychol.* In press.

29. Coltheart M, Patterson K, Marshall JC (eds): *Deep Dyslexia.* London: Routledge, 1980.

30. Saffran EM, Marin OSM: Reading without phonology: Evidence from aphasia. *Q J Exp Psychol* 29:515–525, 1977.

31. Allport DA, Funnell E: Components of the mental lexicon. *Phil Trans R Soc Lond B* 295:397–410, 1981.

32. Coslett HB: Read but not write "idea": Evidence for a third reading mechanism. *Brain Lang* 40:425–443, 1991.

33. Caramazza A, Hillis AE: Where do semantic errors come from? *Cortex* 26:95–122, 1990.

34. Coltheart M: Deep dyslexia: A right hemisphere hypothesis, in Coltheart M, Patterson K, Marshall JC (eds): *Deep Dyslexia.* London: Routledge, 1980.

35. Saffran EM, Bogyo LC, Schwartz MF, Marin OSM: Does deep dyslexia reflect right-hemisphere read-

ing? in Coltheart M, Patterson K, Marshall JC (eds): *Deep Dyslexia.* London: Routledge, 1980.

36. Derouesne J, Beauvois M-F: Phonological processing in reading: Data from alexia. *J Neurol Neurosurg Psychiatry* 42:1125–1132, 1979.

37. Funnell E: Phonological processes in reading: New evidence from acquired dyslexia. *Br J Psychol* 74:159–180, 1983.

38. Bub D, Black SE, Howell J, Kertesz A: Speech output processes and reading, in Coltheart M, Sartori G, Job R (eds): *Cognitive Neuropsychology of Language.* Hillsdale, NJ: Erlbaum, 1987.

39. Friedman RB, Kohn SE: Impaired activation of the phonological lexicon: Effects upon oral reading. *Brain Lang* 38:278–297, 1990.

40. Glosser G, Friedman RB: The continuum of deep/phonological dyslexia. *Cortex* 26:343–359, 1990.

41. Patterson KE: The relation between reading and psychological coding: Further neuropsychological observations, in AW Ellis (ed): *Normality and Pathology in Cognitive Functions.* London: Academic Press, 1982.

42. Friedman RB, Ween JE, Albert ML: Alexia, in Heilman KM, Valenstein E (eds): *Clinical Neuropsychology,* 3d ed. Oxford, England: Oxford University Press, 1993.

43. Shallice T, McCarthy R: Phonological reading: From patterns of impairment to possible procedures, in Patterson KE, Coltheart M, Marshall JC (eds): *Surface Dyslexia.* London: Erlbaum, 1985.

44. Shallice T: *From Neuropsychology to Mental Structure.* Cambridge, England: Cambridge University Press, 1987.

45. Schwartz MF, Saffran EM, Marin OSM: Dissociation of language function in dementia: A case study. *Brain Lang* 7:277–306, 1979.

46. Shallice T, Warrington EK, McCarthy R: Reading without semantics. *Q J Exp Psychol* 35A:111–138, 1983.

47. Howard D, Franklin S: Three ways for understanding written words, and their use in two contrasting cases of surface dyslexia (together with an odd routine for making "orthographic" errors in oral word production), in Allport A, Mackay D, Prinz W, Scheerer E (eds): *Language Perception and Production.* New York: Academic Press, 1987.

48. Coltheart M, Funnell E: Reading writing: One lexicon or two? in Allport DA, MacKay DG, Prinz W, Scheerer E (eds): *Language Perception and Production: Shared Mechanisms in Listening, Speaking,* *Reading and Writing.* London: Academic Press, 1987.

49. Warrington EK: The selective impairment of semantic memory. *Q J Exp Psychol* 27:635–657, 1975.

50. Hodges JR, Patterson K, Oxbury S, Funnell E: Semantic dementia: Progressive fluent aphasia with temporal lobe atrophy. *Brain* 115:1783–1806, 1992.

51. Patterson K, Hodges J: Deterioration of word meaning: Implications for reading. *Neuropsychologia* 30:1025–1040, 1992.

52. Graham KS, Hodges JR, Patterson K: The relationship between comprehension and oral reading in progressive fluent aphasia. *Neuropsychologia* 32:299–316, 1994.

53. Breedin SD, Saffran EM, Coslett HB: Reversal of the concreteness effect in a patient with semantic dementia. *Cog Neuropsychol* 11:617–660, 1994.

54. Cipolotti L, Warrington EK: Semantic memory and reading abilities: A case report. *J Int Neuropsychol Soc* 1:104–110, 1994.

55. Friedman RB, Ferguson S, Robinson S, Sunderland T: Dissociation of mechanisms of reading in Alzheimer's disease. *Brain Lang* 43:400–413, 1992.

56. Raymer AM, Berndt RS: Models of word reading: Evidence from Alzheimer's disease. *Brain Lang* 47:479–482, 1994.

57. Morton J, Patterson KE: A new attempt at an interpretation, or, an attempt at a new interpretation, in Coltheart M, Patterson K, Marshall JC (eds): *Deep Dyslexia.* London: Routledge, 1980.

58. McCarthy RA, Warrington EK: Phonological reading: Phenomena and paradoxes. *Cortex* 22:359–380, 1986.

59. Hillis AE, Caramazza A: Mechanisms for accessing lexical representations for output: Evidence from a category-specific semantic deficit. *Brain Lang* 40:106–144, 1991.

60. Patterson K, Vargha-Khadem F, Polkey CF: Reading with one hemisphere. *Brain* 112:39–63, 1989.

61. Zaidel E: Lexical organization in the right hemisphere, in Buser P, Rougeul-Buser A (eds): *Cerebral Correlates of Conscious Experience.* Amsterdam: Elsevier, 1978.

62. Zaidel E, Peters AM: Phonological encoding and ideographic reading by the disconnected right hemisphere: Two case studies. *Brain Lang* 14:205–234, 1981.

63. Coslett HB, Saffran EM: Preserved object recogni-

tion and reading comprehension in optic aphasia. *Brain* 12:1091–1110, 1989.

64. Coslett HB, Monsul N: Reading and the right hemisphere: Evidence from transcranial magnetic stimulation. *Brain Lang* 46:198–211, 1994.

65. Seidenberg MS, McClelland JL: A distributed, developmental model of word recognition and naming. *Psychol Rev* 96:522–568, 1989.

66. Patterson KE, Seidenberg MS, McClelland JL: Connections and disconnections: Acquired dyslexia in a computational model of reading processes, in Morris RGM (ed): *Parallel Distributed Processing: Implications for Psychology and Neurobiology.* Oxford, England: Oxford University Press, 1989.

67. Plaut D, Shallice T: Deep dyslexia: A case study of connectionist neuropsychology. *Cog Neuropsychol* 10:377–500, 1993.

68. Reggia J, Marsland P, Berndt R: Competitive dynamics in a dual-route connectionist model of print-to-sound transformation. *Complex Systems* 2:509–547, 1988.

69. Coltheart M, Langdon R, Haller M: Simulation of acquired dyslexias by the DRC model, a computational model of visual word recognition and reading aloud, in *Proceedings of the 1995 Workshop on Neural Modeling of Cognitive and Brain Disorders.* College Park, MD: University of Maryland, June 8–10, 1995.

Chapter 14

AGRAPHIA

David P. Roeltgen

Agraphia is traditionally defined as an acquired disorder of writing, although current usage also includes disorders of spelling.[1] Breakdown in writing may occur at any level of production, including the paragraph and sentence level. However, agraphia has typically been studied at the word level. At this level, dysfunction may be the result of either linguistic or motor disturbances. These disturbances may either be unique to the writing or spelling systems (pure agraphia) or more generalized, with associated neuropsychological dysfunction.

HISTORICAL BACKGROUND

Remote History

In 1865, Benedict[2] applied the term *agraphia* to disorders of writing, and many of the current concepts and controversies in the study of writing disorders are actually reflected in the nineteenth-century literature. Ogle[3] found that although aphasia and agraphia usually occur together, they are occasionally separable. He concluded that centers for writing may be separable from centers for speaking. Ogle classified agraphia into two types, amnemonic agraphia and atactic agraphia, a distinction that is still in use today. *Amnemonic agraphia* refers to writing by patients who produce well-formed but incorrect letters. In current terms, this is a linguistic disorder of writing. *Atactic*

agraphia is writing by patients who produce poorly formed letters. In current terms, this is a motor disorder of writing. It is rarely appreciated that the nineteenth-century literature even contains descriptions of different linguistic abilities, that, when dysfunctional, may lead to agraphia. In anticipation of dual route models of coding and writing, Dejerine[4] and Pitres[5] proposed that orthographic or visual word images were important for proper spelling, whereas Grashey[6] and Wernicke[7] postulated that the translation of sound units into letters was important for production of correct spelling. Last, there has always been an interest in the localization of functions for the production of writing. Beginning in the nineteenth century, the angular gyrus[4,5,8–10] and the frontal motor center for writing, "Exner's area,"[8–11] are the areas that have been emphasized the most.

Recent History

In the past decades, two basic approaches have been used in describing agraphias. One of these may be termed the neurologic approach. This emphasizes traditional neurologic disorders and their association with agraphia. These disorders include aphasia, limb apraxia, constructional apraxia, confusion, Parkinson's disease, callosal lesions, and dementia. The second may be termed the neuropsychological or cognitive approach. This approach attempts to examine cognitive processing breakdowns underlying the agraphias.

NEUROLOGIC MODEL

Agraphia and Aphasia

Table 14-1 lists the classic aphasias and their associations with agraphia. Typically, the agraphia is described as being similar to the aphasia.[15] Therefore, the nonfluent agraphias consist of sparse output with effortful processing and agrammatism, while the fluent agraphias consist of normal output, easy production, and normal sentence length. The nonfluent agraphias are usually associated with clumsy calligraphy and the fluent agraphias with well-formed letters.[15] However, some studies[16] have described patients with Broca's aphasia and noted that their agraphia more closely resembled the agraphia of patients with Wernicke's aphasia than the agraphias of other patients with Broca's aphasia. This reflects the dissociation of aphasia and agraphia first described by Ogle.[3]

Agraphia and Alexia

The association between agraphia and alexia has also been noted since the previous century.[4] Benson and Cummings[15] indicate that the agraphia usually resembles that of fluent aphasia and agraphia. Agraphia with alexia has also been called parietal agraphia. Patients with agraphia and alexia who do not have significant aphasia frequently have parietal lobe lesions.[13] However, the category appears to be heterogeneous, and different descriptions of this disorder have been presented. Benson and Cummings's patients produced well-formed letters, while Kaplan and Goodglass's[13] typically made poorly formed letters.

Agraphia and Praxic or Spatial Disturbances

Apraxic agraphia is described as difficulty in writing letters, writing spontaneously, and writing to dictation.[2,12,17,18] Copying or oral spelling are usually less impaired. The lesions causing apraxic agraphia are usually in the parietal lobe, especially the superior parietal lobule[19] opposite the preferred hand (dominant parietal lobe). In contrast, lesions in the parietal lobe ipsilateral to the preferred hand (nondominant parietal lobe) are traditionally associated with spatial agraphia. Patients with this disorder typically duplicate strokes and have spatial disturbances in their writing. This includes trouble writing on a horizontal line and writing only on the right side of the paper. It is frequently associated with the neglect syndrome.[12,17,20,21] With spatial agraphia, there may also be letter omissions or additions within orthographic groupings (e.g., syllables or morphologic units).

Agraphia and Parkinson Disease

Many patients with Parkinson disease have micrographia. This may be one of the earliest findings in Parkinson disease. The writing is not only small but diminishes in size as the patients write across the line. Abnormal kinetics with slower speed and varying force of motor production are associated with this.[22] The micrographia frequently improves with pharmacologic treatment of the parkinsonian patient.[23]

Agraphia and Confusion

Patients with acute confusional states frequently have agraphia.[24] Chedru and Geschwind found agraphia in 33 of 34 cases of acute confusion. Their patients had disruption of linguistic performance with spelling and syntactical disturbances. They also had motor impairment and spatial impairment with poorly formed and improperly placed letters.

Table 14-1
Agraphia and the aphasias

Nonfluent agraphia
    Agraphia and Broca's aphasia[12,13]
        Poor grapheme production
        Agrammatism
    Agraphia and transcortical motor aphasia[14]
Fluent agraphia
    Agraphia and conduction aphasia[12]
    Agraphia and Wernicke's aphasia[12,13]
    Agraphia and anomia[15]

Table 14-2
Callosal agraphias

Callosal region damaged	Type of functional disruption	Type of agraphia
Genu	Verbal motor engrams	Unilateral apraxic agraphia with inability to type
Body	Visual kinesthetic engrams	Unilateral apraxic agraphia with ability to type
Splenium	Linguistic information	Unilateral aphasic agraphia (incorrect spellings)

Agraphia and Callosal Lesions

Spelling and written letter-production systems can access the right hemisphere via the neocommissures. This allows the left hand in a right-handed person with left hemispheric language to write with the left hand. Callosal agraphia occurs when patients have this interhemispheric transfer disrupted. This results in a unilateral agraphia.[25–33] The resultant agraphia from a callosal lesion is, to a degree, variable among patients. Watson and Heilman[33] suggested a model to help explain these variabilities. Some patients may have an apparent apraxic agraphia and inability to type,[27] some may have an apraxic agraphia with preserved ability to type,[33] and others have an agraphia more typical of aphasic agraphia with some preserved ability to produce letters.[26] Watson and Heilman suggested that this related to the location of the callosal lesion and to the subsequent type of information transfer that is disrupted by the callosal lesion (Table 14-2).

Agraphia and Dementia

Agraphia is common in patients with Alzheimer disease.[34–40] Such patients may have a loss of lexical specificity and make semantic errors, such as writing *pencil* for *paper*, or they may have an impaired semantic access to written output, again producing semantic errors or, as frequently tested, homophone errors.[40] (These patients will write *night* when asked to write *knight*, as in "he is a *knight* in shining armor.") Patients may also have a spelling impairment consistent with lexical

breakdown, producing lexical agraphia (see below),[41] and impairment of attentional mechanisms, producing errors consistent with disruption of the graphemic buffer (see below).[42,43] Patients with Alzheimer disease have also been described who produce illegible words and poor spacing, consistent with a spatial agraphia.[44] The findings in patients with Alzheimer disease are consistent with the other cognitive disturbances typically found in Alzheimer patients, including semantic disruption, lexical disruption, and visuospatial dysfunction.

Isolated or Pure Agraphia

This is a writing disorder without other significant language disturbance. These patients produce well-formed letters but make different types of spelling errors that may be dependent upon the lesion location. Multiple lesion sites have been implicated in pure agraphia, including the second frontal gyrus (Exner's area).[12,13,17,45,46] These patients appear to make predominantly linguistic errors.

A second lesion site that has been associated with pure agraphia is the superior parietal lobe.[47–49] Dysfunction from lesions in this region produce varying types of agraphia. The posterior perisylvian region has also been implicated.[50,51] These patients appear to produce predominantly spelling errors. Other lesions that have been associated with pure agraphia are the left occipital lobe,[52] posterior insula and posterior putamen,[50] basal ganglia,[50,53] and left centrum semiovale.[54]

COGNITIVE AND NEUROPSYCHOLOGICAL MODELS

An alternate approach to the neurologic models comprises attempts to analyze the patterns of breakdown in terms of the underlying cognitive processes required for normal performance. This has led to the development of information processing models of writing and its breakdown. Occasionally authors have attempted to assess localization[2,51] or to assess the type of breakdown in specific disorders, such as Alzheimer disease.[40–43] In part, based on studies by Beauvois and Derouesne[55] and Shallice,[56] Ellis[57] developed one of the first information processing models. Others have followed.[16]

A Neuropsychological Model

One model has been described and developed by the author over the past decade[2,16,58] (Fig. 14-1). It divides agraphias into linguistic agraphias and motor agraphias, similar to the classic differentiations. The linguistic agraphias include phonologic agraphia, lexical agraphia, and semantic agraphia. The peripheral agraphias, which are primarily motor, include graphemic buffer agraphia, agraphia from impaired graphemic representations (disruption of graphic programming and disruption of allographic mechanisms), and agraphia from impaired spatial orientation.

Linguistic Agraphias

Phonologic Agraphia Phonologic agraphia is due to a disruption of sound-letter translation.[59] The hallmark of phonologic agraphia is loss of the ability to spell pronounceable nonsense words (i.e., nud) with preserved ability to spell real words, including words that are orthographically irregular (do not correspond to simple sound-letter relationships—i.e., island).[56] Most patients with phonologic agraphia have some impairment of real word spelling (and writing) as well,[59–67] although isolated or pure phonologic agraphia has been described.[55,68] Some patients with impaired non-word-writing ability have additional deficits

including production of semantic paragraphias (i.e., writing *airplane* for *propeller*). This pattern of dysfunction is termed deep agraphia,[59,62,69–73] analogous to deep dyslexia (see Chap. 13). Phonologic agraphia has been associated with midperisylvian lesions, including the insula and the anterior inferior supramarginal gyrus.[58,59,65]

Lexical Agraphia In contrast to phonologic agraphia, lexical agraphia includes preserved ability to spell or write nonsense words but impaired ability to spell irregular words.[55] Patients with this type of dysfunction will regularize irregular words, such as spelling *island* as *iland*.[61,65,74–80] Lexical agraphia appears to be associated with nonperisylvian lesions in multiple sites within the left hemisphere.[58] It has also been described in Alzheimer disease.[41]

Semantic Agraphia Semantic agraphia is due to a disruption of semantic influence on spelling output.[81] Patients with this disorder have trouble incorporating meaning into spelling and writing.[82,83] The error made by these patients is most commonly that of homophone confusions, such as writing *knight* when asked to write *night*, as in "The moon comes out at *night*." Lesion sites associated with semantic agraphia include those regions typically associated with transcortical aphasias with impaired comprehension.[58,77] This type of agraphia also occurs in and may be one of the earliest linguistic disruptions of many Alzheimer disease patients.[40]

Peripheral Agraphias

Graphemic Buffer Agraphia The graphemic buffer is thought to be a temporary working memory store of abstract letters. It was conceptually defined before patients with proposed disruption of this store were described.[57] Disorders within this system produce errors that are not affected by linguistic factors (i.e., words or nonsense words). Errors include letter omissions, substitutions, insertions, and transpositions. The patients usually produce correctly formed letters. There is usually

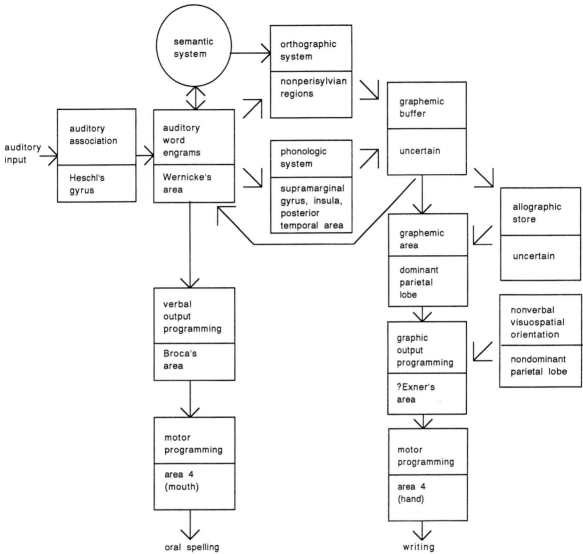

Figure 14-1
A neuropsychological model of writing and spelling. (From Roeltgen,[2] with permission.)

a significant influence of word length, with longer words being written less well than shorter words. Patients with both focal lesions[84–86] and Alzheimer disease[42,43] produce this type of agraphia. Lesion sites associated with impaired attention appear to be associated with this type of agraphia.

Apraxic Agraphia Apraxic agraphia has been described in patients with apraxia as well as in those without apraxia. In the latter case, this has also been termed ideational agraphia. Subjects with apraxic agraphia produce poorly formed letters, spell aloud better than they write, and improve their performance when copying.[87,88] They are usually able to type or use anagram letters.[89] Baxter and Warrington[90] used the term *ideational agraphia* to describe their patient, who produced poor letters but had good praxis and visuospatial skills. A similar patient has been described by Croisile and coworkers.[75]

Allographic Agraphia Patients with agraphia due to disruption of the allographic store spell aloud better than they write, have normal praxis, normal visuospatial ability, and normal letter form, but they make frequent case (lower versus upper) and style (print versus script) errors. Ellis[57] hypothesized the existence of the allographic store on the basis of errors made by normal subjects. Since then, there have been a few reports of patients with apparent disruption of this type.[91–93] The anatomic location of the allographic store is unclear.

Spatial Agraphia In information processing models, this disorder is similar to the agraphia from spatial disturbances described previously in this chapter.

Impaired Oral Spelling The mechanisms for oral spelling are not well defined. Rare patients have been described with good writing but impaired oral spelling.[94] Since oral spelling is not a common behavior and is infrequently examined, further delineation of this potential disorder is difficult.

AGRAPHIAS AND THEIR ASSESSMENT

As indicated previously, agraphia can occur at the paragraph, sentence, and word levels. Spontaneous writing is the most sensitive test for examining all levels of breakdown. With spontaneous writing, both form and content can be judged. However, having the patient write to dictation affords the examiner better control of the stimuli. Using the possible dysfunctions in the models described previously, the dictated stimuli can be varied (short word or long word, real word or nonsense word)

and the errors analyzed. The error analyses include both spelling and letter form. The patients can also be asked to copy and spell aloud. The approach to assessment usually produces sufficient information that the examiner can have an understanding of the agraphia type and its relationship to other neurologic or neuropsychological deficits.[2]

REFERENCES

1. Benedikt M: Uber Aphasie, Agraphie und verwandte pathologische Zustande. *Wien Med Pr* 6:1865.
2. Roeltgen DP: Agraphia, in Heilman KM, Valenstein E (eds): *Clinical Neuropsychology.* 3d ed. New York: Oxford University Press, 1993, pp 63–89.
3. Ogle JW: Aphasia and agraphia. *Report of the Medical Research Counsel of St. George's Hospital (London)* 2:83–122, 1867.
4. Dejerine J: Sur un cas de cecite verbale avec agraphie, suivi d'autopsie. *Mem Soc Biol* 3:197–201, 1891.
5. Pitres A: *Rapport sur la question des agraphies.* Bordeaux: Congres Francais de Medecine Interne, 1894.
6. Grashey H: Uber aphasie und ihre beziehungen zur wahrnehmung, *Arch Psychiatrie Nervenkrankh* 16:654–688, 1885. De Bleser R (trans). *Cogn Neuropsychol* 6:515–546, 1989.
7. Wernicke C: Nervenheilkunde: Die neueren Arbeiten uber Aphasie. *Fortschr Med* 4:463–482, 1886. De Bleser R (trans). *Cogn Neuropsychol* 6:547–569, 1989.
8. Henschen SE: *Klinische und Anatomische Beitrage zur Pathologie des Gehirns: VII. Uber motorische Aphasie und Agraphie.* Stockholm: Nordiska Bokhandel, 1922.
9. Nielsen JM: *Agnosia, Apraxia, Aphasia: Their Value in Cerebral Localization.* New York: Hoeber, 1946.
10. Pick A: Aphasie, in Bumke O, Foerster O (eds): *Handbuch der Normalen und Pathologischen Physiologie.* Berlin: Springer, 1931, vol xv.
11. Exner S: Untersuchungen uber die Lokalization der Funktionen, in *Der Grosshirnrinde des Menschen.* Wien: Wilhelm Braumuller, 1881.
12. Marcie P, Hecaen H: Agraphia, in Heilman KM, Valenstein (eds): *Clinical Neuropsychology.* New York: Oxford University Press, 1979, pp 92–127.
13. Kaplan E, Goodglass H: Aphasia-related disorders,

in Sarno MT (ed): *Acquired Aphasia.* New York: Academic Press, 1981, pp 303–325.

14. Rubens AB: Transcortical motor aphasia, in Whitaker H, Whitaker HA (eds): *Studies in Neurolinguistics.* New York: Academic Press, 1976, vol 1, pp 293–303.

15. Benson DF, Cummings JL: Agraphia, in Vinken PJ, Bruyn GW, Klawans HL, Frederiks JAM (eds): *Clinical Neuropsychology.* New York: Elsevier, 1985, vol 45, pp 457–472.

16. Roeltgen DP, Heilman KM: Review of agraphia and proposal for an anatomically-based neuropsychological model of writing. *Appl Psycholing* 6:205–230, 1985.

17. Hecaen H, Albert ML: *Human Neuropsychology.* New York: Wiley, 1978.

18. Leischner A: The agraphias, in Vinken PJ, Bruyn GW (eds): *Disorders of Speech, Perception and Symbolic Behavior.* Amsterdam: North-Holland, 1969, pp 141–180.

19. Alexander MP, Fischer RS, Friedman R: Lesion localization in apraxic agraphia. *Arch Neurol* 49:246–251, 1992.

20. Ardila A, Rosselli M: Spatial agraphia. *Brain Cogn* 22:137–147, 1993.

21. Benson DF: *Aphasia, Alexia and Agraphia.* New York: Churchill Livingstone, 1979.

22. Margolin DI, Wing A: Agraphia and micrographia: Clinical manifestations of motor programming and performance disorders. *Acta Psychol* 54:263–283, 1983.

23. McLennan JE, Nakano K, Tyler HR, Schwab RS: Micrographia in Parkinson's disease. *J Neurol Sci* 15:141–152, 1972.

24. Chedru F, Geschwind N: Writing disturbances in acute confusional states. *Neuropsychologica* 10:343–354, 1972.

25. Bogen JE: The other side of the brain: I. Dysgraphia and dyscopia following cerebral commissurotomy. *Bull LA Neurol Soc* 34:3–105, 1969.

26. Gersh F, Damasio AR: Praxis and writing of the left hand may be served by different callosal pathways. *Arch Neurol* 38:634–636, 1981.

27. Geschwind N, Kaplan EF: A human cerebral disconnection syndrome. *Neurology* 12:675–685, 1962.

28. Levy J, Nebes RD, Sperry RW: Expressive language in the surgically separated minor hemisphere. *Cortex* 71:49–58, 1971.

29. Liepmann H, Maas O: Fall von Linksseitger agraphie und apraxie bei rechtsseitiger lahmung. *J Psychol Neurol* 10:214–227, 1907.

30. Rubens AB, Geschwind N, Mahowald MW, Mastri A: Posttraumatic cerebral hemispheric disconnection syndrome. *Arch Neurol* 34:750–755, 1977.

31. Sugishita M, Toyokura Y, Yoshioka M, Yamada R: Unilateral agraphia after section of the posterior half of the truncus of the corpus callosum. *Brain Lang* 9:212–225, 1980.

32. Watson RT, Heilman KM: Callosal apraxia. *Brain* 106:391–404, 1983.

33. Yamadori A, Osumi Y, Ikeda H, Kanazawa Y: Left unilateral agraphia and tactile anomia. Disturbances seen after occlusion of the anterior cerebral artery. *Arch Neurol* 37:88–91, 1980.

34. Bayles KA, Tomoeda CK: Caregiver report of prevalence and appearance order of linguistic symptoms in Alzheimer's patients. *Gerontologist* 31:210–216, 1991.

35. Henderson VW, Buckwalter JG, Sobel E, et al: The agraphia of Alzheimer's disease. *Neurology* 42:776–784, 1992.

36. Horner J, Heyman A, Dawson D, Rogers H: The relationship of agraphia to the severity of dementia in Alzheimer's disease. *Arch Neurol* 45:760–763, 1988.

37. Neils J, Boller F, Gerdeman B, Cole M: Descriptive writing abilities in Alzheimer's disease. *J Clin Exp Neuropsychol* 11:692–698, 1989.

38. Neils J, Roeltgen DP: Does lexical dysgraphia occur in early Alzheimer's disease? *J Med Speech Lang Pathol* 2:281–289, 1994.

39. Glosser G, Kaplan E: Linguistic and nonlinguistic impairments in writing: A comparison of patients with focal and multifocal CNS disorders. *Brain Lang* 37:357–380, 1989.

40. Neils J, Roeltgen DP, Constantinidou F: Decline in homophone spelling associated with loss of semantic influence on spelling in Alzheimer's disease. *Brain Lang* 49:27–49, 1995.

41. Rapcsak SZ, Arthur SA, Bliklen DA, Rubens AB: Lexical agraphia in Alzheimer's disease. *Arch Neurol* 46:65–68, 1989.

42. Croisile B, Brabant M, Carmoi T, et al: Comparison between oral and written spelling in Alzheimer's disease. *Brain Lang.* In press.

43. Neils J, Roeltgen DP, Grier A: Spelling and attention in early Alzheimer's disease: Evidence for impairment of the graphemic buffer. *Brain Language* 49:241–262, 1995.

44. LaBarge E, Smith DS, Dick L, Storandt M: Agraphia in dementia of the Alzheimer type. *Arch Neurol* 49:1151–1156, 1992.

45. Aimard G, Devick M, Lebel M, et al: Agraphie pure (dynamique?) origine frontale. *Rev Neurol* 7:505–512, 1975.

46. Vernea JJ, Merory J: Frontal agraphia (including a case report). *Proc Aust Assoc Neurol* 12:93–99, 1975.

47. Auerbach SH, Alexander MP: Pure agraphia and unilateral optic ataxia associated with a left superior parietal lobule lesion. *J Neurol Neurosurg Psychiatry* 44:430–432, 1981.

48. Basso A, Taborielli A, Vignolo LA: Dissociated disorders of speaking and writing in aphasia. *J Neurol Neurosurg Psychiatry* 41:556–563, 1978.

49. Kinsbourne M, Rosenfeld DB: Agraphia selective for written spelling, an experimental case study. *Brain Lang* 1:215–225, 1974.

50. Rosati G, De Bastiani P: Pure agraphia: A discreet form of aphasia. *J Neurol Neurosurg Psychiatry* 44:266–269, 1981.

51. Roeltgen DP: Prospective analysis of a model of writing, anatomic aspects. Presented at the Academy of Aphasia, October 1989, Sante Fe, NM.

52. Kapur N, Lawton NF: Dysgraphia for letters: A form of motor memory deficit. *J Neurol Neurosurg Psychiatry* 46:573–575, 1983.

53. Laine TN, Marttila RJ. Pure agraphia: A case study. *Neuropsychologia* 19:311–316, 1981.

54. Croisile B, Laurent B, Michel D, Trillet M: Pure agraphia after deep left hemisphere haematoma. *J Neurol Neurosurg Psychiatry* 53:263–265, 1990.

55. Beauvois MF, Derouesne J: Lexical or orthographic agraphia. *Brain* 104:21–49, 1981.

56. Shallice T: Phonological agraphia and the lexical route in writing. *Brain* 104:412–429, 1981.

57. Ellis AW: Spelling and writing (and reading and speaking), in Ellis AW (ed): *Normality and Pathology in Cognitive Functions.* London: Academic Press, 1982, pp 113–146.

58. Roeltgen DP, Rapcsak SZ: Acquired disorders of writing and spelling, in Blanken G, Dittmann J, Grimm H (eds): *Linguistic Disorders and Pathologies: An International Handbook.* Berlin: De Gruyter, 1993, pp 262–278.

59. Roeltgen DP, Sevush S, Heilman KM: Phonological agraphia: Writing by the lexical-semantic route. *Neurology* 33:733–757, 1983.

60. Baxter DM, Warrington EK: Category specific phonological dysgraphia. *Neuropsychologia* 23:653–666, 1985.

61. Bolla-Wilson K, Speedie LJ, Robinson RG: Phonologic agraphia in a left-handed patient after a right-hemisphere lesion. *Neurology* 35:1778–1981, 1985.

62. Goodman-Schulman R, Caramazza A: Patterns of dysgraphia and the nonlexical spelling process. *Cortex* 23:143–148, 1987.

63. Hatfield FM: Visual and phonological factors in acquired dysgraphia. *Neuropsychologia* 23:13–29, 1985.

64. Morton J: The logogen model and orthographic structure, in Frith U (ed): *Cognitive Processes in Spelling.* London: Academic Press, 1980, pp 117–133.

65. Nolan KA, Caramazza A: Modality-independent impairments in word processing in a deep dyslexic patient. *Brain Lang* 16:236–264, 1982.

66. Roeltgen DP, Heilman KM: Lexical agraphia, further support for the two-system hypothesis of linguistic agraphia. *Brain* 107:811–827, 1984.

67. Roeltgen DP, Rothi LJG, Heilman KM: Isolated phonological agraphia from a focal lesion. Presented at the Academy of Aphasia, October 1982, New Paltz, NY.

68. Roeltgen DP: Prospective analysis of writing and spelling: Part II. Results not related to localization. *J Clin Exp Neuropsychol* 13:48, 1991.

69. Assal G, Buttet J, Jolivet R: Dissociations in aphasia: A case report. *Brain Lang* 13:223–240, 1981.

70. Bub D, Kertesz A: Deep agraphia. *Brain Lang* 17:146–165, 1982.

71. Marshall J, Newcombe F: Syntactic and semantic errors in paralexia. *Neuropsychologica* 4:169–176, 1966.

72. Saffran EM, Schwartz MF, Marin OSM: Semantic mechanisms in paralexia. *Brain Lang* 13:255–265, 1981.

73. Van Lancker D: A case of deep dysgraphia attributed to right hemispheric function. Presented at the Academy of Aphasia, October 1990, Baltimore, MD.

74. Alexander MP, Friedman R, LoVerso F, Fischer R: Anatomic correlates of lexical agraphia. Presented at the Academy of Aphasia, October 1990, Baltimore, MD.

75. Croisile B, Trillet M, Laurent B, et al: Agraphie lexicale par hematome temporo-parietal gauche. *Rev Neurol (Paris)* 145:287–292, 1989.

76. Friedman RB, Alexander MP: Written spelling agraphia. *Brain Lang* 36:503–517, 1989.

77. Hatfield FM, Patterson KE: *Phonological spelling. Q J Exp Psychol* 35A:451–468, 1983.

78. Rapcsak SZ, Arthur SA, Rubens AB: Lexical

agraphia from focal lesion of the left precentral gyrus. *Neurology* 38:1119–1123, 1988.

79. Rapcsak SZ, Rubens AB, Laguna JF: From Letters to words: Procedures for word recognition in letter-by-letter reading. *Brain Lang* 38:504–514, 1990.

80. Rothi LJG, Roeltgen DP, Kooistra CA: Isolated lexical agraphia in a right-handed patient with a posterior lesion of the right cerebral hemisphere. *Brain Lang* 30:181–190, 1987.

81. Roeltgen DP, Rothi LG, Heilman KM: Linguistic semantic agraphia. *Brain Lang* 27:257–280, 1986.

82. Patterson K: Lexical but nonsemantic spelling? *Cogn Neuropsychol* 3:341–367, 1986.

83. Rapcsak SZ, Rubens AB: Disruption of semantic influence on writing following a left prefrontal lesion. *Brain Lang* 38:334–344, 1990.

84. Badecker W, Hillis A, Caramazza A: Lexical morphology and its role in the writing process: Evidence from a case of acquired dysgraphia. *Cognition* 35:205–243, 1990.

85. Caramazza A, Miceli G, Villa G, Romani C: The role of the graphemic buffer in spelling: Evidence from a case of acquired dysgraphia. *Cognition* 26:59–85, 1987.

86. Hillis AE, Caramazza A: The graphemic buffer and attentional mechanisms. *Brain Lang* 36:208–235, 1989.

87. Heilman KM, Coyle JM, Gonyea EF, Geschwind N: Apraxia and agraphia in a left hander. *Brain* 96:21–28, 1973.

88. Heilman KM, Gonyea EF, Geschwind N: Apraxia and agraphia in a right hander. *Cortex* 10:284–288, 1974.

89. Valenstein E, Heilman KM: Apraxic agraphia with neglect-induced paragraphia. *Arch Neurol* 67:44–56, 1979.

90. Baxter DM, Warrington EK: Ideational agraphia: A single case study. *J Neurol Neurosurg Psychiatry* 49:369–374, 1986.

91. Black SE, Bass K, Behrmann M, Hacker P: Selective writing impairment: A single case study of a deficit in allographic conversion. *Neurology* 37:174, 1987.

92. De Bastiani K, Barry C: A cognitive analysis of an acquired dysgraphic patient with an ''allographic'' writing disorder. *Cogn Neuropsychol* 6:25–41, 1989.

93. Yopp KS, Roeltgen DP: Case of alexia and agraphia due to a disconnection of the visual input to and the motor output from an intact graphemic area. *J Clin Exp Neuropsychol* 9:42, 1987.

94. Kinsbourne M, Warrington EK: A case showing selectively impaired oral spelling. *J Neurol Neurosurg Psychiatry* 28:563–566, 1965.

Chapter 15

ACALCULIA

Jordan Grafman
Timothy Rickard

Acalculia is defined as an impairment of the ability to calculate. It is used interchangeably with the term *dyscalculia,* although some authors have suggested reserving the term *acalculia* for a complete inability to calculate and using the term *dyscalculia* in cases where some ability to calculate remains. In this chapter we use the term *acalculia* to refer to both forms of impairment.

Acalculia is a frequently appearing deficit following damage to the left posterior region of the brain, but it can occur following damage to other brain regions. It is a significant functional deficit for patients, since it may restrict their ability to use a checkbook, pay bills, exchange money, or plan activities. Acalculia is also an opportunity for clinical researchers interested in the organization of cognitive architectures, response execution, lexical-semantic stores, and the cooperation between fact-based and analogue-scaled cognitive processes to study these processes within the context of a relatively narrow domain of knowledge.

In this chapter, we review the contemporary cognitive neuropsychological approach to the study of calculation disorders, discuss current models of normal and abnormal calculation processing, and cautiously attempt to specify which aspects of numeric computation can be mapped to brain regions. These sections are followed by our suggestions for a comprehensive assessment of calculation and number processing disorders.

DESCRIPTION AND INCIDENCE OF ACALCULIA

There are a number of general classification schemes for describing forms of acalculia, which have divided acalculia into three broad types.[1] Type 1 is a secondary form of acalculia due to deficits in verbal processing. Type 2 is also a secondary form of acalculia and is due to deficits in visuospatial processing. Type 3 is the primary form of acalculia, which is independent of (but may coexist with) any other cognitive deficit. A *primary acalculia* has been described in individual cases and made up approximately 6 percent of acalculic patients with right-hemispheric lesions and 23 percent of acalculic patients with left-hemispheric lesions.

DEVELOPMENT OF NUMBER PROCESSING AND CALCULATION SKILLS

Some elements of calculation are preliterate and perhaps innate in origin. People without formal schooling can develop procedural skills related to counting, numerosity, and magnitude estimation. Numerical abilities at very young ages, however, appear to be limited to small numerical values.[2] An example is the ability to *subitize,* or quickly judge the number of a small group of items (e.g., dots on a page) without having to count them. This ability, which has been demonstrated in infants and monkeys as well as in adults, appears to be limited to set sizes of 4 or 5. Other elements of calculation—such as formal calculation procedures, number fact retrieval (e.g., 9 × 9 = ?), and estimation skills for large numbers—are generally learned with formal training. Children initially learn counting strategies for calculation, but these strategies are eventually replaced by fact retrieval skills.[3,4] Educators believe that extensive experience with procedural strategies and representational models of the calculation process is essential for the mastery of calculation. We refer the reader to papers by Dehaene,[5] Nesher,[6] Resnick,[7] and by Siegler and Shrager[8] for a comprehensive look at developmental changes in normal calculation ability, and to Gross and colleagues,[9] Lyytinen and coworkers,[10] Shalev and associates[11] for detailed discussions of developmental acalculia.

HISTORICAL SKETCH OF RESEARCH IN ACALCULIA

Brain-Behavior Correlates

Primary acalculia can take the form of either global or selective deficits in a large number of number processing and calculation abilities, including comprehension of numbers and numerical magnitude, performance on single-digit arithmetic operations, execution of procedures (such as carrying and borrowing, necessary for complex arithmetic), and solving of word problems. A large number of studies have implicated left posterior lesions in primary acalculia, most often in the vicinity of the left angular and supramarginal gyri.[12–15] In particular, the evidence suggests that arithmetic facts and calculation procedures are preferentially stored in that brain region.

Despite the strong association of acalculia and left posterior quadrant lesions, there are certain characteristics of acalculia that have led to the suggestion of a right-hemispheric contribution. The finding that acalculia can result from poor placement of digits in a multidigit problem suggests that right-hemispheric processes contribute to the spatial construction of a problem solution

if not its actual calculation.[15] Other work has suggested that magnitude estimation (e.g., which is larger, 3 or 4?) is a scaling process linked with the right hemisphere.[16] Estimation of magnitude is important in a number of real-world situations where a quick, approximate answer is adequate, and it appears also to provide a way to converge on the exact answer to simple and complex arithmetic problems, particularly when an answer has not been memorized. A contribution of magnitude processes to arithmetic may help explain results of a functional imaging study of Rueckert and colleagues in which a simple subtract-by-7's task activated not only the left angular gyrus and frontal cortex (the latter presumably reflecting a working memory component of the task, see Chaps. 31 and 36) but in most subjects the right parietal region as well.[17]

However, it appears that arithmetic facts and calculation procedures on one hand and spatial and magnitude processes on the other are not completely lateralized to the left and right hemispheres, respectively. Grafman and coworkers[15] found that patients with left-hemispheric lesions also made a large number of spatial errors (e.g., column misalignment). It has been claimed that magnitude estimation might be represented in the right cerebral cortex; however, in a functional neuroimaging study, magnitude estimation has been reported to activate left- as well as right-hemispheric brain regions.[18] To date, carefully controlled structural magnetic resonance imaging studies have not been done to demonstrate a clear effect of right posterior lesions on primary calculation ability.

In conclusion, the overwhelming evidence suggests that arithmetic facts and calculation procedures are stored in the left parietal cortex. However, a contribution of frontal lobe[19] and right parietal processes is also implicated. A more precise delineation of these contributions awaits further investigation.

Associated Deficits

Acalculia is often associated with other cognitive impairment by virtue of the location of the lesions that cause primary acalculia and because of the relationship of the domain-specific calculation procedures to other cognitive processes. Finger agnosia, agraphia, and right-left discrimination are frequently observed together with acalculia following left posterior cortical lesions, but each symptom may occur as frequently with other symptoms. This tetrad of symptoms is known collectively as the Gerstmann syndrome, and its appearance has been associated with lesions of the left angular gyrus.[20,21] Other symptoms associated with primary acalculia have included alexia, visuospatial deficits, and conduction aphasia. On-line serial calculations may involve working memory processes. Thus, a breakdown in serial calculation (as opposed to simple fact retrieval) may be associated with a general deficit in working memory, word fluency, or planning.

The Gerstmann syndrome symptom collection at first may seem like the odd quartet. Odd, that is, until it is remembered that preliterate calculation depended upon counting, numerosity, and magnitude estimation. Since counting often relied upon fingers, with fingers on different hands representing different quantities, it should not be completely surprising that calculation, finger recognition, left-right discrimination, and writing ability could all be impaired following an angular gyrus lesion.

Modular Aspects

Acalculia has been noted to be the initial symptom of degenerative dementias,[22] the outstanding symptom following a stroke, and the main symptom in several developmental disorders. These observations suggest that primary acalculia could be a result of a dysfunction in a modular system, that is, a system that is specialized for calculation. The modules impaired in these cases could be devoted to number fact storage (categorized perhaps by operation), and potentially to the actual calculation procedure (in the case of novel problems). Whether the procedure and the fact-retrieval stores are overlapping, adjacent, or distant remains to be adjudicated.

Numerous case studies indicate that selective fact retrieval for one or more of the basic operations is possible.[23–25] These selective deficits can appear independently of other cognitive impairment, suggesting that the modular approach applies even to the level of the individual arithmetic operation. Indeed, there is even a case study describing a more specific deficit for processing arithmetic problems involving only the numbers 7 or 9.[26] This deficit could not be attributed to a secondary acalculia (such as deficits in auditory lexicon or visual analysis) and were interpreted as reflecting a deficit in the semantic, or abstract, level of representation for those numbers. Whether these sorts of deficits are best understood as reflecting a very fine-grained modularity or as selective damage to parts of larger networks is still an open question. However, these and other data on number processing and calculation tasks do demonstrate, perhaps better than any other neuropsychological data to date, the hyperspecificity of function that can occur in at least some regions of the brain.

The evidence that argues for the modularity of various calculation skills was originally based on rather gross neuropsychological analyses. Over the last 15 years, however, a plethora of cognitive arithmetic models have been developed that offers the clinician and investigator exciting new hypotheses regarding the storage and retrieval of number facts and procedures. A few of these are described broadly in the next section.

CONTEMPORARY COGNITIVE MODELS AND THEIR FRACTIONATION IN ACALCULIA

The empirical research of many investigators, including Warrington, Deloche and Seron, and Mc-Closkey, among others, has now established a solid empiric base on which to build functional cognitive models of number processing and calculation. In a seminal paper, Warrington[27] reported on a patient with a left parietal-occipital lobe lesion who was found to have an outstanding problem in calculation. Warrington noted that the patient had a particular deficit in arithmetic fact retrieval on all operations, even though his arithmetic knowledge—estimation and counting, number reading, and number writing—were all preserved.

At about the same time, Deloche and Seron[28] were conducting analyses of patients' ability to transcode between Arabic numerals and word numbers. Length of the number word but not Arabic numeral was an important factor in producing errors. Morphologic structure appeared to be maintained in the transcoding process. There was some regularity in patient lexical errors in that errors were often only one digit away from the answer. The main types of errors were "stack errors," which resulted in a distorted syntactic frame, such as "2" instead of "12," and "stack position" errors, which involved inappropriate lexical selection, such as "four" instead of "three." Anterior lesions tended to result in stack errors, whereas posterior lesions tended to result in stack position errors. Deloche and coworkers' results demonstrate the importance of evaluating the patient's ability to transcode as part of an overall acalculia test battery.

The work of McCloskey and colleagues has also stimulated much research in acalculia.[29,30] They have been primarily concerned with describing the components required to read, write, and pronounce numbers and to retrieve basic arithmetic facts from memory. In one study—using arithmetic fact verification, magnitude estimation, and matching tasks—they were able to demonstrate that some patients may have difficulty expressing number names even though the comprehension of numbers is intact. In another study, they argued that the word-number and Arabic-number systems could be dissociated. They have also shown that some patients may have more difficulty producing word numbers compared to Arabic numbers despite comprehension of both kinds of number symbols. Errors were similar for writing or speaking numbers. These and other results have led McCloskey and coworkers to argue for a common abstract syntactic frame for both verbal and written number production systems.

A few componential models of number processing and mental calculation now exist, and their underlying assumptions are based largely on the empiric research summarized above.[5,29,31] All models stress that certain operations in arithmetic resemble those processes required for comprehending symbols or information in other domains, such as reading words or understanding logic. For example, number processing probably has at least two routes to a fact lexicon, a direct visual route to a number lexicon and an indirect route that requires phonologic processing. Several other features would appear to be required in a complete model. Numbers, like letters and words, must be perceived as distinct meaningful entities and as orthographic or idiographic symbols. Working memory buffers and executive functioning must hold numeric information until it can be processed directly under an attentional spotlight. The representation of numbers and number facts should be independent of representations for the numeric computational procedures demanded by particular operational symbols. Output mechanisms servicing speech or graphomotor functions should be similar to those imagined for uttering or writing letters and words. In these types of cognitive architectures, a modular design assuming, among other things, a central abstract level of representation of numeric knowledge, is sometimes assumed.[29] On the other hand, based on their experimental paradigms, Campbell and colleagues[31] have argued that there is no abstract level of representation for numbers but rather that numeric cognition involves a *complex encoding* architecture that includes only interconnected, notation-dependent representations of numbers and of arithmetic problems, thus inextricably *linking* number perception and fact retrieval as well as interpenetration of number reading and fact retrieval processes (diminishing their modular characteristics). The issue of whether or not an abstract, semantic level of representation for numbers exists is a central one in this area of research and is an issue with potentially far-reaching implications for representation of knowledge more generally in the human brain.

These types of models, derived initially from empiric data, now make explicit predictions that can be tested in future research. This emerging interplay between theory and data promises to lead to rapid progress in understanding the architecture of number processing and calculation.

METHODOLOGIC ISSUES

Assessment of Acalculia

There are a number of clinical and experimental test batteries currently in use that can aid the clinician or researcher in determining the ability level and intactness of arithmetic cognitive processing of their subjects. These are discussed next.

Clinical Assessment Tools

The most common test used to assess calculation by clinical neuropsychologists has been the Wide Range Achievement Test (WRAT).[32] The arithmetic portion of this test allows for some sense of the subject's operational skills (addition, subtrac-

tion, etc.) but is limited in how it tests subjects and in the space provided for subjects to answer problems. The subtest itself does allow for a grade-equivalent score to be obtained, and results on this subtest can be compared to other language-based subtests from the WRAT. Much better tests, however, are available for the clinician, although many of these were originally designed for use with children. One commonly used test, the Key Math Test,[33] is commercially available; it has grade-equivalent and standardized scores. The test batteries generally sample all the standard arithmetic operations, including addition, subtraction, multiplication, division, fractions, percentages, quantification, algebra, geometric relations, practical use of quantities, etc. The advantage of using these test batteries is that they have been normed on children and adolescents and have all the psychometric and presentation advantages of commercial products. None of the commercially avail-

Table 15-1

Suggested test battery for the evaluation of acalculia

Test	Description
1. Number recognition	Reading arabic numerals and and number words aloud
2. Number writing	Writing arabic numerals and number words to dictation
3. Number transcoding	Transcoding arabic numeral to number word and vice versa
4. Quantification	Estimating the quantity of collections of symbols or objects
5. Magnitude estimation	Deciding which of two arabic numerals or number words is the largest
6. Basic arithmetic operations	Addition, subtraction, multiplication, and division
7. Calculation fact verification	Computer-assisted presentation of calculation facts for response-time verification
8. Multicolumn calculation	All four operations—some problems should involve carry and borrow procedures
9. Magnitude comparison	Computer-assisted presentation of numeric quantities for response-time verification
10. Fractions	Computing percentages and fractions
11. Algebra	Algebraic computations
12. Numeric knowledge	Retrieving numeric knowledge such as "How many inches are there in one yard?"

Note: Single numbers and problems should be varied by the magnitude of the number, the numeric distance between component parts of the problem, the relationship of the error (e.g., test 7) to the correct answer, and by other important variables that can be found in the experimental literature.

able instruments, however, have norms for adults, nor were they specifically designed to test models of number processing and calculation.

Experimental Tasks

A few experimental batteries have been developed in the last 10 years that are based on cognitive models of calculation and number processing and include a variety of tasks not usually available in the clinical batteries referred to above.[34] Such supplemental experimental tasks include number transcoding, fact and operation verification tasks, and timed magnitude-estimation tasks. In addition, many authors have adapted error-analysis systems that may help isolate dysfunctional information-processing components in acalculia patients. Most of the experimental tasks alluded to above are easily programmed for response-time experiments using currently available test-authoring software and with designs that can be guided by articles appearing in experimental and cognitive psychology journals. Since there are a variety of error-analysis systems, we would recommend that readers peruse each author's rationale for his or her scoring system and then decide on the system that appears most convincing and practical to them. In Table 15-1 we suggest a set of tasks and an error-analysis approach that can be used in a general but comprehensive assessment of number processing and calculation.

CONCLUSIONS

Acalculia is a common developmental disorder and is a frequent concomitant of acute and progressive left posterior hemispheric lesions in children and adults. It can affect a patient's ability to balance a checkbook, make change, use a temperature gauge, etc. Clinically, it is important to assess number processing and calculation, and we have made suggestions for such an assessment in this chapter. Studying number processing and calculation in acalculic patients can also teach us about the cognitive architecture and computational demands of a relatively encap-

sulated cognitive function by revealing patterns of spared and impaired abilities across individual patients. Given that numbers and calculation represent a relatively closed information processing system with a limited number of rules and symbols, it makes for an ideal domain of study.

REFERENCES

1. Levin HS, Goldstein FC, Spiers PA: Acalculia, in Heilman K, Valenstein E (eds): *Clinical Neuropsychology.* New York, Oxford University Press, 1993, pp 91–118.
2. Gallistel CR, Gelman R: Preverbal and verbal counting and computation. *Cognition* 44(1–2):43–74, 1992.
3. Siegler RS: Strategy choice procedures and the development of multiplication skill. *J Exp Psychol General* 117:258–275, 1988.
4. Rickard TC, Bourne LE Jr: Some tests of an identical elements model of basic arithmetic skills. *J Exp Psychol Learn Mem Cog.* In press.
5. Dehaene S: Varieties of numerical abilities. *Cognition* 44(1–2):1–42, 1992.
6. Nesher P: Learning mathematics: A cognitive perspective. Special Issue: Psychological science and education. *Am Psychol* 41:1114–1122, 1986.
7. Resnick LB: Developing mathematical knowledge. Special issue: Children and their development: Knowledge base, research agenda, and social policy application. *Am Psychol* 44:162–169, 1989.
8. Siegler RS, Shrager EA: *How Children Discover New Strategies.* Hillsdale, NJ: Erlbaum, 1989.
9. Gross A, Tsur V, Manor O, Shalev RS: Developmental dyscalculia, gender, and the brain. *Arch Dis Child* 68:510–512, 1993.
10. Lyytinen H, Ahonen T, Rasanen P: Dyslexia and dyscalculia in children—Risks, early precursors, bottlenecks and cognitive mechanisms. *Acta Paedopsychiatr* 56:179–192, 1994.
11. Shalev RS, Weirtman R, Amir N: Developmental dyscalculia. *Cortex* 24:555–561, 1988.
12. Ashcraft MH, Yamashita TS, Aram DM: Mathematics performance in left and right brain-lesioned children and adolescents. *Brain Cog* 19:208–252, 1992.
13. Boller F, Grafman J: Acalculia: Historical develop-

ment and current significance. *Brain Cog* 2:205–223, 1983.

14. Rosselli M, Ardila A: Calculation deficits in patients with right and left hemisphere damage. *Neuropsychologia* 27:607–617, 1989.

15. Grafman J, Passafiume D, Faglioni P, Boller F: Calculation disturbances in adults with focal hemispheric damage. *Cortex* 18:37–49, 1982.

16. Dehaene S, Cohen L: Two mental calculation systems: A case study of severe acalculia with preserved approximation. *Neuropsychologia* 29:1045–1054, 1991.

17. Rueckert L, Lange N, Partiot A, et al: Visualizing cortical activation during mental calculation with functional MRI. 1996. Submitted.

18. Dehaene S, Tzourio N, Frak V, et al: Cerebral activations during number multiplications and comparison: A PET study. 1996. Submitted.

19. Tohgi H, Saitoh K, Takahashi S, et al: Agraphia and acalculia after a left prefrontal (F1, F2) infarction. *J Neurol Neurosurg Psychiatry* 58:629–632, 1995.

20. Mazzoni M, Pardossi L, Cantini R, et al: Gerstmann syndrome: A case report. *Cortex* 26:459–467, 1990.

21. Moore MR, Saver JL, Johnson KA, Romero JA: Right parietal stroke with Gerstmann's syndrome: Appearance on computed tomography, magnetic resonance imaging, and single-photon emission computed tomography. *Arch Neurol* 48:432–435, 1991.

22. Grafman J, Kampen D, Rosenberg J, et al: The progressive breakdown of number processing and calculation ability: A case study. *Cortex* 25:121–133, 1989.

23. Pesenti M, Seron X, Van Der Linden M: Selective impairment as evidence for mental organisation of arithmetic facts: BB, a case of preserved subtraction? *Cortex* 30:661–671, 1994.

24. Cipolotti L, Costello AD: Selective impairment for simple division. *Cortex*. In press.

25. Lampl Y, Eshel Y, Gilad R, Sarova-Pinhas I: Selective acalculia with sparing of the subtraction process in a patient with left parietotemporal hemorrhage. *Neurology* 44:1759–1761, 1994.

26. Weddell RA, Davidoff JB: A dyscalculic patient with selectively impaired processing of the numbers 7, 9, and 0. *Brain Cog* 17:240–271, 1991.

27. Warrington EK: The fractionation of arithmetic skills: A single case study. *Q J Exp Psychol* 34A:31–51, 1982.

28. Deloche G, Seron X: Some linguistic components of acalculia. *Adv Neurol* 42:215–222, 1984.

29. McCloskey M, Caramazza A, Basili A: Cognitive mechanisms in number processing and calculation: Evidence from dyscalculia. *Brain Cog* 4:171–196, 1985.

30. McCloskey M, Macaruso P: Representing and using numerical information. *Am Psychol* 50:351–363, 1995.

31. Campbell JI: Architectures for numerical cognition. *Cognition* 53(1):1–44, 1994.

32. Jastak S, Wilkinson GS: *Wide Range Achievement Test—Revised.* Wilmington, DE, Jastak Assessment Systems, 1984.

33. Connolly AJ, Nachtman W, Pritchett EM: *KeyMath Diagnostic Arithmetic Test.* Circle Pines, MN, American Guidance Services, 1976.

34. Deloche G, Seron X, Larroque C, et al: Calculation and number processing: Assessment battery; role of demographic factors. *J Clin Exp Neuropsychol* 16:195–208, 1994.

Chapter 16

DISORDERS OF SKILLED MOVEMENTS: LIMB APRAXIA

Kenneth M. Heilman
Robert T. Watson
Leslie Gonzalez Rothi

Apraxia is an inability to correctly perform learned skilled movements. In part, it is defined by what it is not.[1] Patients with impaired motor performance induced by weakness, sensory loss, tremors, dystonia, chorea, ballismus, athetosis, myoclonus, ataxia, and seizures are not considered apraxic. Patients with severe cognitive, memory, motivational, and attentional disorders may have difficulty performing skilled motor acts because they cannot comprehend, cooperate, remember, or attend, but these deficits are also not considered apraxic.

Limb apraxia may be the most frequently unrecognized behavioral disorder associated with cerebral disease. It is most often associated with strokes and degenerative dementia of the Alzheimer type but also occurs with a variety of other diseases. Apraxia may be the presenting symptom and sign in cortical basal ganglionic degeneration.

Apraxia may go unrecognized for several reasons. The apraxia associated with strokes is often accompanied by weakness of the preferred arm. In attempting to perform skilled acts with the nonpreferred arm, apraxic patients may recognize that they are not performing well, but they may attribute their difficulty in performing skilled acts to the inexperience of this nondominant arm or to premorbid clumsiness of the nonpreferred arm. However, even when using their dominant limb, apraxic patients may be anosognosic for their apraxia[2] and therefore will not complain of a problem in performing skilled movements. Finally, many physicians and other health professionals do not test for limb apraxia and are not aware of the nature of errors that are associated with it or that it may be a disabling disorder.

The subtypes of limb apraxia are defined by the nature of errors made by the patient and the means by which these errors are elicited. Liepmann[3] subdivided limb apraxic disorders into three types: melokinetic (or limb-kinetic), ideomotor, and ideational. In addition to discussing these forms of apraxia, we will also discuss three additional forms of apraxia we have called disassociation apraxia, conduction apraxia, and conceptual apraxia. The apraxias are differentiated by the types of errors made by the patient and the means by which these errors are elicited.

Apraxia Testing

The physician must perform a thorough neurologic examination to be certain that abnormal performance is not induced by the nonapraxic motor, sensory, or cognitive disorders mentioned above. The presence of elemental motor defects does not prohibit apraxia testing; however, the examiner must interpret the results with the knowledge gained from the neurologic examination.

Both the right and left arm and hands should be tested independently. Patients should be requested to pantomime to verbal command (e.g., "Show me how you would use a pair of scissors"). All patients should also be asked to imitate the examiner's motor acts. The examiner may want to perform both meaningful and meaningless gestures for the patient to imitate. Independent of the results of the pantomime and imitation tests, the patient should be given actual objects and tools and asked to demonstrate how to use the tool or object. One should test transitive movements (i.e., using a tool or instrument) and intransitive movements (i.e., communicative gestures not using tools, such as waving good-bye). When having a patient pantomime, in addition to giving verbal commands, the examiner may also want to show the patient a tool or a picture of the tool or object that the patient is required to pantomime. It may be valuable to see if the patient can recognize transitive and intransitive pantomimes performed by the examiner and discriminate between those that are well and poorly performed. The patient should be given a task that requires several motor acts in sequence. Last, one may want to learn if the patient knows what tools operate on what objects (e.g., hammer and nail), what action is associated with each tool or object, and how to fabricate tools to solve mechanical problems.

LIMB KINETIC APRAXIA

In limb kinetic apraxia, there is a loss of the ability to make finely graded, precise, individual finger movements. Limb kinetic apraxia occurs in the limb contralateral to a hemispheric lesion. Lawrence and Kuypers[4] demonstrated that monkeys with lesions confined to the corticospinal system show similar errors. Because limb kinetic apraxia may be an elemental motor disorder rather than a disorder of learned skilled movements, it will not be discussed in this chapter.

IDEOMOTOR APRAXIA

Clinical Findings

Typically, the patient with ideomotor apraxia (IMA) makes the most errors when asked to pantomime transitive acts, typically improves with imitation, and may perform the best when using actual objects.

We classify apraxic errors as errors of content or of production.[5] In order to be considered as having IMA, a patient should make primarily production errors. Content errors occur when a patient substitutes another recognizable pantomime for the target pantomime. For example, when asked to pantomime using scissors, a patient may demonstrate hammering movements. Occasionally, a patient's performance is so profoundly impaired that the examiner cannot recognize the movement. When patients with IMA pantomime, their pantomimes may be incorrectly produced, but the goal or intent of the act can usually be recognized as correct.

Patients with IMA make two major types of production errors: spatial and temporal. Spatial errors can be divided into several subtypes, including postural (or internal configuration), spatial movement, and spatial orientation errors. Regarding postural errors, Goodglass and Kaplan[6] note that when apraxic patients are asked to pantomime, they often use a body part as the tool. For example, when patients with IMA are asked to pantomime using a pair of scissors, they may use their fingers as if they were the blades. Many normal subjects may make a similar error; therefore, it is imperative that the patient be instructed not to use a body part as a tool. Patients with IMA may continue to make errors using body parts as tools in spite of these instructions. Patients with IMA will often fail to position their hands as if they were holding the tool or object they were requested to pantomime.

When normal subjects are asked to use a tool, they will orient that tool to the target of that tool action (whether real or imaginary). Patients with IMA often fail to orient their forelimbs to a real or imaginary target. For example, when asked to pantomime cutting a piece of paper in half with a scissor, rather than keeping the scissors oriented in the sagittal plane, the patient may orient the scissors laterally.[5]

When making spatial movement or trajectory errors, patients with IMA will often make the correct core movement (e.g., twisting, pounding, cutting) but will not move their limb correctly through space.[5,7] These spatial trajectory errors are associated with incorrect joint movements such that frequently the apraxic patients will stabilize a joint that should be moving and move joints that should be stabilized. For example, in pantomiming the use of a screwdriver, the patient with IMA may rotate his arm at the shoulder joint and fix his elbow. Shoulder rotation moves the hand in circles rather than rotating the hand on a fixed axis. When multiple joint movements must be coordinated, the patient may be unable to coordinate the movement to get the desired spatial trajectory. For example, in pantomiming the sawing of wood, the shoulder and elbow joints must be alternatively flexed and extended. When the joint movements are not well coordinated, the patient may make primarily chopping or stabbing movements.

Poizner and colleagues[7] have noted that patients with IMA may make timing errors, including a long delay before initiating a movement and brief multiple stops (stuttering movements). Patients with IMA often do not demonstrate a smooth sinusoidal hand speed when they perform cyclic movements, such as cutting with a knife.

Pathophysiology

Whereas in right-handed individuals, IMA is almost always associated with left-hemisphere lesions, in left-handers IMA is usually associated with right-hemisphere lesions. Ideomotor apraxia can be induced by lesions in a variety of structures, including the corpus callosum, the inferior parietal lobe, and the supplementary motor area. IMA has also been reported with subcortical lesions that involve basal ganglia and white matter. Below, each of these anatomic areas is discussed and an attempt is made to develop a model of how the brain mediates learned skilled motor activity of the limbs.

Corpus Callosum In 1907 Liepmann and Maas[8] described a patient with a right hemiparesis from a lesion of the pons and a lesion of the corpus callosum. This patient was unable to pantomime correctly to command with his left arm. Because this patient had a right hemiparesis, his right hand

could not be tested. Since the work of Broca and Wernicke, we have known that right-handers' left hemisphere is dominant for language. Liepmann and Maas could have attributed their patient's inability to pantomime to a disconnection between language and motor areas, such that the left hemisphere, which mediates comprehension of the verbal command, could not influence the right hemisphere, which is responsible for controlling the left hand. However, this patient could also not imitate gestures or use actual objects correctly, and language-motor disconnection could not account for these findings. Liepmann and Maas therefore posited that the left hemisphere of right-handers contains movement formulas (or spatiotemporal representations of movements) and that the callosal lesion disconnects these movement formulas from the motor areas of the right hemisphere.

Geschwind and Kaplan[9] and Gazzaniga and coworkers[10] found that their patients with callosal disconnection, unlike the callosal patient of Liepmann and Maas, could not correctly pantomime to command with the left hand but could imitate and correctly use actual objects with this hand, suggesting that the apraxia of callosal disconnection in these patients was induced by a language-motor disconnection. In addition, many of the errors made by the patient of Liepmann and Maas appeared to be content errors. However, Watson and Heilman[11] described a patient with an infarction of the body of the corpus callosum. The patient reported by Watson and Heilman had no weakness in her right hand and performed all tasks flawlessly with that hand; with her left hand, however, she could not correctly pantomime to command, imitate, or use actual objects. Although early in her course she made content errors, she subsequently made spatial and temporal errors. Her performance indicated that not only language but also movement representations were stored in the left hemisphere and her callosal lesion disconnected these movement formulas from the right hemisphere.

Inferior Parietal Lobe Whereas Geschwind[1] proposed that the ideomotor apraxia associated with left-sided parietal lesions was inducing a language motor disconnection, Heilman and colleagues[12] and Rothi and coworkers[13] proposed that the movement representations or movement formulas were stored in the left parietal lobe of right-handers and that destruction of the left parietal lobe should induce not only a production deficit (apraxia) but also a gesture comprehension/discrimination disorder. Apraxia induced by premotor lesions, lesions of the pathways that connect premotor areas to motor areas, or the pathways that lead to the premotor areas from the parietal lobe may also cause a production deficit. In contrast to parietal lesions, however, these lesions should not induce gesture comprehension/discrimination disorders. Heilman and colleagues[12] and Rothi and associates[13] tested patients with anterior and posterior lesions and found that while both groups were apraxic, the patients with a damaged parietal lobe had comprehension-discrimination disturbances and those with more anterior lesions did not.

Liepmann proposed that handedness was related to the hemispheric laterality of the movement representation. It is not unusual, however, to see right-handed patients with left-hemisphere lesions who are not apraxic. Although it is possible that these patients' lesions did not destroy a critical left-hemisphere area, it is also possible that not all right-handers have movement formulas entirely represented in their left hemisphere. Some people may have either bilateral movement representations or even right-hemisphere representations. Apraxia from a right-hemisphere lesion in a right-hander is rare but has been reported, suggesting that hand preference is not entirely determined by the laterality of the movement representations and may be multifactorial. Whereas the laterality of the movement formula may be the most important factor, there are other factors including primary motor factors such as strength, speed, precision, attentional factors, and even environmental factors.

Supplementary Motor Area Muscles move joints, and motor nerves from the spinal cord activate these muscles. The motor nerves are activated by corticospinal neurons. The corticospinal tract neurons are, in turn, activated by the premotor areas.

For each specific skilled movement there is a set of spatial loci that must be traversed in a specific temporal pattern. We proposed that movement formulas that are represented in the inferior parietal lobe are stored in a three-dimensional supramodal code. Although Geschwind[1] thought that the convexity premotor cortex was important for praxis, apraxia has not been reported from a lesion limited to this cortex, and its function in the control of praxis remains unknown. The convexity premotor cortex may be important in motor learning or in adapting the program to environmental pertubations.

The medial premotor cortex or supplementary motor area (SMA), however, appears to play an important role in mediating skilled movements. Whereas electrical stimulation of the primary motor cortex induces simple movements, SMA stimulation induces complex movements of the fingers, arms, and hands. The SMA receives projections from parietal neurons and projects to motor neurons. The SMA neurons appear to discharge before neurons in the primary motor cortex. Studies of cerebral blood flow, an indicator of cerebral metabolism, have revealed that a single repetitive movement increases activation of the contralateral motor cortex, but complex movements increase flow in the contralateral motor cortex and bilaterally in the SMA. When subjects remain still and think about making complex movements, blood flow to the SMA but not to the motor cortex is increased. Watson and coworkers[14] reported several patients with left-sided medial frontal lesions that included the SMA who demonstrated an ideomotor apraxia when tested with either arm. Unlike patients with parietal lesions, these patients could both comprehend and discriminate pantomimes.

The model we have discussed so far is illustrated in Fig. 16-1. The praxicon is a theoretical store of the temporospatial representations of learned skill movements. When a skilled act is being performed, these representations are transcoded into innervatory patterns by the SMA.

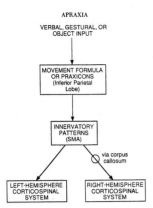

Figure 16-1
Diagrammatic model of ideomotor apraxia. SMA = supplementary motor area. (From Heilman and Rothi,[20] with permission.)

When the right-hand acts, the SMA programs the motor cortex (Brodmann's area 4) of the left hemisphere, and when the left hand acts, these innervatory patterns activate the motor regions of the right hemisphere via the corpus callosum.

DISASSOCIATION APRAXIAS

Clinical Findings

Heilman[15] described several patients who, when asked to pantomime to command, looked at their open hands or would slowly pronate and supinate their arms and hands but would not perform any recognizable action. Unlike the patients with ideomotor apraxia described above, these patients' imitations and use of objects were flawless. DeRenzi and colleagues[16] reported patients similar to those reported by Heilman[15] and also other patients who had a similar defect in other modalities. For example, when asked to pantomime in response to visual or tactile stimuli, they may have been unable to do so, but they could pantomime to verbal command.

Pathophysiology

While callosal lesions may be associated with an ideomotor apraxia, callosal disconnection may also cause disassociation apraxia. The subjects of

Gazzaniga and associates and the patients described by Geschwind and Kaplan had disassociation apraxia. Whereas language in these patients was mediated by the left hemisphere, we posit that movement representations may have been bilaterally represented, and a callosal lesion induced a disassociation apraxia only of the left hand. Whereas the patient with callosal disassociation apraxia will not be able to correctly carry out skilled learned movements of the left arm to command, he or she will be able to imitate and use actual objects with the left hand. Patients with callosal disassociation apraxia will be unable to carry out movements to verbal command because the movement formulas in the right hemisphere have been disconnected from the left hemisphere, which mediates language. The patient with bilateral movement representation can imitate and use actual objects flawlessly with the left hand because these tasks do not require language and the patient's right hemisphere contains the movement formula and the other apparatus needed to transcode the time-space movement representations to motor acts.

Right-handed patients who have both language and movement formula represented in their left hemisphere may show a combination of disassociation and ideomotor apraxia with callosal lesions.[11] When asked to pantomime with their left hands, they may look at them and perform no recognizable movement (disassociation apraxia); but when imitating or using actual objects, they may demonstrate the spatial and temporal errors seen with ideomotor apraxia.

Left-handers may demonstrate an ideomotor apraxia with aphasia from a right-hemisphere lesion. These left-handers are apraxic because their movement representations were stored in their right hemispheres and their lesions destroyed these representations.[17,18] These left-handers were not aphasic because language was mediated by their left hemispheres (as is the case in the majority of left-handers). If these left-handers had a callosal lesion, they may have demonstrated a disassociation apraxia of the left arm and an ideomotor apraxia of the right arm.

The disassociation apraxia described by

Heilman[15] from left-hemisphere lesions was unfortunately incorrectly termed "ideational apraxia." The patients reported by Heilman[15] and those of DeRenzi and associates[16] probably have an intrahemispheric language-movement formula, visual-movement formula, or somesthetic-movement formula disassociation. The locations of the lesions that cause these intrahemispheric disassociation apraxias are not known.

CONDUCTION APRAXIA

Clinical Findings

Ochipa and coworkers[19] reported a patient who, unlike patients with ideomotor apraxia who usually improve with imitation, was more impaired when imitating than when pantomiming to command.

Pathophysiology

Because this patient with conduction apraxia could comprehend the examiner's pantomime and gestures, we believe that the patient's visual system could access the movement representations, or what we have termed praxicons,[20] and that the activated movement representations could activate semantics. It is possible that decoding a gesture requires accessing different movement representations than does programming an action. Therefore, Ochipa and colleagues[19] and Rothi and coworkers[21] suggested that there may be two different stores of movement representations, an input praxicon and output praxicon. In the verbal domain, a disconnection of the hypothetical input and output lexicons induces conduction aphasia; in the praxis domain, a disconnection between the input and output praxicons could induce conduction apraxia.

Whereas the lesions that induce conduction aphasia are usually in the supramarginal gyrus or Wernicke's area, the location of lesions that induce conduction apraxia are unknown.

IDEATIONAL APRAXIA

Unfortunately, there has been much confusion about the meaning of the term *ideational apraxia.* The inability to carry out a series of acts, an ideational plan, has been called ideational apraxia.[22,23] In performing a task that requires a series of acts, these patients have difficulty sequencing the acts in the proper order (for example, instead of cleaning the pipe, putting tobacco in the bowl, lighting the tobacco, and smoking, the patient might attempt to light the empty bowl, put the tobacco in the bowl, and then clean it). Pick[23] noted that most of the patients with this type of ideational apraxia have a dementing disease.

Whereas most patients with ideational apraxia improve when they are using objects. DeRenzi and colleagues[24] reported patients who made errors with the use of actual objects. Although the inability to use actual objects may be associated with a conceptual disorder, a severe production disorder may also impair object use.[25] However, as we will discuss in the next section, production and conceptual disorders may be associated with different types of errors.

CONCEPTUAL APRAXIA

Clinical Findings

To perform a skilled act, two types of knowledge are needed: conceptual knowledge and production knowledge. Dysfunction of the praxis production system induces ideomotor apraxia. Defects in the knowledge needed to successfully select and use the tools and objects we term conceptual apraxia. Whereas patients with ideomotor apraxia make production errrors (e.g., spatial and temporal errors), patients with conceptual apraxia make content and tool-selection errors. The patients with conceptual apraxia may not recall the types of actions associated with specific tools, utensils, or objects (tool-object action knowledge) and therefore make content errrors.[26,27] For example, when asked to demonstrate the use of a screwdriver, either pantomining or using the tool, the patient with the loss of tool-object action knowledge may pantomime a hammering movement or use the screwdrivers as if it were a hammer.

The patient with ideomotor apraxia may make production errors by moving the hand in circles rather than twisting the hand on its own axis. Although such patients make production errors by moving the hand in circles, they are demonstrating knowledge of the turning action of screwdrivers. Content errors (i.e., using a tool as if it were another tool) can also be induced by an object agnosia. However, Ochipa and associates[27] reported a patient who could name tools (and therefore was not agnosic) but often used them inappropriately.

Patients with conceptual apraxia may be unable to recall which specific tool is associated with a specific object (tool–object association knowledge). For example, when shown a partially driven nail, they may select a screwdriver rather than a hammer from an array of tools. This conceptual defect may also be in the verbal domain, such that when an actual tool is shown to a patient with conceptual apraxia, the patient may be able to name it (e.g., hammer); but when the patient is asked to or point to a tool when its function is discussed, he or she cannot. The patient may also be unable to describe the functions of tools.

Patients with conceptual apraxia may also have impaired mechanical knowledge. For example, if they are attempting to drive a nail into a piece of wood and there is no hammer available, they may select a screwdriver rather than a wrench or pliers (which are hard, heavy, and good for pounding).[28] Mechanical knowledge is also important for tool development, and patients with ideational apraxia may be unable to develop tools correctly.[28]

Pathophysiology

Liepmann[3] thought that conceptual knowledge was located in the caudal parietal lobe, and DeRenzi and Luccelli[26] placed it in the temporoparietal junction. The patient reported by Ochipa and coworkers[27] was left-handed and rendered conceptually apraxic by a lesion in the right hemisphere, suggesting that both production and conceptual knowledge have lateralized representations and that such representations are contralateral to the preferred hand. Further evidence that these conceptual representations are lateralized contralateral to the preferred hand comes from the observation of a patient who had a callosal disconnection and demonstrated conceptual apraxia of the nonpreferred (left) hand.[11] However, conceptual apraxia is perhaps most commonly seen in degenerative dementia of the Alzheimer type.[28] Ochipa and colleagues also noted that the severity of conceptual and ideomotor apraxia did not always correlate. The observation that patients with ideomotor apraxia may not demonstrate conceptual apraxia and patients with conceptual apraxia may not demonstrate ideomotor apraxia provides support for the postulate that the praxis production and praxis conceptual systems are independent. However, for normal function, these two systems must interact.

CONCLUSIONS

On the basis of material discussed in this chapter, it appears that movement representations (praxicons) are stored in the left inferior parietal lobe of right-handers. These representations code the spatial and temporal patterns of learned skilled movements. Injury to the parietal lobe induces a production deficit termed ideomotor apraxia. Patients with ideomotor apraxia make spatial and temporal errors. Patients with injury to these representations are not only impaired at pantomiming, imitating, and using actual objects but also cannot discriminate between well- and poorly performed gestures. These patients may also not be able to comprehend gestures.

There are patients who are more impaired at imitation of gestures than they are when gesturing to command (conduction apraxia), suggesting that movement representations (praxicons) may be divided into input and output subdivisions. In conduction apraxia, there is a dissociation between these input and output praxicons.

In order to perform learned skilled acts, these abstract movement representations have to be transcoded into motor programs. This transcoding appears to be performed by a premotor (supplementary motor area)–basal ganglia (putamen-globus pallidus-thalamus) system. Injuries to the brain that interrupt the connections between the movement representations stored in the parietal lobe and the portions of the brain that develop the innervatory patterns or the parts of the brain that allow the innervatory patterns to gain access to the motor system may also produce a praxis production deficit (ideomotor apraxia).

A patient may have intact representations of learned skilled movements but have modality-specific deficits in accessing these representations. For example, a patient with dissociation apraxia may be unable to pantomime to command but be able to pantomime correctly when seeing the tool.

Last, some patients, when pantomiming or using actual tools, may make content errors. Whereas spatial and temporal errors are related to deficits in the praxic production system, content errors are related to deficits in a hypothetical praxis conceptual system or action semantics. Dysfunction of this system, termed conceptual apraxia, may produce deficits of associative knowledge, such as tool-action or tool-object knowledge (i.e., knowing that a hammer is used to pound and that a hammer is associated with a nail). Defects in action semantics may also be associated with deficits in mechanical knowledge (i.e., knowing how to use alternative tools and how to fabricate tools).

REFERENCES

1. Geschwind N: Disconnection syndromes in animals and man. *Brain* 88:237–294, 585–644, 1965.
2. Rothi LJG, Mack L, Heilman KM: Unawareness of apraxic errors. *Neurology* 40(suppl 1):202, 1990.
3. Liepmann H: Apraxia. *Erbgn Ges Med* 1:516–543, 1920.
4. Lawrence DG, Kuypers HGJM: The functional organization of the motor system in the monkey. *Brain* 91:1–36, 1968.
5. Rothi LJG, Mack L, Verfaellie M, et al: Ideomotor apraxia: Error pattern analysis. *Aphasiology* 2:381–387, 1988.
6. Goodglass H, Kaplan E: Disturbance of gesture and pantomime in aphasia. *Brain* 86:703–720, 1963.
7. Poizner H, Mack L, Verfaellie M, et al: Three dimensional computer graphic analysis of apraxia. *Brain* 113:85–101, 1990.
8. Liepmann H, Mass O: Fall von linksseitiger Agraphie und Apraxie bei rechsseitiger Lahmung. *Z Psychol Neurol* 10:214–227, 1907.
9. Geschwind N, Kaplan E: A human cerebral disconnection syndrome. *Neurology* 12:675–685, 1962.
10. Gazzaniga M, Bogen J, Sperry R: Dyspraxia following diversion of the cerebral commisures. *Arch Neurol* 16:606–612, 1967.
11. Watson RT, Heilman KM: Callosal apraxia. *Brain* 106:391–403, 1983.
12. Heilman KM, Rothi LJ, Valenstein E: Two forms of ideomotor apraxia. *Neurology* 32:342–346, 1982.
13. Rothi LJG, Heilman KM, Watson RT: Pantomime comprehension and ideomotor apraxia. *J Neurol Neurosurg Psychiatry* 48:207–210, 1985.
14. Watson RT, Fleet WS, Rothi LJG, Heilman KM: Apraxia and the supplementary motor area. *Arch Neurol* 43:787–792, 1986.
15. Heilman KM: Ideational apraxia—A re-definition. *Brain* 96:861–864, 1973.
16. DeRenzi E, Faglioni P, Sorgato P: Modality-specific and supramodal mechanisms of apraxia. *Brain* 105:301–312, 1982.
17. Heilman KM, Coyle JM, Gonyea EF, Geschwind N: Apraxia and agraphia in a left-hander. *Brain* 96:21–28, 1973.
18. Valenstein E, Heilman KM: Apraxic agraphia with neglect induced paragraphia. *Arch Neurol* 36:506–508, 1979.
19. Ochipa C, Rothi LJG, Heilman KM: Conduction apraxia. *J Clin Exp Neuropsychol* 12:89, 1990.
20. Heilman KM, Rothi LJG: Apraxia, in Heilman KM, Valenstein E (eds): *Clinical Neuropsychology*, 3d ed. New York: Oxford University Press, 1993.
21. Rothi LJG, Ochipa C, Heilman KM: A cognitive neuropsychological model of limb praxis. *Cogn Neuropsychol* 8:443–458, 1991.
22. Marcuse H: Apraktiscke Symotome bein linem Fall von seniler Demenz. *Zentralbl Mervheik Psychiatr* 27:737–751, 1904.
23. Pick A: *Studien über Motorische Apraxia und ihre Mahestenhende Erscheinungen.* Leipzig: Deuticke, 1905.
24. DeRenzi E, Pieczuro A, Vignolo L: Ideational

apraxia: A quantitative study. *Neuropsychologia* 6:41–52, 1968.

25. Zangwell OL: L'apraxie ideatorie. *Nerve Neurol* 106:595–603, 1960.

26. DeRenzi E, Lucchelli F: Ideational apraxia. *Brain* 113:1173–1188, 1988.

27. Ochipa C, Rothi LJG, Heilman KM: Ideational apraxia: A deficit in tool selection and use. *Ann Neurol* 25:190–193, 1989.

28. Ochipa C, Rothi LJG, Heilman KM: Conceptual apraxia in Alzheimer's disease. *Brain* 115:1061–1071, 1992.

Part 3

DISORDERS OF PERCEPTION, ATTENTION, AND AWARENESS

Chapter 17

VISUAL OBJECT AGNOSIA

Martha J. Farah
Todd E. Feinberg

The term *visual object agnosia* refers to the impairment of object recognition in the presence of relatively intact elementary visual perception, memory, and general intellectual function. This chapter reviews the different subtypes of agnosia, their major clinical features and associated neuropathology, and their implications for cognitive neuroscience theories of visual object recognition.

The study of agnosia has a long history of controversy, with some authors doubting that the condition even exists. For example, Bay[1] suggested that the appearance of disproportionate difficulty with visual object recognition could invariably be explained by synergistic interactions between mild perceptual impairments on the one hand and mild general intellectual impairments on the other. The rarity of visual object agnosia has contributed to the slowness with which this issue has been resolved, but several decades of careful case studies have now shown, to most people's satisfaction, that agnosic patients may be no more impaired in their elementary visual capabilities and their general intellectual functioning than many patients who are not agnosic. Therefore, most current research on agnosia focuses on a new set of questions. Are there different types of visual object agnosia, corresponding to different underlying impairments? At what level of visual and/or mnestic processing do these impairments occur? What can agnosia tell us about normal object recognition? What brain regions are critically involved in visual object recognition?

APPERCEPTIVE AGNOSIA

Lissauer[2] reasoned that visual object recognition could be disrupted in two different ways: by impairing visual perception, in which case patients would be unable to recognize objects because they could not see them properly, and by impairing the process of associating a percept with its meaning, in which case patients would be unable to recognize objects because they could not use the percept to access their knowledge of the object. He termed the first kind of agnosia *apperceptive agnosia* and the second kind *associative agnosia*. This terminology is still used today to distinguish agnosic patients who have frank perceptual impairments from those who do not, although the implicit assumption that the latter have an impairment in "association" is now questioned.

Behavior and Anatomy

One might wonder whether apperceptive agnosics should be considered agnosics at all, given that the definition of agnosia cited at the beginning of this article excludes patients whose problems are caused by elementary visual impairments. The difference between apperceptive agnosics and patients who fall outside of the exclusionary criteria for agnosia is that the former have relatively good acuity, brightness discrimination, color vision, and other so-called elementary visual capabilities. Despite these capabilities, their perception of shape is markedly abnormal. For example, in the classic case of Benson and Greenberg,[3] pictures, letters, and even simple geometric shapes could not be recognized. Figure 17-1 shows the attempts of their patient to copy a column of simple shapes. Recognition of real objects may be somewhat better than recognition of geometric shapes, although this appears to be due to the availability of cues such as size and surface properties such as color, texture, and specularity rather than object shape. Facilitation of shape perception by motion of the stimulus has been noted in several cases of apperceptive agnosia. In most cases of apperceptive agnosia, the brain damage is diffuse, often caused by carbon monoxide poisoning. For a review of other cases of apperceptive visual agnosia, see Ref. 4.

Figure 17-1

The attempts of an apperceptive agnosic patient to copy simple shapes. (From Benson and Greenberg,[3] with permission.)

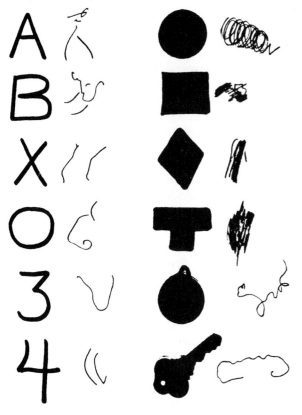

Interpretation of Apperceptive Agnosia

One way of interpreting apperceptive agnosia is in terms of a disorder of grouping processes that normally operate over the array of local features representing contour, color, depth, and so on.[4] Outside of their field defects, apperceptive agnosics have surprisingly good perception of local visual properties. They fail when they must extract more global structure from the image. Motion is helpful because it provides another cue to global structure in the form of correlated local motions. The perception of structure from motion may also have different neural substrates from static contour,[5] and may therefore be spared in apperceptive agnosia.

Relation to Other Disorders

Some authors have used the term *apperceptive agnosia* for other, quite different types of visual disorders, including two forms of simultanagnosia and an impairment in recognizing objects from unusual views or under unusual lighting conditions. *Simultanagnosia* is a term used to describe an impairment in perception of multielement or multipart visual displays. When shown a complex picture with multiple objects or people, simultanagnostics typically describe them in a piecemeal manner, sometimes omitting much of the material entirely and therefore failing to interpret the overall nature of the scene being depicted.

Dorsal simultanagnosia is a component of Balint's syndrome (see Chap. 26), in which an attentional limitation prevents perception of more than one object at a time.[4,6–8] Occasionally attention may be captured by just one part of an object, leading to misidentification of the object and the appearance of perception confined to relatively local image features. The similarity of dorsal simultanagnosia to apperceptive agnosia is limited, however. Once they can attend to an object, dorsal simultanagnosics recognize it quickly and accurately, and even their "local" errors encompass much more global shape information than is available to apperceptive agnosics. Their lesions are typically in the posterior parietal cortex bilaterally.

Despite some surface similarity to apperceptive agnosia and dorsal simultanagnosia, *ventral simultanagnosia* represents yet another disorder.[9] Ventral simultanagnosics can recognize whole objects, but are limited in how many objects can be recognized in a given period of time. Their descriptions of complex scenes are slow and piecemeal, but unlike apperceptive agnosics their recognition of single shapes is not obviously impaired. The impairment of ventral simultanagnosics is most apparent when reading, because the individual letters of words are recognized in an abnormally slow and generally serial manner (letter-by-letter reading, see Chap. 13). Unlike the case with dorsal simultanagnosics, their detection of multiple stimuli appears normal; the bottleneck is in recognition per se. Unlike apperceptive agnosics, they perceive individual shapes reasonably well. Their lesions are typically in the left inferior temporooccipital cortex.

Some patients have roughly normal perception and recognition of objects except when viewed from unusual perspectives or under unusual lighting. Their impairment has also been grouped with apperceptive agnosia by some, but for clarity's sake can also be called *perceptual categorization deficit* because they cannot categorize together the full range of images cast by an object under different viewing conditions. This disorder does not have great localizing value, although the lesions are generally in the right hemisphere and frequently include the inferior parietal lobe.[10]

ASSOCIATIVE AGNOSIA

Behavior and Anatomy

In associative agnosia, visual perception is much better than in apperceptive agnosia. Compare, for example, the copies made by the associative agnosics shown in Figs. 17-2 and 17-3 with the copies shown in Fig. 17-1. Nevertheless, object recognition is impaired. Associative agnosic patients may be able to recognize an object by its feel in their hand or from a spoken definition, demonstrating that they have intact general knowledge of the object in addition to being able to see it well enough to copy it, but they cannot recognize the

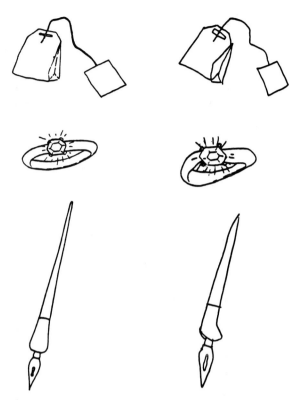

Figure 17-2
The copies of an associative agnosic patient with prosopagnosia and object agnosia. The patient did not recognize any of the original drawings. (From Farah et al.,[27] with permission.)

same object by sight alone. The impairment is not simply a naming deficit for visual stimuli; associative agnosics cannot indicate their recognition of objects by nonverbal means, as by pantomiming the use of an object or by grouping together dissimilar-looking objects from the same semantic category[11–16] (see Ref. 4 for a review of representative cases).

The scope of the recognition impairment varies from case to case of associative agnosia. Some patients encounter difficulty mainly with face recognition (see Chap. 18), while others demonstrate better face recognition than object recognition. Printed-word recognition is similarly impaired in some cases but not others. The selectivity of these impairments suggests that there is more than

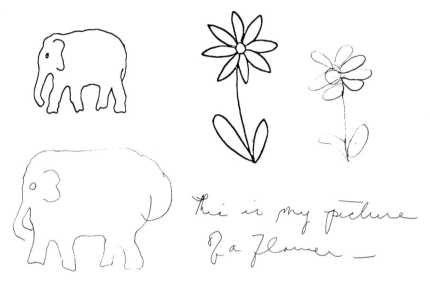

Figure 17-3
The copies of associative visual agnosic patients with alexia and object agnosia. The patients did not recognize the original drawings. Also shown is a sample of a patient's writing to dictation. After a delay, her own handwriting could not be read. (From Feinberg et al.,[16] with permission.)

one system involved in visual recognition. According to one analysis,[17] there are two underlying forms of visual representation, one of which is required for face recognition, used for object recognition but not for word recognition, and the other of which is required for word recognition, used for object recognition and not required for face recognition. Indeed, if one regards associative agnosia as a single undifferentiated category, it is difficult to make any generalizations about the brain regions responsible for visual object recognition. Although the intrahemispheric location of damage is generally occipitotemporal, involving both gray and white matter, cases of associative agnosia have been reported following unilateral right-hemispheric lesions,[18] unilateral left-hemispheric lesions,[15,16,19,20] and bilateral lesions.[21–23] However, if one considers impairments in face and word recognition as markers for different underlying forms of visual recognition disorder, then a pattern emerges in the neuropathology. When face recognition alone is impaired or when face and object recognition are impaired but reading is spared, the lesions are generally either on the right or bilateral. De Renzi has proposed that the degree of right-hemispheric specialization for face recognition may normally cover a wide range, such that most cases of prosopagnosia become manifest

only after bilateral lesions, but in some cases a unilateral lesion will suffice (see Chap. 18). When reading alone is impaired or when reading and object recognition are impaired but face recognition is spared, the lesions are generally on the left. In a series of patients studied by us and additional cases of agnosia sparing face recognition culled from the literature, the maximum overlap in lesion locus was in the left inferior medial region involving parahippocampal, fusiform, and lingual gyri.[16] When recognition of faces, objects, and words is impaired, the lesions are generally bilateral.

Interpreting Associative Agnosia

Is associative agnosia a problem with perception, memory, or both? Associative agnosia has been explained in three different ways that suggest different answers to this question. The simplest way to explain agnosia is by a disconnection between visual representations and other brain centers responsible for language or memory. For example, Geschwind[24] proposed that associative agnosia is a visual-verbal disconnection. This hypothesis accounts well for agnosics' impaired naming of visual stimuli, but it cannot account for their inability to convey recognition nonverbally and may therefore be more suited to explaining *optic aphasia*, a form of anomia limited to impaired naming of visual stimuli (see Chap. 37). Associative agnosia has also been explained as a disconnection between visual representations and medial temporal memory centers.[23] However, this would account for a modality-specific impairment in new learning, not the inability to access old knowledge through vision.

The inadequacies of the disconnection accounts lead us to consider theories of associative agnosia in which some component of perception and/or memory has been damaged. Perhaps the most widely accepted account of associative agnosia is that stored visual memory representations have been damaged. According to this type of account, stimuli can be processed perceptually up to some end-state visual representation, which would normally be matched against stored visual representations. In associative agnosia, the stored representations are no longer available and recognition therefore fails. Note that an assumption of this account is that two identical tokens of the object representation normally exist, one derived from the stimulus and one stored in memory, and that these are compared in the same way as a database might be searched in a present-day computer. This account is not directly disconfirmed by any of the available evidence. However, there are some reasons to question it and to suspect that subtle impairments in perception may underlie associative agnosia.

Although the good copies and successful matching performance of associative agnosics might seem to exonerate perception, a closer look at the manner in which these tasks are accomplished suggests that perception is not normal in associative agnosia and suggests yet a third explanation of associative agnosia. Typically, these patients are described as copying drawings "slavishly"[25] and "line by line."[26] In matching tasks, they rely on slow, sequential feature-by-feature checking. It therefore may be premature to rule out faulty perception as the cause of associative agnosia. Recent studies of the visual capabilities of associative agnosic patients confirm that there are subtle visual perceptual impairments present in all cases studied.[4] If the possibility of impaired

recognition with intact perception is consistent with the use of a computational architecture in which separate perceptual and memory representations are compared, then the absence of such a case suggests that a different type of computational architecture may underlie object recognition. Parallel distributed processing (PDP) systems exemplify an alternative architecture in which the perceptual and memory representations cannot be dissociated (see Chap. 8; see also Ref. 4, Chap. 5, for a discussion of PDP models and agnosia). In a PDP system, the memory of the stimulus would consist of a pattern of connection strengths among a number of neuronlike units. The "perceptual" representation resulting from the presentation of a stimulus will depend upon the pattern of connection strengths among the units directly or indirectly activated by the stimulus. Thus, if memory is altered by damaging the network, perception will be altered as well. On this account, associative agnosia is not a result of an impairment to perception *or* to memory; rather, the two are in principle inseparable, and the impairment is better described as a loss of high-level visual perceptual representations that are shaped by, and embody the memory of, visual experience. It will thus be of great interest to see whether future studies of associative agnosics will ever document a case of impaired recognition with intact perception.

Relation to Other Disorders

As with apperceptive agnosia, a number of distinct disorders have been labeled associative agnosia by different authors. Visual modality–specific naming disorders exist and are usually termed *optic aphasia,* but they may on occasion be called *associative visual agnosia. Impairments of semantic memory* (see Chap. 37) will affect object-recognition ability (as well as entirely nonvisual abilities such as verbally defining spoken words) and perhaps for this reason have sometimes been called *associative visual agnosia.*

REFERENCES

1. Bay E: Disturbances of visual perception and their examination. *Brain* 76:515–530, 1952.

2. Lissauer H: Ein Fall von Seelenblindheit nebst einem Beitrage zur Theori derselben. *Arch Psychiatr Nervenkrankh* 21:222–270, 1890.

3. Benson R, Greenberg JP: Visual form agnosia. *Arch Neurol* 20:82–89, 1969.

4. Farah MJ: *Visual Agnosia: Disorders of Object Recognition and What They Tell Us about Normal Vision.* Cambridge, MA: MIT Press, 1990.

5. Marcar VL, Cowey A: The effect of removing superior temporal cortical motion areas in the macaque monkey: II. Motion discrimination using random dot displays. *Eur J Neurosci* 4:1228–1238, 1992.

6. Williams M: *Brain Damage and the Mind.* Baltimore: Penguin Books, 1970.

7. Girotti F, Milanese C, Casazza M, et al: Oculomotor disturbances in Balint's syndrome: Anatomoclinical findings and electrooculographic analysis in a case. *Cortex* 18:603–614, 1982.

8. Tyler A, Gelade G: A feature-integration theory of attention. *Cog Psychol* 12:97–136, 1980.

9. Kinsbourne M, Warrington EK: A disorder of simultaneous form perception. *Brain* 85:461–486, 1962.

10. Warrington EK: Agnosia: The impairment of object recognition, in Vinken PJ, Bruyn GW, Klawans HL (eds): *Handbook of Clinical Neurology.* Amsterdam: Elsevier, 1985.

11. Rubens AB, Benson DF: Associative visual agnosia. *Arch Neurol* 24:305–316, 1971.

12. Bauer RM, Rubens AB: Agnosia, in Heilman KM, Valenstein E (eds): *Clinical Neuropsychology,* 2d ed. New York: Oxford University Press, 1985.

13. Albert ML, Reches A, Silverberg R: Associative visual agnosia without alexia. *Neurology* 25:322–326, 1975.

14. Hécaen H, de Ajuriaguerra J: Agnosie visuelle pour les objets inanimes par lesion unilaterale gauche. *Rev Neurol* 94:222–233, 1956.

15. McCarthy RA, Warrington EK: Visual associative agnosia: A clinico-anatomical study of a single case. *Neurol Neurosurg Psychiatry* 48:1233–1240, 1986.

16. Feinberg TE, Schindler RJ, Ochoa E, et al: Associative visual agnosia and alexia without prosopagnosia. *Cortex* 30:395–412, 1994.

17. Farah MJ: Patterns of co-occurrence among the associative agnosias: Implications for visual object representation. *Cog Neuropsychol* 8:1–19, 1991.

18. Levine DN: Prosopagnosia and visual object agnosia: A behavioral study. *Neuropsychologia* 5:341–365, 1978.

19. Pilon B, Signoret JL, Lhermitte F: Agnosie visuelle associative rôle de l'hemisphere gauche dans la perception visuelle. *Rev Neurol* 137:831–842, 1981.

20. Feinberg TE, Heilman KM, Gonzalez-Rothi L: Multimodal agnosia after unilateral left hemisphere lesion. *Neurology* 36:864–867, 1986.

21. Alexander MP, Albert ML: The anatomical basis of visual agnosia, in Kertesz A (ed): *Localization in Neuropsychology.* New York: Academic Press, 1983.

22. Benson DF, Segarra J, Albert ML: Visual agnosia-prosopagnosia: A clinicopathologic correlation. *Arch Neurol* 30:307–310, 1973.

23. Albert ML, Soffer D, Silverberg R, Reches A: The anatomic basis of visual agnosia. *Neurology* 29:876–879, 1979.

24. Geschwind N: Disconnexion syndromes in animals and man: Part II. *Brain* 88:585–645, 1965.

25. Brown JW: *Aphasia, Apraxia and Agnosia: Clinical and Theoretical Aspects.* Springfield, IL: Charles C Thomas, 1972.

26. Ratcliff G, Newcombe F: Object recognition: Some deductions from the clinical evidence, in Ellis AW (ed): *Normality and Pathology in Cognitive Functions.* New York: Academic Press, 1982.

27. Farah MJ, Hammond K, Levine DN, et al: Visual and spatial mental imagery. *Cog Neuropsychol* 20:439–462, 1988.

Chapter 18

PROSOPAGNOSIA

Ennio De Renzi

Faces represent a class of stimuli that enjoy a special status in the study of visuoperceptual disorders and have been the subject of a number of investigations unparalleled by any other perceptual category. Historically, the main factors calling attention to them have been reports of patients who, following a brain lesion, manifest a deficit of recognition that is unique to familiar faces, or at least disproportionate with respect to other types of stimuli, and that is not accounted for by loss of knowledge about the biographic features of the unidentified people.

The earliest mention of the symptom was made by A. Quaglino,[1] an Italian ophthalmologist, who, in 1867, reported a patient suffering from left hemianopia, achromatopsia, and inability to recognize familiar faces—problems caused by a cerebrovascular accident. The patient's preserved ability to read words printed in very small type convinced the author that elementary visual deficits played no primary role in the patient's impairment. Although Quaglino recognized the cerebral origin of the disorder, the impact of his paper on the scientific community was practically nil. The symptom had to await Bodamer's report[2] in 1947 to be identified as a distinct form of agnosia, deserving a distinctive name (prosopagnosia, from the Greek word *prosopon*, meaning face).

Since the 1940s, more than a hundred case reports[3] have been published, and some patients have been extensively and repeatedly investigated. Yet it was not so much for its clinical frequency that prosopagnosia raised such a marked interest

as for the light it threw on the organization of the visual recognition system.

THE CLINICAL PICTURE

Patients are usually aware of their deficit and complain of it, although a few of them may be reluctant to speak about it because they feel ashamed of being unable to do such a simple thing as recognizing their closest relatives and friends, all the more as the organic nature of the symptom may go unrecognized. In two patients of mine, the ophthalmologist, to whom they had been referred by the family doctor, diagnosed a psychogenic disorder, baffled by their inability to recognize familiar faces in spite of normal acuity, campimetry, and visual object recognition.

Even upon superficial investigation, it is apparent that the failure to recognize people is restricted to the processing of facial features, and that these patients try to compensate for their handicap by relying on nonfacial cues, such as the subject's voice, gait, clothing, and so on. Sometimes they complain of seeing faces distorted or in a dim light, but they never fail to realize that they are looking at a face. With a few exceptions, they can discriminate its gender, race, and approximate age, although finer age estimation may be impaired.[4] Face recognition disorders do not extend to the identification of emotional expressions, which is preserved in the great majority of prosopagnosics, while it may be impaired in patients who do not have problems in recognizing familiar faces,[5] providing evidence that discrete neural structures subserve the two abilities (see later).

RECOGNITION OF FAMILIAR AND UNFAMILIAR FACES

Bodamer thought that the predominant deficit shown by his patients in recognizing faces justified the inference that these stimuli have a special status in the brain. This hypothesis found some support in subsequent studies, which showed that the processing of unknown faces differs from that of other categories of stimuli in being closely related to right hemispheric functioning. This is the kind of material most suitable for bringing out a right hemispheric advantage in recognizing laterally projected nonverbal stimuli. Interestingly, patients with right posterior lesions are more impaired than any other brain-damaged group in tasks requiring them to match to sample photographs of faces taken from different perspectives or in different conditions of illumination.[6–9] It was at first thought[7] that performance on unknown face matching tasks was strictly correlated with that on familiar face recognition and could represent a reliable index of the patient's skills in processing this unique category of stimuli. However, it was soon discovered that in brain-damaged patients, the correlation between familiar and unfamiliar face recognition is zero,[10] and that there are a few prosopagnosic patients who perform the unknown face tests correctly.[11,12] Morover, right brain–damaged patients who do very poorly on these tests yet have no difficulty in recognizing familiar faces. The conclusion drawn by Benton[13] was that there are two types of disorders related to face recognition—one concerning unknown faces, which is basically perceptual, and the other concerning familiar faces, which also entails an amnestic component.

LEVEL OF IMPAIRMENT IN PROSOPAGNOSIA

There have been several attempts to fractionate prosopagnosia according to the functional level at which face recognition is disrupted. A preliminary broad distinction, similar to that proposed by Lissauer[14] for object agnosia, is between apperceptive and associative (or amnestic) prosopagnosia.[15,16] However, this dichotomous classification can be further fractionated, based on the models recently proposed by cognitive psychologists to analyze how the flow of facial information is processed in normals. The most popular of them, elaborated by Bruce and Young,[17] envisages four stages that can be activated in a bottom-up or a top-down direction. The structural encoding stage represents the final product of perceptual analysis and yields a tridimensional, abstract representation of the stimulus, which is independent of the context and the viewpoint from which it is observed. If the face is known, the product of structural encoding is matched with its representation, stored in recognition units, and gives rise to a feeling of familiarity, though not yet permitting its identification. Recognition occurs when the firing of recognition units activates the identity nodes, a part of the semantic system that stores the information relevant to the identification of a person (when and where that person has been encountered, his or her profession, biography, and so on). Identity nodes can also be accessed from nonfacial inputs, such as the person's voice, way of walking, clothes, and so forth, and they have reciprocal connections with the people/name module. Its independence is shown by the dissociation between the ability to recognize a face and the failure to retrieve the corresponding name, occasionally exhibited by normals and, in a more massive way, by a few brain-damaged patients. In some cases the name is unavailable with any cue, verbal or visual (proper name anomia[18]); in others, the difficulty arises only on visual presentation of the face (prosopanomia[19]).

Damage at the level of structural encoding or at even earlier stages of perceptual processing is obviously implicated in cases where the inability to identify familiar faces appears in the context of a more general deficit of visual perception. Severe apperceptive agnosia[20–25] is always accompanied by prosopagnosia. More problematic is the assessment of the relevance of perceptual deficits to prosopagnosia, when the impairment outside the "face" category is apparent only for objects that are visually homogeneous or on tasks that are perceptually demanding, such as matching stimuli taken from different views, identifying incomplete or overlapping figures, discriminating patterns that differ for minimal features, and so on. When, in the sixties, it was found that right brain–damaged patients were impaired in matching photographs of unknown faces taken from different perspectives, the hypothesis was advanced that prosopagnosia represented the extreme end of a continuum of perceptual disorders, particularly evident for faces, because their physical similarity makes them hard to differentiate. However, as already mentioned, some prosopagnosics perform correctly these tests, possibly because their deficit is mainly amnestic. Also, the score on other tests of perception of facial features and facial configuration may not be predictive of familiar face recognition.[26] There have been attempts to ground the specificity of the patient's perceptual impairment on firmer evidence. Sergent and coworkers[27,28] proposed a sophisticated method to estimate the patient's ability to perform the configurational operations whereby facial features are processed in an interactive manner. De Renzi and coworkers[15] measured, in 100 normal subjects, the difference between the standardized scores of two-face perceptual tests and two-face memory tests and computed the internal and external tolerance limits of the difference in score distribution. These norms make it possible to identify prosopagnosics who are outliers either for an exceedingly poor performance on perceptual tests (apperceptive prosopagnosia), or for an exceedingly poor performance on memory tests (associative prosopagnosia). The question remains whether these measures also differentiate prosopagnosics from right brain–damaged patients who are not impaired in recognizing faces. McNeil and Warrington[26] have warned that scores on tests of facial features and facial configuration may not be predictive of familiar face recognition.

When the impairment of perceptual processing does not account for the inability to recognize familiar faces, a face-specific amnestic deficit must be considered. The identification of the stage at which the recognition process fails rests on performance on tests of familiarity (point to the one face in an array that is known; no recognition is required), of visual-verbal matching (point to the face named by the examiner), and of visual and verbal naming. Instead of the proper name, the knowledge of other semantic features (profession, nationality, and so on) can be required. Visual knowledge must be compared with knowledge elicited by the verbal presentation of information (name or some other qualifying feature) pointing to the same person. Prosopagnosics respond competently to verbal questions and can, therefore, be easily differentiated from patients who do not recognize familiar persons because they suffer from an amnesia specific for people[29–31] and are unable to retrieve information concerning them, no matter whether it is requested through the presentation of a face, name, or voice. The impairment may extend to knowledge about exemplars of other categories that have become famous in their individuality—for example, famous animals (Lassie), buildings (the Kremlin), or products that were much advertised in the past.[29]

Damage to identity nodes without involvement of recognition units should be manifest by the ability to perform familiarity tests, but there is just one case where a dissociation between sense of familiarity and recognition has been found.[32] All other patients fail on both types of tests. Further information on the level of impairment can be drawn from the study of nonconscious recognition.

NONCONSCIOUS FACE RECOGNITION

A fascinating phenomenon that has been pointed out in different neuropsychological domains, from blindsight to amnesia, neglect, and alexia, is the dissociation between what the patients overtly know about a stimulus and the implicit knowledge the patient manifests, through changes in behavior, in response to its presentation. The same holds in prosopagnosia, where patients who deny recognizing a face show a different pattern of physiologic or psychological responses depending on whether the face is familiar or unfamiliar. Among physiological procedures, positive findings have been reported with the galvanic skin reaction,[21,33] eye-movement scan paths,[34] and event-related potentials.[35] For instance, patient LF[21] was unable to choose which of five names successively spoken by the examiner corresponded to a famous face, but his skin conductance responses occurred more often and with a higher amplitude to true than to untrue names.

Paradigms based on psychological parameters have used learning and priming tasks, which have shown an advantage of familiar over unfamiliar faces. For instance, prosopagnosics learn to associate a familiar face with a name or a profession more successfully if the pairs are true than if they are untrue.[27,35–37] The effect, however, depended on the nature of the information provided or of the response required, since it vanished when only the first name instead of the full name of the person was given or when knowledge of specific instead of generic semantic information was required (e.g., not simply whether a face was that of a politician or a nonpolitician, but to what political party the person belonged).[38] Covert effects were also demonstrated by the interference exerted on a name-classification task (politicians versus nonpoliticians) by a distractor face, depending on whether it belonged to the same semantic category of the name[39] and by priming of name recognition by face primes.[36] In the one patient, who could be tested with physiologic as well psychological procedures, covert recognition was demonstrated on both.[40]

These findings provide evidence that some knowledge on faces that are not overtly recognized is still retained by some prosopagnosics and, if properly cued, can be activated. Note that unconscious recognition can also be shown when explicit decisions are requested, as in forced-choice tasks. Though the patients maintain that they are simply guessing, they respond faster in matching different views of familiar than of unfamiliar faces,[36] score above chance on a face-name matching test where the name or profession of a famous face must be chosen among alternatives,[26,27,32,37] and are able to pair two faces of

the same famous person across a 30-year age period much better than normal controls who are unfamiliar with that person.[27] Surprisingly, if the same forced-choice paradigm is used to assess familiarity, they score at chance.

An amazing finding, reported by Sergent and Poncet[27] and partially replicated[32,37] is the capacity shown by some prosopagnosic patients, if they are provided with partial information, to progressively attain a stage of transient recognition of faces they were initially unable to identify. When they were told that a set of nonrecognized faces belonged to the same professional category, they suddenly remembered it and then also succeeded in retrieving the associated names. Yet recognition was contingent on the spontaneous pop out of the category, since, no face could be named if the category was not retrieved or when the same exemplars that had been named were later presented intermingled with faces of other categories.

Implicit knowledge of familiar faces is not found in every prosopagnosic. Negative cases[21,28,41–43] are relevant to understanding the functional level of damage. The absence of covert recognition has been interpreted as evidence that recognition units are damaged, while its presence would indicate that they are intact but can only communicate with the identity nodes via an indirect route, which, though being able to alert the semantic system that the face is familiar, is inadequate to transmit the information needed for conscious recognition.[38,44]

Bauer[21] interpreted the overt-covert recognition dissociation in the light of the anatomic model,[45] which envisages two separate pathways for processing visual information—a ventral one linking the visual association cortex with the temporal limbic cortex and transmitting information about "what" the stimulus is and a dorsal one projecting to the superior temporal sulcus and then to the inferior parietal lobule and concerned with "where" the stimulus is. Lesion to the ventral occipitotemporal pathway would cause loss of conscious recognition but leave patent the dorsal occipitoparietal route, which, thanks to its reciprocal connections with the cingulate cortex, can mediate the emotional reaction to the nonrecognized face.

The same interpretation was extended[46] to the manifestations of covert recognition, disclosed by psychological procedures, attributing to the dorsal system the unconscious processing of the information transmitted by the recognition units. This account, however, leaves unanswered the question of what the anatomic connections are that, in a forced-choice paradigm, make it possible to match a face with a name but not to make a familiarity judgment.

An alternative, simpler interpretation of the dissociation between overt and covert recognition is that a sensory percept reaches awareness only if the output from downstream centers attains a given threshold. Subthreshold information is not, however, lost and may be processed by unconscious mechanisms if we assume that they require a lower level of activation. Damage to the recognition units does not necessarily result in an all-or-none response. Depending on the degree of their impairment, they may either cease to fire (in which case covert recognition will also fail), or they may generate a reduced output that is inadequate to activate the identity nodes to the point of conscious recognition but is sufficient to raise their response above chance. In support of this contention, Farah and coworkers[47] built a computer simulation of face recognition that performed a variety of overt and covert tasks. When visual face perception was degraded by lesioning the model, overt recognition was eliminated, yet the model continued to show priming and interference from faces, facilitation in matching familiar faces, and savings in relearning face-name associations. The quality of covert recognition performance in prosopagnosic patients is also consistent with the hypothesis of a damaged, but not obliterated, face recognition system. The improvement patients show when confronted with familiar faces remains, in most cases, below the level found in normal subjects. Wallace and Farah[48] pointed out that normal subjects showed the same dissociation between overt recognition and savings in relearning, when overt recognition was hindered by delaying it over a 6-month period. Recognition units can also receive top-down information from names, and this may increase their activation.[37]

SPECIFICITY OF FACES

A question that has recurred ever since the earliest report of prosopagnosia is whether the deficit is confined to the category of faces or represents but one aspect of an impairment pervading other gnostic domains (although attention is unavoidably focused on the face recognition disorder because of its social implications). On this view, prosopagnosia would correspond to a mild visual agnosia.[49] Authors advocating the latter position have emphasized some features that would make faces particularly prone to disruption by brain damage. One is the great perceptual similarity of their external configuration and internal structure and the consequent need for a fine-grained discrimination system. The second is the high number—on the order of several hundred and even a few thousand—of unique exemplars of faces that must be stored in memory in order to ensure appropriate social relations. No comparison is possible with what happens with other categories of objects, where it is at most necessary that we recognize the individuality of those exemplars we own—it would be embarrassing to mistake one's own car in a parking lot or one's own overcoat on a coat tree—but we can use most objects interchangeably, without any need to retrieve the context in which we first met them and the network of associations that identifies them. This difference is reflected in the way object and face recognition is tested: the former is assessed by requiring the patient to name or provide semantic knowledge of the category to which the target belongs, the latter by requiring the recognition of that particular face.

From these considerations and from the finding that there are prosopagnosic patients who also show difficulty in recognizing the members of other categories (breeds of dogs, buildings, cars, articles of clothing) that, like faces, have great physical similarity, it has been argued[50,51] that the basic deficit of these patients concerns the identification of an exemplar within a class whose members have great perceptual similarity. If we extend the investigation to perceptual domains that share the same features, it will be apparent that the deficit is not specific for faces. For instance, some patients have been reported who were inpaired in recognizing individual animals.[52,53]

However, there are data in the literature that contradict this assumption. Sergent and Signoret[54] had a patient who was particularly suitable to test it, since he was an expert on car makes and models, having made a hobby of collecting miniature cars. When he was presented with 210 photographs of cars, comprising 14 models from 15 makes, he was able to identify 172 of them correctly; and of the remaining 38, he correctly reported the company name for 31 and the model name for 22. Taking advantage of the fact that their patient was skillful in recognizing sheep faces, McNeil and Warrington[44] contrasted his ability to learn to associate sheep and human faces with arbitrary names and found that, differently from normal controls, he was poorer in learning faces than sheep. Farah and coworkers[55] tested the ability of a prosopagnosic to recognize faces and a variety of nonface objects, including a large set of similar-looking eyeglass frames, and found him to be disproportionately impaired with faces relative to normal subjects' performance. De Renzi[56] tested the hypothesis that if a prosopagnosic is asked to identify a specific object, "he will be just as incapable of evoking the history of a familiar object as he will be of evoking the history of a familiar face"[50] by asking his patient to recognize his own belongings when presented with other exemplars of the same class. The patient, who was a typical amnestic prosopagnosic, showed no difficulty in identifying his own electric razor, glasses, wallet, and necktie from among 6 to 10 exemplars of the same category and his own handwriting from among 9 samples of the same sentence written by other persons. The same behavior has been replicated in a second patient[15] and confirmed by Sergent and Signoret.[54] These authors, however, questioned the cogency of the finding, arguing that in these experiments recognition was contingent on the use of a forced-choice paradigm with a limited number of alternatives, a condition not comparable with that of unexpectedly encountering a familiar person and being unable to recognize him or her. In a forced-choice condition, the prosopagnosic patients did show

correct recognition of the photograph of their own faces or of a close relative from among unknown faces when their names were provided. It must be emphasized, however, that when the same task was given using photographs of famous people as targets instead of those of close relatives, both patients failed. These results were not different from what De Renzi and coworkers[15,56] had reported in their patients when they were requested to point to the one face out of four that was familiar or to that whose name was given. Thus the aid provided by forced recognition was confined to a limited number of very familiar faces (no more than two faces were given to one patient and five to another) and may be related to unconscious rather than to conscious recognition, since, as already mentioned above, prosopagnosic patients score above chance on a forced-choice face-name matching test. It can be added that, were it true that a forced-choice paradigm is sufficient to show preserved knowledge in prosopagnosics, all experiments carried out to show covert recognition would be superfluous.

If faces have something special that deserves a separate organization in the brain, what is the psychological and the biological basis of their discrete treatment by the central nervous system? Farah and coworkers[57] have argued that face recognition differs from object recognition because the representation of the former is mainly based on overall structure, which is not parsed in the component parts, while that of the latter relies mostly on a preliminary decomposition into the local defining features. This hypothesis was borne out by a series of experiments that compared the contribution of part and whole representations to the perception of upright and inverted faces and the detrimental effect that masking parts or wholes exerts on the perception of upright and inverted faces, words, and houses. Thus, faces would lie at the end of a continuum, ranging from parts-based representations used for words to whole-based representations used for faces, with objects occupying an intermediate position and sharing either ability, depending on their structure. Farah[3,58] claimed that the different contribution that the holistic and analytic encoding of information make to these three classes of stimuli is borne out by the patterns of association with which the corresponding disorders appear. In its purest form, the disruption of the ability to decompose a stimulus into its parts results in alexia and that of encoding nondecomposed perceptual wholes in prosopagnosia. Object perception shares either encoding mechanism, depending on the features of the stimulus. It follows that there will never be a case of object agnosia without either alexia or prosopagnosia or a case of alexia associated with prosopagnosia in the absence of object agnosia. Support for this contention was found[3] in a review of the literature, but quite recently a case has been reported[59] that questions the former of the two assumptions. It remains, therefore, an open question whether the prevailing patterns of visual recognition impairment pointed out by the literature are indeed evidence of different encoding procedures depending on the nature of the stimulus or whether they reflect the degree of specialization that the left and right hemispheres have in processing and storing words, faces, and objects.

Face specificity also finds support in neurophysiologic data, which show the presence in the inferior temporal cortex and in the cortex of the superior temporal sulcus of cells that discharge selectively in response to the presentation of a face.[60,61] They may have different functional specification. Those in the inferior temporal cortex would be involved in the identification of single exemplars and would, therefore, be germane to the deficit in face recognition found in humans following damage to the same area. Those in the superior temporal sulcus would be sensitive to emotional expressions and to the direction of gaze,[62] a dimension that plays a paramount role in the social communication of monkeys. The superior temporal sulcus has strong connections with the amygdala, whose injury has been found in humans to cause a severe deficit in the comprehension of facial expressions and gaze directions.[63,64] The discrete anatomic organization of the abilities involved in face recognition and in the recognition of facial expressions is borne out by their dissociation produced by pathology. Most patients with prosopagnosia perform emotion-matching tasks

correctly, while the opposite pattern of impairment has been reported in nonprosopagnosic patients.[5] Two cases with selective impairment in naming and pointing to emotional expressions but integrity in understanding the meaning of facial affect have been reported following right temporal lobe damage;[65,66] this has been interpreted as being due to a category-specific bidirectional visuoverbal disconnection between intact visual semantic and verbal semantic representations for facial expressions. The locus of lesion of these patients (right middle temporal gyrus) tallies with the findings of a study[67] where neurons of the right middle temporal gyrus of epileptic patients showed a specific increase of their activity when the patients had to label facial expressions.

ANATOMIC CORRELATES OF PROSOPAGNOSIA

The ascendancy of the right over the left hemisphere in processing faces is beyond question, having been confirmed by many normal and clinical studies. What is a matter of debate is whether this asymmetry of function is so marked as to cause the inability to recognize familiar faces following a lesion confined to the right side or if bilateral damage is necessary to produce this result.

Bodamer[2] was cautious in drawing anatomic inferences from his cases, since they lacked autopsy, but he remarked that both showed evidence of bilateral lesions. Fifteen years later, a review of the available clinical cases[68] emphasized the presence in a substantial proportion of them of left visual field defects, a sign pointing to right brain damage. It was speculated that damage to this side played a crucial role in causing prosopagnosia. Although this paper was very influential in drawing attention to the possible specialization of the right hemisphere in face processing, its relevance to the anatomic basis of prosopagnosia was questioned by a subsequent review focusing on case reports with necroscopy documentation,[69] which pointed out that all of the patients had bilateral damage. New pathologic studies[70,71] corroborated this finding. Although Meadows[69] was cautious in drawing definite conclusions from his review of the literature—since there were also a few patients in whom surgery had shown a disease confined to the right hemisphere and in some bilateral cases the left lesion was located in areas having no relation to the processing of visual information—the view that bilateral damage is a necessary condition for the occurrence of prosopagnosia[50] gained overwhelming consensus. Yet the exceptions to the "bilaterality of damage" rule remarkably increased with the introduction of neuroimaging procedures, which made it possible to localize the lesion in a much greater number of patients. It must be stressed that while this source of information cannot compete with autopsy in terms of accuracy of localization, it has the great advantage of being available in practically every prosopagnosic, not only in those that come to autopsy (which may represent a biased sample) and that is available at the same time testing is carried out. A review of the pertinent literature published up to 1992[72] brought out 27 patients with evidence on computed tomography (CT) or magnetic resonance imaging (MRI)—complemented in 5 cases by positron emission tomography (PET)—of damage restricted to the right hemisphere, plus 3 cases with surgical documentation and 1 following right hemispherectomy. There is now also a case of prosopagnosia in which autopsy has shown an infarct in the territory of the right posterior cerebral artery.[73]

The pendulum is, therefore, shifting again toward the "unilaterality of lesion" thesis, to the effect that damage to the right brain may be sufficient to cause prosopagnosia. It is fair to recognize, however, that the exclusive specialization of this side of the brain for face recognition is far from attaining the same generality the left hemisphere has for language. For instance, in a consecutive series of 10 patients with an infarct of the right posterior cerebral artery, which supplies the occipitotemporal cortex involved in face recognition, none showed prosopagnosia,[72] while alexia was present in 13 consecutive patients out of 16 who had an infarct of the left posterior cerebral artery.[74] A likely inference suggested by these findings is that the degree of hemispheric asymmetry

in face recognition is a dimension showing a wide range of functional variation in humans, such that only a minority of them have these skills preponderantly represented in the right brain.

The most frequent etiology of prosopagnosia is an infarct in the territory of the posterior cerebral artery, which encroaches upon the medial cortex of the occipital and temporal lobes and the inferior longitudinal fasciculus, running in the subjacent white matter. The role played in face recognition by these structures, in particular those of the right hemisphere, finds support in normal studies, showing that some physiologic parameters recorded from these areas are specifically activated by the presentation of familiar as opposed to unfamiliar faces. An enhancement of the late negative component (wave N500) of event-related cerebral potentials associated with familiar faces was recorded from the right occipital lead;[75] a different pattern of visual evoked potentials—recorded by depth electrodes inserted in the amygdala, hippocampus, and the superior and inferior temporal sulcus—is produced by the presentation of familiar and unfamiliar faces, and the difference is more marked on the right.[76] Two PET studies[77,78] agreed in showing a bilateral increase of cerebral blood flow in the striate and extrastriate cortex (lingual and fusiform gyri) when faces were processed as opposed to a resting condition, but they disagreed as to the side that was more activated when the face task involved memory. In one study,[78] changes were more marked in the right lingual, fusiform, and parahippocampal gyri; in the other[77] they were more marked in the left posterior hippocampus, and there was also a significant decrease of blood flow in the left superior temporal gyrus. Further studies are required to solve this contradiction.

CONGENITAL PROSOPAGNOSIA

Two cases with prosopagnosia dating back to early years of age and without evidence of an acquired cerebral disease have been reported.[41,79,80] Interestingly, both had a relative who complained of the same type of difficulty, which points to the genetic nature of the disorder. The first patient was reported by McConachie,[79] when she was 12 years old; she was tested again by De Haan and Campbell[41] 15 years later. Her disorder was prominent in face recognition, but extended to object recognition in only a minor degree, especially in discriminating items that belonged to a category made up of perceptually similar exemplars and in identifying figures seen from an unusual perspective. She was thought to fail at the stage where a fully specified code of a face must be constructed. Temple's[80] patient, on the contrary, was not impaired at the perceptual level and her deficit was specific for faces. It probably concerned the acquisition of stable stored representations. A third patient[43] with prosopagnosia dating back to childhood, when she incurred a meningoencephalitis, had difficulties similar to those of McConachie's[79] patient.

REFERENCES

1. Quaglino A: Empilegia sinistra con amaurosi- Guarigione- Perdita totale della percezione dei colori e della memoria della configurazione degli oggetti. Annotazione alla medesima di GB Borelli. *Giorn Oftalmol Ital* 10:106–117, 1867.

2. Bodamer J: Die Prosopagnosie. *Arch Psychiatr Nervenkrank* 179:6–53, 1947.

3. Farah M: Visual agnosia: Disorders of object recognition and what they tell us about normal vision. Cambridge, MA: MIT Press, 1990.

4. De Renzi, E, Bonacini MG, Faglioni P: Right posterior patients are poor at assessing the age of a face. *Neuropsychologia* 27:839–848, 1989.

5. Kurucz J, Feldmar G: Prosopo-affective agnosia as a symptom of cerebral organic disease. J Am Geriatric Soc 23:225–230, 1979.

6. Benton AL, Van Allen MW: Impairment in facial recognition in patients with cerebral disease. *Cortex* 4:314–358, 1968.

7. De Renzi E, Faglioni P, Spinnler H: The performance of patients with unilateral brain damage on face recognition tasks. *Cortex* 4:17–34, 1968.

8. De Renzi E, Spinnler H: Facial recognition in brain-damaged patients. *Neurology* 16:145–152, 1966.

9. Milner B: Visual recognition and recall after right temporal lobe excision in man. *Neuropsychologia* 6:191–209, 1968.

10. Warrington EK, James M: An experimental investigation of facial recognition in patients with unilateral cerebral lesions. *Cortex* 3:317–326, 1967.

11. Benton AL, Van Allen MW: Prosopagnosia and facial discrimination. *J Neurol Sci* 15:167–172, 1972.

12. Malone DR, Morris HH, Kay MC, Levin HS: Prosopagnosia: A double dissociation between the recognition of familiar and unfamiliar faces. *J Neurol Neurosurg Psychiatry* 45:820–822, 1982.

13. Benton AL: The neuropsychology of facial recognition. *Am Psychol* 35:176–186, 1980.

14. Lissauer H: Ein Fall von Seelenblindheit nebst einem Beiträge zur Theorie derselben. *Arch Psychiatr* 27:222–270, 1890.

15. De Renzi E, Faglioni P, Grossi D, Nichelli P: Apperceptive and associative forms of prosopagnosia. *Cortex* 27:213–221, 1991.

16. Hécaen H: The neuropsychology of face recognition, in Davies G, Ellis H, Shepherd J (ed): *Perceiving and Remembering Faces*. London: Academic Press, 1981, pp 39–54.

17. Bruce V, Young A: Understanding face recognition. *Brit J Psychol* 77:305–327, 1986.

18. Semenza C, Zettin M: Evidence from aphasia for the role of proper names as pure referring expressions. *Nature* 342:678–679, 1989.

19. Carney R, Temple CM: Prosopanomia? A possible category-specific anomia for faces. *Cogn Neuropsychol* 10:185–195, 1993.

20. Adler A: Course and outcome of visual agnosia. *J Nerv Ment Dis* 111:41–51, 1950.

21. Bauer RM: Autonomic recognition of names and faces in prosopagnosia: A neuropsychological application of the guilty knowledge test. *Neuropsychologia* 22:457–469, 1984.

22. Benson DF, Greenberg JP: Visual form agnosia: A specific defect in visual discrimination. *Arch Neurol* 20:82–89, 1969.

23. Campion J, Latto R: Apperceptive agnosia due to carbon monoxide poisoning: An interpretation based on critical band masking from disseminated lesions. *Behav Brain Res* 15:227–240, 1985.

24. De Renzi E, Lucchelli F: The fuzzy boundaries of apperceptive agnosia. *Cortex* 29:187–215, 1993.

25. Landis T, Graves R, Benson DF, Hebben N: Visual recognition through kinesthetic mediation. *Psychol Med* 12:515–531, 1982.

26. McNeil JE, Warrington EK: Prosopagnosia: A reclassification. *Q J Exp Psychol* 43A:267–287, 1991.

27. Sergent J, Poncet M: From covert to overt recogni-

tion of faces in a prosopagnosic patient. *Brain* 113:989–1004, 1990.

28. Sergent J, Villemure JG: Prosopagnosia in a right hemispherectomized patient. *Brain* 112:975–995, 1989.

29. Ellis AW, Young AW, Critchley EMR: Loss of memory for people following temporal lobe damage. *Brain* 112:1469–1483, 1989.

30. Evans JJ, Heggs AJ, Antoun N, Hodges JR: Progressive prosopagnosia associated with selective right temporal lobe atrophy: A new syndrome? *Brain* 118:1–13, 1995.

31. Kartsounis LD, Shallice T: Modality specific semantic knowledge loss for unique items. *Cortex*. In Press.

32. De Haan EHF, Young AW, Newcombe F: A dissociation between the sense of familiarity and access to semantic information concerning familiar people. *Eur J Cogn Psychol* 3:51–67, 1991.

33. Tranel D, Damasio AR: Knowledge without awareness: An autonomic index of facial recognition by prosopagnosics. *Science* 228:1453–1454, 1985.

34. Rizzo M, Hurtig R, Damasio AR: The role of scanpaths in facial recognition and learning. *Ann Neurol* 22:41–45, 1987.

35. Renault B, Signoret JL, Debruille B, et al: Brain potentials reveal covert facial recognition in prosopagnosia. *Neuropsychologia* 27:905–912, 1989.

35a. Bruyer R, Laterre C, Séron X, et al: A case of prosopagnosia with some preserved covert remembrance of familiar faces. *Brain Cogn* 2:257–284, 1983.

36. De Haan EHF, Young AW, Newcombe F: Face recognition without awareness. *Cogn Neuropsychol* 1:385–415, 1987.

37. Diamond BJ, Valentine T, Mayes AR, Sandel ME: Evidence of covert recognition in a prosopagnosic patient. *Cortex* 30:377–393, 1994.

38. Young AW, De Haan EHF: Boundaries of covert recognition in prosopagnosia. *Cogn Neuropsychol* 5:317–336, 1988.

39. De Haan EHF, Young AW, Newcombe F: Faces interfere with name classification in a prosopagnosic patient. *Cortex* 23:309–316, 1987.

40. De Haan EHF, Bauer RM, Greve KW: Behavioral and physiological evidence for covert recognition in a prosopagnosic patient. *Cortex* 28:27–95, 1992.

41. De Haan EHF, Campbell R: A fifteen year follow-up of a case of developmental prosopagnosia. *Cortex* 27:489–509, 1991.

42. Newcombe F, Young AW, De Haan EHF: Pros-

opagnosia and object agnosia without covert recognition. *Neuropsychologia* 27:179–191, 1989.

43. Young AW, Ellis HD: Childhood prosopagnosia. *Brain Cogn* 9:16–47, 1989.

44. McNeil JE, Warrington EK: Prosopagnosia: A face-specific disorder. *Q J Exp Psychol* 46A:1–10, 1993.

45. Mishkin M, Ungerleider LG, Macko KA: Object vision and spatial vision: Two cortical pathways. *Trends Neurosci* 6:414–417, 1983.

46. De Haan EHF, Young AW, Newcombe F: Covert and overt recognition in prosopagnosia. *Brain* 114:2575–2591, 1992.

47. Farah MJ, O'Reilly RC, Vecera SP: Dissociated overt and covert recognition as an emergent property of a lesioned neural network. *Psychol Rev* 100:571–588, 1993.

48. Wallace MA, Farah MJ: Savings in relearning face-name associations as evidence for "covert recognition" in prosopagnosia. *J Cogn Neurosci* 4:150–154, 1992.

49. Humphreys GW, Riddoch MJ: The fractionation of visual agnosia, in Humphreys GW, Riddoch MJ (eds): *Visual Object Processing: A Cognitive Neuropsychological Approach*. Hillsdale, NJ: Erlbaum, 1987.

50. Damasio AR, Damasio H, Van Hoesen GW: Prosopagnosia: Anatomical basis and behavioral mechanisms. *Neurology* 32:331–341, 1982.

51. Lhermitte F, Pillon B: La prosopagnosie: Rôle de l'hémisphère droit dans la perception visuelle. (A propos d'un cas consécutif à une lobectomie occipitale droite). *Rev Neurol* 131:791–812, 1975.

52. Assal G, Favre C, Anderes JP: Non-reconnaissance d'animaux familiers chez un paysan. *Rev Neurol* 140:580–584, 1984.

53. Bornstein B, Sroka, H, Munitz H: Prosopagnosia with animal face agnosia. *Cortex* 5:164–169, 1969.

54. Sergent J, Signoret JL: Varieties of functional deficits in prosopagnosia. *Cerebral Cortex* 2:375–388, 1992.

55. Farah MJ, Klein KL, Levinson K: Face recognition and within-category discrimination in prosopagnosia. *Neuropsychologia* 33:661–674, 1995.

56. De Renzi E: Current issues on prosopagnosia, in Ellis HD, Jeeves MA, Newcombe F, Young A (eds): *Aspects of Face Processing*. Dordrecht: Nijhoff, 1986, pp 243–252.

57. Tanaka JW, Farah MJ: Parts and wholes in face recognition. *Q J Exp Psychol* 46A:225–245, 1993.

58. Farah M: Patterns of co-occurrence among the associative agnosias: Implications for visual object representation. *Cogn Neuropsychol* 8:1–19, 1991.

59. Rumiani RI, Humphreys GW, Riddoch M: Pure visual agnosia without prosopagnosia or alexia: Evidence for hierarchical theories of visual recognition. *Visual Cognition* 1:181–226, 1994.

60. Desimone R: Face-selectivity cells in the temporal cortex of monkeys. *J Cogn Neurosci* 3:1–8, 1991.

61. Perret DI, Mistlin AJ, Chitty AJ: Visual neurons responsive to faces. *TINS* 10:358–364, 1987.

62. Perret DL, Hietanen JK, Oram MW, Benson PJ: Organization and functions of cells responsive to faces in the temporal cortex. *Phil Trans R Soc Lond B* 335:23–30, 1992.

63. Adolphs R, Tranel D, Damasio H, Damasio A: Impaired recognition of emotions in facial expressions following bilateral damage to the human amygdala. *Nature* 372:369–372, 1994.

64. Young AW, Aggleton JP, Hellawell DJ, et al: Face processing impairments after amygdalotomy. *Brain* 118:15–24, 1995.

65. Rapcsak SZ, Comer JF, Rubens AB: Anomia for facial expressions: Neuropsychological mechanisms and anatomical correlates. *Brain Lang* 45:233–252, 1993.

66. Rapcsak SZ, Kaszniak AW, Rubens AB: Anomia for facial expression: Evidence for a category specific visual-verbal disconnection syndrome. *Neuropsychologia* 27:1031–1041, 1989.

67. Ojemann JG, Ojemann GA, Lettich E: Neuronal activity related to faces and matching in human right nondominant temporal cortex. *Brain* 115:1–13, 1992.

68. Hécaen H, Angelergues R: Agnosia for faces (prosopagnosia). *Arch Neurol* 7:92–100, 1962.

69. Meadows JC: The anatomical basis of prosopagnosia. *J Neurol Neurosurg Psychiatry* 37:489–501, 1974.

70. Cohn R, Neumann MA, Wood DJ: Prosopagnosia: A clinicopathological study. *Ann Neurol* 1:177–182, 1977.

71. Nardelli E, Buonanno F, Coccia G, et al: Prosopagnosia: Report of four cases. *Eur Neurol* 21:289–297, 1982.

72. De Renzi E, Perani D, Carlesimo GA, et al: Prosopagnosia can be associated with damage confined to the right hemisphere: An MRI and PET study and a review of the literature. *Neuropsychologia* 32:893–902, 1994.

73. Landis T, Regard M, Blieste A, Kleihues P: Prosopagnosia and agnosia for noncanonical views: An autopsied case. *Brain* 111:1287–1297, 1988.

74. De Renzi E, Zambolin A, Crisi G: The pattern of neuropsychological impairment associated with left posterior cerebral artery infarcts. *Brain* 110:1099–1116, 1987.

75. Uhl F, Lang W, Spieth F, Deecke L: Negative cortical potentials when classifying familiar and unfamiliar faces. *Cortex* 26:157–161, 1990.

76. Seek M, Mainwaring N, Ives J, et al: Differential neural activity in the human temporal lobe evoked by faces of family members and friends. *Ann Neurol* 34:369–372, 1993.

77. Kapur N, Friston KJ, Young A, et al: Activation of human hippocampal formation during memory for faces: A PET study. *Cortex* 31:99–108, 1995.

78. Sergent J, Ohta S, MacDonald B: Functional neuroanatomy of face and object processing. *Brain* 115:15–36, 1992.

79. McConachie HR: Developmental prosopagnosia: A single case report. *Cortex* 12:76–82, 1976.

80. Temple CM: A case of developmental prosopagnosia, in Campbell R (ed): *Mental Lives: Case Studies in Cognition.* London, Blackwell, 1991.

Chapter 19

DISORDERS OF COLOR PROCESSING (PERCEPTION, IMAGERY, RECOGNITION, AND NAMING)

Daniel Tranel

Disorders of color perception and recognition involve conditions in which patients with previously normal color vision develop an inability to perceive or recognize colors via the visual modality as the result of an acquired cerebral lesion (this chapter does not cover disorders attributable to noncerebral lesions). The defect can set in anywhere along a neural processing stream that runs from perception to recognition, resulting in a variety of different conditions. The unifying theme in these conditions, however, is *an acquired defect in the central (i.e., cerebral) processing of color knowledge.* The principal conditions in which central color processing is impaired—perception, imagery, recognition, and naming—are reviewed below.

TERMINOLOGY AND MEASUREMENT

Terms

At the cerebral level, *color perception* refers to the capacity to perceive color in primary visual cortex and early visual association cortices located in the lingual and fusiform gyri (Fig. 19-1; in Brodmann terms, this region corresponds to parts of areas 17 and 18/19; also known as V1, V2/V3, V4; see Ref. 1). In determining whether a patient has an acquired defect in color perception or recognition, it is critical to establish first whether color perception was normal premorbidly. Congenital (inherited) color "blindness" occurs in a sizable

number of persons, especially in males; it has been estimated that about 1 percent of males are red-blind and about 2 percent are green-blind.[2] Hence, it is important to screen carefully to determine whether such a premorbid condition existed; otherwise, the interpretation of failure on various color-processing tasks is confounded.

A capacity closely related to color perception is *color imagery,* that is, the ability to image colors and to imagine entities in color. (In practice, imagining colors may always require imagining some entity of which color is a feature; it is difficult to think of colors as pure unbounded entities per se.) For example, we use color imagery when we bring into our mind's eye a scene in which blue mountains with white, snow-capped peaks span a green valley dotted with yellow wheat fields.

Color recognition is the assignment of meaning to color information that is perceived by the brain. *Meaning* refers to several psychological capacities, such as knowing the difference between various colors, knowing the colors in which various objects normally appear, and being able to retrieve other pertinent knowledge related to color processing. Again, color knowledge is highly linked to its role as a salient feature of entities.

Color naming is a different capacity, distinct from color perception, imagery, and recognition. The term denotes the retrieval of the lexical form (name) that refers to a particular color, e.g., *purple* for the color purple. Patients may perceive and recognize colors normally and yet be unable to name them. This condition conforms to the desig-

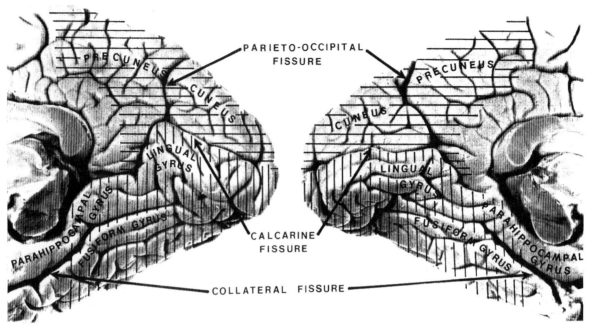

Figure 19-1
*Mesial view of human brain, showing major sulci and gyri. The regions that are important
for various aspects of color processing include the lingual and fusiform gyri, located
below the calcarine fissue in the mesial and ventral aspects of the hemisphere.*

nation of color anomia, and it should be kept separate from disorders of color perception and recognition.

Measurement

Color perception, recognition, and naming can be assessed with several standardized procedures that provide precise quantification of varied color-related capacities (see Ref. 3 for a detailed summary of state-of-the-art testing procedures). Color imagery is subjective, and depends primarily on the self-report of the patient. Different aspects of color processing may be affected in isolation, and care must be taken not to mistake one type of defect for another. However, it should be noted that acquired defects in color perception and color recognition are closely linked to impairments in color imagery. Nonetheless, these capacities can be separated to some extent, as the discussion below indicates.

Perception Color perception is measured with color-plate tests (e.g., the Ishihara Color Plate Test) and color arrangement tests (e.g., the Farnsworth-Munsell 100-Hue Test). Red-green and blue-yellow discriminations should be tested. Normal performance on these procedures does not require accurate color naming, and the tests can be passed even if patients call colors by the wrong names.

Since the most common forms of acquired color imperception affect only part of the visual field (e.g., a quadrant or hemifield), it is important to assess color perception in different quadrants of vision. This can be done by passing a colored chip (we use the distinctively colored chips from the Token Test) slowly from one side of the visual field to the other, in the superior and inferior planes, and from the top to the bottom of the visual field (and bottom to top), in the left and right hemifields. Patients who describe changes in the appearance of the color of a chip as it moves from peripheral to central vision or as it crosses the midline (e.g., "It went from red to pink" or "It's less bright now") should be suspected of having acquired color perception defects.

Recognition Color recognition can be tested with verbal and nonverbal procedures that require the patient to assign colors to objects. In a nonverbal task, for example, the patient is presented plates featuring a black-and-white line drawing of a common object, such as a carrot or a mouse. The patient is required to select from four foils the color that "matches" the object. Verbal tasks involve asking the patient questions about color knowledge. The questions should be given in two forms, one in which a color name constitutes the answer (e.g., "What color is grass?"), and one in which a color name is in the question (e.g., "What are some things that are red?").

Naming Color naming is tested by asking the patient to produce color names to colored stimuli and, given the name, to point to colored stimuli. Naming should be tested in both aural and written formats. Basic color names constitute a relatively "closed class," and it is generally sufficient to probe 6 to 10 basic colors (cf. Ref. 4). In fact, more extensive testing may be problematic, in that large premorbid differences in expertise become the predominant influence in performance. Normal individuals, however, can easily name eight or so basic colors; in fact, this ability enters the cognitive repertoire quite early in development (e.g., Ref. 5).

DISORDERS OF COLOR PERCEPTION (CENTRAL ACHROMATOPSIA)

Central achromatopsia is a defect in color perception caused by an acquired cerebral lesion. The nature of the impairment remains unclear; reduced hue discrimination[6,7] and deficient color constancy[8] have been proposed as explanatory mechanisms, but this issue is unresolved.[3]

Clinical Presentation

A patient with central achromatopsia may complain that colors are "washed out," "dirty," or "faded." It is common for patients to report that the lighting seems poor or that everything looks "dark," even in conditions of bright sunshine. Full-field achromatopsia is possible but rare; more commonly, the defect affects a hemifield or only one quadrant of vision.[3,9–11] Commonly, the portion of visual field near the fovea is spared, and achromatopsia will be evident only in the more peripheral portion of the field.

Neuroophthalmologic and Neuropsychological Findings

Several characteristic neuroophthalmologic and neuropsychological findings accompany central achromatopsia. Blindness is common; for example, a patient may lose form vision in one quadrant and color vision in the other quadrant of the same hemifield. Other aspects of vision, however, are often spared; in the nonblind part of the field, patients generally have normal acuity, spatial contrast sensitivity, and flicker and motion perception.

Two higher-order neuropsychological manifestations are regularly associated with central achromatopsia. One, *acquired alexia,* occurs with left-sided occipital lesions (and hence with right-field achromatopsia); this refers to a defect in reading that is caused by a cerebral lesion. So-called pure alexia (also known as "alexia without agraphia") is the most common form of acquired alexia occurring together with achromatopsia; in this condition, reading is affected but writing is spared. The other higher-order defect is *visual agnosia,* a condition in which patients lose the ability to recognize entities presented visually. The problem may be restricted to certain classes of stimuli, and the most commonly affected class is faces (prosopagnosia). Visual recognition defects for other items are often restricted to certain categories of entities; for instance, the patient may be defective in recognizing animals but may perform normally in recognizing tools.[12–17] The reverse pattern—impaired recognition of tools, and normal recognition of animals—has also been described recently.[16,18]

Neural Correlates

Lesion Studies Full-field achromatopsia is caused by bilateral lesions in the region of the occipitotemporal junction,[9] in the lingual and fusiform gyri. Hemiachromatopsia is associated with a lesion to the contralateral occipitotemporal region. The most common presentation of central achromatopsia involves a combination of quadrantanopia and quadrantachromatopsia in one hemifield. The anopia affects the upper quadrant, contralateral to the lesion, and is caused by the encroachment of the lesion into primary visual cortex in the inferior bank of the calcarine fissure. The achromatopsia affects the lower quadrant, where form vision remains intact. Right-sided lesions may produce a fairly pure form of this condition (as noted above, left-sided lesions usually cause alexia in addition to achromatopsia).[19] The neuroanatomic findings in a typical patient with hemiachromatopsia and associated pure alexia and category-specific visual object agnosia are presented in Fig. 19-2, Plate 5.[20]

The most precise anatomic studies based on the lesion method have indicated that the middle third of the lingual gyrus is the most common site of damage in patients with central achromatopsia,[3,21] followed by damage to the white matter immediately behind the posterior tip of the lateral ventricle. In our experience, lesions confined to the fusiform gyrus or to the white matter beneath the ventricle do not produce achromatopsia.

Functional Imaging Studies Studies using functional neuroimaging techniques have corroborated the lesion-based work. It has been shown that when subjects are given tasks requiring inspection or searching for colored stimuli, there are areas of activation (e.g., increased cerebral blood flow or metabolism) in the region of the lingual and fusiform gyri, or putative human area V4, essentially the same area implicated by lesion work.[22–24] There is some indication that the activation is stronger on the left side.[25] The functional imaging and lesion studies are also consistent with neurophysiology work in animals[26,27] (see Ref. 8 for review) and with ERP studies.[28]

DISORDERS OF COLOR IMAGERY

Color imagery is linked closely to color perception. In fact, the position has been advanced that defective color perception (achromatopsia) invariably results in defective color imagery. The weight of the empirical data supports this position,[29,30] and these findings have been used to argue that imagining an object in color (e.g., a yellow banana) requires at least some of the same neural representations as those required to perceive color.[31] This position has also received support from functional imaging studies, which have shown that imagining and naming the colors associated with various entities activates a region in the fusiform gyrus, bilaterally but more strongly on the left.[32]

Assessment of color imagery depends primarily on the self-report of the patient. Patients may complain that they cannot "remember" the colors that various objects should have (this complaint may also indicate color agnosia; see below). Questions regarding what the world "looks like" in the mind's eye will elicit responses suggestive of absent color information. Another informative approach is to ask the patient questions about entities that do not have a characteristic color; for example, personal items (What color is your car? Your dog? Your favorite hat?) or items whose color is determined by social convention (What color is a yield sign? A mile-marker sign on the interstate? The diamond suit in a card deck?). Since the coloration of such entities is idiosyncratic or arbitrary, persons typically must imagine the items, in color, to produce correct responses to these questions.[33,34] It is also worth asking about dreaming, as patients may note that following a brain lesion, they no longer dream in color (there is wide interindividual variability in this domain, however). Interestingly, it has been suggested that recall of most personal memories depends on color and other visual imagery.[35]

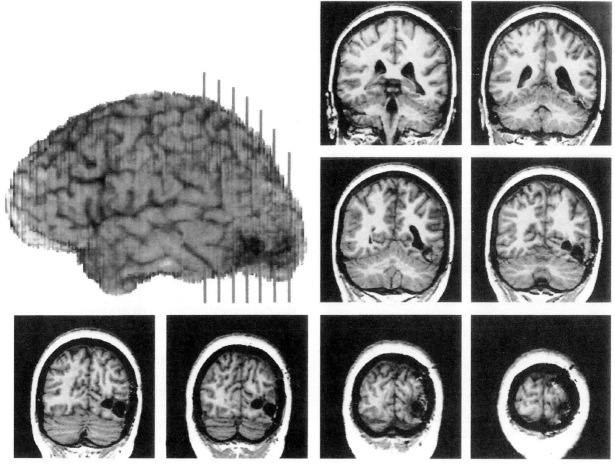

Figure 19-2
Three-dimensional reconstruction (using Brainvox[20]) of a T_1-weighted magnetic resonance imaging in a typical patient with hemiachromatopsia, pure alexia, and category-specific visual object agnosia (animals impaired; tools/utensils normal). The lesion is centered in the left occipitotemporal region and involves parts of the lingual and fusiform gyri.

DISORDERS OF COLOR RECOGNITION (COLOR AGNOSIA)

Following the Teuber[36] (see also Ref. 37) definition of agnosia as a "normal percept stripped of its meaning," *color agnosia* refers to the loss of the ability to retrieve color knowledge pertinent to a given stimulus that is not caused by deficient color perception. The defect should also be distinguished from color anomia and from color imagery impairment. In the latter condition, the patient cannot bring into the mind's eye a particular color, but the patient still knows what the color is and can give verbal or nonverbal testimony to that knowledge—for instance, by performing normally on tasks requiring matching of colors or color names with objects. A patient with color agnosia, by contrast, has lost the "knowing" of colors and will not perform such tasks normally. Color agnosia is rare.

Clinical Presentation

A compelling and elucidating case of color agnosia involved an artist who, premorbidly, was expert in painting with oils. Following bilateral damage to the occipitotemporal region, the patient found that he could no longer mix paints to obtain desired colors. He remained capable of perceiving and naming colors accurately (i.e., neither achromatopsia nor color anomia was present), and he could even articulate in considerable detail the process he should apply to achieve certain colors (e.g., "I need to mix a little of this red with a little of this blue and a hint of black . . ."), but he could not perform the process "intuitively" any longer.

In patients without special expertise in the domain of color, color agnosia may manifest itself in more subtle form. As noted earlier, patients may complain that they cannot remember what colors things should have (e.g., "I can't remember the color of sweet corn."). Errors in matching colors to objects will occur, and patients will not be able to provide accurate information about the colors of arbitrarily colored objects such as road signs, emergency vehicles, and playing cards.

Neuropsychological and Neuroanatomic Findings

Only a few well-studied cases of color agnosia have been reported.[38–41] One reason for this is the confusing and sometimes contradictory way in which the condition has been defined. Some authors have taken a color-naming impairment as evidence of color agnosia and have argued that especially in cases in which the defect is "two-way"—i.e., when the patient cannot name colors from color stimuli and cannot point to colors given the color names—the designation of agnosia is accurate. We disagree, as such a patient may still be entirely capable of retrieving color concepts normally. But such discrepancies abound in the literature, and definitive conclusions regarding neuropsychological and neuroanatomic characteristics of color agnosia are difficult to reach.

The two cases recently described by Luzzatti and Davidoff[40] were carefully studied from a neuropsychological perspective, but the authors provide no anatomic interpretation (one case had a "left temporal" lesion; the other had a "left temporo-parieto-occipital" lesion). The case of Schnider and colleagues[41] was also carefully studied, and the authors attributed the patient's color agnosia to a left "inferotemporo-occipital" lesion. It would appear that the most frequent lesion correlate for color agnosia is occipitotemporal damage (unilateral left or bilateral), but it is unclear how this pattern would differ from that which has been described in connection with achromatopsia (e.g., Ref. 42). A frequent neuropsychological correlate is some degree of visual object agnosia, which usually affects living entities more than artifacts (e.g., Refs. 12 and 13), and possibly some degree of visual confrontation anomia (cf. Refs. 40 and 41).

DISORDERS OF COLOR NAMING (COLOR ANOMIA)

Color naming can be affected independently of color perception, imagery, and recognition.[3,21,43,44] Patients may have impaired perception or recognition of colors and yet have normal color naming, or color naming may be defective in the setting of normal color perception and recognition. As alluded to earlier, however, confusions are frequently made, both in the research literature and in clinical practice, whereby color naming is used inappropriately as an index of color perception or recognition (e.g., Ref. 45). A patient with defective color naming, for example, may be referred to as having "color agnosia." Careful testing may demonstrate that the defect is confined to the lexical retrieval aspect, i.e., coming up with color names, and that recognition of colors is actually intact. The designation of agnosia in this situation is not appropriate; the term *color anomia* should be applied instead.

Color anomia is relatively rare, and, in fact, naming of colors is often relatively spared in patients who have severe naming defects for other classes of stimuli. In one of the largest studies available, Goodglass and coworkers[46] found that color naming was very infrequently impaired in various aphasic patients and was, in fact, one of the categories that tended to stand out as being especially intact—a finding consistent with an older case study.[47] These observations are consistent with our own data, which have suggested very few instances of defective color naming in patients who have severe impairments in the naming of nonunique entities from various categories.[12,48,49]

Clinical Presentation

Our operational definition of color anomia is a *failure to name colors or to point to colors given their names in a nonaphasic patient who has no demonstrable defect in color perception.* In the most common presentation of color anomia, patients have a right homonymous hemianopia and intact color (and form) perception in the left hemifield.

Neuropsychological and Neuroanatomic Findings

The most common neuropsychological correlate of color anomia is pure alexia;[19] in fact, cases of color anomia without alexia are extremely rare.[50,51] As noted, severe aphasia is an exclusion criterion. The most common neuroanatomic correlate of color anomia is a lesion in the left mesial occipitotemporal region, in a subsplenial position,[50,52] which also affects visual cortex or optic radiations in such a way as to produce the right hemianopia. The net effect of the right-field cut is that visual information is circumscribed to the right visual cortex. The left occipitotemporal lesion prevents language areas in left hemisphere from receiving information related to color.

SUMMARY

Disorders of color processing are rare, but their study has provided several important insights into the neural basis of visual functions in the human brain. Studies based on the lesion method have furnished testable hypotheses, which are beginning to be pursued with new functional imaging techniques, including positron emission tomography and functional magnetic resonance imaging. So far, these new approaches have corroborated earlier work that linked color processing to the mesial and ventral occipital and occipitotemporal sectors bilaterally but with some skewing to the left.

ACKNOWLEDGMENT

Supported by NINDS Program Project Grant NS 19632.

REFERENCES

1. Felleman DJ, Van Essen DC: Distributed hierarchical processing in the primate cerebral cortex. *Cereb Cortex* 1:1–47, 1991.
2. Gouras P: The perception of colour, in *Vision and Visual Dysfunction.* London: Macmillan, 1991, vol VI.
3. Rizzo M, Smith V, Pokorny J, Damasio AR: Color perception profiles in central achromatopsia. *Neurology* 43:995–1001, 1993.
4. Berlin B, Kay P: *Basic Color Terms.* Berkeley, CA: University of California Press, 1969.
5. Bornstein MH: On the development of color naming in young children: Data and theory. *Brain Lang* 26:72–93, 1985.
6. Heywood CA, Wilson B, Cowey A: A case study of cortical colour "blindness" with relatively intact achromatic discrimination. *J Neurol Neurosurg Psychiatry* 50:22–29, 1987.
7. Victor J, Maiese K, Shapley R, et al: Acquired central dyschromatopsia with preservation of color discrimination. *Clin Vis Sci* 3:183–196, 1989.
8. Zeki S: A century of cerebral achromatopsia. *Brain* 113:1727–1777, 1990.
9. Damasio AR, Yamada T, Damasio H, et al: Central achromatopsia: Behavioral, anatomic and physiologic aspects. *Neurology* 30:1064–1071, 1980.
10. Kolmel HW: Pure homonymous hemiachromatopsia: Findings with neuro-ophthalmologic examination and imaging procedures. *Eur Arch Psychiatry Neurol Sci* 237:237–243, 1988.
11. Paulson HL, Galetta SL, Grossman M, Alavi A: Hemiachromatopsia of unilateral occipitotemporal infarcts. *Am J Ophthalmol* 118:518–523, 1994.
12. Damasio AR, Damasio H, Tranel D, Brandt JP:

Neural regionalization knowledge access: Preliminary evidence. *Symp Quant Biol* 55:1039–1047, 1990.

13. Farah MJ, Meyer MM, McMullen PA: The living/nonliving dissociation is not an artifact: Giving an a priori implausible hypothesis a strong test. *Cog Neuropsychol* 13:137–154, 1996.

14. Hillis AE, Caramazza A: Category-specific naming and comprehension impairment: A double dissociation. *Brain* 114:2081–2094, 1991.

15. Sartori G, Job R, Miozzo M, et al: Category-specific form-knowledge deficit in a patient with herpes simplex virus encephalitis. *J Clin Exp Neuropsychol* 15:280–299, 1993.

16. Tranel D, Damasio AR, Damasio H, Brandt JP: Separate concepts are retrieved from separate neural systems: Neuroanatomical and neuropsychological double dissociations. *Soc Neurosci* 21:1497, 1995.

17. Warrington EK, Shallice T: Category specific semantic impairments. *Brain* 107:829–853, 1984.

18. Warrington EK, McCarthy RA: Multiple meaning systems in the brain: A case for visual semantics. *Neuropsychologia* 32:1465–1473, 1994.

19. Damasio AR, Damasio H: The anatomic basis of pure alexia. *Neurology* 33:1573–1583, 1983.

20. Damasio H, Frank R: Three-dimensional in vivo mapping of brain lesions in humans. *Arch Neurol* 49:137–143, 1992.

21. Damasio AR, McKee J, Damasio H: Determinants of performance in color anomia. *Brain Lang* 7:74–85, 1979.

22. Lueck CJ, Zeki S, Friston KJ, et al: The colour centre in the cerebral cortex of man. *Nature* 340:386–389, 1989.

23. Corbetta M, Miezin FM, Dobmeyer S, et al: Attentional modulation of neural processing of shape, color, and velocity in humans. *Science* 248:1556–1559, 1990.

24. Zeki S, Watson JDG, Lueck CJ, et al: A direct demonstration of functional specialization in human visual cortex. *J Neurosci* 11:641–649, 1991.

25. Corbetta M, Miezin FM, Dobmeyer S, et al: Selective and divided attention during visual discrimination of shape, color, and speed: Functional anatomy by positron emission tomography. *J Neurosci* 11:2383–2402, 1991.

26. Hubel DH, Livingstone MS: Segregation of form, color, and stereopsis in primate area 19. *J Neurosci* 7:3378–3415, 1987.

27. Livingstone MS, Hubel DH: Anatomy and physiology of a color system in the primate visual cortex. *J Neurosci* 4:309–356, 1984.

28. Rosler F, Heil M, Hennighausen E: Distinct cortical activation patterns during long-term memory retrieval of verbal, spatial, and color information. *J Cog Neurosci* 7:51–65, 1995.

29. Beauvois MF, Saillant B: Optic aphasia for colours and colour agnosia: A distinction between visual and visuo-verbal impairments in the processing of colours. *Cog Neuropsychol* 2:1–48, 1985.

30. DeRenzi E, Spinnler H: Impaired performance on color tasks in patients with hemispheric lesions. *Cortex* 3:194–217, 1967.

31. Farah MJ: Is visual imagery really visual? Overlooked evidence from neuropsychology. *Psychol Rev* 95, 307–317, 1988.

32. Martin A, Haxby JV, Lalonde FM, et al: Discrete cortical regions associated with knowledge of color and knowledge of action. *Science* 270:102–105, 1995.

33. De Vreese LP: Two systems for colour-naming deficits: Verbal disconnection vs colour imagery disorder. *Neuropsychologia* 29:1–18, 1991.

34. Farah MJ: The neurological basis of mental imagery: A componentional analysis. *Cognition* 18:245–272, 1984.

35. Ogden JA: Visual object agnosia, prosopagnosia, achromatopsia, loss of visual imagery, and autobiographical amnesia following recovery from cortical blindness: Case M.H. *Neuropsychologia* 31:571–589, 1993.

36. Teuber HL: Alteration of perception and memory in man, in Weiskrantz L (ed): *Analysis of Behavioral Change.* New York: Harper & Row, 1968, pp 268–375.

37. Tranel D, Damasio AR: The agnosias and apraxias, in Bradley WG, Daroff RB, Fenichel GM, Marsden CD (eds): *Neurology in Clinical Practice,* 2d ed. Stoneham, MA: Butterworth, 1996, pp 119–129.

38. Farah MJ, Levine DN, Calvanio R: A case study of mental imagery deficit. *Brain Cog* 8:147–164, 1988.

39. Kinsbourne M, Warrington EK: Observations on colour agnosia. *J Neurol Neurosurg Psychiatry* 27:296–299, 1964.

40. Luzzatti C, Davidoff J: Impaired retrieval of object-colour knowledge with preserved colour naming. *Neuropsychologia* 32:933–950, 1994.

41. Schnider A, Landis T, Regard M, Benson DF: Dissociation of color from object in amnesia. *Arch Neurol* 49:982–985, 1992.

42. Benton AL, Tranel D: Visuoperceptual, visuospatial, and visuoconstructional disorders, in Heilman

KM, Valenstein E (eds): *Clinical Neuropsychology,* 3d ed. New York: Oxford University Press, 1993, pp 165–213.

43. Geschwind N, Fusillo M: Color naming defects in association with alexia. *Arch Neurol* 15:137–146, 1966.

44. Rizzo M, Damasio AR: Acquired central achromatopsia, in Kulikowski JJ, Dickinson CM, Murray IJ (eds): *Seeing Contour and Color.* Oxford, England: Pergamon Press, 1989, pp 758–763.

45. Pena-Casanova J, Roig-Rovira T: Optic aphasia, optic apraxia, and loss of dreaming. *Brain Lang* 26:63–71, 1985.

46. Goodglass H, Wingfield A, Hyde MR, Theurkauf JC: Category specific dissociations in naming and recognition by aphasic patients. *Cortex* 22:87–102, 1986.

47. Yamadori A, Albert ML: Word category aphasia. *Cortex* 9:83–89, 1973.

48. Damasio AR, Damasio H: Brain and language. *Sci Am* 267:88–95, 1992.

49. Tranel D, Damasio AR, Damasio H: On the neurology of naming, in Goodglass H, Wingfield A (eds): *Anomia.* New York: Academic Press. In Press.

50. Davidoff J, De Bleser R: Impaired picture recognition with preserved object naming and reading. *Brain Cog* 24:1–23, 1994.

51. Mohr JP, Leicester J, Stoddard LT, Sidman M: Right hemianopia with memory and color deficits in circumscribed left posterior cerebral artery territory infarction. *Neurology* 21:1104, 1971.

52. Damasio AR: Disorders of complex visual processing: Agnosias, achromatopsia, Balint's syndrome, and related difficulties of orientation and construction, in Mesulam M-M (ed): *Principles of Behavioral Neurology.* Philadelphia: Davis, 1985, pp 259–288.

Chapter 20

AUDITORY AGNOSIA AND AMUSIA

Russell M. Bauer
Tricia Zawacki

The term *auditory agnosia* refers to an impaired capacity to recognize sounds in the presence of otherwise adequate hearing as measured by standard audiometry. Historically, the term has been used broadly to refer to impaired capacity to recognize sounds in general and in a narrow sense to refer to a selective deficit in recognizing nonverbal sounds only. Terminological confusion abounds, with such terms as *cortical auditory disorder,*[1,2] *auditory agnosia,*[3,4] and *auditory agnosia and word deafness*[5] all being used to describe similar phenomena. In most cases, impairment in the recognition of both speech and nonspeech sounds is present to some degree. The relative severity of these impairments depends on lesion localization, on premorbid lateralization of linguistic and nonlinguistic skills in the individual patient, and on which hemisphere is first or more seriously damaged[6] (but see Ref. 7). Complicating the picture even further is the fact that many patients evolve from one disorder to another as recovery takes place.[8] In regard to generalized auditory agnosia, we prefer the theoretically neutral term *cortical auditory disorder,* and we first discuss this entity together with *cortical deafness.* We then discuss more "selective" deficits, including *pure word deafness* (a selective impairment in speech-sound recognition), *auditory sound agnosia* (selective impairment in recognizing nonspeech sounds), and *paralinguistic agnosias* (in which recognition of prosodic features of spoken language is impaired). Finally, we describe patients with *receptive (sensory) amusia,* loss of the ability to appreciate various characteristics of heard music. Table 20-1 lists the major clinical features of each syndrome.

CORTICAL DEAFNESS AND CORTICAL AUDITORY DISORDER

Patients with cortical deafness show profound impairments in processing auditory stimuli of any kind and often have electrophysiologic signs of primary impairment in auditory-perceptual acuity. The behavior of patients with cortical auditory disorders is similar, though auditory evoked responses are more often normal in this population. Both groups show a range of impairments in auditory perception, discrimination, and recognition that affect verbal and nonverbal material.[9,10] If present, aphasic signs are mild and do not prevent the patient from identifying visual or somesthetic stimuli. Difficulties in elementary auditory function, including temporal auditory analysis and localization of sounds in space, are common.

In our view, cortical auditory disorders and cortical deafness are related in much the same way as visual agnosia is related to cortical blindness. If so, then cortical auditory disorders can take apperceptive or associative[11] forms, though some degree of perceptual deficit is apparent in nearly all cases where the evaluation of auditory abilities has been sufficiently comprehensive. This statement is true even in cases where pure tone audiometry is relatively normal. Jerger and coworkers[12,13] reported impairments in auditory perception (ear

Table 20-1

Clinical features of various forms of auditory agnosia

	Cortical deafness	Cortical auditory disorder	Pure word deafness	Auditory sound agnosia	Sensory/receptive amusia
Audiometric sensitivity	−	+/−	+	+	+
Speech comprehension	−	−	−	+	+
Speech repetition	−	−	−	+	+
Spontaneous speech	+	+[a]	+[a]	+	+
Reading comprehension	+	+	+	+	+
Written language	+	+	+	+	+
Recognition of familiar sounds	−	−	+	−	?
Musical perception	−	−	−[b]	−	+/−
Recognition of vocal prosody	−	−	+	?	−

Key: + = spared ability; − = impaired ability; ? = insufficient information in literature to generalize.

[a]May be some paraphasia.

[b]When tested (rarely), musical perception has been shown to be impaired in these patients.

Sources: Adapted from Buchman et al.[7] and Oppenheimer and Newcombe,[3] with permission.

suppression in dichotic listening, abnormal click fusion thresholds, and impaired discrimination of basic sound attributes) in patients with cortical auditory disorders. These sometimes evolve from a state of cortical deafness, making it difficult to distinguish between the two entities. Michel and colleagues[14] argued that the cortically deaf patient looks and feels deaf, whereas the patient with cortical auditory disorders insists that he or she is not deaf. This turns out to be a poor criterion, because the subjective experience of deafness in the former condition is typically so transient and patients in both groups are "deaf" when subjected to appropriate tests. Although it was once believed that bilateral cortical lesions involving primary auditory cortex resulted in total hearing loss, evidence from animal experiments,[15,16] cortical mapping of the auditory area,[17] and clinicopathologic studies in humans[18,19] indicate that complete destruction of primary auditory cortex does not lead to permanent loss of audiometric sensitivity. Thus, clinical, pathologic, and electrophysiologic data question the distinctive nature of cortical deafness[1,9,10] and

suggest that it is one of a spectrum of auditory impairments that runs from generalized disturbances in detecting and discriminating basic sound attributes to more complex and selective impairments in auditory recognition.

Cortical deafness is most often seen in bilateral cerebrovascular disease. The course is usually biphasic, with an initial deficit (often aphasia and hemiparesis) related to unilateral damage, followed by a second (contralateral) deficit associated with sudden transient total deafness.[12,13,20,21] A biphasic course is also typical of cortical auditory disorders. In cortical deafness, bilateral destruction of the auditory radiations or the primary auditory cortex (Heschl's gyrus) has been a constant finding.[20] The anatomic basis of cortical auditory disorders is more variable. Lesions can be quite extensive,[3] though the superior temporal gyrus and efferent connections of Heschl's gyrus are often involved. Two recent Japanese cases[22,23] suggest that cortical auditory disorders can result from bilateral lesions sparing the cortex entirely. Thus, the lesions in cortical auditory disorders seem to involve either intrinsic or disconnecting lesions of auditory association cortex, with relative sparing of Heschl's gyrus.

PURE WORD DEAFNESS (AUDITORY AGNOSIA FOR SPEECH, AUDITORY VERBAL AGNOSIA)

The patient with pure word deafness is unable to comprehend spoken language although he or she can read, write, and speak in a *relatively* normal manner.[7] Writing to dictation is typically impaired, though copying of written material is not. By definition, comprehension of nonverbal sounds is *relatively* spared, but nonverbal auditory recognition is impaired in the majority of cases in which it has been evaluated.[7] Thus, the syndrome is "pure" in that (1) the patient is *relatively* free of signs of posterior aphasia (see Chap. 9) and (2) the impairment in speech sound recognition is disproportionately severe. The disorder was first described by Kussmaul.[24] Lichteim[25] later defined it as an isolated deficit and postulated a bilateral subcortical interruption of fibers from ascending auditory projections to the left "auditory word center." With few exceptions, pure word deafness has been associated with bilateral, symmetric corticosubcortical lesions of the anterior part of the superior temporal gyri with some sparing of Heschl's gyrus, particularly on the left. Some patients have subcortical lesions of the dominant temporal lobe only, presumably destroying the ipsilateral auditory radiation as well as callosal fibers from the contralateral auditory region.[26–28] It is generally agreed that the lesion profile results in a bilateral disconnection of Wernicke's area from auditory input.[29] The fact that it involves an unusually placed, circumscribed lesion explains the low incidence of pure word deafness. In the review performed by Buchman and colleagues,[7] the lesions in 30 of 37 reviewed cases were of cerebrovascular origin.

When first seen, the patient is often recovering from a Wernicke's aphasia, though occasionally pure word deafness may actually give way to a Wernicke's aphasia.[30–33] As the paraphasias and writing and reading disturbances disappear, the patient still does not comprehend spoken language but can communicate by writing. Deafness can be ruled out by normal audiometric pure-tone thresholds. At this point, the patient may experience auditory hallucinations or may exhibit transient euphoric[34] or paranoid[35] ideation. The inability to repeat poorly comprehended speech stimuli distinguishes pure word deafness from transcortical sensory aphasia; the absence of florid paraphasia and of reading and writing disturbance distinguishes it from Wernicke's aphasia. This having been said, it should be recognized that "aphasic" and "agnosic" symptoms may both be present, though different in degree, in the individual case.[7]

Many patients are responsive to speech input but complain of dramatic, sometimes aversive changes in their subjective experience of speech sounds.[8] The pure word deafness patient may complain that speech is muffled or sounds like a foreign language. Hemphill and Stengel's[36] patient stated that "voices come but no words." Klein and Harper's[31] patient described speech as "an undifferentiated continuous humming noise without any rhythm" and "like foreigners speaking in the distance." Albert and Bear's[30] patient said "words come too quickly" and, "they sound like a foreign language." The speech of these patients is often slightly louder than normal. Performance on speech perception tests is inconsistent and highly dependent upon context[37] and linguistic complexity.[38]

Many studies of pure word deafness have emphasized the role of auditory-perceptual processing in the genesis of the disorder.[1,8,12,30,38] Problems with temporal resolution[30] and phonemic discrimination[39–41] have also received attention. Auerbach and coworkers[38] suggest that the disorder may take two forms: (1) a prephonemic temporal auditory acuity disturbance associated with bilateral temporal lesions or (2) a disorder of phonemic discrimination attributable to left temporal lesions and closely linked to Wernicke's aphasia. Albert and Bear[30] suggest that the problem in pure word deafness is one of temporal resolution of auditory stimuli rather than specific phonetic impairment. Their patient demonstrated abnormally long click-fusion thresholds, and improved in auditory comprehension when speech was presented at slower rates. Saffran and colleagues,[41] on the other hand, showed that informing their patient of the nature of the topic under discussion significantly facilitated comprehension. Thus, the disorder appeared to arise at different levels in these two patients. This variability supports the contention of Buchman and co-workers[7] that pure word deafness describes a spectrum rather than an individual disorder.

On tests of phonemic discrimination, patients with bilateral lesions tend to show distinctive deficits for the feature of place of articulation.[38,39,42] Those with unilateral left hemispheric disease (LHD) show either impaired discrimination of voicing[41] or no distinctive pattern.[40] In dichotic listening, some patients show extreme suppression of right-ear perception,[30,41] suggesting the inaccessibility of the left hemispheric phonetic decoding areas (Wernicke's area) to auditory material that has already been acoustically processed by the right hemisphere. Several studies have reported brainstem and cortical auditory evoked responses in pure word deafness patients.[14] Brainstem auditory evoked potentials (BAEPs) are almost always normal, suggesting intact processing up to the level of the auditory radiations.[30,38,43] Results from studies of cortical auditory evoked potentials (AEPs) more variable, consistent with variable pathology.[38] For example, the patient of Jerger and colleagues[12] had no appreciable AEP, yet heard sounds. The patient of Auerbach and associates[38] showed normal P1, N1, and P2 responses to right-ear stimulation but had minimal response over either hemisphere to left-ear stimulation.

Although patients with pure word deafness are supposed to perform relatively well with environmental sounds, many show subnormal performances when such abilities are formally tested.[7] Similarly, the appreciation of music is often disturbed. Some patients may recognize foreign languages by their distinctive prosodic characteristics, and others can recognize *who* is speaking, suggesting preserved ability to comprehend paralin-

guistic aspects of speech. Coslett and associates[44] described a word-deaf patient who showed a remarkable dissociation between the comprehension of neutral and affectively intoned sentences. He was asked to point to pictures of males and females depicting various emotional expressions. When instructions were given in a neutral voice, he performed poorly, but when instructions were given with affective intonations appropriate to the target face, he performed normally (at a level commensurate to his performance with written instructions). This patient had bilateral destruction of primary auditory cortex with some sparing of auditory association cortex, suggesting at least some direct contribution of the auditory radiations directly to association cortex without initial decoding in Heschl's gyrus.[44] These authors speculate that one reason why pure word deafness patients improve their auditory comprehension with lip reading is that face-to-face contact allows them to take advantage of visual cues (gesture and facial expression) that are processed by different brain systems. Another explanation is that lip reading provides visual information about place of articulation, a linguistic feature that is markedly impaired at least in the bilateral cases.[38] In either case, the preserved comprehension of paralinguistic aspects of speech in pure word deafness patients further reinforces the widely held belief that comprehension of speech and nonspeech sounds are dissociable abilities.

AUDITORY SOUND AGNOSIA (AUDITORY AGNOSIA FOR NONSPEECH SOUNDS)

Patients with auditory sound agnosia have selective difficulty recognizing and identifying nonverbal sounds. The disorder is rare, less common by far than pure word deafness, but its existence has raised interest because it suggests the same type of "domain-specificity" in the auditory system that has received much recent attention in the study of visual recognition disorders.[45–47] The lower incidence of auditory sound agnosia may be due in part to the fact that such patients are less likely to seek medical advice than are those with a disorder of speech comprehension and also because nonspecific auditory complaints may be discounted when pure tone audiometric and speech discrimination thresholds are normal. This is unfortunate, since normal audiometry does not rule out the possibility of primary auditory perceptual defects.[48,49]

Vignolo[9] argued that there may be two forms of auditory sound agnosia: (1) a perceptual-discriminative type associated mainly with right hemisphere damage and (2) an associative-semantic type associated with left hemisphere damage and linked with posterior aphasia. The former group makes predominantly acoustic (e.g., "man whistling" for birdsong) errors on picture-sound matching tasks, while the latter makes predominantly semantic (e.g., "train" for automobile engine) errors. This division follows the original classification of Kliest,[50] who distinguished between the ability to detect/perceive isolated sounds or noises and the inability to understand the meaning of sounds. In the verbal sphere, the analogous distinction (at least on the input side) is between pure word deafness (perceptual-discriminative) and transcortical sensory aphasia (semantic-associative). Relatively few cases of "pure" auditory sound agnosia have been reported.[51–55]

The patient of Spreen and colleagues[54] is a paradigm case. He was a 65-year-old right-handed male who complained of "nerves" and headache when seen 3 years after a left hemiparetic episode. Audiometric testing revealed moderate bilateral high-frequency loss and speech reception thresholds of 12 dB for both ears. The outstanding abnormality was the inability to recognize common sounds. There was neither aphasia nor any other agnosic deficit. Sound localization was normal, but scores on the pitch subtest of the Seashore Tests of Musical Talent were at chance level. The patient performed well on a matching-to-sample test, suggesting that his sound recognition disturbance could not be attributed to serious acoustic disturbance. He claimed no musical experience or talent and refused to cooperate with further testing of musical ability. Postmortem examination revealed a sharply demarcated old infarct of the right hemisphere centering around the parietal lobe and involving the superior temporal and angular gyri as well as a large portion of the inferior parietal, inferior, and middle frontal gyri and the insula. Other cases with unilateral pathology were reported by Fujii and coworkers[52] (small posterior right temporal hemmorhagic lesion of the middle and superior temporal gyri), Neilsen and Sult[53] (right thalamus and parietal lobe), and Wortis and Pfeffer[55] (large lesion of the right temporoparietooccipital junction).

These data suggest that an inability to recognize environmental sounds can occur after unilateral right hemisphere damage. Such a defect is less commonly seen in the context of bilateral disease,[51] but these cases are less "pure" at least in the acute stage. The association of auditory sound agnosia with right hemisphere damage implies that acoustic processors within the right hemisphere are preferentially involved in dealing with nonlinguistic sounds. The left hemisphere is likely involved in providing linguistic labels for identified sounds, and in performing semantic-associative functions supporting sound recognition and identification.

"PARALINGUISTIC AGNOSIAS": AUDITORY AFFECTIVE AGNOSIA AND PHONAGNOSIA

The auditory speech signal conveys not only linguistic meaning but also—through variations in volume, timbre, pitch, and rhythm—information about the emotional state of the speaker (see Chap. 56). Recent clinical evidence suggests that comprehension of affective tone can be selectively impaired. Heilman and coworkers[56] showed that patients with hemispatial neglect from right temporoparietal lesions were impaired in the comprehension of affectively intoned speech (a deficit they called "auditory affective agnosia") but showed normal comprehension of linguistic speech content. Patients with left temporoparietal lesions and fluent aphasia showed normal comprehension of both linguistic and affective (paralinguistic) aspects of speech. Whether this defect is "agnosic" in nature remains to be seen, since auditory sensory/perceptual skills were not assessed. It is possible that auditory affective agnosia is a subtype of auditory sound agnosia (i.e., that it represents a category-specific auditory agnosia), but further studies are necessary before this can be asserted with any certainty.

Recent studies by Van Lancker and associates[57–59] have revealed another type of paralinguistic deficit after right hemisphere damage. In these studies, patients with unilateral right hemisphere damage showed deficits in discriminating and recognizing familiar voices, while patients with left hemisphere damage were impaired only on a task that required a discrimination between two famous voices. Although the exact nature of this distinction is elusive, it seems to parallel that between episodic (personally experienced) versus semantic (generally known) memory in amnesia research. Evidence from computed tomography (CT) suggested that right parietal damage resulted in voice-recognition impairment, while temporal lobe damage in either hemisphere led to deficits in voice discrimination. The authors refer to this deficit as "phonagnosia," but, like auditory affective agnosia, it remains to be seen whether it is truly agnosic in nature.

SENSORY (RECEPTIVE) AMUSIA

The subject of amusia has been reviewed in detail by Wertheim,[60] Critchley and Henson,[61] and Gates and Bradshaw.[62] *Sensory amusia* refers to an inability to appreciate various characteristics of heard music. Impairment of music perception occurs to some extent in all cases of auditory sound agnosia and in the majority of cases of aphasia[62] and pure word deafness, though its exact prevalence in such populations is unknown. Loss of musical perceptual ability is probably underreported because a specific musical disorder rarely interferes with everyday life.

Wertheim[60] believed that receptive amusia occurs more frequently with left hemisphere damage, while expressive musical disabilities are more apt to be associated with right hemisphere damage. More recent evidence suggests that music perception is a multicomponent process to which both hemispheres contribute in complex ways. Dichotic listening studies show that the right hemisphere plays a more important role than the left in the processing of musical and nonlinguistic sound patterns.[63,64] However, the left hemisphere appears to be important in the processing of sequential (temporally organized) material of any kind, including musical series. The dominant hemisphere may process heard music more analytically or with more attention to specific features of the music, such as temporal order or rhythm.[62,65] According to Gordon,[64] melody recognition becomes more dependent on sequential processing as time and rhythm factors become more important for distinguishing tone patterns (see Ref. 66). The multicomponental nature of music perception makes it difficult to define receptive amusia and to localize the deficit to a particular brain region. Further complicating the picture is the fact that pitch, harmony, timbre, intensity, and rhythm may be affected to different degrees and in various combinations in the individual patient.

Many clinical studies distinguish between "instant" perceptual processes governing judgments of pitch, harmony, timbre, and intensity (loudness) and more "sequential," time-dependent processes governing melody recognition and judgments of rhythm and duration. Tentative clinical support for this kind of distinction exists in a double dissociation between the perceptual processing of pitch and the processing of temporal sequences,[67] dissociations that also hold true for reading music and for singing. There is further evidence that aspects of musical denotation (the "real-world" events referred to by lyrics) and musical connotation (the formal expressive patterns indicated by pitch, timbre, and intensity) are selectively vulnerable to focal brain lesions.[68,69] Gordon and Bogen[70] reported that during the right hemispheric anesthesia by the WADA procedure, singing was impaired with disrupted pitch production but preserved rhythmic expression. Hallucinations of voices and musical sounds have been reported with electrical stimulation of the lateral and superior surfaces of the first temporal convolutions in either hemisphere with more frequent occurrence on the nondominant side.[71]

Peretz and colleagues[68] applied comprehensive nonverbal auditory testing to two patients with bilateral lesions of auditory cortex. In their patients, the perception of speech and environmental sounds was spared, but the perception of tunes, prosody, and voice was impaired. Based on these behavioral dissociations, they argue that music processing is distinct from the processing of speech or environmental sounds. Their data led them to argue for a task- and process-specific approach to the analysis of cases of auditory agnosia. They suggest that nominally "auditory" tasks should be broken down into their functional subcomponents and that more extensive component-based analysis of auditory processing deficits is warranted. For example, they distinguish between processes involved in the recognition of specific voices or musical instruments (which is timbre-dependent), and processes involved in recognition of tunes (which is pitch-dependent). The notion that nominally distinct classes of auditory material (e.g., melodies, prosody, and voice) share common processes may be critically important in developing a functional taxonomy of auditory recognition disorders in general and of amusia in particular.

This suggestion points out certain significant deficiencies in the evaluation of amusic patients. Although theories linking brain function to music perception have long been available,[60,72,73] such theories do not often contain sufficient process specificity to guide the clinical evaluation of amusic patients. Thus, for example, relatively little is known regarding which musical features will be most informative in constructing a neuropsychological model of music perception. Another obstacle to systematic study of acquired amusia is the variability of preillness musical abilities, interests, and experience (see Wertheim[60] for a system of classifying musical ability level). The cerebral organization of musical perception has been sug-

gested to be dependent upon on the degree of these preillness characteristics.[72]

SUMMARY

In this chapter, we have briefly reviewed major types of auditory recognition disorders. Although certain identifiable syndromes exist, our review suggests a bewildering array of clinical symptoms and assessment methods. A fundamental problem concerns the lack of a comprehensive theory of auditory cognition. Compared to vision, for example, we know relatively little about the cognitive architecture underlying auditory identification of voices or environmental sounds. This theoretical anarchy has led to terminologic confusion and has slowed development of a cognitive taxonomy of auditory disorders because it has been unsafe to assume that different authors are using such terms in the same way. Another problem is that relatively little agreement exists regarding necessary and sufficient methods of testing in patients with auditory recognition disturbances. Thus, for example, it is not uncommon for claims of a specific defect in one area of auditory processing to be made when, in fact, such specificity is a spurious result of incomplete testing. This problem has been noted by others,[9] and it is obvious that further theoretical development in the area of auditory recognition disturbances will depend on the ability of researchers to devise more comprehensive and theoretically driven assessments of auditory function.[68]

Despite these problems, some progress has been made in identifying potentially important dissociations within auditory recognition disturbances that may eventually reveal the underlying structure of higher auditory processes. Dissociations between verbal (pure word deafness) and nonverbal (auditory sound agnosia) deficits and between perceptual-discriminative and semantic-associative forms of recognition disturbance have been described. Recent findings of impairments in recognizing affective prosody, tunes, and voice are exciting because they raise the further possibility of "category-specificity"[47,74,75] (or process-specificity) in auditory recognition, as has been described for vision (see Chaps. 17 and 18).

It seems clear at this point that further divisions within the concept of auditory agnosia are necessary and that a more comprehensive, process-based approach to evaluating auditory function is required. If this approach is developed further, the important building blocks in the structure of auditory cognition will eventually become apparent through behavioral dissociations.[46] In our view, the clinical approach to a patient suspected of auditory agnosia should consist, at a minimum, of the following steps. First, extensive testing of nonauditory language functions and of general neuropsychological status should be conducted in order to rule out the contribution of aphasia or dementia to the auditory recognition deficit. Second, detailed testing of auditory-perceptual abilities should be conducted, including but not necessarily limited to pure tone audiometry, speech-detection thresholds, temporal auditory acuity (e.g., click fusion thresholds), auditory discrimination,[76] and sound-localization tasks. When possible, brainstem and cortical auditory evoked responses should be evaluated in order to ascertain the "level" at which the patient's deficit occurs. Third, a broad evaluation of auditory capacities should be conducted, including evaluation of the patient's ability to recognize speech, environmental sounds, and music. Performance in other areas not typically assessed in these patients (e.g., voice recognition, singing and related expressive behavior, and evaluation of the patient's ability to recognize linguistic and nonlinguistic prosody) should be assessed. In order to sharpen the hazy distinctions between auditory agnosia (identification and recognition disturbances) and auditory comprehension deficits associated with aphasia, it might also be fruitful to routinely subject aphasic groups to the same kind of comprehensive auditory testing instead of assuming that their impairment in speech comprehension is a straightforward consequence of linguistic impairment. The interested reader should consult Peretz and associates[68] for a useful and reasonably comprehensive instantiation of this kind of approach to the study of auditory agnosias.

REFERENCES

1. Kanshepolsky J, Kelley J, Waggener J: A cortical auditory disorder. *Neurology* 23:699–705, 1973.
2. Miceli G: The processing of speech sounds in a patient with cortical auditory disorder. *Neuropsychologia* 20:5–20, 1982.
3. Oppenheimer DR, Newcombe F: Clinical and anatomic findings in a case of auditory agnosia. *Arch Neurol* 35:712–719, 1978.
4. Rosati G, DeBastiani P, Paolino E, et al: Clinical and audiological findings in a case of auditory agnosia. *J Neurol* 227:21–27, 1982.
5. Goldstein MN, Brown M, Holander J: Auditory agnosia and word deafness: Analysis of a case with three-year follow up. *Brain Lang* 2:324–332, 1975.
6. Ulrich G: Interhemispheric functional relationships in auditory agnosia: An analysis of the preconditions and a conceptual model. *Brain Lang* 5:286–300, 1978.
7. Buchman AS, Garron DC, Trost-Cardamone JE, et al: Word deafness: One hundred years later. *J Neurol Neurosurg Psychiatry* 49:489–499, 1986.
8. Mendez MF, Geehan GR: Cortical auditory disorders: clinical and psychoacoustic features. *J Neurol Neurosurg Psychiat* 51:1–9, 1988.
9. Vignolo LA: Auditory agnosia: A review and report of recent evidence. In Benton AL (ed): *Contributions to Clinical Neuropsychology*. Chicago: Aldine, 1969.
10. Lhermitte F, Chain F, Escourolle R, et al: Etude des troubles per-ceptifs auditifs dans les lesions temporales bilaterales. *Rev Neurol* 128:329–351, 1971.
11. Teuber H-L: Alteration of perception and memory in man, in Weiskrantz L (ed): *Analysis of Behavioral Change*. New York: Harper & Row, 1968.
12. Jerger J, Weikers N, Sharbrough F, Jerger S: Bilateral lesions of the temporal lobe: A case study. *Acta Oto-Laryngologica,* 258(suppl):1–51, 1969.
13. Jerger J, Lovering L, Wertz M: Auditory disorder following bilateral temporal lobe insult: Report of a case. *J Speech Hearing Dis* 37:523–535, 1972.
14. Michel J, Peronnet F, Schott B: A case of cortical deafness: Clinical and electrophysiological data. *Brain Lang* 10:367–377, 1980.

15. Massopoust LC, Wolin LR: Changes in auditory frequency discimination thresholds after temporal cortex ablation. *Exp Neurol* 19:245–251, 1967.

16. Dewson JH, Pribram KH, Lynch JC: Effects of ablation of temporal cortex upon speech sound discrimination in the monkey. *Exp Neurol* 24:279–291, 1969.

17. Celesia GG: Organization of auditory cortical areas in man. *Brain* 99:403–414, 1976.

18. Mahoudeau D, Lemoyne J, Dubrisay J, Caraes J: Sur un cas dagnosie auditive. *Rev Neurol* 95:57, 1956.

19. Wohlfart G, Lindgren A, Jernelius B: Clinical picture and morbid anatomy in a case of "pure word deafness." *J Nerv Ment Dis* 116:818–827, 1952.

20. Leicester J: Central deafness and subcortical motor aphasia. *Brain Lang* 10:224–242, 1980.

21. Earnest MP, Monroe PA, Yarnell PA: Cortical deafness: Demonstration of the pathologic anatomy by CT scan. *Neurology* 27:1172–1175, 1977.

22. Kazui S, Naritomi H, Sawada T, Inque N: Subcortical auditory agnosia. *Brain Lang* 38:476–487, 1990.

23. Motomura N, Yamadori A, Mori E, Tamaru F: Auditory agnosia: Analysis of a case with bilateral subcortical lesions. *Brain* 109:379–391, 1986.

24. Kussmaul A: Disturbances of speech, in von Ziemssien H (ed): *Cyclopedia of the Practice of Medicine.* New York: William Wood, 1877.

25. Lichteim L: On aphasia. *Brain* 7:433–484, 1885.

26. Kanter SL, Day AL, Heilman KM, Gonzalez-Rothi LJ: Pure word deafness: A possible explanation of transient-deterioration after extracranial-intracranial bypass grafting. *Neurosurgery* 18:186–189, 1986.

27. Liepmann H, Storch E: Der mikroskopische Gehirnbefund bei dem Fall Gorstelle. *Monatsschr Psychiatr Neurol* 11:115–120, 1902.

28. Schuster P, Taterka H: Beitrag zur Anatomie und Klinik der reinen Worttaubbeit. *Z Neurol Psychiatr* 105:494, 1926.

29. Geschwind N: Disconnexion syndromes in animals and man. *Brain* 88:237–294, 585–644, 1965.

30. Albert ML, Bear D: Time to understand: A case study of word deafness with reference to the role of time in auditory comprehension. *Brain* 97:373–384, 1974.

31. Klein R, Harper J: The problem of agnosia in the light of a case of pure word deafness. *J Mental Sci* 102:112–120, 1956.

32. Gazzaniga M, Glass AV, Sarno MT: Pure word deafness and hemispheric dynamics: A case history. *Cortex* 9:136–143, 1973.

33. Ziegler DK: Word deafness and Wernicke's aphasia: Report of cases and discussion of the syndrome. *Arch Neurol Psychiatry* 67:323–331, 1942.

34. Shoumaker RD, Ajax ET, Schenkenberg T: Pure word deafness (auditory verbal agnosia). *Dis Nerv Sys* 38:293–299, 1977.

35. Reinhold M: A case of auditory agnosia. *Brain* 73:203–223, 1950.

36. Hemphill RC, Stengel E: A study of pure word deafness. *J Neurol Psychiatry* 3:251–262, 1940.

37. Caplan LR: Variability of perceptual function: The sensory cortex as a categorizer and deducer. *Brain Lang* 6:1–13, 1978.

38. Auerbach SH, Allard T, Naeser M, et al: Pure word deafness: Analysis of a case with bilateral lesions and a defect at the prephonemic level. *Brain* 105:271–300, 1982.

39. Chocholle R, Chedru F, Bolte MC, et al: Etude psychoacoustique d'un cas de surdite corticale. *Neuropsychologia* 13:163–172, 1975.

40. Denes G, Semenza C: Auditory modality-specific anomia: Evidence from a case of pure word deafness. *Cortex* 11:401–411, 1975.

41. Saffran EB, Marin OSM, Yeni-Komshian GH: An analysis of speech perception in word deafness. *Brain Lang* 3:255–256, 1976.

42. Naeser M: The relationship between phoneme discrimination, phoneme/picture perception, and language comprehension in aphasia. Presented at the Twelfth Annual Meeting of the Academy of Aphasia, Warrenton, Virginia, October 1974.

43. Stockard JJ, Rossiter VS: Clinical and pathologic correlates of brainstem auditory response abnormalities. *Neurology* 27:316–325, 1977.

44. Coslett HB, Brashear HR, Heilman KM: Pure word deafness after bilateral primary auditory cortex infarcts. *Neurology* 34:347–352, 1984.

45. Bauer RM: Agnosia, in Heilman KM, Valenstein E (eds): *Clinical Neuropsychology,* 3d ed. New York: Oxford University Press, 1993, pp 215–278.

46. Farah MJ: *Visual Agnosia: Disorders of Object Vision and What They Tell Us about Normal Vision.* Cambridge, MA: MIT Press/Bradford, 1990.

47. Farah MJ, Hammond KM, Mehta Z, Ratcliff G: Category-specificity and modality-specificity in semantic memory. *Neuropsychologia* 27:193–200, 1989.

48. Buchtel HA, Stewart JD: Auditory agnosia: Apperceptive or associative disorder? *Brain Lang* 37:12–25, 1989.

49. Goldstein MN: Auditory agnosia for speech ("pure word deafness"): A historical review with current implications. *Brain Lang* 1:195–204, 1974.

50. Kliest K: Gehirnpathologische und Lokalisatorische Ergebnisse uber Horstorungen, Geruschtaubheiten und Amusien. *Monatsschr Psychiatr Neurol* 68:853–860, 1928.

51. Albert ML, Sparks R, von Stockert T, Sax D: A case study of auditory agnosia: Linguistic and non-linguistic processing. *Cortex* 8:427–433, 1972.

52. Fujii T, Fukatsu R, Watabe S, et al: Auditory sound agnosia without aphasia following a right temporal lobe lesion. *Cortex* 26:263–268, 1990.

53. Nielsen JM, Sult CW Jr: Agnosia and the body scheme. *Bull LA Neurol Soc* 4:69–81, 1939.

54. Spreen O, Benton AL, Fincham R: Auditory agnosia without aphasia. *Arch Neurol* 13:84–92, 1965.

55. Wortis SB, Pfeffer AZ: Unilateral auditory-spatial agnosia. *J Nerv Ment Dis* 108:181–186, 1948.

56. Heilman KM, Scholes R, Watson RT: Auditory affective agnosia. Disturbed comprehension of affective speech. *J Neurol Neurosurg Psychiatry* 38:69–72, 1975.

57. Van Lancker DR, Kreiman J: Unfamiliar voice discrimination and familiar voice recognition are independent and unordered abilities. *Neuropsychologia* 25:829–834, 1988.

58. Van Lancker DR, Kreiman J, Cummings J: Voice perception deficits: Neuroanatomical correlates of phonagnosia. *J Clin Exp Neuropsychol* 11:665–674, 1989.

59. Van Lancker DR, Cummings JL, Kreiman J, Dobkin BH: Phonagnosia: A dissociation between familiar and unfamiliar voices. *Cortex* 24:195–209, 1988.

60. Wertheim N: The amusias, in Vinken PJ, Bruyn GW (eds): *Handbook of Clinical Neurology.* Amsterdam: North-Holland, 1969, vol 4.

61. Critchley MM, Henson RA: *Music and the Brain: Studies in the Neurology of Music.* Springfield, IL: Charles C Thomas, 1977.

62. Gates A, Bradshaw JL: The role of the cerebral hemispheres in music. *Brain Lang* 4:403–431, 1977.

63. Blumstein S, Cooper W: Hemispheric processing of intonation contours. *Cortex* 10:146–158, 1974.

64. Gordon HW: Auditory specialization of the right and left hemispheres, in Kinsbourne M, Smith WL (eds): *Hemispheric Disconnection and Cerebral Function.* Springfield, IL: Charles C Thomas, 1974.

65. Krashen SD: Mental abilities underlying linguistic and nonlinguistic functions. *Linguistics* 115:39–55, 1973.

66. Mavlov L: Amusia due to rhythm agnosia in a musician with left hemisphere damage: A nonauditory supramodal defect. *Cortex* 16:331–338, 1980.

67. Peretz I: Processing of local and global musical information by unilateral brain-damaged patients. *Brain* 113:1185–1205, 1990.

68. Peretz I, Kolinsky R, Tramo M, et al: Functional dissociations following bilateral lesions of auditory cortex. *Brain* 117:1283–1301, 1994.

69. Gardner H, Silverman H, Denes G, et al: Sensitivity to musical denotation and connotation in organic patients. *Cortex* 13:242–256, 1977.

70. Gordon HW, Bogen JE: Hemispheric lateralization of singing after intracarotid sodium amylobarbitone. *J Neurol Neuorsurg Psychiatry* 37:727–738, 1974.

71. Penfield W, Perot P: The brain's record of auditory and visual experience. *Brain* 86:595–696, 1963.

72. Bever TG, Chiarello RJ: Cerebral dominance in musicians and nonmusicians. *Science* 185:137–139, 1974.

73. Hecaen H: Clinical symptomotology in right and left hemispheric lesions, in Mountcastle VB (ed): *Interhemispheric Relations and Cerebral Dominance.* Baltimore: Johns Hopkins University Press, 1962.

74. Warrington EK, Shallice T: Category-specific semantic impairments. *Brain* 107:829–854, 1984.

75. Damasio AR: Category-related recognition defects as a clue to the neural substrates of knowledge. *Trends Neurosci* 13:95–98, 1990.

76. Chedru F, Bastard V, Efron R: Auditory micropattern discrimination in brain damaged subjects. *Neuropsychologia* 16:141–149, 1978.

Chapter 21

TACTILE AGNOSIA AND DISORDERS OF TACTILE PERCEPTION

Richard J. Caselli

Somesthetic processing of form is a necessary but insufficient step for tactile object recognition. The glabrous skin of the digits and palm, which has been called the "fovea" of the human somatosensory system,[1] contains four major types of low-threshold mechanoreceptors, each with its own submodal specificity that contributes in some measure to somesthetic perception. For most types of tactile object recognition, spatial acuity or form perception would seem to be of special importance. The slowly adapting type I (SAI) receptor-afferent unit is the critical peripheral limb of the spatial system concerned with somesthetic processing of form.[1–5] Its responses are isomorphic at the peripheral afferent fiber level[3–5] and produce isomorphic responses in the cortical neurons of area 3b.[6] The sensations evoked by stimulation of such single receptor units alone, however, are not "natural" sensations, and even the most basic somesthetic sensations (like touch) probably result from highly specific combinations of various receptor inputs.[7] In addition, active exploration confers no advantage over passive touch in the spatial resolution of SAI units,[8] despite the fact that most tactile object perception is accomplished using active manual exploration.[9,10] These observations suggest that the spatial properties of tactual stimuli are transduced by the SAI system, which is necessary for the high-fidelity reproduction of form in area 3b, primary somatosensory cortex, but that additional processing in primary and somatosensory association cortices will be required for the somesthetic percept to be incorporated into our ongoing behavior.

SOMATOSENSORY CORTICES

Primary Somatosensory Cortex

All motor and koniocortical sensory systems are made up of multiple cortical areas, each defined by its own somatotopic representations, cytoarchitecture, and thalamocortical/corticocortical connectivity patterns. Within the somatosensory system, the "first somatosensory area," or SI, located on the postcentral gyrus, is considered the primary sensory area. It receives a dense thalamocortical projection from the ventrobasal complex, which contains the somatosensory relay nuclei. Reciprocal corticocortical connections of SI include primary motor cortex (Brodmann area 4) and somatosensory association cortices (see below). Broadly defined, SI has included Brodmann areas 3a, 3b, 1, and 2. It was originally defined as a somatotopically unitary area in laboratory animals[11,12] and subsequently in humans.[13] More recent studies, however, have shown that there are approximate mirror-image somatotopic representations in Brodmann areas 3b and 1 as well as additional somatotopies in Brodmann areas 2 and 3a.[14–16] Though more relative than absolute, there are functional differences between these areas: areas 3b and 1 respond to cutaneous stimuli, and areas 3a and 2 respond to muscle, visceral, and joint afferent stimulation.[16] Area 3b contains the greatest number of neurons with isomorphic responses to peripheral tactual stimulation of SAI afferents and hence the greatest spatial fidelity.[6]

Area 3b also contains some neurons that respond in a nonisomorphic fashion, but these occur in increasing numbers in area 1 (and beyond), suggesting progressively increasing degrees of abstraction as the stimulus moves away from area 3b.[6] With these differences in mind, comparative neuroanatomic studies have led to the more modern interpretation that area 3b is the one and only SI that is homologous in humans, monkeys, and lower mammals.[16]

Somatosensory Association Cortices

The SI is bounded ventrolaterally by SII (parietal operculum), which has been mapped in many animal species[12,16,17] and in humans.[13,18–20] In cats[21–23] and monkeys,[22,25] two other somatosensory areas contiguous to SII have been described and labeled SIII (inferior parietal cortex) and SIV (posterior insula and retroinsular cortex). Each region appears to contain its own somatotopic representations of the body, and the somatotopic patterns differ between regions.

The SI is bounded dorsomedially by another somatosensory association cortex, originally defined by Penfield during intraoperative stimulation studies in humans, which he called the supplementary sensory area.[13] Anatomic studies in monkeys suggest that it encompasses mesial Brodmann area 5 and possibly the anterior portion of mesial area 7.[26–28] Supplementary motor area stimulation[13,29–31] and ablation[32] experiments during brain surgery in humans have sometimes elicited somesthetic sensations, suggesting that this motor association cortex may also be a dorsomedial somatosensory association cortex.

Ventrolateral and dorsomedial somatosensory association cortices are topographically disparate (Fig. 21-1) but share a prokoniocortical cytoarchitecture, bridge a limbic or paralimbic cortex with a koniocortical sensory cortex, and derive phylogenetically from the parainsular/paralimbic growth ring.[33] Ventrolateral somatosensory association cortex, however, phylogenetically derives from olfactocentric paleocortex, while dorsomedial somatosensory association cortex derives from hippocampocentric archicortex.[33] Anatomi-

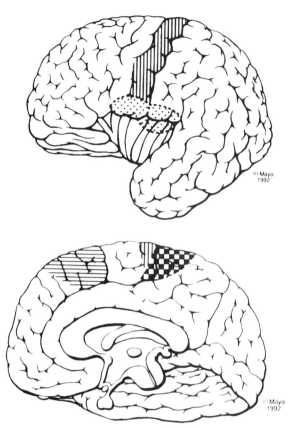

Figure 21-1

Ventrolateral and dorsomedial somatosensory association cortices depicted in a human brain. Homologies between humans and monkeys are inferred (see text). (Top) Small dots demarcate SII and posterior insula. (Bottom) Checkerboard demarcates SSA, and horizontal lines demarcate SMA. Vertical lines in both figures demarcate SI. (© Mayo 1992.)

cally, ventrolateral somatosensory association cortex appears more closely related than supplementary sensory area to SI in terms of corticocortical reciprocity and thalamocortical connectivity,[34] whereas supplementary sensory area is more closely related than ventrolateral somatosensory association cortex to the supplementary motor area[27] and posterior parietal cortices.[35] Physiologic studies have also suggested a strong functional distinction between ventrolateral and dorsomedial somatosensory association cortex. Ablation stud-

Table 21-1

Ventrolateral and dorsomedial somatosensory association cortices

	Ventrolateral somatosensory association cortex	Dorsomedial somatosensory association cortex	
	SII	SSA	SMA
Phylogenetic derivation	Insulolimbic paleocortical	Mediolimbic archicortical	Mediolimbic archicortical
Cytoarchitecture	Prokoniocortex (good lamina iv)	Prokoniocortex (poor lamina iv)	Prokoniocortex
Thalamic projections	VPL, VPM, LP	VL, LP, DM, intralaminar, pulvinar	VL, LP, DM, intralaminar, VA
Corticocortical/reciprocal Motor connections		Premotor and SMA (area 6), area 4	Area 4, premotor, prefrontal (area 9), area 44
Sensory connections	SI, contralateral SII, area 7b (monkey (SIII), retroinsular (monkey SIV)	Area 5	
Corticocortical/afferent Motor connections Sensory connections		Areas 1 and 2	Area 1 SII, insula, superior temporal gyrus
Corticocortical/efferent Motor connections Sensory connections	Area 4		
Somatotropic interface with SI	Face	Hindlimb	None (hindlimb with MI)
Sensory receptive fields	Same size as SI; touch, tap	Larger than SI and SII; touch, pain	
Human stimulation studies	Contralateral and bilateral tingling	Contra- and bilateral tingling, total body aura	Mainly movement-related; some "sensory phenomena"
Human lesion studies	Transient numbness acutely; tactile agnosia	Transient relief of thalamic pain; SSA and SMA combined ablation produces dorsomedial syndrome (see text)	Acute akinesis; bilateral grasp reflex; slowed rapid alternating movement

Abbreviations: DM = dorsal medial nucleus; LP = lateral posterior nucleus; MI = first motor area; SI = first somatosensory area; SII = second somatosensory area; SIII = third somatosensory area; SIV = fourth somatosensory area; SMA = supplementary motor area; VA = ventral anterior nucleus; VL = ventral lateral nucleus; VPL = ventral posterior lateral nucleus; VPM = ventral posterior medial nucleus

ies have shown that SII activity can depend entirely upon SI and not thalamic input, providing evidence for serial cortical processing between SI and SII.[36] Receptive field properties of neurons in SII are similar in size and sensitivity to neurons in SI.[12] Neurons in supplementary sensory area, however, have much larger receptive fields, and some supplementary sensory area neurons are sensitive to pain.[27] Therefore, ventrolateral and dorsomedial somatosensory association cortex have different phylogenetic derivations, anatomic connections, and physiologic properties (Table 21-1).

CLINICAL SOMATOSENSORY ASSESSMENT

Psychophysics has probed the limits of somesthetic perception in neurologically healthy subjects and has demonstrated how slight a stimulus or change in stimulus is required for touch detection,[37,38] two-point discrimination (gap detection),[39] vibratory detection,[40–42] shape recognition,[8,39,41] and texture discrimination (which includes both roughness and hardness),[5,44–46] as well as how one property (such as size) influences the perception of another property (such as shape).[47,48] Behavioral syndromes that we will discuss, like tactile agnosia, have not been defined or studied using psychophysical techniques, although such would represent a logical extension of somesthetic research. Rather, clinical somatosensory disorders have been defined, by and large, with cruder "bedside" techniques that vary somewhat between examiners and are rarely highly standardized.[49–51] Nonetheless these techniques have been used over many years with great practical success.[49]

From a clinical standpoint, somatosensory testing can be classified as outlined below.

Basic Somesthetic Functions

As noted above, microneurographic stimulations of single afferent units result in pure sensations that are not identical to naturally experienced sensations such as light touch.[7] With that caveat in mind, those "basic" somesthetic functions that are tested clinically include light touch (with, for example, a wisp of cotton or von Frey hairs), vibratory sensation (generally over a bony prominence such as a joint), proprioception (the examiner simply moves the patient's joint a small distance and asks the patient to guess the direction of movement), superficial pain (pinprick), temperature (a cold or warm object applied to the skin), and two-point discrimination (generally with a lower limit of 3 mm, which is approximately three times greater than the psychophysical threshold for gap detection).

Intermediate Somesthetic Functions

These include weight discrimination (e.g., differentially weighted objects of identical size, shape, and exterior substance), texture discrimination (e.g., relative grades of sandpaper from very fine to very coarse), dimension perception (e.g., length, width, and height of four rectangular wooden blocks), generic shape recognition (e.g., square, circle, triangle, rectangle, sphere), substance recognition (e.g., plastic, metal, wood, glass, Styrofoam, rubber, paper, wax), and double-simultaneous stimulation (right and left sides of the patient).

Complex Somesthetic Functions

Tactile object recognition requires the use of familiar objects.[51,52] Familiar objects handled unimanually by a blindfolded patient are normally recognized quickly (within 5 s in over 90 percent,[52] accurately, 87 to 99 percent[51,52]) and symmetrically between the two hands.[52] Braille and other types of letter/digit recognition techniques (e.g., Optacon[53]) serve as aids to the visually impaired and can sometimes be used to assess somesthetic perception. Graphesthesia, the recognition of characters and shapes traced on the skin,[49] can also be used but is less reliable than object recognition.

Clinical Laboratory Assessment

Nerve conduction studies and needle electromyography (EMG) are used to evaluate peripheral nerve function and somatosensory evoked potentials to evaluate central somatosensory conduction pathways in patients with somatosensory abnormalities. Computer assisted sensory examinations (CASE) are used occasionally to determine vibratory and temperature thresholds.[54]

CLINICAL SOMATOSENSORY DISORDERS RESULTING FROM CORTICAL LESIONS

Parietal lobe damage is capable of producing a wealth of possible somesthetic problems. Critchley in 1953[55] summarized these based on his own considerable experience and an extensive literature, including the seminal contributions of Head and Holmes:[56] (1) focal sensory epilepsy; (2) tactile perseveration and hallucinations of touch (e.g., feeling two points when only one is applied or feeling a nonexistent object in an anesthetic hand); (3) cortical sensory loss: impaired recognition of objects, texture, two-point discrimination, stimulus localization, barognosis, vibratory sensation, position sense, graphesthesia; (4) hemianesthesia; (5) tactile inattention (to double simultaneous stimulation); (6) altered sensory adaptation time (the time it takes for a continued monotonous somesthetic stimulus, such as clothing, to cease engaging the perceiver's attention); (7) "anaesthoagnosia" (bilateral sensory alterations following a unilateral lesion); (8) asymboly for pain (failure to be bothered by an otherwise correctly perceived painful stimulus); and (9) "pseudothalamic syndrome" (hemianesthesia with spontaneous pain and painful perception of normally nonpainful stimuli in the anesthetic areas, akin to the Roussy-Dejerine thalamic pain syndrome but occurring on a parietal basis).

Following parietal lobe infarction in patients with minimal hemiparesis, a typical, routine neurologic examination is more likely to reveal a more modest number of somesthetic syndromes: (1) faciobrachiocrural elementary sensory loss (or pseudothalamic sensory syndrome), which essentially means impairment of all modalities tested in the face and upper limb contralateral to the side of the stroke; (2) isolated discriminative sensory loss (or cortical sensory syndrome), which means impaired stereognosis (processing of shape; see below), graphesthesia, and position sense in some combination of face and hand; and (3) complete sensory loss with partial distribution (or atypical sensory syndrome), which is the same as the first type but topographically incomplete.[57]

The following classification of cortical somatosensory disorders is based upon modern anatomical concepts and attempts at once to be both simplified and comprehensive.

The SI Syndrome: Astereognosis

An early description of stereognosis as a complex sensory function that perceived images rather than the simple sensory functions of pain, touch, and temperature was that of Verger in 1897.[58] According to an early classification by Delay, astereognosis is a complex somatosensory disorder that has three subsidiary parts: amorphognosia, the inability to recognize size and shape; ahylognosia, the inability to decipher density, weight, thermal conductivity, and roughness; and tactile asymboly, which is the same as tactile agnosia, the inability to identify an object in the absence of amorphognosis and ahylognosis.[59] Because tactile agnosia was disputed and in 1965 disavowed,[60] there has until recently seemed little reason to limit the scope of astereognosis. However, with the reemergence of tactile agnosia as a plausible behavioral entity,[51,61-63] the term *astereognosis* needs limits imposed upon it that will permit distinction from tactile agnosia. Astereognosis should be restricted to mean impaired tactual spatial perception that is due to severe basic somatosensory imperception. In contrast, tactile agnosia is a selective disturbance of tactile object recognition in the absence of more basic somatosensory imperception.[51]

In this revised light, astereognosis reflects cortical deafferentation arising from damage to any level of the somatosensory system including the peripheral nerves (particularly severe large-fiber peripheral neuropathies, such as Guillain-Barré syndrome), spinal cord (especially posterior column pathways), brainstem (interruption of the medial lemniscus), and thalamus (ventral posterior lateral) nucleus, or SI destruction.[51,60,64,65] Patients with astereognosis typically have severe impairment of most of the basic and intermediate sensory modalities listed above and, if this results from a right hemispheric lesion, may also have extinction on the left to double simultaneous stimulation due to concurrent hemineglect (see below). Impairment of tactile object recognition is generally more severe when caused by a cortical lesion than by a peripheral nerve, spinal cord, or thalamic lesion.

The Ventrolateral Somatosensory Association Cortex Syndrome: Tactile Agnosia

Behavioral Considerations *Definition* The selective impairment of tactile object recognition in the absence of more basic somesthetic impairment is called tactile agnosia. The inability to recognize a previously known object must be distinguished from the inability to simply name the object (aphasia)[66] and "tactile inexperience," in which the target object might not be familiar to the subject.[55] Psychophysical analyses are few in tactile agnosia research to date, and the statement that impaired TOR occurs in the *absence* of more basic somesthetic impairment should be modified currently to state that impaired TOR occurs in the absence of *clinically demonstrable* or *clinically significant* basic somesthetic impairment.

Properties Tactile agnosia is a unilateral disorder (it affects only the left or only the right hand) that results from a unilateral lesion.[51,61,63] It is not a source of great disability for the affected patients. For example, one such patient complained that she had to take an object out of her pocket and look at it to be certain it was her key. Several types of misidentifications commonly occur in tactile agnosia. First, an object may be described in spatially approximate terms: "pencillike, with a string" for an artist's paintbrush. Second, an object may be confused with a spatially similar object: "safety pin" for a paper clip. In this example, the patient correctly identified the supraordinate spatial category (small, wiry pinlike items), but misjudged the specific subordinate member. Third, an object may be identified in a more generic way: "a tool" for a wrench. In this example, the supraordinate spatial/functional category was correctly identified, but the patient failed to access the taxonomically deeper subordinate member of that category. Tactile agnosics can draw the object they are feeling (Fig. 21-2), providing further demonstration of their preserved ability to decipher the salient somethetic characteristics of the object they fail to recognize.[67] In tactile agnosia unlike prosopagnosia, the ability to associate tactually defined objects and their parts with episodic memory is preserved. This is based upon the finding that in tactile agnosia, personal items such as the patient's own wallet, hairbrush, and so on are recognized with greater success than other items.[61]

Tactual exploration strategies are normal in tactile agnosics,[61] and, in fact seem unimportant for TOR. Hemiparetic patients without damage to somatosensory-related structures have normal TOR despite an impaired (and in hemiplegic cases, nonexistent) search strategy.[51,63,68]

It should be noted parenthetically that, to date, there has not been a patient studied with normal development who, as an adult, developed selective bilateral damage to ventrolateral association cortices. Before our knowledge of tactile agnosia can be considered complete, such a patient will have to be studied. The resulting somethetic disorder in such a patient might prove far more revealing than the nondisabling unilateral disorder described above.

Figure 21-2

Drawings of a combination lock and can opener made by a tactile agnosic after feeling but not seeing these objects. She was unable to identify these objects tactually. (From Caselli,[67] with permission.)

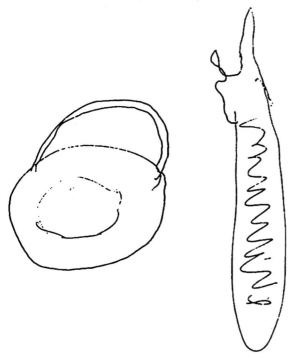

Mechanisms   Based upon lesion studies in monkeys, Mishkin posited a role for the posterior insula in tactile learning and object recognition in which it served to connect SII to mesial temporal limbic structures.[69] From this perspective, tactile agnosia results from an interruption in the flow of information between the somatosensory and memory systems. Behavioral evidence favoring such a role for the anatomically defined somethetic-limbic pathway includes the finding that amnesic subjects have difficulty learning a tactually mediated task (maze learning).[70] However, impaired memory alone is not sufficient to impair TOR in humans, based upon more recent demonstrations that amnesics have no difficulty tactually recognizing familiar objects.[51]

Tactile agnosia seems to reflect a faulty high-level perceptual process. This conclusion stems from three observations. First, tactile agnosia is a unilateral disorder. Patients with unilateral damage to ventrolateral somatosensory association cortex have a contralateral tactile agnosia, with normal tactile object recognition in the ipsilateral hand.[51,61,63] Although lesion studies in monkeys have shown bilateral impairment of shape recognition following unilateral SII ablation,[71–73] bilaterally impaired tactile object recognition in humans

Figure 21-3
Sections by MRI of two patients with tactile agnosia. The patient to the left (T_1-weighted coronal section) had infarction of both the parietal operculum and posterior insula of the right hemisphere. The patient to the right (proton-density-weighted transverse section) had a tiny infarction confined to the left inferior parietal lobule.

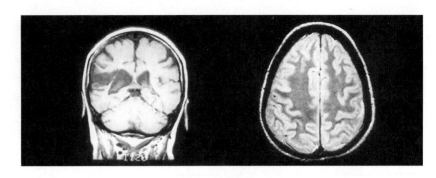

is almost always the result of massive right hemispheric lesions in the setting of left hemineglect.[71] These patients had severe astereognosis in the left hand and tactile agnosia in the right hand. The finding of right-sided tactile agnosia was unexpected but may have reflected transcallosal diaschisis, since the right hemisphere is dominant for cortical arousal and was clinically impaired in these patients.[71,74] One patient has also been described who had a mild bilateral impairment of tactile object recognition following extensive damage to dorsomedial somatosensory association cortices[63] (see "Dorsomedial Syndrome," below). The generally unilateral nature of tactile agnosia implies a perceptual, as opposed to mnemonic, impairment because if memory representations were destroyed, then it should not matter which hand is used to access those representations.

A second reason for attributing tactile agnosia to faulty high-level perception comes from the mental imagery abilities of a recently studied case.[61] Although impaired at the tactile recognition of upright letter shapes, performance declined further when the letters were misoriented in a mental rotation task, which taxes high-level perceptual processes.[75] In contrast, the patient performed normally in a memory imagery task, in which she had to answer questions such as "Which feels smoother, a Styrofoam cup or an orange peel?"

Anatomic Considerations Tactile agnosia results from lesions involving inferior parietal cortices (Fig. 21-3), including Brodmann area 40 and probably area 39.[51,61,63] (SII is an inferior parietal cortical region, but it is defined physiologically.) However, the posterior insula may also play a role: positron emission tomography (PET) studies have shown a somatotopic representation in humans,[20] and lesions causing tactile agnosia have included but were not restricted to the posterior insula.[51,63] The observation that tactile agnosia results from damage to the inferior parietal lobule supports the idea that certain parts of the human inferior parietal lobule are homologous to simian area 7b (area 7 is located in the superior parietal lobule of humans but is inferior to the intraparietal sulcus of monkeys).[61,63]

Based upon behavioral[70] and anatomic[76] studies in monkeys and behavioral-anatomic correlation studies in humans,[63] it has been posited that there are dual streams of somesthetic information processing, including a ventral stream concerned with object recognition, tactual learning, and memory and a dorsal stream possibly concerned with sensorimotor integration and somesthetic spatiotemporal functions. Lesions of the ventral object-recognition pathway result in tactile agnosia, and lesions of the dorsal sensorimotor-integration pathway result in severe apraxia and a type of astereognosis. Neither somatosensory association cortex syndrome reflects damage to SI.

The Dorsomedial Somatosensory Association Cortex Syndrome: Apraxia-Astereognosis Syndrome

An unusual type of astereognosis results from damage to the dorsomedial somatosensory associ-

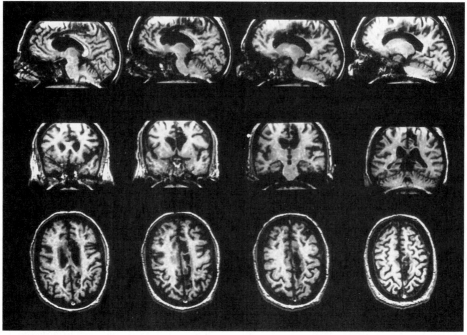

Figure 21-4

T₁-weighted sagittal (top row), *coronal* (middle row), *and transverse* (bottom row) *MRI of a patient with infarction of left mesial frontal and parietal cortices who had the "dorsomedial syndrome" (see text).*

ation cortices,[63] though more cases need to be studied. Patients with extensive damage to SMA and SSA (Fig. 21-4) have moderate to severe impairment of basic, intermediate, and complex somesthetic functions. They have severe limb apraxia with an extremely disordered tactile search strategy. In addition to the faulty spatial and temporal control of movements that characterize the apraxia, they have an analogous spatio-temporal defect of somesthetic perception: they have difficulty localizing a stimulus within a limb or telling whether they have been touched once or twice. Finally, they show surprisingly good recovery in the chronic stages.

Somesthetic Results of Other Behavioral Disorders

Cerebral Commissurotomy Studies of patients with complete separation of the cerebral hemispheres have shown that the somesthetic representation of the limbs is more highly lateralized than that of the trunk.[77] Stimuli presented to the right hand can be described by the perceiving and linguistically eloquent left hemisphere. Objects presented to the left hand are equally well recognized, but cannot be named by the linguistically deprived right hemisphere. The right hemisphere is superior on some perceptual and tactile-memory tasks,[78,79] and children have better left- than right-hand ability in learning Braille.[80]

Amnesia Patients have difficulty with new learning in somatosensory[70] and other[81] modalities.

Tactile Aphasia This is a somatosensory modality–specific naming impairment and therefore a type of aphasia,[66] which should not be confused with tactile agnosia.

Asymboly for Pain   As Critchley states, "there is nothing symbolic about a pain stimulus or the patient's reaction thereto,"[55] so the term itself is unfortunate. Nonetheless, PET studies have demonstrated that painful thermal stimuli activate not only somatosensory cortices but anterior cingulate cortex as well,[82] an area thought to play a role in emotion. Anosognosia (unawareness of illness) and anosodiaphoria (unconcern about illness) lend further credence to the concept of pathologic disregard for the painful nature of a stimulus. Lesion studies of patients with asymboly for pain, however, have implicated the posterior insula as the critical substrate,[83] and such findings have been thought to support Geschwind's theory[84] that asymboly for pain is a disconnection syndrome between the ventrolateral somatosensory cortices and mesial temporal limbic structures.[83]

DEGENERATIVE DISEASES AS A CAUSE OF CORTICAL SENSORY LOSS

Any lesion affecting somatosensory cortices can result in cortical patterns of sensory loss, but the severe cortical somatosensory impairments caused by certain degenerative brain diseases are underrecognized.

Degeneration of primary sensorimotor cortices, or of more posteriorly situated parietal cortices (including mesial hemispheric cortices) causes gradually progressive apraxic disorders (including limb, constructional, dressing, and writing apraxia) as well as astereognosis,[85] consistent with the dorsomedial somatosensory association cortex syndrome (Fig. 21-5). Tactile object recognition occasionally is more severely affected than more basic somesthetic functions, reminiscent of tactile agnosia, though it is rarely pure when it occurs in a degenerative context. Although a tumor or other structural lesion should be sought, severe sensorimotor impairment evolving over a few years in an elderly patient is commonly degenerative. Several pathologic patterns have been described, including corticobasal degeneration with neuronal achromasia, nonspecific degenerative changes, Alzhei-

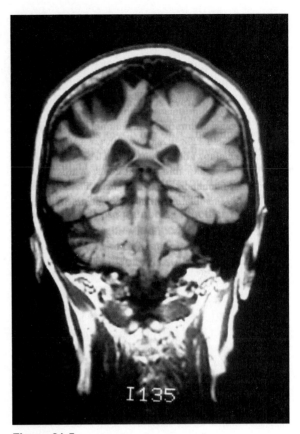

Figure 21-5
T₁-weighted coronal MRI of a patient with corticobasal degeneration primarily involving the right hemisphere who had severe apraxia and astereognosis affecting the left arm.

mer disease, and Pick disease. Clinical features overlap extensively between these varied histologies.

REFERENCES

1. Darian-Smith I: The sense of touch: Performance and peripheral neural processes, in *Handbook of Physiology—The Nervous System III.* Bethesda, MD, American Physiological Society, 1984, pp 739–788.
2. Johansson RS, Vallbo AB: Tactile sensibility in the human hand: Relative and absolute densities of four types of mechanoreceptive units in glabrous skin. *J Physiol Lond* 286:283–300, 1979.

3. Johnson KO, Phillips JR: A rotating drum stimulator for scanning embossed patterns and textures across skin. *J Neurosci Meth* 22:221–231, 1988.

4. Phillips JR, Johansson RS, Johnson KO: Representation of Braille characters in human nerve fibres. *Exp Brain Res* 81:589–592, 1990.

5. Johnson KO, Hsiao SS: Neural mechanisms of tactual form and texture perception. *Ann Rev Neurosci* 15:227–250, 1992.

6. Phillips JR, Johnson KO, Hsiao SS: Spatial pattern representation and transformation in monkey somatosensory cortex. *Proc Natl Acad Sci USA* 85:1317–1321, 1988.

7. Torebjork HE, Ochoa JL: Specific sensations evoked by activity in single identified sensory units in man. *Acta Physiol Scand* 110:445–447, 1980.

8. Vega-Bermudez F, Johnson KO, Hsiao SS: Human tactile pattern recognition: Active versus passive touch, velocity effects, and patterns of confusion. *J Neurophysiol* 65:531–546, 1991.

9. Klatzky RL, McCloskey B, Doherty S, et al: Knowledge about hand shaping and knowledge about objects. *J Mot Behav* 19:187–213, 1987.

10. Lederman SJ, Klatzky RL: Hand movements: A window into haptic object recognition. *Cognit Psychol* 19:342–368, 1987.

11. Marshall WH, Woolsey CN, Bard R: Cortical representation of tactile sensibility as indicated by cortical potentials. *Science* 85:388–390, 1937.

12. Woolsey CN, Fairman D: Contralateral, ipsilateral, and bilateral representation of cutaneous receptors in somatic areas I and II of cerebral cortex of pig, sheep, and other animals. *Surgery* 19:684–702, 1946.

13. Penfield W, Jasper H: *Epilepsy and the Functional Anatomy of the Human Brain.* Boston, Little, Brown, 1954.

14. Kaas JH, Sur M, Nelson RJ, Merzenich MM: The postcentral somatosensory cortex: Multiple representations of the body in primates, in Woolsey CN, (ed): *Cortical Sensory Organization.* Clifton, NJ: *Humana Press,* 1981, vol 1, pp 29–45.

15. Kaas JH: The segregation of function in the nervous system: Why do sensory systems have so many subdivisions?, in Neff WD (ed): *Contributions to Sensory Physiology.* New York, Academic Press, 1982, vol 7, pp 201–240.

16. Kaas JH: What, if anything, is SI? Organization of first somatosensory area of cortex. *Physiol Rev* 63:206–231, 1983.

17. Robinson CJ, Burton H: Somatotopographic organization in the second somatosensory area of *M. fascicularis. J Comp Neurol* 192:43–67, 1980.

18. Lueders H, Lesser RP, Dinner DS, et al: The second sensory area in humans: Evoked potential and electrical stimulation studies. *Ann Neurol* 17:177–184, 1985.

19. Hari R, Karhu J, Hamalainen M, et al: Functional organization of human first and second somatosensory cortices: A neuromagnetic study. *Eur J Neurosci* 5:724–734, 1993.

20. Burton H, Videen TO, Raichle ME: Tactile-vibration-activated foci in insular and parietal-opercular cortex studied with positron emission tomography: Mapping the second somatosensory area in humans. *Somat Mot Res* 10:297–308, 1993.

21. Darian-Smith I, Isbister J, Mok H, Yokota T: Somatic sensory cortical projection areas excited by tactile stimulation of the cat: A triple representation. *J Physiol (Lond)* 182:671–689, 1966.

22. Clemo HR, Stein BE: Somatosensory cortex: A "new" somatotopic representation. *Brain Res* 235:162–168, 1982.

23. Clemo HR, Stein BE: Organization of a fourth somatosensory area of cortex in cat. *J Neurophysiol* 50:910–925, 1983.

24. Burton H, Robinson CJ: Organization of the SII parietal cortex: Multiple somatic sensory representations within and near the second somatic sensory area of cynomologus monkeys, in Woolsey CN (ed): *Cortical Sensory Organization.* Clifton, NJ: Humana Press, 1981, vol 1, pp 67–119.

25. Friedman DP: Body topography in the second somatic sensory area: Monkey SII somatotopy, in Woolsey CN (ed): *Cortical Sensory Organization.* Clifton, NJ: Humana Press, 1981, vol 1, pp 121–165.

26. Blomquist AJ, Lorenzini CA: Projection of dorsal roots and sensory nerves to cortical sensory motor regions of squirrel monkey. *J Neurophysiol* 28:1195–1205, 1965.

27. Bowker RM, Coulter JD: Intracortical connectivities of somatic sensory and motor areas: Multiple cortical pathways in monkeys, in Woolsey CN (ed): *Cortical Sensory Organization.* Clifton, NJ: Humana Press, 1981, vol 1, pp 205–242.

28. Murray EA, Coulter JD: Supplementary sensory area: The medial parietal cortex in the monkey, in Woolsey CN (ed): *Cortical Sensory Organization.* Clifton, NJ: Humana Press, 1981, vol 1, pp 167–195.

29. Penfield W, Welch K: The supplementary motor area of the cerebral cortex: A clinical and experi-

mental study. *AMA Arch Neurol Psychiatry* 66:289–317, 1951.

30. Van Buren JM, Fedio P: Functional representation on the medial aspect of the frontal lobe in man. *J Neurosurg* 44:275–289, 1976.

31. Fried I, Katz A, McCarthy G, et al: Functional organization of human supplementary motor cortex studied by electrical stimulation. *J Neurosci* 11:3656–3666, 1991.

32. Laplane D, Talairach J, Meininger V, et al: Clinical consequences of corticectomies involving the supplementary motor area in humans. *J Neurol Sci* 34:301–314, 1977.

33. Sanides F: Functional architecture of motor and sensory cortices in primates in the light of a new concept of neocortex evolution, in Noback CR, Montagna W (eds): *The Primate Brain: Advances in Primatology.* New York, Appleton-Century-Crofts, 1970, vol 1, pp 137–208.

34. Burton H: Second somatosensory cortex and related areas, in Jones EG, Peters A (eds): *Cerebral Cortex: Sensory-Motor Areas and Aspects of Cortical Connectivity.* New York: Plenum Press, 1985, vol 5, pp 31–98.

35. Cavada C, Goldman-Rakic PS: Posterior parietal cortex in rhesus monkey: I. Parcellation of areas based on distinctive limbic and sensory corticocortical connections. *J Comp Neurol* 287:393–421, 1989.

36. Pons TP, Garraghty PE, Friedman DP, Mishkin M: Physiological evidence for serial processing in somatosensory cortex. *Science* 237:417–420, 1987.

37. Johansson RS, LaMotte RH: Tactile detection of a single asperity on an otherwise smooth surface. *Somat Res* 1:21–31, 1983.

38. Srinivasan MA, Whitehouse JM, LaMotte RH: Tactile detection of slip: Surface microgeometry and peripheral neural codes. *J Neurophysiol* 63:1323–1332, 1990.

39. Johnson KO, Phillips JR: Tactile spatial resolution: I. Two-point discrimination, gap detection, grating resolution, and letter recognition. *J Neurophysiol* 46:1177–1191, 1981.

40. Verrillo RT, Fraioli AJ, Smith RL: Sensation magnitude of vibrotactile stimuli. *Percept Psychophys* 6:366–372, 1969.

41. Mountcastle VB, LaMotte RH, Carli G: Detection thresholds for stimuli in humans and monkeys: Comparisons with threshold events in mechanoreceptive afferent nerve fibers innervating the monkey hand. *J Neurophysiol* 35:122–136, 1972.

42. Mountcastle VB, Steinmetz MA, Romo R: Frequency discrimination in the sense of flutter: Psychophysical measurements correlated with postcentral events in behaving monkeys. *J Neurosci* 10:3032–3044, 1990.

43. Loomis JM: Tactile recognition of raised letters: A parametric study. *Bull Psychosom Soc* 23:18–20, 1985.

44. Lederman SJ: Tactile roughness of grooved surfaces: The touching process and effects of macro- and micro-surface structure. *Percept Psychophys* 16:385–395, 1974.

45. Sathian K, Goodwin AW, Darian-Smith I: Perceived roughness of a grating: Correlation with responses of mechanoreceptive afferents innervating the monkeys fingerpad. *J Neurosci* 9:1273–1279, 1989.

46. Lamb G: Tactile discrimination of textured surfaces: Psychophysical performance measurements in humans. *J Physiol* 338:551–565, 1983.

47. Klatzky RL, Lederman S, Reed C: Haptic integration of object properties: Texture, hardness, and planar contour. *J Exp Psychol: Hum Percep Perf* 15:45–57, 1989.

48. Reed CL, Lederman SJ, Klatzky RL: Haptic integration of planar size with hardness, texture, and planar contour. *Can J Psychol* 44:522–545, 1990.

49. Members of the Department of Neurology Mayo Clinic and Mayo Foundation for Medical Education and Research: *Clinical Examinations in Neurology,* 6th ed. St Louis, Mosby-Year Book, 1991, pp 255–275.

50. Lezak MD: *Neuropsychological Assessment,* 2d ed. New York, Oxford University Press, 1983.

51. Caselli RJ: Rediscovering tactile agnosia. *Mayo Clin Proc* 66:129–142, 1991.

52. Klatzky RL, Lederman SJ, Metzger VA: Identifying objects by touch: An "expert system." *Percept Psychophys* 37:299–302, 1985.

53. Craig JC: Tactile pattern perception and its perturbations. *J Acoust Soc Am* 77:238–246, 1985.

54. Dyck PJ, Karnes J, O'Brien PC, Zimmerman IR: Detection threshold of cutaneous sensation in humans, in Dyck PJ, Thomas PK, Griffin JW (eds): *Peripheral Neuropathy,* 3d ed. Philadelphia, Saunders, 1993, pp 706–728.

55. Critchley M: *The Parietal Lobes.* New York, Hafner, 1971, pp 86–155.

56. Head H, Holmes G: Sensory disturbances from cerebral lesions. *Brain* 34:102–254, 1911–1912.

57. Bassetti C, Bogousslavsky J, Regli F: Sensory syn-

dromes in parietal stroke. *Neurology* 43:1942–1949, 1993.

58. McHenry LC: *Garrison's History of Neurology.* Springfield, IL, Charles C Thomas, 1969, p 297.

59. Delay JPL: *Les Asterognosies, Pathologie du Toucher, Clinique, Physiologique, Topographie.* Paris, Masson, 1935.

60. Teuber HL: Postscript: Some needed revisions of the clinical views of agnosia. *Neuropsychologia* 3:371–378, 1965.

61. Reed CL, Caselli RJ: The nature of tactile agnosia: A case study. *Neuropsychologia* 32:527–539, 1994.

62. Tranel D: What has been rediscovered in "rediscovering tactile agnosia"? (editorial). *Mayo Clin Proc* 66:210–214, 1991.

63. Caselli RJ: Ventrolateral and dorsomedial somatosensory association cortex infarction produce distinct somesthetic syndromes. *Neurology* 43:762–771, 1993.

64. Halpern L: Astereognosis not of cortical origin. *J Neurol Sci* 7:245–250, 1968.

65. Norrsell U: Behavioral studies of the somatosensory system. *Psychol Rev* 60:327–354, 1980.

66. Beauvois MF, Saillant B, Meininger V, Lhermitte F: Bilateral tactile aphasia: A tacto-verbal dysfunction. *Brain* 101:381–401, 1978.

67. Caselli RJ: Somesthetic syndrome (letter). *Neurology* 43:2423–2424, 1993.

68. Caselli RJ: Bilateral impairment of somesthetically mediated object recognition in humans. *Mayo Clin Proc* 66:357–364, 1991.

69. Mishkin M: Analogous neural models for tactual and visual learning. *Neuropsychologia* 17:139–150, 1979.

70. Corkin S: Tactually-guided maze-learning in man: Effects of unilateral cortical excisions and bilateral hippocampal lesions. *Neuropsychologia* 3:339–351, 1965.

71. Garcha HS, Ettlinger G: The effects of unilateral or bilateral removals of the second somatosensory cortex (area SII): A profound tactile disorder in monkeys. *Cortex* 14:319–326, 1978.

72. Garcha HS, Ettlinger G: Tactile discrimination learning in the monkey: The effects of unilateral or bilateral removals of the second somatosensory cortex (area SII). *Cortex* 16:397–412, 1980.

73. Garcha HS, Ettlinger G, Maccabe JJ: Unilateral removal of the second somatosensory projection cortex in the monkey: Evidence for cerebral predominance? *Brain* 105:787–810, 1982.

74. Meyer JS: Does diaschisis have clinical correlates? *Mayo Clin Proc* 66:430–432, 1991.

75. Warrington EK, Taylor AM: The contribution of the right parietal lobe to object recognition. *Cortex* 9:152–164, 1973.

76. Friedman DP, Murray EA, O'Neill JB, Mishkin M: Cortical connections of the somatosensory fields of the lateral sulcus of macaques: Evidence for a corticolimbic pathway for touch. *J Comp Neurol* 252:323–347, 1986.

77. Gazzaniga MS, Bogen JE, Sperry RW: Laterality effects following cerebral commissurotomy in man. *Neuropsychologia* 1:209–215, 1963.

78. Milner B, Taylor L: Right-hemisphere superiority in tactile pattern-recognition after cerebral commissurotomy: Evidence for nonverbal memory. *Neuropsychologia* 10:1–15, 1972.

79. Sperry RW: Cerebral organization and behavior. *Science* 133:1749–1757, 1981.

80. Rudel RG, Denckla MB, Spalten E: The functional asymmetry of Braille letter learning in normal, sighted children. *Neurology* 24:733–738, 1974.

81. Milner B: Visually-guided maze learning in man: Effects of bilateral hippocampal, bilateral frontal, and unilateral cerebral lesions. *Neuropsychologia* 3:317–338, 1965.

82. Talbot JD, Marrett S, Evans AC, et al: Multiple representations of pain in human cerebral cortex. *Science* 251:1355–1358, 1991.

83. Berthier M, Starkstein S, Leiguarda R: Asymbolia for pain: A sensory-limbic disconnection syndrome. *Ann Neurol* 24:41–49, 1988.

84. Geschwind N: Disconnexion syndromes in animals and man. *Brain* 88:237–294, 1965.

85. Caselli RJ, Jack CR Jr: Asymmetric cortical degeneration syndromes: A proposed clinical classification. *Arch Neurol* 49:770–780, 1992.

86. Caselli RJ, Jack CR Jr, Petersen RC, et al: Asymmetric cortical degenerative syndromes: Clinical, planar MRI, MRI-based surface rendering, and SPECT correlations. *Neurology* 42:1462–1468, 1992.

Chapter 22

DISORDERS OF
BODY PERCEPTION

Georg Goldenberg

LEVELS OF INFORMATION ABOUT ONE'S BODY

In this chapter we distinguish three levels at which information about one's body is perceived and represented, as outlined below.

A Body-Centered Reference System for Motor Actions

Information about the current configuration and position of one's body is a necessary prerequisite for the planning and execution of most movements aimed at external targets. Reaching with the hand for a visually presented object requires that the retinotopic coordinates of the perceived object be transformed into body-centered coordinates. This transformation has to take into account the current position of the eyes relative to the head and of the head relative to the trunk. In addition to the representation of the target in body-centered coordinates, the brain must also represent the initial arm configuration in order to plan the trajectory. Single-cell recordings in monkeys have provided evidence that cells in Brodmann's areas 7 and 5 in the posterior parietal lobe are informed about the current position and configuration of the eyes, head, body, and limbs and perform the computations necessary for transforming visually perceived locations into body-centered coordinates.[1–4]

Reaching for an object is a highly automatized task. One need not pay attention to the position and configuration of one's body in order to accurately reach for a seen object. Assessment of the body-centered reference frame and computation of the target's location in body-centered coordinates take place automatically and without necessitating conscious awareness of one's body.

Awareness of One's Own Body

One can, of course, pay attention to the position and configuration of one's own body. Vestibular, kinesthetic, tactile, and visual perceptions provide information about the actual position and configuration of one's body; but even without distinct afferences from these channels, one has a basic "feeling" of where one's body parts are. One can point to the tip of one's nose without a mirror even if the nose does not itch. This basic awareness of the limits and the spatial layout of one's own body has been conceptualized as a mental "body schema."[6]

General Knowledge about the Human Body

General knowledge about human body and body parts can be of different kinds.[6] On the one hand, there is lexical and semantic knowledge, which defines the names, categories, and functions of body parts. This knowledge specifies, for example, that the wrist and ankle are both articulations or that the mouth is for speaking and the ear for hearing. On the other hand, there is topographic knowledge about the spatial layout of body parts.

This knowledge provides information about the positions of individual body parts, the proximity relations that exist between them, and the boundaries that define each body part. For example, it specifies that the nose is in the middle of the face and that its upper end is contiguous to the forehead with the line of the eyebrows marking the border between them.

One's own body is one instance of the general configuration of human bodies. Pointing on command to parts of one's own body therefore assesses both awareness of one's own body and general knowledge about the human body.

With this classification in mind, we will discuss the following neuropsychological symptoms: optic ataxia, body-part phantoms, unilateral neglect, autotopagnosia, finger agnosia, and impaired imitation of gestures in ideomotor apraxia.

OPTIC ATAXIA

Optic ataxia was originally described in association with apraxia of gaze and simultanagnosia but has since then been recognized as an independent symptom that can occur without the other elements of Balint syndrome.[8–11] Patients with optic ataxia cannot accurately reach for visually perceived external targets. They move a hand into the approximate vicinity of the target and then start searching movements with the hand widely opened. Optic ataxia can occur in association with a general disorder of visuospatial perception, but there are patients who can give accurate judgments about the location and orientation of the objects they are unable to find with the hand.[10] By contrast, such a patient can reach without hesitation or error to parts of his or her own body. Asked to touch the tip of the nose or a finger, they do so as fast and accurately as normal persons.

One interpretation of optic ataxia is that the basic disorder concerns the transformation of retinotopic locations into a body-centered reference frame necessary for movement planning. The patients can reach for parts of their own bodies accurately because they are a priori coded in body-

centered coordinates. At the same time, successful pointing to body parts indicates that awareness of the patient's own body is preserved as well as general conceptual knowledge about the human body.

Anatomic data support this interpretation. Lesions in optic ataxia are centered around the intraparietal sulcus and regularly affect human area 5 in the adjacent superior parietal lobe.[9,10] This location coincides with the location of neurons that have been found to be responsible for transformations from retinotopic to body-centered coordinates in monkeys (see above).

BODY-PART PHANTOMS

The occurrence of phantom limbs has been among the first[5] and continues to be among the most impressive arguments for the contention that the brain houses a mental body schema which underlies and modifies the way we experience our own bodies. After an amputation, about 90 percent of adults experience a phantom of the lost limb.[12–14] Initially, the phantom may be experienced in exactly the same way as the true limb was experienced before amputation. Over time, the experience may become less natural. Particularly where there is an upper limb phantom, the representation of the proximal portion may become weaker and eventually vanish, leading to the strange sensation of a hand belonging to one's own body but being disconnected from it. Alternatively, a shrinking of the proximal portions may lead to "telescoping" and give rise to the belief that the phantom arm is shorter than the other arm or even that a phantom hand resides within the amputation stump.[13,15]

Phantom experiences are not restricted to limbs but have also been reported after the loss of eyes,[16] teeth, external genitalia, and the female breast.[14] Phantoms of the amputated breast occur in about 40 percent of women who undergo mastectomy.[17–21] In about one-third of them, the phantom is limited to the nipple.[18] This restriction of the phantom to the most distal portion of the body part resembles the overrepresentation of the hand and fingers in upper limb phantoms.

Phantoms occur not only after amputation but can be caused by nervous system lesions provided that they interrupt all afferents from the affected body part. This may be the case with lesions of the peripheral nerves, the plexus, and the spinal cord but also with subcortical cerebral lesions.[12,14,22] If the deafferented limb is still present and visible, the phantom may be experienced as an additional, supernumerary limb.[14,22]

The occurrence of sensations in phantoms has been discussed in relation to plastic changes in synaptic connectivity of neurons in the primary sensory cortex. It has been demonstrated that phantom limb sensations can be induced by stimulation of the amputation stump or, in the case of upper limb phantoms, the face, and that there is an exact and reproducible correspondence between the locations of the actual and referred sensations leading to a "remapping" of the phantom on either the stump or the face.[15,23–25] Particularly remapping from the face to the hand is a strong argument in favor of the view that the phantom sensation arises in the primary sensory cortex, as the portion of the postcentral sensory cortex devoted to the face is adjacent to that devoted to the fingers and the hand. Converging evidence for neuronal plasticity in the primary sensory cortex has come from magnetencephalographic investigations showing an enlargement of the primary sensory field of the face in patients with upper limb phantoms.[25] Recently, remapping of sensory stimulation has also been demonstrated in patients with breast phantoms.[26] Tactile sensations from the ipsilateral dorsal thorax, the shoulder, and the pinna were referred to the amputated breast, mainly to the nipple. According to Penfield's homunculus, the somatosensory representations of the stimulated regions could be adjacent to the former representation of the amputated breast.

It is important to emphasize that remapping of stimulations concerns phantom sensations and not the very existence of the phantom. The basic experience of the phantom's existence persists even if no stimulation is applied to corresponding zones of intact body. Consequently, the demonstration that the source of phantom sensations resides in the primary sensory cortex does not necessarily indicate that primary sensory cortex is the neural substrate of the phantom itself.

Further insight into the cerebral substrate of body-part phantoms is provided by observation of patients who have lost the basic experience of the phantom after cerebral lesions. There are a few patients on record in whom a cortical lesion of the posterior parietal lobes abolished a phantom limb on the opposite side of the body.[12,27,28] In one of them (case 2), the clinical evidence strongly suggests preservation of the primary sensory cortex.[28] It can be concluded that integrity of the posterior parietal lobes is necessary for phantom limbs and that integrity of the primary sensory cortex is not sufficient. As there are no observations of restricted postcentral regions in patients with phantom limbs, it cannot be said whether integrity of the posterior parietal lobes is sufficient or integrity of the primary sensory area necessary for phantom limbs.

Body part phantoms are the most direct manifestation of a mental body schema that continues to exist even if it has lost its correlate in the real body. One interesting question is whether this mental body schema is innate or acquired by experience. An argument for the native predetermination of the representation of one's own body is the occurrence of limb phantoms in persons with congenital absence of limbs or with amputations in early childhood.[12,13,29] However, the frequency of phantom limbs in persons who lost their limbs before the age of 6 appears to be only some 10 percent as compared to about 50 percent in persons amputated between 6 and 10 years and 90 percent in persons amputated later· (Piorreck, cited in Ref. 13). This increase would suggest that the mental body schema is at least enhanced and made more durable by continuing experience of the intact body. The case for a significant shaping of the body schema by experience is even stronger for breast phantoms. Girls do not have phantoms of their "congenitally absent" future breasts. In adult women, the frequency of breast phantoms diminishes with advancing age at mastectomy.[17–21] This apparent weakening of the mental representation of the breast might reflect the age-related decline of the breasts' volume and tension. Thus, the breasts' mental representations change in accord with the biological changes of the breasts across the life cycle. It would appear highly improbable that the course of these alterations is innately preprogrammed in the neural substrate of the body schema.

NEGLECT OF ONE-HALF OF THE BODY

Patients with hemineglect may neglect not only one-half of external space but also one-half of their own body. When combing, washing, shaving, or dressing, they restrict grooming to the nonneglected half of the body. When asked to indicate with the normal hand the midline of the body, they deviate to the healthy side,[11,30] as if the nonneglected half of the body were thinner or completely absent. When asked to touch the neglected hand with the normal one, the reaching movement may end at the shoulder or even at the midline of the trunk.[31]

Only a few studies have looked for the possibility that personal neglect of one-half of the body dissociates from extrapersonal neglect of one-half of surrounding space. A group study found only 1 out of 97 right-brain-damaged patients in whom personal neglect was not associated with extrapersonal neglect, while the reverse dissociation was far more frequent. Another group study[32] included only right-brain-damaged patients who displayed evidence of neglect on conventional tests like star cancellation. As these tests assess neglect in extrapersonal space, there was a priori no possibility of finding a patient in whom personal neglect was not associated with extrapersonal neglect. However, the authors found that success on tasks sensitive to personal neglect correlated only weakly with success on tasks sensitive to extrapersonal neglect. The same group then published a single case study of a patient who, after a right parietal hemmorhage, displayed conspicuous neglect of the left half of his own body but no sign of neglect of extrapersonal space even in extensive testing.[33]

In view of the paucity of systematic observation, it would be premature to speculate as to the location of lesions responsible for personal as opposed to extrapersonal neglect. It is not even clear whether the preponderance of left-sided hemineglect applies to personal neglect, as the large studies that established this hemispheric asymmetry were all restricted to measures of extrapersonal neglect.

Body part phantoms and neglect of one-half of the body are both disorders that concern the awareness of the patient's own body. Kinematic analyses do reveal abnormalities of reaching to external targets in patients with left hemineglect.[11,34,35] The patients were selected for having neglect of extrapersonal space, and it is not clear whether they had personal neglect at all. In any case, the abnormalities are different from those shown by patients with optic ataxia. Movements toward targets in the neglected half of space are slowed down and the movement path may deviate toward the nonaffected side of space, but the patients ultimately reach visible targets accurately and without searching. Apparently they are able to translate retinotopic localization into body-centered coordinates.

General knowledge about the human body is preserved in patients with phantom limbs or personal hemineglect. They are able to point on command to body parts on a model and even on their own bodies provided that these parts are not amputated or, respectively, neglected.[33] There are, however, reports of impaired performance on visuoconstructional tasks involving the human body, like assembling a human figure from its parts or judging the laterality of rotated hands[33,36] in patients with personal hemineglect. As the affected patients had right brain damage, it is questionable whether these symptoms were due to a lack of topographic knowledge about the human body or an expression of general visuoconstructional difficulties.

AUTOTOPAGNOSIA

Taken literally, the term *autotopagnosia* would indicate an inability to recognize locations on one's own body, but it is generally understood as designating the inability to localize body parts on one's own body as well as on another person or on a model of the human body. The term *somatotopagnosia*[37] would be more appropriate but has not found wide acceptance.

Earlier case reports of autotopagnosia have been criticized as demonstrating nothing more than the effects of general mental deterioration or of aphasia on the task of pointing to body parts on verbal command,[38] but since then several carefully conducted single-case studies have established the independence of autotopagnosia from aphasia and dementia and have drawn a consistent clinical picture of "pure" autotopagnosia:[1,39–41] when asked to point to body parts on themselves, on another person, or on a model of the human body, the patients commit errors. The majority of these errors are "contiguity" errors, in which the patient points to a different body part in the vicinity of the designated one. Less frequent are "semantic" errors which confuse body parts of the same category—as, for example, the elbow and the knee. Errors occur not only when the body parts are designated by verbal command but also when they are shown on pictures or even when the examiner demonstrates correct pointing and the patient tries to imitate. Patients with pure autotopagnosia are able to name the body parts when they are pointed at by someone else or shown on pictures, and although they invariably have left-sided brain lesions (see below), several of them were not aphasic at all.[6,39,40,43] Some patients were asked to give verbal descriptions of body parts. They could describe the function and the individual visual appearance of body parts but got lost when asked to describe their location.[6,39,40] According to the classification proposed in the opening of this chapter, this pattern of deficits would correspond to a selective loss of knowledge about the spatial layout of the human body.

The selectivity of this spatial disturbance has been disputed. It has been found that single patients committed errors also when asked to point to single parts of other multi-part objects than the human body as, for example, a bicycle or a house,[40,43] and it has been concluded that they suffer from a general inability to "analyze a whole into its parts." However, since this proposal was published, additional reports have documented patients with autotopagnosia who could locate the parts of multipart objects other than the human body.[6,39,41]

There are patients with autotopagnosia in whom localizing of individual fingers was found to be preserved.[40,42] We discuss further differences between autotopagnosia and finger agnosia in the next section but want to stress now that the preserved ability to differentiate the individual fingers of the hand is a further argument against a general deficit of "analyzing a whole into its parts."

Reaching to external targets and hence the computation of body-centered coordinates is unimpaired in autotopagnosia. Awareness of one's own body is difficult to assess formally, as autotopagnosia itself affects reaching for body parts. There are, nonetheless, observations suggesting that awareness of the patient's own body is preserved in autotopagnosia. One patient could correctly point to body parts when asked where certain garments are worn.[41] Another patient could locate her body parts when small objects where fixed to them and she was asked to point either to the objects or, after they had been removed, to their remembered locations.[6] Apparently these patients could orient themselves on their own bodies. Autotopagnosia seems to result from the inability to link preserved spatial orientation on one's own body with general knowledge about the human body.

The lesions in cases of pure autotopagnosia are remarkably uniform. They always affect the posterior parietal lobe of the left hemisphere.[39–43] In a group study of patients with left- or right-sided brain damage, errors in pointing to body parts occurred only in left-brain-damaged patients.[44] In this unselected sample, there were no cases of pure autotopagnosia. The patients who committed errors in localizing body parts were all aphasic and had on average larger lesions than patients who performed without error.

FINGER AGNOSIA

Finger agnosia was originally been described as part of the "Gerstmann syndrome,"[45] which is a combination of finger agnosia with right-left confusion, acalculia, and agraphia. However, it has been demonstrated that these are unrelated symptoms, which may or may not happen to occur together.[46]

The value of verbal tasks of finger identification has been called into question because they may be more sensitive to language disorders than to defective orientation on the body.[38,44] However, a considerable number of brain-damaged patients fail on nonverbal tasks of finger localization, like pointing on a drawing of a hand to fingers touched on the patient's own hand.[38,44,47]

Finger agnosia has been considered as a minor form of autotopagnosia,[45] but whereas autotopagnosia as characterized by errors in pointing to proximal body parts has been observed exclusively in patients with left brain damage, finger agnosia occurs with approximately equal frequency in patients with left and right brain damage.[38,44,47,48] We have already mentioned that there are patients with autotopagnosia in whom identification of fingers is preserved. If they are compared with those right-brain-damaged patients who have difficulties with the localization of fingers but not with pointing to proximal body parts,[44] there emerges a double dissociation between autotopagnosia and finger agnosia.

Common neuropsychological wisdom would suggest that a task which is sensitive to both left- and right-hemispheric damage does not tap a single psychological function. Presumably, disturbances of finger localization have different reasons in left- and right-brain-damaged patients.

IDEOMOTOR APRAXIA

Ideomotor apraxia is a symptom of left brain damage, which is usually considered as a disorder of motor control.[49–52] (See Chap. 16.) In particular, defective imitation of gestures has been considered as testifying a deficit of motor execution. In the words of de Renzi, "Since the examiner provides the model and the patient has only to copy it, errors can only be due to a deficit of motor execution."[51] This argument seems to be particularly convincing if novel and meaningless gestures are to be imitated. Whereas imitation of familiar and meaningful gestures could be mediated by preexisting knowledge of the gestures' spatial configuration, imitation of meaningless gestures appears to test a direct route from visual perception to motor execution.[53–55]

There is, however, an alternative interpretation of the task demands of imitation of meaningless gestures. It proposes that general topographic knowledge about the human body mediates the transition from visual perception to motor execution.[56–59] Application of this knowledge reduces the multiple visually perceived details of the demonstrated gesture to simple relationships between a limited number of significant body parts, which can easily be implemented in routine motor programs. As a further advantage, translating the gesture's visual appearance in terms of the human body produces an equivalence between demonstration and imitation that is independent of the particular angle of view under which the demonstration is perceived.

The idea that defective imitation of gestures is due to a lack of topographic knowledge about the human body likens it to autotopagnosia. The parallel between defective imitation of meaningless gestures and autotopagnosia was strengthened by a study by the author who examined imitation of three kinds of gestures: for imitation of hand postures, the patients were required to copy different positions of the hand relative to the head while the configuration of the fingers remained invariant; for imitation of finger postures, patients were asked to replicate different configurations of the fingers, and the position of the whole hand relative to the body was not considered for scoring; for imitation of combined gestures, both a defined position of the hand relative to the body and defined configuration of the fingers were required.[59] Regardless of whether imitations of hand positions and finger configurations were tested each on their own or together, they proved to show differential susceptibility to left and right brain damage. Whereas imitation of finger configurations was about equally impaired in left- and right-brain-damaged patients, defective imitation of hand positions occurred exclusively in left-brain-damaged patients, and whereas controls as well as right-brain-damaged patients committed fewer errors with hand positions than with finger configurations, the reverse was the case in left-brain-damaged patients. This dissociation between gestures requiring orientation relative to the proximal body and gestures requiring orientation within the hand closely resembles the above-mentioned dissociation between autotopagnosia and finger agnosia.

A lack of general knowledge about the human body should lead to errors regardless of whether gestures are to be replicated on another body or on oneself. Indeed, patients who display apraxia on imitation of hand positions commit more errors than either left-brain-damaged patients without apraxia or right-brain-damaged patients when trying to replicate the same positions on a manikin.[57]

REFERENCES

1. Mountcastle VB, Lynch JC, Georgopoulos A, et al: Posterior parietal association cortex of the monkey: Command functions for operations within extrapersonal space. *J Neurophysiol* 38:871–908, 1975.

2. Andersen RA: Visual and eye movement functions of the posterior parietal cortex. *Annu Rev Neurosci* 12:377–403, 1989.

3. Bizzi E, Mussa-Ivaldi FA: Motor control, in Boller F, Grafman J (eds): *Handbook of Neuropsychology.* New York: Elsevier, 1990, vol 2, pp 229–244.

4. Stein JF: The representation of egocentric space in the posterior parietal cortex. *Behav Brain Sci* 15:691–700, 1992.

5. Pick A: Zur Pathologie des Bewußtseins vom eigenen Körper—Ein Beitrag aus der Kriegsmedizin. *Neurol Zentralbl* 34:257–265, 1915.

6. Sirigu A, Grafman J, Bressler K, Sunderland T: Multiple representations contribute to body knowledge processing. *Brain* 114:629–642, 1991.

7. Balint R: Seelenlaehmung des "Schauens," optische Ataxie, räumliche Störung der Aufmerksamkeit. *Monatsschr Psychiat Neurol* 25:51–81, 1909.

8. Rondot P, de Recondo J, Dumas JLR: Visuomotor ataxia. *Brain* 100:355–376, 1977.

9. Damasio AR, Benton AL: Impairment of hand movements under visual guidance. *Neurology* 29:170–178, 1979.

10. Perenin MT, Vighetto A: Optic ataxia: A specific disruption in visuomotor mechanisms: I. Different aspects of the deficit in reaching for objects. *Brain* 111:643–674, 1988.

11. Jeannerod M: *The Neural and Behavioural Organization of Goal-Directed Movements.* Oxford, England: Clarendon Press, 1988.

12. Poeck K: Zur Psychophysiologie der Phantomerlebnisse. *Nervenarzt* 34:241–256, 1963.

13. Poeck K: Phantome nach Amputation und bei angeborenen Gliedmaßenmangel. *Dtsche med Wochensch* 46:2367–2374, 1969.

14. Frederiks JAM: Phantom limb and phantom limb pain, in Frederiks JAM (ed): *Handbook of Neurology:* New York: Elsevier, 1985, vol 1, pp 395–404.

15. Haber WE: Observations on phantom-limb phenomena. *Arch Neurol Psychiatry* 75:624–636, 1956.

16. Cohn R: Phantom vision. *Arch Neurol* 25:468–471, 1971.

17. Simmel ML: A study of phantoms after amputation of the breast. *Neuropsychologia* 4:331–350, 1966.

18. Jarvis JH: Post-mastectomy breast phantoms. *J Nerv Ment Dis* 144:266–272, 1967.

19. Jamison K, Wellisch DK, Katz RL, Pasnau RO: Phantom breast syndrome. *Arch Surg* 114:93–95, 1979.

20. Weinstein S, Vetter RJ, Sersen EA: Phantoms following breast amputation. *Neuropsychologia* 8:185–197, 1970.

21. Kroner K, Krebs B, Skov J, Jorgensen HJ: Immediate and long-term phantom breast syndrome after mastectomy: Incidence, clinical characteristics and relationship to pre-mastectomy breast pain. *Pain* 36:327–334, 1989.

22. Halligan PW, Marshall JC, Wade DT: Three arms: A case study of supernumerary phantom limb after right hemisphere stroke. *J Neurol Neurosurg Psychiatry* 56:159–166, 1993.

23. Ramachandran VS: Behavioral and magnetoencephalographic correlates of plasticity in the adult human brain. *Proc Natl Acad Sci USA* 90:10413–10420, 1993.

24. Ramachandran VS, Rogers-Ramachandran D, Stewart M: Perceptual correlates of massive cortical reorganization. *Science* 258:1159–1160, 1992.

25. Flor H, Elbert T, Knecht S, et al: Phantom-limb pain as a perceptual correlate of cortical reorganization following arm amputation. *Nature* 375:482–484, 1995.

26. Aglioti S, Cortese F, Franchini C: Rapid sensory remapping in the adult human brain as inferred from phantom breast sensation. *NeuroReport* 5:473–476, 1994.

27. Head H, Holmes G: Sensory disturbances from cerebral lesions. *Brain* 34:102–254, 1911.

28. Appenzeller O, Bicknell JM: Effects of nervous system lesions on phantom experience in amputees. *Neurology* 19:141–146, 1969.

29. Melczack R: Phantom limbs and the concept of a neuromatrix. *Trends Neurosci* 13:88–92, 1990.

30. Karnath HO: Subjective body orientation in neglect and the interactive contribution of neck muscle proprioception and vestibular stimulation. *Brain* 117:1001–1012, 1994.

31. Bisiach E, Perani D, Vallar G, Berti A: Unilateral neglect: Personal and extrapersonal. *Neuropsychologia* 24:759–767, 1986.

32. Zoccolotti P, Judica A: Functional evaluation of hemineglect by means of a semistructured scale: Personal and extrapersonal differentiation. *Neuropsychol Rehab* 1:33–44, 1991.

33. Guariglia C, Antonucci G: Personal and extrapersonal space: A case of neglect dissociation. *Neuropsychologia* 30:1001–1010, 1992.

34. Chieffi S, Gentilucci M, Allport A, et al: Study of selective reaching and grasping in a patient with unilateral parietal lesion. *Brain* 116:1119–1137, 1993.

35. Mattingley JB, Phillips JG, Bradshaw JL: Impairment of movement execution in unilateral neglect: A kinematic analysis of directional bradykinesia. *Neuropsychologia* 32:1111–1134, 1994.

36. Coslett HB: The role of the body image in neglect. *J Clin Exp Neuropsychol* 11:79, 1989.

37. Gerstmann J: Problems of imperception of disease and of impaired body territories with organic lesions: Relation to body scheme and its disorders. *Arch Neurol Psychiatry* 48:890–913, 1942.

38. Poeck K, Orgass B: An experimental investigation of finger agnosia. *Neurology* 19:801–807, 1969.

39. Ogden JA: Autotopagnosia: Occurrence in a patient without nominal aphasia and with an intact ability to point to parts of animals and objects. *Brain* 108:1009–1022, 1985.

40. de Renzi E, Scotti G: Autotopagnosia: Fiction or reality? *Arch Neurol* 23:221–227, 1970.

41. Semenza C: Impairment of localization of body parts following brain damage. *Cortex* 24:443–450, 1988.

42. Assal G, Butters J: Troubles du schéma corporel lors des atteintes hémisphériques gauches. *Schweiz Med Rundsch* 62:172–179, 1973.

43. Poncet M, Pellissier JF, Sebahoun M, Nasser CJ: A propos d'un cas d'autotopagnosie secondaire à une lésion pariéto-occipitale de l'hémisphère majeur. *Encephale* 61:1–14, 1971.

44. Sauguet J, Benton AL, Hecaen H: Disturbances of the body schema in relation to language impairment and hemispheric locus of lesion. *J Neurol Neurosurg Psychiatry* 34:496–501, 1971.

45. Gerstmann J: Zur Symptomatologie der Hirnläsionen im Übergangsgebiet der unteren Parietal- und mittleren Occipitalwindung. *Nervenarzt* 3:691–696, 1930.

46. Benton AL: The fiction of the "Gerstmann syndrome." *J Neurol Neurosurg Psychiatry* 24:176–181, 1961.

47. Gainotti G, Cianchetti C, Tiacci C: The influence of the hemispheric side of lesion on nonverbal tasks of finger localization. *Cortex* 8:364–381, 1972.

48. Kinsbourne M, Warrington EK: A study of finger agnosia. *Brain* 85:47–66, 1962.

49. Liepmann H: *Drei Aufsätze aus dem Apraxiegebiet.* Berlin: Karger, 1908.

50. Poeck K: The two types of motor apraxia. *Arch Ital Biol* 120:361–369, 1982.

51. de Renzi E: Apraxia, in Boller F, Grafman J (eds): *Handbook of Neuropsychology.* New York: Elsevier, 1990, vol 2, pp 245–263.

52. Heilman KM, Rothi LJG: Apraxia, in Heilman KM, Valenstein E (eds): *Clinical Neuropsychology.* New York: Oxford University Press, 1993, pp 141–164.

53. Barbieri C, de Renzi E: The executive and ideational components of apraxia. *Cortex* 24:535–544, 1988.

54. Rothi LJG, Ochipa C, Heilman KM: A cognitive neuropsychological model of limb praxis. *Cog Neuropsychol* 8:443–458, 1991.

55. Roy EA, Hall C: Limb apraxia: A process approach, in Proteau L, Elliott D (eds): *Vision and Motor Control* Amsterdam: Elsevier, 1992, pp 261–282.

56. Morlaas J: *Contribution à l'étude de l'apraxie.* Paris: Amédée Legrand, 1928.

57. Goldenberg G: Imitating gestures and manipulating a mannikin—The representation of the human body in ideomotor apraxia. *Neuropsychologia* 33:63–72, 1995.

58. Goldenberg G, Hermsdörfer J, Spatt J: Ideomotor apraxia and cerebral dominance for motor control. *Cog Brain Res.* In press.

59. Goldenberg G: Defective imitation of gestures in patients with left and right hemisphere lesions. *J Neurol Neurosurg Psychiatry.* In press.

Chapter 23

VISUOSPATIAL AND CONSTRUCTIONAL DISORDERS

Ennio De Renzi

Anatomoclinical correlations in patients with brain injury[1] provided the earliest firm evidence that knowledge of the shape of a stimulus is processed separately from knowledge on its spatial properties (location, orientation, space relation with respect to the examiner, and other objects, and so on). This early work in neuropsychology anticipated the view, later suggested by animal work, that there are two functionally and anatomically separate systems processing visual information—one dealing with knowledge of what an object is and the other with knowledge of where it is.[2] The output of primary visual areas is transmitted to higher perceptual centers following two pathways, one directed to the inferomedial temporal cortex, where the meaning of the stimulus is decoded, and the other to the posterior parietal cortex, where its spatial coordinates are analyzed. The evidence from pathology is consistent with the assumption of a discrete organization for the processing of space data, but, when we pass from animal species to humans, a new variable must be taken into account—the functional specialization of the hemisphere—which assigns a prominent role to the left brain in the semantic identification of the stimulus and to the right brain in the analysis of its spatial properties.

DISORDERS OF PERCEPTION

Right brain–damaged (RBD) patients perform more poorly than left brain–damaged (LBD) pa-

tients on a series of elementary space perception tasks, from point localization[3–5] to depth perception[6–8] and detection of line orientation both in a bidimensional[9] and in a tridimensional space.[10] The superiority of the right hemisphere for this kind of task, brought out by cerebral damage, is paralleled by the left visual field advantage, shown by normal subjects in conditions of lateralized tachistoscopic projection.[11] The same hemispheric asymmetry is also found in the haptic modality both in normals[12] and in brain-damaged patients[10,13] and is likely responsible for the prominent contribution of the right hemisphere to tactile nonsense-shape discrimination. Patients with RBD have been found to perform more poorly than patients with LBD on a task where they had to run the forefinger of the ipsilateral hand along the raised outlines of a meaningless block and then to recognize it on a multiple-choice visual display.[14] The same selective impairment of RBD patients was reported when they were asked to manipulate a nonsense shape and then to match it to sample.[15] In keeping with these findings, commissurotomized patients scored better in a matching-to-sample tactile pattern-recognition test, when they used the left hand (controlled by the right hemisphere) than when they used the right hand (controlled by the left hemisphere),[16] and children submitted to dichaptic stimulation with different shapes performed better with the left hand.[17,18] Mental rotation is a more complex spatial task, involving the ability to imagine how a shape appears when it is rotated on a plane. Hemispheric differences have not been generally found on these tasks,[3,19,20] the only exception being the selective impairment shown by right posterior patients when they were required to judge which hand of a schematic figure, presented upside-down, held a flag.[21]

The data pointing to right hemisphere ascendancy in spatial functions derive from group studies. In single patients, errors of space perception become clinically apparent in various conditions showing no particular hemispheric asymmetry. When they are requested to reach out to an object presented at the periphery of the visual field while keeping central fixation, the limb may be misdirected, sometimes overestimating and sometimes underestimating the distance, until it runs by chance into the target. No hemispheric asymmetry has been shown for misreaching, which does not necessarily imply a deficit of perceptual localization, since it can be due to a disconnection between visual and motor centers. Misreaching is a component of the Balint syndrome and is treated in detail in Chap. 24.

Another rare manifestation of defective space perception is loss of stereopsis. Flattened vision "as if in a picture or a photograph"[22] has occasionally been reported following bilateral occipito-temporal damage.[22–24] Holmes and Horrax's[23] patient was unable to say which of two persons was closer or farther away. Milder deficits of depth perception, of which the patient does not spontaneously complain, are more frequent provided that they are assessed with appropriate techniques. Using Julesz's stereograms, which assess retinal disparity in the absence of monocular information, Carmon and Bechtold[7] found an impaired performance of RBD patients. Epileptic patients submitted to temporal lobectomy of either side showed a mild, but significant impairment in detecting the shapes of Julesz's stereograms.[25] However, it remains open to question whether the deficit is specific to the processing of disparity data or reflects a more general deficit in using minimal information to discriminate shapes.[26]

CONSTRUCTIONAL APRAXIA

By far the most common way to demonstrate an impairment of spatial skills in brain-damaged pa-

tients is to ask them to copy drawings or tridimensional patterns, a task that demands accurate analysis and reproduction of the spatial arrangement and the reciprocal relation of the elements (lines, or blocks) composing the model. Copying drawings is a task that enjoys particular popularity in clinical practice because it is easy to administer at the bedside and is the simplest way to bring out constructional apraxia. This symptom, known to neurologists for more than sixty years,[27] consists in the inability to assemble the elements of a bidimensional or tridimensional whole, respecting their orientations and spatial relationships. Constructional skills are required by many mechanical tasks and children's games, and they also enter into a number of nonverbal mental tests, such as the block-design and picture-assembly subtests of the Wechsler Adult Intelligence Scale (WAIS). However, the more complex the task, the less specific its impairment because of the great number of skills it involves; it is, therefore, more appropriate to study constructional apraxia with simpler tests (e.g., copying geometric drawings of increasing complexity, three-dimensional block constructions, and the spatial arrangement of sticks).

Kleist[27] viewed constructional apraxia as a left parietal deficit, due to the disruption of a center (tentatively localized in the left angular gyrus) that would represent the interface between the analysis of visuospatial information and the planning of hand movements. On this assumption, the deficit would be attributable to neither a perceptual nor an executive impairment but to the stage where movement programs, which are organized by the left hemisphere, must be monitored by spatial analysis. However, this hypothesis was abandoned when subsequent studies showed that constructional apraxia is by no means limited to left parietal damage and is indeed as frequent or even more frequent following right brain damage. Since this side of the brain is not involved in the organization of actions, while it plays a prominent role in space perception, it seemed logical to conceive of constructional apraxia associated with right brain damage as dependent on defective visuospatial analysis. What about the nature of constructional apraxia following left brain damage? The discussion revolved around the question of whether it differs from right constructional apraxia in terms of frequency, severity, quality of errors, and impairment of other cognitive abilities with which it is associated. In the sixties, the view prevailed that the deficit underlying constructional apraxia is basically apraxic when the lesion affects the left hemisphere (which is dominant for praxis) and agnosic when it affects the right hemisphere (which is dominant for space perception), and it was proposed[28] to reserve the term *constructional apraxia* for the deficit shown by LBD patients and that of *visuospatial agnosia* for the deficit shown by RBD patients. However, this dichotomy has not passed the test of time.

Let us first address the question of the frequency and severity of constructional apraxia in unselected samples of patients with unilateral hemispheric damage. Contrasting findings have been reported. A scrutiny[11] of the relevant papers has pointed out that, while the incidence of constructional apraxia in RBD patients was approximately the same across the studies (about one-third of patients were impaired), in LBD samples, it was much more variable, ranging from 14 to 37 percent. What made the difference was apparently the type of test employed to assess constructional apraxia: the percentage of LBD patients with constructional apraxia was low when performance was tested with tasks such as block designs, which are part of intelligence scales and involve more than constructional abilities, while it was at the same level as that found in RBD patients when tested with simpler tasks. It is reasonable to suspect that the choice of complex tests entailed the exclusion from the investigation of aphasics with severe comprehension deficits, resulting in a sampling bias that is all the more risky as there is evidence that constructional apraxia is significantly associated with receptive language impairment, even when it is measured with elementary copying tasks.[29,30] Also, differences in the severity of the disorder were remarkably reduced when the hemispheric samples were unselected, and they were seldom consistent enough to reach significance.

If quantitative scores do not reliably discriminate RBD from LBD patients, are there clues in the quality of their performance that suggest whether their disability has a perceptual or motor origin? Early authors[28,31–33] replied in the positive and listed a series of signs that would characterize the performance of RBD and LBD patients, respectively. The drawings of the former are disorganized and made with many strokes, present errors of rotation and show a diagonal orientation. Those of the latter are oversimplified and small in size but with an increased number of right angles and improvement on repetition. The problem with these conclusions is that the distinguishing features are present in only a minority of patients and are therefore difficult to replicate across studies. The only sign that has been consistently verified in RBD patients is failure to reproduce left-sided details, a manifestation of their neglect of the left side of space.

Another approach to the discrimination of the mechanisms underlying constructional apraxia in the two hemispheric groups has been the search for a differential association between constructional disability and the performance on tests taxing manipulative skills and space perception, respectively. It has been hypothesized that left apraxics would score poorly on the former but not on the latter, while right apraxics would show the opposite pattern.

It must be said at once that a strong version of the motor or executive hypothesis, claiming that constructional apraxia in LBD patients is a minor form of ideomotor apraxia (see Chap. 16), is untenable. First, some of these patients do not show limb apraxia; second, and more damaging to the hypothesis, there are also a few limb apraxics who do not manifest constructional apraxia.[34] In a more moderate formulation of the executive hypothesis, constructional apraxia in LBD patients can be construed as consequent to the disruption of the motor abilities required by drawing and other constructional performances. This view predicts that the impairment should be remarkably attenuated when tasks less demanding in terms of motor control are given. The hypothesis was bolstered by a study[35] in which plastic pieces of different form had to be assembled, without time limits, in the shape of an 8-cm square, a task only mildly taxing to manual dexterity. Both hemispheric groups scored less well than normal controls and, in addition, the mean performance of RBD patients was significantly impaired in comparison to that of LBD patients. Further, while in the former group the constructional scores correlated significantly with the scores of two simple visuoperceptual tasks (line-length and angle-size discrimination), correlations were not significant in LBD patients. The results of this study are neat but in need of replication because of the amazingly high number of RBD patients who fell below the cutoff point on the constructional test, while in most investigations no more than one-third of them have been found to suffer from constructional apraxia. Also, the fact that the right-sided group was more impaired than the left-sided group on an elementary visual test, such as line-length discrimination, is not in keeping with previous experience and raises suspicion that the sample was not representative of the corresponding population.

The other prediction made by the dichotomous theory of constructional apraxia (i.e., that its correlation with space perception disability is significant in RBD patients but not in LBD patients) found support in Mack and Levine's[35] study and was replicated with a different procedure by Griffiths and Cook,[36] but it is at variance with other findings, reporting similar degrees of impairment in right and left constructional apraxics on a wide range of space perception tasks: Progressive Matrices,[31,37,38] Minnesota paper formboard,[39] Benton's visual form discrimination test,[29,39] and the recognition of reversed shapes.[3]

In conclusion, the evidence that constructional apraxia reflects the disruption of different abilities, depending on the damaged side, is at most suggestive but has not been unequivocally demonstrated. Although an executive impairment remains a possible component of the defective performance of LBD patients, visuospatial disorders are likely to be influential in both hemispheric groups.

The anatomical correlates of constructional apraxia are in keeping with the assumption that spatial disorders contribute to the difficulty of both hemispheric groups but that executive disorders may also play a role in LBD patients. Parietal damage is a frequent anatomic correlate of constructional apraxia after damage to either hemisphere, although the association is closer in RBD patients than in LBD patients.[34] It must, however, be added that the reproduction of a structured model is a sequential task that requires a certain degree of planning and is, therefore, liable to be sensitive to the functioning of frontal structures.[40] Indeed, there is evidence that frontal damage may result in constructional apraxia[41] and that the performance improves if planning cues are provided.[42] Supportive of the idea that different mechanisms underlie parietal and frontal constructional apraxia is the finding that the disorder is associated with poor performance on a line bisection task in RBD patients having damage to the parietooccipital cortex but not in those with frontal, subcortical damage.[43]

Since the introduction of imaging techniques in clinical practice, it has been increasingly recognized that subcortical structures contribute to cognitive functions, and disorders of language, praxis, lateralized attention, and so on have been reported following damage to basal nuclei. The same holds for constructional apraxia, whose incidence and severity do not differ in subcortical as compared to cortical lesions.[44] Whether the deficit is due to the interruption of pathways connecting cortical areas, resulting in their hypometabolism or to the specific participation of basal nuclei in the performance is a matter of debate for this as well as for other cognitive disorders.

Constructional apraxia is also frequently seen in demented patients and has been claimed to be one of the earliest signs of Alzheimer disease[45] and to progress as the disease worsens. There is, however, no correlation with language and memory performance,[46] and a case of intact constructional performance in a grossly demented patient has been reported.[47]

DISORDERS OF SPATIAL MEMORY

Psychometric Assessment of Spatial Memory

Studies of focal brain lesions provide definite evidence that spatial memory is organized in the brain separately from memory for other kinds of information and that the right hemisphere plays a major role in subserving this ability. Support for this contention comes from two sources of evidence, the differential impairment shown by unselected groups of patients with damage to either hemisphere in performing spatial memory tests and a few case reports showing an inability to navigate through familiar environments in the absence of global amnesia.

A simple and convenient test of spatial memory has been devised by Corsi.[48] It consists of nine cubes glued to a board in an irregular arrangement, which the examiner taps in sequences of increasing length for the patient to reproduce immediately afterwards. Since the cubes have the same size and color, they are identifiable only by their position. Both short-term memory span and the learning of a supraspan sequence can be assessed and results are easily comparable with those obtained with the forward digit span, which is the verbal analogue of the Corsi test. Long-term spatial memory can also be tested[49] with a stepping-stone maze, where the patient is requested to discover and memorize a path hidden in a 10×10 array of boltheads. The correct boltheads are those that, when touched with a stylus, do not produce a loud click, and the subject must proceed by trial and error until criterion (two errorless performances) is reached.

Both RBD and LBD patients with visual field defects have a reduced spatial memory span.[50] The impairment is not attributable to the visual field deficit per se or to scanning and misreaching disorders, since it no longer obtains when a digit sequence is given that must be tapped on cubes having a digit on their upper side. It is, therefore, likely that the presence of visual field defects merely points to the posterior location of lesion. In some patients the spatial short-term memory deficit is so striking as to be also apparent in everyday life. Two of them,[11] as soon as they closed their eyes, were unable to point to the pieces of furniture in the room that they had just named or to find the article they were reading as soon as they folded the page of the newspaper. Although both had serious difficulty in taking their bearings

in familiar surroundings, short- and long-term deficits are usually unrelated, as shown by normal maze-path learning in patients with a spatial span of two[51] and by normal spatial span in patients with topographic disorientation. A patient has, however, been reported[52] with a reduced spatial span who had problems in learning new routes, though she could navigate in surroundings that were familiar before the disease began.

Unlike short-term memory, long-term spatial memory has been found to be associated with right-sided lesions. Patients with right posterior damage of predominantly vascular etiology were impaired in learning a supraspan string on the Corsi block-tapping test[53] and epileptics submitted to right temporal lobectomy, including the hippocampal region, performed poorly on a stepping-stone maze[49] and on a test requiring memory for the relative position of elements in a spatially distributed array.[50] More difficult is the systematic assessment of spatial knowledge that has been acquired before the disease (retrograde amnesia) because of the difference across subjects in traveling experience. The only common background involves the geographic notions learned at school, which are probably related to the level of education. No retrograde deficit was found when patients with unilateral brain damage were requested to say in which direction they would travel in going from an American city to another[54] or when a patient with extensive right temporal lobe removal[55] was given the Fargo Map Test, which required him to locate American cities on a blank map. At variance with these findings, RBD patients scored significantly less well than controls in estimating the distance in miles between two major American cities,[56] a task implying the revisualization of the map of the United States and of the spatial relations among its cities. Unfortunately, the verbal nature of the task prevented its administration to LBD patients and it remains, therefore, open to question whether the impairment is specifically associated with RBD.

Topographical Disorientation

The most striking manifestation of spatial memory deficit is topographic disorientation—namely, the inability to find one's way in a familiar environment and to learn new paths, in the absence of global amnesia, severe mental deterioration, or disorders of visual perception and exploration. The symptom had not escaped the attention of nineteenth-century neurologists and its earliest report probably dates back to Jackson.[57] However, Foerster[58] and Meyer[59] must be credited with having provided the first exhaustive description of its features. In its most severe form, the deficit involves both retrograde and anterograde spatial knowledge, and patients may lose their bearings even at home. With restitution of function or in milder cases from the beginning, navigation is impaired only in environments that the patient has first experienced since the onset of disease.[60]

Meyer's case report provides the guidelines for a thorough examination of the deficit:

1. When the patient left his room in the wards, he was unable to find his way back to it, because he was at a loss any time in the route he had to choose whether to go left, right, downstairs, or upstairs. When he eventually arrived in front of his own room, he did not recognize it by its location, but only if he could rely on some distinguishing feature he perceived inside it (e.g., the black beard of his roommate), a behavior that attested to his preserved visual memory.

2. The same behavior was observed, when he had to take his bearings in sections of the city he was well familiar with before the disease. He tried hard to find landmarks that could give him cues about the place where he was, but their help was limited, because, even when he had recognized them and thus knew that he was close to home, he still did not know what direction to take to get there.

3. Verbal knowledge of spatial relations was good as long as it resorted to rote memory (e.g., he could recite the names of the intermediate stations of the railway he used daily), but was impaired when it had to rely on an internal map depicting how different places of the city were related to each other. For instance, he could not tell how he would walk between two randomly chosen sites in the city.

4. He grossly mislocated cities and countries on a map.

It is apparent that the basic deficit underlying the patient's difficulty is the inability to retrieve an abstract map of the route, which specifies the spatial relationships defining the position of a place with respect to other places and the subject and to transform them in guidelines for walking.

The behavior of Meyer's patient can be usefully contrasted with that of the patient of Pallis,[61] because they epitomize two different forms of topographic disorientation. Pallis's patient too was unable to find his way in familiar surroundings, but he could give a satisfactory description of the paths he had to follow to reach a given place and could draw maps of familiar places. His failure was mainly due to the inability to recognize buildings and places and thus to know exactly where he was. As the patient said: "In my mind's eye I know exactly where places are, what they look like. I can visualize T . . . square without difficulty and the streets that come into it. . . . It is when I'm out that the trouble starts. My reason tells me that I am in a certain place and yet I don't recognize it. . . . My difficulty with buses is to know where to get off." The patient had "an excellent performance in drawing maps of places familiar to him before the illness" and could trace a path on a map. It is apparent that his problem was mainly agnosic and did not concern the ability to retrieve a spatial map of the route. He was able to distinguish different types of buildings, e.g., a terraced council house from a detached villa, but could not identify a unique exemplar of the subcategory (incidentally, he also was prosopagnosic) and consequently could not take advantage of landmarks to find his way out.

Landmark recognition and spatial map construction are the main mental operations that assist navigation through familiar surroundings, and their discrete disruption underlies two forms of route-finding disability, topographic agnosia and topographic amnesia.[62] The nature of topographic agnosia has not been extensively investigated. The failure to identify a specific building might result from perceptual impairment that prevents the appreciation of the small, distinctive features identifying an exemplar of a category whose elements are similar or from the inability to match the perceived building with its representation stored in memory. The problem is whether the agnosia is class-specific or extends to other categories (e.g., faces) that demand the recognition of the stimulus in its uniqueness. Prosopagnosia is a frequent, but not necessary concomitant of topographic agnosia. For instance, Landis and coworkers[63] found it in only 7 of 16 patients suffering from what they called "environmental agnosia." A specific deficit for building memory was advocated by Whiteley and Warrington[64] in their patient, who performed in the normal range on perceptual, spatial, and memory tests but was impaired in learning to recognize photographs of unknown buildings. The critical test would have been, however, recognition of familiar buildings.

Failure to recognize familiar environments is by no means a constant feature of patients with topographic disorientation; even when it is present, it may not be the main reason for route-finding disability. For instance, the patient of De Renzi and Scotti (summarized in Ref. 11) who was unable to identify famous buildings did not improve in taking his bearings when their names were provided by the examiner because he could not remember their position with respect to other sites of the city. The amnestic nature of this form of topographic disorientation is confirmed by the patient's failure to give a verbal description of the route, to trace it on a road map, and to draw a map of a familiar place. Patients endeavor to find salient objects, but these are of little help because they are devoid of orientation value and do not tell them, for instance, whether they must proceed straight ahead, or turn left. The dissociation between topographic amnesia and topographic agnosia is exemplified by patient 5 of Aimard and coworkers,[65] who was unable to find a room in his apartment but, when he eventually opened its door, immediately recognized it. Of course, agnosic and amnesic disorders can coexist in the same patient, as both are dependent on right hemispheric damage.

The elaborate strategies developed by these patients to make up for their disability are revealing. They tend to rely on verbal tags (the room number, the street names) or on salient objects to which they have learned to associate an index value and on a verbal summation of the segments composing the route.[66,67] In neurofunctional terms, this behavior suggests an attempt to compensate for the defective abilities subserved by the right hemisphere by exploiting those mediated by the left hemisphere as much as possible.

The study of the anatomic correlates of topographic disorientation has pointed out the crucial role played by the posterior regions of the brain, especially of the right hemisphere. In some cases damage is bilateral,[58,59,68–70] but in others it is confined to the right side, where the areas more frequently involved are the parietal lobe[62,65,71–73] and the medial occipitotemporal cortex.[22,60,63,65,67,74] The most frequent etiology is an infarct in the territory of the right posterior cerebral artery, which supplies blood to the medial surface of the occipital and temporal lobe. This is the same region whose damage can also cause prosopagnosia, but, as already mentioned, the two deficits are not necessarily associated. From the analysis of the computed tomography (CT) evidence provided by their four cases, Habib and Sirigu[57] argued that the crucial lesion is located in the right parahippocampal gyrus (posterior to the uncus and anterior to the subsplenial region), but it is difficult to reconcile this assumption with the lack of topographic disorientation found in patients submitted to right temporal ablation, although they showed psychometric signs of spatial learning impairment.[48,49,75] More problematic is the role played in route-finding deficit by the parietal lobe. In the animal, parietal area 7, corresponding to the inferior parietal lobule in humans, has strong connections with the posterior parahippocampal gyrus, but the evidence that its damage results in route-finding impairment is meager and based only on the report that monkeys are hesitant and slow in finding their way to the cage after bilateral[76,77] and also unilateral ablation[53] of areas 5 and 7.

Episodes of topographic disorientation are frequently seen in the advanced stages of degenerative dementia of Alzheimer type. More rarely they may be one of the early manifestations of the disease; in such a case, they must be differentiated from episodes of loss of topographic memory that transiently occur in patients without any other sign of brain disease. The latter are reminiscent of episodes of transient global amnesia but are distinguished by the preserved recall of the whole attack. Eleven cases have been reported.[78-80] All were women aged 54 to 81 years at the time of the first episode. During the attack, which lasted from 5 to 40 min, the patients were perfectly aware of what was happening to them and retained the ability to recognize places, shops, streets, and so on, but they could not find their way out. None of them showed signs of mental deterioration or of verbal and spatial dysmnesia when the episode was over. In a few cases attacks recurred, up to a maximum of three. Their interpretation is open to the same questions that are raised by transient global amnesia. A vascular etiology can be occasionally envisaged,[65] but for the great majority of them the only conjecture that can reasonably be advanced is that they reflect a transient dysfunction of unknown origin of the right occipitotemporal region.

Reduplicative Amnesia for Places

Confused and demented patients often fail to identify the place they are in, mistaking, for instance, the hospital room for a home room, unaware or unconcerned of the implausibility of their claim. A different case is that of patients who recognize their whereabouts but maintain that they are located in a different place, familiar to them, which is a duplicate of the original one and may be changed from day to day (e.g., the patient correctly identifies the environment as part of the Massachusetts General Hospital but then adds that it is outside of London, or in Paris, Arizona, etc.).[81] When requested to justify the absurdity of their claims, patients indulge in florid confabulations but are ready to abandon them in the face of the examiner's objections. The disorder was first reported by Pick[82] under the name of reduplicative amnesia in a demented patient and attributed to a memory

deficit, but it was subsequently pointed out[83] that it could persist even when amnesia had recovered and in the absence of errors in orientation to time and persons. Although some of these patients show definite signs of spatial impairment,[84] route-finding difficulty has been only occasionally reported.[85]

Weinstein[86] emphasized the compensatory nature of the mechanism that underlies this as well as other reduplicative phenomena and surmised that it would represent an attempt at coping with stress. Others[83,84] have viewed it as the consequence of an acute brain lesion, disrupting the networks specialized in spatial memory that are located in the frontal and parietal lobe of the right hemisphere.

REFERENCES

1. Newcombe F, Russel WR: Dissociated visual perceptual and spatial deficits in focal lesions of the right hemisphere. *J. Neurol Neurosurg Psychiatry* 32:73–81, 1969.

2. Ungerleider LG, Mishkin M: Two cortical visual systems, in Ingle DJ, Mansfield RJW, Goodale MS (eds): The analysis of visual behavior. Cambridge, MA, MIT Press, 1982, pp 549–586.

3. De Renzi E, Faglioni P: The relationship between visuo-spatial impairment and constructional apraxia. *Cortex* 3:327–342, 1967.

4. Hannay HJ, Varney NR, Benton AL: Visual localization in patients with unilateral brain disease. *J Neurol Neurosurg Psychiatry* 39:307–313, 1976.

5. Tartaglione A, Benton AL, Cocito L, et al: Point localization in patients with unilateral brain damage. *J Neurol Neurosurg Psychiatry* 44:935–941, 1981.

6. Benton AL, Hécaen H: Stereoscopic vision in patients with unilateral cerebral damage. *Neurology* 20:1084–1088, 1970.

7. Carmon A, Bechtold HP: Dominance of the right cerebral hemisphere for stereopsis. *Neuropsychology* 7:29–40, 1969.

8. Hamsher K de S: Stereopsis and unilateral brain disease. *Invest Ophthalmol* 17:336–343, 1978.

9. Benton AL, Hannay J, Varney NR: Visual perception of line direction in patients with unilateral brain disease. *Neurology* 25:907–910, 1975.

10. De Renzi E, Faglioni P, Scotti G: Judgment of spatial orientation in patients with focal brain damage. *J Neurol Neurosurg Psychiatry* 34:489–495, 1971.

11. De Renzi E: *Disorders of Space Exploration and Cognition.* Chichester, England, Wiley, 1982.

12. Benton AL, Varney NR, Hamsher de SK: Visuospatial judgment: A clinical test. *Arch Neurol* 35:364–367, 1978.

13. Fontenot DJ, Benton AL: Tactile perception of direction in relation to hemispheric locus of lesion. *Neuropsychologia* 9:83–88, 1971.

14. De Renzi E, Scotti G: The influence of spatial disorders in impairing tactual discrimination of shapes. *Cortex* 5:53–62, 1969.

15. Bottini G, Cappa S, Sterzi R, Vignolo LA: Intramodal somaesthetic recognition disorders following right and left hemisphere damage. *Brain* 118:395–399, 1995.

16. Milner B, Taylor L: Right hemisphere superiority in tactile pattern recognition after cerebral commissurotomy: Evidence from nonverbal memory. *Neuropsychologia* 10:1–15, 1972.

17. Witelson SF: Hemispheric specialization for linguistic and nonlinguistic tactual perception using a dichotomous stimulation technique. *Cortex* 10:3–17, 1974.

18. Witelson SF: Sex and the single hemisphere: Specialization of the right hemisphere for spatial processing. *Science* 193:425–427, 1976.

19. Butters N, Barton M, Brody BA. Role of the parietal lobe in the mediation of cross modal associations and reversible operations in space. *Cortex* 6:174–190, 1970.

20. Metha Z, Newcombe F, Damasio H: A left hemisphere contribution to visuospatial processing. *Cortex* 23:447–461, 1987.

21. Ratcliff G: Spatial thought, mental rotation, and the right cerebral hemisphere. *Neuropsychologia* 17:49–54, 1979.

22. Gloning K: *Die Cerebralen Bedingten Stoerungen des Raumlichen Sehens und des Raumerlebens.* Vienna, Maudrig, 1965.

23. Holmes G, Horrax G: Disturbances of spatial orientation and visual attention with loss of stereoscopic vision. *Arch Neurol Psychiatry* 1:385–407, 1919.

24. Michel F, Jeannerod M, Devic M: Trouble de l'orientation visuelle dans les trois dimension de l'espace. *Cortex* 1:441–466, 1965.

25. Ptito A, Zatorre RJ, Larson WI, Tosini C: Stereopsis after unilateral temporal lobectomy. *Brain* 114:1323–1333, 1991.

26. Cowey A: Disturbances of stereopsis by brain damage, in Ingle DJ, Jeannerod M, Lee DN (eds): *Brain Mechanisms and Spatial Vision.* Dordrecht, Martinus Nijoff, 1985, pp. 259–278.

27. Kleist K: *Gehirnpathologie.* Leipzig, Barth, 1934.

28. McFie J, Zangwill OLO: Visual-constructive disabilities associated with lesions of the left cerebral hemisphere. *Brain* 83:243–260, 1960.

29. Arena R, Gainotti G: Constructional apraxia and visuoperceptive disabilities in relation to laterality of cerebral lesion. *Cortex* 14:463–473, 1978.

30. Benton AL: Visuoconstructive disability in patients with cerebral disease: Its relationship to side of lesion and aphasic disorder. *Doc Ophthalmol* 34:67–76, 1973.

31. Gainotti G, Tiacci C: Sui rapporti fra aprassia construttiva, agnosia visuo-spaziale e negligenza spaziale unilaterale. *Riv Pat Nerv Ment* 93:103–116, 1970.

32. Piercy M, Hécaen H, de Ajuriaguerra J: Constructional apraxia associated with unilateral cerebral lesions: Left and right sided cases compared. *Brain* 83:225–242, 1960.

33. Warrington EK, James M, Kinsbourne M: Drawing disability in relation to laterality of lesion. *Brain* 89:53–82, 1966.

34. Ajuriaguerra J, Hécaen H, Angelergues R: Les apraxies: Variétés cliniques et latéralisation lésionelle. *Rev Neurol* 102:566–594, 1960.

35. Mack JL, Levine RN: The basis of visual constructional disabilities in patients with unilateral cerebral lesions. *Cortex* 17:515–532, 1981.

36. Griffiths K, Cook M: Attribute processing in patients with graphical copying disability. *Neuropsychologia* 24:371–383, 1986.

37. Arrigoni G, De Renzi E: Constructional apraxia and hemispheric locus of lesion. *Cortex* 1:180–197, 1964.

38. Piercy M, Smyth VOG: Right hemisphere dominance for certain non-verbal intellectual skills. *Brain* 85:775–790, 1962.

39. Dee HL: Visuoconstructive and visuoperceptive deficit in patients with unilateral cerebral lesions. *Neuropsychologia* 8:305–314, 1970.

40. Luria AR, Tsvetkova LS: The programming of constructive activity in local brain injuries. *Neuropsychologia* 2:95–108, 1964.

41. Benton AL: Differential behavioral effects in frontal lobe disease. *Neuropsychologia* 6:53–60, 1968.

42. Pillon B: Troubles visuoconstructifs et méthodes de compensation: Resultats de 85 patients atteints de lésions cérébrales. *Neuropsychologia* 19:375–383, 1981.

43. Marshall RS, Lazar RM, Binder JR, et al: Intrahemispheric localization of drawing dysfunction. *Neuropsychologia* 32:493–501, 1994.

44. Kirk A, Kertesz A: Subcortical contribution to drawing. *Brain Lang* 21:57–70, 1993.

45. Ajuriaguerra J, Muller M, Tissot R: A propos de quelques problèmes posés par l'apraxie dans les démences. *Encéphale* 49:375–401, 1960.

46. Kirk A, Kertesz A: On drawing impairment in Alzheimer's disease. *Arch Neurol.* 48:73–77, 1991.

47. Denes F, Semenza C: Sparing of constructional abilities in severe dementia. *Eur Neurol* 21:161–164, 1982.

48. Milner B: Interhemispheric differences in the localization of psychological processes in man. *Brit Med Bull* 27:272–277, 1971.

49. Milner B: Visually-guided maze learning in man: Effects of bilateral hippocampal, bilateral frontal and unilateral cerebral lesions. *Neuropsychologia* 3:317–338, 1965.

50. De Renzi E, Faglioni P, Previdi P: Spatial memory and hemispheric locus of lesion. *Cortex* 13:424–433, 1977.

51. De Renzi E, Nichelli P: Verbal and non-verbal memory impairment following hemispheric damage. *Cortex* 11:341–354, 1975.

52. Hanley JR, Young AW, Pearson NA: Impairment of the visuo-spatial sketch pad. *Q J Exp Psychol* 43:101–125, 1991.

53. Sugishita M, Ettlinger G, Ridley RM: Disturbance of cage-finding in the monkey. *Cortex* 14:431–438, 1978.

54. Benton AL, Levin HS, Van Allen MW: Geographical orientation in patients with unilateral cerebral disease. *Neuropsychologia* 12:183–191, 1974.

55. Beatty WW, MacInnes WD, Porphyris HS, et al: Preserved topographical memory following right temporal lobectomy. *Brain Cogn* 8:67–76, 1988.

56. Morrow L, Ratcliffe G, Johnston CS: Externalizing spatial knowledge in patients with right hemisphere lesions. *Cogn Neuropsychol* 2:265–273, 1985.

57. Jackson JH: Case of large cerebral tumour with optic neuritis and with left hemiplegia and imperception, in *Selected Writings.* London, Taylor, 1932, pp 146–152.

58. Foerster R: Ueber Rindenblindheit. *Albrecht v. Graefe Arch Ophthalmol* 38:94–108, 1890.

59. Meyer O: Ein- und doppelseitige homonyme Hemianopsie mit Orientierungstoerungen. *Monatschr Psychiatr Neurol* 8:440–456, 1900.

60. Habib A, Sirigu A: Pure topographical disorienta-

61. Pallis CA: Impaired identification of locus and places with agnosia for colours. *J Neurol Neurosurg Psychiatry* 18:218–224, 1955.

62. Paterson A, Zangwill OL: A case of topographical disorientation associated with a unilateral cerebral lesion. *Brain* 68:188–121, 1945.

63. Landis T, Cummings JL, Benson DF, Palmer EP: Loss of topographical familiarity: An environmental agnosia. *Arch Neurol* 43:132–136, 1986.

64. Whiteley AM, Warrington EK: Selective impairment of topographical memory: A single case study. *J Neurol Neurosurg Psychiatry* 41:575–578, 1978.

65. Aimard G, Vighetto A, Confavreux C, Devic M: La désorientation spatiale. *Rev Neurol* 137:97–111, 1981.

66. Clarke S, Assal G, De Tribolet N: Left hemisphere strategies in visual recognition, topographical orientation and time planning. *Neuropsychologia* 31:99–113, 1993.

67. Whitty CWM, Newcombe F: Oldfield's study of visual and topographical disturbances in a right occipito-parietal lesion after 30 years duration. *Neuropsychologia* 11:471–475, 1973.

68. Dunn TD: Double hemiplegia with double hemianopia and loss of a geographical center. *Trans Coll Phys Philadelphia* 17:45–55, 1895.

69. Peters A: Ueber die Beziehungen zwischen Orientierungsstoerungen und ein- und doppelseitiger Hemianopsie. *Arch Augenheilk* 32:175–187, 1896.

70. Wildbrand H: Ein Fall von Seelenblindheit und Hemianopsie mit Sections-Befund. *Dtsch Z Nervenheilk* 2:361–387, 1892.

71. Assal G: Regression des troubles de la reconaissance des physiognomies et de la memoire topographique chez un malade opéré d' un hematome intracérébral pariéto-temporal droite. *Rev Neurol* 121:184–185, 1969.

72. Hécaen H, Penfield W, Bertrand C, Malmo R: The syndrome of apractognosia due to lesions of the minor cerebral hemisphere. *Arch Neurol Psychiatry* 75:400–434, 1956.

73. Newcombe F, Ratcliff G: Disorders of visuospatial analysis, in Boller F, Grafman J (eds): *Handbook of Neuropsychology.* Amsterdam, Elsevier, 1990, vol 2, pp 333–356.

74. Hécaen H, Tzortzis C, Rondot P: Loss of topographical memory with learning deficits. *Cortex* 16:525–542, 1980.

75. Smith ML, Milner B: The role of the right hippocam-

pus in the recall of spatial location. *Neuropsychologia* 19:781–793, 1981.

76. Bates JAV, Ettlinger G: Posterior biparietal ablations in the monkey. *Arch Neurol* 3:177–192, 1960.

77. Ettlinger G, Wegener J: Somaesthetic alternation, discrimination and orientation after frontal and parietal lesions in the monkey. *Q J Exp Psychol* 10:177–186, 1958.

78. Moretti G, Cafarra P, Parma M: Transient topographical amnesia. *Ital J Neurol Sci* 3:361, 1983.

79. Stracciari A: Transient topographical amnesia. *Ital J Neurol Sci* 13:593–596, 1992.

80. Stracciari A, Lorusso S, Pazzaglia P: Transient topographical amnesia. *J Neurol Neurosurg Psychiatry* 57:1423–1425, 1994.

81. Fisher CM: Disorientation for place. *Arch Neurol* 39:33–36, 1982.

82. Pick A: On reduplicative paramnesia. *Brain* 26:242–267, 1903.

83. Benson DF, Gardner H, Meadows JC: Reduplicative paramnesia. *Neurology* 26:147–151, 1976.

84. Ruff RL, Volpe BT: Environmental reduplication associated with right frontal and parietal lobe injury. *J Neurol Neurosurg Psychiatry* 44:382–386, 1981.

85. Vighetto A, Aimard G, Confavreux C, Devic M: Une observation anatomo-clinique de fabulation (ou délire) topographique. *Cortex* 16:501–507, 1980.

86. Weinstein EA: Patterns of reduplication in organic brain disease, in Vinken PJ, Bruyn GW (eds): *Handbook of Neurology*. Amsterdam, North Holland, 1969, vol 3, pp 251–257.

Chapter 24

NEGLECT: CLINICAL AND ANATOMIC ASPECTS

Kenneth M. Heilman
Robert T. Watson
Edward Valenstein

Neglect is a failure to report, respond, or orient to stimuli that are presented contralateral to a brain lesion, when this failure is not due to elementary sensory or motor disorders.[1] Many subtypes of neglect have been described. A major distinction is between neglect of perceptual input, termed *sensory neglect* or *inattention,* and neglect affecting response outputs, termed *motor* or *intentional neglect.* Some further distinctions are outlined below.

Sensory neglect involves a selective deficit in awareness, which may apply to all stimuli on the affected side of space (*spatial neglect*) or be confined to stimuli impinging on the patient's body (*personal neglect*). It may even affect awareness of one side of internal mental images (*representational neglect*). The perceptual modalities affected by neglect may also vary: Subtypes of sensory neglect exist for the visual, auditory, and tactile modalities. The deficit in awareness is accompanied by an abnormal attentional bias. Attention is usually biased toward the ipsilesional side but in rare cases may be contralesional. Once attention is engaged on an ipsilesional stimulus, subjects may have difficulty disengaging their attention to move it to the contralesional side. If the lack of awareness and attentional bias are present only when there is a competing stimulus at a more ipsilateral location, the disorder is termed *extinction.* Many patients with neglect recover and become able to detect isolated contralesional stimuli but continue to manifest extinction.

Motor or *intentional neglect* involves a response failure that cannot be explained by weakness, sensory loss, or unawareness. There may be a failure to move a limb (*limb akinesia*), or the limb can be moved but only after a long delay and strong encouragement (*hypokinesia*). Patients with intentional neglect who can move may make movements of decreased amplitude (*hypometria*). They may also have an inability to maintain posture or movements (*impersistence*). Patients with motor neglect who can move their contralesional limb may fail to move this limb (or have a delay) when they are also required to move their ipsilateral limb (*motor extinction*). Limb akinesia, hypokinesia, hypometria, and motor impersistence can affect some or all parts of the body, including limbs, eyes, or head. The elements of intentional neglect discussed above can be *directional* (toward the contralesional hemispace) or *spatial* (within the contralesional hemispace). Patients with motor neglect may have intentional biases such that there is a propensity to move toward ipsilesional space. There may also be impaired ability to disengage from motor activities (motor perseveration).

TESTING FOR NEGLECT

In this brief review we cannot address all aspects of testing; therefore, for a complete discussion and list of references, the reader is referred to Heilman and coworkers.[1]

Inattention or Sensory Neglect

To test for inattention, the patient is presented with unilateral stimuli on either the ipsilesional or contralesional side in random order. If a patient fails to detect more stimuli on the contralesional side than the ipsilesional side, it would suggest that the patient is suffering from inattention. However, if the patient totally fails to detect any stimuli on the contralesional side, it is often difficult to tell whether or not the patient has inattention or a sensory loss. The auditory modality is the least difficult in which to dissociate inattention and sensory loss because sounds made on one side of the head project to both ears, and each ear projects to both the ipsilateral as well as the contralateral hemisphere. Therefore, if a patient is unaware of noises made on one side of his or her head, this unawareness cannot be explained by a sensory defect and suggests that the patient has inattention. In the visual modality, because unawareness may be hemispatial (body-centered) rather than retinotopic, having the patient deviate the eyes toward ipsilateral hemispace may allow him or her to become aware of stimuli projected to the contralesional portion of the retina. In regard to tactile neglect, one may have to use caloric stimulation of the ear to see if the patient can detect stimuli during such stimulation. One may also use psychophysiologic techniques such as evoked potentials or galvanic skin responses to see whether patients who are unaware of stimuli demonstrate autonomic signs of stimulus detection.[2]

Extinction

To test for extinction, one may randomly intermix the unilateral stimuli described above with bilateral simultaneous stimuli. The stimuli can be given in any modality (e.g., visual, auditory, tactile). When a subject has hemianopia, extinction may even occur within the ipsilesional visual field.

Intentional or Motor Neglect

Patients who have severe limb akinesia may appear to have a hemiparesis. An arm may hang off the bed or wheelchair. Sometimes, with strong encouragement by the examiner, it can be demonstrated that such a patient has normal strength. However, some patients will still not move, and

one may have to rely on brain imaging to learn whether the corticospinal tract is involved. In patients with motor neglect, the lesion should not involve the corticospinal system. Magnetic stimulation may also be helpful in demonstrating that the corticospinal tract is normal.[3] As we discussed, patients with hypokinesia are reluctant to move the affected arm or only move it after delay. However, once they have moved, their strength may be normal. To test for hypometria, the arm is passively moved or the patient is shown a line and asked to make a movement of the same length. Patients with hypometria will undershoot the target. To test for impersistence, the patient is asked to sustain a posture. Patients with impersistence cannot maintain postures. As mentioned, patients can be tested for forms of motor neglect by using the limbs, eyes, or even head. They can be tested in ipsilateral versus contralateral hemispace and in an ipsilesional versus contralesional direction.

Spatial Neglect

Four clinical tests are commonly used to assess for spatial neglect. In the line bisection task, the patient is given a long line and asked to indicate its midpoint (Fig. 24-1). Although horizontal lines are most commonly used (intersection of the coronal and axial planes), neglect has been reported in the vertical dimension (both up neglect and down neglect) and in the radial dimension (near neglect and far neglect).

In general, the longer the line, the greater the percentage of error. Placing the line in contralesional hemispace can also increase the severity of the error, as can putting cues on the ipsilesional side.

In performing the cancellation task, a sheet of paper that contains targets is placed before the patient and the patient is asked to mark out (cancel) all the targets (Fig. 24-2). Increasing the number of targets can increase the sensitivity of this test. Increasing the difficulty with which one discriminates targets from distractors can also increase the sensitivity of this task.

In testing drawing, the patient should be asked to draw spontaneously as well as to copy

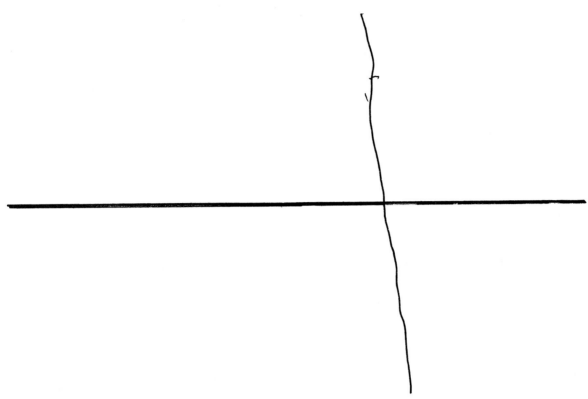

Figure 24-1
Line bisection task performed by a patient with a right hemisphere infarction and left hemispatial neglect. (From Dr. Todd E. Feinberg with permission.)

figures (Figs. 24-3 and 24-4). Copying asymmetrical nonsense figures may be more difficult than copying well-known symmetrical figures.

In testing for representational neglect, one should ask a subject to image a famlar scene and then report what he or she sees. A patient with representational neglect will recall more objects from the ipsilesional than the contralesional part of the image.

At times it may be difficult to dissociate sensory attentional disorders from motor intentional disorders. In general, the best means of doing this is by performing cross-response tasks where the subject responds in one side of space to a stimulus presented on the opposite side. Video cameras, strings and pulley, or mirrors can be used in the performance of a cross response task.

To dissociate intentional from representa-

tional defects, one can use a fixed-aperture technique. To do this, an opaque sheet with a fixed window is placed over a sheet with targets so that only one target can be seen at a time, thereby reducing attentional demands. In one-half the trials, the subject moves the top sheet; in the other trials, the subject moves the target sheet. A failure to explore one portion of the target sheet in both conditions suggests a representational defect, and a failure to explore opposite sides of the target sheet in direct and indirect conditions suggests a motor intentional deficit.[4]

To dissociate neglect of one side of the environment from neglect of one side of the person, one can ask the patient to lie down on his or her side. This decouples the environmental left and right from the body's left and right. If the patient has a right hemispheric lesion, is lying on the right

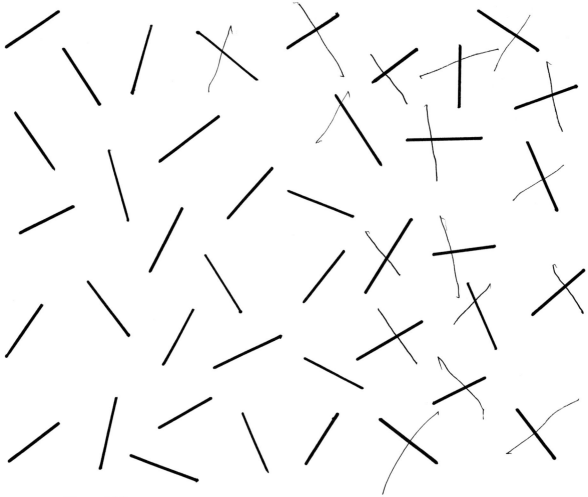

Figure 24-2
Cancellation task of same patient as in Fig. 24-1. (From Dr. Todd E. Feinberg with permission.)

side, and now fails to detect targets toward the ceiling, the neglect is body-centered. However, if the patient continues to neglect targets on his or her left side, the neglect is environmentally centered (see Chap. 21).[5,6]

PATHOPHYSIOLOGY

As the foregoing review suggests, neglect is not a homogeneous syndrome. The neglect syndrome

not only has many manifestations but also many levels of explanation. For a more complete discussion see Heilman and coworkers.[1] The heterogeneity of neglect is apparent on an anatomic level as well.

In humans, neglect is most often associated with lesions of the inferior parietal lobe (IPL), which includes Brodmann's areas 40 and 39. However, neglect has also been reported from dorsolateral frontal lesions, medial frontal lesions that include the cingulate gyrus, thalamic-mesencephalic

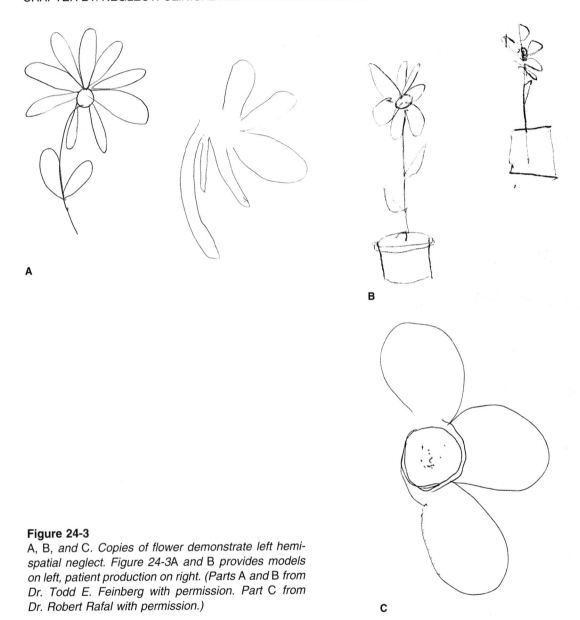

Figure 24-3

A, B, *and* C. *Copies of flower demonstrate left hemi-spatial neglect. Figure 24-3*A and B *provides models on left, patient production on right. (Parts* A *and* B *from Dr. Todd E. Feinberg with permission. Part* C *from Dr. Robert Rafal with permission.)*

lesions, basal ganglia, and white matter lesions. Because there is a limit on the anatomic, physiologic, and behavioral research that can be done in humans, much of what we know about the pathophysiology of the neglect syndrome comes from research on old-world monkeys. Monkeys also have an IPL; however, their IPL is Brodmann's area 7. In humans, the intraparietal sulcus separates the superior parietal area, Brodmann's area 7, from the inferior parietal lobule, Brodmann's areas 40 and 39. Some have thought that the IPL of monkeys is a homologue of the IPL in humans. Others, however, have thought that both banks of the superior temporal sulcus (STS) are the homologue of the inferior parietal lobule in humans. Recently, we[7] demonstrated that neglect in mon-

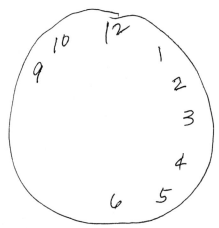

Figure 24-4
*Clock drawn by a patient with left hemispatial neglect.
(From Dr. Robert Rafal with permission.)*

keys is associated with ablation of the STS region and not the IPL. These results suggest that, in regard to neglect, it is the monkeys' STS that is the homologue of the humans' IPL.

Anatomic studies of the STS of monkeys have provided some information as to why this area produces neglect when ablated. The STS is composed of multiple subareas and is one of the sites of multimodal sensory convergence. Visual, auditory, and somatosensory association cortices all project to portions of the STS. In addition, the STS has reciprocal connections to other multi-modal convergence areas such as monkeys' IPL (Brodmann's area 7). Because ablation of area 7 in monkeys, a multimodal convergence area, was not associated with neglect, we do not believe that ablation of a sensory convergence area alone can account for the unawareness that is seen with ne-glect syndrome. Therefore, Watson and coworkers[7] have proposed a role for monkeys' STS or humans' IPL in awareness.

Mishkin and colleagues[8] suggested that the visual system, when presented with stimuli, per-forms dual parallel processes. Whereas the ventral division is important for determining the type of stimulus ("What is it?"), the dorsal system codes the spatial location of the stimulus ("Where is

it?"). In monkeys the "where" system is in part mediated by the posterior portion of Brodmann's area 7 or the monkey's IPL, and the "what" system is in part being mediated by the inferior visual association cortex found in the ventral temporal lobe. It has been long recognized that bilateral ventral temporal lesions in humans and monkeys induce visual object agnosia, a deficit in the "what" system. In contrast, biparietal lesions in monkeys induce deficits of visual spatial localization but not object discrimination. Watson and coworkers[7] posited that these "where" and "what" systems integrate in the banks of monkeys' STS or in the inferior parietal lobule of humans. According to Watson and colleagues,[7] lesions of monkeys' STS and humans' IPL induce unawareness or neglect not only because this is the area that receives poly-modal sensory input but also because it is a conver-gence site of these perceptual-cognitive systems that deal with both the "what" and "where" as-pects of environmental awareness. Both anatomic and electrophysiologic data substantiate the hy-pothesis that monkeys' STS is an area of conver-gence of these two systems (see Watson and co-workers).[7] Watson and colleagues[7] also proposed that similar areas important for spatial localization and object identification may also exist in the audi-tory and tactile systems and that these modalities may also converge in the STS.

Although there is anatomic and physiologic evidence that there is convergence from the Brod-mann's area 7 "where" system and the ventral temporal lobes' "what" system, this cannot ac-count for the observation that ablation of the STS induces unawareness. The STS receives input not only from these "what" and "where" systems but also from the cingulate gyrus and the dorsolateral frontal lobe. In earlier studies, we have demon-strated that lesions in both these areas are also able to induce neglect. The dorsolateral prefrontal region is important in the mediation of goal-di-rected behavior and may provide the STS with information that is not directly stimulus-depen-dent or related to immediate drives and biological needs but rather directed at long-term goals. The cingulate gyrus is part of the limbic system and may provide the STS with information about biological needs and drives. Because monkeys' STS or humans' IPL is supplied with "what" and "where" conative and motivational information, it may be able to make attentional computations.

Monkeys' STS has reciprocal connections with the ventral temporal "what" region and the parietal "where" region. Therefore, after the STS region (or the IPL in humans) performs an attentional computation, it may reciprocally influence the neurons in the ventral temporal lobe and Brodmann's area 7 regions.

Electrical stimulation of the STS is capable of activating the midbrain reticular formation more than stimulation of surrounding posterior regions. Therefore, the superior temporal sulcus appears to be important in the cortical control of arousal, and the supermodal synthesis that we discussed above may also lead to neuronal activation in the ventral temporal "what" and dorsal area 7 "where" systems. Therefore, if the STS in monkeys or the IPL in humans is dysfunctional, it not only fails to make attentional computations but also cannot arouse or activate directly or indirectly those areas that determine both location of objects and their identity. This failure of activation may prevent the monkey or human from being aware that there is a stimulus in the space opposite the STS or IPL (human) lesion.

Bisiach and Luzzati[9] have demonstrated that subjects with neglect may also have an inability to image those objects in scenes that would fall into contralesional hemispace. In addition, Heilman and coworkers[10] have demonstrated a hemispatial antegrade memory deficit associated with neglect. Therefore, lesions of the IPL in humans may be associated with the inability to activate old memory or form new memories of objects that are located in contralesional hemispace. In monkeys, the STS has strong reciprocal connections with the hippocampus. The hippocampus has also been posited to be important in retroactivation of sensory association areas,[11] and a partial (spatial) failure of retroactivation may account for the imagery-memory deficits.

In monkeys and humans, spatial neglect can often be distinguished from deafferentation by observing exploratory behaviors. Deafferented subjects fully explore their environment. However, patients with neglect often fail to fully explore the neglected portion of space. Theoretically, if we ablated both area 7 (the "where" system) and the ventral temporal cortex (the "what" system in monkeys), we suspect that these animals would continue to be able to explore their contralateral hemispace. The failure to explore contralesional space that we observed in animals with STS lesions and humans with IPL lesions may be related to the reciprocal connections that the STS has with the frontal arcuate gyrus region. The frontal arcuate gyrus region or frontal eye field is important for the initiation of purposeful saccades to important visual targets. The periarcuate region is important for the initiation of voluntary arm movements to important visual stimuli. It has been demonstrated that lesions of this region, as well as the basal ganglia and thalamus, which are all part of an intentional functional network, may induce motor intentional neglect. However exploratory defects may be also seen with posterior STS lesions in monkeys or IPL lesions in humans. In monkeys the frontal arcuate area and periarcuate regions have strong connections with both area 7 and the STS. Whereas the STS may be critical in activating both periarcuate and arcuate regions, area 7 may be important for providing these frontal regions with the spatial maps needed to make purposeful exploratory limb and eye movements. In addition to the dorsolateral frontal lobe, the motor intentional network also comprises the medial frontal lobes, including the cingulate gyrus, the basal ganglia, and the thalamic cortical loops as well as input from the STS or IPL. Whereas the attentional and intentional networks are highly interactive, they do not entirely overlap. Therefore one may, as we discussed, see neglect fractionate into motor intentional and sensory attentional components.

Although neglect can be in association with both right and left hemispheric lesions, neglect is in general more severe and frequent with right hemispheric lesions. These asymmetries appear to be related to asymmetrical representations of space and the body. For example, whereas the left hemisphere primarily attends to the right side, the right hemisphere attends to both sides.[12,13] Similarly, while the left hemisphere prepares for right-side action, the right prepares for both.[12]

TREATMENT AND MANAGEMENT OF NEGLECT

Because patients with neglect may be unaware of stimuli, they should avoid both driving and working with tools or machines that might cause injury to themselves or others. Their environment should be adjusted such that interactions with people and objects take place in the space that is ipsilateral to the damaged hemisphere.

Behavioral training paradigms have been used to teach patients with neglect to explore contralateral space. Although these procedures may be successful in the laboratory, they often fail to generalize to the environment. Similarly, prisms may be used to shift images from the contralateral to the ipsilateral side. Again, although this may improve performance on some tasks in the laboratory, these prisms do not seem to dramatically improve quality of life for patients with neglect.

Dynamic novel stimuli strongly summon attention in normal subjects. Butter and colleagues[14] used dynamic stimuli in the contralateral field of patients with neglect. Many patients showed a dramatic improvement following the treatment. However, because even hemianopic patients improved with dynamic stimuli, it is possible that these stimuli activate subcortical structures such as the colliculus. The colliculus receives more ipsilateral than contralateral input from the eyes. Lesions of the ipsilateral colliculus can reduce neglect (see Sprague[15]). Therefore, patching the ipsilateral eye may reduce the severity of neglect because it reduces ipsilateral collicular activation.[16] Irrigating the contralesional ear with cold water (caloric stimulation) may also dramatically improve neglect. Unfortunately, this improvement is only temporary. Last, pharmacologic therapy has been tried. If the dopaminergic system is unilaterally destroyed with toxins, animals may show neglect.[17]

Corwin and associates[18] demonstrated that animals with neglect from frontal lesions improved with dopamine agonists. Fleet and colleagues[19] reported two patients who seemed to improve with dopamine agonist therapy. However, double-blind controlled studies with dopamine agonists must still be performed on subjects with neglect. These studies should also learn whether dopamine therapy helps intentional or attentional neglect or both.

REFERENCES

 1. Heilman KM, Watson RT, Valenstein E: Neglect and related disorders, in Heilman KM, Valenstein E (eds): *Clinical Neuropsychology.* New York: Oxford University Press, 1993.
 2. Valler G, Sandroni P, Rusconi ML, Barberi S: Hemianopia, hemianesthesia, and spatial neglect: A study with evoked potentials. *Neurology* 41:1918–1922, 1991.
 3. Triggs WJ, Gold M, Gerstle G, et al: Motor neglect associated with a discrete parietal lesion. *Neurology* 44:1164–1166, 1994.
 4. Gold M, Shuren J, Heilman KM: Proximal intentional neglect: A case study. *J Neurol Neurosurg Psychiatry* 57:1395–1400, 1994.
 5. Mennemeier MS, Wertman E, Heilman KM: Neglect of near peripersonal space: Evidence for multidirectional attentional systems in humans. *Brain* 115:37–50, 1992.
 6. Ladavas E: Is the hemispatial deficit produced by right parietal damage associated with retinal or gravitational coordinates. *Brain* 110:167–180, 1987.
 7. Watson RT, Valenstein E, Day A, Heilman KM: Posterior neocortical systems subserving awareness and neglect: Neglect after superior temporal sulcus but not area 7 lesions. *Arch Neurol* 51:1014–1021, 1994.
 8. Mishkin M, Ungerleider LG, Macko KA: Object vision and spatial vision: Two cortical pathways. *Trends Neurosci* 6:414–417, 1983.
 9. Bisiach E, Luzzati C: Unilateral neglect of representational space. *Cortex* 14:129–133, 1978.
10. Heilman KM, Watson RT, Schulman H: A unilateral memory deficit. *J Neurol Neurosurg Psychiatry* 37:790–793, 1974.
11. Damasio AR: Time locked multiregional retroactivation: A systems-level proposal for the neural sub-

strates of recall and recognition. *Cognition* 33:25–62, 1989.

12. Heilman KM, Van Den Abell T: Right hemisphere dominance for attention: The mechanisms underlying hemispheric asymmetries of inattention (neglect). *Neurology* 30:327–330, 1980.

13. Pardo JV, Fox PT, Raichle ME: Localization of a human system for sustained attention by positron emission tomography. *Nature* 349:61–64, 1991.

14. Butter CM, Kirsch NL, Reeves G: The effect of lateralized dynamic stimuli on unilateral neglect following right hemisphere lesions. *Restorative Neurol Neurosci* 2:39–46, 1990.

15. Sprague JM: Interaction of cortex and superior colliculus in mediation of visually guided behavior in the cat. *Science* 153:1544–1547, 1966.

16. Posner MI, Rafal RD: Cognitive theories of attention and rehabilitation of attentional deficits, in Mier MJ, Benton AL, Diller L (eds): *Neuropsychological Rehabilitation*. New York: Guilford, 1987.

17. Marshall JF: Somatosensory inattention after dopamine-depleting intracerebral 6-OHDA injections: Spontaneous recovery and pharmacological control. *Brain Res* 177:311–324, 1979.

18. Corwin JV, Kanter S, Watson RT, et al: Apomorphine has a therapeutic effect on neglect produced by unilateral dorsomedial prefrontal cortex lesions in rats. *Exp Neurol* 36:683–698, 1986.

19. Fleet WS, Valenstein E, Watson RT, Heilman KM: Dopamine agonist therapy for neglect in humans. *Neurology* 37:1765–1771, 1987.

Chapter 25

HEMISPATIAL NEGLECT: COGNITIVE NEUROPSYCHOLOGICAL ASPECTS

Robert D. Rafal

This chapter reviews some of what has been learned about the cognitive neuropsychology of visual attention from the study of patients with neglect. The mutually supporting contributions of neurology and psychology have enriched both disciplines. Theories and methods for studying visual attention in normal people have contributed to our understanding of neglect; at the same time, a better understanding of neglect has helped illuminate some of the tougher theoretical issues in cognitive science.

DISENGAGING ATTENTION AND THE MECHANISM OF EXTINCTION

Does the phenomenon of extinction indicate that the parietal lobe is involved in controlling the orienting of attention? It had been argued[1,2] that an attentional explanation is not necessary to explain extinction. Instead, extinction could simply result from sensory competition. That is, although parietal lobe lesions do not produce hemianopia, they might nevertheless cause visual perceptions to be more weakly represented in the contralesional than in the ipsilesional field. Under conditions of sensory competition, the weakest sensory signal might not be perceived.

The most direct evidence for an attentional explanation of extinction was provided in an experiment in which it was shown that attending to the ipsilesional visual field could cause extinction, even under conditions where there was no compet-

ing visual target to be reported in the ipsilesional field.[3] Patients with lesions of the parietal lobe were asked to respond, by pressing a key, to the appearance of a target in the visual field either ipsilateral or contralateral to the lesion. The target was preceded by a cue that could summon attention to target location (valid cue) or to the wrong location (invalid cue). As illustrated in Fig. 25-1, the cue was either a brightening of one of the possible target locations or an arrow in the center of the display instructing the subject where to expect the forthcoming target signal. The results showed that patients with parietal lesions, even those who did not have neglect or show clinical extinction on conventional examination, demonstrated an "extinction-like reaction-time pattern": slow detection of targets in the contralesional field when attention had been summoned to the ipsilesional field. Detection reaction time (RT) in the field opposite to the lesion (contralesional field) was not much slowed (and in some patients not slowed at all compared to the ipsilesional field) if a valid cue was given. Therefore, the patients were able to use the cue to move their attention to the contralesional field; when they did so, their performance for contralesional targets was relatively unimpaired. When, however, a cue summoned attention toward the ipsilesional field and the target subsequently occurred in the opposite, contralesional field (invalid cue), detection RT slowed dramatically. This extinction-like RT pattern occurred even after the cue disappeared. That is, the extinction effect occurred when attention

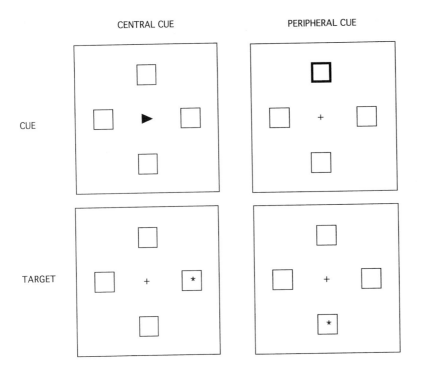

Figure 25-1

The experimental displays used to assess the orienting of spatial attention in a detection reaction time task. The subject's task is to press a button as soon as the target, an asterisk, appears in any of four locations. Preceding the presentation of the target is a cue that directs attention to one particular location. The cue can be central, in the form of an arrow (top left panel), *or peripheral, as when one box brightens* (top right panel). *When the cue directs attention to the location of the target, it is said to be a valid cue* (bottom left panel); *when it directs attention to a different location from the target, it is said to be invalid* (bottom right panel).

was directed ipsilesionally, even though there was no competing target signal to detect there. So it was not sensory competition that caused the extinction-like RT performance, but a difficulty in disengaging attention from the ipsilesional field.

The disengaging of attention has been hypothesized to be one of a number of elementary operations underlying the orienting of spatial attention.[4] Support for this framework comes from a replication of the cued detection RT experiment comparing patients with lesions of the temporoparietal junction (TPJ) to patients with progressive supranuclear palsy (PSP) who have degeneration of the midbrain.[5] Figure 25-2 shows the results of this experiment. The effects of valid and invalid cues are measured by differences in RT between the affected visual hemifield and the more normal hemifield. For TPJ-lesioned patients, this is the difference between ipsilesional and contralesional fields; for patients with PSP, the difference is between vertical and horizontal attention shifts (because PSP affects vertical movements of the eyes

and of attention more than horizontal). Patients with TPJ lesions show the extinction-like RT pattern, with no impairment for valid cues and an impairment for invalid cues only when attention is engaged ipsilesionally. This can be interpreted as an impairment of the *disengage* operation. In contrast, patients with midbrain lesions show a deficit in orienting only with valid cues, reflecting a difficulty in moving attention to its target location. This can be interpreted as an impairment in the *move* operation.

EXTINCTION AND NEGLECT: DISENGAGING ATTENTION DURING VISUAL SEARCH AND EXPLORATION

The foregoing experiments, and a number of others, examined the effect of parietal lesions on detection of a luminance change in a relatively uncluttered field.[6–9] The results show that the extinction phenomenon is caused by a deficit in at-

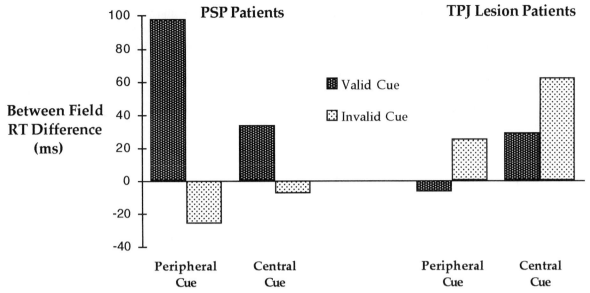

Figure 25-2

Covert orienting in patients with progressive supranuclear palsy and temperoparietal junction lesions. The results are depicted as the difference in detection RT between the more affected and the more normal visual fields. A greater difference in a given condition, thus, indicates a greater impairment in orienting in that condition. For the PSP patients (left) and the TPJ lesion patients (right) the between field detection RT differences are shown (in ms) for valid and invalid peripheral and central cues. The PSP patients are more impaired in the valid cue condition, especially with peripheral cues; whereas the TPJ lesion patients are more impaired in the invalid cue conditon, especially for central cues.

tention. Yet extinction is just one component of the neglect symptom complex. Other symptoms of neglect include defective exploratory behavior as revealed by tasks like line bisection, drawing, and cancellation. To understand how the deficit in disengaging attention can contribute to deficient exploration, we must examine attentional search in a cluttered field, where many objects are competing for attention. This is a more typical situation in the real world.

Eglin and coworkers[10] studied visual search in patients with neglect using a task developed by Treisman.[11] They varied the side of a predesignated conjunction target (one defined by a specific color and shape, requiring the conjunction of more than one feature to identify) among a variable number of distractors and measured the time to find the target. When distractors were present,

they could occur in either the ipsilesional or contralesional field. As long as no distractors appeared on the ipsilesional side of the display, no differences were found in locating a target on the neglected and intact sides. In other words, in displays that were limited to the ipsilesional side of a page, there were no objects to attract attention to the intact side and therefore nothing from which to disengage attention. Under these circumstances, the patients searched the display on the left as readily as they searched displays on the right. In contrast, for bilateral displays, in which distractors were present in both fields, search times increased as a function of the number of distractors or objects in the ipsilesional field. Each distractor on the intact side tripled the search time to locate the contralesional target. That is, the difficulty in disengaging attention from the ipsilesional field of distractors to move attention to the contralesional field depended on the number of items in the display.

Mark and colleagues[12] provide an elegantly simple demonstration that patients with neglect have difficulty in disengaging attention when ipsilesional items are present. They used a line cancellation task, a conventional bedside method for demonstrating and measuring neglect. The patient is shown a page filled with lines and asked to "cross them all out." Typically, a patient with left hemineglect fails to cross out many of the items on the left side of the page. Mark and coworkers[12] compared this conventional cancellation task with another condition in which they asked the patient to erase all the lines. As each line was erased and thus no longer present, the patient no longer had to disengage from it before moving on. Performance was strikingly better in this erasure task than in the conventional line cancellation task.

LOCAL PERCEPTUAL BIASES AFTER LESIONS OF THE RIGHT TEMPOROPARIETAL JUNCTION EXACERBATE VISUAL NEGLECT

Some patients with parietal lobe lesions may have extinction but not exhibit any of the exploratory deficits of neglect on drawing, copying, cancellation, or bisection tasks. In fact, extinction appears to be just as frequent after left as after right hemispheric lesions. However, other components of the syndrome, including deficits in exploration of contralesional space, are much more frequent after right hemispheric lesions, especially those that involve the right temporoparietal junction.[14] So while a deficit in disengaging attention may be a satisfactory explanation for extinction, it seems that other factors, perhaps specific to right hemispheric lesions, are at work in patients with the full-blown syndrome of neglect.

The observations of Eglin and coworkers[10] and Mark and colleagues,[12] discussed in the last section, show that the difficulty in disengaging attention is greater when attention is more actively

engaged. Factors that cause attention to become more actively engaged in the ipsilesional field will exacerbate the problem of disengaging attention and, hence, will exacerbate visual neglect. One effect of a lesion of the right temporoparietal junction (TPJ)—but not the left TPJ—is that it causes attention to become locked onto local perceptual details.[14] Figure 25-3[15] shows the copying of a patient with a large stroke of the right hemisphere and that of a patient with a large stroke involving the left hemisphere. The right hemispheric lesion causes almost complete exclusion of the global organization of the figure, while the left hemispheric lesion causes the exclusion of local detail.

The conjoint effects of the local bias with a difficulty in disengaging attention combine in producing some classic constructional signs of neglect in paper-and-pencil tasks. Consider, for example, a patient writing a number on to a clock face. She will be more successful if, as she is writing each number, she remains oriented to her task with reference to the whole clock. If her attention becomes excessively focused on the number she is writing and she loses sight of the whole clock, she will have more difficulty in disengaging from that number to fill in the rest of the numbers in

Figure 25-3

Drawings of hierarchical stimuli by two patients. A. The figure which the patients were asked to copy is a hierarchical pattern in which the large letter at the global level is an M, constructed from small Z's at the local level. B. Global organization is lost in this drawing by a patient with a right hemispheric lesion. C. Only the global organization of the figure is preserved while the local details are lost in this copy by a patient with a left hemispheric lesion. (From Delis, et al.,[15] with permission.)

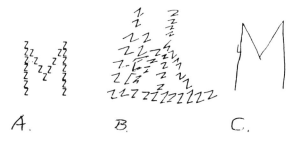

the correct location on the clock face. As she writes a number on the clock face, her attention becomes stuck there, and the difficulty in disengaging attention causes the numbers drawn subsequently to be bunched up together next to it. On the other hand, if the clock face remains uncluttered with other numbers, patients with neglect are better able to remain oriented to the whole clock face. Di Pellegrino[16] showed that neglect patients can put a single number in the appropriate location on a clock face as long as they are given a separate sheet for each number.

Halligan and Marshall[17] have shown the importance of the local bias as a contributor to neglect and how the local bias and the deficit in disengaging attention interact to determine neglect behavior. They asked their patient to bisect a horizontal line. In one condition, they also presented a vertical line at the right end of the line that was to be bisected. Before asking the patient to bisect the horizontal line, they gave their patient a task that required attending to the full extent of the vertical line. This obliged the patient to expand the "attentional spotlight" from the point at the end of the horizontal line, and this improved subsequent bisection performance on the horizontal line. By helping to overcome the tendency of the patient to become hyperengaged in a small focus of attention at the end of the line to be bisected, they were able to mitigate the neglect. Perhaps this expansion of attention to a more global level explains why patients with neglect make less bisection error when bisecting a rectangle than when bisecting a line, and why the higher the vertical extent of the rectangle, the less the bisection error.[19]

ORIENTING BIAS AND HEMISPHERIC RIVALRY

One model of the neurobiological basis of spatial attention postulates that each hemisphere, when activated, mediates an orienting response in the contralateral direction.[19–21] According to this account, neglect results from a unilateral lesion

because of a breakdown in the balance of hemispheric rivalry such that the nonlesioned hemisphere generates an unopposed orienting response to the side of the lesion. Experimental observations in patients with hemineglect provide some support for this view. Ladavas and colleagues[22] showed that, in patients with neglect, detection performance was best for the most ipsilesional targets, and detection of these ipsilesional targets was even better than for normal control subjects. These results suggest that patients with neglect hyperorient toward the ipsilesional field.

One variant of the hemispheric rivalry account emphasizes putative mutually inhibitory callosal connections between the hemispheres. According to this account, when one hemisphere is lesioned, homologous regions of the opposite hemisphere, which normally receive inhibitory projections from the damaged region, become disinhibited and hyperorient attention to the ipsilesional side. A recent study[23] has obtained some support for this hypothesis by examining the effects of transcranial magnetic stimulation (TMS) on thresholds for tactile perception detection in normal subjects. A suprathreshold (i.e., sufficiently strong to activate a twitch in the contralateral thumb when applied over motor cortex) TMS stimulus transiently inactivates subjacent cortex. This study examined whether the hemisphere opposite the TMS stimulus would show signs of disinhibition, manifested as a reduced threshold to detect a tactile stimulus in the thumb *ipsilateral* to the TMS lesion. Results supported the attentional disinhibition account by showing a reduced ipsilateral tactile threshold after parietal (3 or 5 cm posterior to motor cortex) TMS but not when TMS was applied at control locations over the motor cortex or 5 cm anterior to it.

Another mechanism that has been suggested for ipsilesional hyperorienting postulates a corticosubcortical interaction. According to this account, the unlesioned parietal lobe becomes disinhibited tonically increasing activity in the superior colliculus ipsilateral to it; whereas the colliculus on the side of the lesion loses some normally present tonic activation. As a result, parietal lesions also produce an imbalance in the activity of subcortical structures involved in orienting, such as the superior colliculus. The contralesional superior colliculus becomes disinhibited, and this results in exaggerated reflexive orienting to signals in the ipsilesional field.

Sprague's experiments in the cat confirmed that this kind of corticosubcortical interaction is important in regulating visually guided orienting behavior.[24] Cats were first rendered blind in one visual field by removing occipital and parietal cortex. It was then shown that vision in this field improved if the *opposite* superior colliculus were removed. A similar result is obtained if the inhibitory connections are severed between the contralesional substantia nigra pars reticulata and the ipsilesional colliculus.[25,26]

This "Sprague effect" is thought to work in the following way. Parietooccipital projections to the ipsilateral superior colliculus normally exert a tonic facilitation on it. After parietal lesions, the colliculus looses this tonic activation, and at the same time the opposite (contralesional) colliculus is in fact hyperactive due to increased activation from its parietal lobe, which, as we saw earlier, is disinhibited. The unilateral parietal lesion therefore also produces a subcortical imbalance between the two hemispheres. Moreover, this imbalance is sustained and aggravated by the mutually inhibitory connections between the two colliculi themselves. The more active contralesional superior colliculus is released from inhibition. The disinhibited contralesional colliculus produces disinhibited reflexive orienting to ipsilesional signals. Once attention is reflexively drawn to the ipsilesional field, the disengage deficit causes attention to get stuck there—resulting in neglect. If the contralesional superior colliculus is then removed (or the fibers of passage from the substantial nigra pars compacta to the opposite colliculus), the hyperorienting, and hence neglect, is ameliorated.

The Sprague effect demonstrates (at least in cats) that neglect is aggravated by disinhibition of subcortical visual pathways on the side opposite the cortical lesions and that prevention of visual input to this colliculus can alleviate neglect. Are there any practical applications of this phenomenon in rehabilitation? It is obviously not an option to surgically remove the contralesional superior colliculus in humans who have suffered parietal lobe strokes. It is possible, however, to decrease contralesional collicular activation and reflexive orienting by occluding the ipsilesional eye with a patch.[27] Indeed, patching the eye on the side of the lesion has been shown to help reduce symptoms of neglect.[28]

It seems likely that both cortical and subcortical imbalances contribute to the rightward bias of attention in patients with neglect. The subcortical imbalance is presumably more pronounced during the period of extensive diaschisis in the acute stage following the ictus. This imbalance is thought to produce not just a turning bias but also a shift in the spatial frame of reference such that the contralesional space is more weakly represented.[20,29] The effect of the rightward bias on spatial representation can be reduced transiently by production of a countervailing orienting bias through vestibular activation using a caloric stimulus. Vestibular activation can transiently alleviate not only visual[30,31] and somatosensory[32] neglect, but also the lack of awareness of the deficit (anosognosia).[33] A shift in spatial representation by vibration of neck muscles[34] or by optokinetic stimulation[35] can also decrease neglect.

PERCEPTUAL AND MOTOR NEGLECT

As reviewed in Chap. 24, the neural circuitry controlling spatial attention is a distributed network involving cortical and subcortical structures (see also Ref. 36). Within this network, there appear to be several specialized if interconnected circuits for regulating different kinds of behavior. Consider the different kinds of representations of space that would be needed for performing some common, simple tasks. A representation of space for generating an eye movement to a visual signal requires retinotopic coordinates. One for controlling reaching requires an egocentric representation of space—a scene-based representation in which location in the environment is coded and remains constant even if the eyes move. In monkeys, areas of parietal lobe have been identified in which retinotopically mapped information is gated by eye position.[37] For reaching, moreover, this representation must be integrated with a reference frame mapped relative to hand position.[38] This kind of representation of near peripersonal space may not, however, be adequate for throwing, which may require a separate representation of distant space.[39] The representations of space that might be adequate for reaching to a stationary object may not suffice to reach for an object that is moving. For this, one wants an object-based representation that updates the changing location of parts of the object relative to an egocentric reference frame. Finally, consider the problem of remembering the location of a cache of food relative to some geographic landmark or the problem of remembering the locations of cities on a map. For this one wants an allocentric reference frame in which the relative locations of objects are represented in a frame of reference totally independent of the viewpoint of the individual. For navigating while moving in the environment, this allocentric map must be continually updated and integrated with some enduring record of changes in body position with regard to this allocentric reference frame—for example, the "place" cells that have been identified in rat hippocampus.[40]

Given that there may be many such independent circuits that might be affected by some lesions and spared in others, it is not surprising that the manifestations of visual neglect may vary from patient to patient. In some, neglect may be more perceptual; in others, more motor. While this distinction may be better appreciated as a continuum rather than a dichotomy, the distinction between disorders of attention and intention has been a useful one.[41] Some patients with a more pure attentional disorder (typically those with more posterior lesions sparing frontal lobes) may have visual extinction and other perceptual deficits but no motor bias against turning contralesionally, moving the limbs contralateral to the lesion, or reaching into the contralesional field (directional hypokinesia).[42,43] Other patients who do not show extinction or other signs of perceptual neglect may, nevertheless, have a motor bias causing ne-

glect behavior in cancellation and construction tasks. Many patients with neglect have both perceptual and motor components affecting performance in these types of tasks. The relative contributions of these components may vary from patient to patient, depending on the size and location of the lesion in each patient and the task used to assess neglect.

Performance on many of the tests used clinically to diagnose neglect and measure its severity can be influenced by both motor and perceptual factors. Errors in line bisection or missed items in a cancellation task could be caused by perceptual neglect, motor neglect, or a combination of the two. Failure to cross out the leftmost items on a cancellation task, for example, could be due to failure to see the leftmost items or to a motor bias against moving toward the left.

Several ingenious studies have recently dissociated perceptual and motor components of neglect to measure their effects independently. Bisiach[44] first demonstrated this dissociation between perceptual and motor neglect by using a pulley device in a bisection task. Patients with neglect bisected lines under two conditions. In one, movement of the pencil toward the left (contralesional) direction required movement of the hand to the left. In this standard version of the task, a deficit in bisection could be due to perceptual neglect, motor neglect, or a combination of both. In the other version of the task, the pulley device required rightward movement of the hand to move the pencil to the left. Patients in whom neglect was exclusively due to a motor bias against moving the hand toward the left could be expected to improve their bisection performance in this version of the task. Some patients, those in whom neglect was dominantly perceptual, showed an equal amount of neglect in both versions of the task. Some patients showed some improvement in bisection with the pulley, and some, those in whom neglect was dominantly a motor bias, had no neglect under the pulley condition. These patients with more pure motor neglect tended to have more frontal lesions. Similar dissociations between perceptual and motor neglect have been also demonstrated using other devices, such as TV cameras[42] and mirrors[45] to separate out motor bias contributions to neglect. While there are clear tendencies for motor neglect to be more associated with more frontal lesions, the anatomic substrates relating to perceptual and motor neglect remain to be more precisely specified.[46]

Some simple bedside tests have recently been introduced to separate motor bias from perceptual neglect. Gold and colleagues[47] used a fixed-aperture technique in a cancellation task in which an opaque sheet with an aperture is placed over the page. The task can be done in one of two ways. In the standard task, the top sheet with the aperture is moved leftward by the patient during the cancellation task. In this task, both motor and perceptual neglect can influence performance. In the other condition, the bottom sheet is moved to the right by the patient in order to expose items on the left side of the page. In this version of the task, motor bias to the left cannot contribute to neglect performance, allowing for a purer assessment of perceptual contributions to neglect.

An elegant companion test to line bisection has been introduced[48] to determine whether motor neglect is contributing to bisection errors in an individual patient. Patients who manifest bisection errors are shown prebisected lines that may be bisected in the middle or to the left or right of midline. The patients are asked to point to the end of the line that is *closest* to the bisection mark. The critical condition is that in which the line is bisected in the middle. Patients in whom bisection error is due exclusively to a motor bias to the right would be expected to point to the right end of the line in this condition. In fact, several of the patients who were studied pointed to the left end of the line. This result indicates that, in these patients, their bisection errors were not due to a motor bias toward the right. These important observations suggest, in fact, that patients with perceptual neglect perceive the left side of the line as being shorter.

A more recent study has confirmed that neglect reduces perceived length. Milner and co-workers[49] showed patients with neglect two horizontal bars on a sheet of paper, one in each visual field, and asked them to judge which bar was shorter. On the critical trial in which the bars were equal in length, the patients indicated the bars in the left field to be shorter. In a control test in which vertical bars were shown, no such asymmetry in length judgment was evident. These findings indicate that patients with perceptual neglect experience compression of the left side of space.

This result may seem to be contradicted by a recent study of oculomotor behavior in patients with visual neglect.[50] Patients with left hemineglect, when asked to look straight ahead in the dark, deviated their eyes to the right of objective midline. This observation is consistent with the rightward hyperorienting described earlier, when we considered the hemispheric rivalry account of neglect. However, these patients did not show any asymmetry of oculomotor exploration around their subjective midline. That is, although they deviated their eyes rightward of true midline, eye movements to the left of their subjective midline were as great as eye movements to the right of it. This result would seem to indicate that there is a shift in perceived center of the egocentric world but no compression of spatial representation to the left of this center. However, the study of Karnath and associates[50] measured eye movements in the dark, presumably in relation to far extrapersonal space. That of Milner and coworkers[49] examined attention in relation to objects being manipulated in near peripersonal space. In the next section, we will see that neglect can be greatly influenced by the frame of reference in which it is examined and that the operations of visual attention are contingent on the requirements made of it for perception and action.

WHAT IS NEGLECTED IN NEGLECT?

It is now clear that visual neglect is not simply blindness in one visual field or even a lack of attention restricted to one visual field. Although neglect is greater for objects to the left (for right hemineglect) of fixation, it does not have the sharp retinotopic boundaries of hemianopia. Rather, it seems to operate over a gradient.[22] Using the cueing task described earlier, it has been shown, for example, that an extinction-like RT deficit can occur for detecting the leftmost of two stimuli in the right visual field,[7] even though this event is in the "good" field (and is in fact closer to the fovea). In this sense neglect seems to operate as a directional bias independent of visual field. However, neglect does, also, differentially affect the two visual fields. Baynes and coworkers[6] showed that vertical shifts of attention from an invalid cue were slower in the contralesional than the ipsilesional visual field.

So while it is clear that neglect is a deficit in attending to visual information, we still need to consider what it is that is neglected. We have seen that several different representations of space are maintained in the brain. Neglect could result from a degradation of any of these representations or of the ability to attend to any of them. Thus, what is neglected in neglect may differ from patient to patient, depending on which representations of space are involved by the lesion; in any given patient, what is neglected may depend on the requirements of the task at hand.

Reference Frames of Visual Neglect

Extrapersonal space exists independent of the viewpoint of the observer. Even when we are lying down (or standing on our heads), "up" and "down" remain the same, determined by the gravitational field. Ladavas[51] first showed that when patients with neglect tilted their heads, neglect was manifest not in terms of visual field but in terms of "gravitational" coordinates.

However, Fig. 25-4 shows a striking demonstration, using a test devised by Lynn Robertson, that neglect is not always manifest in terms of simple environmental (gravitational) coordinates. The examiner tests for extinction by wiggling a finger on each of his hands. In one condition, the examiner's body and face are rotated to the left (that is, the reference frame is rotated counterclockwise). In this condition the patient detects the upper finger wiggle and extinguishes the lower; that is, there is extinction of the left side of the reference frame. In contrast, when the examiner's body and face are rotated to the right (that is the reference frame is rotated clockwise), the patient

now detects the lower finger wiggle and extinguishes the upper. That is, there is now extinction of the opposite spatial location, but this again is on the left side of the reference frame. In this case, then, neglect is not manifest with reference to gravitational coordinates but with reference to the principal axis of the attended object.

It seems that visual neglect does not simply affect a visual field mapped in retinotopic coordinates nor even simply one side of egocentric space. It can be manifest in object-based coordinates. To understand how neglect can operate in object-based coordinates for objects that are neglected—an apparent contradiction—we must first consider to what degree visual objects can be represented in the neglected field outside of the focus of attention.

Figure-Ground Segregation and Grouping in Visual Neglect

When we look at the two drawings on the left (*A*) and right (*B*) of Fig. 25-5,[52] we normally see bright-green objects on a dim red background (both because the green is brighter and because its area is smaller than that of the dim red). Driver and colleagues[53] showed a patient with left hemineglect figures like these; they asked him to remember the shape of the dividing line between red and green and to then match this line with the probe shapes (shown under the study shapes in Fig. 25-5). Notice that the boundary to be remembered is on the left side of the page in *A* and on the right in *B*; yet for *A*, the boundary to be remembered lies on the right side of the green object, while in *B* it lies on the left side of the green object. The patient's task did not require any judgment about either the perceived object (green) or its ground (red). His task was only to attend to the shape of the line bordering the two colored areas. Were neglect manifest strictly with respect to egocentric space, more errors would have been expected for *A* than for *B*. The results showed the exact opposite pattern. The patient was much more accurate in condition *A*, where the contour to be remembered was on the right side of the object but on the left side of the page, than in condition *B*, where

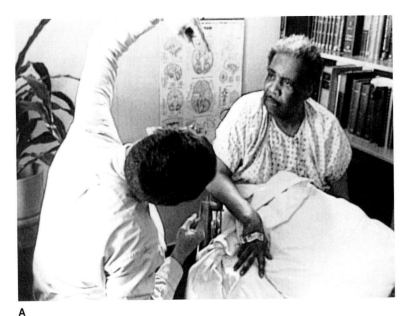

A

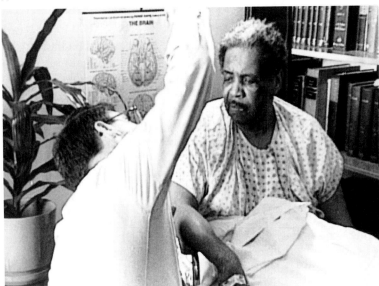

B

Figure 25-4
*Reference frames and neglect. This patient detected a single finger wiggling in his contralesional field but did not see it when a finger was also wiggled simultaneously in the ipsilesional (right) field (extinction). The test illustrated here demonstrates the dependence of extinction on the reference frame of the patient. When the examiner rotates clockwise (A), there is extinction of the lower stimulus, which is still the left side of the object, and the patient looks up. When the examiner rotates counterclockwise (B), there is extinction of the upper stimulus, which is still the left side of the object, and the patient looks down.
(From Rafal,[75] with permission.)*

the contour to be remembered was on the left side of the object but on the right side of the page. Although the green shape on the left side in *A* was in the neglected field and while judgments about the object were not relevant to the task at hand, the patient's attention was nevertheless summoned to it.

In this example, neglect operated with regard to the reference frame of the object. These observations tell us two important things: (1) the processes for segregating figure from ground can operate preattentively in the neglected field and (2) attention operates at a later stage on candidate objects generated by these preattentive processes.

Figure 25-5

A patient with left hemispatial neglect was shown figures like those shown here and asked to report verbally whether the contour dividing red (hatched) and bright-green (white) areas of a rectangle matched the probe line presented immediately below the rectangle following its offset. Normally the small bright-green region is seen as figure against the dim red background. Although not required to identify figure or ground, the patient showed more neglect for the left side of the figure (B), even though this figure was in the right visual field. (Adapted from Driver et al.,[53] with permission.)

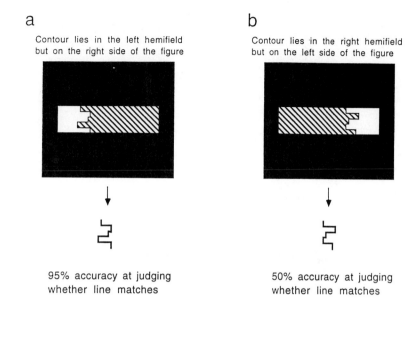

a

Contour lies in the left hemifield but on the right side of the figure

95% accuracy at judging whether line matches

b

Contour lies in the right hemifield but on the left side of the figure

50% accuracy at judging whether line matches

The object-based neglect of objects segregated from ground is nicely shown by the drawings of similar shapes shown in Fig. 25-6.[54]

Another preattentive process that is preserved in patients with unilateral neglect is the segregation of figure from ground based on symmetry. The effect of symmetry in preattentively generating candidate objects was first demonstrated by showing a patient with visual neglect pictures in which isoluminant red and green areas were alternated across a page. Either the red or the green areas on each page were symmetrical. The patient was asked to report simply whether the red or green areas appeared to be "in front." Normal individuals see symmetrical regions as being the figure and report them to be in front of the ground. Like any normal individual, the patient reported symmetrical regions to be in front, indicating that he had perceived the symmetrical objects as the figure. When he was asked to judge whether the shapes were symmetrical or not, he performed at chance. That is, even though his neglect prevented him from reporting whether or not shapes were symmetrical, he nevertheless per-

Figure 25-6

Object-based neglect is demonstrated by the copying performance of a patient with left hemispatial neglect. When asked to copy the black object, the patient did well, since the jagged contour is on the right side of the black object. When asked to copy the white object, the patient was unable to copy the jagged contour, since it is on the left side of the object being attended. (From Marshall and Halligan,[54] with permission.)

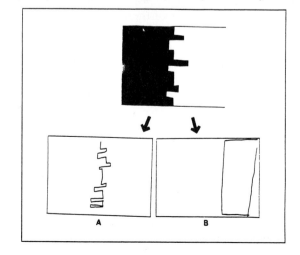

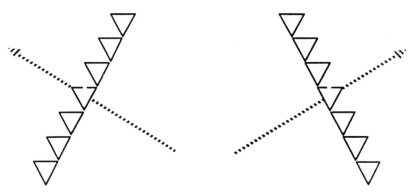

Figure 25-7
The figures used by Driver and coworkers[55] to study axis-based visual neglect. Three patients with left hemispatial neglect were asked to report whether or not the triangle in the center had a gap in it. Because of grouping of the triangles, triangles on the left were seen as pointing toward the northwest, so that the gap in the top of the central triangle is on the right side of its principal axis, whereas the triangles on the right are seen as pointing toward the northeast, so that the gap in the top of the central triangle is on the left side of its principal axis. All three patients had more neglect (missed seeing the gap) in the condition shown on the right than in the condition shown on the left. (From Driver et al.,[55] with permission.)

ceived symmetrical shapes as the objects in the visual scene.

Once candidate objects are preattentively segregated from background, they may then be grouped with other objects based on gestalt principals. Figure 25-7 shows a task used to test whether grouping is preserved in visual neglect.[55] The patient's task was simply to determine whether or not there was a gap in the top of the central triangle. The principal axis of the triangle (i.e., which way it appeared to point) was manipulated by the way in which the central triangle was grouped with the others. In the figure on the right, the alignment of the triangles (from southwest to northeast) causes them to appear to be pointing toward the northwest; the gap in the top of the central triangle is perceived to appear on the right side of its perceived principal axis. In the figure on the left, the alignment of the triangles (from southeast to northwest) causes them to appear to be pointing toward the northeast. The gap in the top of the central triangle is perceived to appear on the left side of its perceived principal axis. Results in three patients with left hemineglect showed that all missed more of the gaps in the condition on the

right, in which the gap was on the perceived left of the triangle. These results demonstrate that grouping is preserved in visual neglect and that attention operates in the reference frame of the group such that visual neglect is determined based on the principal axis of the group.

Object-Centered Neglect

The results of the experiment shown in Fig. 25-7[55] provide a more formal proof of the phenomenon shown in Fig. 25-4. After figure-ground segmentation occurs preattentively, candidate objects become represented to which attention may then be directed. Attention is allocated to the attended object aligned with its principal axis. Neglect is then manifest for parts of the object or other objects contralateral to the primary axis of the attended object. If, as shown in Fig. 25-4, the principal axis of the attended object moves or rotates, neglect moves or rotates with it.[56] Behrman and Tipper showed object-based neglect which actually moved to the ipsilesional side of the object after it rotated. Reaction time was measured to targets appearing in either the left (contralesional) or right (ipsilesional) side of a dumbbell. Patients were slower to respond to targets on the left. If the dumbbell rotated, however, such that the two sides of the dumbbell reversed field, RTs were prolonged for targets on the right.

Object-based neglect has also been inferred from the reading errors of neglect patients. In a striking demonstration of neglect dyslexia,[57] a patient with right hemineglect made more errors at the end of the word regardless of the orientation of the word on the page—that is, even when the word was upside down, such that the right end of the word was in the left visual field. Patients with neglect have also been shown to make more reading errors when they read pronounceable nonwords than when they read words.[58–60] This shows that word forms are preattentively processed and integrate the constituent letters into a single object. The study by Brunn and Farah[59] incorporated cancellation or line bisection tasks along with the reading task. Less neglect was found on these secondary tasks when the primary task required reading a word as opposed to a nonword. This finding suggests that word processing causes an automatic deployment of attention to encompass the word and, in patients with left neglect, this draws their attention to the left.

Not all attempts to identify object-based neglect have been successful; a contrast of the studies that demonstrated object-based neglect and those that did not is instructive. Farah and colleagues[61] asked patients to name colors surrounding pictures of common objects. When the pictures were rotated, the colors neglected did not rotate with the object; that is, neglect remained location-based rather than object-based. Behrman and Moscovitch[62] used the same paradigm and confirmed the lack of object-based neglect with object drawings. However, object-based neglect was manifest in the special case where the objects were asymmetrical letters. That is, object-based neglect was manifest when the object's identity was uniquely defined by its principal axis.

Spatial Representations and Neglect

Neglect can result not only in the failure to perceive or to respond to contralesional signals or objects but also to a lack of conscious access to the contralesional side of visual images stored in memory.[65] Bisiach and Luzzatti[64] asked patients with left hemineglect to imagine themselves in the Piazza del Duomo in Milan. In one condition, they asked the patients to imagine themselves at one end of the square, looking toward the cathedral dominating the other end of the square, and to describe what they would be able to see. In another condition, the patients were asked to imagine themselves standing on the cathedral steps facing the opposite way. In both circumstances, the patients reported fewer landmarks on the contralesional side of the mental image. (For non-Milanese clinicians, a baseball imagery task may be substituted. In one condition, the patient is asked to imagine herself as the catcher and to name the positions of all the players that she would be able to see. Then the patient is told to imagine being in center field and is asked the same question.)

These kinds of observations have engendered an account of neglect in which the parietal lobes are assumed to maintain a representation of space in viewer-centered coordinates, and that parietal lesions produce a degradation of the contralesional representation. In an elegant experimental test of this account, Bisiach and coworkers[65] had patients view cloudlike shapes that were passed slowly behind a slit (so that only part of the shape could be seen at any moment). The task required that a mental image be generated and maintained as the slit moved over the shape they were attempting to remember. The patients were shown two shapes that could be either the same or different, and they were asked to respond whether the shapes were the same or not. On the trials in which the shapes were different, they could be different on the patients' left or right side. The patients made more errors on this task when shapes were different from each other on the contralesional end than on the ipsilesional end.

We need to know more about the neuroanatomic and pathophysiologic basis for the deficit of spatial representation in neglect.[66] Some authors have considered spatial representation in terms of oculomotor coding,[67,68] while others have emphasized spatial working memory.[69] Recent reports show that perceptual neglect and neglect of internal imagery may be dissociated. Two patients with perceptual neglect and mainly parietal lesions did not evidence neglect in visual imagery,[70] whereas a patient with a frontal lesion causing neglect of imagined scenes did not have perceptual neglect.[71]

CONCLUDING REMARKS

In neglect, a constellation of symptoms is seen affecting both perception and exploratory behavior. Which symptoms (and with what severity) occur in any given patient depends upon the extent and location of the lesion, its chronicity, and the premorbid cognitive architecture of the individual. Across the rather heterogeneous population of patients with elements of the neglect syndrome, the pathophysiologic mechanisms underlying each of the component symptoms are diverse. We are just beginning to understand some of these: hyper-reflexive orienting toward the ipsilesional side or to local elements in the visual scene; impaired ability to disengage attention; a deranged internal representation of space, which is not only shifted but contracts contralesionally; impaired voluntary orienting toward the contralesional field; a motor bias toward the ipsilesional side that causes defective contralesional exploratory behavior; deficient ability to generate contralesional voluntary saccades; and failure of contralesional stimuli to produce arousal. The manifestations of neglect in an individual patient may not simply represent the additive contributions of each of these mechanisms, depending on which are affected by the lesion, but rather an interaction between them.[72]

The study of neglect has advanced our understanding of preattentive vision and the functions of attention in object recognition and the control of goal-directed behavior. We have learned that the visual scene is parsed preattentively into candidate objects and that attention then operates on these objects to afford awareness and recognition of them and to guide subsequent action. We are developing a better understanding of the plight of these patients and of their perplexing behavior. These insights can be applied to fashioning more rational approaches to their rehabilitation.[73–75]

REFERENCES

1. Bender MB, Feldman M: The so-called "visual agnosias." *Brain* 95:173–186, 1972.
2. Bay E: Disturbances of visual perception and their examination. *Brain* 76:515–530, 1953.
3. Posner MI, Walker JA, Friedrich FJ, Rafal R: Effects of parietal injury on covert orienting of visual attention. *J Neurosci* 4:1863–1874, 1984.
4. Posner MI, Inhoff AW, Friedrich FJ, Cohen A: Isolating attentional systems: A cognitive-anatomical analysis. *Psychobiology* 15:107–121, 1987.
5. Rafal RD, Posner MI, Friedman JH, et al: Orienting of visual attention in progressive supranuclear palsy. *Brain* 111:267–280, 1988.
6. Baynes K, Holtzman HD, Volpe BT: Components of visual attention: Alterations in response pattern to visual stimuli following parietal lobe infarction. *Brain* 109:99–114, 1986.
7. Posner MI, Walker JA, Friedrich FJ, Rafal RD: How do the parietal lobes direct covert attention? *Neuropsychologia* 25:135–146, 1987.
8. Morrow LA, Ratcliff GCP: The disengagement of covert attention and the neglect syndrome. *Psychobiology* 16:261–269, 1988.
9. Egly R, Driver J, Rafal R: Shifting visual attention between objects and locations: Evidence from normal and parietal lesion subjects. *J Exp Psychol Gen* 123:127–161, 1994.
10. Eglin M, Robertson LC, Knight RT: Visual search performance in the neglect syndrome. *J Cogn Neurosci* 1:372–385, 1989.
11. Treisman A, Gelade G: A feature integration theory of attention. *Cogn Psychol* 12:97–136, 1980.
12. Mark VW, Kooistra CA, Heilman KM: Hemispatial neglect affected by non-neglected stimuli. *Neurology* 38:1207–1211, 1988.
13. Vallar G: The anatomical basis of spatial neglect in humans, in Robertson IH, Marshall JC (ed): *Unilateral Neglect: Clinical and Experimental Studies.* Hillsdale, NJ, Erlbaum, 1993, pp 27–62.
14. Robertson LC, Lamb MR, Knight RT: Effects of lesions of the temporal-parietal junction on perceptual and attentional processing in humans. *J Neurosci* 8:3757–3769, 1988.
15. Delis DC, Robertson LC, Efron R: Hemispheric

specialization of memory for visual hierarchical stimuli. *Neuropsychologia* 24:205–214, 1986.

16. Di Pellegrino G: Clock-drawing in a case of left visu-spatial neglect: A deficit of disengagement. *Neuropsychologia* 33:353–358, 1995.

17. Halligan PW, Marshall JC: Right-sided cueing can ameliorate left neglect. *Neuropsychol Rehabil* 4:63–73, 1994.

18. Vallar G: Left spatial hemineglect: An unmanageable explosion of dissociations? No. *Neuropsychol Rehabil* 4:209–212, 1994.

19. Kinsbourne M: Mechanisms of neglect: Implications for rehabilitation. *Neuropsychol Rehabil* 4:151–153, 1994.

20. Kinsbourne M: Hemi-neglect and hemisphere rivalry, in Weinstein EA, Friedland RP (ed): *Advances in Neurology.* New York, Raven Press, 1977, pp 41–49.

21. Kinsbourne M: Orientational bias model of unilateral neglect: Evidence from attentional gradients within hemispace, in Robertson IH, Marshall JC (ed): *Unilateral Neglect: Clinical and Experimental Studies.* Hillsdale, NJ, Erlbaum, 1993, pp 63–86.

22. Ladavas E, Del Pesce M, Provinciali L: Unilateral attention deficits and hemispheric asymmetries in the control of visual attention. *Neuropsychologia* 27:353–366, 1989.

23. Seyal M, Ro T, Rafal R: Perception of subthreshold cutaneous stimuli following transcranial magnetic stimulation of ipsilateral parietal cortex. *Ann Neurol* 38:264–267, 1995.

24. Sprague JM: Interaction of cortex and superior colliculus in mediation of peripherally summoned behavior in the cat. *Science* 153:1544–1547, 1966.

25. Wallace SF, Rosenquist AC, Sprague JM: Recovery from cortical blindness mediated by destruction of nontectotectal fibers in the commissure of the superior colliculus in the cat. *J Comp Neurol* 284:429–450, 1989.

26. Wallace SF, Rosenquist AC, Sprague JM: Ibotenic acid lesions of the lateral substantia nigra restore visual orientation behavior in the hemianopic cat. *J Comp Neurol* 296:222–252, 1990.

27. Posner MI, Rafal RD: Cognitive theories of attention and the rehabilitation of attentional deficits, in Meir RJ, Diller L, Benton AL (ed): *Neuropsychological Rehabilitation.* London, Churchill Livingstone, 1987.

28. Butter CM, Kirsch NL, Reeves G: The effect of lateralized dynamic stimuli on unilateral spatial ne-

glect following right hemisphere lesions. *Restor Neurol Neurosci* 2:39–46, 1990.

29. Karnath H-O: Disturbed coordinate transformation in the neural representation of space as the crucial mechanism leading to neglect. *Neuropsychol Rehabil* 4:147–150, 1994.

30. Rubens AB: Caloric stimulation and unilateral visual neglect. *Neurology* 35:1019–1024, 1985.

31. Cappa SF, Sterzi R, Vallar G, Bisiach E: Remission of hemineglect and anosognosia after vestibular stimulation. *Neuropsychologia* 25:775–782, 1987.

32. Vallar G, Bottini G, Rusconi ML, Sterzi R: Exploring somatosensory hemineglect by vestibular stimulation. *Brain* 116:71–86, 1993.

33. Bisiach E, Rusconi ML, Vallar G: Remission of somatoparaphrenic delusion through vestibular stimulation. *Neuropsychologia* 29:1029–1031, 1991.

34. Karnath HO, Christ K, Hartje W: Decrease of contralateral neglect by neck muscle vibration and spatial orientation of trunk midline. *Brain* 116:383–396, 1993.

35. Pizzamiglio L, Frasca R, Guariglia C, et al: Effect of optokinetic stimulation in patients with visual neglect. *Cortex* 26:535–540, 1990.

36. Mesulam MM: A cortical network for directed attention and unilateral neglect. *Ann Neurol* 4:309–325, 1981.

37. Zisper D, Anderson R: A back-propagation programmed network that simulates response properties of a subset of posterior parietal neurons. *Nature* 331:679–684, 1988.

38. Graziano MSA, Yap GS, Gross CG: Coding of visual space by premotor neurons. *Science* 266:1054–1057, 1994.

39. Rizzolatti G, Camarda R: Neural circuits for spatial attention and unilateral neglect, in Jeannerod M (ed): *Neurophysiological and Neuropsychological Aspects of Spatial Neglect.* Amsterdam, North-Holland, 1987, pp 289–314. (Stelmach GE, Vroon PA, eds. *Advances in Psychology;* vol 45).

40. O'Keefe J: Hippocampus, theta, and spatial memory. *Curr Opin Neurobiol* 3:917–924, 1993.

41. Heilman KM, Valenstein E, Watson RT: The neglect syndrome, in Fredricks JAM (ed): *Clinical Neuropsychology.* New York, Elsevier 1985, pp 153–183.

42. Coslett HB, Bowers D, Fitzpatrick E, et al: Directional hypokinesia and hemispatial inattention in neglect. *Brain* 113:475–486, 1990.

43. Heilman KM, Bowers D, Coslett HB, et al: Directional hypokinesia: Prolonged reaction times for

leftward movements in patients with right hemi-sphere lesions and neglect. *Neurology* 35:855–859, 1985.

44. Bisiach E, Geminiani G, Berti A, Rusconi ML: Perceptual and premotor factors of unilateral neglect. *Neurology* 40:1278–1281, 1990.

45. Tegner R, Levander M: Through a looking glass: A new technique to demonstrate directional hypokinesia in unilateral neglect. *Brain* 113:1943–1951, 1991.

46. Mattingley JB, Bradshaw JG, Phillips JG: Impairments of movement initiation and execution in unilateral neglect: Directional hypokinesia and bradykinesia. *Brain* 115:1849–1874, 1992.

47. Heilman KM, Valenstein E, Watson RT: The what and how of neglect. *Neuropsychol Rehabil* 4:133–139, 1994.

48. Milner AD, Harvey M, Roberts RC, Forster SV: Line bisection errors in visual neglect: Misguided action or size distortion? *Neuropsychologia* 31:39–49, 1993.

49. Milner AD, Harvey M: Distortion of size perception in visuospatial neglect. *Curr Biol* 5:85–89, 1995.

50. Karnath H-O: Ocular space exploration in the dark and its relation to subjective and objective body orientation in neglect patients with parietal lesions. *Neuropsychologia* 33:371–378, 1995.

51. Ladavas E: Is the hemispatial deficit produced by right parietal damage associated with retinal or gravitational coordinates? *Brain* 110:167–180, 1987.

52. Baylis GC, Driver J: One-sided edge-assignment in vision: 1. Figure-ground segmentation and attention to objects. *Curr Dir Psychol Sci.* In press.

53. Driver J, Baylis G, Rafal R: Preserved figure-ground segmentation and symmetry perception in a patient with neglect. *Nature* 360:73–75, 1993.

54. Marshall JC, Halligan PW: Left in the dark: The neglect of theory. *Neuropsychol Rehabil* 4:161–167, 1994.

55. Driver J, Baylis GC, Goodrich SJ, Rafal RD: Axis-based neglect of visual shapes. *Neuropsychologia* 32:1353–1365, 1994.

56. Behrman M, Tipper SP: Object-based visual attention: Evidence from unilateral neglect, in Umilta C, Moscovitch M (ed): *Attention and Performance: XIV. Conscious and Nonconscious Processing and Cognitive Functioning.* Hillsdale, NJ, Erlbaum, 1994.

57. Hillis AE, Caramazza A: Deficit to stimulus-centered, letter shape representations in a case of "uni-lateral neglect." *Neuropsychologia* 29:1223–1240, 1991.

58. Friedrich FJ, Walker JA, Posner MI: Effects of parietal lesions on visual matching: Implications for reading errors. *Cogn Neuropsychol* 2:253–264, 1985.

59. Brunn JL, Farah MJ: The relationship between spatial attention and reading: Evidence from the neglect syndrome. *Cogn Neuropsychol* 8:59–75, 1991.

60. Sieroff E, Pollatsek A, Posner MI: Recognition of visual letter strings following injury to the posterior visual spatial attention system. *Cogn Neuropsychol* 5:427–449, 1988.

61. Farah MJ, Brunn JL, Wong AB, et al: Frames of reference for allocating attention to space: Evidence from the neglect syndrome. *Neuropsychologia* 28:335–347, 1990.

62. Behrman M, Moscovitch M: Object-centered neglect in patients with unilateral neglect: Effects of left-right coordinates of objects. *J Cogn Neurosci* 6:1–16, 1994.

63. Bisiach E: Mental representation in unilateral neglect and related disorders: The twentieth Bartlett Memorial Lecture. *Q J Exp Psychol* 46A:435–462, 1993.

64. Bisiach E, Luzzatti C: Unilateral neglect of representational space. *Cortex* 14:129–133, 1978.

65. Bisiach E, Luzzatti C, Perani D: Unilateral neglect, representational schema and consciousness. *Brain* 102:609–618, 1979.

66. Kinsella G, Olver J, Ng K, et al: Analysis of the syndrome of unilateral neglect. *Cortex* 29:135–140, 1993.

67. Duhamel JR, Colby CL, Goldberg ME: The updating of the representation of visual space in parietal cortex by intended eye movements. *Science* 255:90–92, 1992.

68. Gianotti G: The role of spontaneous eye movements in orienting attention and in unilateral neglect, in Robertson IH, Marshall JC (ed): *Unilateral Neglect: Clinical and Experimental Studies.* Hillsdale, NJ, Erlbaum, 1993, 107–122.

69. Funahashi S, Bruce CJ, Goldman RP: Dorsolateral prefrontal lesions and oculomotor delayed-response performance: Evidence for mnemonic "scotomas." *J Neurosci* 13:1479–1497, 1993.

70. Anderson B: Spared awareness for the left side of internal visual images in patients with left-sided extrapersonal neglect. *Neurology* 43:213–216, 1993.

71. Guariglia C, Padovani A, Pantano P, Pizzamiglio

L: Unilateral neglect restricted to visual imagery. *Nature* 364:235–237, 1993.

72. Humphreys GW, Riddoch MJ: Interactive attentional systems in unilateral visual neglect, in Robertson IH, Marshall JC (eds): *Unilateral Neglect: Clinical and Experimental Studies.* Hillsdale, NJ, Erlbaum, 1993, pp 139–168.

73. Robertson IH, Halligan PW, Marshall JC: Prospects for the rehabilitation of unilateral neglect, in Rob-

ertson IH, Marshall JC (eds): *Unilateral Neglect: Clinical and Experimental Studies.* Hillsdale, NJ, Erlbaum, 1993, pp 279–292.

74. Diller L, Riley E: The behavioural management of neglect, in Robertson IH, Marshall JC (eds): *Unilateral Neglect: Clinical and Experimental Studies.* Hillsdale, NJ, Erlbaum, 1993, pp 293–310.

75. Rafal RD: Neglect. *Curr Opin Neurobiol* 4:2312–2316, 1994.

Chapter 26

BALINT SYNDROME

Robert D. Rafal

The previous chapters on hemispatial neglect describe the syndrome resulting from *unilateral* lesions of the posterior association cortex. Here we consider the syndrome resulting from *bilateral* parietal damage—Balint syndrome. The Hungarian physician Rezsö Balint first described the fascinating syndrome named after him in 1909. He emphasized, in his patient, the constriction of visual attention resulting in an inability to perceive more than one object at a time, and "optic ataxia," the inability to reach accurately toward an object. Many similar patients have since been reported.[1,4,5,9,15–19]

Figure 26-1 shows simultanagnosia in a patient with Balint syndrome. When I first showed two superimposed objects to this man, he reported seeing the comb; and when asked about the spoon, he denied seeing it. I then set down these objects for a few seconds. When I picked them up and showed them to the patient again, asking him "what do you see now?" he reported seeing only the comb. After setting them down a second time and showing them to the patient a few seconds later, he seemed perplexed and could not seem to make out what he was seeing. When asked if he still saw either the comb or the spoon, he shook his head and said, "I think I see a blackboard with a bunch of writing on it." In fact, there was a blackboard with writing in chalk behind me. He was looking through the comb and the spoon and his attention had become locked on the chalk marks. All other objects, comb and spoon included, were excluded from his awareness.

Patients with simultanagnosia have their at-

tention fixed on a single object or detail in the scene and neglect all other objects except the one they are looking at. This is not due to a constriction of the visual field (tunnel vision); the visual field may be shown to be intact when a single object is presented in the periphery of an otherwise empty visual field. Moreover, the simultanagnosia is independent of the size of the object or the extent to which the object includes the visual periphery. These patients can see an ant or an elephant—but only one object at a time.

The biparietal syndrome of Balint is thus distinguished from hemispatial neglect by a distinctive form of object-based neglect that is independent of spatial location. This constriction of visual attention is accompanied by spatial disorientation, and the conjoint effects of these two symptoms leaves the patient helpless in a visually meaningless and chaotic world. This chapter reviews the clinical and neuropsychological aspects of this intriguing syndrome. It begins with the anatomic basis of the syndrome and some of the diseases that cause it. It then details the independent component symptoms of Balint syndrome. It ends with a provisional synthesis and some conclusions about what Balint syndrome tells us about the role attention and spatial representation in perception and action.

THE MORBID ANATOMY AND ETIOLOGY OF BALINT SYNDROME

The anatomic substrate for Balint syndrome is distinguished from that which causes spatial hemine-

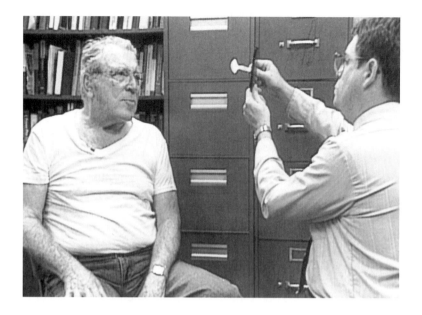

Figure 26-1
Simultanagnosia in patient J.F. He was able to see either the comb or the spoon but not both.

glect not only because the lesions causing Balint syndrome are bilateral but also because the lesions involve different areas of posterior association cortex. Whereas lesions of the temporoparietal junction seem most critical for producing hemispatial neglect, Balint syndrome is produced by bilateral lesions of the parietooccipital junction. Temporoparietal junction involvement by the lesion is not necessary to produce Balint syndrome. Lesions of the occipitoparietal junction that cause Balint syndrome characteristically involve the angular gyrus, the dorsorostral occipital lobe (area 19), and often the precuneus (superior parietal lobe), but they may spare the supramarginal gyrus and the superior temporal gyrus. Figure 26-2 shows a drawing of the lesions in the patient reported by Balint in 1909.[2]

The supramarginal gyrus and the posterior part of the superior temporal gyrus are affected in the right hemisphere but spared on the left. The superior parietal lobule is only minimally involved in either hemisphere. Given the involvement of the superior temporal gyrus on the right in the patient reported by Balint, it is noteworthy that this patient showed left hemispatial neglect in addition to the classic elements of Balint syndrome: "the attention of the patient is always directed [by

approximately 35 or 40°] to the right-hand side of space when he is asked to direct his attention to another object after having fixed his gaze on a first one, he tends to the right-hand rather than the left-hand side."[2]

Balint syndrome may occur, however, unaccompanied by hemispatial neglect and in the absence of temporoparietal junction involvement by the lesion. Figure 26-3 shows the reconstructed magnetic resonance imaging (MRI) brain scan of one of my patients (R.M.) with classic Balint syndrome. The lesion involves the cuneus and precuneus regions of the parietooccipital junction and part of the angular gyrus of both hemispheres but spares the supramarginal and superior temporal gyri. Review of other recent cases of Balint syndrome emphasizes the consistent involvement of the posterior parietal lobe (the angular gyrus) as critical in producing the syndrome.[4–6]

Other adjacent brain regions may contribute to some of the individual component symptoms, especially the lateral occipital gyrus, the cuneus (area 19), and the precuneus (area 7). At this juncture it is not clear that we can relate all the component symptoms of Balint syndrome to a lesion of a specific brain region that causes a deficit in a discrete mechanism underlying all of the compo-

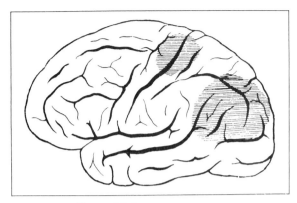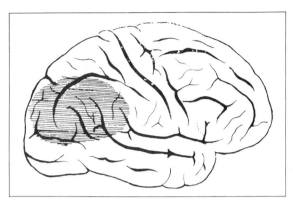

Figure 26-2
Reproduction of Balint's sketches of the brain found at autopsy. (From Husain and Stein,[2] with permission.)

Figure 26-3
Three dimensional neuroimage reconstruction of the MRI of patient R.M. (From Friedman-Hill et al.,[3] with permission.)

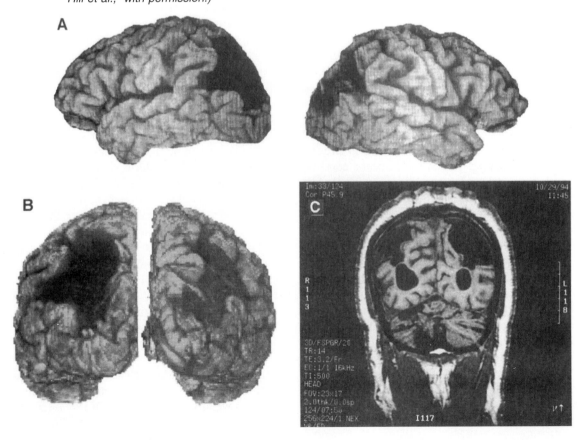

nent symptoms.[7] Rizzo[8] has urged caution in applying the designation of *syndrome* to this constellation of signs, and future research may show further dissociations of the component symptoms based on more discrete lesion analysis. However, it does seem clear that bilateral lesions of the parietooccipital junctions do often lead to a symptom complex that is distinctive and dramatic and that the lesions causing this syndrome may spare brain regions most commonly associated with hemispatial neglect.

Given that Balint syndrome is associated with symmetrical lesions involving the parietooccipital junction, the diseases causing it are those in which symmetrical lesions affecting these areas occur. Penetrating missile wounds from projectiles entering from the side and traversing in the coronal plane through the parietooccipital regions have been reported by Luria[9] and by Holmes and Horax.[10] Strokes, typically due to cardiac emboli, successively insulting both hemispheres in the distribution of posterior parietal branches of the middle cerebral artery are another common cause.[3–5] The parietooccipital junction lies in the watershed between the middle and the posterior cerebral arteries. Therefore watershed infarction due to global cerebral hypoperfusion is perhaps the single entity in which Balint syndrome is most characteristic. While watershed infarction may be seen after cardiac arrest, it is more typically seen in circumstances of reduced rather than absent cerebral blood flow and under conditions in which low blood flow (oligemia) is also associated with reduced oxygen saturation (hypoxia). Hyperglycemia is often an aggravating factor. That is, watershed infarction is associated with conditions predisposing to the development of lactic acidosis in watershed brain regions. Such circumstances arise in patients undergoing surgery requiring cardiopulmonary bypass and in individuals (especially diabetics) suffering from cardiogenic shock producing hypotension accompanied by hypoxia from pulmonary edema. Another symmetrical pathology is the "butterfly" glioma—a malignant tumor originating in one parietal lobe and spreading across the corpus callosum to the other side. Radi-

ation necrosis may develop after radiation of a parietal lobe tumor in the opposite hemisphere in the tract of the radiation port. Cerebral degenerative disease, prototypically Alzheimer disease, may begin, exceptionally, in the parietooccipital regions, and there is now a growing literature reporting cases of classic Balint syndrome due to degenerative diseases.[11–13]

Symmetrical lesions involving the parietooccipital regions and restricted to them will characteristically cause the Balint symptom complex in its pure form. While strokes and head trauma may occasionally cause such discretely restricted and symmetrical lesions (such as those shown in Fig. 26-3), it is more commonly the case that lesions will not respect these territories, and more extensive damage to occipital lobe and other brain regions is more likely. Thus, the elements of Balint syndrome may be dissociable from each other. On the other hand, they may also be discernible in patients whose visual or oculomotor deficits extend beyond those of Balint syndrome per se. Coexisting visual field deficits, apperceptive or associative agnosia, prosopagnosia, alexia, and other cognitive deficits are often present in association with Balint syndrome or some of its constituent elements. The syndrome described in the next section is based on case reports selected for manifesting a more or less "pure" Balint syndrome. It is well to keep in mind that such cases are the exception rather than the rule in clinical practice. The patient reported by Balint,[14] for example, also had left hemispatial neglect, possibly due to extension of the lesion into the right temporoparietal junction, in addition to Balint syndrome as delineated by Holmes and Horax.[10] The next section reviews the component symptoms of Balint syndrome following the analysis of Holmes and Horax, which emphasizes two cardinal symptoms: a constriction of visual attention to one object (simultaneous agnosia) and spatial disorientation. It considers how each of these component symptoms and their interaction contribute to the disability of the patient in everyday tasks such as looking for objects, comparing them, counting them, and reaching for them as well as reading and writing.

THE SYMPTOM COMPLEX OF BALINT SYNDROME

When Balint syndrome is severe, the patient behaves like a blind person. The patient does not blink to a visual threat, bumps into things when walking, and may not turn toward people who approach. If the examiner is calm and forbearing and takes pains to place an object directly at fixation, with no other competing objects present, the patient becomes aware of it and is able to see it clearly, but then becomes locked on it and is unable to see anything else. The degree to which local detail can capture the patient's attention and exclude all other objects from his or her ken can be quite amazing. I was testing a patient one day, drawing geometric shapes on a piece of paper and asking her to tell me what she saw. At one point she shook her head, perplexed, and told me, "I can't see any of those shapes now, doctor, the watermark on the paper is so distracting."

Patients with Balint syndrome can have normal visual acuity, spatial contrast sensitivity, stereopsis, and color vision and have no difficulty in detecting movement or in recognizing not only simple shapes but faces and complex objects as well. They can even recognize a series of individual pictures flashed briefly in a rapid serial visual presentation (RSVP) test.[4] Yet they are severely disabled and functionally blind. The patient is not able to make any sense of the visual world or to interact with it; and as we will see, the patient is lost in space. How are we to understand these difficulties, and what can we learn from them about attention and visual perception?

The 1919 paper of Holmes and Horax[10] stands as definitive in detailing the syndrome and specifying its components. In addition to noting the simultanagnosia and optic ataxia reported by Balint, their analysis emphasized "spatial disorientation" as the cardinal feature of the syndrome.

Constriction of Visual Attention: Simultanagnosia

In their 1919 report of a 30-year-old First World War veteran who had a gunshot wound through the parietooccipital regions, Holmes and Horax observed that "the essential feature was his inability to direct attention to, and to take cognizance of, two or more objects. . . ."[10] They argued that this difficulty "must be attributed to a special disturbance or limitation of attention. . . ."[10] Because of this constriction of visual attention, the patient could attend to only one object at a time regardless of the size of the object. In this report, Holmes and Horax observe that the constriction of visual attention was not location-based but object-based: "In one test, for instance, a large square was drawn on a sheet of paper and he recognized it immediately, but when it was again shown to him after a cross had been drawn in its center he saw the cross, but identified the surrounding figure only after considerable hesitation; his attention seemed to be absorbed by the first object on which his eyes fell."[10]

The visual experience of the patient with Balint syndrome is a chaotic one of isolated snapshots with no coherence in space or time. In a report on their patient, Coslett and Saffran say that "television programs bewildered her because she could only 'see' one person or object at a time and, therefore, could not determine who was speaking or being spoken to: she reported watching a movie in which, after a heated argument, she noted to her surprise and consternation that the character she had been watching was suddenly sent reeling across the room, apparently as a consequence of a punch thrown by a character she had never seen. . . ."[4]

Coslett and Saffran's patient also illustrated how patients with Balint syndrome are confounded in their efforts to read: "Although she read single words effortlessly, she stopped reading because the 'competing words' confused her."[4] Writing was similarly afflicted, as "when creating a letter she saw only the tip of the pencil and the letter under construction and 'lost' the previously constructed letter."[4]

Patients are unable to perform the simplest everyday tasks involving the comparison of two objects. They cannot tell which of two lines is longer or which of two coins is bigger. Holmes and Horax's patient could not tell, visually, which of two pencils was bigger,[10] although he had no difficulty doing so if he touched them. Holmes and Horax made the important observation that, although their patient could not explicitly compare the lengths of two lines or angles of a quadrilateral shape, he had no difficulty distinguishing shapes whose identity is implicitly dependent upon such comparisons: "Though he failed to distinguish any difference in the length of lines, even if it was as great as 50 percent, he could always recognize whether a quadrilateral rectangular figure was a square or not . . . he did not compare the lengths of its sides but 'on the first glance I see the whole figure and know whether it is a square or not'. . . . He could also appreciate . . . the size of angles; a rhomboid even when its sides stood at almost right angles was 'a square shoved out of shape.'"[10] Holmes and Horax appreciated the importance of their observations for the understanding of normal vision: "It is therefore obvious that though he could not compare or estimate linear extensions he preserved the faculty of appreciating the shape of bidimensional figures. It was on this

that his ability to identify familiar objects depended. . . . this is due to the rule that the mind when possible takes cognizance of unities."[10]

The term *simultanagnosia* was originated specifically to describe a defect in integrating complex visual scenes,[20] when shown pictures like that in Fig. 26-4. When Tyler[19] showed this picture to a patient with simultaneous agnosia, she first only reported seeing a mountain. When it was shown to her again, she only noticed a man and did not recognize it as being the same drawing. Only after prolonged examination did she interpret the picture as "a man looking at mountains." She never noticed the camel.

It is important to keep in mind the fact that the term *simultanagnosia*, as operationally defined by Wolpert, is specific to the interpretation of figure drawings and that it includes, but is more general than, the constriction of attention seen in Balint syndrome. It is seen also in conditions other than Balint syndrome. Unilateral lesions of the left temperooccipital cortex can produce simultanagnosia as defined by Wolpert. However, the underlying nature of the deficit in perceiving multi-

Figure 26-4

Tyler's patient initially saw only the man when shown this picture. When shown it a second time, she saw the mountains. Eventually she was able to report seeing a man looking at mountains, but she never did see the camel. (From Tyler,[19] with permission.)

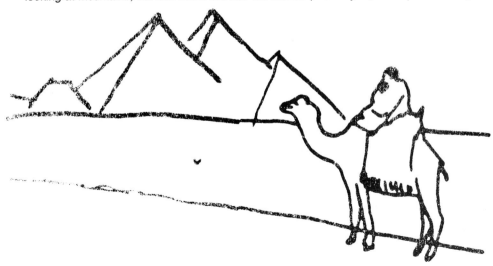

ple objects is different in these cases. Farah[21] has suggested the terms *dorsal* and *ventral simultanagnosia* to distinguish the impairment of patients with Balint syndrome from the impairment that follows left temporooccipital lesions (see Chap. 17). Whereas dorsal simultanagnosia results from an attentional limitation precluding even the detection of multiple objects, ventral simultanagnosia is caused by the slowing of visual processing that results in a bottleneck at the pattern recognition stage of vision.[22,23] Patients with lesions restricted to extrastriate cortex in the occipital lobe may have simultanagnosia, but without the other component symptoms of Balint syndrome or the degree of disability.[24] In Balint syndrome the patient not only cannot attend to more than one object at a time but, as discussed next, is spatially disoriented. He or she does not know where that object is or where to look next.

Spatial Disorientation

Holmes and Horax[10] considered spatial disorientation to be a symptom independent of simultanagnosia and to be the cardinal feature of the syndrome: "The most prominent symptom, however . . . was his inability to orient and localize correctly objects which he saw."[10] Patients with Balint syndrome cannot indicate the location of objects, verbally or by pointing (optic ataxia, to be discussed later). This gentleman was clearly lost in space: "On one occasion, for instance, he was led a few yards from his bed and then told to return to it; after searching with his eyes for a few moments he identified the bed, but immediately started off in a wrong direction." Holmes and Horax emphasized that the defect in visual localization was not restricted to visual objects in the outside world but also extended to a defect in spatial memory: "He described as a visualist does his house, his family, a hospital ward in which he had previously been, etc. But, on the other hand, he had complete loss of memory of topography; he was totally unable to describe the route between the house in a provincial town in which he had lived all his life and the railways station a short distance away, explaining 'I used to be able

to see the way but I can't see it now. . . .' He was similarly unable to say how he could find his room in a barracks in which he had been stationed for some months, or describe the geography of trenches in which he had served."[10]

Holmes and Horax considered spatial disorientation to be the salient feature of the syndrome, and that "The disturbances we have interpreted as a local and special affection of attention [simultanagnosia] . . . do not form an essential part of that complex of symptoms which is of greatest interest in our case, and often occurs apart from and independently of it." Nevertheless, they appreciated that the interaction of simultanagnosia with spatial disorientation combined in contributing to the severe disability in simple, daily tasks like reading and counting. Their patient complained that, " 'When I move my eye from a word I cannot get back to the right place.' " Later, when he became able to read a few words in sequence he could rarely bring his eyes to the left of the succeeding line—" 'That's when I'm done, I can't get my eyes down to the next line.' " "When asked to count a row of coins he became hopelessly confused, went from one end to the other and back again, and often passed over some of the series; but he succeeded in enumerating them correctly when he was allowed to run his fingers over them. . . . he generally stared fixedly for a time at one and then moved his eyes about the surface irregularly and unmethodically without making a systematic attempt to explore the whole. When four or five coins were placed irregularly he generally failed to see them all, frequently included one or more a second time in his count, and eventually became so confused that he gave up the attempt. That this was due to his inability to form a clear picture or idea of the spatial relations of those he perceived was made probable by his own explanation, 'I seem to lose myself when I look from one to the other.' "[10]

Ocular Behavior

Oculomotor behavior is also chaotic in Balint syndrome, with striking disturbances of fixation, saccade initiation and accuracy, and smooth-pursuit eye movements. The patient may be unable to maintain fixation, may generate apparently random saccadic eye movements,[15] and may seem unable to execute smooth-pursuit eye movements. The disorder of eye movement in Balint syndrome is restricted to visually guided eye movements. The patient can program accurate eye movements when they are guided by sound or touch: "When, however, requested to look at his own finger or to any point of his body which was touched he did so promptly and accurately."[10]

Holmes and Horax suggest that the oculomotor disturbances seen in Balint syndrome are secondary to the perceptual derangement: "Some influence might be attributed to the abnormalities of the movements of his eyes, but . . . these were an effect and not the cause." "All these symptoms were secondary to and dependent upon the loss of spatial orientation by vision."[10] Early in the course, some contribution from corticocollicular interactions due to diaschisis may contribute to the severity of the eye movement impairment; even in the chronic stages, the extent of the lesion in some patients may also contribute some additional primary oculomotor disorder.[2,5] However, the oculomotor behavior of Balint syndrome patients is chiefly caused by the failure to see what they are to look at or by uncertainty about the target's location—not necessarily due to deficient oculomotor programming per se. Their eye movements are chaotic because their perceptual experience is chaotic.

Holmes and Horax described the typical behavior of a patient with Balint syndrome when tested for smooth pursuit eye movements: "When an object at which he was staring was moved at a slow and uniform rate he could keep his eyes on it, but if it was jerked or moved abruptly it quickly disappeared. . . ."[10] In the case of patient M.B. shown in Fig. 26-5, she lost the pen after pursuing it only a few degrees, and even though it was still only a few degrees from fixation, it vanished. She stopped pursuing it with her eyes because she could no longer see it. Her eyes then seem to grope randomly for the missed object.

As shown in Fig. 26-6, however, she was able to smoothly and briskly track my face with accurate pursuit eye movements. There is something

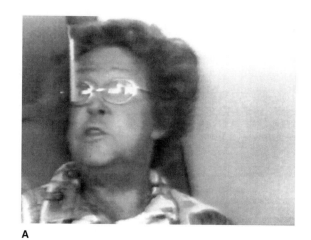

A

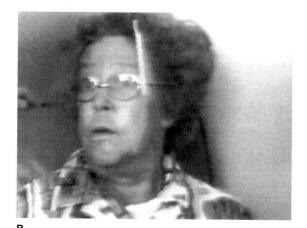

B

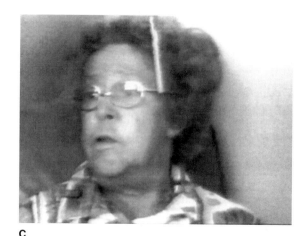

C

Figure 26-5

Impaired pursuit eye movements in patient M.B. After fixating the pen and reporting it (A) *she failed to follow it with her eyes when it moved* (B and C).

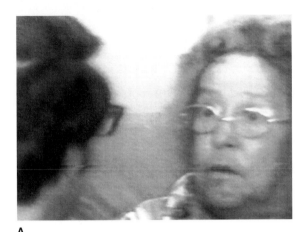

A

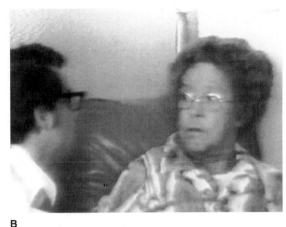

B

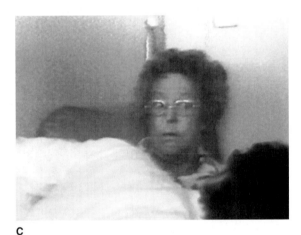

C

Figure 26-6
Preserved pursuit eye movement in patient M.B. when following a face.

special about the human face. Human newborns, in whom visual neocortex has not yet matured, will orient specifically to a face, perhaps reflecting a privileged circuit for faces in the midbrain.[25] As shown in Fig. 26-6, use of a perceptually salient stimulus can serve to demonstrate that, in Balint syndrome, the neural machinery for the generation of smooth-pursuit eye movements is intact.

The neural machinery for executing saccadic eye movements may also be intact. Although the patient is unable to generate accurate saccades when searching strategically, there are occasions, when attention is not engaged on another object, in which reflexive eye movements to a suddenly appearing peripheral target or to a sudden movement may be brisk and accurate. When initially seen, M.B. (the patient shown in Figs. 26-5 and

26-6) was not able to maintain fixation on any object, and she never saw or made a saccade toward any object presented in the peripheral visual field. The sequence shown in Fig. 26-7 was recorded 10 days later, when she had begun to show some signs of improvement. In Fig. 26-7A, she has not yet seen the pipe, even though it is almost right in front of her. It then captures her attention, and in Fig. 26-7B she has made a fast and accurate saccade to it. I put the pipe down for a few seconds and then presented it again in her right visual field. In Fig. 26-7C, she reports seeing "that same old pipe." Then I put the pipe down and presented a pen in her right visual field. In Fig. 26-7D, she sees something there and, obviously puzzled and unable to recognize it, fails spontaneously to look at it, finally saying, "I think that's still a pipe, I'm

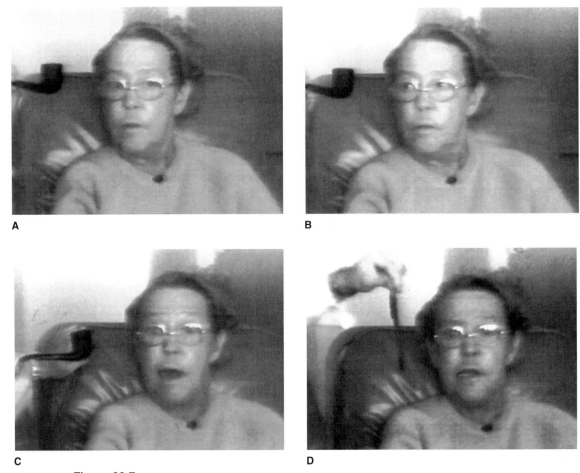

Figure 26-7
Eye movements and perception in patient M.B. (see text).

not sure." When the pen was then briskly moved in front of her (Fig. 26-7*E*), she immediately identified it: "Oh, that's the pen." When the pen was abruptly pulled from fixation, it vanished (Fig. 26-7*F*). When I asked her to "look at it," she responded, "I can't see it, doctor," and began moving her eyes, looking for it (Fig. 26-7*G*). When I wiggled it (Fig. 26-7*H*), it again captured her attention, and she made a saccade directly to it.

Optic Ataxia

Figure 26-8 shows misreaching in Balint syndrome. Even after the patient sees the spoon, he does not look directly at it, and his reaching is inaccurate

in depth as well as being off to the side. He then gropes for the spoon until his hand bumps into it. Given a pencil and asked to mark the center of a circle, the patient with Balint syndrome typically will not even get the mark within the circle. In part this may be because the patient cannot take cognizance, simultaneously, of both the circle and the pencil point; but it is also clear that the patient does not know where the circle is. Holmes and Horax considered optic ataxia, like the oculomotor impairment, to be secondary to "his inability to orient and localize correctly in space objects which he saw. When . . . asked to take hold of or point to any object, he projected his hand out vaguely, generally in a wrong direction, and had

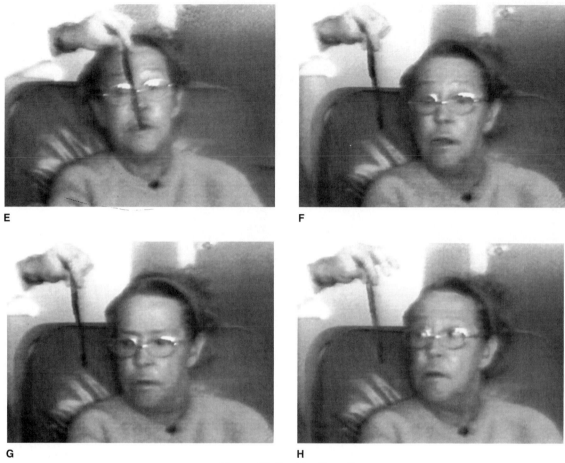

E

F

G

H

Figure 26-7 *(Continued)*

obviously no accurate idea of its distance from him."[10] Figure 26-9, from Holmes and Horax, shows the misreaching in their patient in a perimetric record of their patient's "binocular visual field to represent the false localization of objects. . . ." The roman numerals indicate the location of the target objects and the arabic numbers the point to which the patient reached.

Again, Holmes and Horax[10] observed that the lack of access to a representation of space was selective for vision. Their patient was able to localize sounds and he did have a representation of peripersonal space based on kinesthetic input: "The contrast between the defective spatial guidance he received from vision and the accurate knowledge of space that contact gave him, was

excellently illustrated when he attempted to take soup from a small bowl with a spoon; if he held the bowl in his own hand he always succeeded in placing the spoon accurately in it, . . . but when it was held by an observer or placed on a table in front of him he could rarely bring his spoon to it at once, but had to grope for it till he had located it by touch."[10]

Impaired Depth Perception

Holmes and Horax[10] also incorporated the lack of depth perception within the deficit of spatial disorientation. Although the patient in their 1919 report did have deficient stereoscopic vision, they considered his astereopsis as an incidental associa-

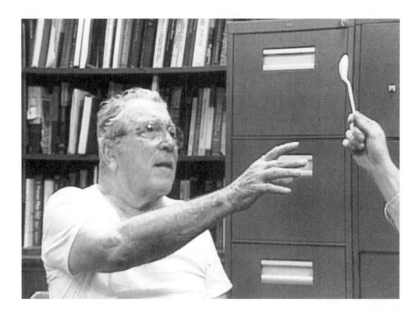

Figure 26-8
Optic ataxia in patient J.F.

tion and not typical of Balint syndrome, since Holmes[26] had reported six different patients with the same syndrome but with preserved stereoscopic fusion. They viewed the loss of depth perception in Balint syndrome as a consequence of the loss of topographic perception and as a failure to have any appreciation of distance.

The lack of depth perception even extends to superimposed objects in line drawings whose relative positions in depth to one another are indicated by occlusion cues. When R.M. was shown drawings like that in Fig. 26-10 by Dr. V. S. Ramachandran,[39] he was unable to tell which was closer to him, the square, or the circle partly occluded by it. Again, the combined deficits of simultanagnosia and spatial disorientation make this seemingly effortless task impossible for the patient with Balint syndrome. Since he could attend to only one, either the square or the circle, he was unable to make a comparative judgment relating them, and he also did not know where either of them were.

This patient did not lack a concept of depth or distance. When shown a single object like a book tilted toward him and asked to judge whether the top or bottom was tilted toward him (no judgment relating the relative locations of two objects is needed here), he was able to do so. The impairment of depth perception in Balint syndrome,

then, seems to be due to a failure to appreciate the relative location of two objects—or of the patient and the object he or she is looking at. Size cues seem not to help the patient judge the distance to an object. However, Holmes and Horax commented that their patient's lack of a sense of distance did not indicate a lack of appreciation of metrics in general, since he could ". . . indicate by his two hands the extension of ordinary standards of linear measurement, as an inch, a foot, or a yard . . . and he could indicate the lengths of familiar objects, as his rifle, bayonet, etc."[26]

Although a patient may not be able to estimate the distance from an object or to report which of two objects is closer, depth cues do influence the perception of individual objects. When Ramachandran showed R.M. the drawings seen in Fig. 26-11, the patient clearly experienced both shape from shading and the sense of depth it imparted. Like normals, he saw the top-lit circles in Fig. 26-11 as "bumps" and those bottom-lit circles as "holes." It was also the case that, although he could not tell if the object he was looking at was behind or in front of any other object, he nevertheless seemed to experience objects as being in front of the background. For drawings like those described in Chap. 25, on hemispatial neglect, normal individuals typically report symmetrical shapes as

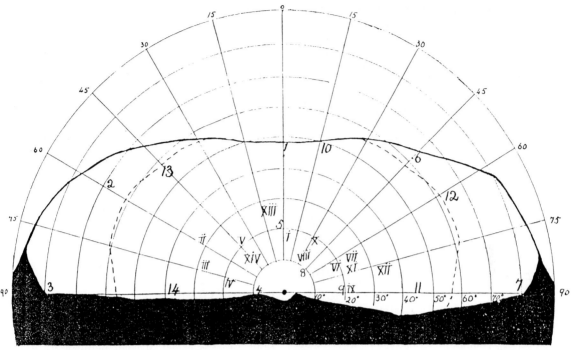

Figure 26-9
Spatial disorientation and optic ataxia in Holmes and Horax's patient. The binocular visual field to represent the false localization of objects seen by extramacular vision. The arabic numerals indicate the true positions of the objects; the roman figures the positions into which the patient projected them. (From Holmes and Horax,[10] with permission.)

"figures" and experience them as being in front of the background. When Diane Beck showed R.M. these figures and asked him to say "which color is in front," he reliably reported the color of the symmetrical shape as being in front.

Figure 26-10
Occlusion cues cause normal individuals to see a circle behind a square. Patient R.M. could not tell which shape was in front of which. (From Ramachandran,[39] with permission.)

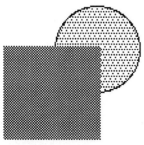

BALINT SYNDROME: THEORETICAL IMPLICATIONS

All of the cardinal features of Balint syndrome can be attributed to two major components and their interaction: (1) a constriction of visual attention to a single object and (2) the lack of conscious access to a topographic representation of visual space for either the external visual field or for topographic memory. The constriction of visual attention causes the patient to become locked on a single object. That object becomes the entire visual world without any relation to other objects—or to its own past or future.

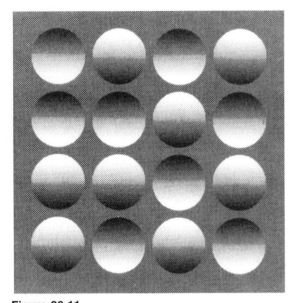

Figure 26-11

Preserved perception of depth from shading in patient R.M. Like normal individuals, he saw the top-lit circles in this figure as "bumps" and the bottom-lit circles as "holes." This percept occurs because the visual system assumes, for purposes of depth computation based on shading, that light is coming from above. (Note that if the page is turned on the side, so that light and dark are on left or right, the perception of depth is absent.) (From Ramachandran,[39] with permission.)

A real object is perceptually distinguished from others based on its unique location; it must be in a different place from any other object. Even if it is superimposed in the retinal image, occlusion cues normally assign each of the two objects to different distances from the observer and will engender an experience of depth. Because patients lack conscious access to a visual representation of topographic space, there is only one "there" out there—and hence there can be only one object.

Even the one object that is seen is experientially mutable. While normal mechanisms of object-based visual attention will follow an "object file" if the object moves,[27,28] for the patient it disappears and the patient's eyes cannot follow. Even if the object stays still, exceptional effort is required for the patient to interact manually with it.

Not knowing where the object is, the patient has to grope for it, as if in the dark.

The reality experienced by the patient with Balint syndrome must inform contemporary theories of attention and perception. This final section considers three major issues: (1) dissociable mechanisms for attending to objects and locations; (2) preattentive perceptual processing, and (3) the role that attention and spatial representation play in integrating the features of objects and of objects with one another into a coherent visual world.

OBJECT-BASED ATTENTION

The Contributions of the Left Hemisphere in Shifting Attention between Objects

Chapter 25, on hemispatial neglect, discussed attention mechanisms for selecting by spatial locations and the effect of right hemispheric lesions on spatially based attention. In this chapter we have seen that the addition of a lesion in the left hemisphere adds an additional deficit in strictly object-based attention.

Egly and coworkers have recently employed the experiment shown in Fig. 26-12 to demonstrate, in patients with focal unilateral lesions[29] and in a split-brain patient,[30] the special contribution of the posterior association cortex of the left hemisphere in shifting attention between objects. The subjects in these experiments made simple reaction-time (RT) key-press responses to the appearance of a target presented at the end of one of two rectangles that were present throughout the trial. At the beginning of each trial, part of an object (in this case one of two rectangles) was cued by brightening the end of it. The cue indicated that a target was likely to occur at the location of the cue. On occasional trials in which the target did not appear at the cued location, it could either appear at the other end of the rectangle that was cued or an equal distance from the cue but in the other rectangle (Fig. 26-12A). Normal subjects showed a "cost" (i.e., slower RT) for detecting a target appearing at an uncued location, providing

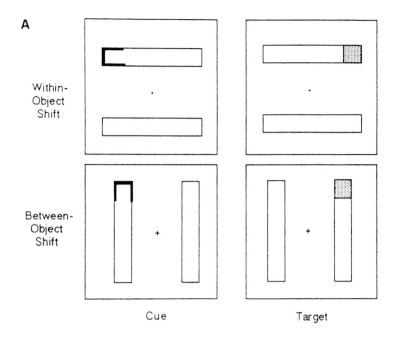

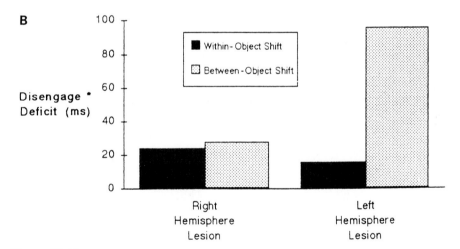

Figure 26-12

Egly's experiment for measuring shifts of attention between objects and locations. Top: One end of a rectangle is cued to indicate the location where a detection target is likely to occur. Occasionally this cue is invalid and the target appears at a different location. The uncued location where this target appears may either be within the same object or may require an attention shift to a different object. Bottom: The results from the experiment in patients with left (n = 5) and right (n = 8) parietal lesions. The size of the disengage deficit (the greater costs in reaction time to reallocate attention from ipsilesional to contralesional field compared to reallocating attention from contralesional to ipsilesional field) is shown in each patient group for the within- and between-object shift conditions. In the right parietal lesion group, the disengage deficit is present in both between- and within-object shift conditions and is not larger in the between-object shift condition. In the left parietal lesion group, the disengage deficit is manifest only in the between-object shift condition. (From Rafal and Robertson,[38] with permission.)

a measure of the time to shift attention to the target from the location where it had been expected. Moreover, cueing effects (or "costs") were greater for shifting attention between than within objects. Thus, this experiment provides a measure of the time to shift attention between objects that is independent of spatial location.

The results in the patients suggested a special role for the left parietal lobe in shifting attention between objects. Both groups of patients with unilateral lesions (left or right hemispheric lesion) had larger costs to respond to targets in their contralesional than ipsilesional fields, replicating the deficit in disengaging spatial attention described in Chap. 25. The important new finding was a difference between the two patient groups in shifting attention between objects (Fig. 26-12B). While both patient groups showed problems in disengaging attention from their intact field, the disengage deficit in patients with left hemispheric lesions only occurred for between-object shifts of attention from the ipsilesional to the contralesional field.[29] This finding suggests that the right parietal lobe may be critical for shifting attention between locations while the left parietal lobe is critical for shifting attention between objects. Converging evidence for a left hemispheric specialization in shifting attention between objects was obtained in a commissurotomized patient with disconnected neocortices.[30] In his right visual field, normal costs for shifting between objects were observed; no object-based costs were observed for attention shifts in the right visual field.

What Is a Visual Object?

Early visual processing parses the visual field into candidate objects based on uniform connectedness[31] and gestalt grouping principles. Our conscious attention is then engaged by objects. In Balint syndrome, the patient can be aware of only one entity, and typically that entity is an object rather than a feature or a constituent part. Thus, the patient of Holmes and Horax was able to see a "square" when shown four dots (: :): ". . . this is due to the rule that the mind when possible takes cognizance of unities."

Luria[9] systematically explored the question of what constitutes an object for a patient with Balint syndrome. Shown a six-pointed star drawn in a single color, Luria's patient saw a star. When the two triangles were drawn in different colors, the patient saw only one triangle.[9] When shown two adjacent circles, the patient saw only one of them; yet when the two circles were connected by a line, the patient saw a single object (a dumbbell or spectacles).

Applying a similar approach, Humphreys and Riddoch[32] have provided elegant experimental evidence demonstrating the object-based restriction of attention in Balint syndrome and the principles operating in early vision for generating objects for attentional selection. Two patients were shown 32 circles that were all red, all green, or half red and half green. The task was simply to report whether each display contained one or two colors. The critical test was when the displays contained two colors. In one condition, the spaces between the circles contained randomly placed black lines. In two further conditions, the lines connected either pairs of same-colored circles or pairs of different-colored circles. Both patients were better at correctly reporting the presence of two colors when the lines connected different-colored pairs of circles. Circles connected by a line are perceived as a single object (e.g., as a dumbbell). When each object contained both red and green, the patients could report the presence of the two colors. When the lines connected circles of the same color such that each object contained only a single color, only one color was perceived.

Of the candidate objects in the visual scene, which will be selected? The chaotic visual experience of the patient might seem to suggest a randomness in the selection process, but this is not always the case. In Fig. 26-13, searching for an O in a field of Qs (*top*) requires effortful search, while a Q in a field of Os pops out and is found effortlessly irrespective of the number of O distractors in the field. When Robertson and Grabowecky showed patient R.M. displays like those in Fig. 26-13 and asked him to tell what he saw, he rarely reported seeing an O for the array on the top and always reported seeing Q for the array on

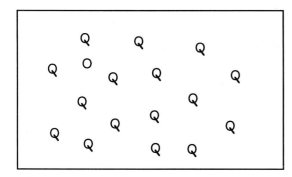

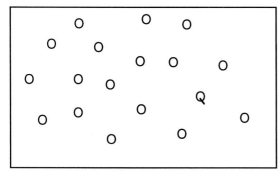

Figure 26-13
Normal individuals find that the search for an O among Qs (top) is effortful, and the more Qs in the field, the longer it takes to find the O. In contrast, a Q pops out in a field of Os (bottom), and the time to find it is independent of the number of O distractors. Patient R.M. never saw an O in the figure on the top, but the Q in the figure on the bottom popped out, just as it does for normal individuals.

the bottom. He could not find an O in a field of Qs, but a Q reliably popped out in a field of Os. The patient reported by Coslett and Saffran similarly experienced a visual pop out when shown a tilted line in a field of straight lines.[4]

Recall the example of the four dots. A patient with Balint syndrome typically will see either a single dot or a square, but he or she will not see four dots. In this example, seeing the square requires that all four dots be processed, but none of them can be "seen"; if the patient becomes aware of any one of them, the square disappears. How does the patient with Balint syndrome cope in a world filled with objects that contain other objects? A house also contains other objects, like

windows, doors, and a roof. The American flag is another example. A patient with Balint syndrome who can see only one object could see the stars, the stripes, or the flag. What determines whether the patient will see a house or a door? A flag? A star or stripe?

Robertson and Grabowecky showed R.M. hierarchical stimuli of the type employed by Navon[33] in which, for example, a large letter H was constructed from small S's (Fig. 26-14, top), and asked him to report what he saw. In every instance he reported the local element first (e.g., "S"). On repeated testing over several months, only twice did he also report the global element ("H") at all. His attention was consistently captured by the local element. When the global letter was made up of several different letters, he reported seeing "the alphabet." This demonstration

Figure 26-14
Hierarchical stimuli in which the local and global levels are incongruent (top) or congruent (bottom). Patient R.M. was almost never aware of the global letter in the figure on the top, but he was slower to report the local letter for this incongruent condition than he was when there was no competition from the global letter (bottom).

Global and Local

		S			S
		S			S
Incongruent		S S S S			S
		S			S
		S			S

		H			H
		H			H
Congruent		H H H H			H
		H			H
		H			H

illustrates the propensity of patients to get perceptually sucked into local details. It is reminiscent of the difficulties of J.F. (Fig. 26-1) getting stuck on the distant chalk marks and those of the lady whose attention got stuck on the watermark.

In Fig. 26-14, top, the elements at the local and global levels were both letters and psychologically equipotential. This will often not be the case with many real hierarchical objects. For example, a patient with Balint syndrome will more typically see a flag rather than a star or a stripe (in contrast to a patient with integrative agnosia, who fails to recognize an object because he gets stuck on a part of it[34]).

Visual Processing Outside of Conscious Awareness

As described in the last section, patient R.M. almost never saw the global stimulus when shown hierarchical letters like a big H made up of little S's (Fig. 26-14, top). Nevertheless, Egly and Robertson showed that R.M. reported the local letter more quickly when the global and local letters were congruent—a big H made of little H's (Fig. 26-14, bottom) than when they were incongruent—a big H made of little S's (Fig. 26-14, top). That is, although the patient was almost never aware of the big H in the latter case, the H was processed outside of his awareness, and it did slow him in reporting the S at the local level.

This finding demonstrates that, as is the case in hemispatial neglect, neglected objects do appear to be processed to a high level of semantic classification in patients with Balint syndrome. Furthermore, although this information is not consciously accessible to the patient, it does influence the perception of other objects that are seen. Coslett and Saffran[4] simultaneously presented pairs of words or pictures briefly to their patient, and asked her to read or name them. When the two stimuli were not related semantically, the patient usually saw only one of them; but when they were related, she was more likely to see them both. Hence, both stimuli must have been processed to a semantic level of representation, and the meaning of the words or objects determined whether one or both would be perceived.

Words are an example of hierarchical stimuli in which letters are present at the local level and the word at the global level. We[35] showed patient R.M. letter strings and asked him to report all the letters he could see. Since he could see only one letter at a time, he found this task difficult and, with the brief exposure durations used in the experiment, usually only saw a few of the letters. However, he was able to report more letters when the letter string constituted a word than when it did not. That is, even when the patient was naming letters and ignoring the word, the word was processed and helped bring the constituent letters to his awareness.

Attention, Spatial Representation, and Feature Integration: Gluing the World Together

I discussed earlier how the single object seen by the patient is experientially mutable in time. It has no past or future. Any object that moves disappears. In addition, objects seen in the present can be perplexing to the patient, because other objects that the patient does not see, and their features, are processed and do impinge upon the patient's experience of the attended object. Normally, the features of an object, such as its color and shape, are correctly conjoined, because visual attention selects the location of the object and combines all the features sharing that same location.[36] For the patient with Balint syndrome, however, all locations are the same, and all the features that impinge on the patient's awareness are perceptually conjoined into that object.

Friedman-Hill and coworkers[3] showed R.M. pairs of colored letters and asked him to report the letter he saw and its color. R.M. saw an exceptional number of illusory conjunctions,[37] reporting the color of the letter that he did not see as being the color of the letter that he did report. Lacking access to a spatial representation in which colocated features could be coregistered by his constricted visual attention, visual features throughout the field are free-floating and conjoined arbitrarily. Even when features of an object are correctly coregistered, I have noted anecdotally that they sometimes do not seem to be fully conjoined experientially. Once, when I showed M.B. (the patient shown in Fig. 26-7) an opaque yellow plastic water pitcher (the kind found in every hospital), she looked at it as if perplexed and finally said that she was not sure but thought that it was "a pitcher of lemonade." She perceived the yellow and the pitcher shape independently and had to venture a guess that it was a glass pitcher filled with lemonade.

CONCLUSION

Lost in space and stuck in a perceptual present containing only one object which he or she cannot find or grasp, the patient with Balint syndrome is helpless in a visually chaotic world. Objects appear and disappear and their features jumble together. Contemporary theories of attention and perception help us to understand the experience of these patients, and their experience provides critical clues for helping us understand the neural basis of visual attention and perception and how they operate together normally to provide a coherence and continuity of perceptual experience.

REFERENCES

1. Williams M: *Brain Damage and the Mind.* Baltimore, Penguin Books, 1970, pp 61–62.
2. Husain M, Stein J: Rezsö Balint and his most celebrated case. *Arch Neurol* 45:89–93, 1988.
3. Friedman-Hill SR, Robertson LC, Treisman A: Parietal contributions to visual feature binding: Evidence from a patient with bilateral lesions. *Science* 269:853–855, 1995.
4. Coslett HB, Saffran E: Simultanagnosia: To see but not two see. *Brain* 113:1523–1545, 1991.
5. Pierrot-Deseillgny C, Gray F, Brunet P: Infarcts of both inferior parietal lobules with impairment of visually guided eye movements, peripheral visual inattention and optic ataxia. *Brain* 109:81–97, 1986.
6. Verfaellie M, Rapcsak SZ, Heilman KM: Impaired shifting of attention in Balint's syndrome. *Brain Cog* 12:195–204, 1990.
7. Damasio AR: Disorders of complex visual processing: Agnosia, achromatopsia, Balint's syndrome, and related difficulties of orientation and construction, in Mesulam MM (ed): *Principles of Behavioral Neurology.* Philadelphia, Davis, 1985.
8. Rizzo M: "Balint's syndrome" and associated visuospatial disorders. *Bailliere's Clin Neurol* 2:415–437, 1993.
9. Luria AR: Disorders of "simultaneous perception" in a case of bilateral occipito-parietal brain injury. *Brain* 83:437–449, 1959.
10. Holmes G, Horax G: Disturbances of spatial orientation and visual attention, with loss of stereoscopic vision. *Arch Neurol Psychiatry* 1:385–407, 1919.
11. Benson DF, Davis RJ, Snyder BD: Posterior cortical atrophy. *Arch Neurol* 45:789–793, 1988.
12. Hof PR, Bouras C, Constantinidis J, Morrison JH: Balint's syndrome in Alzheimer's disease: Specific disruption of the occipito-parietal visual pathway. *Brain Res* 493:368–375, 1989.
13. Hof PR, Bouras C, Constantinidis J, Morrison JH: Selective disconnection of specific visual association pathways in cases of Alzheimer's disease presenting with Balint's syndrome. *J Neuropathol Exp Neurol* 49:168–184, 1990.
14. Balint R: Seelenlahmung des "Schauens," optische Ataxie, raumliche Störung der Aufmerksamkeit. *Monatschr Psychiatrie Neurol* 25:51–81, 1909.
15. Luria AR, Pravdina-Vinarskaya EN, Yarbuss AL: Disorders of ocular movement in a case of simultanagnosia. *Brain* 86:219–228, 1963.
16. Girottin F, Milanese C, Casazza M, et al: Oculomotor disturbances in Balint's syndrome: Anatomoclinical findings and electrooculographic analysis in a case. *Cortex* 16:603–614, 1982.
17. Godwin-Austen RB: A case of visual disorientation. *J Neurol Neurosurg Psychiatry* 28:453–458, 1965.
18. Kase CS, Troncoso JF, Court JE, et al: Global spatial disorientation. *J Neurol Sci* 34:267–278, 1977.
19. Tyler HR: Abnormalities of perception with defective eye movements (Balint's syndrome). *Cortex* 3:154–171, 1968.
20. Wolpert I: Die simultanagnosie: Störung der Geamtauffassung. *Zeitschr Ges Neurol Psychiatrie* 93:397–415, 1924.
21. Farah MJ: *Visual Agnosia.* Cambridge, MA, MIT Press, 1990.
22. Kinsbourne M, Warrington EK: A Disorder of simultaneous form perception. *Brain* 85:461–486, 1962.
23. Kinsbourne M, Warrington EK: The localizing significance of limited simultaneous visual form perception. *Brain* 86:697–702, 1963.
24. Rizzo M, Robin DA: Simultanagnosia: A defect of

sustained attention yields insights on visual information processing. *Neurology* 40:447–455, 1990.

25. Johnson MH, Morton J: *Biology and Cognitive Development: The Case of Face Recognition.* Oxford, England, Blackwell, 1991.

26. Holmes G: Disturbances of visual orientation. *Br J Ophthalmol* 2:449–468, 506–518, 1918.

27. Tipper SP, Brehaut JC, Driver J: Selection of moving and static objects for the control of spatially directed action. *J Exp Psychol Hum Percep Perf* 16:492–504, 1990.

28. Kahneman D, Treisman A, Gibbs BJ: The reviewing of object files: Object-specific integration of information. *Cog Psychol* 24:175–219, 1992.

29. Egly R, Driver J, Rafal R: Shifting visual attention between objects and locations: Evidence from normal and parietal lesion subjects. *J Exp Psychol Gen* 123:127–161, 1994.

30. Egly R, Rafal R, Driver J, Starreveld Y: Hemispheric specialization for object-based attention in a split-brain patient. *Psychol Sci* 5:380–383, 1994.

31. Palmer S, Rock I: Rethinking perceptual organization: The role of uniform connectedness. *Psychonom Bull Rev* 1:29–55, 1994.

32. Humphreys GW, Riddoch MJ: Interactive attentional systems in unilateral visual neglect, in Robertson IH, Marshall JC (eds): *Unilateral Neglect: Clinical and Experimental Studies.* Hillsdale, NJ, Erlbaum, 1993, pp 139–168.

33. Navon D: Forest before trees: The precedence of global features in visual perception. *Cog Psychol* 9:353–383, 1977.

34. Riddoch MJ, Humphreys GW: A case of integrative visual agnosia. *Brain* 110:1431–1462, 1987.

35. Baylis GC, Driver J, Baylis LL, Rafal RD: Perception of letters and words in Balint's syndrome: Evidence for the unity of words. *Neuropsychologia* 32:1273–1286, 1994.

36. Treisman A, Gelade G: A feature integration theory of attention. *Cog Psychol* 12:97–136, 1980.

37. Treisman A, Schmidt N: Illusory conjunctions in the perception of objects. *Cog Psychol* 14:107–141, 1982.

38. Rafal R, Robertson L: The neurology of visual attention, in Gazzaniga MS (ed): *The Cognitive Neurosciences.* Cambridge, MA, MIT Press, 1995, pp 625–648.

39. Ramachandran VS: Perceiving shape from shading. *Sci Am* 259:76–83, 1988.

Chapter 27

PERCEPTION AND AWARENESS

Martha J. Farah
Todd E. Feinberg

Perception and awareness of perception are normally inextricably related. Most people would say that one has not perceived an object if one is not consciously aware of it. Yet, recent findings in behavioral neurology and neuropsychology are forcing us to revise this notion of the relation between perception and conscious awareness. Brain-damaged patients may manifest considerable knowledge of stimuli or particular properties of stimuli of which they deny any conscious perceptual experience. Although these findings challenge the intuitive idea that part and parcel of perceiving something is being aware of it, they also offer us a unique opportunity for investigating the neural bases of consciousness. In this chapter we review six perceptual disorders in which perception and awareness are dissociated and relate these disorders to the three main schools of thought concerning the brain correlates of conscious awareness.

THE NEURAL CORRELATES OF CONSCIOUS AWARENESS: THREE TYPES OF PROPOSAL

A Localized System for Consciousness

The first and most straightforward account of the relation between consciousness and the brain is to conceive of particular brain systems as mediating conscious awareness. The great grandfather of this type of account is Descartes' theory of mind-body interaction through the pineal gland. The most direct and influential descendant of this tradition is the DICE (dissociated interactions and conscious experience) model of Schacter and coworkers shown in Fig. 27-1.[1] According to this account, there is some brain system or systems, the conscious awareness system (CAS), separate from the brain systems concerned with perception, cognition, and action, whose activity is necessary for conscious experience and only for conscious experience. In a variant of this view, a brain system could be necessary for conscious awareness and for other functions as well. For example, Gazzaniga[2] attributes many of the differences between what one would call conscious and unconscious behavior to the involvement of left-hemispheric interpretive mechanisms, closely related to speech.

Consciousness as a State of Integration

In contrast to the first type of proposal, the next two types explain the relations between conscious and unconscious information processing in terms of the dynamic states of brain systems rather than in terms of the enduring roles of particular brain systems themselves. According to Kinsbourne's "integrated field theory," conscious awareness is a brain state in which the various modality-specific perceptions, recollections, current actions, and action plans are mutually consistent.[3] Normally, the interactions among these disparate brain systems automatically bring the ensemble into an integrated state, continually updated to reflect the current information available in all parts of the brain.

357

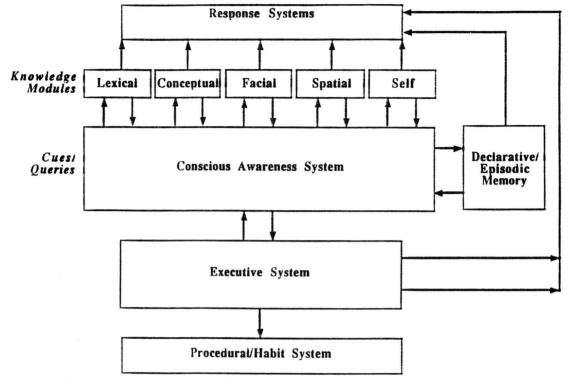

Figure 27-1
The DICE model (dissociated interactions and conscious experience) of Schacter and coworkers. (From Schacter et al.,[1] with permission.)

Integration accounts have also been proposed by Crick and Koch[4] and by Damasio.[5] Crick and Koch limit themselves to the issue of visual awareness and equate the phenomenon of visual awareness with the binding together of the different, separately represented visual properties of a stimulus (e.g., color, shape, depth, motion) into a single integrated percept. They call upon the work of Singer and colleagues (e.g., Engel et al.[6]), who found synchronization of the oscillations of neuronal activity within visual cortex for different parts of the same representation of a stimulus and who suggested that this could be a mechanism for binding together the different parts of the representation. Crick and Koch suggest that synchronization across visual areas could enable both binding and conscious awareness of stimuli. Damasio[5] has proposed a similar identification of binding

with conscious awareness, which in his theory is accomplished via the "convergence zone" to which the separate representations all project.

Consciousness as a Property of Graded Representation

A third account emphasizes the graded nature of representation in neural networks and suggests that consciousness may be associated only with the higher-quality end of the continuum of degrees of representation. Experiments on subliminal perception in normal subjects dissociate perception and awareness by using very brief, masked stimulus presentations or by other experimental manipulations known to degrade the quality of the perceptual representation. According to this account, in both normal and in brain-damaged subjects there is a correlation between the quality of the perceptual representation and the likelihood of conscious awareness (e.g., Farah et al.[7]).

It is worth noting that these different types of explanation are not necessarily mutually exclusive. For example, the idea of a convergence zone fits the criteria for a particular brain area necessary for consciousness, as well as emphasizing integration of different brain areas.

DISSOCIATIONS BETWEEN PERCEPTION AND AWARENESS AFTER BRAIN DAMAGE

In a number of different disorders of perception, special tests have revealed surprisingly preserved visual processing in the absence of conscious awareness. What do these dissociations tell us about the neural correlates of visual awareness? Let us briefly review each dissociation with respect to the three proposals just outlined.

Blindsight

Representative Findings *Blindsight* refers to the preserved visual abilities of patients with damage to primary visual cortex for stimuli presented in regions of the visual field formerly represented by the damaged cortex. In the best-known case of blindsight, case DB, Weiskrantz and colleagues documented relatively preserved ability to point to stimulus locations, detect movement, discriminate the orientation of lines and gratings, and discriminate shapes such as X's and O's despite DB's denial that he was seeing the stimuli.[8] The pattern of preserved and impaired abilities has been found to vary considerably from case to case. Detection and localization of light and detection of motion are invariably preserved to some degree. In addition, many patients can discriminate orientation, shape, direction of movement, and flicker. Color vision mechanisms also appear to be preserved in some cases, as indicated by Stoerig and Cowey's[9] findings of normal-shaped spectral sensitivity functions. A good review of the blindsight literature can be found in Cowey and Stoerig.[10]

Proposed Mechanisms The mechanism of blindsight has been a controversial topic. Some researchers have argued that the phenomenon is mediated, directly or indirectly, by residual functioning of primary visual cortex. For example, Campion and coworkers[11] alleged that blindsight abilities are mediated by primary visual cortex, either indirectly, by light from the scotomatous region of the visual field reflecting off other surfaces into regions of the visual field represented by intact primary visual cortex, or directly, by residual functioning of lesioned areas of primary visual cortex. Fendrich and colleagues[12] have shown that small islands of preserved primary cortex can support certain visual discriminations in the absence of awareness. The explanation of blindsight as residual functioning of damaged primary visual cortex is consistent with the view that conscious awareness is correlated with the quality of a neural representation. However, this explanation meets several difficulties in accounting for the totality of the empirical data now available on blindsight. For example, it is difficult to see how scattered light would enable patient DB to perceive black figures on a bright background, nor how this account could explain the qualitative differences in his performance within his natural blind spot and his acquired blind region. Residual functioning of spared cortex is clearly not a possibility for subjects who show blindsight in one hemifield following hemidecortication, yet they, too, show a wide range of blindsight abilities.[13]

Other than spared primary visual cortex, what other neural systems might mediate the preserved abilities in blindsight? One possibility is the subcortical visual system, which consists of projections from the retina to the superior colliculus, and on to the pulvinar and cortical visual areas, as shown in Fig. 27-2. Evidence in favor of the subcortical mediation hypothesis includes the close functional similarities between the known specializations of the subcortical visual system and many of the preserved abilities in blindsight, such as detection and localization of onsets and moving stimuli, and the asymmetries observed between the nasal-temporal hemifields in some measures of blindsight, consistent with asymmetries in retinal-

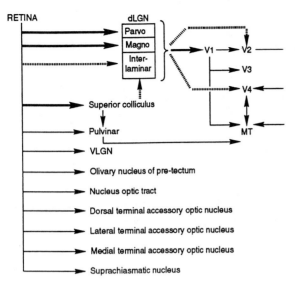

Figure 27-2
Cortical and subcortical visual pathways, including the two that may mediate blindsight: superior colliculus to pulvinar to extrastriate visual cortex, and lateral geniculate nucleus to extrastriate visual cortex.

collicular projections.[14] Thus according to this explanation, awareness is correlated with the activity of the cortical but not the subcortical visual system. This is consistent with the first of the proposals reviewed earlier, that some brain systems are endowed with conscious awareness and others are not.

Cowey and Stoerig have suggested that the cortical visual system, which projects from the retina to cortex by way of the lateral geniculate nucleus (LGN), may also contribute to blindsight.[15] They note that a population of cells in the LGN projects directly to extrastriate visual cortex and could therefore bring stimulus information into such areas as V4 and MT in the absence of primary visual cortex. According to this account, many of the same visual association areas are engaged in blindsight and in normal vision. What distinguishes normal vision and visual performance without awareness is that in the latter only a subset of the normal inputs arrive in extrastriate visual cortex. This type of mechanism fits most naturally with the third hypothesis, that representational

quality is the critical factor for enabling conscious awareness.

Implicit Shape Perception in Apperceptive Visual Agnosia

Representative Findings   In apperceptive visual agnosia, patients are unable to name, copy, or match even the simplest shapes, such as squares or triangles, and cannot discriminate differently oriented line segments despite relatively preserved perception of brightness, color, motion, and acuity (see Chap. 17). Yet in at least one carefully studied case of apperceptive agnosia following carbon monoxide poisoning, good performance in a variety of visuomotor tasks implies the preservation of visual shape representations. Goodale and Milner[16] found that their patient DF reached toward a variety of objects with appropriate hand shapes for grasping. They went on to demonstrate that she could insert cards into slots of differing orientation while being unable to discriminate those orientations in purely perceptual tasks. A review of this work can be found in Milner and Goodale's recent book.[17]

Proposed Mechanism   Goodale and Milner[16] suggest that the dissociation between perception and awareness in their patient may result from an interruption in the flow of information from occipital to ventral visual areas needed for conscious object recognition. They hypothesize that the dorsal visual pathway, needed for spatial and visuomotor processing, normally operates without engendering conscious awareness, and that this pathway is relatively preserved in their patient. Thus, they endorse a variant of the first type of account, according to which conscious awareness accompanies the operation of some brain systems and not others.

Covert Recognition of Faces in Prosopagnosia

Representative Findings   Prosopagnosia is an impairment of face recognition following brain damage, which can occur relatively independently of impairments in object recognition and which is not caused by impairments in lower-level vision or memory (see Chap. 18). In some cases of prosopagnosia, there is a dramatic dissociation between the loss of face recognition ability as measured by standard tests of face recognition, as well as by patients' own introspections and the apparent preservation of face recognition when tested by certain indirect tests.[18]

For example, when prosopagnosics are required to learn to associate the facial photographs of famous people with the names of such people, some have been found to learn correct pairings faster than incorrect pairings.[19] Evidence of preserved recognition has also come from reaction time (RT) tasks in which the familiarity or identity of faces is found to influence processing time. In a visual identity match task with simultaneously presented pairs of faces, De Haan and colleagues[19] found that a prosopagnosic patient was faster at matching pairs of previously familiar faces than unfamiliar faces, as is true of normal subjects, even though he performed poorly at judging the familiarity of the faces. In so-called "priming" studies, photographs of faces have been found to influence the time needed to make decisions about printed names, such as those shown in Fig. 27-3.[19] For example, in deciding whether a name belonged to an actor or a politician, a prosopagnosic was found to be faster when an accompanying face also came from the same occupational category than when it came from another occupational category. Good reviews of research in this area may be found in Bruyer[20] and Young.[21]

Proposed Mechanisms The oldest and still predominant explanation of covert recognition is that the face-recognition system is intact in these patients but has been disconnected from other brain mechanisms necessary for conscious awareness (e.g., the model of De Haan and coworkers,[22] who base their account on the DICE model). Thus, the neural correlate of conscious awareness is taken to be activation of a particular brain system dedicated to conscious awareness.

Tranel and Damasio[23] also interpret covert

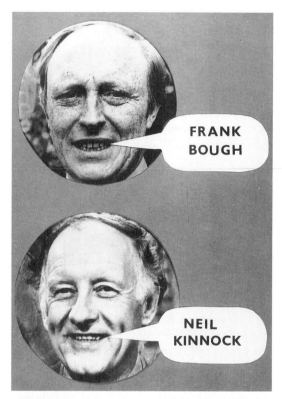

Figure 27-3
Examples of stimuli from the study of De Haan and colleagues. Subjects must classify the names as belonging to an actor or a politician. Their speed is influenced by the occupation of the faces. (From De Haan et al.,[19] with permission.)

recognition as the normal activation of visual face representations, disconnected from the convergence zones from whence representations in other areas of the brain can be activated. A similar idea is embodied in the computer simulation of Burton and colleagues.[24] These interpretations are most consistent with the second type of proposal discussed earlier in suggesting that conscious awareness requires the integration of representations across different brain areas; we cannot be consciously aware of an isolated, modality-specific representation.

It is also possible that covert recognition reflects the residual processing capabilities of a damaged but not obliterated visual face-recognition system. Farah and associates[7] trained a neural network to associate "face" patterns with "semantic" patterns and to associate these, in turn, with "name" patterns. As described in Chap. 8, we found that, at levels of damage to the face representations that led to poor or even chance performance in overt tasks, the network showed all of the behavioral covert recognition effects reviewed above: it relearned correct associations faster than novel ones, completed the visual analysis of familiar faces faster than unfamiliar, and showed priming and interference from the faces on judgments about names.

Unconscious Perception in Neglect and Extinction

Representative Findings Neglect is a disorder of spatial attention that generally follows posterior parietal damage and results in patients' failure to report or even orient to stimuli occurring on the side of space contralateral to the lesion (see Chaps. 24 and 25). Extinction is often viewed as a mild form of neglect, resulting in difficulty with contralateral stimuli only when an ipsilateral stimulus is presented at the same time. The behavior of patients with neglect and extinction suggests that they do not perceive neglected and extinguished stimuli. However, evidence is beginning to accumulate showing that, in at least some cases, considerable information about such stimuli is extracted by patients. As with covert recognition in prosopagnosia, this information is generally only detectable using indirect tests.

The first suggestion that patients with extinction may see more of the extinguished stimulus than is apparent from their conscious verbal report came from Volpe and coworkers.[25] They presented right-parietal-damaged extinction patients with pairs of visual stimuli, including drawings of common objects and three-letter words, one in each hemifield. On each trial, subjects were required to state whether the two stimuli shown were the same or different and to name the stimuli. Figure 27-4 shows the stimuli and results from a typical trial. Subjects did poorly at overtly identifying the stimuli on the left, sometimes remarking that they did not even see anything on the left, but they did well at same/different matching.

Berti and coworkers[26] used the paradigm of Volpe and associates to determine the level of processing to which extinguished stimuli were encoded. They included pairs of pictures that were physically different but depicted either the same object from a different view or different-looking exemplars of the same type of object, and they instructed their subject to say "same" if the two stimuli had the same name. The subject was able to do this, implying that extinguished stimuli are encoded to the level of meaning.

A recent study by McGlinchey-Berroth and colleagues[27] showed semantic priming by neglected pictures in a lexical decision task. On each trial of this experiment, subjects with left neglect viewed a picture in one hemifield, followed by a letter string in central vision to which they made a "word"/"nonword" response. When the picture was semantically related to the word, "word" responses were faster, and this was true even when the picture had been presented on the left side of the display. For a good review of these and other findings of unconscious perception after parietal damage, see Wallace.[28]

Proposed Mechanisms The earliest and most straightforward interpretation of these findings was offered by Volpe and colleagues,[25] who suggested that the stimulus processing was carried out normally and unconsciously in parietal-damaged patients but that the transfer of those representations to other parts of the system needed for conscious awareness was interrupted. This presupposes the first of the three kinds of relations between neural systems and consciousness—namely, the existence of particular localized systems needed for conscious awareness.

An alternative interpretation suggested by Kinsbourne[3] and Bisiach[29] is that the effects of parietal damage are to attenuate the influence of the percept on the rest of the system. This is consistent with the view that integration among neural systems is essential for awareness. However, insofar as the hypothesized failure of integration re-

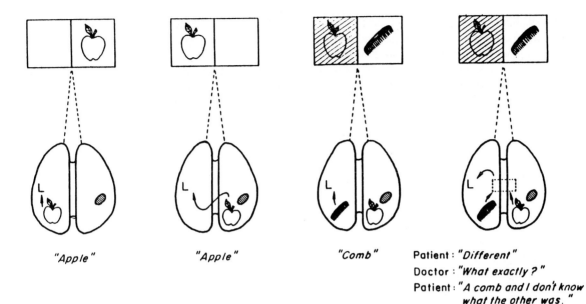

"Apple" "Apple" "Comb" Patient : *"Different"*

Doctor : *"What exactly ?"*

Patient : *"A comb and I don't know what the other was."*

Figure 27-4
Typical trials from the experiment of Volpe and coworkers, showing extinction of the left stimulus with preserved same/different matching. (From Volpe et al.,[25] with permission.)

sults from the poor perception of neglected and extinguished stimuli, this interpretation is also consistent with the third type of proposal outlined earlier.

There is some support for the view that neglect and extinction impair perceptual processing and that the output of impaired perceptual processing can be used for perceptual same/different matching and partially activate appropriate semantic representations. Farah and coworkers[30] demonstrated that the dissociation described by Volpe and colleagues can be obtained with perceptual degradation with normal subjects and that it can be eliminated in patients when the perceptual demands of the same/different and naming tasks are matched. Also relevant is the simulation discussed in the previous section and Chap. 8 of semantic priming by faces after visual system damage. Although initially interpreted with respect to face perception and prosopagnosia, it nevertheless provides a generic demonstration that the output of impaired visual processing can evoke semantic information that will be detectable using indirect

tests such as priming. Berti and associates[26] suggest that priming may underlie the matching performance of their patient, with the nonextinguished stimulus semantically priming the extinguished one.

Implicit Reading in Pure Alexia

Representative Findings Patients with pure alexia are impaired at reading, despite being able to write normally and understand spoken words. To the extent that they can read at all, they appear to do so in a "letter by letter" fashion, spelling the word to themselves before they can recognize it (see Chap. 13).

The first comprehensive investigation to suggest that pure alexics might understand more than they can report was carried out by Shallice and Saffran.[31] Their subject was able to discriminate words from nonword letter strings with relatively high accuracy with stimuli presented too quickly for him to reliably identify the words explicitly. Shallice and Saffran also demonstrated that their subject was able to make reasonably accurate semantic categorizations of briefly presented words, such as *animal* versus *nonanimal.* Coslett and Saffran[32] replicated and extended these findings with additional cases, showing that concrete words were understood better than abstract and that affixes were not processed (e.g., subjects would accept *elephanting* as a word). Perhaps their most striking finding is that their subjects performed the implicit reading tasks more accurately with extremely brief exposures of the words, such as 250 m, than with exposures of 2 s.

Proposed Mechanisms   Although DICE has been applied to implicit reading (see Fig. 27-1), it fails to explain findings such as the concreteness effect, insensitivity to affixes, and improvement in performance with shorter presentations. A quality-of-representation account, whereby implicit reading is mediated by a degraded but not obliterated reading system, seems compatible with the first two findings, but it does not easily accommodate the third.

The most successful account at present attributes implicit reading to the right hemisphere, which is known to be deficient in knowledge of abstract words and morphology.[31,32] According to Coslett and Saffran, brief exposures may be necessary to foil the damaged but still dominant left hemisphere's letter-by-letter strategy. This interpretation implies that awareness of word recognition depends on the involvement of the left hemisphere and is thus an instance of the first type of explanation reviewed at the outset. It should be noted, however, that some implicit readers are aware of the information they glean from words (Shallice and Saffran;[31] personal observations). The core dissociation in implicit reading is between knowledge of certain word properties and knowledge of the specific word (e.g., knowing it is an animal but not knowing it is *camel*). It may be that only when tachistoscopic presentations are necessary to enable implicit reading does word knowledge dissociate from awareness, and this could be by the same mechanisms responsible for tachistoscopic subliminal perception in normal subjects.

Implicit Object Recognition in Associative Visual Agnosia

Representative Findings   Associative visual agnosia is a disorder of visual object recognition not attributable to underlying primary perceptual or linguistic impairments (see Chap. 17). These patients perform adequately on figure copying tasks, thus distinguishing their disorder from apperceptive agnosia, and can name objects to verbal description, thus distinguishing their disorder from aphasia. They cannot demonstrate an object's use nonverbally through pantomime or other means, separating the disorder from optic aphasia.

In spite of their failures on tasks of explicit object recognition, residual object recognition abilities have been found in some of these patients. For instance, Taylor and Warrington[33] reported a patient with severe associative visual agnosia who was nonetheless able to place pictures in their proper orientation and sort pictures into basic categories. Similar abilities were reported in another associative visual agnosic by Jankowiak.[34]

We recently tested a patient with classic associative visual agnosia and alexia due to a dominant medial occipital infarction from a left posterior cerebral occlusion.[35,36] In spite of a severe defect in object naming, describing use, and pantomiming to visually presented objects, she showed a surprising ability to make semantic matches on forced-choice matching tasks with both pictures and words. Figure 27-5 shows an example of the picture-matching task. In an effort to assess the nature of the residual knowledge, we developed two tests of her metaknowledge on these tasks. On every trial, prior to responding, we assessed her "judgment of knowledge" by asking "Do you know what this picture is?" and, after she responded, we assessed her "judgment of accuracy" by asking "Are you sure or are you guessing?" We found three results of interest—first, overall accuracy varied directly with the number of choices, that is the more choices the worse her performance; second, while judgment of knowledge was poor overall, judgment of accuracy varied with performance accuracy. Under conditions of high accuracy (two-choice tasks) and low accu-

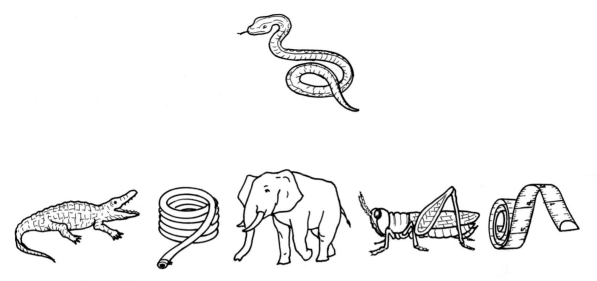

Figure 27-5

Example of five choice picture-to-picture matching tasks. Patient is asked which one is most like or goes with the target. Choices at bottom include two visual and two semantic foils.

racy (unlimited choice), the patient showed significant insight into her knowledge with better than chance judgment of accuracy on both tasks. When her accuracy was intermediate (five-choice tasks), her judgment of accuracy was poor. She thus showed her maximum level of insight when she had very much or very little knowledge. Finally, on the subset of trials in which she claimed no knowledge of the objects' identity during judgment-of-knowledge assessment, though the patient showed better than chance response accuracy, she still showed significant insight on judgment of accuracy, stating she was "sure" of her responses on almost 80 percent of trials where she was accurate, compared to only 25 percent of trials where her responses were inaccurate.

Proposed Mechanisms The findings that our patient's level of awareness was associated with her recognition performance is inconsistent with the view that the systems required for conscious awareness of recognition are disconnected from the recognition systems themselves. This fact coupled with the finding that performance accuracy varied with the number of choices is most consistent with the hypothesis of degraded knowledge. Additionally, while her residual reading abilities were consistent with those subserved by the right hemisphere,[31,32] there was no asymmetry in the accuracy of the patient's performance between the two hands. Our findings overall were most consistent with a degraded object-recognition system, whether left, right, or bilaterally represented, which is nonetheless accessible to either hemisphere.

GENERAL CONCLUSIONS

Heterogeneity at the Level of Phenomena

There are differences in the ways in which awareness is described by patients and operationalized by experimenters in these disorders. Blindsight patients may profess to be guessing on the basis of no subjective awareness or may respond with some confidence on the basis of a subjective experience that is nevertheless nonvisual—for example, sensing movement. In contrast, prosopagnosic subjects typically report absolutely no sense of familiarity when they view a face and have low confidence in their identifications, and apperceptive agnosics guess at shapes with low confidence. Similarly, in neglect and extinction subjects profess no awareness of the stimulus properties assessed in the matching or priming tasks on which they evince perception. Anecdotal evidence suggests that at times they even lack awareness that there was a stimulus. In implicit reading, awareness is not invariably dissociated from reading performance, although subjects who read implicitly under tachistoscopic conditions report being unaware of the information gleaned. Although implicit object recognition appears to occur without awareness, in at least one patient there was a systematic relation between her feeling of confidence in her "guesses" and their accuracy. In sum, the five disorders constitute a somewhat heterogeneous group from the point of view of awareness.

Heterogeneity at the Level of Mechanism

The five disorders also appear to be heterogeneous from the point of view of mechanism. For example, in blindsight, there are two types of mechanism that are currently under consideration, without any intended mutual exclusivity: subcortical mediation and extrastriate cortical mediation. As already discussed, there are consistent with the ideas that certain localized brain systems must be engaged and that a certain minimal quality of representation must be available for conscious awareness to take place. In apperceptive agnosia, preserved shape processing within the visual-motor system is also consistent with the idea that conscious awareness accompanies the functioning of certain localized brain systems and not others, although the empirical support for this interpretation is currently weak because of the diffuse nature of the one subject's brain damage.

The mechanisms responsible for the dissociations observed in covert recognition in prosopagnosia and unconscious perception in neglect and extinction are not well established, and more evidence is needed to distinguish among the possible candidates. However, both syndromes currently seem explainable in terms of the quality of the representations available in each. In prosopagnosia, the poor quality of the representations is presumably due to a loss of stored perceptual knowledge of faces, whereas in neglect and extinction it is due to a more dynamic processing failure of the attention system.

Although the issue of mechanism is also far from settled in the case of implicit reading, the right-hemisphere hypothesis seems most promising at present. This is consistent with the view that certain localized brain systems are needed for normal aware perception. Recall, however, that some implicit readers appear to be aware of the information they perceive; therefore this syndrome may not be as relevant to understanding the neural correlates of conscious awareness as the other four.

General Implications for the Neural Correlates of Awareness

It should be clear that the five syndromes reviewed here are unlikely to share a common explanation. Although there is a family resemblance among them, closer inspection reveals that the kinds of perceptual abilities and the nature of subjective experience are not uniform. We may therefore need to consider the possibility that the relation between conscious awareness and neural systems is itself not explicable by just one of the types of account discussed earlier. For example, on the basis of the present review, it seems plausible that conscious awareness requires certain cortical perceptual regions to be engaged, and that, within these regions, a certain quality of representation is also necessary (thus denying consciousness to both the normal-quality functioning of the superior colliculus and to the impaired functioning of cortical face representations). Furthermore, it is possible that the importance of representational quality derives from the reduced ability of low-quality representations to influence the ambient state of integration across brain areas.

The foregoing conclusion about the neural correlates of awareness is both tentative and rather unconstrained, in that it leaves room for at least some versions of all three types of proposal outlined earlier. However, there is one type of proposal we can reject with reasonable confidence on the basis of the findings reviewed here: proposals that feature some component whose dedicated function is to enable awareness. Among all of the disorders, there is none for which visual perception has been convincingly demonstrated to be normal or near normal. This, in turn, deprives theories featuring a "consciousness awareness system" or "convergence zones" of their basic motivation, which is to explain a straightforward dissociation between perception and awareness of perception. On the basis of the evidence currently available, it seems unlikely that there are any brain systems needed for conscious awareness of perception that do not also play a role in perception per se.

REFERENCES

1. Schacter DL, McAndrews MP, Moscovitch M: Access to consciousness: Dissociations between implicit and explicit knowledge in neuropsychological syndromes, in Weiskrantz L (ed): *Thought without Language.* Oxford, England: Oxford University Press, 1988.

2. Gazzaniga MS: Brain modularity: Towards a philosophy of conscious experience, in Marcel AJ, Bisiach E (eds): *Consciousness in Contemporary Science.* Oxford, England: Clarendon Press, 1988.

3. Kinsbourne M: Integrated field theory of consiousness, in Marcel AJ, Bisiach E (eds): *Consciousness in Contemporary Science.* Oxford, England: Clarendon Press, 1988.

4. Crick F, Koch C: Function of the thalamic reticular complex: The searchlight hypothesis. Semin Neurosci 2:263–275, 1990.

5. Damasio AR: Synchronous activation in multiple cortical regions: A mechanism for recall. Semin Neurosci 2:287–296, 1990.

6. Engel AK, Konig P, Kreiter A, et al: Temporal coding in the visual cortex: New vistas on integration in the visual system. *Trends Neurosci* 15:218–226, 1992.

7. Farah MJ, O'Reilly RC, Vecera SP: Dissociated overt and covert recognition as on emergent property of lesioned attractor networks. *Psychol Rev* 100:571–588, 1993.

8. Weiskrantz L: *Blindsight: A Case Study and Implications.* Oxford, England: Oxford University Press, 1986.

9. Stoerig P, Cowey A: Wavelength sensitivity in blindsight. *Nature* 342:916–918, 1990.

10. Cowey A, Stoerig P: The neurobiology of blindsight. *Trends Neurosci* 14:140–145, 1991.

11. Campion J, Latto R, Smith YM: Is blindsight an effect of scattered light, spared cortex, and near-threshold vision? *Behav Brain Sci* 3:423–447, 1983.

12. Fendrich R, Wessinger CM, Gazzaniga MS: Residual vision on a scotoma: Implications for blindsight. *Science* 258:1489–1491, 1992.

13. Perenin MT: Visual function within the hemianopic field following early cerebral hemidecortication in man: II. Pattern discrimination. *Neuropsychologia* 16:696–708, 1978.

14. Rafal R, Smith J, Krantz J, et al: Extrageniculate vision in hemianopic humans: Saccade inhibition by signals in the blind field. *Science* 250:118–121, 1990.

15. Cowey A, Stoerig P: Projection patterns of surviving neurons in the dorsal lateral geniculate nucleus following discrete lesions of striate cortex: Implications for residual vision. *Exp Brain Res* 75:631–638, 1989.

16. Goodale MA, Milner DA: Separate visual pathways for perception and action. *Trends Neurosci* 15:20–25, 1992.

17. Milner AD, Goodale MA: *The Visual Brain in Action.* New York: Oxford University Press, 1995.

18. Bauer RM: Autonomic recognition of names and faces in prosopagnosia: A neuropsychological application of the guilty knowledge test. *Neuropsychologia* 22:457–469, 1984.

19. De Haan EHF, Young AW, Newcombe F: Face recognition without awareness. *Cog Neuropsychol* 4:385–415, 1987.

20. Bruyer R: Covert recognition of faces in prosopagnosia: A review. *Brain Cog* 15:223–235, 1992.

21. Young A: Covert face recognition, in Farah MJ, Ratcliff G (eds): *The Neuropsychology of High-Level Vision: Collected Tutorial Essays.* Hillsdale, NJ: Erlbaum, 1994.

22. De Haan EHF, Bauer RM, Greve KW: Behavioral and physiological evidence for covert recognition in a prosopagnosic patient. *Cortex* 28:77–95, 1992.

23. Tranel D, Damasio A: Knowledge without awareness: An autonomic index of facial recognition by prosopagnosics. *Science* 228:1453–1454, 1985.

24. Burton AM, Young AW, Bruce V, et al: Understanding covert recognition. *Cognition* 31:129–166, 1991.

25. Volpe BT, LeDoux JE, Gazzaniga MS: Information processing of visual stimuli in an "extinguished" field. *Nature* 22:724, 1979.

26. Berti A, Allport A, Driver J, et al: Levels of processing for visual stimuli in an "extinguished" field. *Neuropsychologia* 30:403–415, 1992.

27. McGlinchey-Berroth R, Milberg WP, Verfaellie M, et al: Semantic processing in the neglected visual field: Evidence from a lexical decision task. *Cog Neuropsychol* 10:79–108, 1993.

28. Wallace MA: Unconscious perception in neglect and extinction, in Farah MJ, Ratcliff G (eds): *The Neuropsychology of High-Level Vision: Collected Tutorial Essays.* Hillsdale, NJ: Erlbaum, 1994.

29. Bisiach E: Understanding Consciousness: Clues from unilateral neglect and related disorders, in Milner AD, Rugg MD (ed): *The Neuropsychology of Consciousness.* San Diego, CA: Academic Press, 1992.

30. Farah MJ, Monheit MA, Wallace MA: Unconscious perception of "extinguished" visual stimuli: Reassessing the evidence. *Neuropsychologia* 29:949–958, 1991.

31. Shallice T, Saffran E: Lexical processing in the absence of explicit word identification: Evidence from a letter-by-letter reader. *J Cog Neuropsychol* 3:429–458, 1086.

32. Coslett HB, Saffran EM: Evidence for preserved reading in "pure alexia." *Brain* 112:327–359, 1989.

33. Taylor A, Warrington EK: Visual agnosia: A single case report. *Cortex* 7:152–161, 1971.

34. Jankowiak J, Kinsbourne M, Shalev RS, Bachman DL: Preserved visual imagery and categorization in a case of associative visual agnosia. *J Cogn Neurosci* 4:119–131, 1992.

35. Feinberg TE, Schindler RJ, Ochoa E, et al: Associative visual agnosia and alexia without prosopagnosia. *Cortex* 30:395–411, 1994.

36. Feinberg TE, Dyckes-Berke D, Miner CR, Roane DM: Knowledge, implicit knowledge and metaknowledge in visual agnosia and pure alexia. *Brain* 118:789–800, 1995.

Chapter 28

ANOSOGNOSIA AND CONFABULATION

Todd E. Feinberg

Unawareness of neurologic defects or illness, also referred to as anosognosia, has many aspects, and consideration of the nature and origin of this complex symptom has engendered many theories. In this chapter I will focus on a few seemingly diverse conditions that entail unawareness of a neurologic defect, namely: unawareness of visual defects including the blind spot, scotomas, hemianopias, and cerebral blindness; issues of unawareness after callosal disconnection; unawareness of hemiplegia; and unawareness of memory defects. In all of these, the role of completion and confabulation in fashioning and sustaining the unawareness is considered. Finally, the viewpoint is presented that two major types of unawareness associated with completion and confabulation can be discerned across all the varieties of unawareness considered.

UNAWARENESS OF VISUAL DEFECTS

Unawareness of the Blind Spot

The physiologic blind spot in the temporal field of each eye is caused by the lack of retinal ganglion cells at the optic disk, located 3 to 4 mm nasal to the fovea. Unawareness of the blind spot was first described by Mariotte in 1668.[1] It is well known that even when viewing with one eye closed, we are generally unaware of our own blind spot unless its presence is specifically sought. Gassell and Williams[2] reviewed Helmholtz's explanation for unawareness of the blind spot, namely that the blind spot was only discovered *negatively* by careful observation of the absent aspects of the stimulus. When these absences were recognized, the gap could be deduced. They suggested that "The discovery is therefore a judgement rather than a direct sensation."

Fuchs[3] explained unawareness of the blind spot on the basis of perceptual completion for certain stimuli such as evenly colored surfaces, printed pages, and continuous lines and circles. This completion is not total, however. For example, as Fuchs points out, if a line enters and ends within the blind spot, it will not be completed. He explained these findings on the basis of gestalt principles, suggesting "completion can and does occur only if the 'seen' part implies a *whole* of which it is a part—i.e., whose law it already contains. . . . The tendency towards wholeness exhibited by an incomplete *part* is a tendency towards simplicity or *Prägnanz*." Only when the missing part enters into a "totalized whole-apprehension" will the stimulus be completed and the blind spot pass unnoticed. Ramachandran[4] has also provided evidence that the filling in of the blind spot is *perceptual* as opposed to *conceptual,* and is a perceptually "primitive" process, occurring at an early stage of visual processing.

Some preliminary physiologic evidence regarding completion of the blind spot has been provided by Gattass and coworkers.[5] They performed unit recordings on neurons in layer 4C of V1 in the area of the representation of the contralateral blind spot. A line stimulus, which exceeded in diameter the blind spot, was swept across it. They found a significant potentiation of the response when both sides of the blind spot were stimulated in this manner as compared with unilateral stimulation of either side alone. The authors suggest that through this process, these cells "interpolated" the area across the blind spot and completed this region of blindness.

Unawareness of Acquired Scotomata and Hemianopias

Unawareness of acquired scotomata and hemianopias has been reported by most investigators to be the rule rather than the exception. Critchley[6] noted that anterior lesions were more likely to be noticed by patients than posterior lesions and that lack of awareness did not correlate with mental confusion. Bender[7] noted that patients with homonymous visual field defects usually do not see the surrounding space as split in the middle, though they may notice blurring of vision. Both of these authors suggested that macula-sparing lesions were more likely to remain unnoticed than those in which the macular was split.

Critchley described two types of experience associated with hemianopia. "Positive hemianopias," in which objects appear bisected with one half obscured, occur rarely in posteriorly situated cerebral lesions. Alternatively, patients may have a "negative hemianopia," in which no obscurity is experienced, though there is the experience of something missing on the impaired side. Critchley terms this the *héminanopsie nulle of Dufour*.[8] Teuber and coworkers[9] found that of 46 persons with visual field defects due to penetrating gunshot wounds of the brain, only 2 experienced positive scotomata, while 44 experienced negative scotomata such as a "blank" or "void." If they were aware of the problems, most patients attributed their visual difficulties to deficits in their eyes—typically the eye contralateral to the occipital lesion. Patients were generally unaware of the ipsilateral (nasal field) defect. Teuber and colleagues[9] suggested that the functional dominance of the crossed temporal field over the uncrossed nasal field accounted for greater subjective awareness

of the disordered temporal field of the contralateral eye.

Another factor related to unawareness of visual defects cited by Bender and Teuber[10] and Critchley[6] is the development of the "pseudofovea." Originally described by Fuchs,[3] the pseudofovea results as an adaptation to hemianopsia in which the patients develops a functional shift in "central" fixation toward the hemianopic side, with the development of a new center of maximal acuity. In this manner, the patient somewhat "automatically" decreases the functional significance of the hemianopia, thus facilitating unawareness of the visual defect.

Another factor undoubtedly significant in unawareness of hemianopias is the presence of perceptual completion. Poppelreuter in 1917[12] reported that if a figure, such as a circle or square, was presented such that a portion of it fell into a hemianopic field, the patient would nonetheless report seeing the whole figure. He also found that even if objectively incomplete figures were presented such that the gap fell within the hemianopic field, perceptual completion would nonetheless occur.

Fuchs[3] found that patients who experience visual blackness in the defective region do not report completion. In those few patients reporting completion, Fuchs found that (1) "simple" geometric figures such as circles and squares could be completed but complex though highly familiar figures such as a dog, face, or bottle—or even symmetrical but complex figures such as a butterfly—would not be completed; (2) simple figures objectively incomplete in the area of visual defect would nonetheless be completed; (3) figures presented in defective fields might be *extinguished* (disappear from awareness) if presented simultaneously with a stimulus in the normal field to which it bore no relation but might enter into completion with the normal field if an appropriate "gestalt" were formed.

Bender and Teuber[10] suggested that completion resulted from residual visual perception occurring in a damaged area of the brain. Completion of a stimulus in an area of perimetric blindness could occur if stimuli were presented briefly enough to prevent the occurrence of extinction. Completion in their view was the "absence of extinction"; it would occur only with objectively intact objects and could not be the result of a "psychological filling in" of a missing part. In agreement, Torjussen[13] demonstrated completion in hemianopic subjects only when using objectively complete stimuli. He suggested that completion resulted from an interaction between the normal and impaired visual areas, in which the normal field facilitated perception in the abnormal field.

It has been suggested by many investigators over the years that insight into hemianopic defects is inversely related to perceptual completion.[2,3,10,11] Fuchs found he could eliminate the completion effect if the patient was encouraged to adopt a "critical attitude" toward his or her perceptual experience. Fuchs[3] and Bender and Teuber[10] found the subjective fields to vary with the extent of completion. Gassel and Williams[2] tested 35 hemianopic patients for perceptual completion. In one condition, patients fixated either to the examiner's nose or to the eye opposite the lesion and were asked whether the whole face was seen. They were tested with and without a black object covering the portion of the face falling in the defective field. The investigators found completion of the face in 28 of the 35 patients. Most important for present purposes, Gassell and Williams made the following observations: (1) completion would occur even when a black object was slowly interposed to cover the completed side of the face, thus making residual perception of that side impossible; (2) encouraging an "analytic attitude" toward perceptions tended to decrease the degree of completion; (3) completion and awareness of defects were inversely related. An additional important issue emphasized by these authors is that gaps in the visual fields have no direct sensory effect but rather are *deduced* when the missing aspects of a stimulus are recognized. In their words: "The hemianopic field is an area of absence which is discovered rather than sensed; it is a negative area whose presence is *judged* from some specific failure in function, rather than directly perceived."

Warrington[14] reported her observations on 20 patients with homonymous hemianopic defects from various etiologies. She observed completion of both whole and half figures and found that of the 20 patients, the 11 who were unaware of their visual defects all showed visual completion, while none of those patients who were aware of their defects demonstrated completion. Completion was found to be associated with parietal lobe damage and tended to be associated with unilateral neglect but not mental deterioration.

In the presence of neglect, therefore, incomplete stimuli may be completed, and this phenomenon cannot be explained by latent perception made explicit via a process of facilitation. Rather, it is more appropriate to describe these patients as having *confabulated* the missing aspects of the stimulus. Significantly, Warrington[14] found this type of completion to be inversely related to awareness of defect and Zangwill[15] surmised that "completion, far from being a compensatory reaction to hemianopia (as Poppelreuter supposed) is in fact a variety of visual confabulation constrained by unawareness or denial of defect." Zangwill attributed this "anosognosic misperception" to parietal lobe pathology.

Unawareness of Divided Visual Fields in Split-Brain Patients

The corpus callosum, anterior commissure, and hippocampal commissure provide the only direct pathways connecting the neocortices of the left and right hemispheres. It is through these connections that unilateral neocortical contributions to sensorimotor functions, learning, and cognition are unified.[16–25] After cerebral commissurotomy, the patient essentially has a fovea-splitting "double hemianopia"[20] with regard to the two hemispheres. As a result, stimuli requiring detailed visual discrimination cannot be compared across the vertical meridian.[19,20,26] In spite of this, it has been repeatedly and somewhat surprisingly noted that these patients may appear (and apparently feel) in most respects quite normal after the acute postoperative period has elapsed.[22,27] Except in cases where intermanual conflict and the alien hand syndrome arise,[28] patients appear to be largely unaware of any change in themselves.

Many mechanisms are available to these patients that allow them to compensate for their deficits and remain subjectively unaware (anosognosic) of any alteration in brain function. Sperry[27,29] points out that a number of sensory projection systems—including tactile representation of the face, crude representation of pain, temperature, and position sense as well as audition—provide bilateral cortical projections, therefore enabling each hemisphere to develop some degree of independent sensory representation. A certain degree of bilateral motor control,[29] including ipsilateral control of eye movements, also provides some unification of action. The emotional tone in response to a unilateral stimulus may spread to the contralateral hemisphere via an intact anterior commissure[16] or remaining brainstem connections[27,29] and provide unification or double representation of an emotional experience.[30,31] Functional adaptations such as exploratory head and eye movements and cross-cueing strategies[24] also provide the disconnected hemispheres with a shared experience. While the split hemispheres are functionally disconnected for detailed visual perception involving foveal geniculostriate vision, Trevarthen has pointed out that ambient nongeniculostriate vision remains undivided after callosal division.[19,25] The speaking left hemisphere may still be able to detect and report the presence of an ipsilaterally presented flash of light or movement and some direction information of a stimulus while also attending to and dealing with ipsilaterally positioned targets. This is particularly true for high-contrast, low-spatial-resolution stimuli.[19] It is also possible that transfer via the anterior commissure may account for the lack of disconnection in some cases.[19,20]

Other factors are important in the lack of divided self-awareness in these patients, however. Levy and colleagues[31] presented to callosally sectioned patients visual "chimeric" figures composed of two different halves joined at the midline. With the patient's gaze fixated centrally, each hemisphere would receive different visual input.

In these investigations it was demonstrated that when a single response was called for, patients typically responded to either the left or right side of the chimeric stimulus, and the side they responded to was to a large extent determined by task requirements.[31,35] Thus, if a verbal response or a match based on semantic knowledge was required, the right half of the chimera presented to the subject's left hemisphere determined the response. If a visual match based on the object's appearance was required, the left half of the chimera presented to the subject's right hemisphere determined the response.

From the standpoint of unawareness, a number of points are pertinent here. First, patients are not aware that they have seen chimeric figures, though both hemispheres have processed, at least partially, the contralateral aspects of the chimeras. Trevarthen pointed out that one of his patients (LB), though able to respond to *both* sides of the chimera simultaneously, never became aware that the stimuli were chimeras.[32] Levy noted that when the patient's left hemisphere responded verbally and even *confabulated* a response to a stimulus that only the right hemisphere knew, the right hemisphere never indicated that it knew via a "frown or head shake" whether the response was in error. Likewise, the patient's left hemisphere did not verbally object to a right hemisphere response.

Second, "completion" of the conflicting or absent aspects of the stimulus probably contributes to this unawareness. Trevarthen noted that when a verbal response was called for, split-brain patients completed the missing left side of objectively partial figures[32] and reported a whole face when shown chimeras with only the right half of a drawing of a face.[16] When shown a chimera with the left side of a tree, the patient's left hand drew a whole tree when instructed to draw what it "saw." Thus, each hemisphere was capable of experiencing a "whole" stimulus, though each actually saw only half.

Third, I suggest that this phenomenon occurs as a result of *confabulatory completion*. As noted previously, the conception of completion developed by Bender and Teuber[10] and Torjussen[13] was that completion resulted from residual visual perception occurring in a damaged area of the brain. According to this view, completion would occur only with objectively intact objects and could not be the result of a "psychological filling in" of a missing part. In split-brain patients, however, the completed aspects of the stimulus that these patients claim to see in the ipsilateral field do not need to be objectively present. This phenomenon, which does not rely on the presence of the actual stimulus in the impaired field, is thus an example of *confabulatory completion* and should be distinguished from the *veridical completion* (a term suggested by Weizkrantz[36]) of objectively complete figures as described by Bender and Teuber[10] and Torjussen.[13,37] It thus may be concluded that the unawareness of defect in split-brain patients depends in part upon the presence of this form of perceptual confabulation.

Unawareness of Blindness

Von Monakow is credited with the first scientific report of unawareness of cortical blindness in patients with bilateral posterior cortical pathology.[38–43] Subsequently, similar cases were described by Müller[44] and Déjerine and Vialet.[45] Gabriel Anton, in a series of papers between 1893 and 1899, presented the first systematic treatment and theoretical discussion of personal unawareness of neurologic signs including visual loss, cortical deafness, and hemiparesis.[42]

Anton is best known for his description of unawareness of cortical blindness, a particular condition that Albrecht[46] suggested be grouped under the rubric *Anton's symptom* in 1918. It is now known as Anton's syndrome. Anton's most widely cited case[47] was a 56-year-old seamstress named Ursula Mercz who, in spite of complete amaurosis of central origin, was unaware of her visual loss.[40,42,43] Neuropathologic findings on autopsy revealed bilateral cystic necrosis of the white matter of the occipital lobes. Though Anton found generalized cognitive impairment in many of his patients with unawareness of deficits, he maintained that these patients lacked sufficient dementia to explain their unawareness. He proposed that they were mentally blind *(seelenblind)* to their neurologic defects.[42] Anton suggested that the destruction of association tracts between primary sensory areas and the remaining brain was necessary to produce unawareness of neurologic deficits.

Neuropathologic Features of Anton's Syndrome

The causes of Anton's syndrome are diverse. The origin of the blindness is most commonly bilateral occipital lobe infarctions.[40,48,49] For instance, Redlich and Dorsey[40] found that 4 of 6 patients with Anton's had bilateral hemianopias. However, they suggested the cause of the blindness was actually not important for the appearance of the Anton's syndrome. In a more recent review of the syndrome,[48] it was also concluded that the blindness may be caused by lesions at any point along the visual pathways. Geschwind[50] suggested that blindness caused by peripheral lesions is much less likely to cause unawareness of deficit in the absence of significant dementia, while patients with occipital infarctions may manifest unawareness without clouding of consciousness.

Previous authors have observed clinical similarities between Anton's and Korsakoff's syndromes.[49] Stuss and Benson[51] noted that bilateral infarction in the posterior cerebral artery distribution is a frequent cause of Anton's syndrome and can produce damage to the hippocampus and limbic structures, which may result in a Korsakoff-like syndrome. In this circumstance, the two syndromes, which involve both unawareness of defects and confabulation, may share a common limbic neuropathology.[52]

Other lines of evidence point to the importance of frontal pathology. Stengel and Steele[53] reported a patient with bilateral optic atrophy and frontal lobe tumors with denial of blindness. Stuss and Benson[51] described a patient with bilateral traumatic optic neuropathy and frontal damage sustained as a result of a motor vehicle accident.

The patient was described as alert, oriented, and without other neurologic deficits. While he readily admitted his blindness, he stated that with the proper illumination he could see perfectly. McDaniel and McDaniel[49] described a similar case of a patient with monocular blindness due to optic nerve pathology and bifrontal encephalomalacia. This patient denied her visual defect and her illness in general. She exhibited visual as well as generalized confabulation. The anosognosia and confabulation persisted after the resolution of an acute confusional state. These authors suggest that a memory defect coupled with a failure of self-monitoring due to frontal pathology produced the denial of blindness and further offered that Bychowki may have been the first to make this suggestion.[54]

Relationship to Cognitive Impairment

The presence of generalized cognitive impairment has been noted in many instances of Anton's syndrome,[11,40,43,48,55,56] particularly, as noted above, when the visual loss is due to peripheral pathology.[50] However, the presence of total denial of blindness in the absence of significant (or presence of only mild) cognitive impairment has suggested to many investigators that cognitive impairment alone does not explain Anton's syndrome.[40,49,50,57]

Relationship to Confabulation

There is frequent if not universal appearance of visual and other forms of confabulation in patients with Anton's syndrome. Redlich and Dorsey[40] found prominent confabulation in their patients, leading them to suggest that "Anton's syndrome may be said to consist of a Korsakoff psychosis in a blind person." Brockman and von Hagen also noted prominent confabulation in Anton's.[58] McDaniel and McDaniel[49] suggested that in virtually all cases of Anton's syndrome, whether due to peripheral or central pathology, confabulation is present in relation to both the visual defect itself as well as to other aspects of the patient's clinical state. They also found confabulation and anosognosia to be closely allied conditions and considered

confabulation to be a necessary accompaniment to Anton's syndrome regardless of the site of damage to the visual system.

UNAWARENESS OF HEMIPLEGIA

Gabriel Anton, in 1893, probably provided the first descriptions of unawareness of hemiplegia.[59] One patient, Wilhelmy H., was reportedly unaware of a left hemiparesis,[43] and a second, Johann K., expressed the belief that his daughter (not his hemiplegic arm) was lying to his left.[41,42] Pick provided an additional report of denial of left hemiparesis in 1898.[60] Babinski, in 1914[61] and 1918,[62] provided additional clinical examples of unawareness of left hemiplegia and coined the term *anosognosia*.

While the diagnosis of anosognosia for hemiplegia (AHP) requires only a simple unawareness of hemiplegia, the actual clinical syndrome is far more complex. While some patients may appear simply unaware of their paralysis, frequently the belief in the normalcy of the limb is quite refractory to correction. In severe AHP, repeated efforts by the examiner to demonstrate the weakness are futile. In these cases, even when the paralyzed limb is dropped limply in the hemispace ipsilateral to the lesion, still no admission of paralysis is obtained. For this reason, anosognosia often appears to be delusional in nature.[63] Even when the patient admits that the limb does not move upon request, excuses such as "laziness" or "tiredness"[64] may be offered as explanations. Alternatively, the patient may *confabulate* that the limb has indeed moved,[61,65–70] as in Babinski's 1914 case, who, when asked to move the arm responded "Voilà, c'est fait."[61,67]

A host of rather unique and colorful clinical findings not directly related to limb movement per se often accompany the anosognosia. Patients may reject the limb entirely—a condition called *asomatognosia*,[71] and attribute its ownership to someone else.[65–67,71–76] Such was the case with a patient of ours who described her limb as belonging to her deceased husband. The limb may be personified with designations such as "Silly Jimmy" or

"Floppy Joe," as described by Critchley.[74,77] Patients may admit the paralysis but appear indifferent to it, a condition first described by Babinski[61] and termed *anosodiaphoria*.[67] Patients may also display hostility toward and hatred of the limb, called *misoplegia*.[77]

Frequency and Laterality of Anosognosia for Hemiplegia

Nathanson and coworkers[78] found 28 of 100 hemiplegic patients had "denial of illness," 48 had full awareness, and 24 had left-hemispheric lesions with severe aphasia that prevented adequate assessment. In the anosognosia group, 69 percent (19 patients) had left hemiplegia, 21 percent (6 patients) had right hemiplegia with aphasia, and 11 percent (3 patients) had right hemiplegia without aphasia. In Cutting's[79] investigation of a series of 100 acute hemiplegics from presumed "cerebrovascular accidents," 30 right hemiplegics were eliminated due to severe aphasia. Of 48 left hemiplegics, 28 (58 percent) demonstrated anosognosia for hemiplegia (AHP); 3 of 52 right-hemiplegic patients (14 percent of the testable right-hemiplegic group) demonstrated anosognosia. Willanger and coworkers[80] found AHP in 25 percent (14/55) and Hier and associates[81] in 36 percent (15/41) of right-hemispheric stroke patients with varying degrees of weakness, and Bisiach and colleagues[82] found moderate or severe AHP in 12 (33 percent) of 36 severe left hemiplegics.

Starkstein and coworkers[83] reported on 80 patients with acute cerebrovascular accidents (CVAs) and found that 8 (10 percent) showed mild, 9 (11 percent) moderate, and 10 (13 percent) severe AHP. Fifty-three (66 percent) showed no anosognosia. The AHP was significantly more common with right-hemispheric lesions even when aphasics were arbitrarily included as "anosognosic." Of 17 moderately or severely anosognosic patients with positive scans, 12 had right-hemispheric lesions compared to 3 with left-hemispheric lesions (2 had bilateral lesions). Finally, Stone and colleagues[84] studied 171 acute stroke patients (69 right, 102 left) and found AHP in 28 percent of right-hemispheric strokes and in 5 percent of left-hemispheric strokes, but 45 percent with left-hemispheric strokes could not be assessed, compared with only 13 percent with right-hemispheric strokes.

The collective impression of these studies is that while AHP is more commonly associated with right-hemispheric lesions, some of this difference may be due to the large number of patients with left-hemispheric stroke excluded from analysis because the presence of aphasia made their examination impossible or unreliable. In order to circumvent to some extent the issue of aphasia, investigators have employed the WADA test and asked patients if they recall the contralateral paralysis after the effects of the injection have passed and speech recovery has occurred.[85–90] Using amobarbital, Terzian[85] found that patients had poor recall of paralysis regardless of the site of injection. Gilmore and coworkers,[86] using the shorter-acting barbiturate methohexital, found recall of paralysis only after left-hemispheric injection. Durkin and coworkers,[87] using amobarbital, found only a small difference in recall favoring the left-hemispheric injections (4 percent recall right; 9 percent recall left) and noted that 85 percent did not recall weakness after either injection. However, Adair and colleagues,[88] using methohexital, found failure to recall paralysis in 97 percent of right-hemispheric injections compared with 48 percent of those in the left hemispheres. Similar results were reported by Breier and coworkers[89] using methohexital, and with amobarbital by Carpenter and associates[90] using amobarbital. Taken together, the data from WADA testing corroborate the clinical studies and suggest that AHP is more common after right-hemispheric lesions, but some of this difference is likely due to the presence of aphasia in the subjects with left-hemispheric lesions.

Anatomic Considerations in Anosognosia for Hemiplegia

Although the various forms of anosognosia may have different anatomic bases, be they focal or diffuse, AHP has traditionally been reported in association with lesions of the nondominant parietal lobe, the thalamus, or their connections to other sites or each other.[6,39,91–94]

Hier and coworkers[81] found anosognosia associated with right-hemispheric strokes only after larger strokes involving the frontal, parietal, and temporal lobes in addition to subcortical involvement. Levine and coworkers[70] also reported AHP associated with large strokes that involved either the cerebral gyri or adjacent corona radiata. Insula and opercular cortex were the most common cortical structures involved. Levine[70] suggested that no particular focal pathology was required to produce AHP beyond that which was necessary to produce severe sensorimotor loss. Feinberg and coworkers reported verbal asomatognosia associated with lesions of the supramarginal gyrus and posterior corona radiata[71] and AHP associated with lesions of the posterior corona radiata, posterior limb of the internal capsule, and the central gyri and insula, but they found involvement of these structures did not distinguish patients with and without AHP.[95] Finally, Starkstein and colleagues[83] found AHP associated with lesions of the right thalamus, temporoparietal cortex, and basal ganglia as well as with bilateral subcortical atrophy.

Sensory Loss

Babinski noted that sensory loss appeared to be a necessary prerequisite for AHP.[62] This is not surprising, since the lesions associated with paralysis are likely to involve primary somatosensory areas as well, were the latter directly related or not. Barré[96] emphasized the proprioceptive loss often seen in AHP, and authors including Barkman,[92] Gerstmann,[39] Schilder,[97] Weinstein and Kahn,[98] and Critchley[6] noted the common association between AHP and sensory loss.

Cutting[79] reported sensory loss in 87 percent of 31 patients with AHP, compared with its presence in only 38 percent of 16 patients without either AHP or other anosognosia-related phenomena. Bisiach and associates[82] found that of 12 patients with moderate or severe AHP, 11 had impairments in light touch to unilateral stimuli. Many cases with severe sensory impairments did not display AHP; one case of moderate AHP had no sensory impairment within the limited testing performed. Levine and coworkers[70] found severe left sensory impairment in all modalities in cases of persistent AHP, and to a greater extent than in those cases without AHP. They concluded that severe hemisensory impairment is necessary but not sufficient to produce AHP.

Relationship to Hemispatial Neglect

While the manifestations of personal and extrapersonal neglect in a certain sense resemble AHP and these conditions frequently co-occur, they are at least partially dissociable and cannot be reduced one to the other. As Table 28-1 demonstrates, however, these conditions appear related. Some 50 to 100 percent (mean 74 percent) of patients with AHP demonstrated extrapersonal neglect; the percentage of patients with personal neglect has not been extensively studied, but numbers have varied from 32 to 72 percent. In those patients without AHP, extrapersonal neglect may occur, though significantly less frequently (average 21 percent), and this includes many more cases with mild neglect. Cutting[79] found no cases of personal neglect in patients without AHP. Although Bisiach and colleagues[82] reported incidence of personal neglect in 6 of 8 (33 percent) non-AHP patients, they found no severe cases and only 1 moderate case of personal neglect in this group. Bisiach found 3 cases of moderate AHP with no personal neglect at all. This finding is compatible with the observation that AHP may persist if the paralysis is demonstrated to the patient in both the abnormal as well as normal hemispace.

Conversely, AHP occurs in 68 to 82 percent of hemineglect patients (Table 28-1) and much less commonly in those without neglect. This overall relationship between AHP and hemineglect is corroborated by the observation of Cappa and coworkers,[99] who reported reversal of AHP in 2 of 4 right-hemispheric hemineglect patients, with remission of personal and extrapersonal neglect during vestibular stimulation.

Table 28-1

Occurrence of left neglect in right-hemisphere-lesioned patients with and without anosognosia for hemiplegia (AHP)

Author	With AHP		Without AHP	
	Extrapersonal neglect, No. (%)	Personal neglect, No. (%)	Extrapersonal neglect, No. (%)	Personal neglect, No. (%)
Cutting[79]	16/31 (52%)	10/31 (32%)	1/16 (6%)	0/16 (0%)
Hier et al.[81]	13/15 (87%)	—	6/26 (23%)	—
Bisiach et al.[82]	14/18 (78%)	—		
Levine[70]	6/6 (100%) (100% severe)	—	4/7 (57%) (14% severe)	—
Starkstein et al.[83]	15/22 (55%)	—	2/53 (4%)	—

Occurrence of AHP in patients with and without left neglect

	With neglect		Without neglect	
	Extrapersonal	Personal	Extrapersonal	Personal
Hier et al.[81]	13/19 (68%)	—	2/22 (9%)	—
Bisiach[82]	14/17 (82%)	13/19 (68%)	4/19 (21%)	5/17 (29% overall) (18% moderate; 12% mild)

Relationship to General Intellectual Functioning

It has long been noted that many anosognosic patients may appear impaired in general intellectual functions. Nathanson and coworkers[78] reported a series of 100 hemiplegic patients, among whom all 28 with AHP showed disorientation; however, only 15 of 40 (31 percent) patients without AHP had an organic mental syndrome. Weinstein and Kahn[98] noted that patients with various forms of anosognosia for a variety of defects, including AHP, had a high incidence of cognitive and memory impairments. The investigators felt that these defects were an insufficient explanation for the anosognosia. Cutting[79] reported that 71 percent of AHP patients showed disorientation and 86 percent showed visuoperceptual defects, compared with a frequency of 6 percent for both of these disorders in hemiplegic patients without AHP. Levine and colleagues also found a greater incidence of impairments in multiple neuropsychological domains in patients with AHP than in those with right-hemispheric lesions without AHP, which they suggest prevented the AHP patients from discovering their hemiplegia.[70]

Anosognosia for Hemiplegia and Confabulation

Confabulation and AHP are frequently if not universally associated.[6,78,95,98] Critchley[6] and others[68–70,100] noted that when some patients with AHP were told to raise their arms and then asked why no movement occurred, these patients might insist that the limb really had moved or moved "less quickly" than the normal limb. The aforementioned phenomena are generally interpreted as instances of "phantom supernumerary limb" or "phantom third hand,"[6,101] as suggested by Critchley, who coined these terms and likened the phenomenon to other instances of phantom limb following amputation or deafferentation from plexus or spinal cord lesions.[102–104] However, the patient with phantom limb from the latter conditions recognizes the unreality of the phantom sensation and will try to clarify his or her perceptions by touching or looking at the limb, while the anosognosic patient claims to be able to move the limb, though he or she may never attempt to do so. In phantom limb from amputation and deafferentation,[102] the physical location of the phantom—as experienced by the patient—extends from the remaining stump in a position where the limb would be normally; the two dissociate only when the patient does not visually observe the limb and the actual limb is moved.

In contrast, in patients with AHP, the illusory limbs and imagined limb movements are delusional in nature. The patient experiences a partial or complete dissociation between the real limb

and the "limb" that performs the "movements"; visual inspection of the actual limb in the AHP patient does not correct the misperception. Indeed, these patients typically deny ownership of the real limb.[71] The supernumerary limb is experienced as healthy by the AHP patient and as intact and possessing normal strength, while phantom limbs are often felt to be missing parts or to be "telescoped" and to possess limited mobility. Based upon these differences, the phenomenon of illusory limb movements and supernumerary limbs in AHP should not be equated with phantom limbs (Table 28-2).

The question naturally arises whether the occurrence of illusory limb movements and supernumerary limbs in AHP can be explained on the basis of perceptual completion.[11] Bender and Teuber,[10] and Torjussen[37] suggested that completion resulted from residual perception occurring

Table 28-2

Comparison of phantom and supernumerary limbs

Characteristics of illusory limb	Phantom limb after amputation	Phantom limb after deafferentation	Supernumerary limb after (nondominant) central lesion
Time of onset	Acute and tends to diminish with time	Frequency increases with time after injury	Acute and tends to resolve rapidly
Duration	Months or years	Typically weeks to months	Rapid resolution usually within weeks
Physical and functional status	Over time becomes incomplete, shrunken, or telescoped	Telescoping may occur but generally does not	Intact and healthy
Willed movements	Limited, effortful	Limited, effortful	Equal or nearly so to intact limb
Effect of visual inspection	Merges with stump	Merges with limb	Remains dissociated from actual limb
Relation to actual limb	Projected from stump Moves in appropriate relation to the body May dissociate if stump deafferented	Usually located within limb; dissociation may occur acutely but typically fades	Always dissociated from actual limb: actual limb denied (asomatognosia)
Confabulation	Absent	Absent	Usually present
Delusional	Typically absent	Typically absent	Usually present
Anosognosia	Absent	Absent	Usually present

in a damaged area of the brain. For amputated limbs, it is clearly not possible for there to be actual perception of the missing part. Even if phantom limbs did derive in part from movements of the stump, this form of projective hallucination would not warrant the designation "perceptual completion" in this sense, since it is not produced by the facilitation of veridical perception in damaged areas of the brain via the activation of intact regions. These considerations also make perceptual completion an unlikely explanation for phantoms occurring after deafferentation.

However, in the presence of right-hemispheric damage and especially left-hemispatial neglect, the presence of an actual stimulus on the completed side may not be necessary. As noted, Warrington[14] reported that patients with hemispatial neglect who had objectively incomplete figures shown tachistoscopically to their normal field would indeed report whole figures, while hemianopics without neglect reported half figures under these circumstances. This phenomenon, which does not depend on the sensory representation of an actual stimulus being present in the impaired field, is another example of confabulatory completion, a term suggested in this context by Geschwind.[50] This suggests that the supernumerary limbs and illusory limb movements in AHP represent a form of confabulatory completion in which the patients confabulate normal limbs. The presence of hemispatial neglect could contribute to this tendency toward the confabulatory completion of the left side of the body.

Taken together with the previously described findings we conclude that the syndromes of unawareness of visual defects in hemianopia, neglect, and split-brain patients and of paralysis in AHP patients all involve confabulation or confabulatory completion. This point of view is supported by the study of Feinberg and coworkers[95] who found that when right-hemisphere-lesioned patients with neglect and AHP were compared with patients without AHP, those with AHP showed a significantly greater tendency toward visuoverbal confabulation for visual objects in the left hemispace that were not perceived. In other words, the presence of AHP was associated with

the occurrence of confabulation in the visual domain as well as with reference to the hemiplegia.

UNAWARENESS OF AMNESIA

There is much written about amnesia and confabulation and their relationship to unawareness of amnesia (UA) and illness in general. Korsakoff[105,106] first observed the tendency of patients with what is now known as Wernicke-Korsakoff syndrome to display both amnesia and confabulation ("pseudoreminiscences"). The co-occurrence of amnesia and confabulation in Korsakoff syndrome was subsequently confirmed by numerous authors.[106–114] Bonhoeffer[107,108] distinguished between "momentary" confabulation due to the patient's efforts to cover a gap in memory and "fantastic" confabulations, which appeared to exceed the need to conceal or excuse such a gap.[109] Berlyne[109] also found this distinction useful and suggested that "momentary" confabulations had to be provoked by questions from the examiner and that the content of such confabulations consisted of true memories that were temporally displaced. The notion of confabulations as temporally displaced veridical memories was previously suggested by van der Horst,[110] Williams and Rupp,[111] and Talland.[112,113] Berlyne[109] found that "fantastic" confabulations were not rooted in true memory and that their content was grandiose and wish-fulfilling.

Stuss and coworkers[114] found spontaneous confabulation of the "fantastical" variety in five patients with either head trauma, subarachnoid hemorrhage, or infarcts and found that this form of confabulation correlated with frontal dysfunction as judged by neurologic examination, computed tomography (CT)/electroencephalography (EEG) and neuropsychological test data. They suggested that this finding was consistent with the study of Mercer and colleagues,[115] who found inability to inhibit and monitor responses and make self-corrections in a mixed group of confabulatory patients, although the latter group displayed essentially provoked forms of confabulations.

Kapur and Coughlan[116] examined a patient

with subarachnoid hemorrhage due to an aneurysmal rupture who, in addition, had a left frontal infarct in the distribution of the anterior cerebral artery. This patient initially displayed both "fantastic" and "momentary" confabulation. During convalescence, the patient eventually displayed only "momentary" confabulation, and this transition was paralleled by improvement in frontal functions. Finally, Koppleman[117] renamed these "provoked" and "spontaneous" confabulations while retaining the essential characteristics of the two types. He found that the provoked confabulatory errors of Korsakoff and Alzheimer patients resembled those of healthy subjects whose memory was tested at prolonged retention intervals.

Neuroanatomic and Clinical Features of Unawareness of Amnesia

The pathology of alcoholic Wernicke-Korsakoff patients involves primarily the dorsomedial nucleus of the thalamus,[106] mamillary bodies,[118] both of these in combination,[119] or other thalamic nuclei.[120,121] As noted above, rupture of aneurysms of the anterior communicating artery (ACoA) have been noted to produce a Korsakoff-like amnesia, which in some cases is accompanied by confabulation,[116,122–131] is often of the "fantastic" or "spontaneous" type. In the ACoA series of Alexander and Freedman,[124] 5 of 11 patients had the most marked and persistent confabulation. Of these 5 patients, 3 had right anterior cerebral artery (ACA) infarcts; a fourth had bilateral ACA territory infarcts (right greater than left); and the fifth had a right parietal infarct. Thus frontal and particularly right-hemispheric regions were implicated. All patients had anterograde and retrograde amnesia. It was suggested that damage to basal forebrain, particularly the septal nuclei, which provide widespread cholinergic projections to cortical sites including hippocampus, might produce the amnesia. Vilkki's series[125] of ACoA patients also provided links between confabulation and frontal lobe damage; of 5 amnesic ACoA patients, 2 had profound confabulation; of these, 1 had bilateral frontobasal infarctions and the other had a right frontobasal subdural empyema treated surgically.

Damasio and coworkers[126] reported on sev-

eral patients with spontaneous, "dreamlike" confabulations, all of whom had basal forebrain lesions including septal nuclei, nucleus accumbens, diagonal band, and medial substantia innominata. It was felt that the nucleus basalis was also probably involved. All patients had unilateral orbitofrontal lesions as well. The septal lesions were believed to be responsible for the amnesia due to interruption of connections with the hippocampus, amygdala, and parahippocampal gyrus. The anatomy of confabulation was not explored in this series. In another series of amnesic patients of mixed etiology, Baddeley and Wilson[127] found that among the 10 amnesics, there were 2 with confabulation. One had an ACoA and the other a head injury; both had bilateral frontal lesions. Interestingly, while neither of these patients differed from nonconfabulators on measures of delayed recall, both did significantly worse on measures of retrograde autobiographical memory. They attributed the confabulation to a *dysexecutive syndrome* due to frontal pathology. Like Baddeley and Wilson,[127] Stuss and associates[114] and Alexander and Freedman[124] also found retrograde memory impairments in their confabulatory patients. This finding concurs with the report of Dall'Ora and coworkers[132] who described a patient with posthypoxic encephalopathy who presented with "wild confabulations" that reportedly tended to cover the period of deepest retrograde amnesia.

Deluca and coworkers[128,129] provided additional support for the role of frontal damage in producing confabulation. Finally, Fischer and associates[131] reported on nine AcoA patients divided into spontaneous (extended, grandiose) and provoked (limited, plausible) groups. While both groups had lesions of basal forebrain and anterograde amnesia, the spontaneous group had more extensive medial frontal and striatal pathology. They also showed more extensive retrograde amnesia and "executive deficits" on frontal-type tasks.

Relationship between Confabulation and Amnesia

Although in many of the aforementioned conditions confabulation and amnesia co-occur, the two conditions are at least partially dissociable. First of all, not all amnesics confabulate. Both Talland[112] and Victor and coworkers[106] noted that in Wernicke-Korsakoff patients, confabulation occurred most notably in the early stages of the disease, and Talland[112] described how, in the chronic phase of the illness, confabulation may recede from the clinical picture while notable memory impairment persists. Similarly, Alexander and Freedman[124] found that in post-AcoA-rupture patients, confabulation cleared after recovery of weeks or months but amnesia might remain, and Vilkki[125] also reported that only some AcoA patients with amnesia confabulate. The study of Mercer and associates[115] also found a lack of correlation between the degrees of amnesia and confabulation in a group of mixed etiologies. Conversely, some authors have suggested that confabulation does not require amnesia. Wyke and Warrington[133] made this argument with reference to a Korsakoff patient who showed visual completion to tachistoscopic stimuli in a fashion not attributable to memory impairment. They interpreted their findings as suggesting that confabulation per se was a primary symptom of Korsakoff's and not a consequence of amnesia. Kapur and Coughlan[116] also reported, of their post-aneurysm frontally damaged patient, that while memory was impaired, confabulation was prominent in spite of normal or near normal scores of tests on verbal and nonverbal recognition and paired-associate learning. In this context, they pointed out that the patients of Berlyne[109] and Stuss and colleagues[114] showed marked confabulation in spite of only slight impairments in memory. On the other hand, Deluca[128] found that among six AcoA patients, only those with amnesia confabulated.

Relationship between Confabulation and Unawareness

Although Talland[112] noted that the chronic Wernicke-Korsakoff amnestic might stop confabulating without return of insight, in general insight into amnesia and confabulation are inversely related. Williams and Rupp[111] noted that with the return of insight, confabulation cleared. Weinstein and Kahn noted prominent confabulation in patients with denial of their impairments in general.[66] Alexander and Freedman[124] reported that in recovery from ACoA rupture, there was a co-occurrence of recovery from confabulation and denial, and Mercer and coworkers[115] also proposed that return of insight related inversely to confabulation. Zangwill[134] and Parkin[135] suggested that the constellation of amnesia, confabulation, and lack of insight was typical of diencephalic amnesia, yet amnesics of temporal lobe origin did not display these additional features. It should be noted, however, that many of the confabulatory "diencephalic" cases had lesions that also involved the inferior frontal regions either by compression, direct invasion, postsurgical changes, or possibly acute hydrocephalus.

Other Forms of Unawareness

Numerous other varieties of conditions producing unawareness have been described. These include unawareness of disability in such neuropsychiatric conditions as Alzheimer disease,[43,136–143] Huntington disease,[144] auditory agnosia,[145] aphasia,[146–148] schizophrenia,[139] and many nonneurologic conditions including cardiac disease, cancer, acquired immunodeficiency syndrome, and many others.[149,150] Interestingly, two studies have found that frontal impairment correlates with unawareness in Alzheimer disease[141,142] and that patients with Pick disease associated with severe and early frontal lobe pathology have an earlier loss of insight than patients with Alzheimer disease.[43,137] Another investigation has found, on single photon emission tomography, evidence for right frontal involvement in Alzheimer disease associated with anosognosia.[143]

UNAWARENESS AND DENIAL

The role of psychological defense, particularly denial, in the production of unawareness syndromes remains unresolved. Schilder[97] was among the first to emphasize motivational factors and coined the term *organic repression* to describe the tendency of hemiplegic patients unconsciously to suppress knowledge of their paralysis. Goldstein[151] interpreted the unawareness of brain-damaged patients in terms of adaptation to deficits and avoidance of the "catastrophic reaction"; a position also favored by Sandifer.[152]

Paterson and Zangwill[153] made many astute observations relevant to this subject when they considered the patterns of disorientation and confabulation in the posttraumatic confusional state. They noted that patients in the early postacute periods would claim they were located in their home town when they were actually many miles away. During the course of recovering, the patients would simultaneously maintain that they were located in both the correct *and* incorrect locations, a condition termed *reduplicative paramnesia*[154] by Pick and linked by Weinstein and coworkers[66] to anosognosia. Paterson and Zangwill noted that patients in large part were oblivious to the conflict presented by their dual orientation and would confabulate explanations when confronted with the disparity. They observed that patients might accept the correct orientation in an "abstract geographical" sense, such as knowing the correct locale "according to the map," but still maintain they "felt" they were located in a different locale (usually closer to home) based more upon "concrete experience." Thus one patient originally from Grimsby but hospitalized in Scotland reported "If it comes to the map this part is the north of Scotland . . . but if people say 'Do you live here?' I say 'yes, Grimsby!' I feel I'm right . . . I know by my own language, by my own town streets." This patient was confabulatory, had left-hemispatial neglect, and was anosognosic for his left hemiparesis. Although amnesia was initially present, the "retention deficit cleared rapidly" and memory was adequate to recall the day's events a full week before correct orientation returned. This suggested to the investigators that affective motivational factors played a role in the persistent disorientation. This particular patient verbally expressed a strong desire to return home (a feature noted in other reduplicative patients[155]). Paterson and Zangwill suggested that, under the conditions of brain damage, this desire was "actively inhibiting the cognitive mechanisms which normally subserve orientation" and accounted for the persistent disorientation when "cognitive recovery had proceeded far enough to permit and sustain proper orientation." They interpreted the disorientation on the basis of both the *negative* features (in a Jacksonian sense[156]) of anterograde and retrograde amnesia, restriction of perception, and a defect in judgment in which there is a failure to correct incompatible interpretations, as well as the *positive* features of affect and motivation. Thus, motivation and affect could play a determining role in what patients might say about their situation.

The above quote of Paterson and Zangwill's patient is astonishingly similar to that of a patient of Olsen's cited by Nielson.[157] This patient had asomatognosia of her left-hemiplegic arm and claimed that the examiner's or another's arm was in bed with her. When confronted with the connection between her left arm and her own body, she stated "But my eyes and my feelings don't agree, and I must believe my feelings. I know they look like mine, [referring to her arm] but I can feel they are not, and I can't believe my eyes." These two patients have in common anosognosia for hemiplegia and confabulation; both patients in different domains (orientation versus limb ownership) were able in one sense to recognize the actual circumstances (correct orientation versus the real arm) yet maintain their false beliefs in spite of this conflict. These patients seem motivated to hold to a personal, idiosyncratic, concrete belief even when the correct information is supplied and even partially admitted.

It is this sort of observation, among others, that led Weinstein, Kahn, and coworkers[64,66,76,98,142,146] to emphasize the positive motivational and adaptive features of anosognosia and to emphasize the role of *denial* in producing unawareness of any of a variety of neurologic defects. Indeed Weinstein suggested these patients tended to deny any of their current personal problems. Weinstein and coworkers also noted the refractoriness of these beliefs to correction, and argued that cognitive defects alone could not explain the unawareness. They also pointed out that patients appeared implicitly aware of their defects.[76] For instance, they described how a patient with AHP, when asked to raise the left arm, might raise the right arm, but perform normally on other tests of right-left orientation. In the course of our investigations we have frequently noted the tendency for patients with AHP, while denying left-limb paralysis, when asked to raise the hemiplegic-left arm, to lift it with the right arm, suggesting they are implicitly aware that they cannot move the left arm normally. In a similar fashion, a patient of ours with Anton's syndrome due to peripheral blindness and frontal lobe lesions, in spite of denying his blindness and confabulating visual experience, would never attempt to read or walk without the help of his companion, and even obtained and used a blind cane.

Finally, Weinstein and coworkers have provided evidence that many of the reduplications and confabulations produced by these patients are "metaphorical or symbolic representations" of the patient's neurologic disabilities or other problems.[76,158] These fictitious accounts or reduplications are accepted over reality because they provide a greater sense of identity and relatedness, create order and unity, and "provide a more vivid *feeling* of reality than a more referential veridical statement."[76]

Striking examples of these confabulatory reduplications can be found throughout the literature and the neurologic wards if one is attuned to see them. Weinstein and Kahn reported the case of a patient with papilledema, bilateral slowing of the EEG, and enlarged ventricles who underwent resection of right cerebellar lung metastasis. She stated that she had two sons, Bill (her actual son) and Willie (a fictitious son). While she denied any illness or operations on herself, she confabulated that Willie was "recuperating from an illness." Weinstein and Kahn suggested the reduplication expressed her own feelings about herself. Another good example of this type of reduplicative confabulation is provided in a case described by Baddeley and Wilson,[127] as follows: RJ, a 42-year-old man who sustained a severe closed head injury, bilateral frontal hematomas, prominent anterograde and retrograde memory impairment, perseveration, and confabulation. He admitted being in a car accident and being "hurt" but "not badly."

He also confabulated, supposedly verbatim, light-hearted conversations, which purportedly took place after the accident and which tended to minimize the seriousness of the event. He produced a reduplicative confabulation claiming that he had two brothers, both named "Martin" (he actually had one living brother named Martin) and that one "Martin" had been "killed in a car accident." We examined a 65-year-old woman who sustained bifrontal infarcts after repair of a ruptured ACoA aneurysm. She displayed retrograde and anterograde amnesia. She initially denied surgery or illness in herself but confabulated that she was visiting her niece who had an aneurysm. Subsequently she would occasionally admit she had surgery for the aneurysm, but confabulated that she had an aunt who "couldn't think straight" because of an aneurysm and a "couple of cousins" who "all came for the same reason, aneurysm on top of the heads." In all these cases we see a constellation of amnesia (both retrograde and anterograde), unawareness, minimization or denial of illness and confabulations that in a certain sense describe many of the problems of which the patient is seemingly unaware. Like confabulations in AHP and Anton's syndrome, these confabulations and beliefs are refractory to correction, and are produced not only *within* a domain of neurologic dysfunction, but are often *about* the defect or illness in question.

TWO TYPES OF CONFABULATION AND UNAWARENESS

The studies reviewed above suggest that there are actually two major varieties of unawareness and that both are linked to different types of completion and confabulation (Table 28-3). One form I suggest be called *neutral* unawareness and confabulation, which may occur in any domain, (e.g., visual, somatosensory, memory) but is usually confined to that domain and represents an exaggerated tendency of the normal sort of "gap-filling" that occurs in normal perception or memory processes in general. Its occurrence is facilitated by impaired self-monitoring, but it is nondelusional

Table 28-3
Two types of unawareness and confabulation

Neutral unawareness and confabulation	Personal unawareness and confabulation
Gap filling	± Gap filling
Impersonal	Self-referential/autobiographical
Unimodal (tied to defect)	Polymodal
Nondelusional (may be corrected)	Often delusional (impervious to correction)
Impaired self-monitoring	Impaired self-monitoring
Personality and motivation not important	Personality and motivation important
Nonsymbolic	May be symbolic/metaphoric
Exaggeration of normal gap filling	Pathologic gap filling
Associated with completion/confabulatory completion	Associated with dissociation/denial
± Implicit knowledge of stimulus	± Implicit knowledge of defect itself

and the material is not self-referential. Hence the designation *neutral*. Visual completion in hemianopics, split-brain patients, and neglect patients, some aspects of AHP, and some varieties of "provoked" confabulation in amnesia are examples.

The second variety is somewhat more complex and difficult to define. I suggest *personal* unawareness and confabulation as a term to describe this type. Weinstein and coworkers provided the best description of this variety. It may occur with or without the first type, and hence the two are potentially dissociable. The content of the confabulation is personal in the sense that the material is about the patient and the patient's defects or problems, not about particular stimuli or word associations that have no personal relevance for the patient. As described by Weinstein and coworkers, Paterson and Zangwill, and others, the confabulations are motivated in the sense that they appear to serve a role in the adaptation to the defect(s) of which the patient is seemingly explicitly unaware. While patients with neutral forms may show implicit knowledge within their sensory or memory defects[159] patients with personal forms may show implicit awareness of the defects themselves.[76] The confabulations are delusional beliefs that cut across sensory domains and are refractory to correction. Impaired self-monitoring may be important in both varieties. Orbital and ventromedial

frontal damage, particularly of the right hemisphere, may contribute to this impairment in the personal form.

The tendency for right-hemispheric lesions to produce neglect and disorders of attention and intention[161] may account for the tendency of the right hemisphere to produce some of the neutral aspects of AHP and confabulation; this in some way might actually facilitate the expression of personal forms of confabulation, which are more dependent on verbal behaviors and hence preserved language mechanisms. The observation that requiring split-brain patients to produce a verbal response facilitates the extinction of the left half of stimuli may also help explain some of the laterality seen in AHP. As far as the personal forms of confabulation and unawareness are concerned, it has been suggested that the greater limbic connections of the right hemisphere may play a role.[160]

CONCLUSION

This chapter has surveyed some varieties of anosognosia and confabulation. It is apparent that multiple forms exist, and an effort has been made to classify these according to the extent that perceptual, memory, and personal and adaptive features are important. While it is suggested that there are two types, they are not mutually exclusive. In fact, both may coexist and may even interact. This dichotomy is offered in the hope that it might provide a framework within which the various issues in unawareness and confabulation may be organized.

REFERENCES

1. Finger S: *Origins of Neuroscience: A History of Explorations into Brain Function.* New York, Oxford University Press, 1994.
2. Gassel MM, Williams D: Visual function in patients with homonymous hemianopia. III. The completion phenomenon; insight and attitude to the defect; and visual functional efficiency. *Brain* 86:229–260, 1963.
3. Fuchs W: Completion phenomena in hemianopic vision, in Ellis WD (ed): *A Source Book of Gestalt Psychology.* London, Routledge & Kegan Paul, 1955.
4. Ramachandran VS: Filling in gaps in perception: Part I. *Curr Dir Psychol Sci* 1:199–205, 1992.
5. Gattass R, Fiorani M Jr, Rosa MGP, et al: Visual responses outside the classical receptive field in primate striate cortex: A possible correlate of perceptual completion, in Lent R (ed): *The Visual System from Genesis to Maturity.* Boston, Birkhauser, 1992.
6. Critchley M: *The Parietal Lobes.* New York, Hafner, 1953.
7. Bender MB: Disorders in visual perception, in Halpern L (ed): *Problems of Dynamic Neurology.* Jerusalem, Jerusalem Post Press, 1963, pp 319–375.
8. Dufour M: Sur la vision nulle dans i'hémianopsie. *Rev Med Suisse Romande* 9:445–451, 1889.
9. Teuber HL, Battersby WS, Bender MB: *Visual Field Defects after Penetrating Missile Wounds of the Brain.* Cambridge, MA, Harvard University Press, 1960, p 87.
10. Bender MB, Teuber HL: Phenomena of fluctuation, extinction and completion in visual perception. *Arch Neurol Psychiatry* 55:627–658, 1946.
11. Levine DH: Unawareness of visual and sensorimotor defects: A hypothesis. *Brain Cogn* 13:233–281, 1990.
12. Poppelreuter W: *Die psychischem Schadigungen durch Kopfschuss im Kriege.* Leipzig, Leopold Voss, 1917.
13. Torjussen T: Visual processing in cortially blind hemifields. *Neuropsychologia* 16:15–21, 1978.
14. Warrington EK: The completion of visual forms across hemianopic field defects. *Neurol Neurosurg Psychiatry* 25:208–217, 1962.
15. Zangwill OL: The completion effect in hemianopia and its relation to anosognosia, in Halpern L (ed): *Problems of Dynamic Neurology.* Jerusalem, Jerusalem Post Press, 1963, pp 274–282.
16. Myers RE, Sperry RW: Interocular transfer of a visual form discrimination habit in cats after section of the optic chiasam and corpus callosum. *Anat Rec* 115:351, 1953.
17. Myers RE: Function of corpus callosum in interocular transfer. *Brain* 79:358–363, 1956.
18. Sperry RW: Cerebral organizations and behavior. *Science* 1749–1757, 1961.
19. Trevarthen C: Integrative functions of the cerebral commissures, in Nebes RD, Corkin S (eds): *Handbook of Neuropsychology.* New York, Elsevier, 1991, pp 49–83.
20. Bogen JE: The callosal syndromes, in Heilman KM, Valenstein E (eds): *Clinical Neuropsychology.* New York, Oxford University Press, 1993, pp 337–407.
21. Gazzaniga MS, Bogen JE, Sperry RW: Some functional effects of sectioning the cerebral commissures in man. *Proc Natl Acad Sci USA* 48:1765–1769, 1962.
22. Sperry RW, Gazzaniga MS, Bogen JE: Interhemispheric relationships: The neocortical commissures; syndromes of hemispheric disconnection, in Vinken PJ, Bruyn GW (eds): *Handbook of Clinical Neurology.* Amsterdam, North-Holland, 1969, pp 273–290.
23. Gazzaniga MS: *The Bisected Brain.* New York, Appleton-Century-Crofts, 1970.
24. Gazzaniga MS, Le Doux JE: *The Integrated Mind.* New York, Plenum Press, 1978.
25. Trevarthen C, Sperry RW: Perceptual unity of the ambient visual field in human commissurotomy patients. *Brain* 96:547–570, 1973.
26. Frendrich R, Gazzaniga MS: Evidence for foveal splitting in a commissurotomy patient. *Neuropsychologia* 27:273–281, 1989.
27. Sperry RW: Consciousness, personal identity and the divided brain. *Neuropsychology* 22:661–673, 1984.
28. Feinberg TE, Schindler RJ, Flanagan NG, Haber

LD: Two alien hand syndromes. *Neurology* 42:19–24, 1992.

29. Sperry RW: Forebrain commissurotomy and conscious awareness, in Trevarthen C (ed): *Brain Circuits and Functions of the Mind.* New York, Cambridge University Press, 1990, pp 371–388.

30. Sperry RW, Zaidel E, Zaidel D: Self-recognition and social awareness in the disconnected minor hemisphere. *Neuropsychologia* 17:153–166, 1979.

31. Levy J, Trevarthen C, Sperry RW: Perception of bilateral chimeric figures following hemispheric disconnection. *Brain* 95:60–78, 1972.

32. Trevarthen C: Functional relations of disconnected hemispheres with the brain stem and with each other: Monkey and man, in Kinsbourne M, Smith WL (eds): *Hemispheric Disconnection and Cerebral Function.* Springfield, IL, Charles C Thomas, 1974, pp 187–207.

33. Levy J, Trevarthen C: Metacontrol of hemispheric function in human split-brain patients. *J Exp Psychol Hum Percept Perform* 2:299–312, 1976.

34. Levy J: Manifestations and implications of shifting hemi-inattention in commissurotomy patients, in Weinstein EA, Friedland RP (eds): *Advances in Neurology.* New York, Raven Press, 1977.

35. Levy J: Regulation and generation of perception in the asymmetric brain, in Trevarthen C (ed): *Brain Circuits and Functions of the Mind.* New York, Cambridge University Press, 1990, pp 231–248.

36. Weizkrantz L: *Blindsight—A Case Study and Implications.* New York, Oxford University Press, 1986.

37. Torjussen T: Residual function in cortically blind hemifields. *Scand J Psychol* 17:320–322, 1976.

38. von Monakow C: Experimentelle und pathlolgisch-anatomische Untersuchungen über die Beziehungen der sogenannten Sehsphäre zu den infracorticalen Opticuscentren und zum N opticus. *Arch Psychiatrie* 16:151–199, 317–352, 1885.

39. Gerstmann J: Problem of imperception of disease and of impaired body territories with organic lesions. *Arch Neurol Psychiatry* 48:890–913, 1942.

40. Redlich FC, Dorsey JF: Denial of blindness by patients with cerebral disease. *Arch Neurol Psychiatry* 53:407–417, 1945.

41. Bisiach E, Geminiani G: Anosognosia related to hemiplegia and hemianopia, in Prigatano GP, Schacter DL (eds): *Awareness of Deficit after Brain Injury: Clinical and Theoretical Issues.* New York, Oxford University Press, 1991.

42. Förstl H, Owen AM, David AS: Gabriel Anton and "Anton's symptom": On focal diseases of the brain which are not perceived by the patient (1898). *Neuropsychiat Neuropsychol Behav Neurol* 1:1–8, 1993.

43. McGlynn SM, Schacter DL: Unawareness of deficits in neuropsychological syndromes. *J Clin Exp Neuropsychol* 11:143–205, 1989.

44. Müller F: Ein Beitrag zur Kenntnis der Seelenblindhert. *Arch Psychiatrie* 24:857–917, 1918.

45. Déjerine, J, and Vialet: Sur un cas de cécité corticale. *Compt Rend Soc de Biol* 11:983–997, 1893.

46. Albrecht O: Drei Fälle mit Anton's symptom. *Arch Psychiatrie* 59:883–941, 1918.

47. Anton G: Über die Selbstwahrnehmung der Herderkrankungen des Gehirns durch den Kranken bein Rindenblindheit und Rindentaubheit. *Arch Psychiatrie* 32:86–127, 1899.

48. Swartz BE, Brust JCM: Anton's syndrome accompanying withdrawal hallucinosis in a blind alcoholic. *Neurology (Cleveland)* 34:969–973, 1984.

49. McDaniel KD, McDaniel LD: Anton's syndrome in a patient with posttraumatic optic neuropathy and bifrontal contusions. *Arch Neurol* 48:101–105, 1991.

50. Geschwind N: Disconnexion syndromes in animals and man. *Brain.* 88:237–294, 585–643, 1965.

51. Stuss DT, Benson DF: *The Frontal Lobes.* New York, Raven Press, 1986, p 144.

52. Benson DF, Marsden DC, Meadows JC: The amnesic syndrome of posterior cerebral artery occlusion. *Acta Neurol Scand* 50:133–145, 1974.

53. Stengel E, Steele GDF: Unawareness of physical disability (anosognosia). *Br J Psychiatry* 92:379–388, 1946.

54. Bychowski Z: Über das fehlen der Wahrnehmung der eigen Blindheit bei zwei Kriegsverletzen. *Neurol Centralbl* 106:354–357, 1920.

55. Hemphill RE, Klein R: Contribution to the dressing disability as a focal sign and to the imperception phenomena. *J Ment Sci* 94:611–622, 1948.

56. Bergman PS: Cerebral blindness. *Arch Neurol Psychiatry* 78:568–584, 1957.

57. Redlich E, Bonvicini G: Über mangelnde Wahrnehmung (Autoanästhesie) der Blindheit bei cerebralen Erkrankugen. *Neurol Centralbl* 20:945–951, 1907.

58. Brockman NW, von Hagen KO: Denial of own blindness (Anton's syndrome). *Bull LA Neurol Soc* 11:178–180, 1946.

59. Anton G: Beiträge zur klinischen Beurthelung und

zur Localisation der Muskelsinnstorungen im Grosshirne. *Zeitschr Heilk* 14:313–348, 1893.

60. Pick A: *Beiträge zur Pathologie und pathologischen Anatomie des Centralnervensystes unit Bemerkungen zur normalen Anatomie desselben.* Berlin, Karger, 1898.

61. Babinski J: Contribution à l'étude des troubles mantaux dans l'hémiplégie organique cérébrale (anosognosie). *Rev Neurol (Paris)* 27:845–848, 1914.

62. Babinski J: Anosognosie. *Rev Neurol (Paris)* 31:365–367, 1918.

63. Sandifer PH: Anosognosia and disorders of body scheme. *Brain* 69:122–137, 1946.

64. Weinstein EA, Cole M: Concepts of anosognosia, in Halpern LE (ed): *Dynamic Neurology.* Jerusalem, Jerusalem Post Press, 1964.

65. Fisher CM: Neurologic fragment: II. Remarks on anosognosia, confabulation, memory, and other topics; and an appendix on self-observation. *Neurology* 39:127–132, 1989.

66. Weinstein EA, Kahn RL: *Denial of Illness.* Springfield, IL, Charles C Thomas, 1955.

67. Friedland RP, Weinstein EA: Hemi-inattention and hemisphere specialization: Introduction and historical review, in Weinstein EA, Friedland RP (eds): *Advances in Neurology.* New York, Raven Press, 1977, pp 1–31.

68. Nielsen JM: *Agnosia, Apraxia, Aphasia: Their Value in Cerebral Localization.* New York, Hoeber, 1936, p 84.

69. Hécaen H, Albert ML: *Human Neuropsychology.* New York, Wiley, 1978, pp 678–682.

70. Levine DH, Calvanio R, Rinn WE: The pathogenesis of anosognosia for hemiplegia. *Neurology* 41:1770–1781, 1991.

71. Feinberg TE, Haber LD, Leeds NE: Verbal asomatognosia. *Neurology* 40:1391–1394, 1990.

72. Ives ER, Nielsen JM: Disturbance of body scheme: Delusion of the absence of part of body in two cases with autopsy verification of lesion. *Bull LA Neurol Soc* 2:120–125, 1937.

73. Wortis H, Datner B: An analysis of a somatic delusion: A case report. *Psychosom Med* 4:319–323, 1942.

74. Critchley M: Personification of paralyzed limbs in hemiplegics. *Br Med J* 30:284, 1955.

75. Ullman M: Motivational and structural factors in denial of hemiplegia. *Arch Neurol* 3:306–318, 1960.

76. Weinstein EA: Anosognosia and denial of illness, in Prigatano GP, Schacter DL (eds): *Awareness of Deficit after Brain Injury: Clinical and Theoretical Issues.* New York, Oxford University Press, 1991, pp 240–257.

77. Critchley M: Misoplegia or hatred of hemiplegia. *Mt Sinai J Med* 41:82–87, 1974.

78. Nathanson M, Bergman PS, Gordon GG: Denial of illness: Its occurrence in one hundred consecutive cases of hemiplegia. *Arch Neurol Psychiatry* 68:380–387, 1952.

79. Cutting J: Study of anosognosia. *Neurol Neurosurg Psychiatry* 41:548–555, 1978.

80. Willanger R, Danielsen VT, Ankerbus J: Denial and neglect of hemiparesis in right-sided apoplectic lesions. *Acta Neurol Scand* 64:310–326, 1981.

81. Hier DB, Mondlock J, Caplan LR: Behavioural abnormalities after right hemisphere stroke. *Neurology* 33:337–344, 1983.

82. Bisiach E, Vallar G, Perani D, et al: Unawareness of disease following lesions of the right hemisphere: Anosognosia for hemiplegia and anosognosia for hemianopia. *Neuropsychologia* 24:471–482, 1986.

83. Starkstein SE, Fedoroff JP, Price TR, et al: Anosognosia in patients with cerebrovascular lesions: A study of causative factors. *Stroke* 23:1446–1453, 1992.

84. Stone SP, Halligan PW, Greenwood RJ: The incidence of neglect phenomena and related disorders in patients with an acute right or left hemisphere stroke. *Age Aging* 22:46–52, 1993.

85. Terzian H: Behavioral and EEG effects of intracarotid sodium amytal injection. *Acta Neurochir (Wein)* 12:230–239, 1964.

86. Gilmore RL, Heilman KM, Schmidt RP, et al: Anosognosia during Wada testing. *Neurology* 42:925–927, 1992.

87. Durkin MW, Meador KJ, Nichols ME, et al: Anosognosia and the intracarotid amobarbital procedure (Wada test). *Neurology* 44:978–979, 1994.

88. Adair JC, Gilmore RL, Fennell EB, et al: Anosognosia during intracarotid barbiturate anesthesia: Unawareness or amnesia for weakness. *Neurology* 45:241–243, 1995.

89. Breier JI, Adair JC, Gold M, et al: Dissociation of anosognosia for hemiplegia and aphasia during left-hemisphere anesthesia. *Neurology* 45:65–67, 1995.

90. Carpenter K, Berti A, Oxbury S, et al: Awareness of and memory for arm weakness during intracarotid sodium amytal testing. *Brain* 118:243–251, 1995.

91. Pötzl O: Über Störungen der Selbstwahrnehmung

bei linksseitiger Hemiplegie. *Zeitschr Neurol Psychiatry* 93:117–168, 1925.

92. Barkman A: De l'anosognosie dans l'hémiplégie cérébrale: Contribution clinique à l'étude de ce symptome. *Acta Med Scand* 62:235–254, 1925.

93. Von Hagen K, Ives FR: Two autopsied cases of anosognosia. *Bull LA Neurol Soc* 4:41–44, 1939.

94. Nielsen JM: Disturbances of the body scheme: Their physiological mechanism. *Bull LA Neurol Soc* 3:127–135, 1938.

95. Feinberg TE, Roane DM, Kwan PC, et al: Anosognosia and visuoverbal confabulation. *Arch Neurol* 51:468–473, 1994.

96. Barré JA, Morin L, Kaiser: Étude clinique d'un nouveau cas d'Anosognosie de Babinski. *Rev Neurol (Paris)* 39:500–503, 1923.

97. Schilder P: *The Image and Appearance of the Human Body.* London, Kegan Paul, 1935.

98. Weinstein EA, Kahn RL: The syndrome of anosognosia. *Arch Neurol Psychiatry* 64:772–791, 1950.

99. Cappa S, Sterzi R, Giuseppe V, Bisiach E: Remission of hemineglect and anosognosia during vestibular stimulation. *Neuropsychologia* 5:775–782, 1987.

100. Von Hagen KO, Ives ER: Anosognosia (Babinski), imperception of hemiplegia. *Bull Los Angeles Neuro Soc* 2:95–103, 1937.

101. Critchley M: A phantom supernumerary limb after a cervical root lesion. *Arch Neuropsic São Paulo* 10:269–275, 1952.

102. Riddoch G: Phantom limbs and body shape. *Brain* 64:197–222, 1941.

103. Bors E: Phantom limbs of patients with spinal cord injury. *AMA Arch Neurol Psychiatry* 66:610–631, 1951.

104. Frederiks JAM: Occurrence and nature of phantom limb phenomena following amputation of body parts and following lesions of the central and peripheral nervous system. *Psychiatr Neurol Neurochir* 66:73–97, 1963.

105. Victor M, Yakovlev PI: SS Korsakoff's psychic disorder in conjunction with peripheral neuritis: A translation of Korsakoff's original article with brief comments on the author and his contribution to clinical medicine. *Neurology* 5:394–406, 1955.

106. Victor M, Adams RD, Collins GH: *The Wernicke-Korsakoff Syndrome and Related Neurologic Disorders Due to Alcoholism and Malnutrition,* 2d ed. Philadelphia, Davis, 1989.

107. Bonhoeffer K: *Die akuten Geisteskrankheiten der Gewohnheitstrinker.* Jena, Gustav Fischer, 1901.

108. Bonhoeffer K: Der Korsakowsche Symptomenkomplex in seinen Beziehungen zu den verschiedenen Krankheitsformen. *Allg Z Psychiatry* 61:744–752, 1904.

109. Berlyne N: Confabulation. *Br J Psychiatry* 120:31–39, 1972.

110. Van Der Horst L: Über die Psychologie des Korsakowsyndroms. *Monatschr Psychiatry Neurol* 83:65–84, 1932.

111. Williams HW, Rupp C: Observations on confabulation. *Am J Psychiatry* 95:395–405, 1938.

112. Talland GA: Confabulation in the Wernicke-Korsakoff syndrome. *Nerv Ment Dis* 132:361–381, 1961.

113. Talland GA: *Deranged Memory.* New York, Academic Press, 1965.

114. Stuss DT, Alexander MP, Lieberman A, Levine H: An extraordinary form of confabulation. *Neurology* 28:1166–1172, 1978.

115. Mercer B, Wapner W, Gardner H, Benson P: A study of confabulation. *Arch Neurol* 34:429–433, 1977.

116. Kapur N, Coughlan AK: Confabulation and frontal lobe dysfunction. *Neurol Neurosurg Psychiatry* 43:461–463, 1980.

117. Koppleman MD: Two types of confabulation. *Neurol Neurosurg Psychiatry* 43:461–463, 1980.

118. Barbizet J: Defect of memorizing of hippocampal-mammillary origin: A review. *Neurol Neurosurg Psychiatry* 26:127–135, 1963.

119. Weiskrantz L: Neuroanatomy of memory and amnesia: A case for multiple memory systems. *Human Neurobiol* 6:93–105, 1987.

120. Mair WGP, Warrington EK, Weiskrantz L: Memory disorder in Korsakoff's psychosis: A neuropathological and neuropsychological investigation of two cases. *Brain* 102:749–783, 1979.

121. Mayes AR, Meudell PR, Mann D, Pickering A: Location of lesions in Korsakoff's syndrome: Neuropsychological and neuropathological data on two patients. *Cortex* 24:367–388, 1988.

122. Talland GA, Sweet WH, Ballantine HT: Amnesic syndrome with anterior communicating artery aneurysm. *Nerv Ment Dis* 145:179–192, 1967.

123. Lindqvist G, Norlen G: Korsakoff's syndrome after operation on ruptured aneurysm of the anterior communicating artery. *Acta Psychiatr Scand* 42:24–34, 1966.

124. Alexander MR, Freedman M: Amnesia after anterior communication artery aneurysm rupture. *Neurology* 34:752–757, 1984.

125. Vilkki J: Amnesic syndromes after surgery of ante-

rior communicating artery aneurysms. *Cortex* 21:431–444, 1985.

126. Damasio AR, Graff-Radford NR, Eslinger PJ, et al: Amnesia following basal forebrain lesions. *Arch Neurol* 42:263–271, 1985.

127. Baddeley AD, Wilson B: Amnesia autobiographical memory and confabulation, in Rubin DC (ed): *Autobiographical Memory.* Cambridge, England, Cambridge University Press, 1986.

128. Deluca J: Predicting neurobehavioral patterns following anterior communicating artery aneurysm. *Cortex* 29:639–647, 1993.

129. Deluca J, Cicerone KD: Confabulation following aneurysm of the anterior communicating artery. *Cortex* 27:417–424, 1991.

130. Deluca J, Diamond BJ: Aneurysm of the anterior communicating artery: A review of neuroanatomical and neuropsychologic sequelae. *Clin Exp Neuropsychol* 17:100–121, 1995.

131. Fischer RS, Alexander MP, D'Esposito M, Otto R: Neuropsychological and neuroanatomical correlates of confabulation. *Clin Exp Neuropsychol* 17:20–28, 1995.

132. Dall'Ora P, Della Sala S, Spinnler H: Autobiographical memory: Its impairment in amnesic syndrome. *Cortex* 25:197–217, 1989.

133. Wyke M, Warrington E: An experimental analysis of confabulation in a case of Korsakoff's syndrome using a tachistoscopic method. *J Neurol Neurosurg Psychiatry* 23:327–333, 1960.

134. Zangwill OL: The amnesic syndrome, in Whitty CWM, Zangwill OL (eds): *Amnesia.* London, Butterworth, 1966.

135. Parkin AJ: Amnesic syndrome: A lesion-specific disorder? *Cortex* 20:479–508, 1984.

136. Gainotti G: Confabulation of denial in senile dementia: An experimental study. *Psychiatric Clin* 8:99–108, 1975.

137. Gustafson I, Nilsson L: Differential diagnosis of presenile dementia on clinical grounds. *Acta Psychiatr Scand* 65:194–209, 1982.

138. Reisberg B, Gordon B, McCarthy M: Insight and denial accompanying progressive cognitive decline in normal aging and Alzheimer's disease, in Stanley B (ed): *Geriatric Psychiatry: Ethical and Legal Issues.* Washington, DC, American Psychiatric Press, 1985, pp 19–39.

139. McGlynn SM, Kaszniak AW: Unawareness of deficits in dementia and schizophrenia, in Prigatano GP, Schacter DL (eds): *Awareness of Deficit after Brain Injury: Clinical and Theoretical Issues.* New York, Oxford University Press, 1991, pp 84–110.

140. Sevush S, Leve N: Denial of memory deficit in Alzheimer's disease. *Am J Psychiatry* 150:748–751, 1993.

141. Michon A, Deweer B, Pillon B, et al: Relation of anosognosia to frontal lobe dysfunction in Alzheimer's disease. *Neurol Neurosurg Psychiatry* 57:805–809, 1994.

142. Weinstein EA, Friedland RP, Wagner EE: Denial/unawareness of impairment and symbolic behavior in Alzheimer's disease. *Neuropsychiatry Neuropsychol Behav Neurol* 7:176–184, 1994.

143. Starkstein SE, Vazquez S, Migliorelli R, et al: A single-photon emission computed tomographic study of anosognosia in Alzheimer's disease. *Arch Neurol* 52:415–420, 1995.

144. Caine ED, Shoulson I: Psychiatric syndromes in Huntington's disease. *Am J Psychiatry* 140:728–733, 1983.

145. Roth N: Unusual types of anosognosia and their relation to the body image. *Nerv Ment Dis* 100:35–43, 1944.

146. Weinstein EA, Cole M, Mitchell MS, Lyerly O: Anosognosia and aphasia. *Arch Neurol Psychiatry* 10:376–386, 1964.

147. Lebrun Y: Anosognosia in aphasics. *Cortex* 23:251–263, 1987.

148. Rubens AB, Garrett MF: Anosognosia of linguistic deficits in patients with neurological deficits, in Prigatano GP, Schacter DL (eds): *Awareness of Deficits after Brain Injury: Clinical and Theoretical Issues.* New York, Oxford University Press, 1991.

149. Lewis L: Role of psychological factors in disordered awareness, in Prigatano GP, Schacter DL (eds): *Awareness of Deficit after Brain Injury: Clinical and Theoretical Issues.* New York, Oxford University Press, 1991.

150. Levine J, Warrenburg S, Kerns R, et al: The role of denial in recovery from coronary artery disease. *Psychosom Med* 49:109–117.

151. Goldstein K: The organism: *A Holistic Approach to Biology Derived from Pathological Data on Man.* New York, American Book, 1939.

152. Sandifer PH: Anosognosia and disorders of body scheme. *Brain* 69:122–137, 1946.

153. Paterson A, Zangwill OL: Recovery of spatial orientation in the post-traumatic confusional state. *Brain* 67:54–68, 1944.

154. Pick A: On reduplication paramnesia. *Brain* 26:260—267, 1903.

155. Ruff RL, Volpe BT: Environmental reduplication associated with right frontal and parietal lobe injury. *Neurol Neurosurg Psychiatry* 44:382–386, 1981.

156. Taylor J: *Selected Writings of John Hughlings Jackson.* New York, Basic Books, 1958.

157. Nielsen JM: Gerstmann syndrome: Finger agnosia, agraphia, confusion of right and left and acalculia: Comparison of this syndrome with disturbance of body scheme resulting from lesions of the right side of the brain. *Arch Neurol Psychiatry* 39:536–559, 1938.

158. Weinstein EA: Linguistic aspects of amnesia and confabulation. *Psychiatr Res* 8:439–444, 1971.

159. Shacter DL, McAndrews MP, Moscovitch M: Access to consciousness: Dissociations between implicit and explicit knowledge in neuropsychological syndromes, in Weiskrantz L (ed): *Thought without Language.* Oxford, England, Clarendon Press, 1988.

160. Feinberg TE, Shapiro RM: Misidentification—Reduplication and the right hemisphere. *Neuropsychiatry Neuropsychol Behav Neurol* 2:39–48, 1989.

161. Heilman KM: Anosognosia: Possible neuropsychological mechanisms, in Prigatano GP, Schacter DL (eds): *Awareness of Deficit after Brain Injury: Clinical and Theoretical Issues.* New York, Oxford University Press, 1991, pp 52–62.

162. Weinstein EA, Friedland RP: Behavioral disorders associated with hemi-inattention, in Weinstein EA, Friedland RP (eds): *Advances in Neurology.* New York, Raven Press, 1977, pp 51–62.

Chapter 29

MISIDENTIFICATION SYNDROMES

Todd E. Feinberg
David M. Roane

Misidentification syndromes, sometimes referred to as delusional misidentification syndromes, describe conditions in which a patient incorrectly identifies and reduplicates persons, places, objects, or events. The most commonly reported form of misidentification for persons is known as *Capgras syndrome.* The syndrome was first reported in 1923 by Capgras and Reboul-Lachaux[1] who described a 53-year-old woman with a chronic paranoid psychosis who became convinced that multiple persons, including members of her family, had been replaced by imposters. She also asserted that there were several duplicates of herself. Since that time, hundreds of cases of Capgras syndrome have been reported. The essence of the disorder lies in the delusional belief that a person or persons, generally close to the patient, have been replaced by "doubles" or imposters.[2]

A related type of misidentification is the *Frégoli syndrome.*[3] First reported in 1927, the syndrome is named after the famous Italian actor Leopoldo Frégoli, who was extremely adept at impersonation. This condition involves the belief that a person who is well known to the patient is really impersonating, and hence taking on the appearance of, a stranger in the patient's environment. Several authors have commented on the relationship between Capgras and Frégoli syndromes.[4–6] Christodoulou[6] suggested that Capgras syndrome is characterized by a "hypoidentification" of a person known by the patient who is felt to be an imposter, while Frégoli syndrome was the manifestation of a "hyperidentification" in which a known person could be seen in the guise of others. The syndrome of *intermetamorphosis,* described by Courbon and Tusques,[7] is a related condition in which persons known to the patient are believed to have exchanged identities with each other. In the delusion of subjective doubles,[8] the patients believe they themselves have been replaced. Other varieties of delusional misidentification syndromes exist, and different varieties may co-occur in any given patient.

The delusional misidentification syndromes are related to the syndrome of reduplicative paramnesia (see Chap. 28). For instance, Alexander and colleagues[9] described a case of Capgras syndrome following a head injury that resulted in a large right frontal subdural hematoma. The patient stated that his wife and five children had been replaced by a nearly identical family, and he persisted in his conviction even when challenged by his examiners. Alexander and associates suggested a similarity between their case and *reduplicative paramnesia,* a syndrome originally described by Pick[10] in 1903. Pick's patient was a 67-year-old woman who confabulated the existence of two clinics, both headed by Professor Pick. While Capgras syndrome had traditionally been considered a psychiatric condition, reduplicative paramnesia had generally been felt to be a neurologic disorder, since it was usually seen in the setting of brain disorders and was often associated with confusion and memory loss. It differed as well from Capgras syndrome in that it typically involved misidentification of places rather than persons. However, the distinction between the two conditions is not entirely clear. Cases of reduplication reported by Weinstein[11] in the setting of brain disease involved duplication of persons, events, body parts, and even the self (see Chap. 28). Furthermore, Weinstein's cases of reduplication were frequently associated with other psychiatric symptoms including other delusions, hallucinations, and mood changes. It has therefore become customary to group delusional misidentification and reduplicative paramnesia together.

The Capgras delusion is most commonly associated with psychiatric illness and is often accompanied by derealization and depersonalization[12,13] and by other paranoid symptomatology.[14,15] Literature reviews of patients with the Capgras delusion have demonstrated the diagnostic heterogeneity of this condition.[14,16,17] Schizophrenia, mood disorders, and organic conditions, including Alzheimer disease,[18] have all been associated with Capgras syndrome.

Misidentification and reduplication in general have been associated with a wide variety of medical and neurologic conditions.[19,20] In a large literature review of cases of reduplication, Signer[19] found cases due to drug intoxication or withdrawal, infectious and inflammatory disease, and endocrine disorders. Neurologic conditions included seizures, cerebral infarction, and head injury. Diffuse brain syndromes including delirium, dementia, and mental retardation accounted for over 40 percent of patients with diagnosable organic conditions. Electroconvulsive therapy has also been implicated in cases of misidentification.[21,22]

NEUROANATOMIC CORRELATES

In a report of 29 personally examined patients with misidentification for person, Joseph[23] found that 16 patients with abnormal computed tomography (CT) scans had bilateral cortical atrophy, including bifrontal atrophy (88 percent), bitemporal atrophy (73 percent), and biparietal atrophy (60 percent). Weinstein and Burnham suggested that bilateral and diffuse brain involvement with right-hemispheric predominance were the most common neurologic findings.[24] Along these lines, Feinberg and Shapiro[25] reviewed the anatomic correlates on a selected series of case reports of patients with misidentification-reduplication. They found that bilateral cortical involvement occurred frequently (62 percent of Capgras patients and 41 percent of reduplication cases). In considering those cases where cerebral dysfunction was unilateral, they found that right-hemispheric pre-

dominance in reduplication was highly significant (52 percent right versus 7 percent left), with a statistical trend for more frequent right-hemispheric damage in the smaller number of Capgras cases (32 percent right versus 7 percent left). Förstl and coworkers[20] grouped together a wide range of misidentification cases and found that 19 of 20 patients with focal lesions on brain CT scans showed right-sided abnormalities. In a subsequent study, Förstl and colleagues[26] focused on patients with dementia of the Alzheimer's type and found that patients with misidentification had significantly greater atrophy in the right frontal lobe than did demented controls. Based on three cases of head trauma, Benson and associates[27] suggested that reduplicative paramnesia occurred in the setting of bifrontal impairment in concert with damage to the posterior portion of the right hemisphere. Hakim and coworkers,[28] in a prospective study of 50 patients with alcoholism, found that 3 of 4 reduplicators had acute right-hemispheric lesions. They presumed all patients to have chronic bifrontal damage on the basis of their chronic alcohol use and neuropsychological test results. Finally, Fleminger and Burns[29] compared right-versus left-hemispheric asymmetries in CT scans of patients with misidentification. In one selected group, asymmetry was found, with greater right-hemispheric damage in the occipitoparietal area. In the analysis of a second group of patients, greater right-hemispheric damage could be detected in frontal, temporal, and parietal lobes.

At present, while some evidence suggests that a right-hemispheric lesion (particularly right frontal impairment[30]) can be both necessary and sufficient to produce misidentification, the bulk of cases support the argument that a right-hemispheric lesion is much more likely to be associated with misidentification in the context of bifrontal or diffuse cortical disturbance. This finding may reflect the greater tendency in these patients to demonstrate confabulation in general (see Chap. 28).

REPRESENTATIVE THEORIES

It has been suggested that delusional misidentification is a symptom, rather than a distinct syndrome, associated with various psychiatric and neurologic diagnoses.[31] Nonetheless, several explanations have attempted to account for a broad range of misidentification phenomena. Anatomic disconnection has been offered as a mechanism by several authors. Joseph[23] theorized that misidentification could result from hemispheric disconnection of cortical areas responsible for orientation. This could result in each hemisphere's maintaining an independent "image" of person, place, and time, which might lead to reduplication of entities in the environment. However, Ellis and colleagues[32] showed that patients with Capgras syndrome could judge face stimuli more rapidly with bilateral than with unilateral presentation, a finding that they suggested was inconsistent with the hemispheric disconnection hypothesis. Staton and coworkers[33] suggested that reduplication could be a failure to integrate previously stored memories and new information resulting from disconnection of the right hippocampus. Alexander and associates[9] considered that a disconnection of the right temporal and limbic area from the frontal lobes could alter the patients' familiarity for people and places and prevent them from utilizing available information appropriately.

The mechanisms proposed by Staton and associates[33] and Alexander and colleagues[9] attribute misidentification particularly to the loss of functions subsumed by the right hemisphere. Several investigators have emphasized other nondominant hemispheric functions, such as disorders of visuospatial orientation,[28,30] problem solving,[30] and the ability to determine the exact identity and uniqueness of stimuli[34] in the origin of delusional misidentification syndromes and reduplication. A recent study by Ellis and coworkers[32] confirmed that three Capgras patients lacked the normal right-hemispheric superiority for visual processing of faces.

A final disconnectionist account, formulated by Ellis and Young,[35] is based on the suggestion that there are two anatomically independent pathways for facial recognition: a "ventral route" subserving explicit recognition and a "dorsal route" responsible for recognition of the emotional significance of faces but not sufficient to allow for conscious identification.[36] While Capgras syndrome has been linked with prosopagnosia,[37–39] Ellis and Young[35] argue that the two are dissociable because they result from separate lesions. The ventral route disconnection causes prosopagnosia while the dorsal route interruption yields Capgras syndrome.

While the above theories emphasize anatomic disconnection, psychiatric factors have often been cited as etiologically significant for the development of Capgras syndrome. For instance, according to Enoch and Trethowan,[31] ambivalence is the "psychodynamic aspect" of Capgras syndrome. Simultaneous conflicting affects toward a significant object exist, and, through the mechanisms of projection and splitting, the actual object is misidentified and devalued while the normal attachment to the "original" is maintained.

Another point of view emphasizes the *interaction* of neurologic and psychiatric factors in DMS. Early important work emphasizing the link between neurologic and psychiatric factors in DMS can be found in the writings of Jacques Vié[4,40–42] who noted that the diverse DMS (*méconnaissance systématique*) such as Capgras and Frégoli syndromes were related to the neurologic syndromes of anosognosia of Babinski (unawareness of hemiplegia) (see Chap. 28) and asomatognosia[43] (denial of ownership of limb). Vié pointed out that in all these conditions, systematic and selective misidentifications occurred that could not be explained solely on the basis of factors such as generalized confusion.

The position of Weinstein and Kahn,[11,24,44] because of its emphasis on psychological denial, is usually taken to represent a psychological theory. In actuality these authors also suggested that DMS occurred through an interaction of neurologic and psychiatric factors. They suggested that misidentification and reduplication were facilitated by brain alteration and that they represented a denial, representation of, or solution to the patient's problems. More recent analysis by other investigators has also suggested an interaction between neurologic and psychiatric factors.[45,46]

An additional link between neurologic and psychiatric causation of delusional misidentification syndromes is provided by the fact that dissociative symptoms occur in delusional misidentification syndromes associated with both neurologic and psychiatric disorders.[24] Capgras, in the original report,[1] emphasized the importance of the *sentiment d'étrangeté* in the production of the syndrome in his chronic paranoid patient. Many authors have provided additional support for the association of depersonalization/derealization with delusional misidentification syndromes (see Christodoulou[5,6,12]). Christodoulou has suggested that depersonalization/derealization symptoms, under certain circumstances (paranoia, cerebral dysfunction, charged emotional circumstances), may evolve into delusional misidentification syndromes. Weinstein and coworkers have noted that patients with retrograde amnesia after head injury may also display elements of depersonalization and derealization.[24,47] Feelings of altered familiarity also occur during psychomotor seizures and with temporal lobe stimulation (see Feinberg and Shapiro[25] for review).

A PROPOSED FRAMEWORK FOR DELUSIONAL MISIDENTIFICATION SYNDROMES

As noted by prior authors, we agree that DMS can be viewed as being especially related to, and perhaps a special instance of, dissociative disorders, and we regard the origin of these symptoms as a perturbation, as opposed to a loss, of personal relatedness. We suggest that DMS cleaves along the dimension of personal relatedness into three basic groups based upon the pattern of relatedness between the object (person, event, or experience) and the self. The various subtypes of DMS and reduplication can thus be characterized as showing a pattern of decreased (withdrawal) or increased

(insertion of) personal relatedness (or both) between the self and the misidentified object or event.

Our basic dichotomization into patterns of withdrawal or insertion of personal relatedness corresponds in part to several previously suggested dichotomies (Table 29-1) and is consistent with the viewpoint that Capgras may be similar to jamais vu phenomena[25,48–51] and that Frégoli[49] and environmental reduplication[25,49–52] are similar to déjà vu phenomena. Our model (Table 29-1), however, differs in two fundamental ways from previously proposed models (see, for example, de Pauw[51]). First of all, as to the basic means of distinguishing Capgras from Frégoli, these syndromes have previously been categorized on the basis of physical versus psychological substitution or hypoidentification versus hyperidentification. In contrast we view the distinguishing feature to be alteration of personal relatedness or significance. Those syndromes exemplified by decreased relatedness may be said to represent a disavowal, estrangement, or alienation from persons, objects, or events, while those with increased relatedness are manifestations of an overrelatedness with elements in the environment.

We prefer the concept of an alteration in relatedness as opposed to an alteration in familiarity because many stimuli that the patient misidentifies, such as hospitals and aneurysms, are not particularly "familiar" in any sense of the word. Rather they are significant and actually do pertain to the self though the patient rejects them in spite of this.

Secondly, we argue that our approach is particularly useful in explaining instances where Capgras- and Frégoli-type misidentifications co-occur

Table 29-1

Prior formulations of basic dichotomization of Capgras and Frégoli syndrome

Author		
Vié[4]	Illusion of negative doubles (Capgras)	Illusion of positive doubles (Frégoli)
Christodoulou[6]	Delusional hypoidentification	Delusional hyperidentification
Christoldoulou[5]	Physically identical, psychologically different	Physically different, psychologically identical
de Pauw[49–51]	Hypoidentification, denial of familiarity, jamais vu (Capgras)	Hyperidentification, affirmation of familiarity, déjà vu (environmental reduplication)
Feinberg and Shapiro[25]	Pathological unfamiliarity, jamais vu, substitute familiar for unfamiliar (Capgras)	Pathological familiarity, déjà vu, substitute unfamiliar for familiar (environmental reduplication)

Table 29-2
Proposed model of common DMS

Examples of misidentified entities	Mechanism supporting misidentification/reduplication and clinical examples		
	Withdrawal of personal relatedness	Insertion of personal relatedness	Combined withdrawal/insertion of personal relatedness
Persons	Misidentifies wife as "impostor" (Capgras–jamais vu)	Misidentifies stranger as son (Frégoli–déjà vu)	Misidentifies personal physician as a friend from home[44,53] (Capgras/Frégoli–jamais vu/déjà vu)
Hemiplegic arm[40,43,44,53] (asomatognosia)	Denies ownership of arm[50,51]		Misidentifies own arm as belonging to close friend[43,44,53]
Hospital[11,24,44,53,54] (environmental reduplication)	Calls the hospital a "branch" or "annex" of actual hospital[44]	Mislocates actual hospital closer to patient's own neighborhood[44,49–51]	Misidentifies hospital as "annex" of actual hospital and locates it closer to patient's own neighborhood[44]
Traumatic events[11,24,53,54] (temporal reduplication) i.e., car accident	Denies accident occurred to patient (jamais vécu)	Claims similar accident happened previously to patient (déjà vécu)	Minimizes own accident but claims reduplicated brother "Martin" killed in (fictitious) car accident[54]
Illness[11,24,44,53]	Denial of illness	Had similar illness previously	Patient denies illness but claims reduplicated child Bill called "Willie" had same illness as patient[44] Patient with aneurysm minimizes it and claims her relatives have aneurysms

within a single misidentification (Table 29-2, column 4). This occurs, for instance, in asomatognosia where the patient simultaneously denies ownership of the arm[43,44,53] (withdrawal of personal relatedness) while identifying the arm as belonging to a friend or relative (insertion of personal relatedness). In a similar fashion, when a patient with environmental reduplication claims he is located in a hospital "annex" in his own neighborhood, he is *both* denying the actual identity of his current location as well as inserting an element of personal relatedness.

The same pattern of withdrawal and insertion of relatedness occurs in reduplication of illness in the context of anosognosia. Thus a patient of Weinstein did not recognize her own illness, but claimed she had two children, Bill (real) and "Willie" (fictitious), and that "Willie" had an illness similar to hers.[44,53] We saw a patient who minimized the problems posed by her own aneurysm but claimed that several of her relatives had aneurysms. Finally, with regard to misidentification of a traumatic event, Baddeley and Wilson[54] described the patient RJ who denied that he was seriously injured in a car accident, yet simultaneously claimed to have two brothers named Martin: a Martin who actually existed and a fictitious "Martin" who was killed in a car accident (see Chap. 28 for further discussion of these cases). In these cases we hypothesize that the neurologic impairment facilitates the derealization/deperson-alization (dissociation) of an actual person, place, or event, which is then replaced by some other personally significant relationship. Motivational factors appear important in determining both the withdrawal and insertion of significance.

CONCLUDING REMARKS

If a perturbation in personal relatedness to oneself or one's environment is an essential ingredient in delusional misidentification syndromes, one may ask whether this distortion is primarily a result of a neurologic lesion, a psychiatric mechanism linked with motivational variables, or both. Many theories emphasizing a neurologic etiology for Capgras syndrome[9,33,46] assert a limbic disconnection of current perceptions from past experience. This causes a reduced feeling of familiarity with environmental stimuli and a confabulation of "doubleness" to explain the disparity between current and past experience. These theories do not account for the selectivity of many cases of Capgras, their delusional nature, the lack of gross neuropathologic lesions in most cases, the occurrence of misidentification of relatively unfamiliar persons in many cases, the occurrence of misidentifications of the hyperfamiliar type, and the role of motivation. For instance, in regard to the last of these, it has been pointed out that in environmental reduplication, while abnormal spatial perception, poor visual memory, and other neuropsychological defects are evident, these patients often show, in addition, a pronounced desire to return home.[55]

Other theories describe the psychoanalytic viewpoint that derealization/depersonalization is the result of psychological defense mechanisms. As noted by Nemiah,[56] "From the earliest period of the development of psychoanalytic concepts, the experience of estrangement that is central to depersonalization phenomena has been viewed as a psychological defense." In this scenario, derealization/depersonalization occurs as a defense against irreconcilable affects or unacceptable and conflicting motivations. The ambivalence produces the delusion of "doubleness" through mechanisms such as "splitting."[31,57] While these theories can account for selectivity, delusional nature and the possibility of hypo- and hyperfamiliar misidentifications, they do not account for delusional misidentification syndromes occurring in the context of neurologic disease.

A mediating point of view is that the neurologic lesion, and certain neurologic lesions in particular, cause a distortion of normal sensation, memory, and awareness. The response to this distortion, particularly when it involves personally significant objects or events, creates the circumstances which, in the susceptible individual, results in derealization/depersonalization. It is upon this substrate that motivational variables may become evident.

REFERENCES

1. Capgras J, Reboul-Lachaux J: L'illusion des "sosies" dans un délire systématisé. *Bull Soc Clin Med Ment* 11:6–16, 1923.
2. Christodoulou GN: The delusional misidentification syndromes. *Br J Psychiatry* 14:65–69, 1991.
3. Courbon P, Fail G: Syndrome "d'illusion de Frégoli" et schizophrenie. *Ann Med Psychol* 85:289–290, 1927.
4. Vié J: Un trouble de l'identification des personnes: L'illusion des sosies. *Ann Med Psychol* 88:214–237, 1930.
5. Christodoulou GN: Delusional hyper-identifications of the Frégoli type. *Acta Psychiatry Scand* 54:305–314, 1976.
6. Christodoulou GN: The syndrome of Capgras: *Br J Psychiatry* 130:556–564, 1977.
7. Courbon P, Tusques J: L'illusion d'intermetamorphose et de charme. *Ann Med Psychol* 90:401–406, 1932.
8. Christodoulou GN: Syndrome of subjective doubles. *Am J Psychiatry* 135:249–251, 1978.
9. Alexander MP, Stuss DT, Benson DF: Capgras syndrome: A reduplicative phenomenon. *Neurology* 29:334–339, 1979.
10. Pick A: Clinical studies. *Brain* 26:242–267, 1903.
11. Weinstein EA, Kahn RL, Sugarman LA: Phenomenon of reduplication. *AMA Arch Neurol Psychiatry* 67:808–814, 1952.
12. Christodoulou GN: Role of depersonalization-derealization phenomena in the delusional misidentification syndromes, in Christodoulou GN (ed): *The Delusional Misidentification Syndromes*. Basel: Karger, 1986.
13. Spier SA: Capgras' syndrome and the delusions of misidentification. *Psychiatr Am* 22:279–285, 1992.
14. Kimura S: Review of 106 cases with the syndrome of Capgras. *Bibl Psychiatry* 164:121–130, 1986.
15. Todd J, Dewhurst K, Wallis G: The syndrome of Capgras. *Br J Psychiatry* 139:319–327, 1981.
16. Merrin EL, Silberfarb PM: The Capgras phenomenon. *Arch Gen Psychiatry* 33:965, 1970.
17. Signer SF: Capgras' syndrome: The delusion of substitution. *Clin Psychiatry* 48:147–150, 1987.
18. Mendez MF, Martin RJ, Symth KA, Whitehouse PJ: Disturbances of person identification Alzheimer's disease: A retrospective study. *J Nerv Ment Dis* 180:94, 1992.
19. Signer SF: Psychosis in neurologic disease: Capgras symptom and delusions of reduplication in neurologic disorders. *Neuropsychiatr Neuropsychol Behav Neurol* 5:138–143, 1992.
20. Förstl H, Almeida OP, Owen A, et al: Psychiatric, neurological and medical aspects of misidentification syndromes: A review of 260 cases. *Psychol Med* 21:905–950, 1991.
21. Weinstein EA, Linn L, Kahn RL: Psychosis during electroshock therapy: Its relation to the theory of shock therapy. *Am J Psychiatry* 109:22–26, 1952.
22. Hay GG: Electroconvulsive therapy as a contributor to the production of delusional misidentification. *Br J Psychiatry* 148:667–669, 1986.
23. Joseph AB: Focal central nervous system abnormalities in patients with misidentification syndromes, in Christodoulou GN (ed): *The Delusional Misidentification Syndromes*. Basel: Karger, 1986, p 68.
24. Weinstein EA, Burnham DL: Reduplication and the syndrome of Capgras. *Psychiatry* 54:78, 1991.
25. Feinberg TE, Shapiro RM: Misidentification-redu-

plication and the right hemisphere. *Neuropsychiatr Neuropsychol Behav Neurol* 2:39–48, 1989.

26. Förstl H, Burns A, Jacoby R, Levy R: Neuroanatomical correlates of clinical misidentification and misperception in senile dementia of the Alzheimer type. *Clin Psychiatry* 52:268, 1991.
27. Benson DF, Gardner H, Meadows JC: Reduplicative paramnesia. *Neurology* 26:147–151, 1978.
28. Hakim H, Verma NP, Greiffenstein MF: Pathogenesis of reduplicative paramnesia. *Neurol Neurosurg Psychiatry* 51:839–841, 1988.
29. Fleminger S, Burns A: The delusional misidentification syndromes in patients with and without evidence of organic cerebral disorder: A structured review of case reports. *Biol Psychiatry* 33:22–32, 1993.
30. Kapur N, Turner A, King C: Reduplicative paramnesia: Possible anatomical and neuropsychological mechanisms. *Neurol Neurosurg Psychiatry* 51:579–581, 1988.
31. Enoch MD, Trethowan WH: *Uncommon Psychiatric Syndromes*. Bristol: John Wright, 1979.
32. Ellis HD, de Pauw KW, Christodoulou GN, et al: Responses to facial and non-facial stimuli presented tachistoscopically in either or both visual fields by patients with the Capgras delusion and paranoid schizophrenics. *Neurol Neurosurg Psychiatry* 56:215–219, 1993.
33. Staton RD, Brumback RA, Wilson H: Reduplicative paramnesia: A disconnection syndrome of memory. *Cortex* 18:23–36, 1982.
34. Cutting J: Delusional misidentification and the role of the right hemisphere in the appreciation of identity. *Br J Psychiatry* 159:70–74, 1991.
35. Ellis HD, Young AW: Accounting for delusional misidentifications. *Br J Psychiatry* 147:239–248, 1900.
36. Bauer RM: The cognitive psychophysiology of prosopagnosia, in Ellis H, Felves M, Newcombe F, et al (eds): *Aspects of Face Processing*. Dordrecht: Nijhoff, 1986.
37. Shraberg D, Weitzel WD: Prosopagnosia and the Capgras syndrome. *Clin Psychiatry* 40:313–316, 1979.
38. Bidault E, Luaute JP, Tzavaras A: Prosopagnosia and the delusional misidentification syndromes. *Bibl Psychiatry* 164:80–91, 1986.
39. Lewis SW: Brain imaging in a case of Capgras' syndrome. *Br J Psychiatry* 150:117–120, 1987.
40. Vié J: Les méconnaissances systématiques. *Ann Med Psychol* (*Paris*) 102:410–455, 1944.
41. Vié J: Le substratum morbide et les stades évolutifs des méconnaissances systématiques. *Ann Med Psychol* (*Paris*) 102:410–455, 1944.
42. Vié J: Étude psychopathologique des méconnaissances systématiques. *Ann Med Psychol* (*Paris*) 102:1–15, 1944.
43. Feinberg TE, Haber LD, Leeds NE: Verbal asomatognosia. *Neurology* 40:1391–1394, 1990.
44. Weinstein EA, Kahn RL: *Denial of Illness: Symbolic and Physiological Aspects*. Springfield, IL: Charles C Thomas, 1955.
45. Gordon MacCallum WA: The interplay of organic and psychological factors in the delusional misidentification syndrome. *Bibl Psychiatry* 164:92–98, 1986.
46. Fleminger S: Delusional misidentification: An exemplary symptom illustrating an interaction between organic brain disease and psychological processes. 27:161–167, 1994.
47. Weinstein EA, Marvin SL, Keller NJA: Amnesia as a language pattern. *Arch Gen Psychiatry* 6:269–270, 1962.
48. Todd J, Dewhurst K, Wallis G: The syndrome of Capgras. *Br J Psychiatry* 139:319–327, 1981.
49. de Pauw KW, Szulecka TK, Poltock TL: Frégoli syndrome after cerebral infarction. *J Nerv Ment Dis* 175:433–438, 1987.
50. de Pauw KW: Delusional misidentification syndromes, in Bizon Z, Szyszkowski W (eds): *Proceedings of the 35th Congress Polish Psychiatrists*. Warsaw: Polish Psychiatric Association, 1989.
51. de Pauw KW: Delusional misidentification: A plea for an agreed terminology and classification. *Psychopathology* 27:123–129, 1994.
52. Sno HN, Linszen DH, DeJonghe F: Déjà vu experiences and reduplicative paramnesia. *Br J Psychiatry* 161:565–568, 1992.
53. Weinstein EA: Patterns of reduplication in organic brain disease, in Vinken PJ, Bruyn GW (eds): *Handbook of Clinical Neurology*. Amsterdam: North Holland Publishing Co., 1969.
54. Baddeley AD, Wilson B: Amnesia autobiographical memory and confabulation, in Rubin DC (ed): *Autobiographical Memory*. Cambridge: Cambridge University Press, 1986.
55. Ruff RL, Volpe BT: Environmental reduplication associated with right frontal and parietal lobe injury. *Neurol Neurosurg Psychiatry* 44:382–386, 1981.
56. Nemiah J: Dissociative disorders, in Kaplan HI, Sadock BJ (eds): *Comprehensive Textbook of Psychiatry*. Baltimore: Williams & Wilkins, 1989, vol 5.
57. Benson RJ: Capgras' syndrome. *Am J Psychiatry* 140:969–978, 1983.

Part 4

FRONTAL, CALLOSAL, AND SUBCORTICAL SYNDROMES

Chapter 30

FRONTAL LOBES: CLINICAL AND ANATOMIC ASPECTS

D. Frank Benson
Bruce L. Miller

FRONTAL LOBES: CLINICAL AND ANATOMIC ASPECTS

For over a century, the frontal lobes have been an enigma to brain scientists. Significant progress has been made in the past several decades, but many anatomic and functional aspects remain mysterious. The frontal lobes, particularly in humans, are massive in relation to other, better understood cortical areas, and it was long considered that the frontal lobes were the seat of human intelligence. This proved untrue, at least as intelligence is defined by psychometric testing. The functions of the frontal lobes in human behavior remain a mystery.

In 1973 the great Russian psychologist A. R. Luria[1] proposed a simple outline of brain functions. He suggested that subcortical structures, particularly the midbrain and diencephalon, functioned to produce *tonic regularity*. He further stated that the posterior cortex—the premotor and motor aspects of the frontal lobe and all cortex posterior to these areas—carried out primary *sensorimotor functions,* and that the comparatively massive prefrontal cortex functioned to *regulate* mental activities. This tripartite description of mental functions was further elaborated by Albert,[2] who suggested the terms *fundamental, instrumental,* and *superordinate* to define the activities of the brainstem, posterior cortex, and prefrontal cortex respectively.

Classic neuroanatomy divides the cortical surface of the frontal lobes into three major segments: (1) *motor*—the narrow strip of cortical tissue located just anterior to the rolandic fissure; (2) *premotor*—the larger area of frontal tissue anterior to the motor strip that acts as a motor association cortex (Brodmann areas 6 and 8); and (3) *prefrontal*—the vast amount of frontal cortex anterior to the premotor cortex, including a significant amount of the anterior/lateral cortex, most of the medial frontal cortex, and the entire orbital frontal cortex. In the classification suggested by Luria,[1] the motor and premotor areas of the frontal lobes would be included in the sensorimotor division and the prefrontal cortex would carry out the regulatory activities. The motor functions of the frontal lobes are adequately reviewed in many neuroanatomy texts. The prefrontal regulatory functions are important for psychology and are the topic of this chapter.

Of considerable significance in discussion of the neural basis of prefrontal psychological functions are the connections of frontal cortex with other brain areas. The prefrontal cortex receives direct or indirect input from most ipsilateral cortical areas and from the opposite hemisphere via callosal connections. In addition, prefrontal cortex receives strong input from a number of significant subcortical sources: (1) the limbic system, (2) the reticular system, (3) the hypothalamus, and (4) neurotransmitter systems. Prefrontal cortex is the only cortical area that receives strong sensorimotor, limbic, and reticular input. Additional input of hypothalamic and autonomic data and the effects of many neurotransmitters place prefrontal cortex in a strong position to monitor both intrinsic and extrinsic stimuli and to exert regulatory control of brain functions.

PREFRONTAL FUNCTIONS

Behavioral functions performed by the prefrontal cortex have proved difficult to delineate. To date, almost all information has been derived from behavioral aberrations seen following frontal brain damage. In the past several decades some psychological tests aimed directly at the assessment of prefrontal function have been devised (see Chapter 31), and, more recently, psychological testing has been combined with functional brain imaging techniques to provide valuable insights. In general, however, psychological tests of prefrontal function demand inferences from data obtained through primary sensorimotor functions, which themselves may be impaired.[3]

A second problem in studying prefrontal function is a lack of clearly delineated neuropathology. Frontal brain tumors tend to become massive, affecting both posterior ipsilateral tissues and tissues in the opposite frontal lobe, before diagnosis can be made. The only vascular lesion confined to prefrontal cortex involves the anterior cerebral artery, a vessel with considerable collaterals; consistent vascular lesions are rare. Prefrontal leukotomies provided clean, relatively precise prefrontal lesions but were performed only in individuals with significant behavioral abnormality; postsurgical testing was often frustrated by the inherent mental disorder.

Perhaps because of these problems, the underlying impairment in frontally damaged patients has yet to be satisfactorily established. A review of current attempts at characterizing prefrontal function and its impairment is presented in the following chapter. Here we note some of the more common effects of prefrontal damage in terms of their clinical manifestations.

Personality changes following frontal lobe lesions are of two main types. One type could be called pseudoretarded or pseudodepressed, and is characterized by apathy, lethargy, little spontane-ity of behavior, unconcern, reduced sexual interest, little overt emotion, and reduced ability to plan ahead. Although such patients appear retarded, their IQs may be normal or near normal. The other type could be called pseudopsychopathic and is characterized by inappropriate social behavior, lack of concern for others, increased motor activity, sexual disinhibition, and *Witzelsucht,* an inappropriately puerile, jocular attitude. There is some suggestion of differential localization for these two types of personality change, the former being associated with dorsolateral lesions and the latter with orbitofrontal lesions. However, because of the nonfocal effects of many frontal lesions, mentioned above, patients will frequently manifest an almost paradoxical mixture of both personality types.

The cognitive impairments of patients with prefrontal damage are apparent in a variety of tasks, some of which are reviewed in the following chapter. The domains affected include complex motor behavior (see also Chap. 16), planning and sequencing, attention, memory, and language (see discussions of Broca's aphasia and transcortical motor aphasia in Chap. 9). Often patients can perform well on standard tests of intelligence but fail miserably in less constrained real-life situations calling for planning and flexibility.

CONDITIONS THAT INFLUENCE FRONTAL LOBE FUNCTION

Vascular

Ischemic Infarction   The vascular territory for the frontal lobes comes from the anterior cerebral artery (ACA) and middle cerebral arteries (MCA), both of which are branches of the internal carotid artery.[4] The anterior and medial portions of the frontal lobes are supplied by the ACA, while the anterior branch of the MCA supplies most of the lateral dorsal frontal cortex. With ACA infarctions (see Fig. 30-1), the eyes tend to deviate toward the injured hemisphere. This conjugate eye deviation occurs following injury to the frontal eye fields in Brodmann area 8 and is accompanied

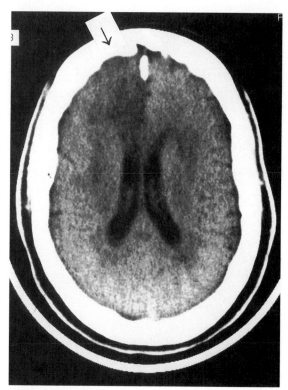

Figure 30-1
Computed tomography scan showing findings of a large anterior cerebral artery infarction involving the medial frontal cortex.

by frontal neglect. Conjugate deviation following from injury to area 8 tends to disappear after a few days, while the frontal neglect often persists. Because the medial portions of the motor strip of the frontal cortex contain fibers for the leg, weakness and sensory loss associated with these infarctions is greatest in the leg, with relative sparing of motor and sensory function in the arm and face. Also, involvement of the supplementary motor area leads to a forced grasp of the contralateral hand. Transcortical motor aphasia is the most common aphasia syndrome seen with ACA occlusion of the dominant hemisphere.[5] Following these infarcts, common behavioral abnormalities include profound apathy and loss of executive control. A manic syndrome may follow acute injury, particularly when the infarction involves the right

hemisphere. Conversely, depression, though more common with left frontal stroke, can occur with injury to either side. Rarely, a single ACA supplies both medial frontal lobes; ACA occlusion can produce bifrontal infarction leading to an akinetic mute state.

Strokes of the dominant hemisphere involving the MCA lead to paralysis of the face and arm on the contralateral side with eyes deviated toward the side of infarction (away from the paralysis). When the stroke is restricted to the anterior MCA branch of the dominant hemisphere, Broca's aphasia occurs; in contrast, complete MCA strokes lead to global aphasia. Loss of sequencing ability and disturbed executive control may be persistent problems. Forced grasp is not a feature of MCA stroke. Neglect may occur following either right- or left-sided MCA occlusion, but denial of illness is more common with right-sided lesions.

Other Vascular Lesions   Other types of vascular injury can also produce frontal dysfunction. A common site for aneurysms is the anterior communicating artery; following rupture, ischemia or infarction within the territory of the ACA often occurs. The sagittal sinus lies adjacent to the medial portions of the frontal lobes, and thrombus formation in this sinus can produce variations on anterior artery syndromes, although seizures and alterations in consciousness are more common with sinus thrombosis than simple arterial infarction. This disease is often idiopathic, although hypercoagulable states are known to cause this disorder.[6]

Trauma

The poles of the frontal lobes lie adjacent to frontal bone while the basal (orbital) frontal regions sit upon the skull's cribriform plate. The frontal lobe's intimate association with bone makes this area particularly prone to injury following trauma (see Fig. 30-2). Patients often recover from the motor and sensory deficits that follow a head injury, only to be left with profound behavioral abnormalities such as disinhibition, apathy, and loss of executive control. Behavioral disinhibition as-

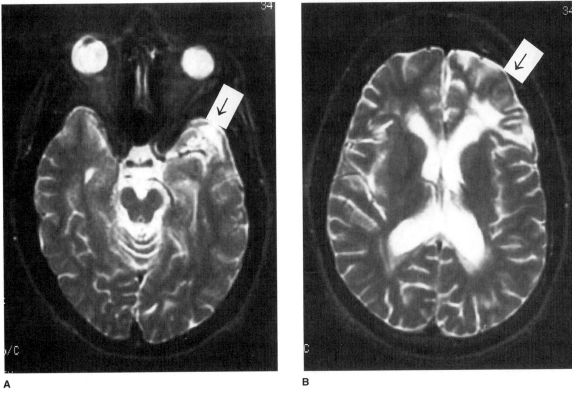

A   B

Figure 30-2
These T_2-weighted MRI scans from the anterior temporal (A) and anterior frontal (B) lobes demonstrate loss of tissue secondary to trauma. The patient was a sexually and verbally disinhibited male with profound frontal-systems deficits on neuropsychological testing.

sociated with head trauma is often also associated with injury of frontal orbitobasal regions; the loss of executive control is a sequela of more widespread frontal damage.[3] Neuropsychological batteries that focus upon executive function can help to identify a frontal injury. When the injury occurs to basofrontal regions, however, neuropsychological test results may be normal, even when there is profound behavioral disinhibition.[7] In these patients, careful questioning and recording of the insights of the family, along with systematic observations by the physician, help delineate the presence and severity of the frontal syndrome.

Documentation of the severity of frontal dysfunction associated with head injury is important,

as therapy for these patients is difficult. A rigidly structured environment can help patients with frontal injury cope with routine daily activities. Unfortunately, current therapies and management of therapies for apathy and loss of executive control have only limited efficacy. Antidepressant medications may help to relieve the depressions that follow frontal injury; tegretol and propranolol have limited efficacy for disinhibition, violence, and irritability.

Tumors

Tumors either intrinsic or extrinsic to the frontal lobes can produce frontal lobe symptomatology.

The most common extrinsic tumors are meningiomas, which typically compress the frontal lobes in either the parasagittal (see Fig. 30-3) or the cribriform plate regions.[8] Parasagittal meningiomas affect the medial aspects of the frontal lobes, so that bilateral leg weakness is a common finding. Once these tumors become sufficiently large, apathy, loss of executive control, or disinhibition can occur. Loss of the sense of smell is a common finding because of the close association of midline frontal tumors to the olfactory nerves. Cribriform plate meningiomas affect the basofrontal lobes, and behavioral disinhibition is common.

Primary brain tumors (gliomas, oligodendrogliomas, etc.) and metastases that involve the frontal lobes also alter frontal function. In current practice, these lesions are easily detected with computed tomography (CT) or magnetic resonance imaging (MRI) and effective surgical and medical therapies can be administered. However, diagnosis is often preceded by vague behavioral alterations that, in retrospect, were caused by frontal dysfunction.

Hydrocephalus

Abnormal absorption of cerebrospinal fluid (CSF) via the arachnoid granulation can cause "normal-pressure hydrocephalus" (NPH). The classic triad of hydrocephalus includes memory disturbance, urinary incontinence, and gait apraxia. Other common findings are profound apathy and even akinetic states. Magnetic resonance imaging typically shows the panventricular dilatation (see Fig. 30-4) as well as extravasated periventricular fluid. Treatment of obstructive hydrocephalus (including NPH) is by shunting CSF from the ventricles to a distant area for absorption. Unfortunately, this therapy is effective in only a minority of cases, and complications of shunt therapy can be troublesome.

Figure 30-3

This T_1-weighted gadolinium-enhanced MRI scan demonstrates a large parasagittal frontal meningioma.

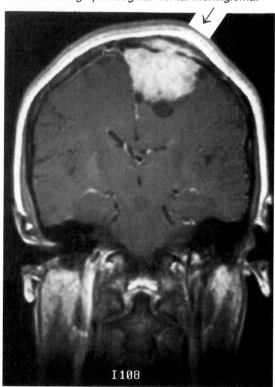

I108

Infections

Many infectious processes can involve frontal cerebral tissues. Bacterial, tuberculous, fungal, and toxoplasmal abscesses can selectively penetrate the frontal regions. Now rare, tertiary syphilis, or "general paresis of the insane" (GPI), showed a predilection to involve the frontal regions.[10] One of the clinical syndromes associated with GPI was characterized by disinhibition and grandiose manic syndromes. Another was characterized by disinterest and slowed cognitive processing. An apathetic frontal lobe syndrome is the most characteristic clinical feature of dementia due to human immunodeficiency virus (HIV). This is probably based on involvement of both subcortical and frontal structures.[11] Often, HIV-dementia responds at least transiently to antiviral therapy.

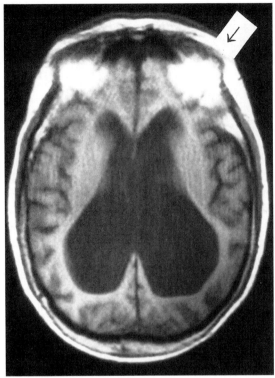

Figure 30-4
A T₁-weighted MRI scan demonstrating hydrocephalus with enlarged frontal and posterior ventricles. There is no periventricular extravasation of fluid.

Degenerative Dementias

Frontotemporal Dementia Although all degenerative brain disorders probably produce frontal dysfunction eventually, several entities show early and selective involvement of the frontal lobes. The frontotemporal dementias (FTDs) are a group of disorders that cause focal degeneration of prefrontal cortex. These are probably the second most common presenile degenerative dementias, ranking only behind Alzheimer disease. The disorders (there are probably several causes) have a mean age of onset in the sixth decade and are slowly progressive; the time from onset to death is typically 7 to 10 years.[12–14] Approximately 50 percent of subjects with FTD have a family history suggesting that FTD is transmitted as an autosomal

dominant trait. In some subjects, amyotrophic lateral sclerosis (ALS) occurs, either preceding or following signs of frontal dysfunction. A linkage with chromosome 17 has been demonstrated.[15] Misdiagnosis is common, but the clinical and imaging features of FTD clearly distinguish FTD from other degenerative dementias, and diagnostic accuracy should be over 90 percent. Initially some mixture of social withdrawal and behavioral disinhibition occurs; as the disease progresses, apathy becomes the dominant finding. Higher cortical deficits include decreased speech output and deficits in judgment, insight, and executive control functions. Antisocial conduct occurs in nearly half of all FTD subjects. Excessive eating and compulsions are common. In the later stages, parkinsonian features and eye-movement abnormalities occur, reflecting degeneration in the midbrain. Eventually profound apathy supervenes and most subjects enter a mute, akinetic state. Visuospatial skills and calculation remain normal or near normal, reflecting the relative sparing of parietal cortex with FTD. Focal presentations of FTD may occur; patients with predominantly left-sided degeneration show progressive aphasia or apraxia, while those with right-sided degeneration suffer profound alterations of social skills. In most FTD patients, MRI shows frontal and anterior temporal atrophy, but generalized atrophy or even normal MRIs may be seen. Functional studies (e.g., single photon emission tomography, or SPECT, and positron emission tomography, or PET) invariably show focal frontal or temporal deficits (see Fig. 30-5, Plate 6).

Histologic studies reveal neuronal loss and gliosis, greatest in the frontal and anterior temporal regions. In about 20 percent of FTD patients, cellular inclusions, so-called Pick bodies, are found. Midbrain cell loss is common, with more variable findings of gliosis in the thalamus and basal ganglia. Severe pre- and postsynaptic deficits in brain serotonin have been reported and may be correlated with the clinical findings of weight gain and compulsions.

Other Degenerative Dementias Most of the degenerative dementias eventually involve the

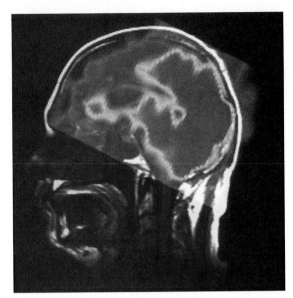

Figure 30-5
This is a xenon-133–corrected-HMPAO SPECT coregistered upon a T$_2$-weighted MRI scan from a patient with frontotemporal dementia. There is profound frontal hypoperfusion.

frontal lobes, even though primary pathology is elsewhere. A few disorders appear to have a selective influence upon frontal lobe function.

Progressive Supranuclear Palsy In this degenerative disorder the primary pathology is located in the midbrain. Extensive frontal connections with midbrain may explain the combination of midbrain and frontal lobe findings. Primary frontal degeneration has not, however, been ruled out. The classical clinical findings in progressive supranuclear palsy (PSP) include frequent falls, axial rigidity, pseudobulbar palsy, dementia, and a loss of vertical gaze. On SPECT, frontal hypoperfusion is seen.[16]

Metachromatic Leukodystrophy This degenerative disorder selectively injures white matter underlying the frontal cortex. A progressive frontal dementia occurs; diagnosis is made by demonstration of an enzymatic abnormality in arylsul-

fatase. Although most cases occur in childhood and early adolescence, late-life onset can occur.[17]

Alcohol Many toxins can affect cerebral cortex, but the symptom picture most often suggests diffuse (toxic) rather than focal abnormalities. The concept of alcohol-induced dementia remains somewhat controversial; in some individuals, chronic alcohol abuse appears to be associated with selective dysfunction of the frontal lobes (apathy and cognitive slowing). In some instances, the frontal symptoms disappear or are considerably improved following abstinence from alcohol; in other cases, permanent dementia seems to develop.[18] The pathology of this dementia is poorly understood, but the presence of frontal symptoms is consistent.

REFERENCES

1. Luria AR: *The Working Brain: An Introduction to Neuropsychology* (Haig B, trans). New York, Basic Books, 1973.
2. Albert ML: Subcortical dementia, in Katzman R, Terry RD, Bick KI (eds): *Alzheimer's Disease, Senile Dementia and Related Disorders.* New York, Raven Press, 1978, pp 173–180.
3. Stuss DT, Benson DF: *The Frontal Lobes.* New York, Raven Press, 1986.
4. Gauthier JC, Mohr JP: Intracranial internal carotid artery disease, in Barnett HJM, Mohr JP, Stein BM, Yatsu FM (eds): *Stroke.* New York, Churchill Livingstone, 1986, pp 337–350.
5. Benson DF: *Aphasia, Alexia, and Agraphia.* New York, Churchill Livingstone, 1979.
6. Tsai FY, Higashida RT, Matovich V, Alrieri K: Acute thrombosis of the intracranial dural sinus: Direct thrombolytic treatment. *Am J Neuroradiol* 13:1137–1141, 1992.
7. Damasio AR: The frontal lobes, in Heilman KM, Valenstein E (eds): *Clinical Neuropsychology.* New York, Oxford University Press, 1979, pp 360–412.
8. Adams RD, Victor M: *Principles of Neurology,* 5th ed. New York, McGraw-Hill, 1993.
9. Hakim S: Biomechanics of hydrocephalus, in Harbert JC (ed): *Cisternography and Hydrocephalus.* Springfield, IL, Charles C Thomas, 1972, pp 22–25.

10. Cummings JL, Benson DF: *Dementia: A Clinical Approach.* Boston, Butterworth-Heinemann, 1992.

11. Price RW, Brew B, Sidtis J, et al: The brain in AIDS: Central nervous system HIV-1 infection and AIDS dementia complex. *Science* 239:286–292, 1988.

12. Brun A: Frontal lobe degeneration of non-Alzheimer type: I. Neuropathology. *Arch Gerontol Geriatr* 6:193–208, 1987.

13. Neary D, Snowden JS, Northen B, Goulding PJ: Dementia of frontal lobe type. *J Neurol Neurosurg Psychiatry* 51:353–361, 1988.

14. Miller BL, Cummings JL, Villanueva-Meyer J, et al: Frontal lobe degeneration: Clinical, neuropsychological and SPECT characteristics. *Neurology* 41:1374–1382, 1991.

15. Wilhelmsen K, Lynch T, Pavlou E, et al: Localization of disinhibition-dementia-parkinsonism-amyotrophy complex to 17q21-22. *Am J Hum Genet* 55:1150–1165, 1994.

16. Johnson KA, Sperling RA, Holman BL, et al: Cerebral perfusion in progressive supranuclear palsy. *J Nucl Med* 33:704–709, 1992.

17. Austin J, Armstrong D, Fouch S, et al: Metachromatic leukodystrophy (MLD). *Arch Neurol* 18:225–240, 1968.

18. Lishman WA: Cerebral disorder in alcoholism: Syndromes of impairment. *Brain* 104:1–20, 1981.

Chapter 31

FRONTAL LOBES: COGNITIVE NEUROPSYCHOLOGICAL ASPECTS

Daniel Y. Kimberg
Mark D'Esposito
Martha J. Farah

As the previous chapter makes clear, prefrontal cortex plays a crucial role in normal intelligent behavior. However, a more precise characterization of the functions of prefrontal cortex has been elusive. In this chapter we provide a brief review of some of the cognitive impairments that often follow prefrontal damage and survey current theoretical claims about the role of the frontal lobes in cognition.

COGNITIVE IMPAIRMENTS FOLLOWING PREFRONTAL DAMAGE

A wide range of tasks have been found to be sensitive to prefrontal damage. Some of the best known are described here for the purpose of illustrating the range and variety of abilities that depend on prefrontal cortex.

Wisconsin Card Sorting Test

In the Wisconsin Card Sorting Test (WCST),[1] patients are given a series of cards and asked to sort them by placing each into one of four piles. The cards vary according to three attributes: the number of objects drawn on the card, the shape of the objects, and their color. The piles are to be started beneath four reference cards, which also vary along these same dimensions, so that each possible value of each attribute will be represented in exactly one pile. The subject is given a deck of cards and asked to place each, in sequence, into one of the four piles. The only feedback given to the subject is the word *right* or *wrong* after each card. Initially, color is the correct sorting category, and the subject is given positive feedback only if the card is placed in the pile of the same color. For example, if the card is red, the subject must place the card next to the reference card that has red objects. However, whenever the subject sorts 10 consecutive cards correctly, the category changes. Only sorts according to the new category will result in positive feedback. The category first changes to shape, then to number, and then repeats in the same order, starting from color. The subject must learn to change sorting categories according to feedback. The test ends after 128 cards or after 6 categories are achieved. Scoring of the test includes two measures: the number of perseverative errors, or failures to change sorting strategy after negative feedback, and the number of categories achieved.

Milner[2,3] tested a variety of neurosurgical patients on the WCST and found that as compared to patients with lesions elsewhere in the brain, patients with damage to the dorsolateral prefrontal cortex made an unusually high number of errors and achieved fewer categories. These differences can be attributed mainly to perseveration. While the dorsolateral prefrontal group committed nonperseverative errors at rates similar to those of the control groups, their rates of perseverative errors were significantly higher. Also striking is Milner's analysis comparing those patients with the smallest dorsolateral frontal lobe removals and those with the largest removals elsewhere (five with parietal-temporal removals and seven with orbitofrontal removals). Whereas the groups performed similarly preoperatively, the dorsolateral prefrontal group performed significantly worse postoperatively, due largely to an increase in perseverative errors. Thus, although patients with many different loci of damage may perform poorly at the WCST, damage to the dorsolateral prefrontal cortex seems closely tied to perseveration at this test. A number of other studies have confirmed the basic finding that the WCST is particularly sensitive to frontal damage[4,5] (but see Ref. 6).

Sequencing Tasks

The term *sequencing* can describe anything from concrete motor sequences, such as sequences of hand motions, to more abstract behavioral sequences, such as the morning routine of preparing to go to work. Of the sequencing errors made by frontal-damaged patients, many but not all are perseverative in nature.[7,8] A number of studies of simple manual and oral movement sequences have indicated that frontal lesions are most disruptive of these abilities.[9–11] Anecdotal reports suggest that the problem extends to the sequencing of more abstract kinds of actions. For example, Penfield and Evans[12] describe a patient who could perform all the individual actions necessary to prepare a meal but could not actually prepare the meal without someone to tell her the order in which to do things.

Tasks that require planning of a sequence in advance may also depend on the frontal areas. Shallice[13] tested frontal-damaged patients on the Tower of London test, a variant of the Tower of Hanoi game, designed specifically to require subjects to use advance planning. Left-frontal-damaged patients showed a disproportionate impairment at this task.

Verbal Fluency

Asked to produce words beginning with a particular letter, frontal-damaged patients (even those with no overt aphasic signs) will typically produce few unique responses, often repeating earlier responses. This frequently reported clinical finding has been supported by a variety of experimental studies.

An early study by Milner[3] demonstrated that patients with left frontal damage were impaired at a written test of verbal fluency when compared to a group with temporal lobe excisions. Benton[14] later confirmed the relative importance of the left frontal areas in the now more common oral version of the test. More recently, Janowsky and coworkers[15] compared verbal fluency in frontal-damaged patients with a variety of control groups and found that patients with left or bilateral frontal lesions but not right frontal lesions were impaired at verbal fluency.

Other fluency tasks have also been found to be sensitive to frontal pathology. Jones-Gotman and Milner[16] have found deficits in design fluency, a nonverbal analogue of the fluency task, in patients with right frontal removals. Similarly, Jason[9] found deficits in gesture fluency in frontal-damaged groups.

Neuroimaging studies have tended to confirm the importance of prefrontal areas in fluency tasks. Parks and coworkers[17] used positron emission tomography (PET) to compare the brain activity of subjects performing a verbal fluency task with controls in a resting state and found increases in activation bilaterally in both the frontal and temporal lobes. Frith and coworkers[18,19] performed PET studies of word finding, comparing the fluency condition to a lexical decision task. They found that "intrinsic" (subject-initiated) generation of a word was associated with increased activity in Brodmann area 46.

Context Memory

Although most frontal-damaged patients are not amnesic, they have nevertheless been found to have impairments on certain memory tasks. The most widely documented impairments involve memory for contextual information, either the source of a correctly recalled fact or its temporal context. Schacter[20] has applied the term *spatiotem-*

poral context to the type of memory that is impaired in frontal-damaged patients.

Janowsky and colleagues[15] investigated memory for recently learned facts and memory for the source of the facts in a group of frontal-damaged patients. Although the patients were normal in their ability to recall the facts, they frequently attributed the facts to incorrect sources. Shimamura and coworkers[21] found that frontal-damaged patients, while unimpaired at recall and recognition of words printed on cards, were impaired at placing the cards in their original sequence of presentation. They also tested the same patients on a similar test of famous events (from 1941 to 1985), also finding that frontal-damaged patients recognized the events but were impaired at judging the decade in which the events occurred.

Similarly, frontal-damaged patients have difficulty identifying which of two items has been presented more recently in a recognition task. Milner and coworkers[22,23] found that left-frontal-damaged patients were most impaired at making recency judgments with verbal materials, while right-frontal-damaged patients were most impaired with nonverbal materials.

Additional support for the role of the frontal lobes in memory for spatiotemporal context comes from studies in which patients with Korsakoff syndrome are compared to non-Korsakoff amnesics. Because Korsakoff syndrome is often accompanied by frontal atrophy, differences between patients with Korsakoff syndrome and those with other amnesias can be used to infer frontal contributions to memory. Disproportionately impaired context memory has been found in this group[24,25] (see Chap. 48).

Go–No-Go Tasks

In tasks designed to elicit false-alarm motor responses, frontal-damaged patients often seem unable to inhibit inappropriate responses. This widely reported clinical sign was confirmed by Drewe,[26] using a version of this test in which subjects were trained to hit a key in response to either of two lights (red and blue). They were then given a test in which they were asked to hit a key only

when they thought it would turn the light off. The key was effective only for the red light, so subjects were supposed to learn not to hit the key in response to the blue light. Drewe reported that frontal-damaged patients made more errors than nonfrontal damaged patient controls and in particular that they made more false-positive responses.

Self-Ordered Tasks

Given a series of cards with multiple stimuli and asked to point to a different item of their choosing on each card, epileptic patients with frontal excisions make more errors than other epileptic patients with temporal lobe excisions,[27] thus failing to monitor a series of self-generated choices. Lesions placed in the mid-dorsolateral prefrontal cortex of nonhuman primates will markedly impair their ability to recall which one of a set of objects they had previously chosen, a process that is critical for successful performance of the self-ordered task.[28] Furthermore, Petrides and colleagues have shown that performance at these self-ordered tasks in normal human subjects activates this same region of the mid-dorsolateral frontal cortex.[29]

Conditional Associative Learning

Frontal-damaged patients are impaired at learning and associating between a set of stimuli (e.g., colored lights) and a set of available responses (e.g., a set of abstract designs).[30,31] Lesions placed in the posterior dorsolateral prefrontal cortex of nonhuman primates (an area adjacent and posterior to the lesions causing impairments in self-ordered tasks) will markedly impair performance on conditional association learning tasks in which the monkey must perform different responses conditional upon the presence of a particular stimulus.[32] Furthermore, Petrides and colleagues have shown that performance of a conditional associative learning task in normal human subjects activates this same region of posterior dorsolateral frontal cortex.[29]

Stroop Task

In this task devised by Stroop,[33] subjects are presented with an array of color names printed in different-colored inks and asked either to name the ink colors or to read the words. Reaction time can be measured either for individual stimuli or for the reading of an entire array. There is a congruent condition, in which the word and the color always agree, and a conflict condition, in which the word and the color always disagree. In addition, control conditions in which the words are replaced with X's or color patches (color-naming control) or in which the words are printed in black ink (word-naming control) are usually used. The general finding is that when naming the color, a conflicting word creates a significant amount of interference, while a congruent word provides a smaller but still notable amount of facilitation.[34] When subjects are reading the word, a similar pattern exists in the reaction times, although the differences between conditions are much smaller.

Perret[35] reported the performance of several patient groups on the Stroop task and found that left-frontal-damaged patients had disproportionate difficulty in the conflict condition, when the dominant response to the word ordinarily causes interference with the color-naming task. Other researchers have replicated this finding.[36,37]

Delayed-Response Tasks

Evidence from infants, monkeys, and adult human subjects using a variety of methodologies has converged to indicate the importance of the prefrontal areas in performing delayed-response tasks (see Ref. 38 for a review). In a typical delayed-response task, the subject is shown some reward (e.g., food for monkeys or a toy for infants) that is placed in one of two locations. The two possible locations are both obscured during a delay period of several seconds, after which the subject is allowed to select one of the two locations (usually by reaching). Many variants of this basic paradigm have been found to depend on the prefrontal cortex.

Jacobsen[39] first established a connection between delayed-response performance and the prefrontal cortex, and the basic facts established in his studies have been well supported by subsequent findings. In his classic study, monkeys with bilateral prefrontal removals were found to be impaired at delayed-response tasks (as well as de-

layed-alternation tasks) but intact at simple visual discriminations. The result has since been confirmed and refined in a variety of studies.[40,41] Evidence from other methodologies has been consistent. Fuster[42] has provided evidence from a variety of methods, including single-unit recording[43,44] and cooling techniques,[45] which converge to implicate the prefrontal areas in the performance of delayed-response tasks.

Freedman and Oscar-Berman[46] found a delayed-response deficit in patients with bilateral frontal lobe lesions as compared to amnesic and alcoholic control groups. And Diamond and Goldman-Rakic[41] have argued that maturation of the prefrontal cortex in human infants underlies the development of competence at delayed-response tasks.

THEORIES OF FRONTAL LOBE FUNCTION

Unified versus Multicomponent Theories

Theories of frontal lobe function vary in the breadth of phenomena they are intended to explain. In some cases they are aimed at explaining performance in just one task, whereas in others they are intended to account for most or all of the cognitive changes that follow prefrontal damage. In this chapter we focus on theories intended to account for more than one isolated phenomenon.

Given the diversity of tasks affected by prefrontal damage, from the execution of simple manual sequences to the sorting of cards according to abstract categories, it might seem unlikely that prefrontal cortex has a single underlying cognitive function. In addition, performance deficits in the "frontal" tasks reviewed above are dissociable. Although most patients who are impaired at one task will also be impaired at some others, across-the-board impairment is rare. Prospects for a unified theory of frontal lobe function seem even slimmer when the known functional anatomy of the frontal lobes is considered. Prefrontal cortex alone includes the frontal eye fields, which are implicated in the control of voluntary eye movements, and Broca's area, which is implicated in language processes. Dorsolateral prefrontal damage is more closely associated with cognitive deficits, while orbitofrontal damage seems to be related to more obvious changes in personality. Consistent and reliable differences in function have been found even between different areas within the dorsolateral areas (e.g., Ref. 29). Finally, hemispheric asymmetries have been widely noted. The left frontal lobe is more strongly and more often implicated in tasks that involve verbal materials, while the right is most clearly implicated in some tasks involving nonverbal materials.[14,16,22,35,47]

Nevertheless, despite the diversity of cognitive changes following frontal damage, their dissociability, and the heterogeneity of the known functional neuroanatomy, unified theories of frontal lobe function are still being sought. What makes the unified theory so irresistible is the sense that many of the distinct and dissociable deficits described above have some underlying commonality. In the eloquent words of Hans-Lukas Teuber:[48] "I started out by trying to find a unitary concept, but as I moved along, it became clear that no single-factor hypothesis could carry one far enough to cover all the manifestations of frontal lesions. And yet the thing that is so tempting to me after this symposium is to think that there may be a family resemblance among symptoms, even among those which seem in part dissociable."

In some cases, the basis of the resemblance is clear. For instance, frontal-damaged patients seem to show perseveration at a variety of tasks, ranging from concrete motor tasks to the sorting of cards into abstract categories.[7,8] The impulsivity that characterizes these patients' failures on the "go–no-go" task is also at times shockingly apparent in their everyday behavior. Impulsivity could also possibly explain their increased susceptibility to interference on the Stroop test. The challenge for unified theories of frontal lobe function is to capture the intuitive commonalities among these signs of frontal damage in an explicit, mechanistic account of frontal lobe function.

Abstract Thinking

Goldstein[49,50] proposed that the frontal lobes were especially important for abstract thought and that the "abstract attitude" could not be adopted by patients with extensive frontal damage. Although it may well be true that many frontal-damaged patients think concretely, this hypothesis does not explain many of the central phenomena of frontal damage. Patients who fail the Wisconsin Card Sorting Test, for example, are often able to describe verbally the different abstract categories into which stimuli might be sorted, but they nevertheless perseverate in using the same categories even after negative feedback.[2] Walsh[51] reports this as well, noting one subject who, after perseverating in grouping several objects according to shape even when asked to form a new grouping, was shown a grouping by color. The subject described the grouping as "one of each shape in each group"—an extremely abstract description— while remaining unable to recognize the new scheme. While not every patient who perseverates on the card sort will produce this kind of behavior, this observation does show that impaired performance on this classic frontal task cannot be attributed to difficulty with abstract thinking. Furthermore, most of the tasks reviewed above do not seem particularly dependent on abstract thought (e.g., sequencing tasks, stroop, go–no-go, context memory).

Error Utilization

Luria[52,53] suggested that frontal patients are impaired in the utilization of errors to guide their behavior. Performance on the WCST is a perfect example of this. While a normal subject would take negative feedback as a cue to switch categories, frontal-damaged patients perseverate in their errors. Another example described by Luria is that frontal patients often fail to concentrate their study time on previously missed items in a memory task. However, most of the tasks reviewed above do not seem to tax error utilization in particular.

Planning

Many authors have attributed a planning function to the frontal lobes,[13,14,53] and Duncan[54] has framed this idea in terms of recent cognitive science models of problem solving. He proposes that human purposive activity requires a list of goals and a set of action structures resembling scripts. Goal-directed behavior is produced by a process similar to that of Newell and Simon's[55] means-end analysis. In effect, the goals inhibit those action structures that are not relevant to their achievement. The authors suggest that a defect in the use of the goal list to constrain behavior is responsible for the behavior of frontal-damaged patients. This account can explain failure on many but not all of the tasks reviewed earlier. For example, it does not explain context memory difficulties. Furthermore, if the notion of goal lists is extended to account for failures in such simple tasks as go–no-go or fluency, then it seems to predict failure at virtually any cognitive task, contrary to the evidence.

Inhibition

The theory that the frontal lobes serve an inhibitory function, suppressing dominant action tendencies in favor of more goal-appropriate behavior, has been proposed recently to account for a variety of data, including normal human development and physiologic experiments with monkeys. Diamond[56] has argued, from the development of reaching behaviors of infants and infant monkeys, that the prefrontal cortex serves such a function in inhibiting inappropriate reaches to formerly rewarded locations. She also suggests that this explanation may generalize to explain frontal deficits at the WCST as well as "capture" behavior, the intrusion of familiar but contextually inappropriate actions that have sometimes been noted after frontal damage. Similarly, Dempster[57] has proposed that inhibitory functions in the frontal cortex, in particular the suppression of irrelevant stimuli or associations, may account for a wide variety of patterns in both cognitive development and cognitive aging as well as data from frontal-damaged patients. And Roberts and coworkers[58] argue that frontal inhibitory processes (as well as working memory) underlie patterns of performance in normal and patient groups at antisaccade tasks. At some level, theories of inhibition are descriptively correct—when a subject produces an inappropriate response, it is true that the response should have been inhibited (at least implicitly). However, since a complex process must underlie the decision to inhibit a prepotent response, it is not clear why the locus of the impairment must be in an inhibitory component. Attributing apparent errors of disinhibition to a malfunctioning inhibitory mechanism raises the equally puzzling question of how the system knows when to inhibit and when to allow a prepotent response. And, as with the other theories so far reviewed, this one fails to explain a number of the phenomena associated with frontal damage in humans (e.g., context memory, self-ordered tasks).

Supervisory Attentional System

According to Shallice,[13,59,60] the frontal lobes instantiate a supervisory attentional system (SAS). Although this system is not needed for routine action, which is controlled by learned associations between stimuli in the environment and possible action, it serves to override these associations when stimuli or goals are novel. Thus, frontal-damaged patients, in whom the SAS is damaged, are no longer able to exert goal-directed control over their actions but simply respond to stimuli. This theory accords well with much of the observed behavior of frontal-damaged patients. For instance, it predicts that they should behave more normally in familiar situations than in unfamiliar ones. It also accords with the slow learning evidenced by many patients in the WCST, as their behavior seems very much like the slow learning of an associative module combined with the tendency of more familiar, routinized responses to emerge even when inappropriate (as in Stroop and go–no-go tasks). However, a number of the other tasks listed earlier do not seem particularly dependent on breaking out of routine action patterns (e.g., verbal fluency, context memory, and conditional associative responses). In addition, compared to the other theories, the SAS could be viewed as less parsimonious in that it represents a new component of the cognitive architecture over and above the components that carry out the tasks, whose sole function is to guide the use of those other components. Last, an impairment to a truly central executive would seem to imply that all frontal signs should always co-occur, which is certainly not the case.

Working Memory

"Working memory" is a form of short-term memory (see Chap. 36) that is often described when the writer wishes to emphasize that the information is being held on line for the purpose of performing computations on it (analogous to a mental scratch pad). Fuster[61,62] provided the first detailed account of the role of working memory in prefrontal processes. He describes the role of the prefrontal cortex as that of integrating temporally distributed information, a complex process which he attributed partly to short-term working memory. Contrasting this view with SAS-like executive accounts of prefrontal function, he writes: "The prefrontal cortex would not superimpose a steering or directing function on the remainder of the nervous system, but rather, by expanding the temporal perspectives of the system, it would allow it to integrate longer, newer, and more complex structures of behavior" (Ref. 62, page 172).

Goldman-Rakic[63] has also proposed a working-memory account of frontal lobe function on the basis of extensive research with nonhuman primates. Building on the well-established relationship between the prefrontal cortex and delayed-response tasks, she argues that the prefrontal cortex is responsible for maintaining information ("representational memory") that is later used to guide action. Funahashi and colleagues[44,64] have carried out a variety of lesion studies and single-unit recording studies to establish the role of prefrontal cortex in working memory, primarily with monkeys trained to perform spatial working-memory tasks. Neuroimaging studies in humans[65–68] suggest that similar working-memory processes are located prefrontally in the human brain. Goldman-Rakic[63] has suggested that the association between prefrontal cortex and working memory can in principle explain a range of human cognitive impairments following focal frontal lesions as well as other nonfocal patholo-

gies affecting prefrontal cortex (e.g., schizophrenia, Huntington disease, Parkinson disease).

The proposal that a working memory impairment could underlie the range of cognitive changes seen after prefrontal damage first found direct support in the work of Cohen and Servan-Schreiber.[69] They built a computational model of some of the cognitive and linguistic tasks that are characteristically failed by schizophrenic patients, including the Stroop task, lexical disambiguation, and the Continuous Performance Test. When the model's representation of context—held in working memory—is degraded, the model simulates the behavior of schizophrenic patients in these tasks.

Kimberg and Farah[70] selected four seemingly disparate tasks from those discussed in the previous section and modeled their performance computationally. When the strength of working memory associations was attenuated, the model perseverated on the WCST, made perseverative and nonperseverative sequencing errors on a simple motor sequencing task, showed source amnesia with relatively preserved recognition memory, and tended to read words rather than name colors in the Stroop task.

We favor working-memory accounts of prefrontal function for a number of reasons. First, they are parsimonious, in that working-memory theories contain only the individual processing components needed to perform the task without needing a central executive (such as the SAS) to coordinate these components (and to serve as the locus of damage when explaining patient behavior). Second, they have proven capable of explaining a wider range of seemingly disparate impairments than other nonexecutive theories.[69,70] Third, they are supported by a wealth of evidence from monkey neurophysiology[42,44,63,64] and, increasingly, from neuroimaging studies in humans.[65–68] Fourth, they suggest a way of resolving what is perhaps the central problem of the neuropsychology of frontal lobe function: the paradox of dissociable impairments with an untuitively compelling "family resemblance." If we assume that working memory is compartmentalized in prefrontal cortex according to what is being represented in memory (for which evidence exists—see

Refs. 66, 71, and 72), then performance in different tasks can be impaired or spared depending on which types of working memory have been damaged. Nevertheless, according to working-memory accounts, there is an underlying commonality among the tasks sensitive to prefrontal damage—namely, their dependence on working memory.

REFERENCES

1. Grant AD, Berg EA: A behavioral analysis of reinforcement and ease of shifting to new responses in a Weigl-type card sorting. *J Exp Psychol* 38:404–411, 1948.

2. Milner B: Effects of different brain lesions on card sorting. *Arch Neurol* 9:90–100, 1963.

3. Milner B: Some effects of frontal lobectomy in man, in Warren J, Akert K (eds): *The Frontal Granular Cortex and Behavior.* New York: McGraw-Hill, 1964.

4. Drewe EA: The effect of type and area of brain lesion on Wisconsin Card Sorting Test performance. *Cortex* 10:159–170, 1974.

5. Nelson HE: A modified card sorting test sensitive to frontal lobe defects. *Cortex* 12:313–324, 1976.

6. Anderson SW, Damasio H, Jones RD, Tranel D: Wisconsin card sorting test performance as a measure of frontal lobe damage. *J Clin Exp Neuropsychol* 13:909–922, 1991.

7. Luria AR: Two kinds of motor perseveration in massive injury of the frontal lobes. *Brain* 88:1–10, 1965.

8. Sandson J, Albert M: Varieties of perseveration. *Neuropsychologia* 22:715–732, 1984.

9. Jason GW: Manual sequences learning after focal cortical lesions. *Neuropsychologia* 23:483–496, 1985.

10. Kimura D: Left-hemisphere control of oral and brachial movements and their relation to communication. *Philos Trans R Soc Lond B* 298:135–149, 1982.

11. Kolb B, Milner B: Performance of complex arm and facial movements after focal brain lesions. *Neuropsychologia* 19:491–503, 1981.

12. Penfield W, Evans J: The frontal lobe in man: A clinical study of maximum removals. *Brain* 58:115–133, 1935.

13. Shallice T: Specific impairments of planning. *Philos Trans R Soc Lond B* 298:199–209, 1982.

14. Benton AL: Differential behavioral effects of frontal lobe disease. *Neuropsychologia* 6:53–60, 1968.

15. Janowsky JS, Shimamura AP, Squire LR: Source memory impairment in patients with frontal lobe lesions. *Neuropsychologia* 27:1043–1056, 1989.

16. Jones-Gotman M, Milner B: Design fluency: The invention of nonsense drawings after focal cortical lesions. *Neuropsychologia* 15:653–674, 1977.

17. Parks RW, Loewenstein DA, Dodrill KL, et al: Cerebral metabolic effects of a verbal fluency test: A PET scan study. *J Clin Exp Neuropsychol* 10:565–575, 1988.

18. Frith CD, Friston KJ, Liddle PF, et al: A PET study of word finding. *Neuropsychologia* 29:1137–1148, 1991.

19. Friston KJ, Frith CD, Liddle PF, et al: Investigating a network model of word generation with positron emission tomography. *Proc R Soc Lond B Biol Sci* 244:101–106, 1991.

20. Schacter DL: Memory, amnesia, and frontal lobe dysfunction. *Psychobiology* 15:21–36, 1987.

21. Shimamura AP, Janowsky JS, Squire LR: Memory for the temporal order of events in patients with frontal lobe lesions and amnesic patients. *Neuropsychologia* 28:803–813, 1990.

22. Milner B, Corsi P, Leonard G: Frontal-lobe contribution to recency judgements. *Neuropsychologia* 29:601–618, 1991.

23. McAndrews MP, Milner B: The frontal cortex and memory for temporal order. *Neuropsychologia* 29:849–859, 1991.

24. Schacter DL, Harbluk JL, McLachlan DR: Retrieval without recollection: An experimental analysis of source amnesia. *J Verb Learn Verb Behav* 23:593–611, 1984.

25. Squire LR: Comparisons between forms of amnesia: Some deficits are unique to Korsakoff's syndrome. *J Exp Psychol Learning, Memory, Cognition* 8:560–571, 1982.

26. Drewe EA: Go–no-go learning after frontal lobe lesions in humans. *Cortex* 11:8–16, 1975.

27. Petrides M, Milner B: Deficits on subject-ordered tasks after frontal- and temporal-lobe lesions in man. *Neuropsychologia* 20:249–262, 1982.

28. Petrides M: Monitoring of selections of visual stimuli and the primate frontal cortex. *Proc R Soc Lond B Biol Sci* 246:293–298, 1991.

29. Petrides M, Alivisatos B, Evans AC, Meyer E: Dissociation of human mid-dorsolateral from posterior dorsolateral frontal cortex in memory processing. *Proc Natl Acad Sci USA* 90:873–877, 1993.

30. Petrides M: Deficits on conditional associative learning tasks after frontal- and temporal-lobe lesions in man. *Neuropsychologia* 23:601–614, 1985.

31. Petrides M: Nonspatial conditional learning impaired in patients with unilateral frontal but not unilateral temporal-lobe excisions. *Neuropsychologia* 28:137–149, 1990.

32. Petrides M: Deficits in non-spatial conditional associative learning after periarcuate lesions in the monkey. *Behav Brain Res* 16:95–101, 1985.

33. Stroop JR: Studies of interference in serial verbal reactions. *J Exp Psychol* 18:643–662, 1935.

34. MacLeod CM: Half a century of research on the Stroop effect: An integrative review. *Psychol Bull* 109:163–203, 1991.

35. Perret E: The left frontal lobe of man and the suppression of habitual responses in verbal categorical behavior. *Neuropsychologia* 12:323–330, 1974.

36. Regard M: Cognitive Rigidity and Flexibility: A Neuropsychological Study. Unpublished doctoral dissertation: University of Victoria, British Columbia.

37. Stuss DT, Benson DF: Neuropsychological studies of the frontal lobes. *Psychol Bull* 95:3–28, 1984.

38. Oscar-Berman M, McNamara P, Freedman M: Delayed-response tasks: Parallels between experimental ablation studies and findings in patients with frontal lesions, in Levin HS (ed): *Frontal Lobe Function and Dysfunction.* New York: Oxford University Press, 1991, pp 230–255.

39. Jacobsen CF: Studies of cerebral functions in primates: I. The function of the frontal association areas in monkeys. *Comp Psychol Monogr* 13:1–60, 1936.

40. Goldman PS, Rosvold HE: Localization of function within the dorsolateral prefrontal cortex of the rhesus monkey. *Exp Neurol* 27:291–304, 1970.

41. Diamond A, Goldman-Rakic PS: Comparison of human infants and rhesus monkeys on Piaget's AB task: Evidence for dependence on dorsolateral prefrontal cortex. *Exp Brain Res* 74:24–40, 1989.

42. Fuster JM: *The Frontal Lobes.* New York: Raven Press, 1989.

43. Fuster JM, Alexander GE: Neuron activity related to short-term memory. *Science* 173:652–654, 1971.

44. Funahashi S, Bruce CJ, Goldman-Rakic PS: Mnemonic coding of visual space in the monkey's dorsolateral prefrontal cortex. *J Neurophysiol* 61:331–349, 1989.

45. Bauer RH, Fuster JM: Delayed-matching and delayed-response deficit from cooling dorsolateral prefrontal cortex in monkeys. *J Comp Physiol Psychol* 90:293–302, 1976.

46. Freedman M, Oscar-Berman M: Bilateral frontal lobe disease and selective delayed response deficits in humans. *Behav Neurosci* 100:337–342, 1986.

47. Petrides M, Alivisatos B, Meyer E, Evans AC: Functional activation of the human frontal cortex during the performance of verbal working memory tasks. *Proc Natl Acad Sci USA* 90:878–882, 1993.

48. Teuber H-L: The riddle of frontal lobe function in man, in Warren JM, Akert K (eds): *The Frontal Granular Cortex and Behavior.* New York: McGraw-Hill, 1964.

49. Goldstein K: Mental changes due to frontal lobe damage. *J Psychol* 17:187–208, 1944.

50. Goldstein K, Scheerer M: Abstract and concrete behavior: An experimental study with special tests. *Psychol Monogr* 43:1–151, 1941.

51. Walsh KW: *Neuropsychology: A Clinical Approach.* New York: Churchill Livingstone, 1987.

52. Luria AR: *Higher Cortical Functions in Man.* London: Tavistock, 1966.

53. Luria AR, Homskaya ED: Disturbance in the regulative role of speech with frontal lobe lesions, in Warren JM, Akert K (eds): *The Frontal Granular Cortex and Behavior.* New York: McGraw-Hill, 1964, pp 353–371.

54. Duncan J: Disorganisation of behaviour after frontal lobe damage. *Cog Neuropsychol* 3:271–290, 1986.

55. Newell A, Simon HA: *Human Problem Solving.* Englewood Cliffs, NJ: Prentice Hall, 1972.

56. Diamond A: Developmental progression in human infants and infant monkeys, and the neural bases of inhibitory control of reaching, in Diamond A (ed): *The Development and Neural Bases of Higher Cognitive Functions.* New York: NY Academy of Science Press, 1989.

57. Dempster FN: The rise and fall of the inhibitory mechanism: Toward a unified theory of cognitive development and aging. *Dev Rev* 12:45–75, 1992.

58. Roberts RJ, Hager LD, Heron C: Prefrontal cognitive processes: Working memory and inhibition in the antisaccade task. *J Exp Psychol Gen* 123:374–393, 1994.

59. Shallice T: *From Neuropsychology to Mental Structure.* Cambridge, England: Cambridge University Press, 1988.

60. Shallice T, Burgess P: Higher-order cognitive impairments and frontal lobe lesions in man, in Levin HS, Eisenberg HM, Benton AL (eds): *Frontal Lobe*

Function and Dysfunction. New York: Oxford University Press, 1991.

61. Fuster JM: *The Prefrontal Cortex: Anatomy, Physiology, and Neuropsychology of the Frontal Lobe.* New York: Raven Press, 1980.

62. Fuster JM: The prefrontal cortex and temporal integration, in Jones EG, Peters A (eds): *Cerebral Cortex:* Vol 4. *Association and Auditory Cortices.* New York: Raven Press.

63. Goldman-Rakic PS: Circuitry of primate prefrontal cortex and regulation of behavior by representational memory, in Plum F, Mountcastle V (eds): *Handbook of Physiology, The Nervous System: V.* Bethesda, MD: American Physiological Society, 1987.

64. Funahashi S, Bruce CJ, Goldman-Rakic PS: Dorsolateral prefrontal lesions and oculomotor delayed-response performance: Evidence for mnemonic "scotomas." *J Neurosci* 13:1479–1497, 1993.

65. Cohen J, Forman S, Braver T, et al: Activation of prefrontal cortex in a nonspatial working memory task with functional MRI. *Hum Brain Mapping* 1:293–304, 1994.

66. D'Esposito M, Shin RK, Detre JA, et al: Object and spatial working memory activates dorsolateral prefrontal cortex: A functional MRI study. *Soc Neurosci Abstr* 21:1498, 1995.

67. D'Esposito M, Detre J, Alsop D, et al: The neural basis of the central executive system of working memory. *Nature* 378:279–281, 1995.

68. Jonides J, Smith E, Koeppe R, et al: Spatial working memory in humans as revealed by PET. *Nature* 363:623–625, 1993.

69. Cohen JD, Servan-Schreiber D: Context, cortex, and dopamine: A connectionist approach to behavior and biology in schizophrenia. *Psychol Rev* 99:45–77, 1992.

70. Kimberg DY, Farah MJ: A unified account of cognitive impairments following frontal lobe damage: The role of working memory in complex, organized behavior. *J Exp Psychol Gen* 122:411–428, 1993.

71. Smith E, Jonides J, Koeppe RA, et al: *J Cog Neurosci* 7:337–356, 1995.

72. Wilson F, Scalaidhe S, Goldman-Rakic P: Dissociation of object and spatial processing domains in prefrontal cortex. *Science* 260:1876, 1993.

Chapter 32

CALLOSAL DISCONNECTION

Kathleen Baynes
Michael S. Gazzaniga

BRIEF HISTORICAL BACKGROUND

Demonstration of Hemispheric Independence Requires Appropriate Techniques

Patients who have undergone cortical disconnection have been primary to the evolution of our understanding of localized brain function. The hypothesis that disconnection of neural transmission between the centers of comprehension and language production would cause problems with repetition was central to Wernicke's prediction that conduction aphasia should exist. Callosal disconnection from naturally occurring lesions plays a role in the explanation of a number of syndromes including limb apraxia (Chap. 16), pure alexia (Chap. 13), and unilateral agraphia (Chap. 14). However, the most systematic investigation of hemispheric specialization and hemispheric integration in cases of callosal disconnection has been carried out with patients who have undergone callosotomy for control of intractible epilepsy. These so-called split-brain patients are the focus of this chapter.

In his early work with split-brain patients, Akelaitis failed to discover cognitive sequelae of the surgery using standard neuropsychological procedures.[1,2] It was the Bogen group that recognized the importance of providing a nonverbal means of response to demonstrate the presence of two independent cognitive systems within the same subject.[3,4] The presentation of stimuli to one hemifield using brief (tachistoscopic) displays and

the use of manual responses (Fig. 32-1) opened the way to exploration of each hemisphere's unique properties. Initial studies confirmed neurologists' assertions that the left hemisphere was dominant for language whereas the right could neither name nor describe objects presented to it visually or tactually, although it could perform certain visuospatial tasks. Current techniques permit visual displays with extended durations, thus allowing more precise observations. Further-refined experiments continue to develop our understanding of perceptual, cognitive, mnemonic, and linguistic processes and their integration into coherent thought and behavior. Such techniques continue to provide a unique means of testing hemispheric hypotheses and enriching our understanding of neurological and neuropsychological symptoms, from alexia to alien hand sign.

LANGUAGE

Variability of Right Hemispheric Language Representation

Perhaps the most striking observation regarding split-brain subjects is the presence of complex, generative language in only one hemisphere. Nonetheless, the series of patients operated on by Bogen demonstrated a well-developed right hemispheric lexicon in the majority of patients examined, although that lexicon appeared to be limited to simple auditory and visual comprehension and some written output.[4-6] The Wilson-Roberts se-

419

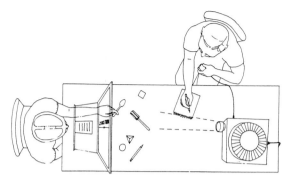

Figure 32-1

Visual information can be presented to one hemisphere at a time in split-brain patients by flashing the stimulus to one side or the other of a fixation point, for less time than is required to make an eye movement from the fixation point to the stimulus. Responses made with one hand favor the contralateral hemisphere, although some ipsilateral control is possible. (From Gazzaniga,[7] with permission.)

ries, however, demonstrated much less frequent right hemispheric participation in even rudimentary language processing. By 1983, of the 28 completed callosotomies, only 3 patients had a documented right hemispheric lexicon.[7] Moreover, there was considerable variation in the quality and sophistication of the language available to the right hemisphere.[8]

In those patients with right hemispheric language capability, semantic and conceptual information appear to be more adequately represented in the right hemisphere than is phonologic and syntactic information. The visual and auditory lexicons of the right hemisphere (RH) appear to be similar to, albeit somewhat smaller than, the corresponding left hemispheric lexicons.[9] Both hemispheres can make a variety of semantic judgments, recognizing categorical, functional, and associative relations.[9] The ability to discriminate word from nonword letter strings is limited but possible,[10–12] which suggests that the visual word form is represented in the RH of these patients.

Limited Control of Speech and Grammar in the Isolated Right Hemisphere

Phonologic information is difficult for the RH to manipulate, although it may possess limited pho-

nologic competence and be able to produce speech. Sidtis[8] assessed discrimination of phonemes (such as "ba" versus "pa") in two callosotomy patients. The RH of one patient was able to discriminate but not identify phoneme contrasts and was also able to identify rhyming words. Not surprisingly, this patient was able to produce some verbal responses to left visual field (LVF) stimuli within a year of her completed surgery.[9] The other patient had more difficulty with the discrimination task and refused to respond to the identification task. His right hemisphere was also unable to identify rhyming words.[8] This patient's RH remained mute until more than 10 years after his surgery; he has now gained rudimentary control of speech within the RH.[13,14] Although he remained unable to make accurate judgments that require moving from letter to sound,[13] he was able to integrate visual and auditory phonologic information within his RH.[15] This remarkable development has implications for the limits of functional plasticity and for the role of the RH in long-term recovery from aphasia (Chap 11).

The linguistic prowess of the RH does not appear to extend to the use of grammatical rules for comprehension or the production of sentences. The ability to use grammatical information to guide comprehension is limited,[9,16] although the RH can distinguish between grammatical and ungrammatical sentences,[16] possibly on the basis of prosodic cues. In a left-handed patient with right hemispheric language dominance, comprehension of grammatical relations appears to be possible only for the RH.[17] Even when the RH is able to make a verbal response to a LVF word or picture, it appears to lose control of speech output rapidly as the LH takes over and expands in a confabulatory fashion on the RH's utterance,[14] perhaps because it lacks the ability to generate more complex, sentence-length responses.

Right Hemispheric Reading

Right hemispheric reading proceeds more slowly than left hemispheric reading and may use a different mode of processing,[12] as has been reported for some deep dyslexic patients. Likewise, a right hemispheric lexicon with more diffuse or associative organization than that of the left hemisphere has been suggested as the source of certain reading errors in deep dyslexic[18,19] and pure alexic patients[20] (Chap. 13). Although insensitivity to grammar and poor print-to-sound skills in the RH of these patients is consistent with some aspects of those claims, both hemispheres appear to be capable of generating the range of error types found in deep dyslexia.[13] The language profile seen in callosotomy patients is more consistent with the profile reported by Coslett and Saffran for the preserved reading of their pure alexic patient than with that reported for deep dyslexic patients.

MEMORY

Recall and Recognition Memory Following Callosotomy

Changes in mnemonic capacity after callosotomy may reflect discrete processing capacities in the isolated hemispheres. Loss of general memory capacity as measured by standardized tests has been reported for some patients,[21,22] while Clark and Geffen[23] suggested that discrepancies in memory function reported after callosotomy might be due to involvement of the hippocampal commissure. Phelps and coworkers[24] have observed a decrement in both visual and verbal recall following posterior callosal section, which may damage the hippocampal commissure, but preserved or even improved memory after anterior callosal section, which does not. Recognition memory was relatively intact in both groups. Kroll and colleagues[24a,b] reported that complete callosotomy interferes with the binding of visual and verbal material yielding error patterns similar to those of hippocampally lesioned patients.

There appear to be hemisphere-specific changes in the accuracy of memory processes that may be useful in understanding the behavior of some neurologically impaired patients. The left hemisphere (LH) appears to make greater use of general knowledge schemas to explain perceptions and experiences and to use them to "interpret" events[25] than does the RH, and this predilection has an impact on the accuracy of memory.[26] When subjects were presented with a series of pictures that represented common events (i.e., getting up in the morning or making cookies) and were then asked, several hours later, to identify whether pictures in another series had appeared in the first, both hemispheres were equally accurate in recognizing the previously viewed pictures and rejecting unrelated ones. Only the RH, however, correctly rejected pictures in the second set that were not previously viewed but were semantically congruent with pictures from the first set. The LH incorrectly "recalled" significantly more of these pictures as having occurred in the first set, presumably because they fit into the schema it had constructed regarding the event. This finding is consistent with the view of a LH "interpreter" that constructs theories to assimilate perceived information into a comprehensible whole. In doing so, however, the elaborative processing involved has a deleterious effect on the accuracy of perceptual recognition. This result has been confirmed by Metcalfe and coworkers[27] and extended to include verbal material.

HEMISPHERIC DOMINANCE

The Left Hemisphere as Interpreter

The LH is considered to be the "dominant" hemisphere in most right-handed people. The term *dominant* is usually taken to mean language-dominant, but Gazzaniga[28] has suggested that the LH is not only superior in terms of language function but also in the ability to make simple inferences and to interpret its own behavior and emotions.[29] It is unclear whether these functions are dependent upon the development of generative language skills or if the two arise independently. Nonetheless, such observations strongly suggest that the LH is not only more able than the right to express itself verbally but that it plays a dominant role in interpreting behavior and providing a rationale for events in the world.

These observations can also yield insight regarding the confabulatory behavior seen in some amnesic patients who are unable to encode new information. Finding themselves in situations for which they cannot remember the antecedents, they may be compelled to explain them in the same way that the LH explains behavior motivated by the RH.

Visuospatial Functions

There are other areas that demonstrate differential hemispheric contributions. The expected right hemispheric superiority in visuospatial function has been demonstrated in callosotomy patients.[3,30] In contrast, superior use of visual imagery has been demonstrated in the LH, using a letter-based task.[31] The use of tactile information to build spatial representations of abstract shapes also appears to be better developed in the RH.[30] Tasks such as Block Design from the Wechsler Adult Intelligence Scale (WAIS), however, which are typically associated with the right parietal lobe, appear to require integration between the hemispheres in some patients.[32] Furthermore, while the RH is better able to analyze unfamiliar facial information than the LH[33,34] and the left is better able to generate voluntary expressions,[35] both hemispheres share in the management of facial expression when spontaneous emotions are expressed.

Although the RH demonstrates superior levels of performance on a variety of perceptual and spatial tasks, the LH appears to have at least some competence in most areas and in some cases is essential for the solution of complex visual problems. The LH is superior at all language tasks and in a variety of tasks that require inferences. Moreover, verbal IQ appears to be stable following callosotomy, although performance IQ may decline.[22] Gazzaniga[36] suggests that the LH is also dominant for intelligent behavior, although that conclusion assumes a contemporary concept of intelligence that rests heavily on verbal abilities.

INTERHEMISPHERIC INTEGRATION OF PERCEPTION AND ATTENTION

Hemispheric Isolation of Visual and Tactile Information

When appropriate lateralization procedures are followed (see Fig. 32-1), visual and tactile perception are isolated in each hemisphere. Although, subjects can independently report visual material that has been isolated to one hemisphere or the other, they cannot make comparisons between the two hemifields. Performance is at or near chance levels in simple same/different comparisons when items are presented in different visual fields.[13,37,38] Despite reports of integration of higher-order information following callosotomy,[39,40] such results have not always been replicated or have proved explicable through the patient's strategic maneuvers.[37,41,42] At present, it appears that if visual or tactile information is presented so that it is initially perceived by only one hemisphere, the perception remains isolated within that hemisphere.

The animal literature, however, has documented that information from areas close to the visual midline is shared by both hemispheres.[43,44] It appears that this observation is also true for the human species in an area no more than 2° from the vertical meridian.[45] Although represented, the visual information in this area has little utility, as neither detailed shape comparisons nor brief displays could be reliably compared across the meridian.[46]

Sharing of Attentional Control

Although both higher cognitive function and basic perceptual information appear to be isolated within each hemisphere, there is some evidence for sharing of control of visual attention. The hemispheres appear to share control of the "attentional spotlight" via their subcortical connections. That is, if attention is directed to a particular position in the visual field by a cue in one field, that information can be used by both hemispheres.[38,47] Nonetheless, explicit interfield comparisons of spatial location cannot be made accurately,[38] nor can attention be simultaneously directed to different points in each visual field.[48]

It also appears that attentional resources are limited despite the "splitting" of consciousness. Holtzman demonstrated that increasing processing demands in one hemisphere had a deleterious effect on performance in the other hemisphere.[49] Nonetheless, in comparison with normal subjects, there was less decrement in a dual-task condition for callosotomized subjects.[50] Thus, although the two hemispheres may compete for cognitive resources, there is evidence for independence of function. This latter finding is consistent with the observation of Luck and coworkers[51] that visual search is independently mediated by both hemispheres. Using a standard spatial cueing paradigm that incorporated a bilateral cue to assess the influence of information presented to one hemisphere on the performance of the other, Mangun and colleagues[52] demonstrated differential processing of spatial cues, with only the LVF (right-hand) trials yielding an advantage for validly cued trials. Although the failure to find a right visual field (RVF) advantage for valid trials is at odds with the other split-brain results,[47,53] it is consistent with a view of the RH as dominant in terms of spatial attention (Chap. 24).

SPECIFICITY OF CALLOSAL FIBERS

Observations regarding functional specificity come from two sources in human studies. First, sections are completed in two stages, usually anterior first, allowing for observation of functional differences. Second, development of improved imaging techniques such as magnetic resonance imaging (MRI) has allowed for verification and definition of the fibers resected during callosotomy.

It has long been noted that separating up to two-thirds of the anterior callosum leads to little if any change in ability.[54] If the anterior split continues far enough, disruption of the ability to transfer sensory and position information from hand to hand will be observed. In contrast, the section of the splenium disrupts the transfer of visual information between the hemispheres, which isolates lateralized visual input. After posterior section, although explicit identification and naming of LVF stimuli is not possible, some transfer of higher-order information may occur.[55]

In cases with inadvertent surgical sparing, very specific transfer of information has been found. Patient V.P. has sparing of fibers in the rostrum and splenium of the callosum. Although she cannot make explicit visual comparisons between fields, she was able to integrate visual and auditory information to make accurate between-field rhyme judgments when words both looked and sounded alike (i.e., between *boat* and *goat,* but not between *boat* and *note*).[56] Occasionally, strokes yield partial callosal lesions as well; one such patient with damage to the body of the corpus callosum demonstrates left-hand tactile anomia and agraphia[57] showing the importance of the fibers of the body of the callosum for the transfer of language information between the hemispheres.

CONCLUSIONS

Although the behaving being is remarkably intact following callosotomy, investigation reveals hemispheric capacities that refine and confirm hypotheses based on normal subjects and patients with focal lesions. The isolated RH usually cannot read, write, or speak, despite displaying a variety of conscious behaviors. Dissociations like left-handed tactile anomia or agraphia may be an indication of less language-competent right hemispheres. However, the ability to comprehend auditory and visual language may be present and can contribute to the presentation of aphasic and alexic patients. Recent observations indicate that the RH may participate in long-term recovery from aphasia. Perhaps of greater interest, however, is the study of callosotomy patients to investigate the hemispheric bases of cognition and the integration of diverse perceptual, sensory, and emotional information into a single behavioral plan. This population was the first in which independent function of the hemispheres was demonstrated as a result of which the important role played by the verbal left hemisphere in allowing the organism to observe and interpret its own actions and emotional states was recognized. Insights regarding the components of perception, memory, attention, and language continue to arise from this population and to inform models of normal perceptual and cognitive processing.

ACKNOWLEDGMENTS

Supported in part by NIH/NIDCD grant number R29 DC00811 to KB and NIH/NINDS grant number P01 NS17778 to MSG and the McDonnell-Pew Foundation.

REFERENCES

1. Akelaitis AJ: Studies on the corpus callosum: Higher visual functions in each homonymous field following complete section of corpus callosum. *Arch Neurol Psychiatry* 45:788–796, 1941.

2. Akelaitis AJ: A study of gnosis, praxis, and language following section of the corpus callosum and anterior commissure. *J Neurosurg* 7:94–102, 1944.

3. Bogen JE, Gazzaniga MS: Cerebral commissurotomy in man: Minor hemisphere dominance for certain visuospatial functions. *J Neurosurg* 23:394–399, 1965.

4. Sperry RW, Gazzaniga MS, Bogen JE: Interhemispheric relationships: The neocortical commissures: Syndromes of hemisphere disconnection, in Vinken PJ, Bruyn GW (eds): *Handbook of Clinical Neurology.* New York: Wiley, 1969, vol 4, pp 273–290.

5. Gazzaniga MS, Bogen JE, Sperry RW: Some functional effects of sectioning the cerebral commissures in man. *Proc Natl Acad Sci USA* 48:1765–1769, 1962.

6. Levy J, Nebes RB, Sperry RW: Expressive language in the surgically separated minor hemisphere. *Cortex* 7:49–58, 1971.

7. Gazzaniga MS: Right hemisphere language following brain bisection: A twenty year perspective. *Am Psychol* 38:525–549, 1983.

8. Sidtis JJ, Volpe BT, Wilson DH, et al: Variability in right hemisphere language function after callosal section: Evidence for a continuum of generative capacity. *J Neurosci* 1:323–331, 1981.

9. Gazzaniga MS, Smylie CS, Baynes K, et al: Profiles of right hemisphere language and speech following brain bisection. *Brain Lang* 22:206–220, 1984.

10. Eviatar Z, Zaidel E: The effects of word length and emotionality on hemispheric contribution to lexical decision. *Neuropsychologia* 29:415–428, 1991.

11. Baynes K, Tramo MJ, Gazzaniga MS: Reading with a limited lexicon in the right hemisphere of a callosotomy patient. *Neuropsychologia* 30:187–200, 1992.

12. Reuter-Lorenz PA, Baynes K: Modes of lexical access in the callosotomized brain. *J Cogn Neurosci* 4:155–164, 1992.

13. Baynes K, Wessinger CM, Fendrich R, Gazzaniga MS: The emergence of the capacity to name left visual field stimuli in a callosotomy patient: implica-

14. Gazzaniga MS, Nisenson L, Eliassen JC, et al: Collaboration between the hemispheres of a callosotomy patient: Emerging right hemisphere speech and the left hemisphere interpreter. Submitted.

15. Baynes K, Funnell MG, Fowler CA: Hemispheric contributions to the integration of visual and auditory information in speech perception. *Percept Psychophys* 55:633–641, 1994.

16. Baynes K, Gazzaniga MS: Right hemisphere language: Insights into normal language mechanisms? in Plum F (ed): *Language, Communication, and the Brain.* New York: Raven Press, 1987, pp 117–126.

17. Lutsep HL, Wessinger CM, Gazzaniga MS: Cerebral and callosal organisation in a right hemisphere dominant "split-brain" subject. *J Neurol Neurosurg Psychiatry* 59:50–54, 1995.

18. Schweiger A, Zaidel E, Dobkin B: Right hemisphere contribution to lexical access in an aphasic with deep dyslexia. *Brain Lang* 37:73–89, 1989.

19. Coltheart M: Deep dyslexia: A right hemisphere hypothesis, in Coltheart M, Patterson KE, Marshall JC (eds): *Deep Dyslexia.* London: Routledge, 1980.

20. Coslett HB, Saffran EM: Evidence for preserved reading in "pure alexia." *Brain* 112:327–359, 1989.

21. Zaidel D, Sperry RW: Memory impairment after commissurotomy in man. *Brain* 97:263–272, 1974.

22. Zaidel E: Language functions in the two hemispheres following complete cerebral commissurotomy and hemispherectomy, in Boller F, Grafman G (eds): *Handbook of Neuropsychology.* New York: Elsevier, 1990, vol 4, pp 115–150.

23. Clark CR, Geffen GM: Corpus callosum surgery and recent memory. *Brain* 112:165–175, 1989.

24. Phelps EA, Hirst W, Gazzaniga MS: Deficits in recall following partial and complete commissurotomy. *Cereb Cortex* 1:492–498, 1991.

24a. Kroll NEA, Knight RT, Metcalfe J, et al: Cohesion failure as a source of memory illusions. *Memory and Language.* In press.

24b. Jha AP, Kroll NEA, Baynes K, Gazzaniga MS: Memory encoding following complete callosotomy. *J Cogn Neurosci.* In press.

25. Gazzaniga MS: *The Social Brain.* New York: Basic Books, 1985.

26. Phelps EA, Gazzaniga MS: Hemispheric differences in mnemonic processing: The effects of left hemisphere interpretation. *Neuropsychologia* 30:293–297, 1992.

27. Metcalfe J, Funnell M, Gazzaniga MS: Right hemi-

sphere memory superiority: Studies of a split-brain patient. *Psychol Sci* 6:157–164, 1995.

28. Gazzaniga MS: *Consciousness and the Cerebral Hemispheres. The Cognitive Neurosciences.* Cambridge, MA: MIT Press, 1995, pp 1391–1400.

29. Gazzaniga MS, Smylie CS: Dissociation of language and cognition. *Brain* 107:145–153, 1984.

30. Milner B, Taylor L: Right hemisphere superiority in tactile pattern recognition after cerebral commissurotomy: Evidence for non-verbal memory. *Neuropsychologia* 10:1–15, 1972.

31. Farah MJ, Gazzaniga MS, Holtzman JD, Kosslyn SM: A left hemisphere basis for visual mental imagery? *Neuropsychologia* 23:115–118, 1985.

32. Gazzaniga MS: Organization of the human brain. *Science* 245:947–952, 1989.

33. Levy J, Trevarthen CB, Sperry RW: Perception of bilateral chimeric figures following hemispheric deconnection. *Brain* 95:61–78, 1972.

34. Gazzaniga MS, Smylie CS: Facial recognition and brain asymmetries: Clues to underlying mechanisms. *Ann Neurol* 13:536–540, 1983.

35. Gazzaniga MS, Smylie CS: Hemispheric mechanisms controlling voluntary and spontaneous facial expressions. *J Cogn Neurosci* 2:239–245, 1990.

36. Gazzaniga MS: Principles of human brain organization derived from split-brain studies. *Neuron* 14:217–228, 1995.

37. Seymour S, Reuter-Lorenz PA, Gazzaniga MS: The disconnection syndrome: Basic findings reaffirmed. *Brain* 117:105–115, 1994.

38. Holtzman JD, Sidtis JJ, Volpe BT, et al: Dissociation of spatial information for stimulus localization and the control of attention. *Brain* 104:861–872, 1981.

39. Sergent J: Unified response to bilateral hemispheric stimulation by a split-brain patient. *Nature* 305:800–802, 1983.

40. Sergent J: Furtive incursions into bicameral minds. *Brain* 113:537–568, 1990.

41. Corballis MC: Can commissurotomized subjects compare digits between the visual fields? *Neuropsychologia* 32:1475–1486, 1994.

42. Kingstone A, Gazzaniga MS: Higher-order subcortical processing in the split-brain patient: More illusory than real? *Neuropsychologia* 9:321–328, 1995.

43. Stone J: The naso-temporal division of the monkey retina. *J Comp Neurol* 136:585–600, 1966.

44. Fukuda Y, Sawai H, Watanabe M, et al: Nasotemporal overlap of crossed and uncrossed retinal gan-

glion cell projections in the Japanese monkey (Macaca fuscata). *J Neurosci* 9:2353–2373, 1989.

45. Fendrich R, Wessinger CM, Gazzaniga MS: Nasotemporal overlap at the retinal vertical meridian: Investigations with a callosotomy patient. *Neuropsychologia.* In press.

46. Fendrich R, Gazzaniga MS: Evidence of foveal splitting in a commissurotomy patient. *Neuropsychologia* 27:273–281, 1989.

47. Holtzman JD, Volpe BT, Gazzaniga MS: Spatial orientation following commissural section, in Parasuraman R, Davies DR (eds): *Varieties of Attention.* New York: Academic Press, 1984, pp 375–394.

48. Holtzman JD: Interactions between cortical and subcortical visual areas: evidence from human commissurotomy patients. *Vision Res* 24:801–813, 1984.

49. Holtzman JD, Gazzaniga MS: Dual task interactions due exclusively to limits in processing resources. *Science* 218:1325–1327, 1982.

50. Holtzman JD, Gazzaniga MS: Enhanced dual task performance following callosal commissurotomy in humans. *Neuropsychologia* 23:315–321, 1985.

51. Luck SJ, Hillyard SA, Mangun GR, Gazzaniga MS: Independent hemispheric attentional systems mediate visual search in split-brain patients. *Nature* 342:543–545, 1989.

52. Mangun GR, Plager R, Loftus W, et al: Monitoring the visual world: Hemispheric asymmetries and subcortical processes in attention. *J Cogn Neurosci* 6:265–273, 1994.

53. Reuter-Lorenz P, Fendrich R: Orienting attention across the vertical meridian: Evidence from callosotomy patients. *J Cogn Neurosci* 2:232–238, 1990.

54. Risse GL, Gates J, Lund G, et al: Interhemispheric transfer in patients with incomplete section of the corpus callosum: Anatomic verification with magnetic resonance imaging. *Arch Neurol* 46:437–443, 1989.

55. Sidtis JJ, Volpe BT, Holtzman JD, et al: Cognitive interaction after staged callosal section: Evidence for transfer of semantic activation. *Science* 212:344–346, 1981.

56. Gazzaniga MS, Kutas M, Van Petten C, Fendrich R: Human callosal function: MRI-verified neuropsychological functions. *Neurology* 39:942–946, 1989.

57. Baynes K, Tramo MJ, Reeves AG, Gazzaniga MS: Isolation of a right hemisphere cognitive system in a patient with anarchic hand syndrome. Submitted.

Chapter 33

SYNDROMES DUE TO ACQUIRED BASAL GANGLIA DAMAGE

Bruce Crosson

The most commonly studied lesions of the basal ganglia are vascular, and this chapter concentrates primarily on the effects of vascular lesions. Prior to doing so, however, we must briefly address mechanisms of vascular lesions to the basal ganglia. The lenticulostriate arteries, supplying a large portion of the basal ganglia and surrounding white matter, originate from the M1 segment of the middle cerebral artery (MCA; see schematic diagram in Fig. 33-1). Ischemic lesions of the basal ganglia are often the result of occlusion of the MCA, from blockage at the bifurcation of the internal carotid artery or blockage of the M1 segment of the MCA. Less often, blockage of the internal carotid artery may be the culprit. In such cases, the function and integrity of cortices supplied by the MCA depend on anastomotic circulation[1,2] (Fig. 33-1). These anastomoses may vary widely in patency; in many cases, circulation is adequate to prevent cystic infarction, though not other changes. Although cortical infarcts may not be identified on computed tomography (CT) or magnetic resonance imaging (MRI) in cases of basal ganglia infarction, inadequate anastomotic circulation may cause structural (ischemic neuronal loss) or functional changes (inadequate neuronal function without cell death) in inadequately supplied cortical areas. When these circumstances are present, the symptoms may be determined more by which cortical areas experience unidentified structural or functional changes than by which subcortical structures demonstrate damage on CT or MRI.[1–3] Cerebral blood flow images from single photon emission computed tomography (SPECT) may be useful in determining the full extent of cortical and subcortical dysfunction.[2] It is worth noting as an exception to these vascular dynamics that since lacunar infarctions frequently result from small-vessel as opposed to large-vessel disease,[4] cortical dysfunction is not necessarily expected to accompany subcortical lacunar infarction. Thus, these smaller lesions may be more useful in exploring structural-functional relationships.

Hemorrhagic lesions can be complicated in a slightly different fashion by ischemic effects not seen on CT or MRI. Large hemorrhagic lesions of the basal ganglia will leave a hematoma that radiates pressure effects. In such cases, pressure may cause temporary or permanent ischemic effects in surrounding areas, including perisylvian language cortex and the thalamus.[1,3] Other space-occupying lesions, such as tumors, may also cause pressure ischemia, resulting in temporary functional effects or permanent structural changes. Again, in such cases the location of cortical or subcortical ischemia may affect symptom presentation. Keeping these thoughts in mind, we can now explore symptom complexes seen after lesions of the basal ganglia identified by CT or MRI.

APHASIA AFTER LESION OF THE BASAL GANGLIA

The incidence of aphasia in larger lesions including the dominant basal ganglia can be substantial.

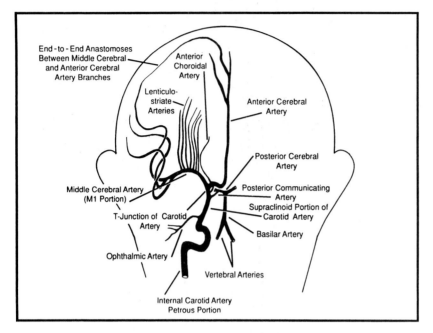

Figure 33-1
Schematic diagram showing the internal carotid artery branching into the middle and anterior cerebral arteries. The lenticulostriate arteries, which supply much of the basal ganglia and surrounding white matter, emerge from the M1 segment of the middle cerebral artery. End-to-end anastomoses between branches of the middle and anterior cerebral arteries are also depicted. (From Nadeau and Crosson,[1] with permission of Academic Press.)

Crosson[5] found the rates of aphasia in vascular lesions involving the dominant basal ganglia to vary between 20 and 83 percent; however, Nadeau and Crosson[1] have noted that the rate of aphasia in cases of smaller lesions confined to the caudate head may be negligible.

When aphasia is present after a lesion of the dominant basal ganglia, the symptoms vary considerably. Crosson[5] reviewed the literature on aphasia after vascular lesion of the dominant basal ganglia and rated reported cases on four dimensions: fluent versus nonfluent output, severity of comprehension deficit, severity of repetition deficit, and predominance of phonemic versus semantic paraphasias. The picture was rather different for hemorrhagic lesions versus infarctions. For aphasia after hemorrhage, the dominant putamen was most frequently involved and aphasia was primarily of a fluent variety. Repetition and comprehension were usually impaired to some degree, often severely. Paraphasias were predominantly semantic as opposed to phonemic. While hemorrhagic cases seemed, at least loosely, to fit a syndrome, cases of infarction did not cohere into a syndrome. Speech/language output could be fluent

or nonfluent. Comprehension was usually impaired to at least some degree, but repetition ranged from unimpaired to severely impaired. When one type of paraphasia predominated for an individual case, it could be phonemic or semantic. No syndrome emerged whether the infarct included the putamen, caudate head, or the globus pallidus. The weakness in this analysis was that lesions frequently included multiple structures, and it was difficult to parcel out the effects on one structure versus another.

For this reason, Nadeau and Crosson[1] reviewed a single type of lesion, dominant striatocapsular infarcts. These lesions have a characteristic comma shape (Fig. 33-2) and most often include the putamen, anterior limb of the internal capsule, and caudate head. Since the structures included are fairly consistent, this type of lesion should produce a characteristic syndrome if the basal ganglia are involved in language. According to this review, patients with dominant striatocapsular infarcts may ($n = 33$) or may not ($n = 17$) have aphasia. When aphasia is reported, levels of impairment are quite variable for fluency, comprehension, repetition, naming, and paraphasia. Articulation is

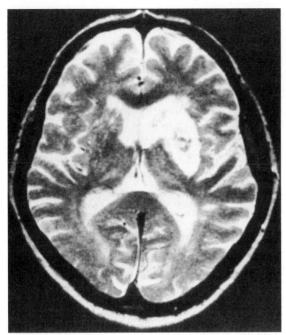

Figure 33-2
T₂-weighted MRI of striatocapsular infarction. Note the comma-shaped appearance. (From Weiller et al.,[2] with permission of Oxford University Press.)

most often moderately impaired. Similarly, Weiller and colleagues[2] studied 57 consecutive cases of striatocapsular infarction. When the lesion involved the dominant hemisphere, patients might or might not be aphasic. Of 15 cases with aphasia, the initial syndrome was Broca's aphasia in 4, Wernicke's aphasia in 3, amnesic aphasia in 4, global aphasia in 2, residual symptoms in 1, and unclassifiable in 1. Thus, consistent with the review of Nadeau and Crosson,[1] no coherent syndrome emerged. For the aphasic patients of Weiller and coworkers,[2] the prognosis was generally good: 9 of 14 patients seen at 1-year follow-up had no or minor language symptoms. Recanalization occurred later, if at all, in patients with aphasia as opposed to those without aphasia; patients with aphasia as opposed to those without aphasia had poor anastomotic circulation.

In summary, patients with sizable hemorrhages in the dominant basal ganglia tend to have

fluent aphasias with semantic paraphasias and at least some impairment of comprehension and repetition. Patients with infarction of the dominant basal ganglia, including those with characteristic striatocapsular lesions, may or may not demonstrate aphasia. When aphasia is present, it may be of almost any variety. Available evidence suggests that in cases of infarction of the dominant basal ganglia, the adequacy of anastomotic circulation to the cortex may determine whether aphasia is seen, and the type of aphasia will depend on which cortical regions cannot function properly.[1,2] For hemorrhagic lesions of the dominant basal ganglia, symptoms may be related to compressive ischemia of the cortex, the thalamus, or the connections between them.[1] On the basis of these data, a subtle or supportive role of the basal ganglia in language cannot be ruled out; if it exists, however, it appears to be obscured after vascular lesion of the dominant basal ganglia by ischemic effects on other structures, primarily the perisylvian cortex.

APRAXIA AFTER LESION OF THE BASAL GANGLIA

Apraxia involves deficits in the execution of learned, skilled movements.[6] The literature on acquired basal ganglia lesions and praxis is problematic.[7] As with aphasia, ischemic phenomena accompanying cystic infarction or large hemorrhages may cause cortical dysfunction, and the cortical dysfunction, in turn, could cause deficits in praxis. A second problem is that different investigators have used different definitions of praxis, with some testing already learned skilled movements and others testing novel movements or postures that have not been learned. The presence of preexisting representations of the movements for the already *learned*, skilled movements could make a large difference in the performance of the appropriate actions. These caveats must be kept in mind in examining the literature on apraxia after acquired lesion of the basal ganglia.

Some studies suggest that apraxia after lesion to the dominant basal ganglia and/or surrounding white matter is less frequent than after lesions to the cortex.[8] Most commonly, apraxia with basal ganglia lesion occurs after dominant-hemisphere lesion, though apraxia has been reported after nondominant-hemisphere lesion as well.

As with aphasia, the pattern of apraxia can be examined to determine whether it coheres into a consistent syndrome and whether the pattern of deficits is unique. A consistent pattern of deficits with at least some unique features relative to cortical apraxia would argue in favor of a role for the basal ganglia in praxis. Unfortunately, such studies have barely begun. Rothi and coworkers[9] reported three cases of striatocapsular infarction, two of which were severely apraxic. In general, these patients made spatial errors on a praxis task similar to those made by patients with cortical apraxias. One patient made perseverative errors that were generally not made by patients with apraxia after cortical lesions. Thus, in this small sample, no consistent syndrome with unique features was found, and no good case for the involvement of the basal ganglia in praxis can be made at this time. As with aphasia after lesion of the dominant basal ganglia, it is a safe bet that the existence, severity, and character of apraxia is determined largely by structural changes or dysfunction in the cortex not seen on structural images.

NEGLECT AFTER LESION OF THE BASAL GANGLIA

The term *neglect* can be used to refer either to sensory-perceptual phenomena or to movement-related phenomena.[10] On the sensory-perceptual side, *neglect* refers to a tendency not attributable to primary sensory deficit to ignore or neglect visual, auditory, and/or tactile stimuli contralateral to a brain lesion. It may be unimodal or multimodal. In addition to affecting the ability to process incoming sensory information, neglect may also affect internal representations of space.[11] Although sensory neglect is more common with right-hemispheric lesions in right-handed patients, more subtle forms of neglect can appear after left-hemispheric lesion in dextrals.[12] On the movement-related side, *neglect* refers to disorders of the inten-

tion to act; the term *akinesia* has been used to describe these disorders. With respect to unilateral lesions affecting intention, patients can have a defect in initiating movement with a limb on one side of the body (limb akinesia), a defect initiating movement in one hemispace (hemispatial akinesia), or a defect initiating movement toward one side of space (directional akinesia).[13] The analysis of Watson and colleagues[14] suggests that dysfunction of the basal ganglia is more likely to produce akinesia than sensory-perceptual neglect. (See also Ref. 10.)

Case reports suggest that neglect is frequently found in cases where scans have identified structural lesions in the basal ganglia and surrounding white matter. Some reports have focused on sensory-perceptual neglect,[15] though others have not distinguished sensory-perceptual from intentional neglect.[16] Neglect appears to be more common with right- than left-hemispheric lesions of the basal ganglia. Weiller and colleagues[2] found that striatocapsular infarct patients with neglect or aphasia showed later or lesser recanalization of the middle cerebral artery and poorer anastomotic circulation than striatocapsular infarct patients without aphasia or neglect. They concluded that when neglect occurred, cortical dysfunction accounted for it in striatocapsular infarct patients. If the analyses of Watson and coworkers[14] are correct, then patients with acquired lesions of the basal ganglia should experience primarily akinesia as opposed to sensory-perceptual neglect. Unfortunately, the descriptions of most studies are not adequate to make the distinction, but the existence of sensory-perceptual neglect in many cases[15] suggests that Weiller and colleagues' conclusions regarding cortical dysfunction accounting for neglect may be accurate.

EMOTIONAL CHANGES AFTER LESION OF THE BASAL GANGLIA

Cummings[17] has reviewed much of the literature regarding emotional changes that accompany subcortical lesions, including those of the basal ganglia. Such alterations are apparently common. One report by Mendez and associates[18] is of particular interest, because the vast majority of the 12 cases reported had unilateral lacunar infarcts of the caudate head, suggesting that concomitant cortical ischemia was not a factor in all of them. Emotional changes were dependent on location of the infarct within the caudate head. Lesions of the dorsolateral caudate head resulted in apathy with decreased spontaneous verbal and motor behavior. This area of the caudate head is involved in a corticostriatopallidothalamocortical loop that terminates in the dorsolateral frontal cortex.[19] Patients with lesions of the ventromedial caudate head demonstrated disinhibition, impulsivity, and inappropriate behavior. This area of the caudate head is in a corticostriatopallidothalamocortical loop that terminates in the orbitofrontal cortex,[19] thus the resemblance to behavior resulting from orbitofrontal lesions. Lesions involving most of the caudate head plus surrounding white matter produced affective symptoms with psychotic features. Effects did not depend upon lateralization. A study by Starkstein and coworkers[20] indicated that lesions of the left basal ganglia (hemorrhage or infarction) resulted in significantly greater depression than lesions of the right basal ganglia or of the left or right thalamus. The heterogeneity of lesions and the inclusion of larger lesions in this latter study suggest that many patients may have had cortical dysfunction, as detailed above.

SUMMARY AND CONCLUSIONS

For large lesions of the basal ganglia, such as striatocapsular infarction, significant dysfunction may occur because of reduced blood flow to various areas of the cortex. This dynamic relates to blockage of the proximal MCA and the adequacy of anastomotic circulation to the various cortical regions supplied by the MCA. In such lesions, the cognitive symptoms in all probability are determined by which areas of the cortex are functionally or structurally compromised in a way that is not detectable by structural imaging techniques. This phenomenon accounts for the wide variety of aphasic symptoms in striatocapsular infarction,

sensory-perceptual neglect in striatocapsular infarction, and the similarity of apraxic symptoms in lesions of the cortex and basal ganglia. Further, any function that depends upon cortex in the distribution of the MCA might be affected after striatocapsular infarction. For example, executive functions involving dorsolateral prefrontal functions and visuospatial functions have been reported to be impaired after infarction of the basal ganglia.[15,18]

Hemorrhage of the basal ganglia, because of the pressure effects surrounding an intracerebral hematoma, and tumors of the basal ganglia, for similar reasons, are likely to cause some pressure ischemia, which will affect the cortex. Thus, symptoms accompanying these types of lesions may also involve cortical dysfunction. Since lacunar infarcts are frequently caused by small-vessel as opposed to large-vessel disease, these smaller lesions may be more useful in determining function when they occur in the basal ganglia. Some evidence exists that such lesions may cause significant cognitive or emotional dysfunction.[18]

REFERENCES

1. Nadeau SE, Crosson B: Subcortical aphasia. *Brain Lang.* In press.
2. Weiller C, Willmes K, Reiche W, et al: The case of aphasia or neglect after striatocapsular infarction. *Brain* 116:1509–1525, 1993.
3. Skyhoj Olsen T, Bruhn P, Oberg RGW: Cortical hypoperfusion as a possible cause of "subcortical aphasia." *Brain* 109:393–410, 1986.
4. Poirier J, Gray F, Escourolle R: *Manual of Basic Neuropathology.* Philadelphia: Saunders, 1990.
5. Crosson B: *Subcortical Functions in Language and Memory.* New York: Guilford Press, 1992.
6. Heilman KM, Rothi LJG: Apraxia, in Heilman KM, Valenstein E (eds): *Clinical Neuropsychology,* 3d ed. New York: Oxford, 1993, pp 141–164.
7. Crosson B: Subcortical limb apraxia, in Rothi LJG, Heilman KM (eds): *Apraxia.* Hillsdale, NJ: Erlbaum. In press.
8. Basso A, Luzzatti C, Spinnler H: Is ideomotor apraxia the outcome of damage of well-defined regions of the left hemisphere? *J Neurol Neurosurg Psychiatry* 43:118–126, 1980.

9. Rothi LJG, Kooistra C, Heilman KM, Mack L: Subcortical ideomotor apraxia. *J Clin Exp Neuropsychol* 10:48, 1988.

10. Heilman KM, Watson RT, Valenstein E: Neglect and related disorders, in Heilman KM, Valenstein E (eds): *Clinical Neuropsychology,* 3d ed. New York: Oxford University Press, 1993, pp 279–336.

11. Bisiach E, Luzzatti C: Unilateral neglect of representational space. *Cortex* 14:129–133, 1978.

12. Maeshima S, Shigeno K, Dohi N, et al: A study of right unilateral spatial neglect in left hemispheric lesions: The difference between right-handed and non-right-handed post-stroke patients. *Acta Neurol Scand* 85:418–424, 1992.

13. Heilman KM, Bowers D, Valenstein E, Watson RT: Hemispace and hemispatial neglect, in Jeannerod M (ed): *Neurophysiological and Neuropsychological Aspects of Spatial Neglect.* Amsterdam: Elsevier, pp 115–150.

14. Watson RT, Valenstein E, Heilman KM: Thalamic neglect: Possible role of the medial thalamus and nucleus reticularis in behavior. *Arch Neurol* 38:501–506, 1981.

15. Bladin PF, Berkovik SF: Straitocapsular infarction: Large infarcts in the lenticulostriate arterial territory. *Neurology* 34:1423–1430, 1984.

16. Fromm D, Holland AL, Swindell CS, Reinmuth OM: Various consequences of subcortical stroke: Prospective study of 16 consecutive cases. *Arch Neurol* 42:943–950, 1985.

17. Cummings JL: Frontal-subcortical circuits and human behavior. *Arch Neurol* 50:873–880, 1993.

18. Mendez MF, Adams NL, Lewandowski KS: Neurobehavioral changes associated with caudate lesions. *Neurology* 39:349–354, 1989.

19. Alexander GE, DeLong MR, Strick PL: Parallel organization of functionally segregated circuits linking basal ganglia and cortex. *Annu Rev Neurosci* 9:357–381, 1986.

20. Starkstein SS, Robinson RG, Berthier ML, et al: Differential mood changes following basal ganglia vs thalamic lesions. *Arch Neurol* 45:725–730, 1988.

Chapter 34

SYNDROMES DUE TO ACQUIRED THALAMIC DAMAGE

Neill R. Graff-Radford

When the thalamus is damaged, the resulting types of deficits can be thought of in terms of the afferent and efferent connections of the affected thalamic nuclei (Table 34-1).[1] Certain nuclei have both afferent input from primary sense organs and efferent output to primary cortices. Damage to these nuclei causes primary sensory deficits. The best clinical examples are damage to the ventroposterolateral (VPL) and ventroposteromedial (VPM) thalamic nuclei, resulting in sensory loss on the opposite side of the body, and damage to the lateral geniculate, causing a contralateral visual field cut. The motor-related thalamic nuclei receive afferent input from the basal ganglia, the substantia nigra, and the cerebellum and give efferent projections to the primary motor and premotor cortices. Damage to these nuclei cause contralateral motor deficits such as an emotional facial weakness and, in the dominant thalamus, a language difficulty. Limbic-related thalamic nuclei recieve input from the hippocampus via the fornix and the medial temporal cortex and amygdala via the inferior thalamic peduncle. The output is to the cingulate gyrus and frontal lobes. Damage to these pathways may cause a permanent amnesia. Damage to nuclei with connections to cortical association areas may conceivably result in deficits of higher cortical functions; examples described include neglect[2] and aphasia,[3] but these abnormalities are less well characterized as to their anatomic basis.

A further constraint in understanding disorders related to thalamic damage is the blood supply of the thalamus. There are 16 named arteries that supply blood to the thalamus, most of which are not end arteries, and the nuclei supplied by one artery differ in different individuals.[4] Thus, knowing both the nuclei that these arteries commonly supply and the arterial territory affected does not necessarily translate into deducing which nuclei are damaged. To establish this, one has to analyze the lesion and plot it in three-dimensional spade, using an atlas such as that of Schaltenbrand and Wahren.[5] Infarctions in four arterial territories commonly occur, can be recognized, and are described in this chapter. The anatomic basis of amnesia and aphasia following thalamic damage will also be addressed.[3,6,7]

SYNDROMES RELATED TO INFARCTION IN DIFFERENT ARTERIAL TERRITORIES

Infarction in the Territory of the Geniculothalamic Artery

The geniculothalamic artery is a branch of the posterior cerebral artery and may be affected by posterior cerebral occlusion.[8] Figure 34-1A shows a typical infarction in this territory. It commonly supplies part of the following thalamic nuclei: dorsomedial, posterolateral, reticular, parafascicular, and lateral geniculate (Fig. 34-1B). Infarction in this territory may cause the Dejerine-Roussy syndrome,[9] characterized by a fleeting

Table 34-1
Thalamic connections[a]

Afferent connections	Thalamic nucleus	Efferent connections
Mammillothalamic tract Fornix	Anterior group (AV)	Cingulate gyrus
Globus pallidus Substantia nigra	Anterior ventral (VA)	Area 6 Diffuse frontal
Dentate nucleus Globus pallidus Substantia nigra	Ventrolateral (VL)	Area 4
Medial lemniscus Spinothalamic tract Trigeminothalamic tract	Ventroposterolateral (VPL) Ventroposteromedial (VPM)	Areas 1, 2, and 3
	Lateral dorsal (LD)	Cingulate Medial parietal
	Lateral posterior	Superior parietal
Areas 18 and 19 Inferior parietal lobule	Pulvinar	Areas 18 and 19 Inferior parietal lobule
Optic tract	Lateral geniculate	Area 17
Inferior colliculus Lateral lemniscus	Medial geniculate	Areas 41 and 42
Amygdaloid complex Temporal neocortex	Dorsomedial nucleus	Prefrontal cortex
	Midline nuclei	Amygdaloid nuclei Anterior cingulate cortex
Reticular formation Spinothalamic tract Dentate nucleus Areas 4, 6, 8, and 9 Globus pallidus Substantia reticulata	Intralaminar nuclei	Putamen Caudate nucleus

[a]Numbers in table refer to Brodmann's cortical areas.

hemiparesis, persistent hemianesthesia to touch, hyperesthesia and paroxysmal pain, slight ataxia, asterognosis, and choreoathetosis. Development of this syndrome does not invariably result from infarction in this territory; some may develop this syndrome and some may not. The Dejerine-Roussy syndrome is more common with right- than with left-sided thalamic infarction. The hallmark of geniculothalamic infarction is loss of sensation in all primary modalities on the contralateral side. Cognitive deficits do not characteristically occur with infarction in this territory un-less there is associated posterior cerebral artery infarction. Sensory evoked potentials show absence of all waves after the positive wave at about 14 ms when the contralateral arm is stimulated.[7]

A geniculothalamic lacune (Fig. 34-1C) in the primary sensory nuclei causes the so-called pure hemisensory loss syndrome with contralateral pain and touch loss but no proprioception or vibration sense deficit.[7,10] There may be some dysesthesia but there is no concomitant neuropsychological deficit.

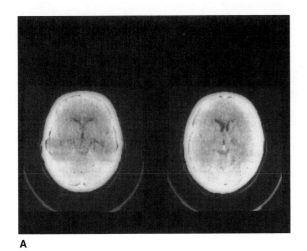

A

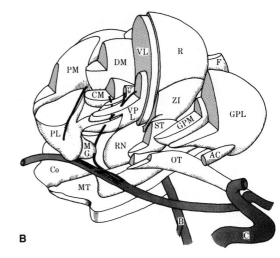

B

Figure 34-1

A. *Computed tomography scan showing infarction in the geniculothalamic arterial territory. B. Territory of the geniculothalamic artery. This is based upon Figs. 27-4 and 27-5 in the Schlesinger atlas.[4] C. Lacune in the geniculothalamic territory. This patient had contralateral hemisensory loss to pinprick and light touch sensations. A = anterior nucleus; AC = anterior commissure; AV = anterior ventral nucleus; B = basilar artery; C = carotid artery; CM = centrum medianum; Co = colliculi; DM = dorsomedial nucleus; DP = deep interpeduncular profundus artery; F = fornix; GPL = globus pallidus (lateral); GPM = globus pallidus (medial); LG = lateral geniculate; LP = lateral posterior nucleus; MG = medial geniculate; MAM = mammillary bodies; MT = midbrain tegmentum; MTT = mammillothalamic tract; OT = optic tract; PCe = posterior cerebral artery; PCo = posterior communicating artery; PL = pulvinar (lateral); PM = pulvinar (medial); R = reticular nucleus; RN = red nucleus; ST = subthalamic nucleus; Tt = tuberothalamic artery; VL = ventrolateral nucleus; VPL = ventral posterolateral nucleus; VPM = ventral posteromedial nucleus; ZI = zona inceta. (From Graff-Radford et al.,[7] with permission.)*

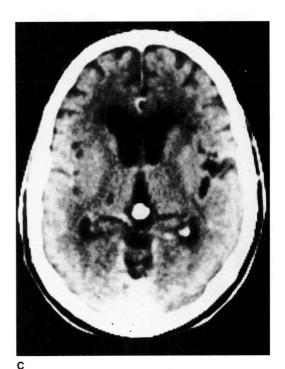

C

INFARCTION IN THE TERRITORY OF THE TUBEROTHALAMIC ARTERY

The tuberothalamic artery (also called the polar artery, the anterior internal optic artery, and the premammillary pedicle) is a branch of the posterior communicating artery. It supplies the anterolateral quadrant of the thalamus. Figure 34-2A shows a typical infarction in this territory, and the nuclei it typically supplies are seen in Fig. 34-2B. Circumstances in which there is infarction in this arterial territory include clipping of a posterior communicating aneurysm and a watershed infarction. As a branch of the posterior

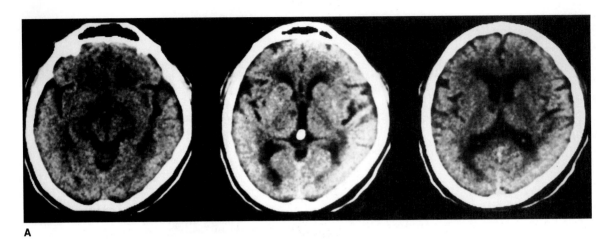

A

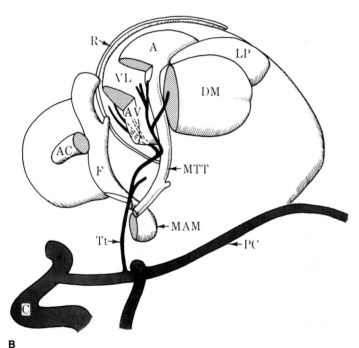

B

Figure 34-2
A. *Computed tomography showing a typical infarction in the tuberothalamic arterial territory.* B. *Territory of the tuberothalamic artery. This is based on Fig. 28-4 of the Schlesinger atlas.[4] Abbreviations as in Fig. 34-1. (From Graff-Radford et al.,[7] with permission.)*

communicating artery, this artery is between the anterior and posterior circulations, possibly making it vulnerable during the circumstances of a watershed infarction, such as a cardiac arrest. Patients with infarction in this territory often have an emotional facial paresis and sometimes have an hemiparesis if the infarction extends into the internal capsule, but they do not have sensory loss. In those with left-sided lesions,

aphasia is frequent, along with impaired intellect, visuospatial abilities, memory, and temporal orientation. Patients with right-sided lesions have impaired nonverbal intellect, visual perceptual discrimination, spatial judgment, visual memory, and constructional praxis. In contrast, they have preserved verbal intellect, verbal memory, and speech and language. Over time, patients improve substantially, but the pattern of deficits remains.

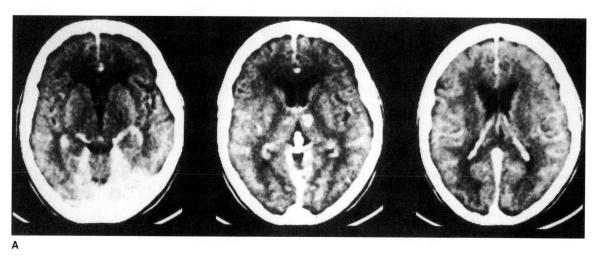

A

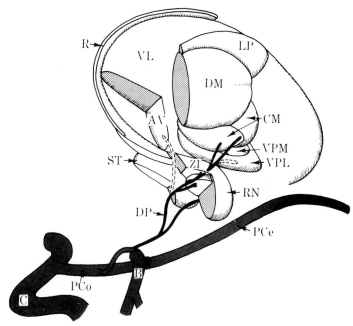

Figure 34-3
A. *Computed tomography showing bilateral infarction in the interpeduncular arterial territory. B. Territory of the interpeduncular profundus artery. The dotted line indicates other areas that may be supplied by this artery. Based on Figs. 28-6 and 28-7 of the Schlesinger atlas.[4] Abbreviations are as for Fig. 34-1. (From Graff-Radford et al.,[7] with permission.)*

B

Figure 34-2*B* shows the brain of a patient with infarction in this territory.

INFARCTION IN THE TERRITORY OF THE INTERPEDUNCULAR PROFUNDA ARTERY

This artery (also called the paramedian thalamic, the internal optic, and thalamoperforating pedi-

cle) is a branch of the basilar portion of the posterior cerebral artery. It originates soon after the basilar artery bifurcates and may come off as one branch supplying both sides of the medial thalamus or as two separate branches. A typical infarction in this territory is seen in Fig. 34-3*A*. The typical nuclei it supplies can be seen in Fig. 34-3*B*. As the tuberothalamic artery may be small or even absent, the interpeduncular profunda may supply the dorsomedial, ventrolateral, and anteroventral thalamic nuclei; in addition, it has been described as supplying the dorsolateral, posterolateral, ventroposteromedial, and ventroposterolateral thalamic nuclei. In the majority of cases, part of the dorsomedial, the centrum medianum, and parafascicular nuclei make up its main territory of supply. The clinical picture of patients with infarction in this territory includes drowsiness in the early stages after the infarction and a vertical supranuclear gaze paresis.[11] At this stage, clinicians have difficulty diagnosing patients with infarction in this territory because there are usually no motor or sensory deficits and acute computed tomography (CT) is often normal. The vertical gaze paresis is probably related to infarction in the rostral part of the medial longitudinal fasciculus. As the patient improves, deficits can be found in intellect, memory, visuospatial processing, and orientation. Following these patients over time reveals that they either recover fairly well or have a permanent amnesia. The anatomic basis of this is discussed below.

INFARCTION IN THE TERRITORY OF THE ANTERIOR CHOROIDAL ARTERY

The anterior choroidal artery supplies part of the amygdala, medial temporal lobe, globus pallidus, posterior limb of the internal capsule, and lateral thalamus. A typical infarction in this territory is shown in Fig. 34-4A. The thalamic nuclei that have been reported to receive blood supply from the anterior thalamic artery are the lateral geniculate, reticular, pulvinar, and ventroposterolateral (Fig. 34-4B). Patients with infarction in this territory have a hemiparesis; a few have minor sensory deficits (to pinprick and light touch but not proprioception and vibration sensation). Rarely they may have a contralateral visual field cut because the artery does provide some supply to the optic tract and lateral geniculate body. Most have some neuropsychological deficit. Patients with left-sided lesions do not have an aphasia but may have a

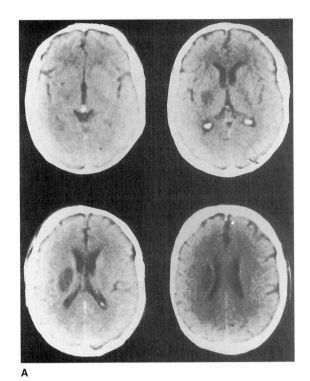

A

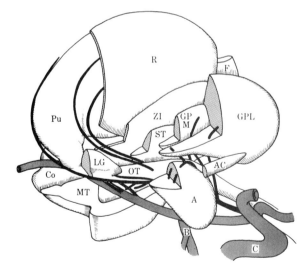

B

Figure 34-4
A. Computed tomography showing infarction in the anterior choroidal territory. B. The territory of the anterior choroid is based on Fig. 27-2 of the Schlesinger atlas.[4] Abbreviations as in Fig. 34-1. (From Graff-Radford et al.,[7] with permission.)

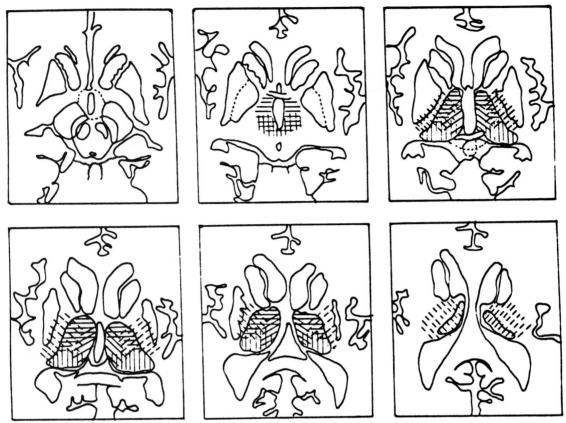

Figure 34-5
Templates (4 mm) through the thalamus depicting the following four arterial territories: Vertical hatching = geniculothalamic territory; horizontal hatching = tuberothalamic territory; unbroken diagonal hatching = interpeduncular profundus territory; broken diagonal hatching = anterior choroidal territory. (From Graff-Radford et al.,[7] with permission.)

dysarthria, difficulty with verbal fluency, and impaired reading comprehension. Upon testing, there might be a mild verbal memory deficit, but this does not translate into a clinically significant amnesia. Visual memory may also be defective despite normal visual perception. Right-sided lesions impair visual perception, visual memory, and nonverbal intellect. Patients with infarction in this territory are often left with a significant hemiparesis.[12]

Figure 34-5 summarizes the sections of the thalamus where infarction in the above four arterial territories occurs.

DIENCEPHALIC AMNESIA

Anatomic Basis

From the classic case of H.M., it became clear that the medial temporal lobes are important in memory[13] (see Chap. 35). After numerous experiments in the primate, Mishkin[14] proposed that the structures involved in medial temporal lobe amnesia were the amygdala and hippocampus, and combined damage to these structures or their connections resulted in a severe amnesia. This work was further refined by Zola-Morgan and cowork-

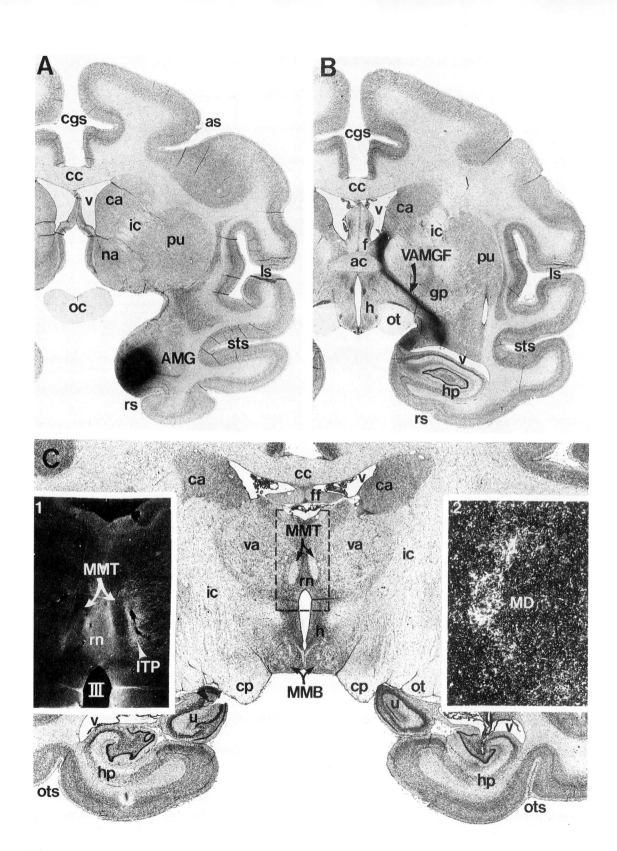

ers,[15,16] who have shown that the crucial areas in the medial temporal lobe which, when damaged, result in a severe amnesia are the hippocampus and the perirhinal cortex. Lesions to both these areas together increase the severity of the amnesia. Keeping this in mind, let us now look at the anatomy of the diencephalic lesions that result in amnesia.

Patients with bilateral infarction in the interpeduncular territory may be left with a permanent disabling amnesia. Lesions situated anteriorly cause an amnesia, whereas those situated posteriorly do not.[17] We believe that the crucial locus of the lesion that results in amnesia is where the mammillothalamic artery is adjacent to the ventroamygdalofugal pathway[6] (also called the inferior thalamic peduncle (Fig. 34-6). A major hippocampal pathway to the thalamus is the fornix, which goes to the mammillary bodies from which the mammillothalmic tract arises and then goes to the anteprior thalamic nucleus. We also know that the amygdala sends a pathway through the ventroamygdalofugal pathway to the dorsomedial nucleus.[6] Although it has not yet been proved, it is

likely that the ventroamygdalofugal pathway contains a pathway connecting the perirhinal cortex and the dorsomedial thalamic nucleus. Thus damage in the anterior thalamus may affect both hippocampal (mammillothalamic tract) and perirhinal (ventroamygdalofugal) pathways with small, strategically located bilateral lesions. This is analogous to the work of Zola-Morgan and colleagues, mentioned above. Further, there is an experimental primate model of this combination of lesions. Bachevalier and colleagues[18] reported on the effects of separate versus combined transection lesions of the fornix and amygdalofugal pathway. They found that the combined but not the separate lesions resulted in a severe recognition deficit in monkeys. We believe that this is analogous to the anatomic damage in our amnestic patients.

Other thalamic nuclei that, by their connections, may be involved in memory, are the midline thalamic nuclei, such as nucleus reunions. These nuclei have both afferent and efferent projections to the hippocampus and other medial temporal lobe structures.[1]

Figure 34-6

A. *Nissl-stained transverse section from the rhesus monkey brain, developed from autoradiography showing the location of tritiated amino acids injected into the medial parts of the basolateral amygdaloid nuclei and the deep layers of the entorhinal cortex. B. Transverse section from the same animal demonstrating the ventroamygdalofugal pathway (VAMGF) in its course from the posterior amygdala beneath the globus pallidus (gp) to the bed nucleus of the stria terminalis at the base of the body of the lateral ventricle (v). C. Nissl-stained transverse section from the same case at the level of the uncus (u) and mammillary bodies (MMB). Note the midline region of the thalamus (outlined rectangle) and the position of the mammillothalamic tracts (MMT). Inset 1 is a dark-field photomicrograph of the rectangular area that demonstrates tritium-labeled axons in the inferior thalamic peduncle (ITP), immediately lateral to the mammillothalamic tract ipsilateral to the amygdaloid injection. As shown in inset 2, these axons follow a posterior intrathalamic course where they terminate in the dorsomedial thalamic nucleus. Note that a selective vascular lesion at the level of inset 1 would disrupt both the mammillothalamic tract and the inferior thalamic peduncle. Other abbreviations: ac = anterior commissure; as = arcuate sulcus; ca = caudate nucleus; cc = corpus callosum; cgs = cingulate sulcus; cp = cerebral peduncle; h = hypothalamus; hp = hippocampal formation; ic = internal capsule; ls = lateral sulcus; na = nucleus accumbens; oc = optic chiasm; ot = optic tract; ots = occipitotemporal sulcus; pu = putamen; rn = nucleus reunions; rs = rhinal sulcus; sts = superior temporal sulcus. (From Graff-Radford et al.,[7] with permission.)*

Neuropsychological Features

The amnesia in these patients is characterized by severe anterograde memory loss, preservation of motor learning, and—in some patients—impaired retrograde memory.[6] In one of our patients whom we followed for 8 years, there was a temporal gradient to the memory loss.[6] Malamut and colleagues[19] reported a young postman who developed a disabling amnesia from bilateral thalamic infarction but was still able to sort the mail for the people and addresses on his route (except for the new persons added since his stroke). It is unclear if this represents preservation of retrograde memory or preservation of overlearned retrograde memories. Further patients should be studied in this regard.

DISTURBANCES OF SPEECH AND LANGUAGE ASSOCIATED WITH THALAMIC DYSFUNCTION

In an analysis of reported cases, we found that there were probably two kinds of thalamic language disturbance.[3] The first is associated with damage to the ventrolateral and anterioventral nuclei and is characterized by decreased but fluent speech output with paraphasias but no neologisms (see Chap. 9). An alternative anatomic explanation is that damage in this area might affect the reticular nucleus, which could influence the frontal lobes' input to the thalamus and in this way affect language.[20] The second type is characterized by normal or increased speech output and neologisms. The anatomic correlate is possibly damage in the pulvinar and posterolateral thalamic nucleus, but the anatomic evidence for this is not as convincing as that for the first hypothesis.

Whether or not these disturbances should be called aphasia is a matter of opinion. The fact that there are nonlinguistic disturbances in most of these patients distinguishes them from other aphasic patients in whom attention and memory are intact. However, these disturbances contain all the symptomatology of an aphasia and occur exclusively with lesions in the dominant thalamus in a set of nuclei that is closely interconnected with the language cortices. The similarity with transcortical aphasia is striking. Many of these patients have a good prognosis, improving considerably over time.[3]

ACKNOWLEDGMENTS

This work was supported in part by a National Institute of Aging grant AG08031-06S1 and the State of Florida Alzheimer's Disease Initiative.

REFERENCES

1. Carpenter BM, Sutin J: *Human Neuroanatomy,* 8th ed. Baltimore: Williams & Wilkins, 1983.
2. Watson RT, Valenstein E, Heilman KM: Thalamic neglect: Possible role of the medial thalamus and nucleus reticularis in behavior. *Arch Neurol* 38:501–506, 1981.
3. Graff-Radford N, Damasio A: Disturbances of speech and language associated with thalamic dysfunction. *Semin Neurol* 4:162–168, 1984.
4. Schlesinger B: *The Upper Brainstem in the Human.* Berlin: Springer-Verlag, 1976.
5. Schaltenbrand G, Wahren W: *Atlas for Stereotaxy of the Human Brain.* Stuttgart, Germany: Thieme, 1977.
6. Graff-Radford N, Tranel D, Van Hoesen G, Brandt J: Diencephalic amnesia. *Brain* 113:1–25, 1990.
7. Graff-Radford N, Damasio H, Yamada T, et al: Non-hemorrhagic thalamic infarctions: Clinical, neuropsychological and electrophysiological findings in four anatomical groups defined by CT. *Brain* 108:485–516, 1985.
8. Goto K, Tagawa K, Uemura K, et al: Posterior cerebral artery occlusion: Clinical, computed tomographic, and angiographic correlation. *Radiology* 132:357–368, 1979.
9. Dejerine J, Roussy G: Le syndrome thalamique. *Rev Neurol* 14:521–532, 1906.
10. Fisher CM: Thalamic pure sensory stroke: A pathological study. *Neurology* 32:871–876, 1978.
11. Buttner-Ennever JA, Buttner U, Cohen B, Baumgartner G: Vertical gaze paralysis and the rostral interstitial nucleus of the medial longitudinal fasciculus. *Brain* 105:125–149, 1982.

12. Bruno A, Graff-Radford N, Biller J, Adams H: Anterior choroidal artery territory infarction: A small vessel disease. *Stroke* 20:616–619, 1989.
13. Corkin S: Lasting consequences of bilateral medial temporal lobectomy: Clinical course and experimental findings in H.M. *Semin Neurol* 4:249–259, 1984.
14. Mishkin M: A memory system in the monkey. *Phil Trans Royal Soc Lond* B298:85–95, 1982.
15. Zola-Morgan S, Squire LR, Amaral DG: Human amnesia and the medial temporal region: Enduring memory impairments following a bilateral lesion limited to field CA1 of the hippocampus. *J Neurosci* 6:2950–2967, 1986.
16. Zola-Morgan S, Squire LR, Amaral DG, Suzuki WA: Lesions of perirhinal and parahippocampal cortex that spare the amygdala and hippocampal formation produce severe memory impairment. *J Neurosci* 9:4355–4370, 1989.
17. Cramon DYV, Hebel N, Schuri U: A contribution to the anatomical basis of thalamic amnesia. *Brain* 108:993–1008, 1985.
18. Bachevalier J, Parkinson JK, Mishkin M: Visual recognition in monkeys: Effects of separate vs combined transection of fornix and amygdalofugal pathways. *Exp Brain Res* 57:554–561, 1985.
19. Malamut B, Graff-Radford N, Chawluk J, Gur R: Preserved and impaired memory function in a case of bilateral thalamic infarction. *Neurology* 42:163–169, 1992.
20. Nadeau SE, Crosson B: Subcortical aphasia. *Brain Lang.* In press.

Part 5
MEMORY AND AMNESIA

Chapter 35

AMNESIA: NEUROANATOMIC AND CLINICAL ASPECTS

Stuart Zola

A BRIEF HISTORY OF IDEAS ABOUT LOCALIZATION OF MEMORY

Ideas about the localization of memory in the brain can be divided roughly into three eras. The first era spans the period from antiquity to about the second century A.D. During this era, debate focused not on the issue of memory explicitly but on the location of the soul—i.e., what bodily organ was the source of all mental life. As recounted in Chap. 1, the two leading contenders were the heart and brain. By the time of Galen, in the second century A.D., the brain had been widely accepted as the organ of the mind. From the second to the eighteenth centuries, the issue was whether cognitive functions were localized either in the ventricular system of the brain or in the brain matter itself. Ventricular hypotheses had the support of the church, as the empty spaces of the ventricular system could contain ethereal spirits, and mind-brain dualism could therefore be maintained. Eventually, however, empirical science upheld the alternative view, according to which brain tissue itself was the material substrate of the mind. The third and current era of ideas about localization of brain function ranges from the nineteenth century to the present time. During this era, the debate has focused on how mental activities are organized in the brain. An early idea, which came to be known as the localizationist view, was that specific mental functions were carried out by specific parts of the brain. An alternative idea was that all parts of the brain were equally involved

in all mental activity and there was no specificity of function with respect to particular brain areas. This idea became known as the equipotential view.

Some of the most influential ideas about localization of brain function came from early-nineteenth-century localizationist Franz Joseph Gall (for a recent review of Gall's contributions to understanding brain organization, see Ref. 6). Two assumptions made by Gall are germane to the present discussion. They were that (1) the brain is the organ of all faculties, tendencies, and feelings ("the organ of the soul")[7] and (2) the brain is composed of as many particular organs as there are faculties, tendencies, and feelings. According to Gall, for a particular individual, the specific regions of the brain associated with especially prominent behaviors were enlarged, and these brain enlargements could be detected by prominences on the individual's cranium. Memory and other higher cognitive functions, for example, were located in the anterior portion of the brain (Fig. 35-1). As it turned out, Gall was wrong about most or all of the details regarding the regions of the brain associated with particular cognitive functions. He was correct, however, in his fundamental idea that specific parts of the brain support specific functions. A substantial portion of contemporary neuroscientific research and neuropsychological practice continues to be guided by this fundamental idea.

Nearly 100 years after Gall proposed that particular regions of the brain were specialized for processing particular kinds of information, evi-

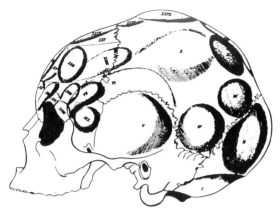

Figure 35-1

Gall's system of organology seen from the left side of the head. The organs were, for the most part, bilateral. Gall's 27 organs representing specific functions of the mind were divided into two groups. There were 19 organs common to humans and animals. Organ 11, the memory of things, memory of facts, refers to the ability to recall specific details of an event or item that distinguishes it from another event or item. Overall, Gall viewed memory not as a separate and fundamental faculty, but as secondary to each of the 27 faculties and organs. (From Zola-Morgan,[6] with permission.)

dence began to accumulate that linked a particular region of the brain, the medial temporal lobe, to memory function. Von Bechterew (1900)[8] presented postmortem neuropathologic findings from the brain of a 60-year-old man who had memory problems during the last part of his life. The patient's brain showed pathologic changes in the medial temporal lobe, including the hippocampal formation.

Following von Bechterew's finding, several other case studies were published that linked defects in memory to damage in the medial temporal lobe (e.g., Refs. 9 and 10). One of the best-known of these cases, that of patient H.M., was published during the 1950s.[11,12] Patient H.M. developed severe impairment in new learning following bilateral removal of the medial temporal lobe regions of his brain in order to treat intractable seizures. He has been studied extensively during the last 40 years. During this interval, his memory impairment has remained stable, and work with this pa-

tient has contributed substantially to our understanding of how memory is organized in the brain. Recent findings from magnetic resonance imaging studies of H.M. (at the age of 66) have determined that the bilateral lesion does not extend as far posteriorly as originally supposed; nevertheless, substantial portions of the hippocampal formation together with perirhinal cortex and entorhinal cortex are damaged bilaterally.[13]

NEUROPSYCHOLOGICAL ASPECTS OF AMNESIA

The impairment of new learning, or *anterograde amnesia*, is a defining attribute of organic amnesia. Severe anterograde amnesia will prevent patients from learning the facts of their hospitalization, the names and faces of clinical staff, and the routes linking their rooms and other locations around the hospital. Yet amnesic patients may have intact intellect as measured by standard psychometric tests (other than memory tests). Recently, it has also been established that certain forms of learning may be intact in amnesic patients, although conscious, explicit recollection is impaired. In addition to anterograde amnesia, most amnesic patients have some degree of *retrograde amnesia,* that is, impairment for memories acquired before their brain damage. The retrograde component of amnesia is most often temporally graded, with recently acquired memories more vulnerable than remote memories. The following chapter includes discussion of the nature of the information processing impairment in amnesia, including the nature of preserved learning in the anterograde component of amnesia and the temporal gradient in the retrograde component.

Assessment of memory impairment normally includes tests of verbal and nonverbal memory, which may be differentially affected in patients with unilateral lesions. Tests of new learning of verbal information generally take the form of lists that must be recalled or recognized (e.g., the California Auditory Verbal Learning Test[14]) or stories that must be recalled (e.g., the Logical Memory subtest of the Wechsler Memory Scale—Revised[15]). Visual learning is generally tested with either recall (by drawing) or multiple choice recognition of abstract designs (e.g., Benton Visual Retention Test[16]). For a fuller discussion of neuropsychological assessment of memory, see Ref. 17.

Development of an Animal Model of Human Amnesia

In 1978, an important study by Mishkin (1978)[18] signaled the development of a model of human amnesia in nonhuman primates. Work with the animal model has allowed us to identify with certainty structures within the medial temporal lobe that are important for memory and to begin to determine systematically how individual structures within the medial temporal lobe contribute to memory function.[19–22] In parallel with this work in monkeys, extensive neuropathologic information has recently been obtained from several well-studied amnesic patients whose damage was limited to the medial temporal lobe. The remainder of this chapter describes the findings from work in monkeys as well as from amnesic patients with medial temporal lobe damage and presents the implications of these findings for the organization of memory in the medial temporal lobe. The role in memory of other regions of the brain (e.g., the diencephalon) has recently been reviewed[23] and is not addressed here. In addition, findings from work with rats have been recently reviewed[24,25] and are also not addressed here.

In monkeys, bilateral lesions of the medial temporal lobe, intended to reproduce the surgical lesion sustained by amnesic patient H.M., produced many of the features of memory impairment in human amnesia.[22] As in human amnesia, the memory deficit in monkeys with damage to the medial temporal lobe occurred in both visual and tactual modalities,[26,27] and the deficit was exacerbated by distracting the animals during the retention interval.[28] Moreover, as in human amnesia, the monkeys with bilateral medial temporal lobe lesions showed certain preserved learning abilities.[29]

Trial-Unique Delayed Nonmatching-to-Sample

Task The work with monkeys has depended on several tasks known to be sensitive to human am-

nesia,[22] including retention of simple object discriminations and the simultaneous learning of multiple pairs of objects (eight-pair concurrent discrimination learning). The most widely used memory task has been trial-unique delayed nonmatching to sample.[30] In this test of recognition memory, the monkey first sees a sample object. Then, after a delay, the original object and a novel object are presented together, and the monkey must displace the novel object to obtain a food reward. New pairs of objects are used on each trial.

The validity of this task as a test of recognition memory was recently questioned, on the grounds that medial temporal lesions seemed to affect performance as much at short delays as at long delays (whereas a memory impairment should be manifest primarily at long delays).[31] However, this conclusion was not based on studies designed to compare short and long retention intervals. When appropriate experimental designs are used, the impairment is indeed confined to long-delay conditions, consistent with the memory performance of amnesic patients.[31a,31b]

Identification of a Memory System in the Medial Temporal Lobe

A difficulty in the work with both monkeys and humans has been a long-standing imprecision with respect to the terminology used to describe the components of the medial temporal lobe. In particular, the term *hippocampus* is sometimes used interchangeably to refer to the cell fields of the hippocampus proper and sometimes to a more extensive region that includes the hippocampus proper as well as the dentate gyrus or the subicular complex. In the present chapter, the following terminology is used in reference to particular components of the medial temporal lobe memory system in both monkeys and humans: The term *hippocampus* includes the cell fields of the hippocampus proper and the dentate gyrus; the term *hippocampal region* includes the hippocampus proper, the dentate gyrus, and the subicular region; and the term *hippocampal formation* includes the hippocampal region and the entorhinal cortex.

Research in monkeys and humans has identified a system of anatomically related structures in the medial temporal lobe that is important for memory (for reviews, see Refs. 19, 21, 23, 32). The medial temporal lobe system is necessary for establishing long-term declarative memory—i.e., the capacity for conscious recollection of facts and events[33] (another term used to describe this kind of memory is *explicit memory*). This system is not required for short-term memory or for a variety of nondeclarative (or implicit) forms of learning, whereby acquired information is expressed through performance (see Chap. 36). This system comprises the hippocampal region and cortical areas adjacent to the hippocampal region (Fig. 35-2). The cortex adjacent to the hippocampal region includes the entorhinal, perirhinal, and parahippocampal cortices. All of these cortical areas are anatomically related to the hippocampal re-

Figure 35-2

A schematic view of the medial temporal lobe memory system. The entorhinal cortex is the major source of projections to the hippocampal region. Nearly two-thirds of the cortical input to the entorhinal cortex originates in the adjacent perirhinal and parahippocampal cortices, which, in turn, receive projections from unimodal and polymodal areas in the frontal, temporal, and parietal lobes. The entorhinal cortex also receives other direct inputs from orbital frontal cortex, cingulate cortex, insular cortex, and superior temporal gyrus. All these projections are reciprocal. (From Zola-Morgan et al.,[42] with permission.)

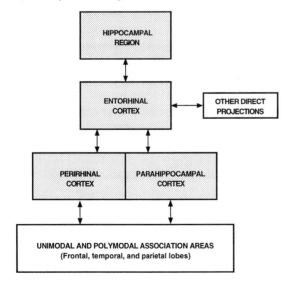

gion.[34–39] In particular, the perirhinal cortex and the parahippocampal cortex provide nearly two-thirds of the cortical input to the entorhinal cortex.[38,39] The entorhinal cortex, in turn, provides the major source of cortical projections to the hippocampus and dentate gyrus.[35,39]

The following sections briefly review the findings that have led to three important and interrelated ideas about the role of the medial temporal lobe system in memory function: (1) the severity of memory impairment depends on the locus and extent of damage within the medial temporal lobe memory system, (2) the hippocampal region is itself important for memory, and (3) the cortical regions of the medial temporal lobe memory system (i.e., the entorhinal, perirhinal, and parahippocampal cortices) themselves play an essential role in memory.

1.   Relation between severity of memory impairment and the locus and extent of damage within the medial temporal lobe memory system.

Work with monkeys and humans has led to the idea that the severity of memory impairment increases as more components of the medial temporal lobe memory system are damaged. This idea has been supported by a large number of individual studies in monkeys where performance on memory tasks by groups of monkeys with varying damage to the medial temporal lobe has been compared (for example, see Refs. 18, 40, and 41). We recently took advantage of cumulated data from more than 10 years of testing monkeys to examine the relationship between severity of memory impairment and extent of damage in the medial temporal lobe.[42] The memory performance in three groups of monkeys with differing extents of damage to the medial temporal lobe memory system was compared to the memory performance in a group of 10 normal monkeys (Fig. 35-3). All of the monkeys had completed testing on our standard memory battery, and all monkeys had been tested on the tasks in the same order. Performance measures from each of the 30 monkeys were converted to *z* scores, so that different performance measures could be averaged together.

The main finding was that the severity of memory impairment depended on the locus and

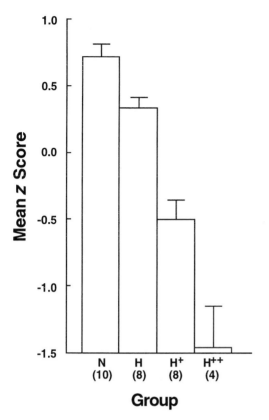

Figure 35–3

Mean z scores based on the data from four measures of memory for 10 normal monkeys (group N); 8 monkeys with damage limited to the hippocampus proper, the dentate gyrus, and the subicular complex (group H); 8 monkeys with damage that also included the adjacent entorhinal and parahippocampal cortices (group H+); and 4 monkeys in which the H+ lesion was extended forward to include the anterior entorhinal cortex and the perirhinal cortex (group H++). As more components of the medial temporal lobe were included in the lesion, the severity of memory impairment increased. All between-group comparisons were statistically significant. Group H consisted of monkeys from two different studies, i.e., 4 monkeys with ischemic damage limited to the hippocampal region[47] and 4 monkeys with stereotaxic radiofrequency lesions limited to the hippocampal region.[41] Both groups exhibited significant and long-lasting memory impairment when evaluated in their respective studies using our standard battery of memory tasks; both groups performed better overall than the H+ group, and the two H groups were not statistically different from each other.[42] Error bars indicate standard errors of the mean. (From Zola-Morgan et al.,[42] with permission.)

extent of damage within the medial temporal lobe memory system (Fig. 35-3). Damage limited to the hippocampal region (group H) caused significant memory impairment. More severe memory impairment occurred following H damage that included the adjacent entorhinal and parahippocampal cortex (group H+). The severity of impairment was greater still following H damage that also included all the adjacent cortical regions—i.e., the perirhinal, entorhinal, and parahippocampal cortices (group H++).

The finding that monkeys with damage that included the hippocampal region together with adjacent cortical regions (groups H+ and H++) exhibited more severe impairment than monkeys with damage limited to the hippocampal region (group H) emphasizes the importance for memory function of the adjacent cortical regions. Indeed, the damage to these cortical regions likely contributes substantially to the severe memory impairment produced by medial temporal lobe lesions in monkeys and in humans.[23] It is important to note that the findings just described cannot be attributed to a principle like mass action.[43] That is, the severity of memory impairment exhibited by the monkeys with H++ lesions was not simply due to the fact that they had more damage overall than the monkeys with H+ lesions. When the H+ lesion was extended forward to include the amygdala (the H+A lesion), the memory impairment associated with the H+ lesion was not increased.[57] Thus, it is not just the extent of damage in the medial temporal lobe that is critical but which specific structures are damaged.[41]

2.   The role in memory of the hippocampal region.

In the retrospective study just described, the finding of impairment in monkeys in group H supports the view that the hippocampus itself is critical for memory function. The finding of impaired memory following bilateral damage limited to the hippocampal region in monkeys is consistent with findings from human amnesia. As described later in this chapter, during the last several years, post-mortem material from four well-studied cases of human amnesia associated with damage limited to the hippocampal region or damage limited to the hippocampal formation (i.e., the hippocampal region together with the entorhinal cortex) have become available.[44–46a]

An important issue about ischemic or anoxic damage is whether the damage indentifiable in histopathologic examination provides an accurate estimate of direct neural damage. For instance, additional direct damage might be present that is sufficient to disrupt neuronal function in areas important for memory and sufficient to impair behavioral performance but not sufficient to progress to cell death and to be detectable in histopathology. In our work with monkeys we have been able to address this issue directly by developing an animal model of cerebral ischemia in the monkey using a noninvasive technique that involves 15 min of carotid occlusion together with pharmacologically induced hypotension. This procedure reliably produced detectable damage only in the CA1 and CA2 cell fields of the hippocampus and in the hilar region of the dentate gyrus. There was no detectable damage elsewhere in the brain.[47] The behavioral result was that the ischemic group performed similarly to a group with a known surgical lesion of the hippocampal region (the H lesion) and significantly better than the H[+] and H[++] lesion groups. Thus, the available data do not support the idea that covert damage occurs sufficiently following global ischemia to contribute to memory impairment. The data suggest instead that the severity of memory impairment in monkeys and humans with ischemic damage is about what would be predicted from the damage that can be detected histopathologically and can be comparable to the impairment that results from histopathologically similar neurosurgical lesions.

The finding of impaired memory following bilateral damage limited to the hippocampal region and the hippocampal formation has also been reported for rats (for reviews see Refs. 25 and 48). Accordingly, the finding from rats, monkeys, and humans, are in good correspondence.[33] Damage limited to the hippocampal region and the hippocampal formation in all three species can produce significant and long-lasting memory impairment.

3. Memory and the entorhinal, perirhinal, and parahippocampal cortices.

Work with monkeys has led to the idea that the cortical regions of the medial temporal lobe (i.e., the perirhinal, entorhinal, and parahippocampal cortices), either separately or together, must themselves contribute to memory function, presumably by virtue of their extensive reciprocal connections with widespread regions of neocortex.[35–37,39,49] Straightforward evidence for the possible importance of the cortical regions came from studies in which direct circumscribed damage has been caused to the perirhinal, entorhinal, or parahippocampal cortices, either separately or in combination.[27,40,50–53] For example, monkeys with combined lesions of the perirhinal and parahippocampal cortices (the PRPH lesion) exhibited severely impaired performance on both a visual[27,40] and tactual[27] version of the delayed nonmatching-to-sample task. Moreover, the monkeys with PRPH lesions continued to exhibit impaired performance when retested on the visual version of the delayed nonmatching-to-sample task approximately 2 years after surgery.[27]

More limited lesions of the cortical regions also produce memory impairment. Monkeys with bilateral lesions limited to the perirhinal cortex exhibit impaired memory.[52,54] Moreover, damage to perirhinal cortex can produce more substantial impairment on the delayed nonmatching-to-sample task than damage to any other single component of the medial temporal lobe memory system.[52,53] In addition, the memory impairment following perirhinal lesions is long-lasting.[54]

Monkeys with bilateral lesions limited to the entorhinal cortex exhibited impaired memory,[50,52,53] and the impairment occurred in both visual and tactile modalities.[50] Overall, however, the impairment following entorhinal damage was less severe than that following perirhinal damage. In addition, the impairment following entorhinal damage is transient. Monkeys with bilateral entorhinal lesions were impaired on the delayed nonmatching-to-sample task when tested postoperatively, but they were not impaired when they were retested on the same task 9 to 14 months after surgery.[53] This finding suggests that while entorhinal cortex may normally participate in tasks that are dependent on the medial temporal lobe system, entorhinal cortex might not, in itself, be essential for the kinds of memory tasks used in the studies just described—e.g., the delayed nonmatching-to-sample task.

The effects in monkeys of damage limited to the parahippocampal cortex have not yet been systematically studied. Preliminary work from monkeys with bilateral parahippocampal cortex lesions has suggested that the parahippocampal cortex might not play an important role in object-recognition memory as measured by the delayed nonmatching-to-sample task or in other visual memory tasks.[54,55]

It is useful to note that the findings from monkeys with circumscribed lesions of the cortical regions need to be evaluated in the context of their neuroanatomic connectivity. That is, it is reasonable to suppose that the individual cortical regions might make different contributions to memory. This idea follows from the fact that information from neocortex enters the medial temporal lobe memory system at different points. For example, perirhinal cortex, unlike parahippocampal cortex, receives rather strong projections from unimodal visual area TE.[39,56] Parahippocampal cortex, but not perirhinal cortex, receives inputs from parietal cortex.[31,39] In this sense it could be supposed that perirhinal cortex might play a greater role than parahippocampal cortex in visual memory, while parahippocampal cortex might play a greater role than perirhinal cortex in spatial memory.

By this view, the finding that lesions of the perirhinal cortex have thus far been reported to have a greater disruptive effect on memory than lesions of the entorhinal or parahippocampal cortex must be tempered by the fact that most of the tasks that have been used to evaluate the effects of damage to the cortical regions have been tasks of visual object memory. While recent findings point to the importance of the cortical regions adjacent to the hippocampal region, it will be important to evaluate the effects of damage to these cortical regions using a variety of tasks in addition to visual object memory.

It is instructive at this point to address the role of two additional brain regions that have been linked to memory function, i.e., the amygdala and the temporal stem. A major point of view during the last decade was that both the hippocampal formation and the amygdala had to be damaged conjointly to produce severe and long-lasting memory impairment in human and monkeys (e.g., Ref. 18). During the last decade, a different conclusion has been reached, based on experimental work.[21,32] A key breakthrough was the development of a procedure for making circumscribed bilateral lesions of the amygdala by a stereotaxic approach that spared surrounding cortex (i.e., the entorhinal and perirhinal cortices). Complete bilateral lesions of the amygdala made by this method did not impair performance on four different memory tasks, including delayed nonmatching to sample.[57] Moreover, extending a lesion of the hippocampal formation forward to include circumscribed damage to the amygdala did not exacerbate the memory impairment that followed lesions of the hippocampal formation alone.[57]

These findings showed that severe memory impairment, of the kind exhibited in human amnesia, depends on damage to the hippocampal formation and adjacent anatomically related cortex (specifically, the perirhinal, entorhinal, and parahippocampal cortices; see Fig. 35-2). One or more of these cortical regions had always been damaged in the earlier studies during the surgical approach ordinarily used to remove the amygdala. A consensus has now been reached about the role of the amygdala.[23,32] (It is also important to note that this consensus is compatible with the idea that the amygdala plays an important role in certain kinds of memory, including conditioned fear and other forms of affective memory;[58–62] see Chap. 54.)

Separate studies in monkeys have also evaluated the effects on memory of separate lesions of the "temporal stem," a fiber system that lies superficial to the hippocampal region. This fiber system links temporal neocortex with subcortical regions, and it had been proposed to be the critical structure damaged in temporal lobe amnesia.[63] However, monkeys with lesions of the temporal stem were not amnesic.[64] Moreover, the recent imaging study of patient H.M.[13] indicates that the temporal stem was not damaged, as originally supposed.[65]

New Cases of Human Amnesia with Lesions Limited to the Hippocampal Formation

As described previously, the findings from formal memory testing of patient H.M., as well as from other patients with less extensive bilateral medial temporal lobe removal, led to the view that damage to the medial temporal lobe and, in particular, the region of the hippocampus was responsible for the amnesia.[66] Damage to the hippocampus was also linked to memory impairments associated with a variety of neurologic conditions, including viral encephalitis,[67,68] posterior cerebral artery occlusion,[69] and hypoxic ischemia.[70] In addition, several single case studies had attributed impaired memory to hippocampal damage (e.g., Refs. 71–75). However, in these cases memory function was sometimes not assessed in a systematic way, and damage often extended beyond the hippocampus and involved other medial temporal lobe regions. Thus, although these cases in humans substantiated the importance in memory functions of the medial temporal lobe, they left some uncertainty as to whether lesions limited to the hippocampus were sufficient to cause amnesia. In the following sections, several new case studies are described where damage has been limited either to the hippocampal region or to the hippocampal formation.

Damage Restricted Primarily to the Hippocampal Region In 1986, we reported a case of amnesia in a patient (R.B.) who developed memory impairment following an episode of ischemia associated with cardiac surgery.[76] Following this episode, patient R.B. exhibited a marked anterograde memory impairment that remained unchanged until his death 5 years later. He showed minimal retrograde amnesia and no signs of cognitive impairment other than memory. Thorough histologic examination revealed that the only damage that could reasonably be associated with the memory defect was a circumscribed bilateral lesion involving the entire CA1 field of the hippocampus. This was the first reported case of amnesia following a lesion limited to the hippocampus in which extensive neuropathologic and neuropsychological information was available.

Recently, an additional case of amnesia with damage limited to the CA1 field of the hippocampus has become available (patient G.D.[45,46,46a]). Patient G.D. became amnesic in 1983 at the age of 43. The event that precipitated his amnesia was a hypotensive episode that occurred during major

---

Figure 35–4

(Top left panel) *Coronal section through the left hippocampal region of a normal human brain stained for Nissl bodies.* (Top right panel) *Coronal section through the left hippocampal region of patient G.D. The lesion includes most of the cells in the CA1 region (marked by arrowheads). The subiculum sustained slight cell loss bilaterally.* (Bottom left panel) *Coronal section through the right hippocampal region of patient L.M. Note the complete loss of CA3 pyramidal cells and the nearly complete loss of CA1 pyramidal cells. The CA2 field is partially intact (arrowheads). There was also extensive loss of cells in the hilar region of the dentate gyrus (arrows), and the entorhinal cortex demonstrated some cell loss.* (Bottom right panel) *Coronal section through W.H.'s right hippocampal region. Extensive pyramidal cell loss is evident in cell fields CA1 and CA3. Less substantial cell loss occurred in field CA2. The dentate gyrus appears very abnormal, with dispersion of the granule cells and complete loss of polymorphic cells. Patchy cell loss is evident in the subiculum and there was patchy cell loss in the entorhinal cortex as well.* Abbreviations: *CA1, CA2 CA3 = cell fields of the hippocampus; DG = dentate gyrus; EC = entorhinal cortex; gl = granular layer; ml = molecular layer; PaS = parasubiculum; pl = polymorphic layer; PrS = presubiculum; S = subiculum.*

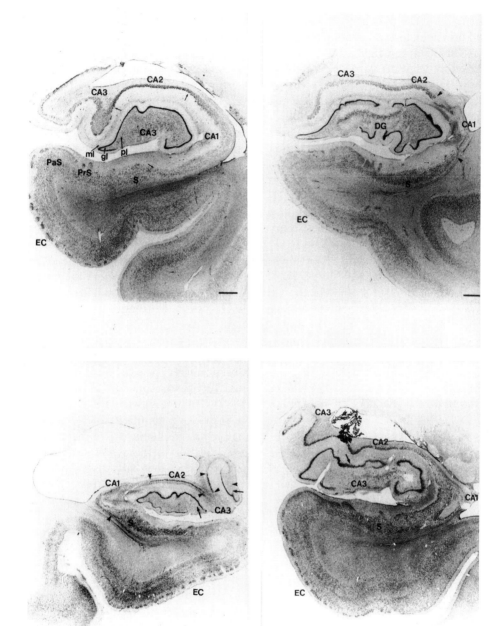

surgery. Patient G.D., like patient R.B., had damage restricted primarily to the CA1 region of the hippocampus (Fig. 35-4, top right panel). Patient G.D. was studied for 9.5 years until his death from congestive heart failure.

Patients R.B. and G.D. exhibited about the same degree of memory impairment in the anterograde domain. Their scores were similar across a range of anterograde memory tasks, including paired associate learning, where subjects were given three consecutive trials to learn 10 unrelated word pairs (maximum score = 30; R.B. = 1, G.D. = 5; and control subjects = 22) and diagram recall where subjects first copied a complex figure and then, without forewarning, were asked to reproduce it from memory 10 to 20 min later (maximum score for delay test = 36; R.B. = 3; G.D. = 7; and control subjects = 20.6).

Retrograde memory—i.e., memory for events that occurred before the onset of amnesia—was also evaluated in the patients. Descriptions of the tests of retrograde memory and the data for the patients described here have been published previously.[76,77–81] Overall, patients R.B. and G.D. exhibited little evidence of retrograde amnesia.[45,46,46a,76]

Finally, Victor and Agamanolis reported another case of amnesia which developed after a series of generalized seizures, the lesion involved all the fields of the hippocampus and the dentate gyrus.[81] Little neuropsychological data concerning anterograde and retrograde deficits were provided for this case, but the severity of memory impairment described in the report seemed greater than that observed in patients R.B and G.D.

Damage Involving the Hippocampal Formation   Patient L.M. became amnesic in 1984 at the age of 54.[46,46a,47] The precipitating event was a series of closely occurring generalized seizures and associated respiratory distress and respiratory acidosis. Patient L.M. had more extensive damage to the hippocampal region than did patients R.B. or G.D. His lesion involved all of the CA fields of the hippocampal region as well as the dentate gyrus (Fig. 35-4, lower left panel). In addition, patient L.M. evidenced some loss of cells in entorhinal cortex. Patient L.M. was studied for 6 years follow-

ing the onset of his amnesia until his death from lung cancer.

Patient L.M.'s performance on individual tests of anterograde memory was similar to the performance of the other two patients (paired associate learning = 5; delay test for diagram recall = 6). However, because patient G.D. had the least education and a low IQ, it was not possible to rank order with confidence the severity of anterograde amnesia in R.B., G.D., and L.M.

On tests of retrograde amnesia, patient L.M. showed a clearly different pattern of performance than the other two patients. While patients R.B. and G.D. evidenced little retrograde memory impairment, patient L.M. demonstrated extensive retrograde amnesia. For example, in a test of autobiographical memory where memories were produced in response to 75 single-word cues,[78] patient G.D. produced episodes from both recent and remote decades in a pattern similar to the responses of normal subjects and showed no evidence of retrograde amnesia. Patient L.M., however, produced mostly episodes from before 1950, and he had very few recollections from the 1960s to the 1980s. The findings from this test and other tests of retrograde memory indicate that patient L.M. had extensive, temporally graded retrograde amnesia (i.e., his memory was poorer for events close to the time of the onset of his amnesia and better for events more remote from the time of onset of amnesia), and his retrograde memory deficit extended back for at least 15 years.[45,46,46a]

Patient W.H. became amnesic during several days in March 1985 at the age of 63.[46,46a] The precise etiology of his amnesia is not clear. The damage in patient W.H. was more extensive than in the previously described patients and involved all of the components of the hippocampal region including the subicular complex (Fig. 35-4, lower right panel). In addition, W.H.'s entorhinal cortex sustained some cell loss. W.H. was studied for 7.5 years until he developed end-stage emphysema in 1993.

Patient W.H.'s anterograde memory impairment was somewhat greater than that of the other patients. On paired associate learning, he obtained a score of 0, and on the delay test of diagram recall he obtained a score of 1. On tests of retrograde

Figure 35-5
(Left panel) *Summary of overall findings from patients R.B., G.D., L.M., and W.H. on tests of anterograde memory (anterograde amnesia) and retrograde memory (retrograde amnesia).* (Right panel) *Summary of brain damage in the medial temporal lobe for each patient.*

	Anterograde Amnesia	Retrograde Amnesia	Damage to the Hippocampal Formation
RB	moderate	minimal	CA1 field
GD	moderate	minimal (?)	CA1 field
LM	moderate	extensive	CA1, CA2, CA3 fields, dentate gyrus (entorhinal cortex)
WH	severe	extensive	CA1, CA2, CA3 fields, dentate gyrus, subiculum, entorhinal cortex

memory, patient W.H. performed like patient L.M. That is, he had a severe retrograde memory deficit, and he demonstrated temporally graded retrograde amnesia that extended back at least 15 years.[45,46,46a]

Anterograde Amnesia: The Relationship between Severity of Impairment and Extent of Damage in the Medial Temporal Lobe

Figure 35-5 summarizes the neuropsychological and the neuropathologic information for patients R.B., G.D., L.M., and W.H. The findings from these patients make two important points with respect to anterograde amnesia. First, the findings from patients R.B., G.D., and L.M. underscore the fact that damage limited mainly to the hippocampal region is sufficient to produce clinically significant and long-lasting anterograde memory impairment. (L.M. did have some cell loss in entorhinal cortex.) As described in previous sections, significant memory impairment has also been shown in monkeys and rats when damage is limited to the hippocampal region.[41,47,48] These findings, therefore, support the long-standing idea that the hippocampal region itself is important for memory.

Second, patients R.B., G.D., and L.M. , with damage limited primarily to the hippocampal region, demonstrated less severe memory impairment overall than patient W.H. or patient H.M., both of whom sustained additional damage. In the case of W.H., the additional damage involved the subicular complex; in the case of H.M., the addi-

tional damage involved the entorhinal and perirhinal cortices.[65] The findings from work with amnesic patients, like the findings in work with monkeys with medial temporal lobe lesions,[42] indicate that memory impairment can be exacerbated when damage includes cortical regions adjacent to the hippocampal region. Thus, findings from the work with amnesic patients are consistent with ideas that have been developed from work with monkeys—i.e., that the severity of memory impairment depends on the locus and extent of damage to the medial temporal lobe and that the cortical regions adjacent to the hippocampal region are themselves important for memory.[42,82]

Retrograde Amnesia: The Relationship between Severity of Impairment and Extent of Damage in the Medial Temporal Lobe

It has rarely been possible to study retrograde amnesia in patients with selective, histologically confirmed damage. The findings from the several patients described here provide important information about several aspects of retrograde amnesia. With respect to the relationship between severity of retrograde amnesia and the extent of damage in the medial temporal lobe, it appears that damage limited to the CA1 field does not produce severe or temporally graded retrograde amnesia (patients R.B. and D.G.). When the damage involves more than the CA1 field, however, extensive, temporally graded retrograde amnesia can occur (patients L.M., W.H., and the case report of Victor and Agamanolis,[81] as well as case H.M.[12]).

The findings from the patients described here also begin to address long-standing questions about the relationship between retrograde amnesia and anterograde amnesia. The impairments in the patients presented here as well as findings from other amnesic patients suggest that retrograde amnesia and anterograde amnesia can be caused by damage to the same region—i.e., the hippocampal formation. While anterograde and retrograde memory are both normally dependent on the integrity of the hippocampal formation, it appears that anterograde memory can be more easily disrupted than retrograde memory (e.g., a lesion of the CA1 field is sufficient to produce significant anterograde memory impairment). As described above, retrograde amnesia, like anterograde amnesia, can vary in its severity as a function of the extent of damage to the hippocampal formation.

Finally, the finding that very remote memories are typically preserved in amnesic patients means that the site of permanent memory storage cannot be the hippocampal formation or any of the other damaged structures in the medial temporal lobe. Thus, while the hippocampal formation is critically involved in the formation of new memories, it has been supposed that the hippocampal formation and related structures must have only a temporary role in memory storage.[23,33,83] That is, the medial temporal lobe memory system has only a temporary role in the formation and maintenance of declarative memory. After learning, memory is gradually reorganized over time. It is initially dependent on this system, but its role diminishes as more permanent memory is established elsewhere, presumably in neocortex.[83]

It is important to note that some memory-impaired patients have extensive retrograde amnesia with no evidence of a temporal gradient.[84] In such cases, remote memory appears to be severely and similarly impaired across all time periods. One possibility is that severe and ungraded retrograde amnesia requires damage in addition to (or different from) that to the medial temporal lobe structures associated with circumscribed amnesia. This additional damage might impair performance on remote memory tests without contributing propor-

tionally to anterograde amnesia. Additional neuropsychological and anatomic information will be needed to identify the determinants of ungraded retrograde amnesia and to confirm that ungraded forms of retrograde amnesia are dissociable from anterograde memory impairment.

OVERVIEW

In concluding, it is useful to underscore that work in monkeys (specifically, the finding that the severity of memory impairment increases as more components of the medial temporal lobe memory system are damaged) is fully consistent with findings from human amnesia. The moderately severe memory impairment in the patients described above who had damage limited to the hippocampal formation can be contrasted with the more severe memory impairment observed in patient H.M., who sustained bilateral resection of the medial temporal lobe, including the hippocampal region and adjacent cortical regions.[65]

For the last 100 years, amnesia has been associated with damage to several regions of the brain. Among these are the amygdala, hippocampal region, and cortex adjacent to the hippocampal region in the medial temporal lobe, and the mammillary nuclei and medial thalamus in the diencephalon. Until recently, it has remained unclear, however, whether damage confined to any of these structures would produce a clinically significant memory impairment. At the present time, the findings from work in three species—rats, monkeys, and humans—share many points of correspondence with the findings from monkeys with medial temporal lobe lesions. In particular, the findings show that circumscribed bilateral lesions limited to the hippocampal region are sufficient to produce amnesia. Additional findings indicate that the cortical regions adjacent to and anatomically linked to the hippocampal region—i.e., the perirhinal, entorhinal, and parahippocampal cortices—are also important for memory function.

ACKNOWLEDGMENTS

This work was supported by the Medical Research Service of the Department of Veterans Affairs and

NIH Grant 19063. I thank Larry R. Squire for his contributions to this work.

REFERENCES

1. McHenry LC Jr: *Garrison's History of Neurology.* Springfield, IL, Charles C Thomas, 1969.
2. Finger S: *Origins of Neuroscience: A History of Explorations into Brain Function.* New York, Oxford University Press, 1994.
3. Gross CG: Early history of neuroscience, in Edelman G (ed): *Encyclopedia of Neuroscience.* Boston, Birkhauser, 1987.
4. Baader J: Observationes medicae, incisionibus cadaverum anatomicis illustrae, in Sandifort E (ed): *Thesaurus Dissertationum* 3:1–62, 1762 (in Latin).
5. Clendening L: *Source Book of Medical History.* New York, Dover, 1942.
6. Zola-Morgan S: Localization of brain function: The legacy of Franz Joseph Gall (1758–1828). *Annu Rev Neurosci* 18:359–383, 1995.
7. Gall FJ: *Sur les Fonctions du Cerveau.* Paris, Shoell, 1822 (in French).
8. von Bechterew W: Demonstration eines Gehirns mit Zerstörung der vorderen und inneren Theile der Hirnrinde beider Schlaffenlappen. *Neurol Zentralb* 19:990–991, 1900.
9. Grunthal E: Über das klinische Bild nach umschriebenem beiderseitigam Ausfall der Ammonshornrinde. *Monatsschr Psychiatrie Neurol* 113:1–16, 1947.
10. Glees P, Griffith HB: Bilateral destruction of the hippocampus (cornu ammonis) in a case of dementia. *Psychiatry Neurol Med Psychol (Leipz)* 123:193–204, 1952.
11. Scoville WB: The limbic lobe and memory in man. *J Neurosurg* 11:64, 1954.
12. Scoville WB, Milner B: Loss of recent memory after bilateral hippocampal lesions. *J Neurol Neurosurg Psychiatry* 20:11–21, 1957.
13. Corkin S, Amaral DG, Johnson KA, Kyman BT: H.M.'s MRI scan shows sparing of the posterior half of the hippocampus and parahippocampal gyrus. *J Neurosci.* In press.
14. Deus DC, Kramer JH, Kaplan E, Ober BA: *California Verbal Learning Test Manual.* San Antonio, The Psychological Corporation, 1987.
15. Wechsler D: *Wecshsler Memory Scale—Revised.* New York, The Psychological Corporation, 1987.
16. Benton AL: *The Revised Visual Retention Test,* 4th ed. New York, The Psychological Corporation, 1974.
17. Lezak MD: *Neuropsychological Assessment,* 2d ed. New York, Oxford University Press, 1987.
18. Mishkin M: Memory in monkeys severely impaired by combined but not separate removal of the amygdala and hippocampus. *Nature* 273:297–298, 1978.
19. Mishkin M: A memory system in the monkey. *Phil Trans R Soc Lond* 98:85–95, 1982.
20. Mahut H, Moss M: Consolidation of memory: The hippocampus revisited, in Squire LR, Butters N (eds): *Neuropsychology of Memory.* New York, Guilford, 1984, pp 297–315.
21. Squire LR, Zola-Morgan S: The medial temporal lobe memory system. *Science* 253:1380–1386, 1991.
22. Squire LR, Zola-Morgan S, Chen K: Human amnesia and animal models of amnesia: Performance of amnesic patients on tests designed for the monkey. *Behav Neurosci* 11:210–221, 1988.
23. Zola-Morgan S, Squire LR: Neuroanatomy of memory. *Annu Rev Neurosci* 16:547–563, 1993.
24. Eichenbaum H, Otto T, Cohen NJ: The hippocampus—What does it do? *Behav Neural Biol* 57:2–36, 1992.
25. Jarrard LE: On the role of the hippocampus in learning and memory in the rat. *Behav Neural Biol* 60:9–26, 1993.
26. Murray EA, Mishkin M: Severe tactual as well as visual memory deficits follow combined removal of the amygdala and hippocampus in monkeys. *J Neurosci* 4:2565–2580, 1984.
27. Suzuki WA, Zola-Morgan S, Squire LR, Amaral DG: Lesions of the perirhinal and parahippocampal cortices in the monkey produce long-lasting memory impairment in the visual and tactual modalities. *J Neurosci* 13:2430–2451, 1993.
28. Zola-Morgan S, Squire LR: Medial temporal lesions in monkeys impair memory on a variety of tasks sensitive to human amnesia. *Behav Neurosci* 99:22–34, 1985.
29. Zola-Morgan S, Squire LR: Preserved learning in monkeys with medial temporal lobe lesions: Sparing of motor and cognitive skills. *J Neurosci* 4:1072–1085, 1984.
30. Mishkin M, Delacour J: An analysis of short-term visual memory in the monkey. *J Exp Psychol* 1:326–334, 1975.
31. Ringo JL: Memory decays at the same rate in macaques with and without brain lesions when expressed in d' or arcsine terms. *Behav Brain Res* 42:123–134, 1991.
31a. Alvarez-Royo P, Zola-Morgan S, Squire LR:

Impairment of long-term memory and sparing of short-term memory in monkeys with medial temporal lobe lesions: A reply to Ringo. *Behav Brain Res* 52:1–5, 1992.

31b. Alvarez-Royo P, Zola-Morgan S, Squire LR: The animal model of human amnesia: Long-term memory impaired and short-term memory intact. *Proc Nat Acad Sci* 91:5637–5641, 1994.

32. Murray EA: Medial temporal lobe structures contributing to recognition memory: The amygdaloid complex versus the rhinal cortex, in Aggleton JP (ed): *The Amygdala: Neurobiological Aspects of Emotion, Memory, and Mental Dysfunction.* New York, Wiley-Liss, 1992, pp 453–470.

33. Squire LR: Declarative and nondeclarative memory: Multiple brain systems supporting learning and memory. *J Cogn Neurosci* 4:232–243, 1992.

34. Van Hoesen G: The parahippocampal gyrus: New observations regarding its cortical connections in the monkey. *Trends Neurosci* 5:345–350, 1982.

35. Van Hoesen GW, Pandya DN: Some connections of the entorhinal (area 28) and perirhinal (area 35) cortices of the rhesus monkey: I. Temporal lobe afferents. *Brain Res* 95:1–24, 1975.

36. Van Hoesen GW, Pandya DN: Some connections of the entorhinal (area 28) and perirhinal (area 35) cortices of the rhesus monkey. III. Efferent connections. *Brain Res* 95:39–59, 1975.

37. Van Hoesen GW, Pandya DN, Butters N: Some connections of the entorhinal (area 28) and perirhinal (area 35) cortices of the rhesus monkey. II. Frontal lobe afferents. *Brain Res* 95:25–38, 1975.

38. Insausti R, Amaral DG, Cowan WM: The entorhinal cortex of the monkey: II. Cortical afferents. *J Comp Neurol* 264:356–395, 1987.

39. Suzuki WA, Amaral DG: Perirhinal and parahippocampal cortices of the macaque monkey: Cortical afferents. *J Comp Neurol* 350:497–533, 1994.

40. Zola-Morgan S, Squire LR, Amaral DG, Suzuki WA: Lesions of perirhinal and parahippocampal cortex that spare the amygdala and hippocampal formation produce severe memory impairment. *J Neurosci* 9:4355–4370, 1989.

41. Alvarez P, Zola-Morgan S, Squire LR: Damage limited to the hippocampal region produces long-lasting memory impairment in monkeys. *J Neurosci* 15:3796–3807, 1995.

42. Zola-Morgan S, Squire LR, Ramus SJ: Severity of memory impairment in monkeys as a function of locus and extent of damage within the medial temporal lobe memory system. *Hippocampus* 4:483–494, 1994.

43. Lashley KS: *Brain Mechanisms and Intelligence: A Quantitative Study of Injuries to the Brain.* Chicago, University of Chicago Press, 1929.

44. Zola S, Squire LR: Human amnesia and the medial temporal lobe, in Kato N (ed): *Functions and Clinical Relevance of the Hippocampus.* New York, Elsevier, 1996.

45. Rempel-Clower NL, Zola-Morgan S, Squire LR: Damage to the hippocampal region in human amnesia: Neuropsychological and neuroanatomical findings from two new cases. *Soc Neurosci Abstr* 24:1975, 1994.

46. Rempel-Clower NL, Zola-Morgan S, Squire LR: Importance of the hippocampal region and entorhinal cortex in human memory: Neuropsychological and neuropathological findings from a new patient. *Soc Neurosci Abstr* 25:1493, 1995.

46a. Rempel-Clower N, Zola-Morgan S, Squire LR, Amaral DG: Three cases of enduring memory impairment following bilateral damage limited to the hippocampal formation. *J Neurosci* Submitted.

47. Zola-Morgan S, Squire LR, Rempel NL, et al: Enduring memory impairment in monkeys after ischemic damage to the hippocampus. *J Neurosci* 9:4355–4370, 1992.

48. Jaffard R, Meunier M: Role of the hippocampal formation in learning and memory. *Hippocampus* 3:203–217, 1993.

49. Witter MP, Groenewegen HJ, Lopes da Silva FH, Lohman AHM: Functional organization of the extrinsic and intrinsic circuitry of the parahippocampal region. *Prog Neurobiol* 33:161–254, 1989.

50. Moss M, Mahut H, Zola-Morgan S: Concurrent discrimination learning of monkeys after hippocampal, entorhinal, or fornix lesions. *J Neurosci* 1:227–240, 1981.

51. Gaffan D, Murray EA: Monkeys (*M. fascicularis*) with rhinal cortex ablations succeed in object discrimination learning despite 24-hour intertrial intervals and fail at matching to sample despite double sample presentation. *Behav Neurosci* 106:30–38, 1992.

52. Meunier M, Bachevalier J, Mishkin M, Murray EA: Effects on visual recognition of combined and separate ablations of the entorhinal and perirhinal cortex in rhesus monkeys. *J Neurosci* 13:5418–5432, 1993.

53. Leonard BW, Amaral DG, Squire LR, Zola-Morgan S: Transient memory impairment in monkeys with bilateral lesions of the entorhinal cortex. *J Neurosci* 15:5637–5659, 1995.

54. Ramus SJ, Zola-Morgan S, Squire LR: Effects of lesions of perirhinal cortex or parahippocampal cor-

tex on memory in monkeys. *Soc Neurosci Abstr* 24:1074, 1994.

55. Horel JA, Pytko-Joiner E, Voytko ML, Salsbury K: The performance of visual tasks while segments of the inferotemporal cortex are suppressed by cold. *Behav Brain Res* 23:29–42, 1991.

56. Webster MJ, Ungerleider LG, Bachevalier J: Connections of inferior temporal areas TE and TEO with medial temporal-lobe structures in infant and adult monkeys. *J Neurosci* 11:1095–1116, 1991.

57. Zola-Morgan S, Squire LR, Amaral DG: Lesions of the amygdala that spare adjacent cortical regions do not impair memory or exacerbate the impairment following lesions of the hippocampal formation. *J Neurosci* 9:1922–1936, 1989.

58. Davis M: Pharmacological and anatomical analysis of fear conditioning using the fear-potentiated startle paradigm. *Behav Neurosci* 100:814–824, 1986.

59. Gallagher M, Graham PW, Holland P: The amygdala central nucleus and appetitive Pavlovian conditioning: Lesions impair one class of conditioned behavior. *J Neurosci* 10:1906–1911, 1990.

60. Kesner RP: Learning and memory in rats with an emphasis on the role of the amygdala, in Aggleton J (ed): *The Amygdala.* New York, Wiley, 1992, pp 379–400.

61. LeDoux J: Emotion, in Brookhart JM, Mountcastle VB (eds): *Handbook of Physiology: The Nervous System:* V. *Higher Functions of the Nervous System,* 5th ed. Bethesda, MD, American Physiological Society, 1987, pp 419–460.

62. McGaugh JL: Involvement of hormonal and neuromodulatory systems in the regulation of memory storage. *Annu Rev Neurosci* 12:255–287, 1989.

63. Horel JA: The neuroanatomy of amnesia. *Brain* 101:403–445, 1978.

64. Zola-Morgan S, Squire LR, Mishkin M: The neuroanatomy of amnesia: Amygdala-hippocampus versus temporal stem. *Science* 218:1337–1339, 1982.

65. Corkin S, Amaral DG, Johnson KA, Hyman BT: HM's MRI scan shows sparing of the posterior half of the hippocampus and parahippocampal gyrus. *J Neurosci.* In press.

66. Scoville WB, Milner B: Loss of recent memory after bilateral hippocampal lesions. *J Neurol Neurosurg Psychiatry* 20:11–21, 1957.

67. Damasio AR, Eslinger PJ, Damasio H, et al: Multimodal amnesic syndrome following bilateral temporal and basal forebrain damage. *Arch Neurol* 42:252–259, 1985.

68. Rose FC, Symonds CP: Persistent memory defect following encephalitis. *Brain* 83:195–212, 1960.

69. Benson DF, Marsden CD, Meadows JC: The amnesic syndrome of posterior cerebral artery occlusion. *Acta Neurol Scand* 50:133–145, 1974.

70. Volpe BT, Hirst W: The characterization of an amnesic syndrome following hypoxic ischemic injury. *Arch Neurol* 40:436–440, 1983.

71. Cummings JL, Tomiyasu U, Read S, Benson DF: Amnesia with hippocampal lesions after cardiopulmonary arrest. *Neurology* 34:679–681, 1984.

72. DeJong RN, Itabashi HH, Olson JR: "Pure" memory loss with hippocampal lesions: A case report. *Trans Am Neurol Assoc* 93:31–34, 1968.

73. Duyckaerts C, Derouesne C, Signoret JL, et al: Bilateral and limited amygdalohippocampal lesions causing a pure amnesic syndrome. *Ann Neurol* 18:314–319, 1985.

74. Muramoto O, Kuru Y, Sugishita M, Toyokura Y: Pure memory loss with hippocampal lesions: A pneumoencephalographic study. *Arch Neurol* 36:54–56, 1979.

75. Woods BT, Schoene W, Kneisley L: Are hippocampal lesions sufficient to cause lasting amnesia? *J Neurol Neurosurg Psychiatry* 45:243–247, 1982.

76. Zola-Morgan S, Squire LR, Amaral DG: Human amnesia and the medial temporal region: Enduring memory impairment following a bilateral lesions limited to field CA1 of the hippocampus. *J Neurosci* 6:2950–2967, 1986.

77. Squire LR, Haist F, Shimamura AP: The neurology of memory: Quantitative assessment of retrograde amnesia in two groups of amnesic patients. *J Neurosci* 9:828–839, 1989.

78. MacKinnon DF, Squire LR: Autobiographical memory and amnesia. *Psychobiology* 17:247–256, 1989.

79. Salmon DP, Lasker BR, Butters N, Beatty WW: Remote memory in a patient with circumscribed amnesia. *Brain Cogn* 7:201–211, 1988.

80. Beatty WW, Salmon DP, Bernstein N, Butters N: Remote memory in a patient with amnesia due to hypoxia. *Psychol Med* 17:657–665, 1987.

81. Victor M, Agamanolis D: Amnesia due to lesions confined to the hippocampus: A clinico-pathologic study. *J Cogn Neurosci* 2:246–257, 1990.

82. Mishkin M, Murray EA: Stimulus recognition. *Curr Opin Neurobiol* 4:200–206, 1994.

83. Alvarez P, Squire LR: Memory consolidation and the medial temporal lobe: A simple network model. *Proc Nat Acad Sci USA* 91:7041–7045, 1994.

84. Squire LR, Alvarez P: Retrograde amnesia and memory consolidation: A Neurobiological perspective. *Curr Opin Neurobiol* 5:169–177, 1995.

Chapter 36

AMNESIA: COGNITIVE NEUROPSYCHOLOGICAL ASPECTS

Tim Curran
Daniel L. Schacter

Research in cognitive neuroscience has inspired the view that distinct neural systems are differentially involved in various aspects of memory. While most or all information processing systems in the brain are capable of using past information to influence current behavior, there is a great deal of functional heterogeneity in the aspects of learning and memory that are supported by different neural mechanisms. This chapter provides an overview of cognitive neuroscience research on the principal brain mechanisms of memory. We start with a discussion of research that has attempted to evaluate the contribution of the medial temporal lobe and related structures to memory by investigating the amnesic syndrome. This research has inspired new perspectives on the storage and retrieval of information in long-term memory. Findings of preserved learning and memory in amnesic patients have suggested that some brain mechanisms support forms of memory that can operate unconsciously (implicit memory) and have also pointed toward distinct short-term forms of memory (working memory). Finally, the contribution of the prefrontal cortex to long-term memory and working memory are discussed.

AMNESIA AND MEDIAL TEMPORAL LOBE FUNCTION: COGNITIVE NEUROPSYCHOLOGICAL PERSPECTIVES

Patients with organic amnesia show profound learning and memory impairments that are typi-cally attributable to medial temporal lobe and/or diencephalic damage (see Chaps. 35 and 48) for a review of these impairments). Research investigating the functional deficit(s) underlying organic amnesia have been strongly influenced by theories of normal learning and memory. Models of human memory that posit a distinction between short- and long-term memory[1] generally have been supported by the finding that amnesic patients show normal retention of small amounts of information (about seven items) across short temporal durations (less than about 30 s). As discussed below, short-term or working memory is supported by neurocognitive processes that are separable from long-term forms of retention. We now consider the component processes of long-term retention that may be compromised in organic amnesia.

Cognitive psychologists generally distinguish between three different information processing stages of memory: encoding, storage, and retrieval. The integrity of each of these stages has been investigated in order to understand the memory impairment resulting from organic amnesia. The observation that amnesic patients can show normal levels of memory when certain retrieval cues are provided (e.g., a three-letter word stem, *tru*, to cue memory for *truck*) led to the hypothesis that amnesia results from a retrieval deficit. Because interference, or competition among similar memories, is considered to be a primary determinant of retrieval failure in normal subjects, retrieval-deficit theories predicted abnormally high levels of interference in amnesic patients. Contrary to this prediction, direct tests of this hypothesis found that amnesic and control subjects were similarly susceptible to interference.[2,3]

Retrieval-deficit theories of amnesia suffered from another, more fundamental flaw that does not relate to interference. The ability to retrieve information encountered prior to the onset of amnesia can remain intact (especially if the information was learned long before the onset of amnesia) despite profound impairments in retaining new information[4] (see Chap. 35). That is, anterograde amnesia can exist without retrograde amnesia. If amnesia involved only a general retrieval deficit, it should affect the retrieval of old and new information equally. The separability of anterograde and retrograde amnesia suggests that the amnesic deficit is likely attributable (at least in part) to an impairment at the time of learning. For this reason among others, encoding deficit theories of amnesia have been proposed.

The levels-of-processing framework[5] has greatly influenced cognitive psychologists' ideas about the manner in which information is encoded into memory. Simply stated, this framework describes the fact that information is remembered more accurately when semantic rather than superficial aspects of stimuli are encoded. Thus, amnesic patients' memory impairments have been hypothesized to reflect a deficit in encoding to-be-remembered information at a semantic level. Semantic coding deficit theories received initial support when Korsakoff's amnesics failed to show a normal levels-of-processing effect,[6] but subsequent studies have found normal levels-of-processing effects with other amnesic patients.[7] Other studies suggested that amnesic patients did not spontaneously use semantic information to organize and encode information in memory[8] but that they could encode semantic aspects of stimuli when properly instructed.[9] Ultimately, semantic coding deficits cannot entirely explain the memory deficit of patients with anterograde amnesia. Besides the evidence that amnesics can properly encode semantic attributes, any theory that focuses purely on encoding processes has difficulty explaining the differential effectiveness of different retrieval cues or the fact that anterograde amnesia

is typically associated with some retrograde memory loss.[4]

Cognitive theories of encoding (e.g., levels-of-processing) and retrieval (e.g., interference theory) have generally been unsuccessful in explaining the amnesic syndrome. Storage-deficit theories, rather than being directly borrowed from cognitive psychology, exemplify how neuropsychological evidence has influenced the evolution of psychological theories. In particular, cognitive neuroscience research on amnesia has revolutionized our ideas about the storage process known as consolidation. Consolidation was originally conceptualized as the process by which information is transferred from short- to long-term memory. More recent theories posit that consolidation is a longer-term process by which memories are integrated with existing knowledge over a time course that lasts from minutes to years. According to consolidation theories,[4,10] memories initially depend on an interaction between the temporal lobe/diencephalon and the cerebral cortex. Over time, the learned representations become integrated with other knowledge in the cerebral cortex and no longer depend on the medial temporal lobe or diencephalon. Evidence for this view is derived from the observation that (1) retrograde and anterograde amnesia are typically correlated and (2) retrograde amnesia follows a temporal gradient. The temporal gradient of retrograde amnesia refers to the finding that retrograde amnesia is typically most severe for information that was encountered immediately prior to the onset of amnesia but is progressively less severe for remote events[4] (see Chap. 35). According to consolidation theories, remote memories have already been completely consolidated with information in the cerebral cortex, so they are no longer dependent on the brain regions affected in amnesia (i.e., medial temporal lobes and/or diencephalon). More recent memories, for which retrograde amnesia is most severe, have not been consolidated, so they are most likely to be lost upon the onset of amnesia.

Another proposed function of the medial temporal lobes—related to consolidation—is the binding of distinct memory attributes that are represented in distributed cortical areas.[10,11] By this view, different stimulus attributes are ultimately represented and stored in dedicated cortical areas: visual features in occipitotemporal cortex, spatial information in parietal cortex, auditory information in superior temporal cortex, and so on. Medial temporal lobe mechanisms interact with these cortical representations to bind them into a coherent memory of the remembered episode. Through consolidation, these cortical representations become directly associated with each other and are no longer dependent upon medial temporal lobe binding.

The previously discussed theories of the amnesic deficit can be collectively referred to as process theories because they try to relate medial temporal lobe function to a particular memory process (e.g., encoding, binding, consolidation, retrieval). Another general class of theories, content theories, have posited that the memory deficits of amnesic patients involve only certain types of information. One example of such a theory posits that amnesics' memory for information about individual items is normal, but amnesics' deficit is specific to contextual or associative information. Other theories hold that the performance of amnesic patients is impaired on tests that require conscious recollection of a previous episode ("explicit memory") but is spared on tasks in which memory influences behavior without conscious recollection ("implicit memory"). As will be seen, these dichotomies (item information versus contextual/associative information, explicit versus implicit) are orthogonal to the process theories, and it is reasonable to combine the two approaches. That is, if amnesics' memory deficits are confined to associative information, this associative-memory deficit could be attributable to a certain stage of information processing. Furthermore, these content dichotomies are not mutually exclusive, so, for example, it is important to consider implicit memory for item information as well as implicit memory for associative information.

Context-memory deficit hypotheses suggest that memory for individual stimuli is spared by organic amnesia, but memory for contextual information (e.g., time, place, and so on) within the learning episode is impaired.[12] A related idea holds that damage to medial temporal lobe structures has little effect on memory for individual stimuli but impairs the ability to remember complex associative or relational information about multiple stimuli.[13,14] A central issue in evaluating context-memory deficit theories is whether or not amnesics' recognition abilities (i.e., the ability to discriminate studied from nonstudied items) is relatively spared in comparison with free or cued recall. The importance of recall versus recognition performance is derived from the fact that recall is typically more context-dependent than recognition. Some studies have found that recognition is spared relative to recall in patients with organic amnesia[15] but others have shown that recall and recognition are similarly impaired.[16] Even if amnesics do show a greater deficit on recognition than recall, context-deficit theories have difficulty explaining the fact that recognition—though better than recall—is not normal in amnesic patients. Such an explanation requires more detailed theories of the conditions in which context-memory influences item recognition.

There is an important relationship between content theories positing an amnesic deficit in associative/contextual memory and process theories positing that the medial temporal lobes act as a binding mechanism. The ability to remember associations between stimuli or to remember the episodic context in which a stimulus was encountered clearly depends on the associative binding of information in memory. Theories that posit a medial temporal lobe (and diencephalic) contribution to consolidation and binding appear to be very promising. Below, we discuss the capacity for other types of learning and memory that do not depend on these mechanisms.

IMPLICIT MEMORY

In considering evidence for retrieval-deficit theories of amnesia, we discussed the finding that amnesic patients' memory can appear normal when tested with appropriate cues like word stems. Graf and coworkers[17] showed that the instructions given to subjects may be just as important as the physical retrieval cue in determining how the memory performance of amnesic patients will compare to that of control subjects. When subjects were asked to intentionally recall a studied word that completes the stem (a direct test of explicit memory), control subjects outperformed amnesic patients. However, when subjects were simply asked to respond with the first correct completion that came to mind (an indirect test of implicit memory), amnesic and control subjects performed equivalently. Both groups of subjects showed superior completion rates for studied compared to nonstudied words (this effect is typically called "priming"), so it is clear that both groups were being influenced by memory for the studied words. This finding of spared priming on implicit tasks has been well replicated (for reviews, see Refs. 18 and 19). Thus, implicit memory does not seem to depend on the medial temporal and diencephalic brain areas that are damaged in organic amnesia.

Implicit memory is observed in tasks in which previous experience can influence behavior in the absence of conscious recollection (for review, see Ref. 20). Research on normal subjects has distinguished between two types of implicit memory tasks: (1) perceptual tasks in which the retrieval cue is perceptually related to the target item (e.g., stem completion, *tru—*) and (2) conceptual tasks in which the retrieval cue is conceptually related to the target item (e.g., category exemplar generation, *vehicle-?*). We will focus on perceptual forms of priming because more is known about the underlying brain mechanisms. In general, performance on perceptual implicit memory tasks is unaffected by semantic variables that greatly influence explicit memory. For example, in our discussion of encoding theories of amnesia, we noted that explicit memory normally benefits from semantic encoding compared to an encoding strategy that emphasizes physical characteristics of the studied stimulus.[5] In contrast, perceptual priming shows little benefit from semantic encoding. Unlike explicit memory, perceptual priming is sensitive to the perceptual compatibility between study and test conditions. On a visual stem completion task, for example, priming is superior when the

study list is presented visually rather than auditorally.[21]

The semantic independence and perceptual sensitivity of implicit memory has suggested that it reflects the influence of previous experience on presemantic brain mechanisms that are normally involved in perception. Cognitive neuroscience studies of perception indicate that different cortical areas are involved in the perception of different kinds of stimuli, such as visual words, auditory words, or visual objects (see Chaps. 10, 13, and 17). For example, evidence from neuropsychology and neuroimaging has converged on the idea that perception of visual words relies on mechanisms in occipitotemporal cortex.[22]

Schacter[23] has suggested that implicit memory is driven by modality-specific perceptual systems. This view has been supported by positron emission tomography (PET; see Chap. 6) studies of the functional anatomy of stem-completion priming.[24,25] Activation by PET in bilateral occipitotemporal regions was stronger when word stems were completed with nonstudied words compared to previously studied words. This is consistent with the idea that priming reflects an influence of previous experience on the mechanisms that underlie visual word perception such that word perception is made easier by previously studying the word. Other PET evidence suggests that similar conclusions apply in the domain of visual object processing.[26]

Converging evidence for a contribution of visual cortical areas to implicit memory has been provided by a study of memory and priming in a patient, M.S., who had most of his right occipital lobe removed in order to alleviate intractable epilepsy.[27] M.S. showed normal explicit memory on a variety of tests but impaired perceptual priming on word-stem completion and word-identification tasks. Further evidence for the visuoperceptual nature of his priming impairment was obtained by demonstrating normal priming when words were studied auditorally rather than visually and normal priming on a conceptual test of implicit memory.

In summary, neuropsychological and neuroimaging studies of visual word priming have strongly implicated visual perceptual mechanisms in occipitotemporal cortex. Other evidence suggests that distinct perceptual mechanisms contribute to implicit memory for auditory words and visual objects.[23] Similarly, brain areas controlling perceptuomotor coordination can implicitly learn information that helps to guide subsequent behavior (often referred to as "procedural learning").[28] These results support the general conclusion that implicit learning and memory reflect the effects of experience on the brain mechanisms that normally support perception and guide behavior. These same information processing mechanisms likely form the cortical storage sites that are bound by medial temporal lobe mechanisms to support explicit recollection of coherent memory episodes. In this light, it is interesting to note that memory for novel associations between multiple stimuli cannot be implicitly retrieved by amnesic patients except under conditions of very extensive training.[29] This is consistent with the notion that conscious recollection and associative binding are dependent on the medial temporal lobe, but unbound cortical memories can still have an unconscious influence on behavior.

PREFRONTAL CONTRIBUTIONS TO LONG-TERM MEMORY

Neuropsychological studies of patients with frontal lobe damage have traditionally suggested that prefrontal cortex plays only a subsidiary role in normal memory functioning. This view has been derived from the observation that patients with frontal lesions typically show memory deficits only for certain types of information (e.g., source memory and memory for temporal context). The term *source amnesia* refers to cases in which a person can normally remember some previously learned information yet cannot remember the source of that information (where or when it was learned or who taught it).[30] For example, Janowsky and colleagues[31] taught subjects some new trivia facts (e.g., "The name of the dog on the Cracker Jack box is Bingo"). Patients with frontal lobe lesions were able to answer correctly questions based on

the newly learned information (e.g., "What is the name of the dog on the Cracker Jack box?") as well as control subjects, yet they showed an impaired ability to remember where they learned the information or when they had most recently encountered it. Impaired memory for temporal information has been demonstrated in experiments in which subjects are asked to remember the order in which items appeared on a studied list. Patients with frontal lobe lesions can demonstrate normal recognition memory but impaired temporal memory for the same stimuli.[32]

Other evidence suggests that the prefrontal cortex is more intimately involved with normal memory functioning than merely supporting memory for circumscribed types of information such as temporal or source memory. Explicit memory studies using PET have found that activity in the right prefrontal cortex is consistently associated with the retrieval of information from memory (for review, see Ref. 33). These results suggest that prefrontal mechanisms may play a more central role in memory retrieval than previously believed.

Recent neuropsychological work has sought to better understand the contribution of prefrontal cortex to memory retrieval. Shimamura and colleagues[34,35] have suggested that patients with frontal lobe lesions have difficulty disregarding or inhibiting irrelevant information. Shimamura and coworkers[34] had subjects learn consecutive lists with competing paired associates (e.g., *lion-hunter* in list 1 and *lion-circus* in list 2). Patients with frontal lobe lesions showed impaired memory when asked to recall the list 2 associations (*lion-*?) because of high levels of interference from the pairs in list 1.

Unlike patients with the classic amnesic syndrome, patients with memory problems associated with frontal lobe damage often confabulate.[34] Confabulation can be characterized as "honest lying"[36] (see Chap. 28), in which patients present inaccurate and sometimes bizarre "memories" of previous events. Other patients with frontal lobe lesions, who do not spontaneously confabulate about their life experiences, exhibit an intriguing form of false memory on recognition tests.[37-39] For example, one patient with a right frontal lesion, B.G., has been tested in a large number of recognition memory experiments in our laboratory.[39] He classifies nonstudied test items as "studied" at a rate that consistently exceeds the false recognition of control subjects. Furthermore, like other frontal patients exhibiting false recognition, he shows an abnormally high degree of confidence in the accuracy of his false memories.

One experiment was particularly informative for understanding the possible basis of B.G.'s false recognition and shedding some light on prefrontal contributions to memory (Ref. 39, experiment 7). B.G. studied a list of pictures that were selected from a limited number of categories (e.g., furniture, tools, and so on). In the recognition test, nonstudied pictures were either members of the studied categories or not members of categories that were tested (e.g., animals). Figure 36-1 shows the percentage of times that subjects called pictures "studied" in each condition. The error bars represent the range of eight control subjects. As seen in Fig. 36-1, B.G. shows a heightened sensitivity to the category membership of the nonstudied pictures. His false recognition rate was near normal when nonstudied pictures were taken from nonstudied categories but was drastically higher when they were taken from studied categories. This suggests that B.G. may be more reliant on a general match between study-list characteristics and test items than are normal subjects. Hence, his right frontal lesion may make him less able to retrieve item-specific information from memory and force him to depend more on general representations of the target episode.[40] This pattern might also be interpreted within Shimamura's[34,35] theory that patients with frontal lobe lesions have difficulty suppressing interfering information—the categorical structure of the list may indiscriminately bring all members of the studied categories to mind, but he may be unable to pick out the pictures that were actually studied.

Other theories of prefrontal contributions to memory emphasize its general involvement in the high-level control of cognition and behavior. Such high-level, or executive, control processes are thought to guide memory functioning just as they

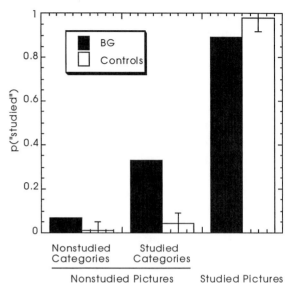

Figure 36-1

Recognition memory performance of patient B.G., who has a right frontal lobe lesion. The dependent measure is the proportion of pictures that subjects classified as "studied" from each condition. Subjects studied a list of pictures from six distinct categories (e.g., furniture, tools, etc.), followed by a recognition test with nonstudied pictures from different categories (left bars), nonstudied pictures from the studied categories (middle bars), and studied pictures (right bars). Error bars represent the range of eight control subjects. The results indicate that B.G. has an abnormal tendency to falsely recognize nonstudied pictures that are categorically consistent with studied pictures.

guide other cognitive processes. Executive processes may strategically guide memory search processes, or they may be used to monitor the information that is retrieved from memory and verify its accuracy.[41,42] Either of these proposals could potentially account for the false recognition pattern exhibited by patient B.G. B.G. may falsely recognize pictures that are related to actually studied pictures because he fails to search for memory attributes that will successfully discriminate between studied and nonstudied pictures. In addition, B.G. may have a deficit in verifying the information that is retrieved from memory in order to avoid false recognition.[38]

WORKING MEMORY

Baddeley[43,44] has hypothesized that an executive control process (the "central executive") forms the centerpiece of a tripartite working memory system that allows for the temporary maintenance and manipulation of information. In addition to the central executive (similar to the frontal executive processes discussed above), two modality-specific slave systems—the "phonological loop" and "visuospatial scratch pad"—are hypothesized to temporally store and manipulate speech-based and visuospatial information respectively. Working memory is typically normal in patients with the amnesic syndrome discussed at the opening of this chapter, so it is considered to be independent from the medial temporal lobe and diencephalic memory system that is required for normal long-term memory. In addition, phonologic and visuospatial working memory appear to be functionally and neuroanatomically distinct, because brain-injured patients with working memory deficits have shown impairments for either speech-based or visuospatial information but never both. In general, these modality-specific subsystems appear to operate in conjunction with the brain mechanisms that are involved in the perception of speech and visuospatial information.

A number of patients have been described who show impaired verbal short-term memory but normal long-term memory (for review, see Ref. 45). The possibility of normal long-term with impaired short-term memory contradicted early information-processing models of memory, which supposed that normal short-term memory processing is a necessary antecedent of normal long-term memory.[1] Such patients may have a phonologic loop impairment, and their lesions are typically near the left supramarginal gyrus (inferior parietal lobe). A recent PET study has also found activation of the supramarginal gyrus in a phonologic working memory task.[46]

Other neuropsychological patients appear to have deficits in visuospatial working memory but preserved verbal working memory (for review, see Ref. 47). The anatomic origins of these impairments have not been well localized beyond the predominance of right-hemispheric damage. Better information about the functional anatomy of visuospatial working memory has been provided by a PET study of visuospatial working memory.[48] Consistent with the existing neuropsychological evidence, activity related to visuospatial working memory was confined to the right-hemispheric regions, including prefrontal, premotor, parietal, and occipital cortices. A prefrontal contribution to spatial working memory has also been suggested by single-unit recording in monkeys performing a task that requires short-term memory of visuospatial stimuli.[49] Within the framework of Baddeley's working memory model, it is unclear whether this prefrontal activity reflects the central executive or the visuospatial scratch pad (see Chap. 31 for further discussion of the choice between central executive and working memory accounts of prefrontal function). Given the well-established role of the parietal and occipital cortices in processing spatial and visual information, it seems clear that activity in these areas uniquely reflects the maintenance of visuospatial information—much like the hypothesized visuospatial scratch pad.

SUMMARY

Cognitive neuroscience research has inspired the view that memory is supported by multiple neural systems. Research on implicit memory and perceptual priming suggests that cortical information-processing modules are capable of some rudimentary forms of learning and memory. Experience shapes the operation of these perceptual mechanisms in a manner that can influence subsequent behavior without conscious recollection. The medial temporal lobe acts to bind information from these diverse cortical modules into a coherent memory episode that can be consciously recollected. Over time, these bound representations become consolidated into a distributed memory trace that is integrated with other information in long-term memory and is no longer dependent upon medial temporal lobe binding. Mechanisms of the prefrontal cortex interact with these core memory mechanisms in a manner that is just beginning to be elucidated. Prefrontal mechanisms may be necessary for establishing effective retrieval strategies, monitoring the quality of retrieved information, and inhibiting irrelevant information. More generally, the prefrontal cortex may act as a central executive that allows for strategic control of long-term memory systems as well as control of modality-specific working memory mechanisms that temporarily hold and manipulate information.

REFERENCES

1. Atkinson RC, Shiffrin RM: Human memory: A proposed system and its control processes, in Spence KW, Spence JT (eds): *The Psychology of Learning and Motivation.* New York: Academic Press, 1968, vol 2, pp 89–105.
2. Kinsbourne M, Winocur G: Response competition and interference effects in paired-associate learning by Korsakoff's amnesics. *Neuropsychologia* 18:541–548, 1980.
3. Warrington EK, Weiskrantz L: Further analysis of prior learning on subsequent retention in amnesic patients. *Neuropsychologia* 16:169–177, 1978.
4. Squire LR: Memory and the hippocampus: A synthesis of findings with rats, monkeys, and humans. *Psychol Rev* 99:195–231, 1992.
5. Craik FIM, Lockhart RS: Levels of processing: A framework for memory research. *J Verbal Learn Verbal Behav* 11:671–684, 1972.
6. Cermak LS, Reale L: Depth of processing and retention of words by alcoholic Korsakoff's patients. *J Exp Psychol Hum Learn Mem* 4:165–174, 1978.
7. Myers A, Meudell P, Neary D: Do amnesics adopt inefficient encoding strategies with faces and random shapes? *Neuropsychologia* 18:527–540, 1980.
8. Cermak LS, Butters N, Moreines J: Some analyses of the verbal encoding deficit of alcoholic Korsakoff patients. *Brain Lang* 1:141–150, 1974.
9. Winocur G, Kinsbourne M, Moscovitch M: The effect of cueing on release from proactive interference in Korsakoff amnesic patients. *Exp Psychol Hum Learn Mem* 7:56–65, 1981.
10. McClelland JL, McNaughton BL, O'Reilly RC: Why there are complimentary learning systems in the hippocampus and neocortex: Insights from the successes and failures of connectionist models of learning and memory. *Psychol Rev* 102:419–457, 1995.
11. Squire LR: Declarative and nondeclarative memory: Multiple brain systems supporting learning and memory, in Schacter DL, Tulving E (ed): *Memory Systems 1994.* Cambridge, MA: MIT Press, 1994, pp 203–231.
12. Mayes AR, Meudell PR, Pickering A: Is organic amnesia caused by a selective deficit in remembering contextual information? *Cortex* 21:167–202, 1985.
13. Cohen NJ, Eichenbaum H: Memory, amnesia, and the hippocampal system. Cambridge, MA: MIT Press, 1993.
14. Rudy JW, Sutherland RJ: The memory-coherence problem, configural associations, and the hippocampal system, in Schacter DL, Tulving E (ed): *Memory Systems 1994.* Cambridge, MA: MIT Press, 1994, pp 119–146.
15. Hirst W, Johnson MK, Phelps EA, Volpe BT: More on recognition and recall in amnesics. *J Exp Psychol Learn Mem Cogn* 14:758–762, 1988.
16. Haist F, Shimamura AP, Squire LR: On the relationship between recall and recognition memory. *J Exp Psychol Learn Mem Cogn* 18:691–702, 1992.
17. Graf P, Squire LR, Mandler G: The information that amnesic patients do not forget. *J Exp Psychol Learn Mem Cog* 10:164–178, 1984.
18. Moscovitch M, Vriezen E, Goshen-Gottstein Y: Implicit tests of memory in patients with focal lesions or degenerative brain disorders, in Spinnler H, Boller F (ed): *Handbook of Neuropsychology.* Amsterdam: Elsevier, 1993, vol 8, pp 133–173.
19. Schacter DL, Chiu CYP, Ochsner KN: Implicit memory a selective review. *Annu Rev Neurosci* 16:159–182, 1993.
20. Roediger HL, McDermott KB: Implicit memory in normal human subjects, in Spinnler H, Boller F (eds): *Handbook of Neuropsychology.* Amsterdam: Elsevier, 1993, vol 8, pp 63–131.
21. Graf P, Shimamura AP, Squire LR: Priming across the modalities and priming across category levels: Extending the domain of preserved function in amnesia. *J Exp Psychol Learn Mem Cogn* 11:386–396, 1985.
22. Posner MI, Carr TH: Lexical access and the brain: Anatomical constraints on cognitive models of word recognition. *Am J Psychol* 105:1–26, 1992.
23. Schacter DL: Priming and multiple memory systems: Perceptual mechanisms of implicit memory, in Schacter DL, Tulving E (eds): *Memory Systems 1994.* Cambridge, MA: MIT Press, 1994, pp 233–268.

24. Buckner RL, Peterson SE, Ojeman JG, et al: Functional anatomical studies of explicit and implicit memory retrieval tasks. *J Neurosci* 15:12–29, 1995.

25. Schacter DL, Alpert N, Savage C, et al: Conscious recollection and the human hippocampal formation: Evidence from positron emission tomography. Proceedings of the *National Academy of Sciences.* In press, 1996.

26. Schacter DL, Reiman E, Uecker A, et al: Brain regions associated with the retrieval of structurally coherent information. *Nature* 376:587–590, 1995.

27. Gabrieli JDE, Fleischman DA, Keane MM, et al: Double dissociation between memory systems underlying explicit and implicit memory in the human brain. *Psychol Sci* 6:76–82, 1995.

28. Willingham DB: Systems of motor skill, in Squire LR, Butters N (eds): *Neuropsychology of Memory.* New York: Guilford Press, 1992, pp 166–178.

29. Bowers J, Schacter DL: Priming of novel information in amnesic patients: Issues and data, in Graf P, Masson M (eds): *Implicit Memory.* Hillsdale, NJ: Erlbaum, 1993, pp 303–326.

30. Schacter DL, Harbluk JL, McLachlan DR: Retrieval without recollection: An experimental analysis of source amnesia. *Verbal Learn Verbal Behav* 23:593–611, 1984.

31. Janowsky JS, Shimamura AP, Squire LR: Source memory impairments in patients with frontal damage. *Neuropsychologia* 27:1043–1056, 1989.

32. Milner B, Corsi P, Leonard G: Frontal-lobe contribution to recency judgments. *Neuropsychologia* 29:601–618, 1991.

33. Buckner RL, Tulving E: Neuroimaging studies of memory: Theory and recent PET results, in Boller F, Grafman J (eds): *Handbook of Neuropsychology.* Amsterdam: Elsevier, 1995, vol 10, pp 439–466.

34. Shimamura AP, Jurica PJ, Mangels JA, et al: Susceptibility to memory interference effects following frontal damage: Findings from tests of paired-associate learning. *J Cog Neurosci* 7:144–152, 1995.

35. Shimamura AP: Memory and frontal lobe function, in Gazzaniga MS (ed): *The Cognitive Neurosciences.* Cambridge: MIT Press, 1995, pp 803–813.

36. Moscovitch M: Confabulation, in Schacter DL, Coyle JT, Fischbach GD, et al (eds): *Memory Distortion.* Cambridge, MA: Harvard University Press, 1995, pp 226–251.

37. Delbecq-Derouesné J, Beauvois MF, Shallice T: Preserved recall versus impaired recognition. *Brain* 113:1045–1074, 1990.

38. Parkin AJ, Bindschaedler C, Harsent L, Metzler C: Verification impairment in the generation of memory following ruptured aneurysm of the anterior communicating artery. *Brain Cog.* In press.

39. Schacter DL, Curran T, Galluccio L, et al: False recognition and the right frontal lobe: A case study. *Neuropsychologia.* In press, 1996.

40. Norman KA, Schacter DL: Implicit memory, explicit memory, and false recognition: A cognitive neuroscience perspective, in Reder L (ed): *Implicit Memory and Metacognition.* In press.

41. Moscovitch M: Memory and working with memory: Evaluation of a component process model and comparisons with other models, in Schacter DL, Tulving E (eds): *Memory Systems 1994.* Cambridge, MA: MIT Press, 1994, pp 269–310.

42. Shallice T: *From Neuropsychology to Mental Structure.* Cambridge, England: Cambridge University Press, 1988.

43. Baddeley A: *Working Memory.* Oxford, England: Claredon Press, 1986.

44. Baddeley A: Working memory: The interface between memory and cognition, in Schacter DL, Tulving E (ed): *Memory Systems 1994.* Cambridge, MA: MIT Press, 1994, pp 351–367.

45. Vallar G, Shallice T: *Neuropsychological Impairments of Short-Term Memory.* Cambridge, England: Cambridge University Press, 1990.

46. Paulesu E, Frith CD, Frackowiak RSJ: The neural correlates of the verbal component of working memory. *Nature* 362:342–345, 1993.

47. Della Sala S, Logie RH: When working memory does not work: The role of working memory in neuropsychology, in Boller F, Grafman J (eds): *Handbook of Neuropsychology.* Amsterdam: Elsevier, 1993, vol 8, pp 1–62.

48. Jonides J, Smith EE, Koeppe RA, et al: Spatial working memory in humans as revealed by PET. *Nature* 363:623–625, 1993.

49. Goldman-Rakic PS: Cellular and circuit basis of working memory in prefrontal cortex of nonhuman primates, in Uylings HBM, Van Eden CG, De Bruin JPC, et al (eds): *Progress in Brain Research.* Amsterdam: Elsevier, 1990, vol 85, pp 325–336.

Chapter 37

SEMANTIC MEMORY IMPAIRMENTS

Martha J. Farah
Murray Grossman

The term *semantic memory* refers to our general knowledge of the objects, people, and events of the world.[1] The facts that Paris is the capital of France, birds have feathers, and a desk is a piece of furniture are examples of semantic memory. More particular knowledge, tied to an individual's personal experience, is considered *episodic memory* rather than semantic memory. Examples of the latter include the facts that you bought this book at a certain store or ate a certain food for breakfast this morning. Neurologic disease and damage can affect semantic memory disproportionately. In this chapter the different forms of semantic memory impairment are reviewed, with attention to their etiologies, major behavioral features, and implications for the neural substrates and functional organization of semantic memory in the normal brain.

GENERALIZED IMPAIRMENT OF SEMANTIC MEMORY

Warrington[2] first documented a pattern of preserved and impaired performance indicative of semantic memory impairment in a series of three patients suffering from progressive degenerative brain disease. Her subjects were relatively preserved on most measures of language and cognitive function but did poorly on tasks dependent on semantic memory, including confrontation naming, word-picture matching, and a verification task in which subjects were shown pictures or words and asked questions such as "Is it a bird?" or "Is it heavy?" In subsequent years a number of similar cases were reported, and the term *semantic dementia* was coined in the context of one such report.[3] Hodges and coworkers[4] presented a wide-ranging study of five new cases of semantic dementia, reviewed the literature, and drew a number of useful generalizations concerning the condition. A summary of their conclusions is presented here.

Semantic dementia may present initially as a language disorder whose most prominent feature is vocabulary loss, both expressive and receptive. Naming is minimally aided by phonemic cues, and naming errors tend to share a semantic relation with the correct name (e.g., *violin* for *accordion,* or *animal* for *fox*). In production, category fluency is severely impaired, and word definitions are impoverished or wrong. Such patients have sometimes been described as having a fluent form of primary progressive aphasia (see Chaps. 9 and 10), but additional language testing and nonverbal semantic memory testing suggest that the underlying impairment is one of semantic memory knowledge rather than language. Syntax and phonology tend to be preserved, whereas entirely pictorial tasks that depend on knowledge of the depicted objects, such as sorting together semantically related objects or distinguishing real from imaginary objects, are failed. Although the formal assessment of episodic memory is difficult because of the loss of knowledge of word and picture meanings, Hodges and coworkers[4] observe that at least some patients show significant preservation of autobiographical memories and practical day-to-day memory. The neuropathologic changes in semantic dementia are focused in the temporal lobes, often affecting the left more than the right. A small number of brains have come to autopsy with Pick's disease.

Another degenerative condition affecting semantic memory is Alzheimer disease[5-10] (AD), although semantic memory is just one of many aspects of cognition impaired in AD (see Chap. 42), and initially some cases may present with only episodic memory impairment. To the extent that semantic memory is impaired in AD, pathologic changes in temporal cortex are responsible.

In sum, semantic memory is at least partially dissociable from other forms of memory, language, and cognition, generally as a result of degenerative diseases. It appears to depend on temporal cortex, with some degree lateralization to the left suggested.

SELECTIVE IMPAIRMENTS OF SEMANTIC MEMORY

In addition to the generalized impairments of semantic memory described above, particular aspects of semantic memory can be disproportionately impaired. These disorders are potentially informative about the internal organization of semantic memory in the brain, although their proper interpretation and even their existence have been issues of controversy.

Category-Specific Semantic Memory Impairment

In some cases it appears that knowledge from certain semantic categories is disproportionately impaired, suggesting that the neural bases of semantic memory are subdivided by semantic category. Category-specific semantic memory impairments are sometimes confused with category-specific impairments in name retrieval and visual recognition. The "fruit and vegetable" impairment observed in two cases[11,12] affects naming only; the face-specificity of prosopagnosia (see Chap. 18) affects visual

recognition only. In contrast, category-specific semantic memory impairments are manifest in all tasks that require knowledge of the object, whether they involve vision, language, or other modalities of stimulus and response. The most common category-specific semantic memory impairment affects knowledge of living things.

The first report of impaired knowledge of living things was made by Warrington and Shallice,[13] who described three patients who had survived herpes encephalitis. Although the patients were impaired across the board at tasks such as picture naming and defining words, they were dramatically worse when the pictures or words represented animals and plants than when they represented artifacts. In subsequent years numerous other reports appeared of similar cases, generally suffering damage to temporal cortex from herpes encephalitis, closed head injury or, less frequently, cerebrovascular or degenerative disease. Category-specific disorders of semantic memory are distinct from the disorders described in the previous section, despite the implication of temporal brain regions in both, as neither semantic dementia[4] nor Alzheimer disease[14] routinely affect knowledge of living things more than nonliving.

The idea that certain brain regions are specialized for representing knowledge about living things has naturally aroused some skepticism and prompted a search for alternative explanations of apparently impaired knowledge of living things. The simplest alternative explanation is that the impairment is an artifact of the greater difficulty of retrieving knowledge about living things. It has been suggested that when difficulty is equated across living and nonliving test items, the selectivity of the semantic memory impairment disappears.[15,16] However, the selectivity has also been shown to be reliable in two cases when multiple measures of difficulty are accounted for,[17] and the null results in other controlled studies are likely due to insufficient statistical power, as our reliable findings disappeared when we reduced our data set to the size of the other studies' data sets.[18]

Cases of impaired knowledge of nonliving things with relatively spared knowledge of living things are rarer but have also been described.[19–23] The lesions in these cases are confined to the left hemisphere. A precise intrahemispheric localization is not possible, as the lesions are typically large and relatively few cases have been reported, although the left temporal region again seems involved.[23] These patients provide the other half of a double dissociation with impaired knowledge of living things, thus adding further support to the hypothesis that category-specific semantic memory impairments are not simply due to the differential difficulty of particular categories.

Building on the hypothesis of Allport,[24] that semantic memory is subdivided into different sensorimotor modalities (e.g., visual knowledge, tactile knowledge, and motor knowledge; see Fig. 37-1 for an illustration of this idea), Warrington and Shallice[13] proposed a different kind of alternative explanation for category-specific knowledge deficits. They suggested that living and nonliving things may differ from one another in their reliance on knowledge from different sensorimotor modalities, with living things being known predominantly by their visual and other sensory attributes. Impaired knowledge of living things could result from an impairment of visual knowledge. Similarly, nonliving things might be known predominantly by their function, an abstract form of motoric representation, and impaired knowledge of nonliving things could result from an impairment of functional knowledge. This interpretation has the advantage of parsimony, in that it invokes a type of organization already known to exist in the brain—modality-specific organization—rather than invoking an organization based on semantic categories such as aliveness. A computer simulation of semantic memory and its impairments has shown that a modality-specific organization can account for category-specific impairments, even the finding that functional knowledge of living things is impaired after visual semantic damage.[25] The latter finding is explained by the need for a certain "critical mass" of associated knowledge to help activate collaterally any one part of a distributed representation; if most of the representation of living things is visual and visual

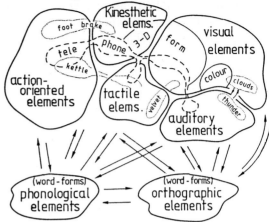

Figure 37-1

A modality-specific organization for semantic memory. Rather than hypothesize a store of knowledge in the brain separate from the various sensorimotor modalities used in perception and action, semantic memory is hypothesized to consist of representations in sensorimotor systems themselves. (From Allport,[24] with permission.)

knowledge is damaged, then the remaining functional knowledge cannot be activated.

Modality-Specific Semantic Memory Impairment

There is a second way in which the phrase *modality-specific semantic memory* has been used in neuropsychology, and that is for components of semantic memory that are accessed *through* a particular input or output modality. According to this usage, visual semantics refers not to semantic knowledge of the visual appearance of objects but to the semantic knowledge of appearance, function, and so on that is accessed when an object is seen. Whether semantic memory has a modality-specific organization in this sense is not clear, although such an organization has been hypothesized for purposes of explaining "optic aphasia."

Optic aphasia is a puzzling disorder, consisting of an impairment in naming visually presented stimuli in the face of relatively preserved naming of nonvisual stimuli and relatively preserved nonverbal demonstrations of visual recognition. It seems reasonable to assume that visual confrontation naming requires three major stages of processing: vision, semantics, and lexical retrieval. That is, it requires seeing the object clearly enough to access semantic knowledge of it, and using that semantic knowledge of what the object is to retrieve its name. Paradoxically, the preserved nonvisual naming and nonverbal recognition performance of optic aphasics seem to exonerate all three stages.

A variety of attempts have been made to explain how an anomia could exist for visual stimuli only, although none has been thoroughly tested or gained wide support (see Ref. 26 for a review). One of these accounts invokes a modality-specific semantic memory system in which visual semantics (i.e., the semantic knowledge accessed by visual inputs) has been disconnected from verbal semantics (i.e., the semantic knowledge necessary to access a verbal output).[27,28] This hypothesis was formulated to explain the major features of optic aphasia and is successful in so doing, although converging evidence from other sources is now desirable.

REFERENCES

1. Tulving E: Episodic and semantic memory, in Tulving E, Donaldson W (eds): *Organization of Memory.* New York: Academic Press, 1972.

2. Warrington EK: The selective impairment of semantic memory. *Q J Exp Psychol* 27:635–657, 1975.

3. Snowden JS, Goulding PJ, Neary D: Semantic dementia: A form of circumscribed cerebral atrophy. *Behav Neurol* 2:167–182, 1989.

4. Hodges JR, Patterson K, Oxbury S, Funnell E: Semantic dementia. *Brain* 115:1783–1806, 1992.

5. Martin A, Fedio P: Word production and comprehension in Alzheimer's disease: The breakdown of semantic knowledge. *Brain Lang* 19:124–141, 1983.

6. Bayles KA, Tomoeda CK, Trosset MW: Naming and categorical knowledge in Alzheimer's disease: The process of semantic memory deterioration. *Brain Lang* 39:498–510, 1990.

7. Chertkow H, Bub D: Semantic memory loss in dementia of Alzheimer's type: What do various measures measure? *Brain* 113:397–417, 1990.

8. Hodges JR, Salmon DP, Butters N: Semantic memory impairment in Alzheimer's disease: Failure of access of degraded knowledge? *Neuropsychologia* 30:301–314, 1992.

9. Nebes RD: Cognitive dysfunction in Alzheimer's disease, in Craik FIM, Salthouse TA (eds): *The Handbook of Aging and Cognition.* Hillsdale, NJ: Erlbaum, 1992.

10. Grossman M, Mickanin J: Picture comprehension and probable Alzheimer's disease. *Brain Cogn* 26:43–64, 1994.

11. Hart J, Berndt RS, Caramazza A: Category-specific naming deficit following cerebral infarction. *Nature* 316:439–440, 1985.

12. Farah MJ, Wallace MA: Semantically bounded anomia: Implications for the neural implementation of naming. *Neuropsychologia* 30:609–621, 1992.

13. Warrington EK, Shallice T: Category specific semantic impairments. *Brain* 107:829–854, 1984.

14. Tippett LJ, Grossman M, Farah MJ: The semantic memory deficit of Alzheimer's disease: Category-specific? *Cortex* 31, 1995.

15. Funnell E, Sheridan J: Categories of knowledge? Unfamiliar aspects of living and non-living things. *Cogn Neuropsychol* 9:135–154, 1992.

16. Stewart F, Parkin AJ, Hunkin NM: Naming impairments following recovery from herpes simplex encephalitis: Category specific? *Q J Exp Psychol* 44A:261–284, 1992.

17. Farah MJ, McMullen PA, Meyer MM: Can recognition of living things be selectively impaired? *Neuropsychologia* 29:185–193, 1991.

18. Farah MJ, Meyer MM, McMullen PA: The living/nonliving dissociation is not an artifact: Giving an a priori implausible hypothesis a strong test. *Cogn Neuropsychol* 13:137–154, 1996.

19. Warrington EK, McCarthy R: Category specific access dysphasia. *Brain* 106:859–878, 1983.

20. Warrington EK, McCarthy R: Categories of knowledge: Further fractionations and an attempted explanation. *Brain* 110:1273–1296, 1987.

21. Hillis A, Caramazza C: Category-specific naming and comprehension impairment: A double dissociation. *Brain* 114:2081–2094, 1991.

22. Sacchett C, Humphreys GW: Calling a squirrel a squirrel but a canoe a wigwam: A category-specific deficit for artifactual objects and body parts. *Cogn Neuropsychol* 9:73–86, 1992.

23. Tippett LJ, Glosser G, Farah MJ: A category-specific naming deficit after temporal lobectomy. *Neuropsychologia.* 34:139–146, 1996.

24. Allport DA: Distributed memory, modular subsystems and dysphasia, in Newman S, Epstein R (eds): *Current Perspectives in Dysphasia.* Edinburgh: Churchill Livingstone, 1985.

25. Farah MJ, McClelland JL: A computational model of semantic memory impairment: Modality-specificity and emergent category-specificity. *J Exp Psychol Gen* 120:339–357, 1991.

26. Farah MJ: *Visual Agnosia: Disorders of Object Recognition and What They Tell Us about Normal Vision.* Cambridge, MA: MIT Press/Bradford Books, 1990.

27. Beauvois MF: Optic aphasia: A process of interaction between vision and language. *Philos Trans R Soc Lond* B298:35–47, 1982.

28. Shallice T: Impairments of semantic processing: Multiple dissociations, in Coltheart M, Sartori G, Job R (eds): *The Cognitive Neuropsychology of Language.* London: Erlbaum, 1987.

Chapter 38

MEMORY DYSFUNCTION AFTER HEAD INJURY

Harvey S. Levin

Memory impairment is a common and debilitating result of closed head injury (CHI). This chapter will review research on both the acute effects of head injury on memory and posttraumatic amnesia and its chronic effects in CHI patients.

POSTTRAUMATIC AND RETROGRADE AMNESIA

Definition and Description

Posttraumatic amnesia (PTA) is a term introduced by Russell and Nathan[1] to refer to the period of disturbed consciousness after head injury. Russell and Smith[2] later refined the concept of PTA to focus on impaired storage of information about ongoing events. In the terminology of cognitive neuropsychology, PTA is a disturbance of episodic memory typically associated with disorientation and confusion if not confabulation. Behavioral correlates of PTA can also include agitation, disinhibition, and lethargy, depending on the individual patient and the phase of recovery.

Assessment of Posttraumatic Amnesia

To obtain a stable measure of PTA and retrograde amnesia (RA) duration, Russell and Nathan[1] relied on retrospective estimates, which he determined by interviewing recovered head-injured patients. Russell questioned the patients about the first event after injury that they clearly recalled

and that was followed by continuous memory for events, whereas he estimated RA by asking the patient to report the last event that occurred before the injury. Russell has contended that retrospective estimates of PTA and RA indicate the severity of a previous closed head injury (CHI), and this has received support;[3] however, more recent studies[4] that prospectively assessed orientation and memory for ongoing events have questioned the intrasubject reliability of this method. Confabulation persisting after resolution of PTA could potentially contaminate retrospective estimates of PTA duration. Moreover, retrospective estimates are potentially biased by reports from family members, which are difficult for the patient to isolate from memory for actual events during the early stage of recovery. Consequently, several brief tests designed for bedside examination of PTA have been introduced for investigative and clinical purposes.[5-8] All of these tests assess orientation and autobiographical memory, and two of the instruments also evaluate new learning for material such as pictures and the examiner's name. The assessment of new learning is potentially useful because of evidence that disorientation may resolve prior to restoration of memory for ongoing events. Based on the distribution of scores obtained in normal subjects, PTA is considered to resolve when the patient's performance consistently improves to within the normal range.

Retrograde amnesia (RA) is the loss of memory for events preceding the injury; it was described by Russell and Nathan[1] as often extending

All Closed Head Injured Patients (n=84)

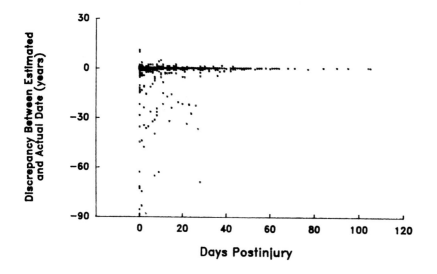

Figure 38-1
Scatterplot of discrepancy between current date and date given by head-injured patients plotted against days postinjury (n = 84). There is a trend for estimates initially displaced to the past to shift toward the present as the patient recovers over days. (From High et al.,[10] with permission.)

to events that occurred months or years prior to the injury and then "shrinks" to an amnesic interval that is typically far briefer (e.g., <30 min) than the duration of PTA.[9] As shown in Fig. 38-1, High and coworkers[10] found that patients evaluated during their initial hospitalization for CHI gave an estimate of the current date that was initially displaced to the past and gradually shifted toward the present. This pattern of serial estimates of RA is consistent with Ribot's law (see Ref. 11 for a historical review), which posits that older memories are more resilient to disruption by cerebral insult than more recent memories.

In contrast to Russell's estimate of RA duration based on the period of total abolition of past memory reported by the recovered patient, Levin and coworkers[12] administered a memory recognition test for titles of television programs that had previously been broadcast to a group of young adult CHI patients who were in PTA and a second group of CHI patients whose PTA had resolved. Although the television program test disclosed a partial disturbance of remote memory that was more severe in the patients tested during PTA, there was no evidence of a temporal gradient.

However, an autobiographical questionnaire divided into various epochs of the patients' lives revealed relative preservation of the oldest memories and more severe disruption of memory for recent events (Fig. 38-2).

Features of Memory during Posttraumatic Amnesia

By serially testing recognition memory, Levin and colleagues[13] found that the rate of forgetting during PTA was more rapid in CHI patients as compared to normal controls and CHI patients who were no longer in PTA. The accelerated forgetting during PTA was found despite presenting stimuli initially to the patients at longer exposure durations than were given to the controls. Apart from rapid forgetting, PTA is also characterized by inactive encoding and retrieval strategies. Gasquonine[14] found that survivors of severe CHI who were in PTA exhibited a flat learning curve for the same list of 12 words presented over five sessions. In the same study Gasquonine[14] also observed that patients in PTA did not cluster words belonging to the same category.

In contrast to the marked impairment of declarative memory during PTA, procedural memory (i.e., for visuomotor skills, visual pattern analysis, and visual maze learning) are relatively preserved. Ewert and coworkers[15] found that CHI patients tested over three sessions while they were in PTA displayed relatively normal procedural learning and retention across sessions, whereas their declarative memory was impaired. Consistent with relative preservation of pattern-analysis skills, the latencies of head-injured patients for reading words presented in mirror orientation decreased across sessions (Fig. 38-3). In contrast, the patients had considerable difficulty recognizing the words that they had learned to read in mirror orientation. An implication of the study by Ewert and associates[15] is that head-injured patients are capable of learning motor and perceptual skills despite severe impairment of declarative memory.

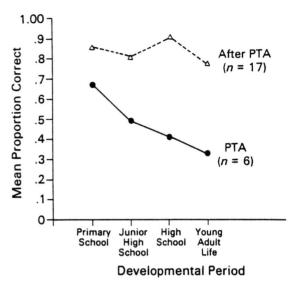

Figure 38-2

Mean proportion of autobiographical events correctly recalled by head-injured patients during the developmental periods during and after PTA. (From Levin et al.,[13] with permission.)

RESIDUAL DISTURBANCE OF MEMORY

Frequency of Memory Deficit

Russell[16] reported that residual memory disturbance was present in 23 percent of over 1000 servicemen who were convalescing from CHI and in 50 percent of severely injured patients. However, these early clinical observations did not differentiate relatively specific memory disorder from global cognitive impairment. To address the specificity of memory disorder in chronic survivors of moderate to severe CHI, Levin and colleagues[17] studied 87 patients at intervals of 5 to 15 months ($n = 65$) and 16 to 42 months ($n = 42$) after injury. By transforming verbal selective reminding[18] and visual recognition memory[19] test scores into standard scores with a mean of 100 and a standard deviation of 15, the investigators selected those patients who had verbal and performance IQs within the normal range of 85 or higher.

Figure 38-4 displays box plots depicting the distribution of IQ and transformed memory scores for controls, moderate, and severe head-injured patients who met this criterion of normal IQ. In contrast to memory deficits involving verbal recall and visual recognition memory, the head-injured patients exhibited intellectual functioning comparable to the normal controls. A similar dissociation between relatively preserved intellectual level and impaired memory was present in the 29 CHI patients who were studied at 16 to 42 months after injury. Disproportionate memory deficit, which was defined by standard scores on both memory tests below 85 and at least 15 points less than the corresponding verbal or performance IQ score, was present in 21 percent of the patients studied between 5 and 15 months after injury and 42 percent of the patients who were studied at 16 to 42 months after injury. In comparison with patients who had global cognitive impairment, the CHI patients who exhibited disproportionate memory deficit had less severe and briefer impairment of consciousness. However, a higher proportion of the memory-impaired CHI patients had nonreactive pupils as compared to the patients whose memory function approximated their intellectual level, which was within the normal range.

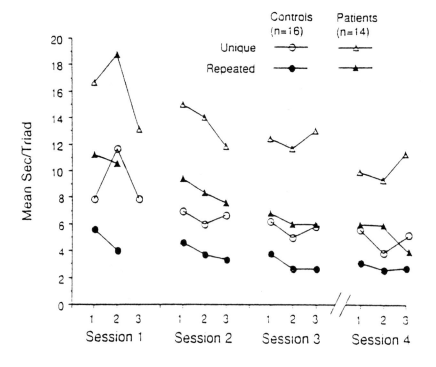

Figure 38-3
Decline in latencies for reading words presented in backward orientation across three sessions during posttraumatic amnesia and a fourth session after return of orientation and memory for ongoing events. (From Ewert et al.,[15] with permission.)

Figure 38-4
Distribution of IQ and transformed memory scores for controls, moderate, and severe head-injured patients who obtained IQ scores within the normal range at 5 to 15 months after injury. The median is indicated by an asterisk, whereas the upper and lower horizontal lines of each bar indicate, respectively, the 75th and 25th percentile scores. The maximum and minimum scores are depicted by the letter x. (From Levin et al.,[17] with permission.)

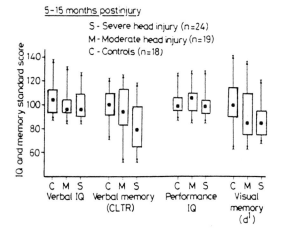

Impact of Memory Deficit on Functional Outcome

Brooks and coworkers[20] investigated the relationship of various neuropsychological test scores to return to work at 7 years following severe CHI. Regression analyses disclosed that verbal memory was the strongest predictor of return to work. Consistent with this finding, an earlier study[21] of young adults examined 1 year after severe CHI indicated that verbal memory measured by the selective reminding test was strongly related to the Glasgow Outcome Scale.

Features of Episodic Memory Deficit

Recovery Curve　　Serial changes in memory following severe CHI were assessed in two studies emanating from the Coma Data Bank.[22,23] Ruff and colleagues[23] administered the verbal selective reminding test and the Benton Visual Retention Test[24] when PTA resolved (i.e., baseline), at 6 and 12 months after injury. The histograms (Fig. 38-5), which plot total consistent long-term retrieval scores on the selective reminding test for

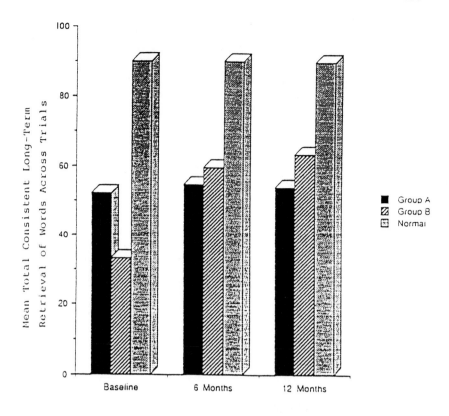

Figure 38-5
Long-term retrieval of words (mean total consistent) recorded in trials with 59 patients at baseline and at 6 and 12 months posttrauma. (From Ruff et al.,[23] with permission.)

the 40 patients comprising group B (who completed all three evaluations), reflect improvement from baseline to 6 months followed by minimal change from 6 to 12 months. Plotting individual recovery curves for the 40 patients in group B disclosed that all but one case could be classified into one of three subtypes. The "peak drop" subtype (one-third of the patients) was characterized by improvement from baseline to 6 months followed by a drop in verbal memory at 12 months; the "flat" subtype, which comprised 17 percent of the patients, exhibited no gains in performance from baseline to 12 months; the third subtype, which consisted of about 50 percent of the patients, was characterized by linear improvement from baseline to 12 months. Similar to the trend over time seen in Fig. 38-5 for consistent long-term retrieval, Fig. 35-6 shows that changes in the number of words recalled after a 30-min delay exhibited a corresponding pattern for the three subtypes. To summarize, longitudinal studies of episodic mem-

ory following severe CHI indicate heterogeneity in the pattern of recovery, which is obscured by averaging data for consecutive patients.

Characteristics of Verbal Memory Deficit

Using a serial recall technique, Brooks[25] asked patients who had sustained CHI of varying severity (PTA duration ranged from <24 h to more than 40 days) to recall a list of words in any order immediately after presentation in a fixed order on repeated trials. Findings on this task in normal subjects characteristically reflect a "recency effect" in which the probability of recall is highest for the terminal items and decreases rapidly the further the item is from the end of the list, with the exception that items at the beginning of the list are more likely to be recalled than items in the middle of the list. Recall of the terminal items has been traditionally attributed to short-term memory, whereas long-term memory has been im-

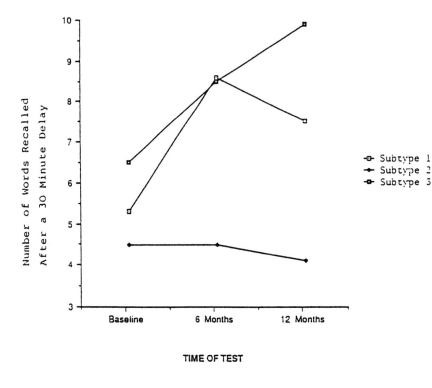

Figure 38-6
Verbal learning data based on selective reminding delayed free recall in 59 patients. Mean value of control group for delayed free recall = 9.85. (From Ruff et al.,[23] with permission.)

plicated in recall of earlier items on the list. As shown in Fig. 38-7, the portion of the curve reflecting recall of words at the beginning of the list indicates a greater disparity in performance between the CHI patients and controls as compared to the relatively slight separation of the curves for recall of items at the end of the list. Classification of the words on the list as short-term versus long-term based on the number of intervening items revealed that the CHI and control groups differed in their recall for the long-term but not the short-term component of memory. Apart from the short-term versus long-term distinction, the CHI patients' memory for words in the middle of the list may have been more vulnerable to interference effects from items occupying earlier and later positions on the list. Brooks[25] found that the recency portion of the curve was relatively preserved in patients who had sustained a severe CHI, whereas these patients exhibited difficulty in recalling the middle portion of the word list (Fig. 38-7).

More recent studies of verbal memory have characterized the processing strategies employed by head-injured patients. Utilizing the levels of processing technique that involved intrasubject comparison of recognition memory for words presented by asking physical (i.e., lower- versus upper-case letters), acoustic (rhyme), or semantic (e.g., "Is it a tool?") questions, Goldstein and coworkers[26] found that chronic survivors of severe CHI showed less improvement under the semantic condition relative to normal controls (Fig. 38-8).

Organization of Verbal Memory

Consistent with this evidence for relatively inactive (or at least ineffective) semantic encoding, there is also evidence that long-term survivors of severe CHI have difficulty in organizing their verbal output. In a study that employed various word list conditions, Goldstein and Levin[27] found that both chronic survivors of CHI and normal controls exhibited facilitation in recalling nouns that were presented in a clustered format (e.g., fruits, parts of a house). However, under a condition in which

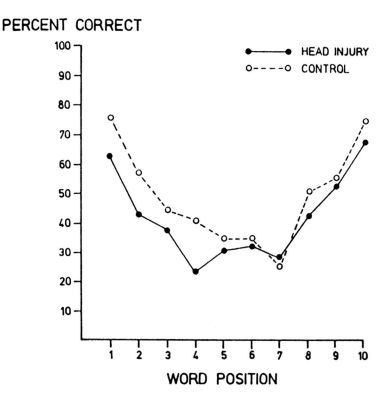

PERCENT CORRECT

Figure 38-7
Mean percentage of correct recall as a function of word position for closed head injured and control patients with recall tested immediately after presentation of the words. (From Brooks,[25] with permission.)

words drawn from three categories were presented in a randomly interspersed order, survivors of severe CHI exhibited a lower-than-normal level of spontaneous clustering in their recall. Figure 38-9 shows the proportion of categorical clustering in spontaneous recall by CHI patients and controls for a list of related words (drawn from three categories) presented at the beginning of each trial by the examiner in an unclustered manner (i.e., words from the three categories were randomly interspersed). The index of clustering depicted in Fig. 38-9 is adjusted for the absolute number of words recalled, thus permitting a comparison of memory organization despite differences in overall performance.

Visual Memory

Based on the extensive literature concerning the effects of right temporal lobectomy, it might be anticipated that a traumatic mass lesion (hema-

toma) situated in the right temporal region would result in a visual memory deficit. This prediction assumes that the effects of temporal lobectomy in epileptic patients correspond to the sequelae of focal mass lesions following head injury. However, few studies have employed appropriate tasks for detecting visual memory deficit following a CHI. Comparisons of visual memory for relatively nonverbal material with verbal memory are frequently complicated by variation in the procedures used for testing memory (recall versus recognition) and the level of difficulty.

Brooks[28] studied visual memory following resolution of PTA in 27 CHI patients by evaluating reproduction of geometric designs following a 10-s exposure, reproduction of the Rey complex design from memory, and performance on the Kimura continuous recognition memory task, which consisted of both geometric and nonsense designs. In comparison with an orthopedic control group, the CHI patients exhibited a visual memory deficit on

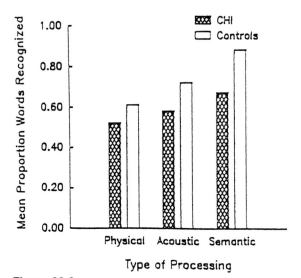

Figure 38-8

Mean proportion of words recognized as a function of type (i.e., physical feature, acoustic, semantic) of processing (collapsed across yes and no responses) for closed head injured patients and control subjects. (From Goldstein et al.,[26] with permission.)

Figure 38-9

Categorical clustering in recall by patients with closed head injuries by controls on the related unclustered list. (From Levin and Goldstein,[35] with permission.)

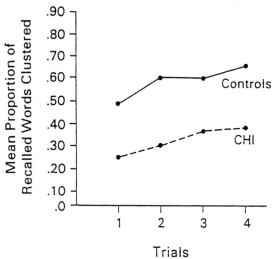

the Rey design and the continuous recognition memory task, whereas short-term visual memory of simple geometric designs did not differ between the two groups. Brooks found that the duration of PTA was related to the degree of impairment on all tasks. In an extension of his first study of visual recognition memory, Brooks[29] administered the continuous recognition memory task to 34 patients following clearing of PTA and again compared the results to findings in orthopedic patients. The results of the later study confirmed the presence of a visual recognition memory deficit related to the duration of PTA in CHI patients who were 30 years of age or older, but not in younger patients. However, Brooks found no relationship between the presence and location of focal brain lesions detected by computed tomography and visual memory performance.

Using a continuous visual recognition memory task based on familiar categories of living things and objects (e.g., flowers, birds), Hannay and associates[30] compared the performance of patients who sustained CHI of varying severity (following resolution of PTA) to normal controls. An increased rate of false-positive errors (i.e., misidentifying a new stimulus as one that had been presented repeatedly) primarily differentiated the severe injuries from the mild CHI and control groups. False-negative errors (i.e., misidentifying a repeatedly presented stimulus as one that was not presented previously) was less frequent and generally confined to the most severely injured patients. Hannay and coworkers[30] found that duration of coma was correlated with the total number of correct responses but not with either type of error taken individually. The sensitivity of this measure of continuous visual recognition memory was supported by the finding that more than two-thirds of the cases with severe CHI obtained a total score that fell below the range of scores in the control group. In addition, the investigators reported no relationship between educational level and any of the visual memory performance measures. In summary, visual recognition and visual recall procedures are a useful adjunct to the assessment of memory in patients who have sustained a CHI. Further research is necessary to ascertain the frequency of identifying patients with specific visual memory disturbances who have otherwise preserved retention of visual material.

Contribution of Frontal Lobe Damage

The postulation that frontal lobe damage contributes to memory deficit after head injury stems from studies that have assessed metamemory, source amnesia, and release from proactive interference. Metamemory, which refers to knowledge about memory skills and self-awareness of memory efficiency, was compared by Volpe and Hirst[31] in patients with frontal damage (including CHI cases) and patients with memory disorder ostensibly due to temporal lobe damage who had no evidence of frontal lobe lesions. Although this study was limited to small samples, Volpe and Hirst[31] were able to demonstrate that metamemory skills were impaired in the patients with frontal lesions, whereas their performance on measures of declarative memory were comparable to or surpassed that of the amnesics with temporal lobe pathology.

Impaired recognition memory following severe CHI is also characterized by difficulty in memory for source (i.e., source amnesia), which refers to the inability to report when or where information was initially encountered. The concept of source amnesia implies that the impairment of memory for source contrasts with the relatively preserved access to information about an experience. Although source amnesia has been attributed to confabulation associated with frontal lobe dysfunction,[32] elucidation of the mechanism awaits confirmation. Dywan and colleagues[33] studied source amnesia in 13 adults who were chronic survivors of CHI of varying severity. On a baseline test involving the discrimination of names of famous persons from those of nonfamous persons, the CHI group performed as well as undergraduate students. To evaluate source amnesia, the subjects were asked to read aloud a list of unfamiliar names, half of which were later interspersed with names of persons who were actually famous. Despite the preserved ability of the head-injured

group in discriminating famous versus nonfamous names in the initial phase of the study, they incurred a higher rate of false-positive errors in misclassifying the nonfamous names they had read earlier in the session as famous. The source amnesia of the CHI group was attributable in part to poor recognition memory, as reflected by difficulty in differentiating the names of nonfamous persons which had been presented in an earlier phase of the study from nonfamous names presented for the first time. However, an index of recognition memory accounted for a small percentage of the variance in source memory errors, thus lending support to the distinctiveness of this deficit. Dywan and coworkers[33] evaluated the postulated role of frontal lobe damage in source amnesia and found no relationship between the presence of frontal lesions (structural imaging) and the degree of source errors. In contrast, the duration of coma was related to the rate of source errors. In view of the small sample size and lack of functional brain imaging, these negative findings concerning the role of frontal dysfunction should be interpreted cautiously.

The role of frontal lobe lesions in the memory deficit of CHI patients was also investigated by Goldstein and colleagues,[26] who used a release from proactive interference procedure that compared recall of word triads after a shift in taxonomic category versus a nonshift condition. Contrary to expectations, the subgroup of patients who had frontal lesions on magnetic resonance imaging exhibited as much release from proactive interference as patients with diffuse cerebral insult.

SUMMARY

In summary, memory deficit is the most frequent neurobehavioral sequel of CHI and is often implicated in chronic disability. Tasks that engage long-term memory processes and require the learning of material that exceeds the limit of immediate span impose demands on effortful processing and tend to be particularly sensitive to the severity of CHI. Although the degree of memory deficit is generally related to the severity of impaired consciousness, further research is indicated to elucidate the mechanisms of injury (e.g., hippocampal versus frontal lobe damage) that contribute to persistent problems in retention.

ACKNOWLEDGMENTS

This chapter was supported in part by NIH grant NS-21889. The author would like to thank Amy Yerkes for assistance in preparing the manuscript for publication.

REFERENCES

1. Russell WR, Nathan PW: Traumatic amnesia. *Brain* 69:183–187, 1946.
2. Russell WR, Smith A: Post-traumatic amnesia in closed head injury. *Arch Neurol* 5:4–17, 1961.
3. Teasdale G, Jennett B: Assessment and prognosis of coma after head injury. *Acta Neurochir* 34:45–55, 1976.
4. Gronwall D, Wrightson P: Duration of post-traumatic amnesia after mild head injury. *J Clin Neuropsychol* 2:51–60, 1980.
5. Artiola i Fortuny L, Briggs M, Newcombe F, et al: Measuring the duration of post traumatic amnesia. *J Neurol Neurosurg Psychiatry* 43:377–379, 1980.
6. Levin HS, O'Donnell VM, Grossman RG: The Galveston orientation and amnesia test: A practical scale to assess cognition after head injury. *J Nerv Ment Dis* 167:675–684, 1979.
7. Shores EA, Marosszeky JE, Sandanam J, Batchelor J: Preliminary validation of a clinical scale for measuring the duration of post-traumatic amnesia. *Med J Aust* 144:569–572, 1986.
8. Russell WR: Cerebral involvement in head injury. *Brain* 55:549–603, 1932.
9. Benson DF, Geschwind N: Shrinking retrograde amnesia. *J Neurol Neurosurg Psychiatry* 30:539–544, 1967.
10. High WM Jr, Levin HS, Gary HE Jr: Recovery of orientation and memory following closed head injury. *J Clin Exp Neuropsychol* 12:703–714, 1990.
11. Levin HS, Peters BH, Hulkonen DA: Early concepts of anterograde and retrograde amnesia. *Cortex* 19:427–440, 1983.
12. Levin HS, High WM Jr, Meyers CA, et al: Impairment of remote memory after closed head injury. *J Neurol Neurosurg Psychiatry* 48:556–563, 1985.
13. Levin HS, High WM Jr, Eisenberg HM: Learning and forgetting during posttraumatic amnesia in head injured patients. *J Neurol Neurosurg Psychiatry* 51:14–20, 1988.
14. Gasquonine PG: Learning in post-traumatic amnesia following extremely severe closed head injury. *Brain Inj* 5:169–175, 1991.
15. Ewert J, Levin HS, Watson MG, Kalisky Z: Procedural memory during posttraumatic amnesia in survivors of severe closed head injury: Implications for rehabilitation. *Arch Neurol* 46:911–916, 1989.
16. Russell WR: *The Traumatic Amnesias.* New York: Oxford University Press, 1971.
17. Levin HS, Goldstein FC, High WM Jr, Eisenberg HM: Disproportionately severe memory deficit in relation to normal intellectual functioning after closed head injury. *J Neurol Neurosurg Psychiatry* 51:1294–1301, 1988.
18. Buschke H, Fuld PA: Evaluating storage, retention, and retrieval in disordered memory and learning. *Neurology* 24:1019–1025, 1974.
19. Hannay HJ, Levin HS, Grossman RG: Impaired recognition memory after head injury. *Cortex* 15:269–283, 1979.
20. Brooks N, McKinlay W, Simington C, et al: Return to work within the first seven years of severe head injury. *Brain Inj* 1:5–19, 1987.
21. Levin HS, Grossman RG, Rose JE, Teasdale G: Long-term orientation and amnesia test: A practical scale to assess cognition after head injury. *J Nerv Ment Dis* 167:675–684, 1979.
22. Levin HS, Gary HE Jr, Eisenberg HM, et al: Neurobehavioral outcome 1 year after severe head injury: Experience of the Traumatic Coma Data Bank. *J Neurosurg* 73:699–709, 1990.
23. Ruff RM, Young D, Gautille T, et al: Verbal learning deficits following severe head injury: Heterogeneity in recovery over 1 year. *J Neurosurg* 75:S50–S58, 1991.
24. Benton AL: *The Visual Retention Test: Clinical and Experimental Applications.* New York: The Psychological Corporation, 1974.
25. Brooks DN: Long and short term memory in head injured patients. *Cortex* 11:329–340, 1975.
26. Goldstein FC, Levin HS, Boake C, Lohrey JH: Facilitation of memory performance through induced

semantic processing in survivors of severe closed head injury. *J Clin Exp Neuropsychol* 58:93–98, 1990.

27. Goldstein FC, Levin HS: Intellectual and academic outcome following closed head injury in children and adolescents: Research strategies and empirical findings. *Dev Neuropsychol* 1:195–214, 1985.

28. Brooks DN: Memory and head injury. *J Nerv Ment Dis* 155:350–355, 1972.

29. Brooks DN: Recognition memory after head injury: A signal detection analysis. *Cortex* 10:224–230, 1974.

30. Hannay HG, Levin HS, Grossman RG: Impaired recognition memory after head injury. *Cortex* 15:269–283, 1979.

31. Volpe BT, Hirst W: The characterization of an amnesic syndrome following hypoxic ischemic injury. *Arch Neurol* 40:436–440, 1983.

32. Janowsky JS, Shimamura AP, Squire LR: Source memory impairment in patients with frontal lobe lesions. *Neuropsychologia* 8:1043–1056, 1989.

33. Dywan J, Segalowitz SJ, Henderson D, Jacoby L: Memory for source after traumatic brain injury. *Brain Cogn* 21:20–43, 1993.

34. Goldstein FC, Levin HS, Boake C: Conceptual encoding following severe closed head injury. *Cortex* 25:541–554, 1989.

35. Levin HS, Goldstein FC: Organization of verbal memory after severe closed head injury. *J Clin Exp Neuropsychol* 8:643–656, 1986.

Chapter 39

REHABILITATION OF MEMORY DYSFUNCTION

Elizabeth L. Glisky

As advances in medical procedures and technologies have dramatically raised the numbers of people surviving brain injury and disease, the demand for rehabilitation services has similarly grown. This demand has been particularly urgent with respect to memory impairment because of its effects on the rehabilitation of all other cognitive deficits and its wide-ranging impact on virtually all aspects of daily life. Because of this urgency to provide services, initial attempts at therapy were not always carefully considered or systematically tested, and outcomes were unreliable. Recently, however, researchers have been testing some new methodologies that appear to yield more consistent benefits.

As yet, there are no well-specified theories of memory rehabilitation, but there are broadly differing approaches to the problem. These approaches differ in terms of their goals, the theoretical mechanisms they propose to account for change, the methods they use to achieve their goals, and the extent to which their techniques are based on well-established cognitive or neuropsychological principles.

GOALS OF MEMORY REHABILITATION

Rehabilitation of memory dysfunction generally focuses on one of two goals: (1) repair of damaged memory processes or (2) alleviation of functional disabilities.[1–3] The first goal assumes that if damaged processes are repaired, general memory *ability* will be reestablished and memory functioning will return to normal. The second goal is less ambitious: to overcome problems caused by memory deficits and improve *performance* on specific everyday memory tasks. The assumption here is that performance might be improved even though the underlying memory ability remains unchanged. Although both goals represent desirable outcomes for therapeutic intervention, the first has so far remained elusive. The bulk of the successful remedial work has been in the area of functional improvement.

THEORIES OF MEMORY REHABILITATION

Although the field of rehabilitation has been criticized as lacking a comprehensive theory of remediation,[4] there are nevertheless some theoretical perspectives that have guided the development of rehabilitation methodologies. Most of these are formulated at a cognitive level, although they often include implicit assumptions concerning the neural underpinnings of cognitive change. Each of the views is associated with one of the above goals and with different methods for achieving those goals.

Restoration of Damaged Function

This approach assumes that damaged memory processes can be restored through stimulation or activation and that premorbid memory ability can thereby be regained. Rehabilitation techniques developed within this framework have focused primarily on memory practice or on retraining of general memory skills.[5] Implicit in this view is the assumption that stimulation of damaged memory processes through exercise, practice, or retraining will result in neural as well as cognitive changes, although the nature of these changes is unclear. As yet, however, there is little evidence to suggest that significant neural regeneration occurs beyond the stage of spontaneous recovery.[6]

Compensation for Lost Function

An alternative approach to the treatment of memory problems assumes that, at least in some cases, cognitive and neural mechanisms cannot be restored and therefore interventions should focus on achieving functional outcomes. In this approach, no attempt is made to restore damaged memory processes. Instead, the need for memory is bypassed by the provision of external supports in the form of environmental restructurings and compensatory devices. This purely pragmatic approach, although a part of many therapies, is often thought to be the only course of treatment for patients with extensive brain damage and severe memory loss.[7]

Optimization of Residual Function

Another theory of rehabilitation assumes that, in many cases, memory processes are not lost entirely but may be reduced in efficiency. Such may be the case in normal aging, for example, or in milder forms of head injury. Under these conditions, rehabilitation may be focused on optimizing the use of residual function. The goal of this approach may be either enhanced performance on specific tasks or the improvement of general memory ability. It usually involves training in the use of mnemonic strategies or skills that were available premorbidly.[8]

Substitution of Intact Function

A final approach to memory remediation assumes that the cognitive and neural mechanisms normally involved in memory may no longer be available but that other *intact* processes can be recruited to assist with memory function. Although the therapeutic goal in this case is improved performance, there is an underlying assumption that change may occur as a result of reorganization at both the cognitive and neural levels.[2,9] This approach may be appropriate when the memory deficit is severe and memory function is minimal.

METHODS OF MEMORY REHABILITATION

Associated with each of the above approaches to rehabilitation are a number of different methodologies, which have proved variously effective. Some of these are based on common sense, others on findings from the normal cognitive literature, and still others on consideration of neuropsychological factors. Their success has been primarily in the achievement of improved behavior or performance; there is, as yet, little evidence that memory ability can be affected in any general sense.

Exercises and Drills

A procedure frequently advocated as a way to restore memory ability has been the use of exercise and drill regimens. It is still common practice in many rehabilitation settings to seat patients in front of computer screens and have them repeatedly practice trying to remember arbitrary lists of words, digits, numbers, locations, or shapes. Although this commonsense method may have face validity, there is no evidence that it leads to any general improvements in memory ability. Patients may learn the specific information that they practice (which often is not very useful), but benefits do not generalize beyond the training context.[3,10,11]

External Aids

A way to compensate for the loss of memory is to use a variety of memory aids, such as notebooks, diaries, alarm watches, calendars and so forth.[10,12] Many of these have been incorporated effectively into the everyday lives of memory-impaired individuals, although considerable training in their use is often required.[13] Recently, micro- and pocket computers have begun to be used as cuing devices[14] and as external supports for a variety of everyday activities,[15–17] but as yet their potential as prosthetic devices has gone largely untapped.

Mnemonic Strategies

A variety of mnemonic strategies, including visual imagery and semantic elaboration, have been adapted from cognitive psychology, where they have proven effective in enhancing the memory performance of normal individuals. With neurologic patients, however, they have been useful only in limited circumstances. For example, patients with unilateral lesions may benefit from a strategy that makes use of the preserved hemisphere.[8,18] Patients with bilateral lesions or severe memory impairments, however, tend not to be able to learn or use these strategies effectively.[8] This finding is consistent with the notion that mnemonic strategy training relies on the use of residual memory function. Even those patients who can learn the techniques, however, do not use them spontaneously; therefore general memory improvements are not observed. Despite this lack of generalization, mnemonic strategies are often effective in helping patients learn specific information that may be relevant in their everyday lives, such as people's names.[8,19,20]

Spaced Retrieval

Another method borrowed from cognitive psychology that has been found to be particularly effective with memory-impaired patients is a rehearsal technique referred to as *spaced retrieval*.[21] This method requires patients to rehearse information at gradually increasing time intervals. Using this technique, patients with memory disorders of varying severity and etiology, including Alzheimer's disease, have been able to learn particular

pieces of information such as name-face associations,[22,23] the location of objects,[24] and items of orientation.[25] The method may rely on residual memory function or it may tap into other preserved processes. Camp and McKitrick[24] have noted that acquisition of new information through spaced retrieval appears to occur effortlessly, and they have speculated that it may involve intact implicit memory systems.

Errorless Learning

Baddeley[26] and Wilson[18] have suggested that memory-impaired patients have a problem with error correction. They have proposed that avoiding early errors during the learning process might facilitate learning. In a series of studies, memory-disordered patients were found to benefit substantially from errorless learning and were able to acquire information such as names and other items of general knowledge important for their daily functioning.[27,28] The authors proposed that patients were relying on implicit learning processes to acquire new information and that these processes were particularly susceptible to interference caused by initial errors. Baddeley[29] has suggested that learning is one of the key components of rehabilitation and that principles of learning should be incorporated into any theory of remediation.

Vanishing Cues

This method, like the previous two, focuses on the learning of specific information rather than on the restoration of memory ability; it has been used primarily for teaching large amounts of complex domain-specific knowledge such as that required to maintain a job or manage a home. The training technique involves the provision of partial information as a cue or prompt, which is then gradually withdrawn as learning progresses. The methodology has been used effectively with a range of memory-disordered patients who have learned vocational tasks such as computer data entry[30,31] and more general skills such as computer programming[32] and word processing.[16] The vanishing cues methodology has been hypothesized to tap into preserved implicit memory processes such as those involved in priming and procedural memory.

IMPACT OF COGNITIVE NEUROPSYCHOLOGY ON REHABILITATION

Much of the recent research in memory rehabilitation has suggested that memory-impaired patients may be learning new information through different processes and structures than those used by normal subjects.[33] So, for example, even patients with very severe disorders can acquire knowledge using spaced retrieval, errorless learning, and vanishing cues; the latter two methods seem not to provide any special benefits to normal subjects. Further, although patients are able to acquire new information, they often cannot access it flexibly and cannot recollect the occasions of learning.[16,31] Nevertheless, they are often able to use recently acquired knowledge in an implicit fashion to carry out various tasks in their daily lives.[16,30]

Recent theoretical work in cognitive neuropsychology has provided a framework for understanding these rehabilitation findings and a direction for future research. Schacter and Tulving[34] have proposed that there may be at least five different memory systems, only one of which—the episodic system—may be significantly damaged in amnesia. Three of the other systems—semantic memory, procedural memory, and perceptual representation—may subserve the kind of implicit memory and learning that has been observed in the rehabilitation studies. (The primary memory system is a short-term system used only for temporary holding and manipulation of information.) Empirical findings supporting the existence of alternate memory systems have provided new impetus to rehabilitation approaches that attempt to take advantage of spared functions. By continuing to explore the extent and characteristics of new learning that can be achieved by memory-impaired patients, rehabilitation research may be able to assist the basic research enterprise in specifying the properties of these alternate memory systems as well as improve the remedial services and treatment outcomes for memory-impaired patients.

ACKNOWLEDGMENTS

Preparation of this manuscript was supported by Grant AG 09195 from the National Institute on Aging.

REFERENCES

1. Harris JE: Methods of improving memory, in Wilson B, Moffat N (eds): *Clinical Management of Memory Problems.* London: Aspen, 1984, pp 46–62.
2. Rothi LJ, Horner J: Restitution and substitution: Two theories of recovery with application to neurobehavioral treatment. *J Clin Neuropsychol* 5:73–81, 1983.
3. Schacter DL, Glisky EL: Memory remediation: Restoration, alleviation, and the acquisition of domain-specific knowledge, in Uzzell B, Gross Y (eds): *Clinical Neuropsychology of Intervention.* Boston: Nijhoff, 1986, pp 257–282.
4. Caramazza A, Hillis A: For a theory of remediation of cognitive deficits. *Neuropsychol Rehabil* 3:217–234, 1993.
5. Sohlberg MM, Mateer CA: *Introduction to Cognitive Rehabilitation.* New York: Guilford, 1989.
6. Meier MJ, Strauman S, Thompson WG: Individual differences in neuropsychological recovery: An overview, in Meier MJ, Benton AL, Diller D (eds): *Neuropsychological Rehabilitation.* London: Guilford, 1987, pp 71–100.
7. Kirsch NL, Levine SP, Fallon-Krueger M, Jaros LA: The microcomputer as an "orthotic" device for patients with cognitive deficits. *J Head Trauma Rehabil* 2(4):77–86, 1987.
8. Wilson B: *Rehabilitation of Memory.* New York: Guilford, 1987.
9. Luria AR: *Restoration of Function after Brain Injury.* New York: Macmillan, 1963.
10. Godfrey HPD, Knight RG: Cognitive rehabilitation of memory functioning in amnesiac alcoholics. *J Consult Clin Psychol* 53:555–557, 1985.
11. Berg IJ, Koning-Haanstra M, Deelman BG: Long-

term effects of memory rehabilitation. *Neuropsychol Rehabil* 1:97–111, 1991.

12. Harris JE: Ways to help memory, in Wilson BA, Moffat N (eds): *Clinical Management of Memory Problems,* 2d ed. London: Chapman & Hall, 1992, pp 59–85.

13. Sohlberg MM, Mateer CA: Training use of compensatory memory books: A three stage behavioral approach. *J Clin Exp Neuropsychol* 11:871–887, 1989.

14. Kirsch NL, Levine SP, Lajiness-O'Neill R, Schnyder M: Computer-assisted interactive task guidance: Facilitating the performance of a simulated vocational task. *J Head Trauma Rehabil* 7(3):13–25, 1992.

15. Cole E, Dehdashti P, Petti L: Design and outcomes of computer-based cognitive prosthetics for brain injury: A field study of three subjects. *NeuroRehabil* 4(3):174–186, 1994.

16. Glisky EL: Acquisition and transfer of word processing skill by an amnesic patient. *Neuropsychol Rehabil* 5(4):299–318, 1995.

17. Glisky EL: Computers in memory rehabilitation, in Baddeley AD, Wilson BA, Watts FN (ed): *Handbook of Memory Disorders.* New York: Wiley, 557–575, 1995.

18. Wilson B: Rehabilitation and memory disorders, in Squire LR (ed): *Neuropsychology of Memory,* 2d ed. New York: Guilford, 1992, pp 315–321.

19. Thoene AIT, Glisky EL: Learning of name-face associations in memory impaired patients: A comparison of different training procedures. *J Int Neuropsychol Soc* 1(1):29–38, 1995.

20. Wilson B: Success and failure in memory training following a cerebral vascular accident. *Cortex* 18:581–594, 1982.

21. Landauer TK, Bjork RA: Optimum rehearsal patterns and name learning, in Gruneberg MM, Morris PE, Sykes RN (eds): *Practical Aspects of Memory.* London: Academic Press, 1978, pp 625–632.

22. Camp CJ: Facilitation of new learning in Alzheimer's disease, in Gilmore GC, Whitehouse PJ, Wykle ML (eds): *Memory, Aging, and Dementia.* New York: Springer-Verlag, 1989, pp 212–225.

23. Schacter DL, Rich SA, Stampp MS: Remediation of memory disorders: Experimental evaluation of the spaced-retrieval technique. *J Clin Exp Neuropsychol* 7:79–96, 1985.

24. Camp CJ, McKitrick LA: Memory interventions in Alzheimer's-type dementia populations: Methodological and theoretical issues, in West RL, Sinnott JD (eds): *Everyday Memory and Aging: Current Research and Methodology.* New York: Springer-Verlag, 1992, pp 155–172.

25. Moffat N: Strategies of memory therapy, in Wilson BA, Moffat N (eds): *Clinical Management of Memory Problems,* 2d ed. London: Chapman & Hall, 1992, pp 86–119.

26. Baddeley AD: Implicit memory and errorless learning: A link between cognitive theory and neuropsychological rehabilitation, in Squire LR, Butters N (eds): *Neuropsychology of Memory,* 2d ed. New York: Guilford, 1992, pp 309–321.

27. Baddeley AD, Wilson BA: When implicit learning fails: Amnesia and the problem of error elimination. *Neuropsychologia* 32:53–68, 1994.

28. Wilson BA, Baddeley AD, Evans J, Shiel A: Errorless learning in the rehabilitation of memory impaired people. *Neuropsychol Rehabil* 4:307–326, 1994.

29. Baddeley A: A theory of rehabilitation without a model of learning is a vehicle without an engine: A comment on Caramazza and Hillis. *Neuropsychol Rehabil* 3:235–244, 1993.

30. Glisky EL, Schacter DL: Acquisition of domain-specific knowledge in organic amnesia: Training for computer-related work. *Neuropsychologia* 25:893–906, 1987.

31. Glisky EL: Acquisition and transfer of declarative and procedural knowledge by memory-impaired patients. *Neuropsychologia* 30:899–910, 1992.

32. Glisky EL, Schacter DL, Tulving E: Computer learning by memory-impaired patients: Acquisition and retention of complex knowledge. *Neuropsychologia* 24:313–328, 1986.

33. Glisky EL, Schacter DL, Butters MA: Domain-specific learning and remediation of memory disorders, in Riddoch MJ, Humphreys GW (eds): *Cognitive Neuropsychology and Cognitive Rehabilitation.* Hove, England: Erlbaum, 1994, pp 527–548.

34. Schacter DL, Tulving E: What are the memory systems of 1994? in Schacter DL, Tulving E (eds): *Memory Systems 1994.* Cambridge, MA: MIT Press, 1994, pp 1–38.

Part 6
DEMENTIA AND DELIRIUM

Chapter 40

DEMENTIA AND DELIRIUM: AN OVERVIEW

Daniel I. Kaufer
Jeffrey L. Cummings

Dementia and delirium are distinctive clinical syndromes based on central nervous system dysfunction. Both syndromes have enormous social, economic, and epidemiologic ramifications, particularly with respect to the elderly. Almost four million Americans are currently afflicted with Alzheimer disease, a number which will more than double in less than fifty years as longevity increases.[1,2] Aside from the incalculable toll it exacts on individuals and families, the overall cost to society approaches $60 billion annually. Delirium, in contrast to the typically insidious nature of dementia syndromes, poses a more immediate threat in terms of morbidity and mortality. Delirium in elderly general hospital patients is a common problem, although studies based on systematic assessment suggest that up to two-thirds of these cases go unrecognized.[3–6] The failure to detect or the misdiagnosis of delirium may have serious consequences, as delirium is associated with increased rates of other medical complications, institutionalization, and death.[5] Delirium prolongs the length of hospitalization and may dramatically increase the cost of care.[7] Although dementia and delirium syndromes may occur at any time in the life span and have many shared and independent risk factors, the strongest risk factor for both is advancing age.[1,3] Increased awareness and early recognition of these disorders in community, ambulatory, and inpatient settings may help ameliorate their devastating impact.

Dementia and delirium both involve acquired cognitive impairment and behavioral alterations involving multiple cognitive domains. Each is a clinical syndrome with characteristic but variable patterns of expression. The multiplicity of clinical subtypes within each syndrome reflects the wide range of etiologies and pathophysiologic mechanisms underlying these disorders. Dementia and delirium are fundamentally distinguished by the clinical hallmarks of primary memory and attentional deficits, respectively.[8,9] Beyond these core deficits, considerable overlap in the clinical manifestations of these disorders can lead to diagnostic confusion. This highlights the need for valid and reliable definitional guidelines and a systematic approach to assessment. Accurate clinical characterization and distinction of dementia and delirium syndromes is essential to differential diagnosis. Knowledge of respective risk factors and etiologies, in turn, is crucial for guiding relevant laboratory diagnostic evaluation and therapeutic intervention.

As subsequent chapters provide a comprehensive survey of dementing disorders, a more detailed treatment of delirium is presented. The overview of dementia syndromes emphasizes general principles of classification, etiology, pathophysiology, and management. A principal focus is to elaborate a systematic and integrative approach to etiologic diagnosis based on recognizable constellations of brain-behavior relationships evident across a variety of conditions that impair cognition.

DEFINITIONS

Delirium

Historically, more than thirty different terms have been used to describe delirium.[10] The term *acute confusional state* (ACS) is commonly used by neurologists; some authors reserve use of the term *delirium* for the syndrome of agitation, psychosis, and autonomic instability associated with alcohol withdrawal.[11] Use of *confusion* per se as a clinical descriptor is discouraged due to its lack of behavioral specificity. One of the major pitfalls in the assessment of delirium has been the absence of validated diagnostic criteria and rating instruments.[12] This problem has gradually been addressed by the increased availability of standardized definitions, operational criteria, and validated assessment tools.[8,13,14] The first widely used standardized criteria for delirium were presented in the *Diagnostic and Statistical Manual of Mental Disorders*, 3d ed. (DSM-III), published in 1980.[15] The nebulous term *clouding of consciousness* used as the anchoring criterion in DSM-III was replaced in subsequent editions by the term *disturbance of consciousness*.[8,16] The current definitional criteria for delirium presented in DSM-IV are outlined in Table 40-1. The core phenomenologic features of delirium are a disturbance in consciousness, attentional deficits, brief duration of symptoms, and fluctuation in symptoms over time.[8] The principal exclusionary criterion involves distinguishing delirium from a dementia syndrome, although the

two disorders may frequently coexist. Patients with dementia are often more susceptible to delirium-producing insults,[17] but the initial diagnosis of a dementia cannot reliably be made in the presence of a delirium.

Dementia

As with delirium, the first widely applied standardized guidelines for the diagnosis of dementia were contained in DSM-III.[15] The two essential diagnostic features of dementia as defined by DSM-III have been preserved in DSM-IV and include (1) an impairment in social and occupational functioning and (2) memory and other cognitive deficits.[8] Specific domains of cognitive disturbance embraced by the definition include aphasia, apraxia, agnosia, and disturbances in executive functions such as planning, organizing, and abstract thinking. Additional requirements include the exclusion of a delirium or inability to better account for the symptoms by an axis I psychiatric disorder. Classification of dementia syndromes depends on evidence linking the clinical process to one or more medical etiologies (i.e., hypothyroidism), cerebrovascular disease (i.e., vascular dementia), or excluding other medical conditions (i.e., Alzheimer disease).

Cummings and Benson[18] proposed alternative criteria for dementia, highlighting the clinical and topographic heterogeneity of dementia syndromes. These are contrasted with DSM-IV criteria in Table 40-2. They define dementia as an acquired persistent impairment of intellectual function with compromise in at least three of the following spheres of mental activity: language, memory, visuospatial skills, emotion or personality, and cognition (abstraction, calculation, judgment, executive function, and so forth).[18] In contrast to DSM-IV criteria, this definition allows for the possibility that memory disturbance may not be a presenting feature of a dementing illness, as is not infrequently the case with Pick's disease and other frontotemporal dementias (see Chap. 41).[1] The DSM-IV stipulation of a decline in social or occupational functioning provides a measure of ecologic validity, but neurobiologic sensitivity is

Table 40-1
DSM-IV criteria for delirium

Disturbance in consciousness impairing awareness of the environment

Reduced ability to focus, sustain, or shift attention

Cognitive or perceptual disturbance not attributable to dementia

Acute to subacute onset (hours to days)

Diurnal fluctuations

Clinical/laboratory evidence relating the disturbance to a general medical condition

Table 40-2

Comparison of DSM-IV criteria for dementia and Cummings and Benson definition of dementia

DSM-IV	Cummings and Benson
Multiple cognitive deficits including: 　Memory impairment 　One or more of the following: 　　Aphasia 　　Apraxia 　　Agnosia 　　Executive dysfunction	Acquired, persistent intellectual impairment involving at least three of the following domains: 　Language 　Memory 　Visuospatial skills 　Emotion or personality 　Cognition/executive functions
Impairment in social or occupational functioning	
Decline from a previous level of functioning	
Clinical/laboratory evidence relating the disturbance to a general medical condition	
Deficits do not occur exclusively in the course of a delirium	

Sources: DSM-IV[8] and Cummings et al.,[18] with permission.

lost due to the variable social and functional demands an individual may face. Emphasis placed by DSM-IV on the "cortical" deficits of aphasia, apraxia, and agnosia may further diminish its sensitivity to other common manifestations of dementing illnesses, including apathy, psychosis, and other neuropsychiatric symptoms.[19] Despite these differences, most patients meeting the Cummings and Benson criteria for dementia would also be identified as demented using the DSM-IV approach.

DELIRIUM

Clinical Features

Attentional Dysfunction Attentional impairment, the principal manifestation of delirium or ACS, is not a unitary phenomenon (see Chaps. 2 and 4).[9,20] The severity of attentional disturbance may vary from a marked decrease in level of consciousness (i.e., stupor or coma) to a deficient performance of attentionally demanding tasks in a seemingly alert subject. Determining level of alertness is a requisite first step of assessment. In awake

or arousable subjects, simple bedside tests of attention and vigilance include digit span (the number of random, sequential spoken digits the subject is able to repeat) and a continuous performance test (e.g., subject identifies a target stimulus such as the letter *A* among a series of randomly presented target and nontarget stimuli).[21] Both tests have been shown to be as sensitive as formal instruments for detecting delirium.[22] More subtle deficits may be elicited by tests of divided attention such as reversing the sequence of spoken digits, spelling a word backwards, or performing serial subtractions. Numerical scoring of these tests may be augmented informally by noting the degree of effort or length of time required to complete the task.

Nonattentional Cognitive Deficits Attentional deficits are associated with and contribute to other intellectual disturbances.[23] Thought form may be rambling and incoherent, with bizarre content. When there is an associated language comprehension deficit, delirious speech may be confused with a Wernicke-type fluent aphasia (see Chap. 9). Delirium can usually be distinguished from the latter by the relative absence of paraphasic errors and better-preserved ability to repeat.[20] Anomia is common and may be manifest as the syndrome of nonaphasic misnaming.[24,25] Nonaphasic misnaming is characterized by a stilted or pedantic style, facetiousness, and a tendency for misidentifications along a particular theme. Anomia in delirium compared to anomia in Alzheimer disease patients is associated with more perseverative and visual perceptive errors.[26] Writing disturbances include poor legibility, spatial misalignment, agrammatism, and spelling errors, particularly at the ends of words, and are among the most sensitive indicators of delirium.[27] Similarly, mechanical, organizational, and spatial deficits may be apparent in figure copying and drawing. Learning and memory are virtually always affected, often reflecting the inability to encode or register new material. The inability to immediately recall newly presented information confounds formal testing of memory and may help distinguish delirium from a primary amnestic disorder. Confabulation (see Chap. 28) has been observed in 15 percent of delirium patients.[28–30] Disorientation to time and place are commonly present but are neither invariant nor pathognomonic features of delirium. Other cognitive abnormalities include concrete thinking, calculation errors, and perseverative tendencies in thinking, speech, and motor behavior.[23]

Neuropsychiatric Features Neuropsychiatric symptoms are frequent manifestations of delirium. Hallucinations tend to be visual, although auditory and tactile hallucinations may also be present; the latter are particularly common in alcohol and drug withdrawal syndromes.[28] Delusional beliefs may be simple or complex and occasionally take on specific forms, such as the belief that significant others have been replaced by others who appear similar (Capgras syndrome) or the belief that one is simultaneously in two locations (reduplicative paramnesia).[31,32] Psychotic symptoms may sometimes be florid, accompanied by persecutory fear and agitation. Emotional lability, hyperexcitability, and euphoria may produce a manialike state, or the patient may appear depressed, apathetic, or perplexed.[3,28] The polarity of these features has led to subtyping of delirium into "hyperactive-hyperalert" and "hypoactive-hypoalert"[3] or "activated" and "somnolent"[33] variants. Ross and colleagues[33] observed paranoia, agitation, and psychosis much more frequently in patients with "activated" delirium, although admixtures of or alternations between these symptom complexes may occur in the same individual during the course of a delirious episode.[34]

Movement Disorders A variety of movement disorders may accompany delirium, particularly toxic-metabolic encephalopathies. A tremor may be present when the arms are held in extension or during movement.[23,35] Generalized tremulousness often accompanies withdrawal states. Asterixis is the brief, repetitive cessation of muscle activity best observed when the arms are held in a fixed posture extended at the elbow and wrist. Although this is colloquially referred to as the "liver flap" due to its association with hepatic encephalopathy,[36] a wide variety of toxic and metabolic conditions may produce asterixis.[37] Myoclonus, like asterixis, is associated with drug toxicity and metabolic derangements, particularly uremia, but is otherwise a nonspecific finding. Generalized increased motor tone, hyperreflexia, and extensor plantar responses may also occur in delirium. The term *catatonia* refers to a number of abnormal movements, commonly including stereotyped mannerisms and bizarre posturing,[23,38] which occur in an association with a wide variety of conditions including idiopathic psychiatric illnesses (schizophrenia and mood disorders), metabolic and toxic encephalopathies, and structural lesions of the limbic system and basal ganglia.

Sleep-Wake Cycle Disturbances Disturbances of the sleep-wake cycle are a consistent feature of delirium. Sleep patterns may become fragmented, with an overall trend toward diminished physiologic sleep.[3] The normal circadian cycle may be reversed, with daytime somnolence and nocturnal restlessness and agitation.[39]

Course and Prognosis

Delirium frequently prompts admission to an acute care setting or develops during hospitalization for other reasons. Epidemiologic studies may reflect only cases severe enough to warrant hospitalization, thereby underestimating the true incidence and prevalence. The estimated prevalence of delirium in elderly hospitalized patients varies between 11 and 16 percent, with incidence rates ranging between 3 and 31 percent.[40–43] Both rates are typically higher in surgical patient populations.[44] Advanced age, illness severity, fever, infection, and exposure to anticholinergic or sedative drugs are among the strongest risk factors for delirium, and the overall risk is amplified by the number of risk factors present. Dementia increases the risk of delirium two- to threefold, and up to half of all patients with delirium have preexisting or newly acquired dementia.[45]

Short-term morbidity is increased in delirium patients, reflected by longer hospitalizations and an increased number of complications, such as infections and decubitus ulcers.[41,42,45] Elderly patients with delirium are at higher risk for not being able to live independently; in more severe cases, they may require nursing home placement.[45,46] One month mortality rates of 15 to 30 percent have been reported in patients admitted to hospital in a delirium.[3,47] Recovery from a delirium may be protracted and incomplete; intellectual and neuropsychiatric disturbances were noted to persist for more than 6 months in a majority of patients studied.[46] In some cases, further deterioration in functional or intellectual status after an acute delirium-provoking insult may reflect the unmasking of a subclinical dementia.[45,48]

Laboratory Features

General Guidelines The laboratory evaluation of delirium is guided by clinical history, predisposing factors, and initial assessment. A toxicology panel and routine blood chemistries (electrolytes, blood glucose, blood urea nitrogen, creatinine, liver function tests) are appropriate screening tests. In certain situations, vitamin B_{12}, thyroid function tests, and screening for collagen vascular disease may be useful. If respiratory status is compromised, an arterial blood gas is indicated. Focal or asymmetrical neurologic signs suggest an intra-cranial lesion and require radiographic evaluation. If a hemorrhagic process is suspected by a history of apoplectic onset, severe, acute headache, or significant head trauma, a computed tomography (CT) scan is indicated. Cranial nerve abnormalities indicated by pupillary or oculomotor dysfunction and other lesions implicating brainstem involvement are better assessed with magnetic resonance imaging (MRI). The presence of a fever dictates systemic evaluation, including a lumbar puncture, for an infectious process.

Electroencephalography The electroencephalogram (EEG) is often useful in identifying the presence of a metabolic encephalopathy.[49] More recently, quantitative EEG methods have also been demonstrated to be useful in evaluating delirium.[50] Metabolic conditions are typically associated with diffuse slowing of background activity in the theta and delta range in proportion to the severity of cognitive impairment.[51] Triphasic waves are commonly seen in hepatic encephalopathy but are also variably present in uremic and anoxic encephalopathy.[52] Withdrawal states, particularly alcohol withdrawal, are associated with low-voltage fast (beta) activity, but this pattern is also seen with barbiturate and benzodiazepine use. Focal structural or space-occupying lesions typically exhibit localized slowing or, less often, periodic lateralized epileptiform discharges.[49]

Etiologies

Acute disruption of central nervous system (CNS) function can result from a wide variety of etiologic factors, acting alone or in combination. The etiologic potential of a deliriogenic agent or condition is modified by a number of host and environmental factors. Advanced age, preexisting brain disease, constitutional compromise, absence of orienting stimuli in the environment, and sleep deprivation all may render an individual more susceptible.[3] Within the CNS, lesions producing delirium may be broadly categorized into those with diffuse or multifocal involvement and those with more localized topography. Focal intracranial, multifocal to diffuse intracranial, and systemic etiologies of delirium are shown in Table 40-3.

Table 40-3
Etiologies of delirium

Systemic	Intracranial
Metabolic conditions	Multifocal/diffuse CNS
Cardiac, pulmonary, renal, hepatic disease	Head trauma
Glucose and electrolyte disturbances	Encephalitis
Systemic inflammatory disorders	Epilepsy (ictal and postictal)
Hypoxia	Hypertensive encephalopathy
Anemia	Vasculitis
Porphyria	Migraine
Infection	Subdural hematoma
Systemic with fever	Neoplasm
Endocrine dysfunction	Cerebrovascular accident (acute phase)
Thyroid, parathyroid, adrenal, pituitary	Focal CNS
Nutritional deficiency	Right hemisphere
Thiamine (Wernicke encephalopathy)	Temporal (medial)
B_{12}, folate, biotin, niacin	Parietal (inferior)
Protein-calorie malnutrition	Frontal (inferior)
Intoxications	Occipitotemporal (bilateral or left)
Drugs (therapeutic and abused)	Caudate
Alcohol	Thalamus (paramedian)
Withdrawal syndromes	Midbrain (rostral)
Heavy metals, industrial solvents, pesticides	Internal capsule (genu)

Systemic The principal systemic etiologies of delirium include metabolic disturbances or the toxic effects of exogenous chemicals. Metabolic abnormalities arising from organ failure, endocrinopathies, nutritional deficiencies, infection, hypoxia, and withdrawal states may produce delirium.[3,10,23] Dehydration and electrolyte abnormalities, particularly low sodium levels,[42] are common precipitants of delirium in the elderly. Cardiac and respiratory compromise may have a generalized deleterious effect on neuronal aerobic metabolism secondary to hypoxemia. Renal and hepatic failure result in the accumulation of endogenous toxic metabolites. Therapeutic drugs are the most common cause of delirium in the elderly, whether iatrogenic, abused, or taken in standard doses by hypersensitive individuals.[45] Although virtually any class of drug in sufficient doses can produce a delirium, anticholinergic agents, sedative-hypnotics, and narcotic analgesics are among the most frequent offenders. The relatively high incidence of delirium postoperatively is multifactorial and includes routine use of drugs from one or more of these classes.[53,54]

Multifocal/Diffuse Central Nervous System
A number of intracranial disorders may present as a delirium. Insults commonly resulting in diffuse or multifocal disturbances in CNS function include head trauma, encephalitides, epilepsy, hypertensive encephalopathy, vasculitis, migraine, subdural hematoma, neoplasms, and the acute phase of cerebrovascular accidents. Postictal confusion is common after partial or generalized tonic-clonic seizures and may persist after repeated seizures despite a normal EEG.[55] Basilar migraine may produce delirium in children and adolescents.[56] In many instances, a delirium is present at the onset of a cerebrovascular accident, possibly due to the acute disruption of intrinsic neurovascular regulatory mechanisms.

Focal Central Nervous System In specific circumstances, focal cerebrovascular insults may result in a confusional state.[57,58] Delirium states with or without agitation have been observed with acute cerebrovascular lesions in the inferior division of the right middle cerebral artery and in the posterior circulation territories of the basilar and more distal posterior cerebral arteries.[59–67] Radiographic and pathologic studies have implicated lesions in the right inferior parietal, right mediobasal temporal, right inferior frontal, unilateral or bilateral lingual and fusiform gyri, rostral midbrain, and paramedian thalamic nuclei as areas most strongly associated with delirium. A confusional state with or without agitation has also been observed in some patients with infarcts principally involving the caudate nucleus.[68,69] Acute infarctions of the genu of the internal capsule may present with fluctuating attention and psychomotor slowing.[70] Mori and Yamadori[65] have suggested that right hemispheric lesions involving frontostriatal regions are responsible for quiet delirium states, whereas confusional states marked by agitation are more intimately associated with right medial temporal involvement. This view is consistent with the dominant role of the right hemisphere in attentional processes (see Chaps. 7 and 21).

Management

Medical The first and most critical step in the management of delirium is to identify and address the underlying etiology. Once a delirium has been documented by history and appropriate assessment, the potentially causal factor or factors must be evaluated systematically. In many instances, a reversible toxic or metabolic disturbance will become apparent from the history, examination, and routine laboratory studies. A careful history may suggest the possibility of drug intoxication, alcoholism, or environmental toxin exposure. In the elderly, particular attention to alcohol and sedative-hypnotic withdrawal is necessary, as autonomic signs may be minimal or absent.[45] Electrolyte disorders, hepatic and renal dysfunction, serum glucose abnormalities, endocrinopathies,

and hypoxia can all be identified by appropriate laboratory studies and treated accordingly. Febrile illnesses require identifying the source of infection for empiric treatment. Although many elderly patients with delirium will have structural abnormalities evident on MRI, brain imaging has the highest yield in patients with focal neurologic signs or in whom trauma is suspected.[45,47] All prescribed medications known to cause delirium, including those taken on an "as needed" basis, should be scrutinized and adjusted if indicated.[71]

Pharmacologic Severe agitation impedes evaluation and treatment and increases the risk of self-harm. A general principle for the pharmacologic management of behavioral symptoms in the delirious patient is to use the lowest effective dose for the shortest possible time. Parenteral delivery is often necessary due to poor patient cooperation and has the advantage of rapid onset. High-potency neuroleptics such as haloperidol are generally favored due to their lack of cardiac, pulmonary, hypotensive, and anticholinergic side effects.[72] Droperidol can be administered intravenously and has a more rapid onset than haloperidol; it also has more sedative and hypotensive side effects. Both agents can cause extrapyramidal side effects and akathisia; the latter may be misinterpreted as worsening agitation.

Benzodiazepines are the drugs of choice for treating alcohol and sedative drug withdrawal; they are also useful when sedation is desirable or extrapyramidal symptoms make use of neuroleptics impossible.[73] Lorazepam is generally favored over diazepam, due to its relatively shorter half-life and lack of active metabolites.[72] Midazolam has a very short half-life but is not recommended as first-line therapy due to the risk of precipitating benzodiazepine withdrawal symptoms.

The cholinesterase-inhibitor physostigmine has produced mixed results but may have a limited role in the treatment of anticholinergic intoxications.[74] Flumazenil, a benzodiazepine receptor antagonist, has also been used with variable success in the treatment of overdose from this class of drugs.[75]

Nonpharmacologic Beyond identifying and correcting a specific etiology of delirium, the mainstay of care is supportive therapy. Careful attention to nutritional status, hydration, electrolyte balance, and sleep needs may ameliorate the risk or symptoms of delirium. Environmental manipulation to avoid sensory deprivation or overload is an important aspect of care, particularly in the setting of the intensive care unit. Orienting stimuli such as a nightlight or pictures of loved ones may also be helpful. Nursing staff have a preeminent role in serial assessment of the patient's status and providing reassurance and reorienting information. In many instances, the need for sedating medications and restraints can be minimized or eliminated when such measures are put into effect.

DEMENTIA

Etiologic Classification

Degenerative and Nondegenerative The term *dementia* refers to a clinical *syndrome* of acquired intellectual disturbances encompassing a large number of *disease* processes. The key features distinguishing delirium and dementia syndromes are the primary attentional deficits associated with the former and the chronicity of the latter. These distinctions are more relative than absolute. Virtually all etiologies producing delirium may also result in a dementia. Reversibility of either syndrome is principally determined by the specific etiology.

Dementias may result from a wide variety of disorders including degenerative, vascular, traumatic, demyelinating, neoplastic, infectious, inflammatory, hydrocephalic, systemic, and toxic conditions. Etiologies of dementia may be classified into two broad categories, degenerative and nondegenerative. Collectively, degenerative brain diseases are the most common etiology of dementia, with Alzheimer disease accounting for about half of all cases.[1] Each degenerative dementia has a characteristic topography of involvement, although the nature of the underlying pathologic alterations are variable. Several degenerative brain diseases are associated with specific histo-

pathologic markers in affected regions: Alzheimer disease, cortical neuritic (senile) plaques and neurofibrillary tangles; Parkinson disease (PD), brainstem Lewy bodies; progressive supranuclear palsy, subcortical neurofibrillary tangles (distinct from those of Alzheimer disease); and corticobasal ganglionic degeneration, cortical and subcortical achromatic inclusion bodies. Lewy body dementia is a nosologically controversial degenerative condition exhibiting variable degrees of pathologic features common to Alzheimer disease and Parkinson disease.[76,77] Other degenerative conditions, such as Huntington disease and spinocerebellar degeneration, have regionally selective but nonspecific pathologic characteristics of neuronal loss and gliosis. Frontotemporal dementia involves a syndrome of selective frontal and anterior temporal lobe atrophy formerly known as "Pick disease"; the presence of Pick bodies is a variable feature.[78] Hereditary forms or predisposing genetic factors have been identified in the majority of degenerative dementias; heritability is an uncommon feature of nondegenerative dementias. Wilson disease (an autosomal recessive disorder of copper metabolism) and the most common forms of adult leukodystrophy—metachromatic adrenoleukodystrophy (autosomal recessive) and adrenoleukodystrophy (X-linked)—are metabolic-degenerative disorders usually expressed in youth or young adulthood. Similarly, autosomal dominant degenerative conditions—such as Huntington disease, some forms of spinocerebellar degeneration, and familial variants of Alzheimer disease and frontotemporal dementia—tend to have earlier ages of onset. The apolipoprotein E type-4 allele is a marker for earlier onset in sporadic forms and higher incidence in late-onset familial forms of Alzheimer disease.[79,80]

Clinical Pathophysiology

Neuroimaging In contrast to the frequently "global" impact of attentional disturbances on intellectual functioning in delirium, dementing processes usually entail selective involvement of CNS areas.[1] The differential nature and topography of involved neuronal systems results in distinctive patterns of intellectual and behavioral disturbances. The pathologic processes in dementia are diverse, ranging from intrinsic molecular ultrastructural or metabolic defects to exogenous neuronal toxins to gross alterations in brain structure. From a clinical perspective, structural imaging techniques such as CT or MRI will often inform the evaluation and differential diagnosis of disorders with gross structural changes. Pertinent examples include mass lesions, cerebrovascular disease, demyelination, and focal or regional atrophy as seen in Huntington disease (caudate), progressive supranuclear palsy (midbrain), and frontotemporal dementia (frontal and anterior temporal lobes). In the absence of radiographically demonstrable lesions, the underlying metabolic or cerebral perfusion derangements may, in some cases, be detectable by MRI spectroscopy or with functional neuroimaging techniques such as single-photon emission tomography (SPECT) and positron emission tomography (PET).[81] Two burgeoning clinical applications of functional imaging in dementia are the identification of symptom-specific[82,83] and disease-specific[84,85] patterns of altered cerebral perfusion (SPECT) or metabolism (PET). In the latter case, preclinical detection of genetically determined dementias may be possible.[86,87]

Neurochemistry A broad range of neurochemical lesions may produce or contribute to dementia. Nutritional deficiencies of vitamin B_{12}, niacin, or—in the the case of Wernicke encephalopathy—thiamine, typically have systemic and CNS manifestations due to their widespread roles as essential cofactors in intermediate metabolism. Disturbances in thyroid and pituitary function may also have pervasive deleterious effects on both peripheral and CNS metabolic pathways. Chronic exposure to alcohol, illicit substances such as cocaine, or heavy metals such as lead, mercury, or aluminum (chronic renal dialysis) may produce characteristic syndromes of dementia. Prolonged episodes of hypoxia and carbon monoxide poisoning may result in dementia syndromes that reflect the inherent vulnerabilities of the hippocampus and globus pallidus, respectively. The basal ganglia are particularly susceptible to injury due to abnormal metabolism or toxic levels of metallic substances. In Wilson disease, selective deposition of unbound copper in the putamen occurs due to a deficiency in ceruloplasmin, the copper transport protein. Hallervorden-Spatz disease, Fahr disease, and manganese encephalopathy are associated with abnormal accumulations of iron, ferrocalcific aggregates, and manganese, respectively, in the basal ganglia. Deficiency of the myelin synthetic enzyme arylsulfatase A underlies the dysmyelinating dementia of metachromatic leukodystrophy. In many cases, etiologically based treatments of dementing disorders produced by specific neurochemical or biochemical alterations effect a reversal or retard the progression of the dementia.

Neurochemical deficits typically have a less well-defined etiologic role in most degenerative dementias. However, a variety of central neurotransmitter abnormalities may contribute to the clinical manifestations of many degenerative conditions. There are two general types of central neurotransmitter systems: (1) local or intrinsic neurotransmitters, such as gamma-aminobutyric acid (GABA) and glutamate, and (2) projection or extrinsic neurotransmitters, including acetylcholine, dopamine, serotonin, and norepinephrine.[88] Glutamate and GABA are the principal excitatory and inhibitory neurotransmitters of the CNS, respectively, and generally mediate neuronal information transfer along discrete channels in local corticocortical and corticosubcortical circuits. The localized topography and channel specificity of these amino acid neurotransmitters reflect their integral role in neocortically based intellectual functions but render them less susceptible to pharmacologic manipulation.

Projection neurotransmitter systems arise from subcortical and brainstem nuclei and primarily exert a modulatory influence on widely distributed neuronal networks.[88,89] Cholinergic projections from the brainstem reticular system (lateral dorsal tegmentum and pedunculopontine nucleus) terminate in nonspecific thalamic nuclei and basal forebrain regions, activating cortical arousal and attentional mechanisms. Basal forebrain cholinergic nuclei have diffuse projections to neocortical and limbic areas such as the amygdala and hippocampus; disruption of these cholinergic efferents is implicated in the pathogenesis of defects in memory and other intellectual disturbances seen in Alzheimer disease. Dopaminergic projections from the substantia nigra to the putamen are disrupted in Parkinson disease, producing the characteristic motor disturbances of tremor, rigidity, and bradykinesia. Dopaminergic efferents from the ventral tegmental area to the nucleus accumbens, septal area, amygdala (mesolimbic pathway) and to the anterior cingulate, medial temporal, and frontal lobe regions (mesocortical pathway) are affiliated with cognitive functioning and neuropsychiatric disturbances such as depression, mania, and psychosis.[90,91] The locus ceruleus is the origin of two primary ascending noradrenergic projections: (1) a dorsal pathway arising from midbrain nuclei and terminating in neocortical, thalamic, basal forebrain, and medial temporal regions and (2) a ventral pathway arising from lower brainstem areas that project to the hypothalamus and midbrain reticular nuclei. These noradrenergic projections are thought to influence arousal, selective attention, and anxiety states.[89,92] Serotonergic projections arise from median and paramedian raphe nuclei in the brainstem and are widely distributed throughout the cerebral hemispheres. Serotonin principally acts as an inhibitor of diffuse neuronal systems; anxiety, disinhibition, and aggression are associated with altered serotonergic function.[92,93] Together, these diffusely projecting neurotransmitter systems regulate the excitatory and inhibitory tone of multiple, discrete neural circuits underlying specific domains of intellectual function. Regional variations in receptor density and receptor subtypes superimpose a response topography on these "diffuse" systems. Their generally indirect influence on cognition is paralleled by their integrated role in the modulation of behavioral states. Selective disturbances in this regulatory mosaic may produce characteristic patterns of neuropsychological and neuropsychiatric symptoms.

Clinical Features

Cortical and Subcortical Syndromes Dementia has many different etiologies, each with its own range of symptoms. In addition, a multitude of individual-specific factors—including genetic predisposition, education, gender differences, age-related changes, preexisting brain disease, environmental exposures, and medical and psychiatric comorbidity—may impinge on the expression of a dementing illness. Despite the etiologic and individual heterogeneity of dementing illnesses, two basic patterns of neurobehavioral features have been observed and named according to the predominant neuroanatomic regions involved.[1] One syndromic constellation includes *cortical* dementias such as Alzheimer disease. Cerebral cortical regions are the primary locus of involvement in Alzheimer disease, although restricted pathologic alterations in subcortical regions are also present. *Subcortical* dementias—including extrapyramidal disorders such as Parkinson disease, Huntington disease, progressive supranuclear palsy, subcortical vascular disease, white matter diseases, and hydrocephalus—are distinguished by clinical symptoms principally referable to involvement of basal ganglia, limbic-related thalamic nuclei, and portions of the brainstem. From a functional anatomic perspective, striatum, globus pallidus, anterior and medial thalamus, and substantia nigral portions of the midbrain are interconnected with prefrontal cortical regions in a series of circuits with unique neurobehavioral affiliations.[94,95] Similar clinical deficits may result from lesions anywhere in these circuits or reflect circuit dysfunction at both cortical and subcortical levels, as in frontotemporal dementia. A third category, *mixed,* includes conditions such as Lewy body dementia, corticobasal ganglionic degeneration, some vascular dementias, and slow-virus infections, which typically produce symptoms attributable to dysfunction of both cortical and subcortical structures.

From a clinical viewpoint, distinguishing cortical and subcortical patterns of signs and symptoms facilitates a systematic approach to differential diagnosis. A classification of dementia based on degenerative versus nondegenerative etiology and cortical or subcortical type is presented in Table 40-4.

The clinical features of cortical and subcorti-

Table 40-4
Etiological classification of dementias based on cortical and subcortical features

Degenerative	Nondegenerative
Cortical dementias	
Alzheimer disease	Multiple cortical infarcts
	Angular gyrus syndrome
Subcortical dementias	
Extrapyramidal syndromes	Vascular dementias
Parkinson disease	Binswanger disease
Progressive supranuclear palsy	Lacunar state
Striatonigral degeneration	Infectious dementia
Shy-Drager syndrome	HIV dementia
Spinocerebellar degeneration	Whipple disease
Idiopathic basal ganglia calcification	Neurosyphillis
Wilson disease	Demyelinating dementia
Huntington disease	Multiple sclerosis
Neuroacanthocytosis	Miscellaneous dementias
Hallervorden-Spatz	Symptomatic hydrocephalus
Progressive subcortical gliosis	Dementia syndrome of depression
Mixed cortical/subcortical dementias	
Frontotemporal dementia (includes amyotrophic lateral sclerosis with dementia)	Multiple cerebral infarctions
Lewy body dementia	Toxic/metabolic disorders
Corticobasal ganglionic degeneration	Deficiencies (B_{12}, niacin, etc.)
Leukodystrophies	Endocrinopathies (thyroid, etc.)
Metachromatic leukodystrophy	Chronic alcohol/drug abuse
Adrenoleukodystrophy	Marchiafava-Bignami disease
	Industrial/environmental toxins
	Posttraumatic encephalopathy
	Vasculitides (systemic and CNS)
Miscellaneous	
Prion (slow virus) diseases	
Schizophrenia (developmental)	

cal dementias arise from differential involvement of neural components underlying specific cognitive and behavioral functions. The neuropsychological and neurobehavioral concomitants of cortical dementias generally reflect the functional specificities of pathologically disturbed neocortical regions. Cerebral cortex can be viewed as consisting of functionally specialized domains that are linked together in serial and parallel modular networks for information processing.[89] Structural or functional disturbances in these cortically based networks may produce deficits in instrumental intellectual skills such as language, visuospatial functions, and mathematical abilities. Elementary sensory and motor functioning is typically preserved. Subcortical dementias, in contrast, are characterized by slowing and dilapidation of executive functions, affective and personality disturbances, forgetfulness, and movement disorders.[96,97] These features are attributable to disruption of one or more of the structures participating in the frontal subcortical circuits, the nodes of which are less functionally specialized than those of neocortical neural regions. Some features of subcortical dementias are reminiscent of delirium. A comparison between the features of cortical and subcortical dementias and their relationship to delirium is presented in Table 40-5.

Table 40-5
Clinical features of cortical and subcortical dementias and delirium

Feature	Cortical dementia	Subcortical dementia	Delirium
Onset	Insidious	Insidious	Sudden
Duration	Months to years	Months to years	Hours to days
Course	Progressive	Progressive or constant	Fluctuating
Attention	Normal	Normal (slow response time)	Fluctuating arousal and inattention
Speech	Normal	Hypophonic, dysarthric, mute	Slurred, incoherent
Language	Aphasic	Normal or anomic	Anomia, dysgraphia
Memory	Learning deficit (AD)[a]	Retrieval deficit	Encoding deficit
Cognition	Acalculia, concrete (AD)	Slow, dilapidated	Disorganized
Awareness	Impaired	Usually preserved	Impaired
Demeanor	Unconcerned, disinhibited	Apathetic, abulic	Apathetic, agitated
Psychosis	May be present	May be present	Often florid
Motor signs	None	Tremor, chorea, rigidity, dystonia	Tremor, asterixis
EEG	Mild diffuse slowing	Normal or mild slowing (diffuse or focal)	Moderate to severe diffuse slowing

[a]AD = Alzheimer disease.

Differential Diagnosis

Detailed information pertaining to the major classes of dementing illnesses is provided in subsequent chapters. As a prelude to these expositions, salient examples of differential diagnosis related to cortical, subcortical, and mixed dementias are highlighted. Table 40-6 presents a summary of clinical pathoanatomic profiles for the major causes of degenerative and other dementias. Attention to concomitant features such as extrapyramidal and focal or lateralizing neurologic signs complements a systematic approach to the differential diagnosis of dementia syndromes based on the cortical-subcortical organizing principle. Identifying reversible or treatable etiologies of dementia is a preeminent concern.

Cortical Dementia Alzheimer disease is the prototype cortical dementia syndrome. Deficits in short-term memory, visuospatial functions, naming, and verbal fluency are the common initial manifestations of Alzheimer disease. Apathetic indifference, diminished insight or lack of awareness

of deficits, and poor abstract thinking frequently accompany the core neuropsychological deficits. Insidious onset is the rule, although the initial clinical symptoms may be precipitated by a surgical procedure, infection, or minor head injury. Focal neurologic signs are conspicuously absent early in the course; later on, motor dysfunction, myoclonus, and seizures may develop (see Chap. 48).

The principal distinguishing features of Alzheimer disease are the nature of the memory deficits, the presence of other intellectual disturbances, and the absence of neurologic signs. Primary attentional functions are preserved in Alzheimer disease, distinguishing it from toxic and other systemic etiologies of delirium. More isolated disturbances in language or visuospatial functions may reflect cerebrovascular insults or focal cortical degenerative syndromes. The angular gyrus syndrome is a symptom complex of fluent aphasia, constructional disturbances, and elements of the Gerstmann syndrome (acalculia, finger agnosia, dysgraphia, and right-left disorientation).[98] It may result from left hemispheric cerebrovascular lesions in the distribution of the posterior

Table 40-6
Differential diagnostic profiles of clinicopathoanatomic features of dementia

Etiology	Clinical features	Pathoanatomical correlates
Cortical dementias		
Alzheimer disease	Memory deficit (learning)	Hippocampus, nucleus basalis (cholinergic)
	Aphasia, apraxia, agnosia	Temporal and parietal neocortex
	Apathy/indifference	Anterior cingulate, parietal neocortex
Mixed dementias		
Frontotemporal dementia	Memory deficit (retrieval)	Dorsolateral prefrontal cortex
	Speech/language stereotypes	Frontal/temporal neocortex
	Disinhibition	Orbitofrontal cortex
	Hyperorality (Kluver-Bucy)	Amygdala/anterior temporal cortex
Lewy body dementia	Memory deficit (learning)	Nucleus basalis, hippocampal formation
	Aphasia, apraxia, agnosia	Temporal and parietal neocortex
	Extrapyramidal signs	Substantia nigra (dopamine)
	Fluctuating attentional deficits	Pedunculopontine nucleus (cholinergic)?
	Visual hallucinations, delusions	Neocortex (serotonin/cholinergic imbalance)?
Corticobasal ganglionic degeneration	Unilateral limb signs (dystonia, clumsiness, myoclonus)	Subthalamic nucleus, thalamus, globus pallidus
	Cortical sensory loss, apraxia, alien hand phenomena	Parietal and frontal neocortex (asymmetrical)
	Rigidity	Substantia nigra (dopamine)
	Supranuclear gaze palsy (late)	Midbrain
Subcortical dementias		
Progressive supranuclear palsy	Supranuclear gaze palsy	Midbrain
	Dysarthria/dysphagia	Bulbar cranial nerves
	Gait/balance disturbances, axial rigidity	Globus pallidus, subthalamic nucleus, substantia nigra
	Pseudobulbar palsy	Brainstem, prefrontal cortex
Parkinson's disease	Memory deficit (retrieval)	Caudate; nucleus basalis (cholinergic)
	Executive dysfunction	Caudate nucleus
	Tremor, rigidity, bradykinesia	Substantia nigra, putamen (dopamine)
Huntington's disease	Memory deficit (retrieval)	Caudate nucleus
	Executive dysfunction	Caudate nucleus
	Choreiform movements	Putamen, subthalamic nucleus, globus pallidum
Symptomatic hydrocephalus	Gait disturbance	Midline subcortical structures and connections
	Memory deficit (retrieval)	
	Executive dysfunction	
	Incontinence	
Dementia syndrome of depression	Memory deficit (retrieval)	Subcortical white or gray matter
	Impaired concentration/attention	
	Executive dysfunction	
	Parkinsonian features (except tremor)	
Vascular dementia (multiple lacunar strokes or Binswanger disease)	Memory deficit (retrieval)	Thalamic or basal ganglia—frontal disconnection
	Executive dysfunction	Location-dependent
	Focal or asymmetrical elementary neurologic signs	

branches of the middle cerebral artery and is distinguished from Alzheimer disease by its abrupt onset and the relative absence of nonverbal memory deficits. Focal degenerative conditions such as primary progressive aphasia and corticobasal ganglionic degeneration are also characterized by asymmetrical hemispheric involvement and relatively preserved memory but, as with Alzheimer disease, have a more insidious onset and progressive course.[99,100] In corticobasal ganglionic degeneration, unilateral sensory and motor disturbances including apraxia, astereognosis, dystonia, myoclonus, and the "alien hand" syndrome are often present.

Subcortical Dementias Extrapyramidal system involvement is a common feature of subcortical dementias. Parkinsonian features concurrent with a dementia syndrome characterized by retrieval memory deficits, cognitive slowing, and executive dysfunction have a wide differential diagnosis.[1] Parkinson disease, progressive supranuclear palsy, multiple system atrophies, the rigid form of Huntington disease, and many secondary disorders of the basal ganglia produce Parkinson disease with dementia. Most patients with idiopathic Parkinson disease exhibit some degree of intellectual impairment; 20 to 30 percent will have deficits severe enough to meet criteria for dementia.[101] The subcortical dementias of Parkinson disease and progressive supranuclear palsy exhibit overlapping executive deficits[102,103] and are both associated with reductions in frontal lobe metabolism or blood flow.[104,105] Progressive supranuclear palsy is principally distinguished by the early features of gait imbalance and bulbar symptoms (dysarthria and pseudobulbar affect), axial rigidity, and a supranuclear vertical gaze palsy.[106]

Communicating or "normal pressure" hydrocephalus is an uncommon but potentially reversible syndrome produced by impaired egress of cerebrospinal fluid via arachnoid granulations from the intracranial compartment (see Chap. 47). A subcortical dementia syndrome of apathy, psychomotor slowing, retrieval memory deficits, and executive dysfunction may develop over a period of months and is typically preceded by a characteristic "magnetic" or "apraxic" gait.[107] Incontinence generally appears later if at all. The rapidity of decline and prominent gait and balance disturbances help distinguish normal pressure hydrocephalus from Parkinson disease and other extrapyramidal syndromes. Panventricular enlargement is often shown by CT or MRI, particularly in the anterior ventricular regions, out of proportion to the degree of cortical gyral atrophy. However, these radiographic findings lack absolute specificity, which emphasizes the diagnostic primacy of clinical features. Radionuclide cisternography may lend support to the diagnosis.

Depression may influence the symptomatic expression of dementia or may cause a syndrome of dementia (dementia of depression). About 40 percent of Parkinson disease patients exhibit significant depressive symptoms; degree of memory impairment distinguishes them from Parkinson disease patients without depression.[108,109] Depression is also common in Huntington disease, vascular dementia, and other subcortical syndromes. The dementia syndrome of depression is a reversible dementia most commonly seen in elderly patients with a history of severe or psychotic depression. Impaired attention and concentration, forgetfulness, psychomotor slowing, decreased motivation, and impaired ability to grasp the meaning of situations are characteristic features.[110,111]

Vascular dementia is a heterogenous syndrome with multiple clinical presentations, depending on lesion type and location (see Chap. 42). Whereas infarctions in the territory of large cerebral vessels produce characteristic syndromes of cortically based higher intellectual functions, diffuse or multifocal small-vessel ischemic disease affecting periventricular white matter or basal ganglia and thalamic nuclei results in a classic subcortical dementia syndrome. Dementia arising from multiple lacunar infarcts is associated with a preponderance of lesion sites in the frontal lobe white matter, implicating disruption of frontal-subcortical circuit pathways as the relevant pathologic mechanism.[112] More diffuse involvement of subcortical white matter secondary to small-vessel ischemia (Binswanger disease) also functionally disconnects cortical and subcortical regions. Hypertension and other risk factors for vascular disease are commonly present. The vascular dementia syndromes are radiographically distinguishable by characteristic MRI findings on T_2-weighted images.

Huntington disease is a hyperkinetic extrapyramidal syndrome with choreiform movements and a subcortical dementia. The genetic defect in Huntington disease is an autosomal dominant trinucleotide repeat mutation on chromosome 4. Severe atrophy of the caudate nuclei is the pathologic feature accompanying the frequently prominent behavioral and mood disturbances, including depression, irritability, and impulsivity.

Human immunodeficiency virus (HIV) infection is the most common cause of infectious dementia (see Chap. 44). Typical manifestations reflect subcortical dysfunction—psychomotor slowing, memory and concentration impairment, and apathy—due to direct CNS invasion by the virus.[113] Gait, motor, and sensory disturbances may be present due to a vacuolizing myelopathy. Opportunistic infections such as toxoplasmosis and progressive multifocal leukoencephalopathy may produce superimposed deficits.

Mixed Cortical and Subcortical Dementias

Lewy-body dementia involves one or more clinical syndromes with overlapping features of Alzheimer disease and Parkinson disease.[76,77] A characteristic clinical profile—including fluctuating cognitive impairments, prominent psychiatric features (hallucinations, delusions, and depression), gait and balance difficulties, and unexplained loss of consciousness—has been suggested.[114] Neuropsychological disturbances are variable but may reflect more severe deficits in attention, verbal fluency, and visuospatial processing compared to "pure" Alzheimer disease patients.[77] Extrapyramidal signs are a common but not invariable feature and the presentation may be dominated by neuropsychiatric symptoms.[115] Alzheimer disease patients with either extrapyramidal signs or psychotic symptoms have been reported to have more rapid cognitive decline than Alzheimer disease patients without either feature.[116,117] As many patients with

Lewy-body dementia meet research criteria for the diagnosis of Alzheimer disease, the clinical distinction between Alzheimer disease with extrapyramidal signs and psychotic symptoms and Lewy-body dementia is presently unclear. Genetic, biochemical, and neuropathologic variables may help discriminate the clinicopathologic relationship of Lewy-body dementia to Alzheimer disease and to Parkinson disease with dementia.[118,119]

Frontotemporal dementia entails a dementia syndrome with variable pathologic features involving selective frontal and anterior temporal degeneration (see Chap. 41). The core features of frontotemporal dementia are primarily neuropsychiatric and may include behavioral disinhibition, apathy, inappropriate behavior, lack of social awareness, distractibility, impulsivity, and stereotyped or perseverative behaviors.[78] Behavior and personality changes often appear many years before the appearance of frank neuropsychological deficits.[84] Memory function, calculation abilities, and visuospatial skills are preserved early in the course, contrasting with the initial manifestations of Alzheimer disease. The presence of nonfluent speech and language disturbances, motor and verbal stereotypies, hyperorality or change in dietary habits, and earlier age of onset may also help to distinguish frontotemporal dementia from Alzheimer disease.[120] Pathologic involvement is concentrated in frontal lobe cortical areas, with differential involvement of limbic temporal cortex and subcortical basal ganglia structures, particularly the striatum. Gliosis and regional atrophy are typical features; the presence of Pick bodies and swollen neurons may be associated with more severe white matter involvement and more pronounced atrophic changes. Characteristic clinical and pathologic features of frontotemporal dementia may occur with motor neuron disease, with additional degenerative changes in lower brainstem and spinal cord motor neurons.

Treatment and Management of Dementia

Disease-Specific Therapy Etiologically based treatment is not available for any of the degenerative dementias, although treatments informed by disease pathophysiology have recently become available. In Alzheimer disease, the profound reduction in basal forebrain and neocortical acetylcholine, together with evidence linking cholinergic deficits to memory dysfunction, have motivated intensive efforts directed toward enhancing central cholinergic function (see Chap. 39).[121] To date, acetylcholinesterase inhibitors such as tacrine have been the most successful in ameliorating some of the cognitive deficits of Alzheimer disease.[122,123] Other cholinergic-enhancing agents are currently undergoing clinical trials.

Therapeutic strategies in cerebrovascular disease are aimed at both limiting the acute damage of cerebral ischemia and secondary prevention. Excitotoxic mechanisms have been widely implicated in neuronal damage produced by acute ischemia and other neurologic conditions and may prove amenable to intervention.[124] The progression of vascular dementia may be impeded by aggressive control of risk factors such as hypertension and by the use of platelet antiaggregating agents such as aspirin and ticlopidine.

Selegiline is a monoamine oxidase B inhibitor commonly used as an adjunctive treatment of Parkinson disease. Selegiline has a modest impact on the symptoms of Parkinson disease, although it may also have a neuroprotective effect in delaying its progression.[125] The potential neuroprotective benefits of selegiline are currently being assessed in other neurodegenerative conditions such as Alzheimer disease.

The dementia syndrome of depression is potentially reversible with standard antidepressant therapies, including tricyclic antidepressants and selective serotonin reuptake inhibitors. Refractory cases may benefit from electroconvulsive therapy.

Transient improvement in the symptoms of hydrocephalic dementia (particularly gait) following lumbar puncture helps to confirm the diagnosis and may have prognostic significance. The response to shunting in normal pressure hydrocephalus is highly variable but is usually beneficial if there is an identifiable cause and symptom duration has been brief.[126,127]

Toxic and metabolic dementias often respond to removal of the offending agent or reversal of the metabolic abnormality. Steroid and other immunosuppressive agents may ameliorate the cognitive and neuropsychiatric disturbances associated with vasculitis and other CNS inflammatory disorders. The dementia and movement disorders of Wilson disease may be prevented or reversed with penicillamine treatment. Improved cognitive functioning in symptomatic HIV infection may accompany the use of zidovudine.[128] Evacuation of subdural hematomas and surgical resection of CNS neoplasms produce variable improvement, depending on the size, location, and nature of the mass lesion.

Nonspecific Therapy   Neuropsychiatric disturbances are a frequent accompaniment of dementia syndromes and are often a major source of distress to caregivers. Psychotic and agitated behaviors are commonly treated with antipsychotic agents such as haloperidol, although extrapyramidal side effects and the risk of tardive movement disorders limit their application and utility. Newer antipsychotic agents such as risperidone and clozapine may offer advantages in terms of reduced parkinsonian side effects. In Alzheimer disease, there is evidence suggesting that cholinergic agents may ameliorate agitated and psychotic behaviors.[129] Trazodone, in doses up to 300 to 400 mg/day, may have a beneficial effect on insomnia and agitated symptoms. Propanolol and benzodiazepines may help relieve symptoms of anxiety and agitation but are occasionally associated with behavioral complications—depression and paradoxical agitation, respectively. Apathy may be a prominent feature of Alzheimer disease, frontotemporal dementia, Parkinson disease, progressive supranuclear palsy, and Huntington disease[130] but is generally poorly responsive to treatment. Preliminary evidence suggests that apathy may be the target symptom most responsive to tacrine in Alzheimer disease.[131] Depressive symptoms and signs contribute to cognitive and functional morbidity and often respond to pharmacologic treatments. Aggressive behaviors may respond to serotonergic-enhancing agents or, when sexual in nature, to estrogen or anti-testosterone therapy. Supportive care for progressive dementias includes maintenance of adequate nutrition, dietary modification when aspiration risk is present, surveillance for signs of intercurrent respiratory or urinary tract infections, mobilization when possible, and skin care for patients who are bedridden.

Conclusions and Directions

The terms *delirium* and *dementia* respectively denote acute and chronic disorders of brain function producing cognitive impairment. They are common nemeses of aging but differ in their temporal course and the nature of the core neuropsychological deficit—attention in the case of delirium and memory disturbance in dementia. The clinical distinction between attentional and memory dysfunction has important neuroanatomic and etiologic implications. Attention forms the substrate of memory and is subserved by a hierarchical network linking brainstem, thalamic, basal forebrain, and neocortical areas. The broadly distributed nature of pathways subserving attentional function renders it susceptible to a wide variety of toxic and metabolic insults as well as strategically located lesions, particularly those involving the right cerebral hemisphere.

Dementia syndromes may also be produced by a large number of brain diseases. Degenerative dementing illnesses have selective and characteristic topographies of pathologic involvement and associated biochemical lesions. Memory processes disturbed in dementia are mediated by distributed cortical and subcortical networks, and two general clinical patterns of dementia can be distinguished on the basis of a cortical or subcortical locus of primary involvement. Cortical dementias such as Alzheimer disease produce impaired learning of new information and other deficits in intellectual domains associated with dysfunction of cortically based neural networks. Retrieval memory deficits characterize the subcortical dementia syndrome, which is associated with less discretely localized executive and neuropsychiatric disturbances. The subcortical dementia syndrome results from lesions disrupting the integrity of functional circuits linking prefrontal, basal ganglia, and thalamic areas. By distinguishing between subcortical and cortical syndromes of dementia, the etiologic differential diagnosis of dementing disorders is facilitated and insight into functional clinicopathological relationships is provided. Improved accuracy in the diagnosis of degenerative and other dementias will derive from a more precise understanding of how genetic determinants influence the appearance of pathologic disturbances in brain function and lead to the associated clinical manifestations. Integrated knowledge of these relationships provide the basis for unraveling the mechanisms of dementing brain diseases and may help identity therapeutic targets to reverse or prevent these ravaging disorders.

ACKNOWLEDGMENTS

This project was supported by the Department of Veterans Affairs and a National Institute on Aging Core Center Grant (AG10123).

REFERENCES

1. Cummings JL, Benson DF: *Dementia: A Clinical Approach,* 2d ed. Boston: Heinemann-Butterworth, 1992.
2. Max W: The economic impact of Alzheimer's disease. *Neurology* 43(suppl 4):S6–S10, 1993.
3. Lipowski ZJ: *Delirium: Acute Confusional States.* New York: Oxford University Press, 1990.
4. Francis J: Delirium in older patients. *J Am Geriatr Soc* 40:829–838, 1992.
5. Inouye SK: The dilemma of delirium: Clinical and research controversies regarding diagnosis and evaluation of delirium in hospitalized elderly medical patients. *Am J Med* 97:278–288, 1994.
6. Rockwood K, Cosway S, Stolee P, et al: Increasing the recognition of delirium in elderly patients. *J Am Geriatr Soc* 42:252–256, 1994.
7. Francis J, Hilko E, Kapoor W: Delirium and prospective payment: The economic impact of acute confusion. *J Amer Geriatr Soc* 41:SA9, 1993.
8. *Diagnostic and Statistical Manual of Mental Disorders,* 4th ed. Washington, DC: American Psychiatric Association, 1994.
9. Geschwind N: Disorders of attention: A new fron-

tier in neuropsychology. *Philos Trans R Soc Lond [Biol]* 298:173–185, 1982.

10. Liston EH: Delirium in the aged. *Psychiatr Clin North Am* 5:49–66, 1982.

11. Adams RD, Victor M: *Principles of Neurology,* 4th ed. New York: McGraw-Hill, 1989.

12. Liptzin B, Levkoff SE, Cleary PD, et al: An empiric study of diagnostic criteria for delirium. *Am J Psychiatry* 148:454–457, 1991.

13. Trzepacz P, Baker RW, Greenhouse J: A simple rating scale for delirium. *Psychiatry Res* 23:89–97, 1988.

14. Inouye SK, van Dyck CH, Alessi CA, et al: Clarifying confusion: The Confusion Assessment Method: A new method for detection of delirium. *Ann Intern Med* 113:941–948, 1990.

15. *Diagnostic and Statistical Manual of Mental Disorders,* 3d ed. Washington, DC: American Psychiatric Association, 1980.

16. *Diagnostic and Statistical Manual of Mental Disorders,* 3d ed, rev. Washington, DC: American Psychiatric Association, 1987.

17. Sunderland T, Tariot P, Cohen RM, et al: Anticholinergic sensitivity in patients with dementia of the Alzheimer type and age-matched controls. *Arch Gen Psychiatry* 44:418–426, 1987.

18. Cummings JL, Benson DF, LoVerme S Jr: Reversible dementia. *JAMA* 243:2434–2439, 1980.

19. Cummings JL, Victoroff JI: Noncognitive neuropsychiatric syndromes in Alzheimer's disease. *Neuropsychiatry Neuropsychol Behav Neurol* 3:140–158, 1990.

20. Mesulam M-M: Attention, confusional states, and neglect, in Mesulam M-M (ed): *Principles of Behavioral Neurology.* Philadelphia: Davis, 1985, pp 125–168.

21. Strub RL, Black FW: *The Mental Status Examination in Neurology,* 3d ed. Philadelphia: Davis, 1993.

22. Pompei P, Foreman M, Cassel CK, et al: Detecting delirium among hospitalized older patients. *Arch Intern Med* 155:301–307, 1995.

23. Cummings JL: *Clinical Neuropsychiatry.* Orlando, FL: Grune & Stratton, 1985.

24. Weinstein EA, Kahn RL: Nonaphasic misnaming (paraphasia) in organic brain disease. *Arch Neurol Psychiatry* 67:72–79, 1952.

25. Cummings J, Hebben NA, Obler L, Leonard P: Nonaphasic misnaming and other neurobehavioral features of an unusual toxic encephalopathy. *Cortex* 16:316–323, 1980.

26. Wallesch CW, Hundsalz A: Language function in

delirium: A comparison of single word processing in acute confusional states and probable Alzheimer's disease. *Brain Lang* 46:592–606, 1994.

27. Chedru F, Geschwind N: Writing disturbances in acute confusional states. *Neuropsychologia* 10:343–353, 1972.

28. Wolff HG, Curran D: Nature of delirium and allied states. *Arch Neurol Psychiatry* 33:1175–1215, 1935.

29. Mercer B, Wagner W, Gardner H, et al: A study of confabulation. *Arch Neurol* 34:429–433, 1977.

30. Stuss DT, Alexander MP, Lieberman A, Levine H: An extraordinary form of confabulation. *Neurology* 28:1166–1172, 1978.

31. Cummings JL: Organic delusions: Phenomenology, anatomic correlations, and review. *Br J Psychiatry* 46:184–197, 1985.

32. Alexander MP, Stuss DT, Benson DF: Capgras syndrome: A reduplicative phenomenon. *Neurology* 29:334–339, 1979.

33. Ross CA, Peyser CE, Shapiro I, et al: Phenomenologic and etiologic subtypes. *Int Psychogeriatr* 3:135–147, 1991.

34. Liptzin B, Levkoff SE: An empirical study of delirium subtypes. *Br J Psychiatry* 161:843–845, 1992.

35. Jankovic J, Fahn S: Physiologic and pathologic tremors. *Ann Intern Med* 93:460–465, 1980.

36. Adams RD, Foley JM: The neurological changes in the more common types of liver disease. *Trans Am Neurol Assoc* 74:217–219, 1949.

37. Young RR, Shahani BT: Asterixis: One type of negative myoclonus, in Fahn S, Marsden CD, Van Woert M (eds): *Advances in Neurology: Vol 43. Myoclonus.* New York: Raven Press, 1986, pp 137–156.

38. Taylor MA: Catatonia: A review of a behavioral neurologic syndrome. *Neuropsychiatry Neuropsychol Behav Neurol* 3:48–72, 1990.

39. Henry WD, Mann AM: Diagnosis and treatment of delirium. *Can Med Assoc J* 93:1156–1166, 1965.

40. Erkinjuntti T, Wikstrom J, Palo J, et al: Dementia among medical inpatients: Evaluation of 2000 consecutive admissions. *Arch Intern Med* 146:1923–1926, 1986.

41. Rockwood K: Acute confusion in elderly medical patients. *J Am Geriatr Soc* 37:150–154, 1989.

42. Francis J, Martin D, Kapoor WN: A prospective study of delirium in the elderly. *JAMA* 263:1097–1101, 1990.

43. Schor JD, Levkoff SE, Lipsitz LA, et al: Risk factors for delirium in hospitalized elderly. *JAMA* 267:827–831, 1992.

44. Gustafson Y, Berggren D, Brannstrom B, et al: Acute confusional states in elderly patients treated for femoral neck fractures. *J Am Geriatr Soc* 36:525–530, 1988.

45. Francis J, Kapoor W: Prognosis after hospital discharge of older medical patients with delirium. *J Am Geriatr Soc* 40:601–606, 1992.

46. Levkoff SE, Evans DA, Liptzin B, et al: Delirium: the occurrence and persistence of symptoms among elderly hospitalized patients. *Arch Intern Med* 152:334–340, 1992.

47. Beresin EV: Delirium in the elderly. *J Geriatr Psychiatry Neurol* 1:127–143, 1988.

48. Koponen H, Stenback U, Mattila L, et al: Delirium among elderly persons admitted to a psychiatric hospital: Clinical course during the acute stage and one-year follow-up. *Acta Psychiatr Scand* 79:579–585, 1989.

49. Brenner RP: Utility of EEG in delirium: Past views and current practice. *Int Psychogeriatr* 3:211–229, 1991.

50. Leuchter AF, Jacobsen SA: Quanitative measurement of brain electrical activity in delirium. *Int Psychogeriatr* 3:231–247, 1991.

51. Engel GL, Romano J: Delirium: A syndrome of cerebral insufficiency. *J Chronic Dis* 9:260–277, 1959.

52. Brenner RP: The electroencephalogram in altered states of consciousness. *Neurol Clin* 3:615–631, 1985.

53. Tune L, Carr S, Cooper TC, et al: Association of anticholinergic activity of prescribed medications with postoperative delirium. *J Neuropsychiatry Clin Neurosci* 5:208–210, 1993.

54. Marcantonio ER, Juarez G, Goldman L, et al: The relationship of postoperative delirium with psychoactive medications. *JAMA* 272:1518–1522, 1994.

55. Engel J Jr: *Seizures and Epilepsy.* Philadelphia: Davis, 1989.

56. Bickerstaff ER: Impairment of consciousness in migraine. *Lancet* 2:1057–1059, 1961.

57. Krasuki JS, Gaviria M: Neuropsychiatric sequelae of ischaemic cerebrovascular disease: Clinical and neuroanatomic correlates and implications for the concept of dementia. *Neurol Res* 16:241–250, 1994.

58. Trzepacz PT: The neuropathogenesis of delirium: A need to focus our research. *Psychosomatics* 35:374–391, 1994.

59. Horenstein S, Chamberlain W, Conomy J: Infarction of the fusiform and calcarine regions: Agitated delirium and hemianopia. *Trans Am Neurol Assoc* 92:85–88, 1967.

60. Medina JL, Rubino FA, Ross E: Agitated delirium caused by infarctions of the hippocampal formation and fusiform and lingual gyri: A case report. *Neurology* 24:1181–1183, 1974.

61. Mesulam M-M, Waxman SG, Geschwind N, Sabin TD: Acute confusional states with right middle cerebral artery infarctions. *J Neurol Neurosurg Psychiatry* 39:84–89, 1976.

62. Caplan LR: "Top of the basilar" syndrome. *Neurology* 30:72–79, 1980.

63. Caplan LR, Kelly M, Kase CS, et al: Infarcts of the inferior division of the right middle cerebral artery: Mirror image of Wernicke's aphasia. *Neurology* 36:1015–1020, 1986.

64. Katz DI, Alexander MP, Mandell AM: Dementia following strokes in the mesencephalon and diencephalon. *Arch Neurol* 44:1127–1133, 1987.

65. Mori E, Yamadori A: Acute confusional state and agitated delirium: occurrence after infarction in the right middle cerebral artery territory. *Arch Neurol* 44:1139–1143, 1987.

66. Devinsky O, Bear D, Volpe BT: Confusional states following posterior cerebral artery infarction. *Arch Neurol* 45:160–163, 1988.

67. Mehler MF: The rostral basilar artery syndrome. *Neurology* 39:9–16, 1989.

68. Mendez MF, Adams NL, Lewandowski S: Neurobehavioral changes associated with caudate lesions. *Neurology* 39:349–354, 1989.

69. Caplan LR, Schahmann JD, Kase CS, et al: Caudate infarcts. *Neurology* 47:133–143, 1990.

70. Tatemichi TK, Desmond DW, Prohovnik I, et al: Confusion and memory loss from capsular genu infarction: A thalamocortical disconnection syndrome. *Neurology* 42:1966–1979, 1992.

71. Drugs that cause psychiatric symptoms. *Med Lett* 31:113–118, 1989.

72. Fish DN: Treatment of delirium in the critically ill patient. *Clin Pharm* 10:456–466, 1991.

73. Menza MA, Murray GB, Holmes VF, Rafuls WA: Controlled study of extrapyramidal reactions in the management of delirious, medically ill patients: Intravenous haloperidol vs. haloperidol plus benzodiazepines. *Heart Lung* 17:238–241, 1988.

74. Koppel C, Wiegreffe R, Tenczer J: Clinical course, therapy, outcome, and analytical data in amitriptiline and combined amitriptiline/chlordiazepoxide overdose. *Hum Exp Toxicol* 11:458–465, 1992.

75. Haverkas GP, Disalvo RP, Imhoff TE: Fatal sei-

zures after flumazenil administration in a patient with mixed overdose. *Ann Pharmacother* 28:1347–1349, 1994.

76. Perry R, Irving D, Blessed G, et al: Senile dementia of the Lewy body type: A clinically and neuropathologically distinct form of dementia in the elderly. *J Neurol Sci* 95:119–139, 1990.

77. Hansen L, Salmon D, Galasko D, et al: The Lewy body variant of Alzheimer's disease: A clinical and pathological entity. *Neurology* 40:1–8, 1990.

78. Lund and Manchester Groups: Clinical and neuropathological criteria for frontotemporal dementia. *J Neurol Neurosurg Psychiatry* 57:416–418, 1994.

79. van Duijn CM, de Knijff P, Cruts A, et al: Apolipoprotein E4 allele in a population-based study of early-onset Alzheimer's disease. *Nat Genet* 7:74–78, 1994.

80. Strittmatter WJ, Saunders AM, Schmechel D, et al: Apolipoprotein E: high-avidity binding to beta-amyloid and increased frequency of type 4 allele in late-onset familial Alzheimer's disease. *Proc Natl Acad Sci USA* 90:1977–1981, 1993.

81. Prichard JW, Brass LM: New anatomical and functional imaging methods. *Ann Neurol* 32:395–400, 1992.

82. Mayberg HS: Neuro-imaging studies of depression in neurological diseases, in Starkstein Se, Robinson RG (eds): *Depression in Neurological Diseases.* Baltimore: Johns Hopkins University Press, 1993, pp 186–216.

83. Sultzer D, Levin HS, Mahler ME, et al: A comparison of psychiatric symptoms in vascular dementia and Alzheimer's disease. *Am J Psychiatry* 150:1806–1812, 1993.

84. Miller BL, Cummings JL, Vilanueva-Meyer J, et al: Frontal lobe degeneration: Clinical, neuropsychological, and SPECT characteristics. *Neurology* 41:1374–1382, 1991.

85. Jagust WL, Eberling JL, Richardson BR, et al: The cortical topography of temporal lobe hypometabolism in early Alzheimer's disease. *Brain Res* 629:189–198, 1993.

86. Grafton ST, Mazziota JC, Pahl JJ, et al: A comparison of neurological, metabolic, structural, and genetic evaluations in persons at risk for Huntington's disease. *Ann Neurol* 28:614–621, 1990.

87. Small GW, Mazziota JC, Collins MT, et al: Apolipoprotein E type 4 allele and cerebral glucose metabolism in relatives at risk for familial Alzheimer's disease. *JAMA* 273:942–947, 1995.

88. Cummings JL, Coffey CE: Neurobiological basis of behavior, in Coffey CE, Cummings JL (eds): *Textbook of Geriatric Neuropsychiatry.* Washington DC: American Psychiatric Association Press, 1994, pp 72–96.

89. Mesulam M-M: Large scale neurocognitve networks and distributed processing for attention, language, and memory. *Ann Neurol* 28:597–613, 1990.

90. Wolfe N, Katz DI, Albert ML, et al: Neuropsychological profile linked to low dopamine: In Alzheimer's disease, major depression, and Parkinson's disease. *J Neurol Neurosurg Psychiatry* 53:915–917, 1990.

91. Cummings JL: Behavioral complications of drug treatment of Parkinson's disease. *J Am Geriatr Soc* 39:708–716, 1991.

92. Hoehn-Saric R: Neurotransmitters in anxiety. *Arch Gen Psychiatry* 39:735–742, 1982.

93. Palmer AM, Stratmann GC, Procter AW, Bowen DM: Possible neurotransmitter basis of behavioral changes in Alzheimer's disease. *Ann Neurol* 23:616–620, 1988.

94. Alexander GE, Delong MR, Strick PL: Parallel organization of functional circuits linking basal ganglia and cortex. *Annu Rev Neurosci* 9:357–381, 1986.

95. Cummings JL: Frontal-subcortical circuits and human behavior. *Arch Neurol* 50:873–880 1993.

96. Albert ML, Feldman RG, Willis AL: The "subcortical dementia" of progressive supranuclear palsy. *J Neurol Neurosurg Psychiatry* 37:121–130, 1974.

97. Cummings JL, Benson DF: Subcortical dementia. *Arch Neurol* 41:874–879, 1984.

98. Benson DF, Cummings JL, Tsai SY: Angular gyrus syndrome simulating Alzheimer's disease. *Arch Neurol* 39:616–620, 1982.

99. Mesulam M-M: Slowly progressive aphasia without generalized dementia. *Ann Neurol* 11:592–598, 1982.

100. Gibb WRG, Luthert PJ, Marsden CD: Clinical and pathological features of corticobasal degeneration, in Streifler MB, Korczyn AD, Melamed ED, Youdim MBH (eds): *Advances in Neurology:* Vol 53. *Parkinson's Disease: Anatomy, Pathology, and Therapy.* New York: Raven Press, 1990, pp 51–54.

101. Cummings JL: Intellectual impairment in Parkinson's disease: Clinical, pathological, and biochemical correlates. *J Geriatr Psychiatry Neurol* 1:24–36, 1988.

102. Robbins TW, James M, Owen AM, et al: Cognitive deficits in progressive supranuclear palsy, Parkin-

son's disease, and multiple system atrophy in tests sensitive to frontal lobe dysfunction. *J Neurol Neurosurg Psychiatry* 57:79–88, 1994.

103. Pillon B, Gouider-Khouja N, Deweer B, et al: Neuropsychological pattern of striatonigral degeneration: comparison with Parkinson's disease and progressive supranuclear palsy. *J Neurol Neurosurg Psychiatry* 58:174–179, 1995.

104. Foster NL, Gilman S, Berent S, et al: Cerebral hypometabolism in progressive supranuclear palsy studied with positron emission tomography. *Ann Neurol* 24:399–406, 1988.

105. Sawada H, Udaka F, Kameyama M, et al: SPECT findings in Parkinson's disease associated with dementia. *J Neurol Neurosurg Psychiatry* 55:960–963, 1992.

106. Collins SJ, Ahlskog JE, Parisi JE, Maraganore DM: Progressive supranuclear palsy: Neuropathologically based diagnostic clinical criteria. *J Neurol Neurosurg Psychiatry* 58:167–173, 1995.

107. Benson DF: Hydrocephalic dementia, in: Fredericks JAM (ed): *Handbook of Clinical Neurology: Neurobehavioral Disorders.* New York: Elsevier, 1985, vol 2, pp 323–333.

108. Cummings JL: Depression and Parkinson's disease: A review. *Am J Psychiatry* 149:443–445, 1992.

109. Tröster AI, Paolo AM, Lyons KE, et al: The influence of depression on cognition in Parkinson's disease: A pattern of impairment distinguishable from Alzheimer's disease. *Neurology* 45:672–676, 1995.

110. Folstein MF, McHugh PR: Dementia syndrome of depression, in Katzman R, Terry RD, Bick KL (eds): *Alzheimer's Disease, Senile Dementia and Related Disorders.* Raven Press: New York, 1978, pp 87–93.

111. Caine ED: Pseudodementia: Current concepts and future directions. *Arch Gen Psychiatry* 38:1359–1364, 1981.

112. Ishii N, Nishihara Y, Imamura T: Why do frontal lobe symptoms predominate in vascular dementia with lacunes? *Neurology* 36:340–345, 1986.

113. Navia B, Jordan BJ, Price RW: The AIDS dementia complex: I. Clinical features. *Ann Neurol* 19:514–517, 1986.

114. McKeith IG, Perry RH, Fairbarn AF, et al: Operational criteria for senile dementia of the Lewy body type. *Psychol Med* 22:911–922, 1992.

115. McKeith IG, Fairbarn AF, Bothwell RA, et al: An evaluation of the predictive validity and inter-rater reliability of clinical diagnostic criteria for senile dementia of Lewy body type. *Neurology* 44:872–877, 1994.

116. Chui HC, Lyness SA, Sobel E, Schneider LS: Extrapyramidal signs and psychiatric symptoms predict faster cognitive decline in Alzheimer's disease. *Arch Neurol* 51:676–681, 1994.

117. Stern Y, Albert M, Brandt J, et al: Utility of extrapyramidal signs and psychosis as predictors of cognitive and functional decline, nursing home admission, and death in Alzheimer's disease: Prospective analyses from the predictors study. *Neurology* 44:2300–2307, 1994.

118. Harrington CR, Louwagie J, Rossau R, et al: Influence of apolipoprotein E genotype on senile dementia of the Alzheimer's and Lewy body types: Significance for etiological theories of Alzheimer's disease. *Am J Pathol* 145:1472–1484, 1994.

119. Perry EK, Morris CM, Court JA, et al: Alteration in nicotine binding sites in Parkinson's disease, Lewy body dementia and Alzheimer's disease: Possible index of early neuropathology. *Neuroscience* 64:385–395, 1995.

120. Mendez MF, Selwood A, Mastri AR, Frey WH II: Pick's disease versus Alzheimer's disease: A comparison of clinical characteristics. *Neurology* 43:289–292, 1993.

121. Schneider LS: Clinical pharmacology of aminoacridines in Alzheimer's disease. *Neurology* 43(suppl 4):S64–S79, 1993.

122. Farlow M, Gracon S, Hershey L, et al: A controlled trial of tacrine in Alzheimer's disease. *JAMA* 268:2523–2528, 1992.

123. Knapp MJ, Knopman DS, Solomon PR, et al: A 30-week randomized controlled trial of high-dose tacrine in patients with Alzheimer's disease. *JAMA* 271:985–991, 1994.

124. Lipton SA, Rosenberg PA: Excitatory amino acids as a final common pathway for neurological disorders. *N Engl J Med* 330:613–622, 1994.

125. Parkinson Study Group: Effects of tocopherol and deprenyl on the progression of disability in early Parkinson's disease. *N Engl J Med* 328:176–183, 1993.

126. Graff-Radford NR, Godersky JC, Jones MP: Variables predicting surgical outcome in symptomatic hydrocephalus in the elderly. *Neurology* 39:1601–1604, 1989.

127. Clarfield AM: Normal-pressure hydrocephalus: Saga or swamp? *JAMA* 262:2592–2593, 1989.

128. Sidtis JJ, Gatsonis C, Price RW, et al: Zidovudine treatment of the AIDS dementia complex: Results

of a placebo-controlled trial. *Ann Neurol* 33:343–349, 1993.

129. Cummings JL, Gorman DG, Shapira J: Physostigmine ameliorates the delusions of Alzheimer's disease. *Biol Psychiatry* 33:536–541, 1993.

130. Kaufer DI, Cummings JL: "Personality alterations in degenerative brain disorders," in Ratey J (ed): *Neuropsychiatry of Personality Disorders.* Cambridge, MA: Blackwell, 1995, pp 172–209.

131. Kaufer DI, Cummings JL: Does dementia severity predict response to tacrine in Alzheimer's disease (abstr)? *Neurology* 45(suppl 4):A471–A472, 1995.

Chapter 41

ALZHEIMER DISEASE:
Clinical and
Anatomic Aspects

François Boller
Charles Duyckaerts

Alzheimer disease (AD) is a degenerative disease of the central nervous system (CNS), characterized clinically by progressive dementia and, histologically, by senile plaques (SP) and neurofibrillary tangles (NFT). The disease usually starts after the age of 40, and its incidence increases with age. Despite a marked sharpening of diagnostic criteria and some new ancillary tests, the diagnosis is still based on the exclusion of other conditions and on probability.

Strange as it may seem today, AD was long considered a rare disorder. Until about 20 to 30 years ago, classic textbooks either failed to mention it[1] or dismissed it in a few lines.[2] According to Medline, only 42 papers including AD as a key word were published in 1975. This long oblivion was followed by a major upsurge and, since the 1980s, a very large number of articles on AD have been appearing in medical journals (over 1282 entries in Medline for the first 6 months of 1995) as well as in the lay press. In the near future, however, the pendulum may be swinging back, since there are at present several questions about the homogeneity of AD and even about its usefulness as a single nosologic entity.[3–5]

The entrance of dementia and AD into behavioral neurology and neuropsychology has been even slower. In the "classic" age, there had been very important clinical observations: Pick's 1892 paper is an outstanding early example of single case description[6] and Alzheimer's patient[7] had been well studied. Seglas's careful study of the language disorders of the "insane"[8] also goes back to 1892. In later years, however, particularly after World War II, when neuropsychology arrived or rather returned on the scientific scene, AD was strangely absent from the picture. It was as if diseases that produce dementia were not considered worthy of investigation, perhaps because the lesions were considered too "diffuse."* Of course, the disease is not diffuse, clinically or neuropathologically, and important dissociations and "focal signs" can be observed in behavior and cognition. Our knowledge concerning the neuropsychology of memory and attention, among others, has expanded greatly thanks to the study of patients with AD and other degenerative disorders.

In this chapter, we first define AD putting the condition in its historical context, past and present, and review the diagnostic criteria currently in use. After a description of the clinical picture, we outline the known and supposed risk

---

*There were a few noticeable exceptions. Sjögren and colleagues included results of neuropsychological tests in their masterful description of AD and Pick disease.[176] Language disorders in dementia were studied by Pichot, by Critchley, and in a more complete and systematic fashion by De Renzi and Vignolo and by Irigaray.[177–180] Other aspects of behavior and dementia had also been studied sporadically.[181,182] In North America, Benson was probably one of the first to make patients with dementia "acceptable" for systematic neuropsychological studies. Currently, 80 percent of behavioral neurology fellowship programs in the United States include dementia as a major part of their teaching.[183]

factors of AD as well as current laboratory tests, including positron emission tomography (PET) and single photon emission tomography (SPECT). The neuropathology of AD is then presented in detail. The chapter concludes with a review of the "borderland" of AD, particularly diffuse Lewy-body disease (DLBD). In recent years, the so-called non-Alzheimer degenerative dementias (NADD) including progressive aphasia, have been isolated from AD. These are also briefly discussed.

HISTORICAL BACKGROUND OF ALZHEIMER DISEASE

Until recently, the term *AD* applied only to progressive dementias starting in the presenile years.[9] This distinction is still thought to be valid by some researchers;[10] in the past 20 years or so, however, it has become customary, following Katzman and coworkers,[11] to deemphasize the distinction, "since the two conditions, except for their age of onset, are clinically and pathologically indistinguishable."[12]

The diseases that may produce dementia obviously existed long before Alois Alzheimer's short description of the condition that bears his name. On the other hand, many prominent people were actively involved in that area of research not only in Munich (Fig. 41-1) but also in other centers. The Prague group, led by Arnold Pick, came very close to getting the credit for first describing the disease, mainly thanks to the work of Pick's assistant, Oskar Fischer. Following Perusini's work,[13] which confirmed that SP represented "a specific finding in senile dementia cases," the name *Fisher's plaques* started appearing in the literature. As for Nissl, he had worked with Alzheimer since 1889 and their professional relationship was so close that it was impossible to decide which of them owed more to the other.[14] While the work of Nissl and Perusini[15] was important, one gets the feeling that Alzheimer was the driving force of the group and therefore deserves most of the credit and the eponym designating this most common form of dementia. The historic development of studies related to dementia and AD is outlined elsewhere.[16]

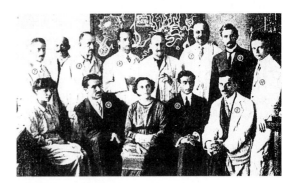

Figure 41-1
Picture of Alois Alzheimer (7) and his coworkers taken in about 1907 at what is today the Max Planck Institute of Munich. The head of the group, Kraepelin, is in the center, smoking a cigar. The picture also includes Cerletti (4), who was to become responsible for the introduction of electroshock; Bonfiglio (6) and Perusini (9), both responsible for the publication of cases of presenile dementia; and Lewy (10), after whom the Lewy bodies are named. Numbers refer to those printed on the picture. Reproduced from,[15] by permission of the authors and of the publishers of Aging.

DIAGNOSTIC CRITERIA

The diagnostic criteria for dementia proposed by the *Diagnostic and Statistical Manual*[17] are presented in detail elsewhere (Chap. 40). In 1984, a consensus conference met in Bethesda, Maryland, under the auspices of the Neurology Institute of the National Institutes of Health (then called NINCDS) and the Alzheimer Association (ADRDA). The so-called NINCDS/ADRDA criteria defined at that conference[18] remain quite valid today. They are now in use in many countries around the world. One of their merits is to have introduced the notion of probable and possible AD, the diagnosis being proved only in cases where neuropathology (i.e., an autopsy or biopsy) confirms the clinical findings. The validity of the NINCDS/ADRDA criteria has been demonstrated by clinical studies and by clinicopathologic correlations.[19,20]

Criteria of the Consortium to Establish a Registry for Alzheimer Disease

Soon after the creation in the United States of the first 10 Alzheimer Disease Research Centers

(ADRC) by the National Institute on Aging in 1985, it was felt that there was a need and an opportunity to establish standardized diagnostic criteria that could be used not only in North America, but in other countries as well. The Consortium to Establish a Registry for Alzheimer Disease (CERAD) criteria were therefore proposed in the late eighties under the leadership of different centers, particularly those of Duke University in Durham, North Carolina, and Washington University in St. Louis, Missouri.[21]

The CERAD criteria are for the most part an operational adaptation of those proposed by NINCDS-ADRDA[18] and lead into one of three diagnoses: no dementia, possible AD, and probable AD. The clinical evaluation battery includes a semistructured interview with the patient and with another person who knows the patient well (if possible, a close family member). The CERAD examination includes general physical and neurologic examinations as well as laboratory tests aimed especially at ruling out other conditions such as thyroid disease or vitamin B_{12} deficiency. A depression scale is also administered. As originally proposed, the neuropsychological battery consisted of the seven tests listed in Table 41-1 (J1 to J7). This short battery was shown to have high interrater and retest reliability.[21] The study of Morris and colleagues[21] also found that the battery discriminated all of 350 AD patients from 275 controls. Another study[22] found that it can distinguish even the mildest cases of AD from nondemented controls. Nevertheless the battery has been augmented by the addition of further measures (L1 to L7), including delayed verbal recall, Trails A and B, and a simple test of verbal intelligence aimed at estimating the subject's premorbid IQ. In addition, finger tapping and clock drawing (which were already part of the neurologic examination) are now considered part of the battery.

An estimate of the overall degree of deterioration is provided by the Mini-Mental Status Examination (MMS),[23] the Blessed test score[24] and the Clinical Dementia Rating Scale (CDR),[25] which relies on subjective assessment by the clinician. Administration of the CDR requires training, for which video cassettes have been developed in the United States; these are also available in other

Table 41-1

Neuropsychological tests of CERAD[a]

J 1: Word fluency (category-animal)

J 2: Boston Naming Test

J 3: MMSE

J 4: Word list memory

J 5: Constructional praxis

J 6: Word list—delayed recall

J 7: Word list—recognition

L 1: Shipley-Hartford Vocabulary

L 2: Verbal Paired Associate learning test (from WMS-R)

L 3: Recall of constructional praxis items

L 4: Verbal Paired Associate Recall

L 5: Trails A and B

L 6: Nelson Adult Reading Test (NART)

L 7: Word fluency (letter: "F" and "P")

Finger tapping

Clock drawing

[a]The "J" tests are those included in the earliest version of the battery.

countries. Its scoring has been simplified by using the "sum of boxes." Recent studies have shown an 83 percent rate of agreement among users of the CDR.

The introduction of the criteria listed above may be responsible for the marked improvement in diagnostic accuracy witnessed in recent years. If the "golden rule" is provided by an autopsy with positive findings for AD, the percentage of accurate diagnosis during the 1970s may have been as low as 50 percent.[26] According to a more recent study,[27] this percentage had reached around 80 percent. Two studies based on small series[28,29] reported 100 percent accuracy, a rather unlikely score. The lastest CERAD data[30] indicate a reliability of the order of 85 percent.

CLINICAL PICTURE

Thanks to personal experience or reading of the literature, most people are aware of what the "typical" picture of AD looks like and how it evolves. Very schematically, one can distinguish three stages. The first (*amnestic*) is dominated by disorders of memory, particularly episodic, but also semantic memory, with therefore a fairly frequent impairment in language even in the initial stages. In the second stage (*dementia*), the loss of intellectual abilities is reflected in everyday life and the patient's independent living becomes more and more difficult. Each of these two stages lasts an average of 2 years, but there is, of course, considerable variation from patient to patient. Even within the same patient, the course may fluctuate a great deal, with relatively long stable periods alternating with precipitous declines.[31] The third stage (known by the unpleasant name of *vegetative stage*) is characterized by the patients' inability to take care of themselves, to feed, and to communicate. One of the tragic aspects of AD is that with proper care, this stage can go on for many years. Patients with AD do not die *of* the disease, they die *with* it from some other cause. It has been shown that survival is affected more by loss of autonomy than by the severity of the dementia.[32]

This brief outline of the clinical picture belies the fact that no two patients are alike, as there is an almost infinite number of combinations of clinical symptoms of varying severity, particularly in the early stages. Among the most atypical forms are those where a specific symptom—for instance, language impairment or apraxia—dominates the picture for a long time. Some of these forms are discussed below. The early phases of AD may also be dominated by noncognitive disorders such as agitation, hallucinations, sleep disturbances or, on the contrary, apathy and depression. This extremely important aspect of AD has been reviewed by Absher and Cummings.[33] Details concerning cognitive changes of AD are found elsewhere (Chap. 42).

RISK FACTORS

Age is, of course, the main "risk factor" for AD, even though we hesitate to qualify as such a process that can hardly be dissociated from life itself. Alzheimer disease can start at age 45 or even earlier, but it is mainly after the age of 60 to 65 that the proportion of AD patients becomes sizable. The proportion increases up 80 to 90 years of age and then seems to become stable.

Chromosomal Abnormalities, Genetics, and Family History

Even though it had been known for years that patients with trisomy 21 (Down syndrome) develop AD-like neuropathologic changes after the age of 40, it was only in the mid- to late 1980s that the first reports of genetic abnormality associated with AD were published.[34] These reports indicated an association with the gene of the amyloid precursor protein (APP). It became apparent shortly thereafter that chromosome 21 is not the only chromosome where abnormalities can be found. A tie between early-onset forms and chromosome 14 (S182) was established by the Seattle group.[35] Implication of chromosome 19 has also been shown, particularly in familial forms with late onset.[36] The latest episode in the chromosomal "saga" comes again from the Seattle group. Studies of a special form of familial Alzheimer disease (FAD) known as the Volga Germans reveals the presence of an AD locus on chromosome 1 (STM2).[37]

An association has been found between AD and the locus of the gene coding for apolipoprotein E, located on chromosome 19. A particular allele of the gene, the Apo ε4, responsible for the synthesis of the ApoE4 phenotype, is genetically associated not only with familial[38] but also with sporadic forms of the disease.[39] It has been shown that as the number of Apo ε4 alleles (which code for the ApoE4 protein) increases (from 0 to 2), so does the risk of developing the disease. According to one group, octogenarians with AD carry the genotype 4/4 three times more often than healthy octagenarians.[40]

After age, ApoE4 is the most significant risk factor for AD. It is not yet clear to what extent these genetic associations are reflected in the course, severity, and other clinical aspects of the disease.[41,42] They might increase Aβ deposition even in intellectually normal subjects.[43] The specificity of ApoE is also the subject of an ongoing debate. ApoE ε4 alleles are reported to be associated not only with AD but also with other conditions, particularly progressive supranuclear palsy (PSP), Pick disease, corticobasal ganglionic degeneration (CBD or CGD),[44] amyloid angiopathy,[45] Down syndrome,[46] and possibly Creutzfeldt-Jakob disease.[47] However, one report indicates no association with Parkinson disease (PD) without or with dementia.[48]

Cases of FAD have been known for many years (see Ref. 49 for a review), and in some families, several dozens of members have been studied, with unequivocal demonstration of autosomal dominant pattern of transmission. This has also been found in a series of unselected cases.[50] A study based on twins aged 62 to 73 years shows high concordance for subjects who are ε4 homozygous, but it also shows that in early-onset AD patients without the ε4 allele, there is little genetic influence.[51]

Families where genetic transmission is apparent are, however, exceptional; in clinical practice, it is quite rare to obtain a positive family history. The discrepancy between research and clinical data is probably related to the fact that AD is almost unique in having such a late clinical expression. Meanwhile there is no question that having a case in a family considerably increases the chances that other family members will develop it. Epidemiologic studies have also shown associations of AD with Parkinson disease[52] and Down syndrome,[53] even though the latter finding has been contradicted.[54]

Geographic Distribution

Available epidemiologic data suggest that AD has a similar incidence everywhere in the world. There may be two exceptions to this rule. In Japan, numerous cases of dementia appear to be caused not by AD but by cerebrovascular diseases. It has been said that in some African countries, AD is much less frequent than in industrialized areas, but this remains to be verified.

Sex

In clinical practice, one is struck by a marked sex difference: there seem to be many more women than men affected. This, however, is probably an artifact, since life expectancy is longer among women. In addition, survival to AD is shorter for males than for females.[32]

Level of Instruction

Several studies have shown that the prevalence of dementia is related to the level of instruction and is much greater among illiterate subjects.[55–57] This finding has yet to receive a clear explanation. The possibility of a bias related to the difficulty of administration and interpretation of cognitive tests in patients with no or little instruction has not been entirely ruled out. On the other hand, one can also hypothesize that education actually increases neocortical synaptic density, allowing for the accumulation of "reserves" and therefore delaying the appearance of dementia.[58] Paradoxically, there is increased risk of mortality in AD patients with more advanced educational and occupational attainment.[59] It is felt that this is because lower education is accompanied by an earlier expression and therefore a longer survival after the first symptoms.

Other factors including parental age at birth, some thyroid diseases, depression, and head injuries are thought by many to be associated with an increased incidence of AD, but these effects cannot be said to have been demonstrated with certainty. The possible protective role of tobacco and alcohol consumption[60,61] could be due to a side effect of the ApoE4 genotype, which is also a significant risk factor for vascular diseases. The proportion of old smokers and drinkers with the ApoE4 genotype could be abnormally low, due to attrition by death from vascular causes.

LABORATORY TESTS

Until fairly recently, no laboratory test could be used to diagnose AD. In routine clinical use, neurophysiologic tests can help corroborate a diagnosis of dementia and rule out some other conditions. The use of more sophisticated techniques, such as the study of P300, has been advocated in the detection of early cases.[62] The new imaging techniques provided by computed tomography (CT) and magnetic resonance imaging (MRI) have been found to be invaluable not only in ruling out other conditions but also in pointing out some specific features such as atrophy of the temporal lobe,[63] of the hippocampal formation,[64] and of the amygdala.[65] Magnetic resonance spectroscopy has shown anomalies that may reflect lesions of the neuronal membrane.[66]

Metabolic abnormalities associated with AD are reflected in positron emission tomography (PET) and single photon emission computed tomography (SPECT) studies. While PET studies remain limited to few patients by practical considerations, SPECT has reached a level of practical interest because it is relatively cheap and, with the use of technetium 99mTc-hexamethyl propyleneamine oxime (HMPAO), is said to have demonstrated between 90 and 100 percent ability to detect AD.[67] In most cases (around 80 percent), one can demonstrate a "characteristic" pattern of bilateral parietotemporal perfusion deficit. The SPECT and PET changes have been shown to correlate with different cognitive profiles[68–71] and even possibly to precede the clinical changes.[72]

The neurochemical changes that accompany AD are described in detail elsewhere (Chap. 43).

NEUROPATHOLOGY OF ALZHEIMER DISEASE

Anatomy

Alzheimer disease affects the very structure of the brain; unlike tumors, it does not invade the parenchyma or destroy it, as infarcts do. The disease affects cerebral organization without causing much destruction or inflammation. In order to comprehend the pathology of AD and its progression, it may therefore be useful to discuss some points concerning the anatomic organization of the brain. In the following section, we distinguish schematically the cortex and the subcortex; in the cortex, we recognize three main divisions: the *hippocampus* (including the dentate gyrus and the subiculum) necessary to normal memory acquisitions (Fig. 41-2, Plate 7); the *isocortex* (sometimes also called neocortex), which covers most of the brain surface; and finally the interface region between the hippocampus and isocortex—i.e., the *entorhinal area,* limited by the rhinal sulcus (*ento-* is the Greek word for "inside" or "limited by"). The neocortex may be subdivided into broad categories depending on their functions.[73] The sensory inputs (somesthetic, auditory, visual) reach areas known as primary. At this stage, the signal is still gross, close to its physical origin. Its main characteristics are extracted in specialized cortical areas.

Figure 41-2
Atrophy of the hippocampus: The upper section comes from a control without neurologic symptoms. The hippocampus has a normal volume. The two other sections come from patients with Alzheimer disease at various stages. Maximal atrophy is seen in the lowest section.

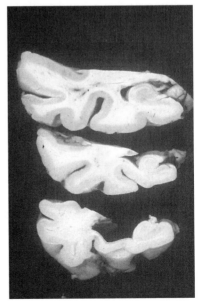

In the visual mode, for example, color, movement, and three-dimensional perception are selectively analyzed in so-called association cortices that are said to be unimodal, since only one type of signal—visual, somesthetic, auditory—is treated in each one.[74] The unimodal association cortical areas are connected with large multimodal areas, located mainly in the prefrontal and parietotemporal regions. From there, the information is funneled onto the entorhinal area, which receives signals that have been processed through the various association cortices. This set of corticocortical connections from the primary to the entorhinal areas ("feed-forward") is paralleled by connections that go back from the multimodal areas to the primary cortex ("feed-backward") (see Ref. 75 for review). These corticocortical connections are thought to play a major role in memory processes by providing the necessary relays between the hippocampus and the isocortex.

The laminar organization of the cortex may give some insight into the preferential topography of the microscopic lesions (SPs and NFTs).[76] The isocortex is made up of six layers. Layer IV consists of small neurons, known as granules, which receive sensory inputs, coming, for example, from the thalamus. The output of the cortex stems from pyramidal neurons. Those located in layer II and, to a greater extent, layer III project to other cortical areas, some through the corpus callosum. This is the layer where SPs are found, as will be seen later. The large pyramidal neurons of layer V send the majority of their axons to subcortical targets such as the lenticular nucleus, the brainstem nuclei, or the spinal motor neuron. The NFTs mainly involve middle-sized pyramidal neurons of layers III and V. The spindle-shaped cells of layer VI contribute to transcortical connections. Layer I contains mainly dendritic expansions from the underlying layers. This brief outline is highly schematic, but it emphasizes the hierarchical organization of the cortex, through corticocortical connections, in which layer III plays a major role.

Main Lesions and Diagnosis

We shall now consider how the two major lesions seen in AD—the SP and the NFT—become integrated within these complex circuitries. Senile plaques and NFTs (Fig. 41-3, Plate 8) differ in shape, topography, and both biochemical and immunohistochemical markers. This has led some authors to consider that only one type of alteration has a diagnostic or pathogenetic meaning. Several diagnostic criteria only take SPs into account,[77,78] the tangles being considered poorly specific; but it has also been said that the clinical symptoms are more tightly linked to the NFTs than to the SPs.[79]

It is probably artificial to consider the plaques and tangles separately, since no case of AD has been published without NFTs in the entorhinal and hippocampal regions, although they may be absent in the isocortex.[80] At the same time, it would be unwise to accept the diagnosis of Alzheimer disease in the absence of SPs in the isocortex, because the two lesions are linked in a rather stereotyped way.

Figure 41-3

The two main lesions of Alzheimer disease: (1) neurofibrillary tangles are located in the neuronal cell body and appear in black; (2) senile plaques are seen as spheres made of entangled neurites. Bielschowsky silver impregnation counterstained by cresyl violet. Staining performed by Dr. Joachim Kauss. Initial magnification: ×750.

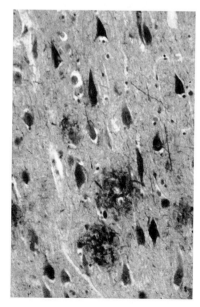

Senile Plaques   Senile plaques are composite and complex lesions. That complexity makes them difficult to analyze, and their density, as evaluated on microscopic sections, is highly dependent on the staining technique. These may reveal more specifically one or more of the three main components of the plaque:[81] (1) extracellular deposits, (2) neurites, or (3) cells (macrophages and astrocytes). The deposits make up the core of the plaque, and the neurites form a crown around it. The astrocytes surround the plaques with their processes, whereas the macrophage is usually located in the core or close to it[82] (Fig. 41-4, Plate 9).

Extracellular Deposits   A number of proteins have been recognized in the core of the plaque: globulins, complement factors,[83] P component, and, most significantly, Aβ and apolipoprotein E.

Aβ   "Birefringence" (light reflected in two directions) and "dichroism" (change of color of the reflected beam) after Congo red staining have

Figure 41-4
Senile plaques. The plaque in the center of the picture, is a composite lesion. Its center, stained gray, consists of amorphous extracellular material mainly composed of Aβ peptide. Other stains, such as Congo red, would show its "amyloid" nature. A crown of degenerating neurites is seen around the amyloid center. The nuclei that are in contact with the plaque belong, for the most part, to microglial cells. Initial magnification: ×1200.

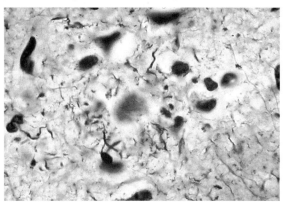

been used to define the amyloid substance. They are thought to be related to the highly repetitive 3D structure of the proteins when they exhibit the β-pleated sheet arrangement. Many proteins or peptides may take this 3D structure and become "amyloid." Proteins with the β-pleated sheet structure become highly insoluble and therefore difficult to isolate and to analyze. This is why the nature of the amyloid protein remained unknown until 1984, when Glenner and Wong[84] described a hitherto unknown peptide they named A4 peptide (A for amyloid and 4 for its weight of 4 kDa). It is also known as Aβ peptide (β stands for β-pleated sheet). It was rapidly found that the peptide came from a large and ubiquitous protein, the APP (amyloid precursor protein),[85] which is probably located across cellular membranes. It has a hydrophobic moiety located between two hydrophilic extremities. The neuron itself contains high amounts of mRNA coding for APP. The enzyme responsible for the cleavage of APP into Aβ is still unknown. Immunohistochemistry has shown that some Aβ deposits are not amyloid; they are not stained by Congo red and can be observed in AD patients as well as in old and apparently normal cases,[86,87] in young patients with trisomy 21, and possibly after a severe head trauma,[88] although this has been contradicted.[89] These nonamyloid deposits are usually larger and less dense than the plaque cores and are called diffuse deposits. They should be clearly distinguished from SPs: they are devoid of neurites and may be seen in intellectually normal persons. It is established that at least some of these diffuse deposits will never mature into true SPs.

APOLIPOPROTEIN E   The presence of proteins linked with the inflammatory process (immunoglobulins, complement factors) has been known for a long time. Apolipoprotein E has been more recently detected in the core of the SPs.[90] The significance of this finding has been more actively investigated since it was discovered, as stated above, that a phenotype of ApoE (known as ApoE4) was a significant risk factor for AD. The ApoE is also present in some nonamyloid deposits. It could play a role in the abnormal folding of

Aβ into a β-pleated, unsoluble, protein—a role described by the term *chaperone protein*. The cell responsible for the presence of ApoE in the plaque core has not yet been determined convincingly. It could be the astrocyte, the microglial cell, or the neuron.[82]

Neurites The neurites are a major component of the SPs and probably participate to the development of the amyloid core, although Aβ deposits have occasionally been found in the white matter without neurites.[91] Most clinicopathologic studies have demonstrated that the density of SP with neurites ("true SP") is correlated with dementia. The correlation is absent or much lower when only the deposits (stained, for example, by Aβ immunohistochemistry) are taken into account. However, the nature (dendritic or axonal) and origin of the neurites involved in the plaque are not very well known. They are usually revealed by silver methods, which show a crown of darkly stained, sometimes dilated fibers coming into contact with the deposit. Electron microscopy has shown that some of the neurites contained presynaptic vesicles, indicating their axonal origin.[80] One study has suggested that they could stem from nearby pyramidal neurons.[92] Some dendritic elements may also be present in the plaques. Many axonal and possibly dendritic processes involved in the plaque contain "paired helical filaments" (PHF), bearing abnormally phosphorylated tau, a structure characteristic of the NFTs, to be described below. The detailed morphologic analysis of the plaque suggest that it should not be considered as a "scar" of some unusual type but rather as a living set of abnormal nervous connections. There must be some relationship between NFTs and plaques. The presence of PHF in the plaque demonstrates the intricacy of the relationship between these two lesions, but it is not yet known whether SPs are physically connected with tangle-bearing neurons.

Cells When looking at sections stained with the usual hematoxylin-eosin (H&E) stain, good evidence of the presence of SPs is the microglial cell. It is usually found close to the amyloid core deposit. Microglial cells can be considered the histiocytes of the brain. Under some circumstances, they become activated and exhibit a phagocytic activity. They belong to the macrophage system, although their origin is still debated. Microglial cells have attracted much attention because the macrophages play a major role in amyloid formation outside the brain during chronic inflammation.[93] The macrophages initiate amyloid formation by cleaving a large precursor protein, which then produces amyloidogenic fragments. This has led to the suggestion that the microglial cell could also be responsible for the cleavage of the APP. Amyloid has indeed been seen in the microglial cell, but its presence could be related as well to its production as to phagocytosis of the deposit.

Astrocytes are also found in the vicinity of SPs. Immunohistochemistry of the glial fibrillary acid protein (GFAp), specific for astrocytes, reveals a meshwork of astrocytic filaments surrounding the SP. The role played by astrocytes is unknown. It could produce significant components—it has been said that it could synthesize ApoE[94]—of the plaque or circumscribe the lesion and limit its extent.

Plaques are often in close contact with capillaries. Some authors suggest that a capillary is always present in the plaque,[95] while others believe that they are topographically unrelated.[96]

Neurofibrillary Tangles and Neuropil Threads
The term *neurofibrillary tangles* denotes fibrillary material in the neuronal cell body, or "perikaryon" (Fig. 41-5, Plate 10). These tangles were first described by Alzheimer himself,[97] using a (then new) silver technique (Bielschowsky method). With this technique, the ionic silver, soluble and invisible, is "reduced" to metallic silver that precipitates on the section. The technique is quite similar to the photographic processing of a black-and-white picture: the silver precipitate appears brown to black, depending on the size of the crystals of metallic silver. The precipitation of silver occurs on fibrillary materials either normal (as in normal axons) or abnormal (as in tangles). Since the time of Bielschowsky, the silver impregnations

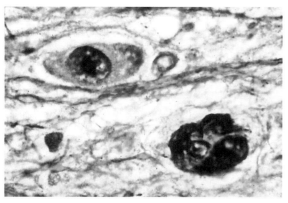

Figure 41-5
Neurofibrillary tangles. This high-power view of the nucleus basalis of Meynert shows two neurons; the cytoplasm of the normal neuron appears light brown. The second neuron contains a neurofibrillary tangle consisting of deep black fibrils surrounding and partly overlapping the nucleus. Bodian silver impregnation. Initial magnification: ×2500.

have improved in specificity: one of the techniques, described by Gallyas, stains only the abnormal neurofibrillary structures. When they are examined with electron microscopy, the NFTs appear to be made of a helicoidal structure—either paired helical filaments (PHFs) or perhaps, as new data would suggest, twisted ribbons.[98]

It has been possible to isolate PHFs and to inject them into animals in order to obtain antibodies. Various anti-NFTs have been produced in this way, but a major step was taken when it was shown that the tangles were specifically stained by an antibody directed against a group of proteins associated with neurotubules and resistant to heat ("tau proteins"[99]). Tau has several phosphorylation sites; in tangles, it appears to be "abnormally phosphorylated," meaning that tau has bound too many phosphate radicals.[100–102] The very existence of this hyperphosphorylation in vivo has been challenged: it could be an artifact due to the relative inefficiency of phosphatases, postmortem or after sampling, in patients with Alzheimer disease.[103] The kinases and the phosphatases implicated in both the normal and abnormal metabolism of tau are currently investigated but are still largely unknown. Tau antibodies have provided a very useful tool to study all types of neurofibrillary pathology.

Tau is actually present in normal brain parenchyma, but after the usual histologic techniques (formalin fixation, alcoholic dehydration, toluene or xylene, paraffin) becomes undetectable except in NFTs, not only seen in AD but also in PSP and CBD.[104]

Tau immunocytochemistry has clearly demonstrated that neurofibrillary pathology is not limited to the cell body but also involves neuronal processes, which indeed contain PHF. In AD brains, tau antibodies (as Gallyas stain) show a great number of small, fragmented, tortuous processes weaving between the cell bodies (i.e., in the "neuropil"—that part of the brain tissue which is not the cell bodies or the white matter tracts). These "tortuous fibers"[105] could be axons or dendrites containing PHF. They are called "neuropil threads"[106] and invariably accompany tangles and plaques when they are numerous.

It is important to stress that the difference between SPs and NFTs is not only morphologic but also topographic. Both lesions are exclusively found in the gray matter, although a few nude $A\beta$ deposits have been found in the white matter.[82] The great majority of plaques is found in the isocortex; the hippocampus is relatively spared, and true plaques are exceptional in the subcortex except for the amygdala. Plaques are never seen in the brainstem and cerebellum, where only diffuse deposits may occasionally occur. In the isocortex, the plaques are diffusely distributed: they are present in primary areas as well as in unimodal and multimodal cortical areas.[107] However, they do not involve all the layers of the cortex evenly. They are much more numerous in layer III,[76] implicated, as we have seen, in the corticocortical connection. The density of the SPs in the isocortex is loosely linked with the cognitive status.

The NFTs involve very specifically some neurons and some areas.[108] The medium-sized pyramidal neurons are electively affected.[107,109] These are located in layers III and V. The granule cells—e.g., of the dentate gyrus or layer IV—are largely spared, as are the giant pyramidal cells of Betz, in area 4. The islands of pyramidal cells in the entorhinal cortex are the most sensitive. They contain tangles, in all the cases of AD.[109] The pyramidal layers of the hippocampus and adjoining subiculum are the next most sensitive areas. It has been noticed that when tangles were present in those areas, they were also present in the previously mentioned entorhinal region. Finally, in advanced cases, one can find numerous tangles in layers III and V of the isocortical associative areas. In those cases, as might be expected, the tangles are also numerous in the entorhinal area, hippocampus, and subiculum. The primary isocortical areas may be devoid of tangles even in far advanced cases.

The distribution of SPs and of NFTs can thus be clearly contrasted. Senile plaques involve all the isocortical areas, and their density increases with the severity of the disease. Neurofibrillary tangles involve an increasing number of areas in a stereotyped order: entorhinal area, hippocampus-subiculum, isocortex. Figure 41-6, Plates 11 and 12, which displays the distribution of NFTs when compared with a map of the functional organization of the cortical areas (see Chap. 4, Fig. 4-1), shows that there is a high degree of concordance between the two maps. Primary areas are devoid of NFTs. Their density is low in unimodal association cortices, increases in multimodal association cortices, and reaches a peak in the paralimbic areas.

All this explains why two systems of criteria may be used with similar efficiency: the *counting* of plaques in the isocortex (CERAD criteria[78]) or the *mapping* of the areas involved by the neurofibrillary pathology (Braak stages[109]). The opposite distribution of the lesions may also explain some of the apparent paradoxes of the clinicopathologic correlations; severe memory disorders may be observed in the absence of isocortical SPs. At this stage, NFTs may be numerous in the entorhinal-hippocampal region;[110] this stage has been described as "limbic."[109] Isocortical plaques may be seen in the isocortex at a stage where tangles involve only the entorhinal-hippocampal region ("plaque-only AD"). In addition, were the plaques the main cause of the deficit, all cortical functions would have to be affected simultaneously, since SPs tend to be diffusely spread over the neocortex. The march of the tangles' progression—first limbic and later isocortical in multimodal and then unimodal association cortices—more clearly follows the usual course of the

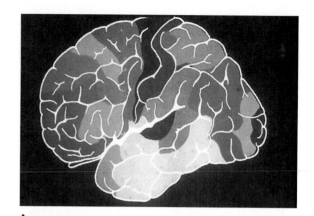

A

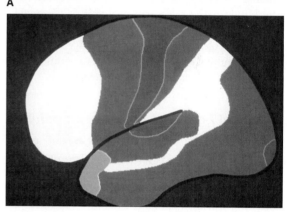

B

Figure 41-6

Comparison of the distribution of neurofibrillary tangles (NFT) with the functional organization of the cortical areas. A. Distribution of the cortical neurofibrillary tangles. The density of lesions is indicated by the following color scale: dark blue (no lesion); light blue, green, yellow and orange (maximal density of lesions). (From Arnold et al.,[107] with permission.) B. Schematic cytoarchitectonic map showing primary cortex (blue), unimodal association areas (green), multimodal association areas (yellow) and paralimbic cortex (red). There is a clear overlap between the density of NFT and the hierarchy of connections from primary (low density) to multimodal association and paralimbic cortex (high density).

symptoms: memory systems are usually affected first; deterioration of other cognitive domains follows, starting with the most complex ones.

The tangles could be the main cause of the synaptic loss, which has recently been extensively studied[111,112] and appears, at least in some areas, to be the most sensitive correlate of dementia.

Neurofibrillary tangles may also be located outside of a neuron, whose shape they keep. These "ghost tangles" are thought to be direct evidence of neuronal death, leaving the tangle in the extracellular space.[113] The cell is easily resorbed by the phagocytic system, but the tangle is not cleaned away.

The atrophy of the cortex also seems better correlated with the presence of tangles than with plaques. As gross atrophy is the direct consequence of neuronal loss, one may conclude that the tangle is the main cause of cell death in AD. It should, however, be added that some cell populations devoid of tangles, most noticeably in the retina, could also be reduced.[114] This could imply other mechanisms of neuronal death.

Neuronal Loss and Neuronal Atrophy

Much has been written about neuronal loss in aging and AD and extreme values have been suggested: for some authors, neuronal loss is the main determinant of dementia:[115] for others, neuronal loss does not even exist.[116] Such discrepancies reflect the methodologic difficulties involved in evaluating the number of neurons in the cortex. This number is much too high for direct assessment. Results are extrapolated from samples on which the density of neurons (i.e., their number by unit volume) has been measured. The mean neuronal density evaluated in the samples is then multiplied by the volume of the cortex. The procedure implies two different types of quantitative evaluation, both of which are subject to error: one of neuronal density and one of cortical volume. Both measures are necessary, as one may indeed imagine extreme and ideal situations in which the volume of the cortex does not change but the neuronal density drops or, on the contrary, the volume of the cortex shrinks and the neuronal density remains the same.[117] Atrophy seen in AD shows that this last mechanism indeed occurs. The reader may imagine that the death of a neuron leaves a hole in the cortex. It would then suffice to count the number of the neurons in the sample to detect the presence

of "holes," responsible for a drop in neuronal density. In fact, the death of a neuron is immediately followed by shrinkage of the neuropile, which, so to speak, fills the holes. Shrinkage has two consequences: the number of neurons per unit volume (i.e., neuronal density) remains the same; the volume of a small part of the cortex decreases, a process which, repeated, leads to what is known as cortical atrophy.[118] Cortical atrophy explains why neuronal density is only slightly affected in Alzheimer disease: the shrinkage of the cortex masks the neuronal loss on the microscopic sections.

On the other hand, the counting of neurons in a microscopic sample does not provide a correct evaluation of neuronal density because it is influenced not only by the density of the neurons in the sample volume but also by their size. To understand this last point, one may consider that the microscopic section is a haphazard hit by the blade of the microtome: the large neurons are more likely to be hit. They are thus oversampled and their density is overestimated. If a population of neurons changes size, its probability of being hit by the microtome blade also changes: for example, if some neurons have become smaller (have shrunk), they are less often cut by the microtome and appear less numerous: however, their number is in fact not reduced and there is no loss. This process, described as "pseudoloss,"[105] should throw some doubt on the notion that the neuronal loss involves the large neurons selectively. It may, in fact, be explained by neuronal atrophy occurring in aging, without actual loss. Various methods have been devised to avoid the interference of pseudoloss in the assessment of neuronal density. The most celebrated is the technique of cell counting known as the "disector":[119] it consists in using two real or virtual ("optical") sections (hence *di-*, for two sections). Only the cells visible in the first section and absent from the second are counted. In so doing, one actually counts one of the poles of the cell, a structure whose presence on the section is said to be independent of cell size. Using this technique, Regeur and coworkers (1994)[116] were unable to detect neuronal loss in AD cases. This result is, in our opinion, not fully convincing, since the presence of ghost tangles is direct and unquestionable evidence of neuronal loss. However it might indicate that it is of a smaller magnitude than previously thought. Neuronal loss is therefore of no diagnostic value and is not included in any of the diagnostic criteria.

CLINICOPATHOLOGIC FRONTIERS OF ALZHEIMER DISEASE

The Lewy-Body Variant of Alzheimer Disease or Diffuse Lewy-Body Disease

In recent years, there has been an increasing number of papers describing an apparently new entity characterized by progressive dementia and parkinsonian symptoms, usually referred to as diffuse Lewy-body disease (DLBD). Although the disease was first described in two American patients,[120] most of the cases initially were found in Japan;[121] more recently, however, there have been reports from other countries, particularly the United Kingdom[122,123] and the United States.[124,125]

Lewy bodies are spherical inclusions found mainly in pigmented neurons of the substantia nigra, in the locus ceruleus, and in the dorsal vagal nucleus of patients who die with Parkinson disease (PD). They are usually located close to the nucleus and appear bright red after routine H&E stain. In recent years, there has been increasing awareness that they can also be found in the cerebral cortex. These cortical Lewy bodies are not as easily recognizable as their subcortical counterparts: they are paler and are not surrounded by a halo. Antiubiquitin immunohistochemistry has made their identification easier.*

Cortical Lewy bodies are found mainly in two different contexts. The first is that of PD patients who have had the disease for many years. The second is that of patients presenting with severe, rapidly evolving dementia. In the latter situation, Lewy bodies tend to be associated with numerous SPs, thus warranting the diagnosis of AD according to current criteria.

The term *DLBD* as applied to cases with numerous cortical Lewy bodies[126] probably encompasses several conditions. This heterogeneity is reflected by the number of names applied to cases with numerous Lewy bodies. These include, besides DLBD, Lewy-body dementia,[122] senile dementia of the Lewy-body type,[127] and Lewy-body variant of AD.[125] All these names refer mainly to cases with rapidly progressing dementia and numerous SPs. The clinical picture of this condition has been better defined in recent years. It has been claimed that the dementia has special features that may help to identify it in vivo.[128] The most frequently observed characteristics include fluctuation of symptoms, severe psychiatric symptoms—particularly hallucinations—and extrapyramidal symptoms and signs.

The prevalence of this type of dementia varies considerably from one geographic area to another and can reach one-third of the cases in some centers, whereas it amounts only to a small percentage in others. A report by Hansen[125] has stated that of 36 patients with dementia fulfilling AD criteria (which exclude patients presenting with parkinsonism), 13 (36 percent) had Lewy bodies. A report based on 150 unselected cases[129] and a review by Lennox[130] have presented data suggesting that close to 20 percent of patients with dementia may have cortical Lewy bodies. This would make DLDB, or rather the Lewy-body variant of AD, the most frequent cause of primary dementia after AD. Some data indicate that the disease is more frequent among males, thus following the pattern of PD rather than AD. The average duration of the disease, about 6 years, tends to be shorter than that of either AD or PD. It parallels, however, the duration found in PD patients with dementia and AD-like neuropathologic changes.[131]

Focal Cortical Atrophies

Diffuse Lewy-body disease and the Lewy-body variant of AD were first defined on the basis of autopsy findings. Other types of dementia have

---

*This antibody is not specific for Lewy bodies and also stains the tangles, which usually can be recognized on account of their shape.

been defined by their clinical peculiarities rather than by their pathology. As if often the case, the features of these clinical syndromes are determined by the topography of the lesions, irrespective of their nature. They do not fully correspond to the pathologic classification of the dementias. It may be useful, at the present time, to keep separate the clinical and the pathologic classifications in order to correctly apprehend the complexity of these diseases. Cases of "typical" AD, where the symptoms suggest a limbic and parietotemporooccipital location of lesions, have been separated from cases with a preponderant aphasia, apraxia, semantic disorder, frontal syndrome, or major visual-perceptive disturbances.[132,133] On the other hand, pathologic classifications rely on the presence of morphologic markers: NFT and SP for AD, Pick bodies in Pick disease (see Chap. 44), chromatolytic neurons and cytoskeletal pathology in corticobasal ganglionic degeneration (CGD), Lewy bodies in the just discussed DLBD, and so on. In other instances, no specific pathologic markers can be found. The status of these cases is presently controversial. Some authors believe they belong to the Pick realm;[134,135] this is the classic conception of type B or C of Pick disease [i.e., Pick disease lacking Pick bodies (B) or Pick bodies and chromatolytic neurons (C)].[136] Others have referred to cases without Pick bodies such as dementia lacking distinctive histology (DLDH).[137,138] Actually, our current ignorance about the causes of these focal degenerations of the cortex could lead to two contrasted attitudes: (1) Either group them in a large chapter and call it Pick disease, which covers all the circumscribed atrophy; this was really the point of view of Pick himself, who used only gross examination to describe the first cases of focal cortical degenerations. Or (2) use an analytical point of view, trying to distinguish by clinical and pathologic means what appears similar at first sight. We would favor this approach, which, historically, was followed by Alzheimer himself, who was the first to describe the inclusion bodies that ironically now bear the name of Pick.

In the following sections, we use the clinical syndromes as the main thread and try to correlate them with the pathologic data.

Primary Progressive Aphasia   In 1982, Mesulam[139] described six patients with a slowly progressive aphasia without obvious dementia. No pathology was available (except for a biopsy in one case, which had yielded no specific findings). Mesulam pointed out the differences with other known pathologic entities and thought that, together with a few cases described previously,[140,141] this could represent a new entity.* Since that time, many more cases have been described. (See summary of 63 cases in Ref. 142.)

The diagnostic criteria proposed by the group of Mesulam[142] emphasize three points:

1.   Language disturbances may or may not be accompanied by a disorder of speech; their onset is insidious and their progression is gradual.

2.   This deficit must remain isolated or nearly so for at least 2 years.

3.   It may, however, coexist with disorders such as constructional apraxia and acalculia.

In the majority of the clinicopathologic cases that have been published up to now, no pathologic markers have been found: neuronal loss and gliosis, poorly specific laminar spongiosis (different from the status spongiosus of Creutzfeldt-Jakob disease), and some chromatolytic neurons were present in large cortical regions, encompassing the language areas. In a high proportion of cases, AD pathology was the main finding, and this suggests that it may be localized for a long period of time, although no neuropathologic evidence of focal AD pathology has been published. Finally, Pick bodies have been found in some cases,[134,135,143] justifying the diagnosis of Pick disease. In view of the focal nature of Pick pathology, the latter findings are less surprising than those of AD-like pathology. These findings do not contradict the existence of primary progressive aphasia (PPA) as a real clinical entity. The relationship of PPA with "hereditary dysphasic dementia"[144] remains unclear.

---

*To these, one should add the carefully documented case of Wechsler;[184] it has been argued that the composer Maurice Ravel who suffered from a neurodegenerative disease in the last years of his life may also have had an early progressive aphasia.[16]

Frontal Lobe Degeneration or Dementia of Frontal Lobe Type and Other Lobar Atrophies

Frontal lobe degeneration (FLD) was first described in southern Sweden in 1987 as a pathologic entity[145] with matching neuropsychiatric and cerebral blood flow changes. Neary and colleagues in Manchester[146] had previously pointed out that cerebral atrophy and cognitive changes need not be synonymous with AD or with Pick disease. Since that time, both groups have written extensively on these topics, pointing out that other parts of the nervous system may also be involved. Frontal lobe dementia (FLD), also called dementia of frontal lobe type (DFT), occurs more often in males below the age of 65, and about half the cases have a positive family history. Initial symptoms include mainly personality, social conduct, and language or speech disorders often evolving toward mutism. Later, neurologic signs such as primitive reflexes and extrapyramidal signs (mainly akinesia and rigidity) emerge. Electroencephalography (EEG) and SPECT tend to show changes in the frontal regions. Frontal lobe dementia and other lobar atrophies are discussed in detail in a recent issue of the journal *Dementia.*[147] In a review article, Neary[148] summarizes the relationships between the above entities. As is the case with practically all neurologic syndromes, the clinical picture found in patients with this pathology reflects the topographic distribution of the lesions rather than the specific histologic features. Bilateral frontal lobe lesions are related to the syndrome of DFT. When the left cerebral hemisphere is predominantly affected, the clinical picture is mainly characterized by nonfluent aphasia. Fluent aphasia and visual agnosia are associated with bilateral involvement of the temporal lobes.

Progressive Apraxia (Corticobasal Degeneration)

Isolated, sometimes unilateral apraxia, usually accompanied by extrapyramidal symptoms, may develop over years. Neuropathologic examination often discloses neuronal loss in the substantia nigra. Some remaining neurons contain a fibrillary tau-positive inclusion. Neuronal loss and gliosis are marked in the parietal lobe and large "achromatic" neurons are seen: this condition, first described by Rebeiz and coworkers,[149] under the name of corticodentatonigral degeneration, is now more often identified as corticobasal degeneration (*basal* stands for the lesions of the substantia nigra located at the base of the brain). However, the pathology typical of Steele-Richardson-Olzewski syndrome has also been seen in similar cases. In addition, the predominant sign of AD at onset may also be apraxia, as documented by many authors.[150,151] It should be stressed that not all cases of progressive apraxia are CBD.[152]

NORMAL AGING

Not all those who develop AD are old, yet AD is a typical example of age-associated disease. The symptoms of AD are so closely tied to age that it has been hard to separate AD from "senility." It was long thought normal for elderly persons to lose their memory, and AD was long confused with senile dementia, which is why the rather awkward term *senile dementia of the Alzheimer type* was used for several years. The opposite attitude is now prevailing, AD being considered a disease whatever its age of onset. Is that fully justified? Actually, AD and senescence are also linked from a pathologic point of view. It is therefore necessary to include descriptions of AD in the context of the changes that accompany normal aging.

Several factors complicate the study of normal aging. Clinicians and researchers alike are aware that the variability in intellectual functioning found in normal adults greatly increases with age.[153] This is probably because age is often accompanied by other events (arterial hypertension, diabetes, traumas, etc.) that may affect the brain to a greater or lesser extent. The methods used in selecting subjects included in studies of aging are a major factor of bias in research, and it is necessary to stress that all studies on "normal" aging must be interpreted in the light of the selection of the subjects involved. *Longitudinal* studies use a group of the same individuals who are followed for as long as the study lasts. Limitations of this approach include, obviously, their cost and logistic difficulties. In addition, the sample is bound to dwindle more or less rapidly because of death, loss of motivation, and so on. Examples of large and fruitful longitudinal studies include the Seattle Longitudinal Study[154,155] and the Framingham Study.[156,157]

On the other hand, *cross-sectional* studies are performed at a given time (sometimes, when the question concerns the prevalence of a given disorder, on a single day) and often use several groups of different ages. Obviously these cross-sectional studies do not suffer from a loss of sampled subjects. They are, however, faced with another drawback, the so-called *cohort effect*. This refers to the changes in performance related to the different socioeconomic and educational characteristics of people of different ages (presumably more important for younger people) and differences in number of relevant medical events (usually greater for older persons). It is not surprising that longitudinal studies tend to show a lesser decline of performance with age than cross-sectional studies. Cohort effects also apply to other aspects of the study of aging, such as the study of brain weight in relation to aging.[158]

Neuropathology and Normal Aging

To include in one title the words *normal* and *pathology* may appear to be an oxymoron. However, even when the methodologic problems mentioned above are taken into account, the great majority of research confirms the intuitive notion that intellectual abilities deteriorate with age, at least to some extent (see Refs. 159 and 160 for a review). It is therefore necessary to attempt to establish the morphologic basis of these changes. Two categories of alterations have been identified: AD-like lesions and cerebral atrophy with neuronal loss. The latter have been extensively studied, with contrasting results.

Atrophy and Neuronal Loss   Macroscopically, the most "obvious" changes concern loss of volume and weight, which have been said to affect up to 15 percent of total brain weight between 20 and 90 years of age. Here again, the cohort effect must be taken into account, and more recent studies indicate that after the age of 60, the mean loss of brain weight is only 2 percent per decade.[161]

This cerebral atrophy seems to be due mainly to a reduction of white matter. This, in turn, is attributed to myelin loss, which is more pronounced in regions where myelination occurs late, such as the limbic and association cortex (see Ref. 161 for a review).

The microscopic changes that accompany aging vary and are often controversial. Neuronal loss, when it occurs, is not uniform. The substantia nigra (SN) is probably the anatomic structure where such loss is best documented.[162] The cellular loss observed in the pars compacta of the SN could be responsible for motor changes often observed in the elderly, such as postural rigidity, tremor, flexed posture, and gait difficulties.[163]

It was long thought that a progressive loss of neurons at the level of the cerebral cortex occurs soon after birth, especially at the level of the superior gyri of the frontal and temporal lobes and in the visual cortex.[164] Recent research has specified that changes occur in these structures, with a decrease in large neurons and a relative increase of small neurons, without clear-cut changes in the total neuronal density.[165,166]

Alzheimer-Like Changes   Microscopic changes —SPs and NFTs—are often found in the cortex of old individuals considered to be intellectually normal. Neurofibrillary tangles tend to increase with age and can be observed in most individuals past the seventh decade, localized mainly in the hippocampus and the entorhinal cortex.[167,168]

The SPs and NFTs have been interpreted as being part of normal aging or as evidence of presymptomatic AD. Current diagnostic criteria[77,78] support the "normal aging interpretation" and adjust the diagnostic weight of a given density of neocortical SPs to the age of the patient. Braak's stages[109] would rather favor the "preclinical disease interpretation," according to which analysis of the topography of neurofibrillary pathology shows no difference between early AD and "normal aging," suggesting that it is just the transentorhinal stage of the disease. Only the distribution of the NFTs and the density of SPs are correlated with dementia: there is a threshold value beyond which these alterations have a clinical expression.

Table 41-2
Location of neurofibrillary tangles and senile plaques in normal aging and Alzheimer disease

Structure	NFT/Aging	NFT/AD	SP/Aging	SP/AD
Hippocampus and entorhinal cortex	+ +	+ + +	+ +	+ + +
Parahippocampal gyrus	+	+ + +	±	+ +
Amygdala	+	+ + +	+ +	+ + +
Neocortex	±	+ +	+	+ + +
Subcortical gray nuclei	±	+ +	±	+ +

Key: ±, minimal or borderline lesions; +, moderate lesions; + +, clear-cut lesions; + + +, severe lesions.
Abbreviations: NFT = neurofibrillary tangles; AD = Alzheimer disease; SP = senile plaques.
Source: Adapted from Hauw and Delaère,[169] with permission.

What are the mechanisms underlying the appearance of these modifications? Are they, like cataracts, an inescapable consequence of time? Are they evidence of a disease against which most individuals have efficient barriers (like rubella in young children)? Are they the stigmata of the early phases of a disease, which would have been full blown if the patient had survived long enough? These three possibilities remain open at the present time. It is, however, important to stress that while these lesions can be found in both normal aging and AD, their location tends to be different, as shown in Table 41-2.

Another argument in favor of a dissociation between normal and pathologic aging can be drawn from data based on the study of 12 well-documented centenarians.[170] Lesions characteristic of AD were, of course, often found in that sample, but no more than in elderly but not so old persons.

Data of another nature may be mentioned here. As pointed out in a previous section, AD is accompanied by fairly typical functional neuro-imaging (PET and SPECT) changes, mainly located in the temporooccipital areas bilaterally. Studies involving normal elderly subjects do not usually show this pattern but rather a decreased metabolism mainly located in the cingulate, parahippocampal, superior temporal, and posterofrontal cortex.[171–173]

As can be seen, several arguments militate against the view that AD is an exaggeration of

normal aging. The similarities and differences between AD and aging have also been discussed by Berg[174] and by Drachman.[175]

CONCLUSIONS

What is the position of AD in current nosology? It has been thought by some to be inevitable, as if it were part of the history of the human race, an unavoidable scourge of phylogeny. However, recent studies have shown that AD may well represent a stereotyped mode of reaction of the brain to different types of aggression—a syndrome rather than a disease. Such a stereotyped reaction of the nervous system is probably due to the fact that it is deeply linked to normal functioning of the brain. In AD, the pathologic process dissects, within the nervous parenchymas, networks of neurons and fibers connected with the hippocampal-entorhinal complex.[185] According to our present knowledge, these connections are mainly involved in the "making of memories" at all levels, including the neocortex, where they are stored. The pathology of AD may then not be adequately covered by our usual neurologic reasoning in terms of "areas" of the cortex, since it rapidly implicates a great number of them and does not fully abolish their functions—as infarcts, for instance, would do. Alzheimer disease can therefore be said to be "transareal"; i.e., it probably implicates the same network within different cortical regions. This naturally leads us to consider that the functions of the brain are distributed following two contrasted systems of organization: one is areal, corresponding to the old concept of "cerebral localization," and the other is transareal or laminar and involves the linkage of different cortices within a given domain such as memory. These questions concerning the mechanisms of AD relate to the functioning of the brain itself. Solving the problems that they raise may unveil some of the mysteries of the most complex object of the known universe: the human brain.

REFERENCES

1. Walshe F: *Diseases of the Nervous System.* London, Livingstone, 1958.
2. Merritt H: *A Textbook of Neurology,* 4th ed. Philadelphia, Lea & Febiger, 1967.
3. Boller F, Forette F, Khatchaturian Z, et al: *Heterogeneity of Alzheimer's Disease.* Berlin, Heidelberg, New York, Springer-Verlag, 1992.
4. Ritchie K, Touchon J: Heterogeneity in senile dementia of the Alzheimer type: Individual differences, progressive deterioration or clinical subtypes. *J Clin Epidemiol* 45:1391–1398, 1992.
5. Hardy J, Duff K: Heterogeneity in Alzheimer's disease. *Ann Med* 25:437–440, 1993.
6. Pick A: Über die Beziehungen der senilen Hirnatrophie zur Aphasie. *Prager Med Wochenschr* 17:165–167, 1892.
7. Alzheimer A: Über eine eigenartige Erkrankung der Hirnrinde. *Allgemeine Zeitschrift für Psychiatrie und Psychisch-Gerichtliche Medizin* 64:146–148, 1907 [pp 41–43 in Rottenberg DA, Hochberg FH (eds): *Neurological Classics in Modern Translation.* New York, Hafner, 1977].
8. Seglas J: *Les troubles du langage chez les aliénés.* Paris, Rueff, 1892.
9. Amaducci L, Rocca W, Schoenberg B: Origin of the distinction between Alzheimer's disease and senile dementia: How history can clarify nosology. *Neurology* 36:1497–1499, 1986.
10. Roth M: Aging of the brain and dementia: An overview, in Amaducci L, Davison A, Antuono P (eds): *Aging of the Brain and Dementia.* New York, Raven Press, 1980, pp 1–21.
11. Katzman R, Terry R, Bick K (eds): *Alzheimer's Disease: Senile Dementia and Related Disorders.* New York, Raven Press, 1978, p 595.
12. Adams RD, Victor M: *Principles of Neurology,* 5th ed. New York, McGraw-Hill, 1993.
13. Perusini G: Sul valore nosografico di alcuni reperti istopatologici caratteristici per la senilità. *Riv Ital Neuropatolo Psichiatr Elettroter* 4:145–151, 1911.
14. Lewey F: Alois Alzheimer, in Haymaker W, Schiller F (eds): *The Founders of Neurology.* Springfield, IL, Charles C Thomas, 1970, pp 315–319.
15. Pomponi M, Marta M: "On the suggestion of Dr. Alzheimer I examined the following four cases." Dedicated to Gaetano Perusini. *Aging* 5:135–139, 1993.
16. Boller F, Lunardelli A: Historique de la démence, in Forette F, Christen Y, Boller F (eds): *La démence; pourquoi?* Paris, Fondation Nationale de Gérontologie, 1996.
17. American Psychiatric Association: *Diagnostic and Statistical Manual of Mental Disorders,* 4th ed. Washington, DC, American Psychiatric Association, 1994.
18. McKhann G, Drachman D, Folstein M, et al: Clinical diagnosis of Alzheimer's disease: Report of the NINCDS-ADRDA Work Group under the auspices of the Department of Health and Human Services Task Force on Alzheimer's Disease. *Neurology* 34:939–944, 1984.
19. Huff FJ, Becker JT, Belle SH, et al: Cognitive deficits and diagnosis of Alzheimer's disease. *Neurology* 36:1198–1214, 1987.
20. Tierney MC, Fisher RH, Lewis AJ, et al: The NINCDS-ADRDA Work Group criteria for the clinical diagnosis of probable Alzheimer's disease: A clinicopathological study of 57 cases. *Neurology* 38:359–364, 1988.
21. Morris JC, Heyman A, Mohs RC, et al: The Consortium to Establish a Registry for Alzheimer's Disease (CERAD): Part I. Clinical and neuropsychological assessment of Alzheimer's disease. *Neurology* 39:1159–1165, 1989.
22. Welsh KA, Butters N, Hughes JP, et al: Detection of abnormal memory decline in mild cases of Alzheimer's disease using CERAD neuropsychological measures. *Arch Neurol* 48:278–281, 1991.
23. Folstein MF, Folstein SE, McHugh PR: "Mini Mental State": A practical method for grading the cognitive state of patients for the clinician. *J Psychiatr Res* 12:189–198, 1975.
24. Blessed G, Tomlinson BE, Roth M: The association between quantitative measures of dementia

and senile change in the cerebral grey matter of elderly subjects. *Br J Psychiatry* 114:797–811, 1968.

25. Hughes CP, Berg L, Danziger WL, et al: A new clinical scale for the staging of dementia. *Br J Psychiatry* 140:566–572, 1982.

26. Todorov A, Go R, Constantinidis J, Elston R: Specificity of the clinical diagnosis of dementia. *J Neurol Sci* 26:81–98, 1975.

27. Boller F, Lopez OL, Moossy J: Diagnosis of dementia: Clinicopathologic correlations. *Neurology* 39:76–79, 1989.

28. Martin EM, Wilson RS, Penn RD, et al: Cortical biopsy results in Alzheimer's disease: Correlation with cognitive deficits. *Neurology* 37:1201–1204, 1987.

29. Morris JC, Berg L, Fulling K, et al: Validation of clinical diagnostic criteria in senile dementia of the Alzheimer type. *Ann Neurol* 22:122, 1987.

30. Mirra SS, Gearing M, McKeel DW, et al: Interlaboratory comparison of neuropathology assessments in Alzheimer's disease: A study of the consortium to establish a registry for Alzheimer's disease (CERAD). *J Neuropathol Exp Neurol* 53:303–315, 1994.

31. Bracco L, Gallato R, Lippi A, et al: Factors affecting course and survival in Alzheimer's disease: A nine-year longitudinal study. *Arch Neurol* 51:1213–1219, 1994.

32. Hébert M, Parlato V, Lese GB, et al: Survival in institutionalized patients: Influence of dementia and loss of functional capacities. *Arch Neurol* 52:469–476, 1995.

33. Absher JR, Cummings J: Noncognitive behavioral alterations in dementia syndromes, in Boller F, Grafman J (eds): *Handbook of Neuropsychology.* Amsterdam, Elsevier, 1993, pp 315–338.

34. Hyslop PHS, Tanzi RE, Polinsky RJ, et al: The genetic defect causing familial Alzheimer's disease maps on chromosome 21. *Science* 235:885–890, 1987.

35. Schellenberg GD, Bird TD, Wijsman EM, et al: Genetic linkage evidence for a familial Alzheimer's disease locus on chromosome-14. *Science* 258:668–671, 1992.

36. Pericak-Vance MA, Bebout JL, Gaskell PC, et al: Linkage studies in familial Alzheimer disease— Evidence for chromosome-19 linkage. *Am J Hum Genet* 48:1034–1050, 1991.

37. Levy-Lahad E, Wijsman E, Nemens E, et al: A familial Alzheimer's disease locus on chromosome 1. *Science* 269:970–972, 1995.

38. Corder EH, Saunders AM, Strittmatter WJ, et al: Gene dose of apolipoprotein E type 4 allele and the risk of Alzheimer's disease in late onset families. *Science* 261:921–923, 1993.

39. Saunders AM, Schmader K, Briether JC, et al: Apolipoprotein E e4 allele distribution in late-onset Alzheimer's disease and other amyloid-forming diseases. *Lancet* 342:710–711, 1993.

40. Poirier J, Davignon J, Bouthillier D, et al: Apolipoprotein E polymorphism and Alzheimer's disease. *Lancet* 342:697–699, 1993.

41. West H, Rebeck G, Growdon J, Hyman B: Apolipoprotein E4 affects neuropathology but not clinical progression in Alzheimer's disease (abstr). *Neurobiol Aging* 15(suppl 1):S28–S29, 1994.

42. Bird T: Apolipoprotein E genotyping in the diagnosis of Alzheimer's disease: A cautionary view. *Ann Neurol* 38:2–4, 1995.

43. Berr C, Hauw JJ, Delaère P, et al: Apolipoprotein E allele epsilon 4 is linked to increased deposition of the amyloid beta-peptide (A-beta) in cases with or without Alzheimer's disease. *Neurosci Lett* 178:221–224, 1994.

44. Schneider J, Gearing M, Robbins R, et al: Apolipoprotein E genotype in diverse neurodegenerative disorders. *Ann Neurol* 38:131–135, 1995.

45. Greenberg S, Rebeck G, Vonsattel JPG, et al: Apolipoprotein E e4 and cerebral hemorrhage associated with amyloid angiopathy. *Ann Neurol* 38:254–259, 1995.

46. vanGool W, Evenhuis H, vanDuijn C: A case-control study of apolipoprotein E genotypes in Alzheimer's disease associated with Down's syndrome. *Ann Neurol* 38:225–230, 1995.

47. Amouyel P, Vidal O, Launay J, Laplanche J: The apolipoprotein E alleles as major susceptibility factors for Creutzfeldt-Jakob disease. *Lancet* 344:1315–1318, 1994.

48. Marder K, Maestre G, Cote L, et al: The apolipoprotein e4 allele in Parkinson's disease with and without dementia. *Neurology* 44:1330–1331, 1994.

49. Rossor M, Kennedy A, Newman S: Heterogeneity in familial Alzheimer's disease, in Boller F, Forette F, Khatchaturian Z, et al (eds): *Heterogeneity of Alzheimer's Disease.* Berlin, Springer-Verlag, 1992, pp 81–87.

50. Huff F, Auerbach J, Chakravarti A, Boller F: Risk of dementia in relatives of patients with Alzheimer's disease. *Neurology* 38:786–790, 1988.

51. Breitner J, Welsh K, Gau B, et al: Alzheimer's disease in the National Academy of Sciences—

National Research Council Registry of Aging Twin Veterans. *Arch Neurol* 52:763–771, 1995.

52. Hofman A, Schulte W, Tanja T, et al: History of dementia and Parkinson's disease in 1st-degree relatives of patients with Alzheimer's disease. *Neurology* 39:1589–1592, 1989.

53. Heyman A, Wilkinson W, Hurwitz B, et al: Alzheimer's disease: Genetic aspects and associated clinical disorders. *Ann Neurol* 14:507–515, 1983.

54. Berr C, Borghi E, Rethoré M, et al: Absence of familial association between dementia and Down syndrome. *Am J Med Genet* 33:545–550, 1989.

55. Dartigues JF, Gagnon M, Michel P, et al: Le programme de recherche PAQUID sur l'épidémiologie de la démence: Méthodes et résultats initiaux. *Rev Neurol* 147:225–230, 1991.

56. Katzman R, Zhang M, Qu W, et al: A Chinese version of the Mini-Mental State examination: Impact of illiteracy in a Shangai dementia survey. *J Clin Epidemiol* 41:971–978, 1988.

57. Rocca W, Bonaiuto S, Lippi A, et al: Prevalence of clinically diagnosed Alzheimer's disease and other dementing disorders: A door-to-door survey in Appignano, Macerata Province, Italy. *Neurology* 40:626–631, 1990.

58. Katzman R: Education and the prevalence of dementia and Alzheimer's disease. *Neurology* 43:13–20, 1993.

59. Stern Y, Tang M, Denaro J, Mayeux R: Increased risk of mortality in Alzheimer's disease patients with more advanced educational and occupational attainment. *Ann Neurology* 37:590–595, 1995.

60. Letenneur L, Dartigues J, Commenges D, et al: Tobacco consumption and cognitive impairment in elderly people. A population-based study. *Ann Epidemiol* 4:449–454, 1994.

61. Letenneur L, Dartigues J, Orgogozo J: Wine consumption in the elderly. *Ann Intern Med* 118:317–318, 1993.

62. Polich J, Laish C, Bloom F: P300 assessment of early Alzheimer's disease. *Electroencephalogr Clin Neurophysiol* 77:179–189, 1990.

63. George AE, De Leon MJ, Stylopoulous LA, et al: CT diagnostic features of Alzheimer disease: Importance of the choroidal/hippocampal fissure complex. *AJNR* 11:101–107, 1990.

64. Jack CR Jr, Petersen RC, O'Brien PC, Tangalos EG: MR-based hippocampal volumetry in the diagnosis of Alzheimer's disease. *Neurology* 42:183–188, 1992.

65. Cuénod CA, Denys A, Michot JL, et al: Amygdala atrophy in Alzheimer's disease: An in vivo magnetic resonance imaging study. *Arch Neurol* 50:941–945, 1993.

66. Cuénod C, Kaplan D, Michot J, et al: Phospholipid abnormalities in early Alzheimer's disease: In vivo 31P NMR spectroscopy. *Arch Neurol* 52:89–94, 1995.

67. O'Brien J, Eagger S, Syed G, et al: A study of regional cerebral blood flow and cognitive performance in Alzheimer's disease. *J Neurol Neurosurg Psychiatry* 55:1182–1187, 1992.

68. Foster NL, Chase TH, Fedio P, et al: Alzheimer's disease: Focal cortical changes shown by positron emission tomography. *Neurology* 33:961–965, 1983.

69. Haxby J: Cognitive deficits and local metabolic changes in dementia of the Alzheimer type, in Rapoport S, Petit H, Leys D, Christen Y (eds): *Imaging, Cerebral Topography and Alzheimer's Disease.* Berlin, Springer-Verlag, 1990, pp 109–119.

70. Steinling M, Leys D: Patterns of dementia in Alzheimer's disease. *J Nucl Med* 33:1431–1432, 1992.

71. Keilp J, Prohovnik I: Intellectual decline predicts the parietal perfusion deficit in Alzheimer's disease. *J Nucl Med* 36:1347–1354, 1995.

72. Grady L, Rapoport S: Métabolisme cérébral: Étude de la consommation du glucose par tomographie par émission de positons, in Signoret J-L, Hauw J-J (eds): *Maladie d'Alzheimer et autres démences.* Paris, Médecine-Sciences, Flamarion, 1991, pp 169–176.

73. Mesulam M-M: *Principles of Behavioral Neurology.* Philadelphia, Davis, 1985.

74. Zeki S: *A Vision of the Brain.* Oxford, England, Blackwell, 1993.

75. Delacoste MC, White CL: The role of cortical connectivity in Alzheimer's disease pathogenesis—A review and model system. *Neurobiol Aging* 14:1–16, 1993.

76. Duyckaerts C, Hauw JJ, Bastenaire F, et al: Laminar distribution of neocortical plaques in senile dementia of the Alzheimer type. *Acta Neuropathol (Berl)* 70:249–256, 1986.

77. Khachaturian ZS: Diagnosis of Alzheimer's disease. *Arch Neurol* 42:1097–1105, 1985.

78. Mirra SS, Heyman A, McKeel D, et al: The consortium to establish a registry in Alzheimer's disease (CERAD): Part II. Standardization of the neuropathologic assessment of Alzheimer's disease. *Neurology* 41:479–486, 1991.

79. Wilcock GK, Esiri MM: Plaques, tangles and de-

mentia: A quantitative study. *J Neurol Sci* 57:407–417, 1982.

80. Terry RD, Hansen LA, DeTeresa R, et al: Senile dementia of the Alzheimer type without neocortical neurofibrillary tangles. *J Neuropathol Exp Neurol* 46:262–268, 1987.

81. Lamy C, Duyckaerts C, Delaère P, et al: Comparison of seven staining methods for senile plaques and neurofibrillary tangles in a prospective study of 15 elderly patients. *Neuropath Appl Neurobiol* 15:563–578, 1989.

82. Uchihara T, Duyckaerts C, He Y, et al: ApoE immunoreactivity and microglial cells in Alzheimer's disease brain. *Neurosci Lett* 195:5–8, 1995.

83. Eikelenboom P, Stam FC: An immunohistochemical study on cerebral vascular and senile plaque amyloid in Alzheimer's dementia. *Virchows Arch [Cell Pathol]* 47:17–25, 1984.

84. Glenner GG, Wong CW: Alzheimer's disease: Initial report of the purification and characterization of a novel cerebrovascular amyloid protein. *Biochem Biophys Res Commun* 120:885–890, 1984.

85. Kang J, Lemaire H-G, Unterbeck A, et al: The precursor of Alzheimer's disease amyloid A4 protein resembles a cell-surface receptor. *Nature* 325:733–736, 1987.

86. Delaère P, Duyckaerts C, Masters C, et al: Large amounts of neocortical βA4 deposits without Alzheimer changes in a nondemented case. *Neurosci Lett* 116:87–93, 1990.

87. Delaère P, He Y, Fayet G, et al: βA4 deposits are constant in the brain of the oldest old: An immunocytochemical study of 20 French centenarians. *Neurobiol Aging* 14:191–194, 1993.

88. Roberts G, Gentleman S, Lynch A, Graham D: Beta A4 amyloid protein deposition in brain after head trauma. *Lancet* 338:1422–1423, 1991.

89. Adle-Biassette H, Duyckaerts C, Vasowicz M, et al: Beta amyloid protein diffuse deposits and head trauma. *Neurobiol Aging*. In press.

90. Wisniewski T, Frangione B: Apolipoprotein E: A pathological chaperone protein in patients with cerebral and systemic amyloid. *Neurosci Lett* 135:235–238, 1992.

91. Uchihara T, Kondo H, Akiyama H, Ikeda K: White matter amyloid in Alzheimer's disease brain. *Acta Neuropathol* 90:51–56, 1995.

92. Probst A, Basler V, Bron B, Ulrich J: Neuritic plaques in senile dementia of the Alzheimer type: A Golgi analysis in the hippocampal region. *Brain Res* 268:249–254, 1983.

93. Glenner GG: Amyloid deposits and amyloidosis: The β-fibrilloses. *N Engl J Med* 302:1283–1292; 1333–1343, 1980.

94. Pitas RE, Boyles JK, Lee SH, et al: Astrocytes synthesize apolipoprotein E and metabolize apolipoprotein E-containing lipoproteins. *Biochem Biophys Acta* 917:148–161, 1987.

95. Miyakawa T, Shimoji A, Kuramoto R, Higuchi Y: The relationship between senile plaques and cerebral blood vessels in Alzheimer's disease and senile dementia. *Virchows Arch* 40:121–129, 1982.

96. Kawai M, Cras P, Perry G: Serial reconstruction of β-protein amyloid plaques: Relationship to microvessels and size distribution. *Brain Res* 592:278–282, 1992.

97. Alzheimer A: Über eigenartige Krankheitsfälle des späteren Alters. *Zentralbl Ges Neurol Psychiatr* 4:356–385, 1911.

98. Pollanen P, Markiewicz P, Bergeron C, Goh MC: Twisted ribbon structure of paired helical filaments revealed by atomic force microscopy. *Am J Pathol* 144:869–873, 1994.

99. Brion JP, Passareiro H, Nunez J, Flament-Durand J: Mise en évidence immunologique de la protéine tau au niveau des lésions de dégénérescence neurofibrillaire de la maladie d'Alzheimer. *Arch Biol (Brux)* 95:229–235, 1985.

100. Flament S, Delacourte A, Hemon B, Defossez A: Démonstration directe d'une phosphorylation anormale des protéines microtubulaires tau au cours de la maladie d'Alzheimer. *CR Acad Sci (Paris)* 208:77–82, 1989.

101. Flament S, Delacourte A: Abnormal tau species are produced during Alzheimer's disease neurodegenerating process. *FEBS Lett* 247:213–216, 1989.

102. Delacourte A: Pathological Tau proteins of Alzheimer's disease as a biochemical marker of neurofibrillary degeneration. *Biomed Pharmacother* 48:287–295, 1994.

103. Matsuo ES, Shin RW, Billingsley ML, et al: Biopsy-derived adult human tau is phosphorylated at many of the same sites as Alzheimer's disease paired helical filament tau. *Neuron* 13:989–1002, 1994.

104. Feany M, Ksiezak-Reding H, Liu W, et al: Epitope expression and hyperphosphorylation of tau protein in corticobasal degeneration: Differentiation from progressive supranuclear palsy. *Acta Neuropathol (Berl)* 90:37–43, 1995.

105. Duyckaerts C, Llamas E, Delaère P, et al: Neuronal loss and neuronal atrophy: Computer simula-

tion in connection with Alzheimer's disease. *Brain Res* 504:94–100, 1989.

106. Braak H, Braak E, Grundke-Iqbal I, Iqbal K: Occurrence of neuropil threads in the senile human brain and in Alzheimer's disease: A 3rd location of paired helical filaments outside of neurofilament tangles and neuritic plaques. *Neurosci Lett* 65:351–355, 1986.

107. Arnold SE, Hyman BT, Flory J, et al: The topographical and neuroanatomical distribution of neurofibrillary tangles and neuritic plaques in the cerebral cortex of patients with Alzheimer's disease. *Cereb Cortex* 1:103–116, 1991.

108. Delaère P, Duyckaerts C, Brion JP, et al: Tau, paired helical filaments and amyloid in the neocortex: A morphometric study of 15 cases with graded intellectual status in aging and senile dementia of Alzheimer type. *Acta Neuropathol* 77:645–653, 1989.

109. Braak H, Braak E: Neuropathological staging of Alzheimer-related changes. *Acta Neuropathologica (Berl)* 82:239–259, 1991.

110. Bancher C, Jellinger KA: Neurofibrillary predominant form of Alzheimer's disease: A rare subtype in very old subjects. *Acta Neuropathol (Berl)* 88:565–570, 1994.

111. Terry RD: The pathogenesis of Alzheimer's disease: What causes dementia? in Christen Y, Churchland P (eds): *Neurophilosophy and Alzheimer's Disease*. Berlin, Springer-Verlag, 1992, pp 123–130.

112. Masliah E, Terry R: Role of synaptic pathology in the mechanisms of denervation in Alzheimer's disease. *Clin Neurosci* 4:192–198, 1993.

113. Cras P, Smith MA, Richey PL, et al: Extracellular neurofibrillary tangles reflect neuronal loss and provide further evidence of extensive protein cross-linking in Alzheimer disease. *Acta Neuropathol (Berl)* 89:291–295, 1995.

114. Blanks J, Hinton D, Sadun A, Miller C: Retinal ganglion cell degeneration in Alzheimer's disease. *Brain Res* 501:364–372, 1989.

115. Mann DMA: Pathological correlates of dementia in Alzheimer's disease. *Neurobiol Aging* 15:357–360, 1994.

116. Regeur L, Badsberg Jensen G, Pakkenberg H, et al: No global neocortical nerve cell loss in brains from patients with senile dementia of Alzheimer's type. *Neurobiol Aging* 15:347–352, 1994.

117. Hauw J-J, Duyckaerts C, Partdrige M: Neuropathological aspects of brain aging and SDAT, in *Modern Trends in Aging Research: Colloque Inserm-Eurage.* London, John Libbey Eurotext, 1986, pp 435–442.

118. Duyckaerts C, Hauw J-J, Piette F, et al: Cortical atrophy in senile dementia of the Alzheimer type is mainly due to a decrease in cortical length. *Acta Neuropathol (Berl)* 66:72–74, 1985.

119. Sterio DC: The unbiased estimation of number and sizes of arbitrary particles using the disector. *J Microsc* 134:127–136, 1984.

120. Okasaki H, Lipkin LE, Aronson SM: Diffuse intracytoplasmatic ganglionic inclusions (Lewy type) associated with progressive dementia and quadriparesis in flexion. *J Neuropathol Exp Neurol* 20:237–244, 1961.

121. Kosaka K: Diffuse Lewy body disease in Japan. *J Neurol* 237:197–204, 1990.

122. Gibb WRG, Luthert PJ, Janota I, Lantos PL: Diffuse Lewy body dementia: Clinical features and classification. *J Neurol Neurosurg Psychiatry* 52:185–192, 1989.

123. Byrne EJ, Lennox G, Lowe J, Godwen-Austen RB: Diffuse Lewy body disease: Clinical features in 15 cases. *J Neurol Neurosurg Psychiatry* 52:709–717, 1989.

124. Dickson DW, Wu E, Crystal HA, et al: Alzheimer's disease and age-related pathology in diffuse Lewy body disease, in Boller F, Forette F, Khatchaturian Z, et al (eds): *Heterogeneity of Alzheimer's Disease.* Berlin, Springer-Verlag, 1992, pp 168–186.

125. Hansen L, Salmon D, Galasko D, et al: Lewy body variant of Alzheimer's disease: A clinical and pathological entity. *Neurology* 40:1–8, 1990.

126. Kosaka K: Dementia and neuropathology in Lewy body disease, in Narabayashi H, Nagatsu T, Yanagisawa N, Mizuno Y (eds): *Parkinson's Disease: From Basic Research to Treatment.* New York, Raven Press, 1993, pp 456–463.

127. Perry EK, Marshall E, Perry RH, et al: Cholinergic and dopaminergic activities in senile dementia of Lewy body type. *Alzheimer Dis Assoc Disord* 4:87–95, 1990.

128. McKeith IG, Perry RH, Fairbairn AF, et al: Operational criteria for senile dementia of Lewy body type (SDLT). *Psych Med* 22:911–922, 1992.

129. Joachim CL, Morris JH, Selkoe DJ: Clinically diagnosed Alzheimer's disease: Autopsy results in 150 cases. *Ann Neurol* 24:50–56, 1988.

130. Lennox G: Lewy body dementia, in Rossor MN (ed): *Baillière's Clinical Neurology.* London, Baillière Tindall, 1992, pp 653–676.

131. Boller F, Mizutani T, Roessmann U, Gambetti PL: Parkinson disease, dementia and Alzheimer disease: Clinico-pathological correlations. *Ann Neurol* 7:329–335, 1980.

132. Benson DF: Posterior cortical atrophy: A new entity or Alzheimer's disease? *Arch Neurol* 46:843–844, 1989.

133. Jacquet MF, Boucquey D, Theaux R, et al: L'atrophie corticale postérieure: Variante anatomo-clinique de la maladie d'Alzheimer. *Acta Neurol Belg* 20:265–273, 1990.

134. Fustinoni O, Mangone CA, Abiusi GRP, et al: Primary progressive aphasia: Clinical subtypes, with one postmortem study (abstr). *Neurology* 44:A387, 1994.

135. Kertesz A, Munoz DG: The pathology and nosology of primary progressive aphasia. *Neurology* 44:2065–2072, 1994.

136. Constantinidis J, Richard J, Tissot R: Pick's disease: Histological and clinical correlations. *Eur Neurol* 11:208–217, 1974.

137. Knopman DS: Overview of dementia lacking distinctive histology: Pathological designation of a progressive dementia. *Dementia* 4:132–136, 1993.

138. Hauw J-J, Duyckaerts C, Seilhean D, et al: The neuropathologic diagnostic criteria of frontal lobe dementia revisited: A study of ten consecutive cases. *J Neural Transm.* In press.

139. Mesulam MM: Slowly progressive aphasia without generalized dementia. *Ann Neurol* 11:592–598, 1982.

140. Déjerine J, Sérieux P: Un cas de surdité verbale pure terminée par aphasie sensorielle suivie d'autopsie. *Comptes Rendus Société Biol* 49:1074–1077, 1897.

141. Cole M, Wright D, Banker BQ: Familial aphasia due to Pick's disease. *Ann Neurol* 6:158, 1979.

142. Weintraub S, Mesulam MM: Four neuropsychological profiles in dementia, in Boller F, Grafman J (eds): *Handbook of Neuropsychology.* Amsterdam, Elsevier, 1993, pp 253–282.

143. Holland AL, McBurney DH, Moossy J, Reinmuth OM: The dissolution of language in Pick's disease with neurofibrillary tangles: A case study. *Brain Lang* 24:36–58, 1985.

144. Morris JC, Cole M, Banker BQ, Wright D: Hereditary dysphasic dementia and the Pick-Alzheimer spectrum. *Ann Neurol* 16:455–466, 1984.

145. Brun A: Frontal lobe degeneration of non-Alzheimer type: I. Neuropathology. *Arch Gerontol Geriatr* 6:193–208, 1987.

146. Neary D, Snowden JS, Bowen DM, et al: Neuropsychological syndromes in presenile dementia due to cerebral atrophy. *J Neurol Neurosurg Psychiatry* 49:163–174, 1986.

147. Brun A: Frontal lobe degeneration of non-Alzheimer type revisited. *Dementia* 4:126–131, 1993.

148. Neary D, Snowden JS, Mann DMA: The clinical pathological correlates of lobar atrophy. *Dementia* 4:154–159, 1993.

149. Rebeiz J, Kolodney E, Richardson E: Corticodentatonigral degeneration with neuronal achromatasia. *Arch Neurol* 18:20–33, 1968.

150. Crystal HA, Horoupian DS, Katzman R, Jotkowitz S: Biopsy-proved Alzheimer disease presenting as right parietal lobe syndrome. *Ann Neurol* 12:186–188, 1981.

151. Jagust W, Davies P, Tiller-Borcich J, Reed B: Focal Alzheimer's disease. *Neurology* 40:14–19, 1990.

152. Léger J-M, Levasseur M, Benoit M, et al: Apraxie d'aggravation lentement progressive: Étude par IRM et tomographie à positons dans 4 cas. *Rev Neurol* 147:183–191, 1991.

153. Thuillard F, Assal G: Données Neuropsychologiques chez le sujet agé normal, in Habib M, Joanette Y, Puel M (eds): *Démences et Syndromes Démentiels.* Paris, Masson, 1991, pp 125–133.

154. Schaie K: The Seattle Longitudinal Study: A 35 year inquiry of adult intellectual development. *Zeitschr Gerontol* 26:129–137, 1993.

155. Willis S, Schaie W: Cognitive training in the normal elderly, in Forette F, Christen Y, Boller F (ed): *Plasticité Cérébrale et Stimulation Cognitive.* Paris, Fondation Nationale de Gérontologie, 1993, pp 91–113.

156. Bachman DL, Wolf PA, Linn R, et al: Prevalence of dementia and probable senile dementia of the Alzheimer's type in the Framingham Study. *Neurology* 42:115–119, 1992.

157. Linn R, Wolf PA, Bachman DL, et al: The "preclinical phase" of probable Alzheimer's disease. *Neurology* 52:485–490, 1995.

158. Miller A, Corsellis J: Evidence for a secular increase in human brain weight during the past century. *Ann Hum Biol* 4:253–257, 1977.

159. Corkin S: Aging, age-related disorders and dementia, in Boller F, Grafman J (ed): *Handbook of Neuropsychology.* Amsterdam, Elsevier, 1991, vols 4, 5.

160. Boller F, Marcie P, Traykov L: La Neuropsychologie du vieillissement normal, in Botez MI (ed): *Neuropsychologie Clinique et Neurologie du Com-*

portement. Paris and Montreal, Masson & Presse Universitaire du Québec, 1996, pp 527–592.

161. Kemper T: Neuroanatomical and neuropathological changes in normal aging and in dementia, in Albert ML (ed): *Clinical Neurology of Aging.* New York, Oxford University Press, 1984, pp 9–52.

162. McGeer E: Aging and neurotransmitter metabolism in the human brain, in Katzman R, Terry R, Bick K (ed): *Alzheimer's Disease: Senile Dementia and Related Disorders.* New York, Raven Press, 1978, pp 427–440.

163. Pirozzolo F, Mahurin R, Swihart A: Motor function in aging and neurodegenerative disease, in Boller F, Grafman J (eds): *Handbook of Neuropsychology.* Amsterdam, Elsevier, 1991, pp 167–194.

164. Brody H: Structural changes in the aging nervous system. *Interdisc Top Gerontol* 7:9–21, 1970.

165. Terry RD, DeTeresa R, Hansen LA: Neocortical cell counts in normal human adult aging. *Ann Neurol* 21:530–539, 1987.

166. Peters A: The absence of significant neuronal loss from cerebral cortex with age. *Neurobiol Aging* 14:657–658, 1993.

167. Arriagada PV, Marzloff K, Hyman BT: Distribution of Alzheimer-type pathologic changes in nondemented elderly individuals matches the pattern in Alzheimer's disease. *Neurology* 42:1681–1688, 1992.

168. Frigard B, Vermersch P, David JP, et al: Le processus neurodegeneratif au cours du vieillissement cerebral et de la maladie d'Alzheimer, in Albarède JL, Vellas P, Garry PJ (eds): *L'Année Gérontologique: Facts and Research in Gerontology.* New York, Springer, 1994, pp 257–269.

169. Hauw J, Delaère P: Topographie des lésions, in Signoret J, Hauw J (eds): Maladie d'Alzheimer et autres démences. Paris, Flammarion, 1991, pp 23–38.

170. Hauw JJ, Vignolo P, Duyckaerts C, et al: Étude neuropathologique de 12 centenaires: La fréquence de la démence sénile de type Alzheimer n'est pas particulièrement élevée dans ce groupe de personnes très âgées. *Rev Neurol* 142:107–115, 1986.

171. Kuhl DE, Metter EJ, Riege WH, Phelps ME: Effects of human aging on patterns of local cerebral glucose metabolism determined by the ^{18}F fluoro-deoxyglucose method. *J Cereb Blood Flow Metab* 2:163–171, 1982.

172. Yamaguchi T, Kanno I, Uemura K, et al: Reduction in regional cerebral metabolic rate of oxygen during human aging. *Stroke* 17:1220–1228, 1986.

173. Martin AJ, Friston KJ, Colebatch JG, Frackowiak RSJ: Decreases in regional cerebral blood flow with normal aging. *J Cereb Blood Flow Metab* 11:684–689, 1991.

174. Berg L: Does Alzheimer's disease represent an exaggeration of normal aging? *Arch Neurol* 42:737–739, 1985.

175. Drachman DA: If we live long enough, will we all be demented? *Neurology* 44:1563–1565, 1994.

176. Sjögren T, Sjögren H, Lindgren A: Morbus Alzheimer and Morbus Pick: A genetic, clinical and pathoanatomical study. *Acta Psychiatr Neurol Scand Suppl* 82:1–152, 1952.

177. Pichot P: Language disturbances in cerebral disease. *Arch Neurol Psychiatry* 74:92–96, 1955.

178. Critchley M: The neurology of psychotic speech. *Br J Psychiatry* 110:353–364, 1964.

179. De Renzi E, Vignolo L: I disturbi del linguaggio nei dementi. *Il Lavoro Neuropsichiatrico,* 12:1–18, 1966.

180. Irigaray L: Approche psycholinguistique du langage des déments. *Neuropsychologia* 5:25–52, 1967.

181. Ajuriaguerra JD, Strejilevitch M, Tissot R: À propos de quelques conduites devant le miroir de sujets atteints de syndrome démentiels du grand âge. *Neuropsychologia* 1:59–73, 1963.

182. Pollock M, Hornabrook RW: The prevalence, natural history and dementia of Parkinson's disease. *Brain* 89:429–448, 1966.

183. Green R, Benjamin S, Cummings J: Fellowship programs in behavioral neurology. *Neurology* 45:412–415, 1995.

184. Wechsler AF: Presenile dementia presenting as aphasia. *J Neurol Neurosurg Psychiatry* 40:303–305, 1977.

185. Duyckaerts C, Delaère P, Hauw JJ: Alzheimer's disease and neuroanatomy: Hypotheses and proposals, in Boller F, Forette F, Khachaturian Z, et al (eds): *Heterogeneity of Alzheimer's Disease.* Berlin, Heidelberg, New York, Springer-Verlag, 1992, pp 144–155.

Chapter 42

ALZHEIMER'S DISEASE: COGNITIVE NEUROPSYCHOLOGICAL ASPECTS

Robert D. Nebes

Much of the psychological research on Alzheimer's disease (AD) has had a clinical focus in that the main goal has been to discriminate AD from normal aging and from other conditions, such as depression, that are often confused with early stage AD (see Chap. 41). Since this approach is generally concerned with diagnosis, it necessarily uses tasks that are clinically validated and standardized. Recently, however, researchers have begun to apply the theories and methodologies of cognitive psychology to AD. The main goal of this approach is to understand the mechanisms underlying the cognitive dysfunctions present in AD. Thus, for example, rather than investigating which memory task best differentiates early AD from normal aging, the cognitive neuropsychology approach is more concerned with whether the memory loss in AD is due to an impairment in the initial encoding of information into memory, a loss of information from the memory store, or a retrieval deficit. It is this cognitive neuropsychology of AD that is briefly reviewed in this chapter.

Alzheimer's disease is a dementing condition that produces severe decrements in multiple areas of cognition, from visual perception to problem solving. Because the decrements are so diverse, most studies restrict themselves to examining relatively discrete aspects of cognition (e.g., short-term memory, syntax, etc.). This has produced a somewhat fragmented literature in which patients' performance in one cognitive domain is investigated without regard to possible interactive effects produced by concurrent problems in other cognitive

operations. Also, there has been little attempt to determine whether changes in one or more fundamental processing mechanisms may be responsible for the large number of apparently independent cognitive deficits seen in AD. That is, it is possible that most or all of the diverse deficits seen in AD patients may arise from a dysfunction in one basic mechanism. The present chapter briefly reviews what is known about the nature of the decrements produced by AD (see Ref. 1 for a more extensive review) in three areas of cognition: attention, memory, and language. From this review, it becomes clear that not all cognitive operations are equally disrupted by AD. The chapter then discusses several of the broader theoretical constructs that have recently been advanced to explain why some mental operations are grossly impaired by AD while others appear to be relatively spared.

ATTENTION

The term *attention* has been applied to a number of very different mental functions, some of which are severely impaired in AD while others remain intact.[2] One major sense of attention involves selection. Humans can process only a limited amount of information at any one time; thus they must select which information they will fully process. Limitations of selective attention are of two types: divided attention and focused attention. To the degree that persons cannot process multiple sources of information as efficiently as they can process one source, they show a limitation in divided attention. Similarly, to the extent that they find it difficult to ignore (i.e., not process) information they know is irrelevant, they show a limitation in focused attention.

Patients with AD have severe problems dividing their attention, but focused attention appears to be less disrupted. One study[3] examined AD patients' ability to divide and focus their attention within the same stimulus. The stimulus was a large digit made up of smaller digits (e.g., a large 1 made up of small 2s). In the focused-attention condition, subjects were told before each trial to direct their attention either to the large digit or to its smaller component digits and to decide whether a 1 or a 2 was present. In the divided-attention condition, they had to attend to both the large digit and its smaller component digits to see if a 1 or a 2 was present in either. In comparison to normals, AD patients were much more impaired in dividing than in focusing their attention. What might be the cause of this problem? In order to attend to multiple sources of information, it is necessary to disengage from one stimulus, shift to the next, and then refocus on this new stimulus. The AD patients' main difficulty appears to lie in disengaging from a currently attended stimulus. This was shown by a study[4] in which subjects were to respond to a stimulus that appeared on either the right or left side of a computer screen. Before each trial, subjects were given a cue that told them on which side the stimulus would appear, thus allowing them to shift the focus of their attention to the proper side of the screen before the stimulus appeared. On most trials this cue was valid (i.e., correct), but on certain trials it was invalid, leading them to shift their attention to the wrong side of the screen. Thus, when the stimulus appeared on those trials with invalid cues, subjects had to disengage their attention from the incorrect side of space and shift to the side on which the stimulus had actually appeared. This disengagement operation was dramatically slower in the AD patients. Therefore, AD patients appear able to focus attention but have trouble disengaging in order to flexibly redeploy their attentional focus.

The other major sense of the term *attention* is alertness—an individual's readiness to process external information and to respond. Fluctuations in alertness can be divided into (1) phasic changes—the rapid mobilization of resources to process an expected input and (2) tonic changes— the slow decline in performance across a long, repetitive task. Phasic changes in alertness are evident in the way a warning signal facilitates subjects' response time (RT) to a later stimulus by allowing them to maximize their alertness for the upcoming stimulus. Not only do AD patients respond faster to a stimulus when given a warning, but the time the patients need to reach maximal alertness (i.e., the optimal delay between the warning and stimulus) is no longer than that required by the normal old.[5] This suggests that AD does not grossly impair patients' ability to mobilize their attentional resources to prepare for an upcoming stimulus. Studies of tonic alertness have found that this component of alertness is also relatively preserved in AD. Tonic alertness is typically tested by giving subjects a long, unbroken period of repetitive testing. A decrease in tonic attention is evident as a decline in response accuracy or RT across time on task. Several studies[3,5] have shown that the performance of AD patients declines no more rapidly than does that of the normal old. Thus, the attentional deficit in AD is most evident in divided-attention situations. Focused attention and tonic and phasic alertness are much less impaired in these patients.

LANGUAGE

Language deficits are among the most prominent early symptoms of AD. However, not all aspects of language are disrupted.[6] AD causes only minimal deficits in syntax, as patients' speech generally remains grammatically correct. However, AD patients often perform badly on tests involving semantics—the production and comprehension of meaning. They have difficulty finding the appropriate word both in spontaneous speech and in formal tests such as object naming. Their speech is littered with indefinite terms such as "stuff" and "things" and thus often conveys little information.

Their comprehension of language, especially of complex sentences and stories, can be quite poor. These patients also have difficulty searching semantic categories and producing semantic associates to a given stimulus.

One explanation for these problems is that AD disrupts patients' knowledge of concept meaning (see Chap. 37). It has been suggested that AD patients no longer know the distinctive semantic attributes of concepts, such as their physical features and functions. A loss of basic perceptual and abstract knowledge about concepts could explain the problems AD patients have in finding the appropriate word or name, understanding and using language, dealing with abstract concepts, etc. It could even contribute to the patients' problems in a variety of other cognitive areas, since humans tend to use language and symbols extensively when storing and manipulating information. Many investigators feel that this semantic dysfunction is one of the core deficits of AD that differentiates it from other dementing diseases.[7]

It is still not clear, however, whether semantic information is actually lost in AD or whether the problems these patients have on semantic tasks spring from failures of more general-purpose cognitive operations such as those involved in accessing and evaluating information. This possibility is raised by studies that have found relatively normal performance by AD patients on some semantic tasks. For example, one recent study[8] presented AD patients with a target word (e.g., *fish*) followed by a stimulus word and measured how accurately and rapidly they could decide whether the stimulus was related to the target. On some of the trials, the stimulus was a semantic attribute of the target (e.g., *fins*), while on others it was not (e.g., *laces*).

In this study, AD patients were extremely accurate in their decisions about the relationship between a target and its attributes. This study also looked at how decision time varied as a function of the relative importance that the attribute had for the meaning of the target. Attribute importance reflects the likelihood that a particular attribute comes to mind when a target concept is presented. For example, when given "airplane" and

asked to name its attributes, people are more likely to think of wings than of wheels, even though both are physical features of an airplane. In this study, the decision time of normals was inversely related to attribute importance—that is, the more important the attribute, the faster their decision. This same pattern was found in the AD patients. These results suggest that not only do AD patients retain knowledge of concept attributes, but they still know the relative importance that different attributes of a concept have for concept meaning.

Overall, investigations into AD patients' semantic abilities have produced a multitude of contradictory results. The underlying cause of their deficits on some semantic tasks—loss of semantic knowledge versus inability to use intact semantic knowledge—is one of the more controversial issues in the cognitive neuropsychology of AD.

MEMORY

While AD causes major deficits in most areas of cognition, the symptom that people commonly associate with this disease is a loss of memory. However, even memory is not uniformly impaired.[1,9] Memory has multiple components and processes, some of which are more disrupted by AD than others. Primary or short-term memory is viewed as a limited-capacity temporary store of information held in consciousness, while secondary or long-term memory is an unlimited-capacity permanent store. There is no question that AD severely disrupts secondary memory. Alzheimer patients have great difficulty recalling any substantial amount of information for more than a few minutes, especially if they engage in any interfering cognitive activity prior to recall. Even if the stimuli are repeated several times or memory cues or possible answers in the form of a recognition test are provided, AD patients still perform quite poorly[10] on tests of secondary memory. By contrast, primary memory seems less affected by AD, although it is not normal. For example, when given a list of words to remember, AD patients tend to recall only the last few items they heard—i.e., what they do recall appears to come from primary memory.

What might be the source of the secondary-memory problems in AD? In order to remember a stimulus, it must be encoded into memory, maintained in storage, and later retrieved. There is a great deal of evidence for a major dysfunction in AD patients' initial processing of information (i.e., encoding). Stimulus factors known to affect encoding in normals (e.g., word familiarity) do not influence encoding in AD patients. Also, in AD patients, unlike normals, semantic knowledge about the stimulus or the context in which the stimulus appears does not always facilitate memory encoding. As for storage, if the level of initial learning is equated in AD patients and normals (a difficult feat), the rate at which information is lost from secondary memory appears to be approximately the same in the two groups. That is, the rate of forgetting may be relatively normal in AD patients. The effect that AD has on memory retrieval is unclear due to the severity of the encoding deficit. One way of demonstrating that a retrieval defect contributes to memory problems is to show that the problems decrease when the demand on retrieval is minimized, either by giving memory cues or by using a recognition task. However, as stated above, such approaches do not help AD patients. But it is possible that memory encoding is so deficient in AD patients that the resultant memory trace is impoverished to the point that cues and recognition choices cannot activate it.

While secondary memory performance is very poor in AD, there are other constituents of memory that appear to be much less disrupted. One is memory for distant events (remote memory). The normal old tend to remember information from the remote past better than more recent events (i.e., their memory accuracy shows a temporal gradient). Remote memory has been assessed by such tests as memory for important public events (John F. Kennedy's death), famous faces from a particular era (e.g., Harry S. Truman), or personal events in an individual's life. While AD patients do not perform as well as normals in such tasks, their memory does show a temporal gradient in that they recall distant information better than more recent information, suggesting a relative preservation of remote memory.

A second aspect of memory that may be at least partially preserved in AD is implicit memory (see Chap. 36). Unlike the memory described up to this point (so-called explicit memory), implicit-memory tasks do not require intentional recollection of prior information. Rather, they measure the facilitation that prior experience has on a subject's performance. For example, if subjects are shown a series of stimulus words and later given the first few letters of those words (word stem), being asked to complete each stem with one of the previously presented stimulus words, this is a measure of explicit memory. By contrast, if, when given the word stem, they are just asked to complete the stem with the first word that comes to mind (no mention being made of any relationship to the prior stimulus words), this is a measure of implicit memory. In such an implicit-memory task, the subjects' previous experience with the stimulus words is evident as an increased likelihood that they will complete the stems with words from the stimulus list (in comparison to a baseline condition where they did not experience the stimuli). The effect of prior experience with the stimuli is thus evident implicitly as a change in the subjects' behavior rather than as explicit recall. This distinction between explicit and implicit memory has generated a great deal of interest because patients with organic amnesias (e.g., Korsakoff patients) can show normal implicit-memory performance despite a total inability to recall the stimuli explicitly. What about AD patients? At present the evidence is mixed. Some studies have shown the implicit memory of AD patients to be grossly defective. However, other researchers[11] argue that normal implicit memory can be demonstrated in AD if the study design ensures that the patients adequately attend to and encode the initial stimulus material. That is, if their initial processing of the stimuli is successful, it may be possible to demonstrate relatively normal implicit memory.

DISCUSSION

From this brief review it is clear that while AD patients have multiple deficits, not all aspects of cognition are equally impaired. Several theoretical mechanisms have been proposed to explain this variability. Some investigators have suggested that the attentional capacity of AD patients is severely diminished. If so, then AD patients should perform poorly on any task that makes a major demand on attentional capacity while performing relatively normally on tasks that require only automatic processes.[12] Attentional capacity has been conceptualized as the mental energy necessary for the active and intentional manipulation of information. By contrast, automatic processes require neither conscious awareness nor intention and place little demand on attentional capacity. For example, actively searching through your memory for a particular piece of information to answer a question is thought to require substantial attentional capacity. By contrast, retrieval of a word's phonology and meanings is thought to be automatic. Unfortunately, there is little direct evidence supporting this attractive hypothesis. One problem is that criteria for what constitutes an automatic process have been specifically defined in only a few experimental paradigms, and AD patients do not always perform normally in these paradigms. For example, the incidental encoding into memory of certain types of information (e.g., the sensory modality in which a stimulus was presented or its frequency of presentation) meets some investigators' criteria for automaticity. However, AD patients' memory for such information is quite poor.[13] Thus, a reduction in attentional capacity seems unlikely to be the sole explanation for the variability seen in AD patients' cognitive performance.

Recently, a variant of the attentional-capacity model has been suggested in which AD patients' deficits are hypothesized to arise from a failure of inhibitory processes.[14] It is argued that AD patients fail to inhibit partially activated but incorrect information. This would result in their processing capacity being swamped by unimportant information that normal individuals would suppress. Evidence for this hypothesis comes from a variety of sources. Alzheimer patients tend to make many intrusion errors (e.g., when remembering a story, they will incorporate information from

outside the story into their recall). They also have difficulty inhibiting the irrelevant meanings of ambiguous words. When normal individuals encounter a word with multiple distinct meanings in a sentence, those meanings that are irrelevant to that particular context are rapidly inhibited. For example, when normal individuals see the word *bank* in the context of a sentence about a river, both senses of the word (i.e., one relevant to money, the other to a river) are automatically activated. However, in normals, within a half second or so, the irrelevant sense of the word (i.e., a place that holds money) is inhibited. By contrast, in AD patients, both the relevant and irrelevant senses of *bank* tend to remain active.[15] Such a failure to inhibit contextually irrelevant information would not only overload AD patients' processing capacity but also interfere with their understanding of the sentence's meaning. A breakdown in inhibitory control in AD patients could contribute to many of their cognitive deficits, including memory, language, problem solving, etc. While the evidence for this model is still limited, it may turn out to be an important mechanism underlying the cognitive deficits of AD.

Another theoretical construct that shows promise for explaining the pattern of cognitive deficits in AD is the central executive system. The central executive system is conceived of as the mechanism that organizes and coordinates simultaneously active processing programs. It resolves scheduling conflicts and orchestrates the operation of concurrent processes. Any central executive system dysfunction would make it difficult for AD patients to intentionally manipulate and process stimulus information, especially in complex tasks where multiple mental operations must be carried out either simultaneously or in the proper sequence.[16] For example, in order to comprehend and remember a sentence, it is necessary to coordinate the decoding of language symbols with the encoding of this information into memory. At the present time, however, it is difficult to evaluate whether a central executive system dysfunction could account for the full array of deficits found in AD, because the nature of the central executive system has not been clearly defined, nor have comparatively pure measures of central executive system function been devised.

SUMMARY

While substantial progress has been made in characterizing the types of mental operations impaired in AD, the mechanisms underlying these deficits are still not clear. Are we dealing with an accumulation of many discrete deficits, such as would result from numerous focal brain lesions, or are only a few basic cognitive dysfunctions responsible for the total array of impairments in AD? To some extent the answer to this question may depend on future advances in cognitive psychology, as it is this area of research that has provided the theoretical frameworks and methodologies underlying the cognitive-neuropsychological approach to AD.

REFERENCES

1. Nebes RD: Cognitive dysfunction in Alzheimer's disease, in Craik FIM, Salthouse TA (eds): *The Handbook of Aging and Cognition.* Hillsdale, NJ, Erlbaum, 1992, pp 373–446.
2. Parasuraman R, Haxby JV: Attention and brain function in Alzheimer's disease: A review. *Neuropsychology* 7:242–272, 1993.
3. Filoteo JV, Delis DC, Massman PJ, et al: Directed and divided attention in Alzheimer's disease: Impairment in shifting attention to global and local stimuli. *J Clin Exp Neuropsychol* 14:871–883, 1992.
4. Parasuraman R, Greenwood PM, Haxby JV, Grady CL: Visuospatial attention in dementia of the Alzheimer type. *Brain* 115:711–733, 1992.
5. Nebes RD, Brady CB: Phasic and tonic alertness in Alzheimer's disease. *Cortex* 29:77–90, 1993.
6. Nebes RD: Semantic memory in Alzheimer's disease. *Psychol Bull* 106:377–394, 1989.
7. Martin A: Degraded knowledge representations in patients with Alzheimer's disease, in Squire LR, Butters N (eds): *Neuropsychology of Memory.* Amsterdam, North-Holland, 1992, pp 220–232.
8. Nebes RD, Brady CB: Preserved organization of semantic attributes in Alzheimer's disease. *Psychol Aging* 5:574–579, 1990.
9. Carlesimo GA, Oscar-Berman M: Memory deficits in Alzheimer's patients: A comprehensive review. *Neuropsychol Rev* 3:119–169, 1992.
10. Weingartner H, Kaye W, Smallberg SA, et al: Memory failures in progressive idiopathic dementia. *J Abnorm Psychol* 90:187–196, 1981.
11. Grosse DA, Wilson RS, Fox JH: Preserved word-stem-completion priming of semantically encoded information in Alzheimer's disease. *Psychol Aging* 5:304–306, 1990.
12. Jorm AF: Controlled and automatic information processing in senile dementia. *Psychol Med* 16:77–88, 1986.
13. Grafman J, Weingartner H, Lawlor B, et al: Automatic memory processes in patients with dementia—Alzheimer's type. *Cortex* 26:361–371, 1990.
14. Spieler DH, Balota DA, Faust ME: Stroop performance in younger adults, healthy older adults and individuals with senile dementia of the Alzheimer type. *J Exp Psychol: Hum Percept Perform.* In press.
15. Balota DA, Duchek JM: Semantic priming effects, lexical repetition effects and contextual disambiguation effects in healthy aged individuals and individuals with senile dementia of the Alzheimer type. *Brain Lang* 40:181–201, 1991.
16. Becker JT: Working memory and secondary memory deficits in Alzheimer's disease. *J Clin Exp Neuropsychol* 10:739–753, 1988.

Chapter 43

ALZHEIMER DISEASE:
Biochemical and
Pharmacologic Aspects

William Samuel
Douglas Galasko
Leon J. Thal

Nearly a century ago, Alzheimer described diseased-appearing neurons as well as extracellular deposits in the cerebral cortex of a 55-year-old woman who suffered from severe dementia.[1] It was assumed that such neuropathology was only rarely associated with senility in the general population, but we now know that the neurofibrillary tangles and senile plaques that he observed are in fact commonly found in the brains of elderly persons with declining cognitive function. When seen in the context of a slowly progressive dementia, these lesions are diagnostic of Alzheimer disease (AD).[2,3] Our increased understanding of AD neuropathology and biochemistry has suggested various pharmacologic treatment strategies, some of which have already found practical clinical applications.

STRUCTURAL LESIONS CHARACTERISTIC OF ALZHEIMER DISEASE

Grossly, the volume of brain parenchyma typically shrinks in AD, while the volume of the fluid spaces expands. These volumetric changes are paralleled on the microscopic level by neuronal loss, intra-neuronal neurofibrillary tangles and extracellular senile plaques, and a reduced density of synaptic contacts between neurons in both cortical and subcortical regions. A subset of patients meeting clinical and pathologic criteria for AD also have a neuronal inclusion called a Lewy body that was previously thought to be exclusively associated with idiopathic Parkinson disease. We will discuss the role these lesions play in AD and the biochemical changes associated with them, emphasizing their implications for treating AD.

The Senile Plaque

Structure of Senile Plaques The major component of the senile plaque is the β-amyloid protein, whose fibrils aggregate themselves into pleated sheets that bind with high avidity to Congo red stain and which, due to their amyloid conformation, have the property of birefringence when viewed under polarized light.[4] All pathologically confirmed AD patients by definition have senile plaques, and nearly all will have deposits of β-amyloid in the walls of cerebral blood vessels,[5] but some degree of cerebral vascular amyloidosis is seen in up to one-third of otherwise normal elderly persons coming to autopsy.[6]

There are two main varieties of senile plaques: (1) the *diffuse* type, which consists mainly of β-amyloid, and (2) the *neuritic* type, which includes nerve cell processes called neurites. Many investigators presume that there is a progression from the first to the second type that roughly parallels the increasing severity of AD and that the most "mature" plaque is neuritic, with a very dense core of β-amyloid. The dystrophic neurites may contain paired helical filaments characteristic of neurofibrillary tangles and may show signs of regenerative as well as degenerative change.[7] An example of the microscopic appearance of senile plaques is shown in Fig. 43-1A.

Biochemistry of Senile Plaques The β-amyloid protein is 39 to 43 amino acids long[8] and is derived from a much larger amyloid precursor protein (APP) that has three major forms, with lengths of 695, 751, or 770 amino acids.[9] The β-amyloid fragment is generated by a cleavage of the APP molecule at amino acid 670 and a more variable cleavage of the molecule at about amino acid 712 (numbering based on APP 770). The en-

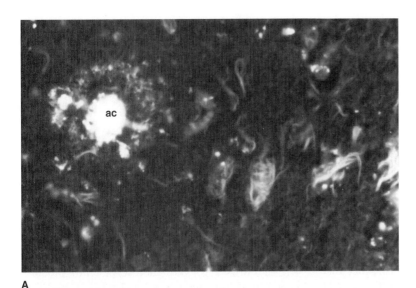

A

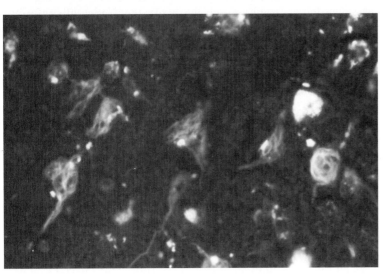

B

Figure 43-1

The classical lesions of Alzheimer disease, as seen using thioflavin S staining and fluorescent microscopy. A. Mature plaque with dense amyloid core (ac). B. Neurofibrillary tangles in the entorhinal cortex. (Photographs provided by Dr. Robert D. Terry.)

zymes required to make these cuts are called *secretases,* and the APP molecule on which they act normally spans the neuronal membrane. It is thought that most of this processing occurs at the cell surface and within organelles such as endosomes and lysosomes[10,11] and that the generation of β-amyloid from APP occurs in normal cells.[12,13] The more common form of secreted β-amyloid and that which predominates in vascular amyloidosis ends at amino acid 40.[14]

It remains controversial whether the deposition of β-amyloid in senile plaques is merely a marker for AD or a causative agent. However, much indirect evidence supports β-amyloid as an injurious substance in AD, since β-amyloid 40 (Aβ40) has been shown to cause neuronal loss and gliosis when applied to neuronal cells grown in culture and when injected in solubilized form into rat or monkey cortex. Even a fragment of the β-amyloid peptide from the 25th to 35th amino acid had a neurotoxic effect.[15] Some laboratories have experienced difficulty in replicating these results (e.g., Refs. 16 and 17), which led Yankner[18] to conclude that the final configurational state of the β-amyloid peptide was a critical factor in its toxicity. Only when β-amyloid or the amino acids 25 to 35 fragment aggregated into insoluble beta pleated sheets could neurotoxicity be reliably demonstrated. The current view is that β-amyloid in soluble form or deposited as amorphous aggregates does not significantly damage neurons, but that β-amyloid in fibrillar form may be neurotoxic.[19] The varieties of β-amyloid that end at amino acids 42 or 43 are much more likely than β-amyloid 39 or β-amyloid 40 to come out of solution and aggregate into a fibrillar structure, and prior deposition of the relatively insoluble longer forms can "seed" subsequent fibrillar aggregation and deposition of the more soluble shorter forms.[20,21] Regardless of the possibilities for seeding, however, the β-amyloid in the senile plaques of AD patients appears to be predominantly longer forms of β-amyloid, ending at amino acids 42 or 43.[14] A key question, as yet unanswered, is whether AD patients suffer from overproduction or impaired clearance of β-amyloid.

The mechanism by which fibrillar β-amyloid might inflict neuronal damage is a subject of much speculation and research. The aggregated peptide could directly damage cell membranes and so cause cell death. More subtly, fibrillar β-amyloid may interfere with ion channels that regulate calcium influx, leading to excess intracellular calcium, vulnerability to excitotoxicity, and cell death.[22,23] Aside from excitatory amino acids, other chemical mechanisms have been proposed for the neurotoxicity of fibrillar β-amyloid, including free radicals and damage to mitochondria. Many proteins are found associated with β-amyloid deposits or with senile plaques, and these may play roles in β-amyloid solubility, inflammation, or neuronal sprouting. Examples of plaque-associated proteins are α-1-antichymotrypsin and proteoglycans, which, along with complement protein suggestive of an inflammatory reaction, have been found within the amyloid component.[24–27] Fibroblast growth factor[28] and apolipoprotein E[29] are also found in the senile plaques. Neuritic senile plaques are typically surrounded by reactive astrocytes and microglial cells which, like complement, are suggestive of an inflammatory process.[30] Plaque neurites contain APP,[31,32] epidermal growth factor receptor,[33] the GAP 43 growth-associated protein,[34] ubiquitin,[35] neurofilaments,[36] and neurotransmitters.[37] Mechanisms underlying the apparent neurotoxicity of β-amyloid 42/43 and interventions by which its aggregation into senile plaques might be stopped are issues consuming much of the ongoing research in AD.

β-Amyloid in Familial Alzheimer Disease

Some of the most impressive evidence for a causative role of β-amyloid is provided by a small number of families who suffer from a strong hereditary predisposition to AD, apparently due to specific point mutations in APP. Affected members of these families typically develop the disease early, often before the age of 50. Mutations in the APP gene that flank the DNA sequence coding for β-amyloid are associated with familial AD, including point mutations at amino acid 717[38,39] and a double mutation at the 670/671 position.[40,41] Though identification of these mutations has not as yet had any clinical impact on treatment of either familial or sporadic AD, it has promoted research into an animal model of the disease. Transgenic mice have been produced that express high levels of protein derived from the human APP gene with a mutant codon 717. The brains of these animals show extensive senile plaques comprising β-amyloid, synapse loss, and inflammatory changes.[42] It is hoped that transgenic models will facilitate the search for effective therapeutic interventions, perhaps through precise characterization of the secretases involved in β-amyloid cleavage and selective inhibition of their mechanisms of action.

Another genetically related observation that points to a central role of β-amyloid in AD pathogenesis is the striking similarity between the cerebral amyloid deposits seen in AD and Down syndrome.[43,44] Down syndrome is most often caused by trisomy of chromosome 21 and is associated with mental retardation and the formation of senile plaques (and of neurofibrillary tangles) in the same brain regions commonly affected in AD. Many Down syndrome patients undergo cognitive decline in their sixth or seventh decade, indicating dementia. The senile plaques seen in Down syndrome are also primarily composed of β-amyloid 42, particularly in the earlier stages of plaque formation, though β-amyloid 40 may also be seen in older plaques, perhaps because its deposition has been promoted by the prior accumulation of β-amyloid 42.[45] Since the gene coding for APP is located on chromosome 21, it is likely that an extra copy of this gene in Down syndrome leads to overproduction of β-amyloid, including β-amyloid 42.

Distribution of Senile Plaques   Senile plaques are rarely found in the cerebellum and are relatively infrequent in the primary sensory cortices in AD; they predominate in parietal and temporal association cortices, in laminae of the frontal neocortex involved in corticocortical connections, in subregions of the hippocampal formation, and in structures of the limbic system.[46] Whether or not senile plaques appear prior to NFT in AD remains controversial, but 15 to 30 percent of clinically demented and pathologically confirmed AD cases

will have only plaques in the neocortex and few if any NFT.[47] Senile plaques often appear in neocortical regions before they are seen in the hippocampus.[48–50]

The Neurofibrillary Tangle

Structure of Neurofibrillary Tangles   Neurons depend on three types of cytoskeletal filament systems to maintain their shape and to assist with the internal transport of nutrients and the constituents of cell products such as neurotransmitters: (1) microfilaments, (2) intermediate filaments oriented longitudinally within axons and dendrites, and (3) microtubules with side-arm projections, to which microtubule-associated proteins can bind. In AD, cytoskeletal derangement results in the formation of neurofibrillary tangles,[51] which are found within the neuronal perikarya and consist of fibrils, pairs of which are twisted into paired helical filaments that fluoresce bright green when stained with thioflavin S. They may be either flame-shaped or globose, modeling the shape of the neuron in which they reside (see Fig. 43-1B).

Biochemistry of Neurofibrillary Tangles   Neurofibrillary tangles are made up of paired helical filaments whose main constituent, a protein called tau,[51] is normally bound to microtubules and appears to assist with their proper bundling and with intracellular transport. When highly phosphorylated at specific sites, tau becomes incapable of binding microtubules, at least in vitro, resulting in an accumulation of tau in dendrites, which is followed by self-aggregation into paired helical filaments.[19] The loss of tau's normal functions is likely to be severely disruptive to the microtubule system, ultimately leading to cell death. In its initial stages of phosphorylation, tau colocalizes with another microtubule-associated protein (MAP-2) that normally plays a role in the proliferation and sprouting of basal dendrites and dystrophic neurites. Later on, MAP-2 expression declines and is followed by neuronal reactivity to ubiquitin, a protein expressed by neurons under stress that binds other proteins designated for degradation.[52] Exposure of hippocampal neurons in culture to fibrillar β-amyloid induces tau phosphorylation and a loss of binding to microtubules, an observation that provides further evidence for a pathogenetic role of β-amyloid in AD.[19]

Neurofibrillary tangles express a protein antigen (A-68) that is thought to be a phosphorylated form of tau, whose presence may be detected using a monoclonal antibody called Alz 50.[53,54] There is little if any staining of neurons from nondemented elderly controls, but in AD patients Alz 50 often labels neurons that appear morphologically normal, which suggests that subtle disturbances in the neuronal cytoskeleton precede signs of degeneration. A subsequently developed antibody called AT8 is even more sensitive in detecting AD pathology, as it does not bind to normal tau epitopes and preferentially labels the phosphorylated tau found in paired helical filaments, dystrophic neurites, and neuropil threads.[55] These studies have demonstrated that disruption of cytoskeletal elements occurs early in the development of AD. The critical phosphorylation sites on tau and the enzymes (kinases and phosphatases) that regulate them are still being defined.

Distribution of Neurofibrillary Tangles In contrast with senile plaques, neurofibrillary tangles have clearly focal concentrations and seem to have a stepwise progression in their distribution, based on comparisons of tissue from patients at various stages of the disease course. This progression has been described by Braak and Braak,[56] who observed neurofibrillary tangles in early AD in perirhinal and entorhinal cortices. Accumulation of neurofibrillary tangles in moderate AD cases was observed in the hippocampus proper, particularly the cornu ammonis (CA) subregions, and in other structures of the limbic system. Later stages were characterized by the appearance of neurofibrillary tangles in the neocortex. Within the neocortex, neurofibrillary tangles are concentrated in the larger pyramidal neurons in layer 3, which are extensively involved in corticocortical connections both within the same hemisphere and across the corpus callosum to the opposite hemisphere, and in layer 5, which send extensive efferents to subcortical structures like the amygdala,

striatum, and brainstem.[57] Neurofibrillary tangles are also prominent in the subcortical nucleus basalis of Meynert and in the locus ceruleus, substantia nigra, and dorsal raphe nuclei.[58,59] These accumulations of neurofibrillary tangles and the neuronal loss that accompanies them would be anticipated to impair the integrity of neurotransmitter systems dependent on the affected populations of nerve cells. As one would expect, premortem impairment of scores on neuropsychological tests has been found to correlate significantly with the frequency of neurofibrillary tangles in the neocortex,[60] hippocampus,[61] nucleus basalis,[58,59] and the locus ceruleus.[62] The frequency of senile plaques, by contrast, correlates poorly or not at all with dementia severity, especially in the most recent studies.[58,59,60–64] Compared to the senile plaques, the lesion progression observed for neurofibrillary tangles better parallels the clinical course of AD, which typically begins with memory deficit suggestive of hippocampal dysfunction.

Atrophy and Neuron Loss

Gross atrophy of the brain is a hallmark of AD, although such changes are seen among the cognitively normal elderly as well (see Fig. 43-2A). Terry and coworkers[65] reported the average brain weight of 14 AD patients as 1055 g and that of 10 age-matched controls as 1152 g; the difference between these groups was statistically significant, but in both the weight was somewhat lower than the 1450 g expected for a normal 30-year-old. Cerebral atrophy can be visualized on computed tomography (CT) or magnetic resonance imaging (MRI) of the living patient.[66–69] Paralleling this decline in brain size is a loss of neocortical large neurons[70] and thinning of the cortical ribbon, which also occur in normal aging but are accelerated in AD.[71] Patients with AD suffer focal losses of pyramidal neurons in the hippocampal formation[72,73] and of neurotransmitter producing cells in the nucleus basalis,[74] the locus ceruleus,[75] and the dorsal raphe nuclei.[76]

Synapse Loss

Given the prominent changes in brain structure and physiology already described as manifesta-

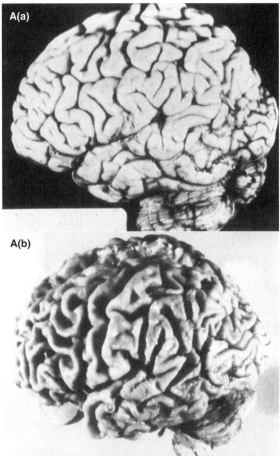

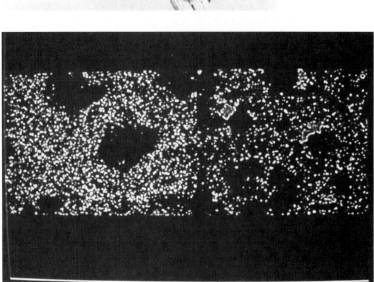

Figure 43-2
Gross and microscopic brain atrophy in Alzheimer disease. A. Gross appearance of the brain of a normal elderly person (a) *and that of an AD patient* (b), *the latter showing gyral atrophy. B. Synapses in the frontal cortex, immunolabeled with an antibody to a protein integral to the presynaptic nerve ending and imaged using a laser scanning confocal microscope. The high synapse density in the neocortex of a normal elderly person* (a) *is easily distinguished from the synaptic loss characteristic of AD* (b). *(Photographs provided by Dr. Robert D. Terry.)*

tions of AD, it would be expected that even the smallest structural components of brain function—the synapses between neurons—would also be impaired. Electron microscopic (EM) studies confirm this expectation and report a 30 to 40 percent relative reduction in synapses in the frontal and temporal cortices of AD patients versus controls, concentrated in layers 2, 3, and 5 and often accompanied by pathologic changes in the synapses themselves.[77–80] Studies of synaptic density in AD using antibodies against synaptic vesicle proteins confirmed the decrease in cortical synapses (see Fig. 43-2B).[81] A lesser degree of synaptic loss was found in the hippocampus and entorhinal cortex, probably due to compensatory sprouting of new neurites. The nucleus basalis and locus ceruleus also showed synaptic loss. It is not known whether synaptic pathology in AD precedes cytoskeletal changes or is related to β-amyloid deposition. However, this loss of synapses is relevant to neurotransmitter-based therapies in AD; for example, loss of neurons in a subcortical center with widespread neocortical projections such as the nucleus basilis could cause a loss of synapses throughout its projection zone. Alternatively, synapse loss might precede neuron loss and perhaps even the appearance of senile plaques and neurofibrillary tangles.

Lewy Bodies

A subgroup comprising 15 to 30 percent of AD patients is afflicted with extensive neocortical senile plaques sufficient to meet pathologic criteria for AD but few if any neurofibrillary tangles.[82] Subcortical and neocortical Lewy bodies are present in at least 75 percent of this "plaque predominant" form of AD.[83] Though AD-type dementia is the presenting complaint of patients with the "Lewy-body variant" of AD, these patients typically develop some parkinsonian features, including bradykinesia, rigidity, and masklike facies.[84] The neocortical Lewy bodies had previously been overlooked because they are not well visualized using routine hematoxylin and eosin stains; instead, antibodies to ubiquitin protein immunostain the Lewy bodies. Lewy bodies are found in subcor-

tical nuclei (nucleus basalis, locus ceruleus, substantia nigra) as well as in the hippocampus, cingulate gyrus, and neocortex. The frequency of neocortical Lewy bodies has been found to correlate significantly with the severity of neuropsychological impairment among Lewy-body variant patients.[85,86]

THERAPEUTIC IMPLICATIONS OF ALZHEIMER DISEASE PATHOPHYSIOLOGY

Our increasing level of understanding of AD pathophysiology is reflected in both current and prospective therapeutic interventions. One approach toward treatment of AD aims at symptomatic relief of its primary manifestations (e.g., memory impairment) or secondary ones (e.g., depression, or agitation) without influencing the basic neurodegenerative process; neurotransmitter-based therapies fall into this category. A second approach aims at slowing disease progression or delaying disease onset and is based on knowledge of AD pathogenetic mechanisms.

Therapies Aimed at Symptomatic Relief

Modulation of Neurotransmitters and Neuropeptides Table 43-1 lists several neurotransmitter systems that are dysfunctional in AD and indicates presently available or prospective therapies for these deficits. Medications are commonly used to treat the secondary neuropsychiatric manifestations of AD; these are presumed to achieve their effects through modulation of neurotransmitter systems.

Acetylcholine The nucleus basalis provides the major source of cholinergic innervation for the cerebral cortex,[87] and AD is associated with a significant depletion of cortical acetylcholinesterase (AChE) and choline acetyltransferase (ChAT),[88] both of which are markers of cholinergic activity. In addition, the nucleus basalis is commonly afflicted by neurofibrillary tangle and senile plaque deposition, by neuron and synapse loss, and

Table 43-1
Major neurotransmitters and neuropeptides involved in Alzheimer disease

Neurotransmitter or neuropeptide	Main sites of production	Main axonal projections relevant to AD	Current or potential therapies
Acetylcholine (ACh)	Nucleus basalis of Meynert Septal nuclei	Neocortex, thalamus, striatum Hippocampus	1. Acetylcholinesterase inhibition: tetrahydro-aminoacridine 2. Induce ACh release: DUP 996 3. Selective agonists of brain muscarinic receptors 4. Trophic support: nerve growth factor
Norepinephrine (NE)	Locus ceruleus	Neocortex, thalamus, limbic mesocortex	1. Tricyclics and some SSRI agents increase NE availability 2. MAO-B inhibition with L-deprenyl yields a small NE increase
Dopamine (DA; deficiency seen in Lewy-body variant of AD)	Substantia nigra Ventral tegmental nuclei	Striatum Neocortex, limbic mesocortex	1. Sinemet (L-dopa) provides a precursor 2. MAO-B inhibition with L-deprenyl yields a small DA increase
Serotonin (5-HT)	Midbrain raphe nuclei	Neocortex, thalamus, reticular formation	1. Reuptake inhibition: SSRIs, trazodone 2. Precursor loading: tryptophan
Amino acid agonists of N-methyl-D-aspartate (NMDA) receptor	Pyramidal neurons in neocortex and hippocampus	Neocortex, striatum, hippocampus	Modulation of NMDA receptor activation
Somatostatin (neuropeptide)	Inhibitory neurons, widely distributed	Neocortex, hippocampus	None yet available

Abbreviations: MAO = monoamine oxidase; SSRI = selective serotonin reuptake inhibitor.

(in Lewy-body variant) by Lewy-body formation. Patients with Lewy-body variants have even lower levels of neocortical ChAT than the pure AD patients.[89] The degree of decline in cholinergic markers has been found to correlate significantly with dementia severity in AD.[90] Animals in whom the nucleus basalis is selectively lesioned show impairments in attention, learning, and memory that appear analogous to the deficits seen in AD patients.[91-93]

Based on the above findings, the cholinergic deficit in AD is a logical target of treatment aimed at improving memory and cognition, and this has been achieved through inhibition of AChE, the enzyme that breaks down acetylcholine (ACh). Tetrahydroaminoacridine (THA) was approved for use in AD after three double-blind placebo-controlled multicenter trials showed small but statistically significant benefits for the THA-treated as compared to the placebo-treated group in terms of the Alzheimer Disease Assessment Scale—Cognitive Component (ADAS-Cog) scores and global ratings of functional ability.[94–96] About 15 to 20 percent of the AD patients treated with this drug improved by four or more points on the ADAS-Cog, which was felt to be clinically significant. Unfortunately, nearly 50 percent of those receiving THA developed liver toxicity, but transaminases returned to normal when the drug was stopped. Treatment with THA is believed to be of greatest benefit early in the disease course, when surviving cholinergic neurons retain some ACh output. The effects of THA are dose-dependent and are more noticeable at higher doses of 160 mg/day. Numerous other AChE inhibitors are currently undergoing clinical trials. Ironically, many of the medications used to treat the secondary neuropsychiatric manifestations of AD have anticholinergic side effects and therefore can worsen cognitive function; these include tricyclic antidepressants and neuroleptics.

Alternative approaches toward correcting the cholinergic deficit have been ineffective: (1) precursor loading with lecithin (a source of choline) or (2) direct stimulation of postsynaptic muscarinic acetylcholine receptors (relatively preserved in AD) with pilocarpine or by intraventricular delivery of bethanechol. Use of muscarinic agonists has been limited by their nonspecific stimulation of all muscarinic receptor subtypes, with consequent development of systemic toxicity. More selective muscarinic agonists for brain m1 and m3 receptors are currently under development. Enhancement of ACh release at the presynaptic terminal by oral administration of a drug called DUP 996 is being studied in clinical trials.

Monoamines Norepinephrine (NE) and dopamine (DA) are produced at different steps along the same metabolic pathway beginning with tyrosine. Because AD lesions often affect the brainstem centers producing these neurotransmitters (locus ceruleus for NE, substantia nigra for DA), it is not surprising that monoamine deficiency is frequently present in AD and that it may be responsible for some of the symptomatology. Norepinephrine is an active transmitter in the medial forebrain bundle, where a deficiency could undermine the attention and activation needed for effective problem solving. It is also deficient in the temporal lobe[97] and putamen[98] of AD patients relative to controls. Dopamine is present in the basal ganglia, where it is involved in the initiation of movement, and in a mesocortical projection system thought to be important for rapidity of thinking, responsiveness to rewards, planning and initiation, and switching mental sets.[99] Dopamine is deficient in the caudate and putamen of Lewy-body variants but not pure AD patients relative to controls,[98] and there may be smaller DA deficiencies in the neocortex among pure AD patients as well.

Both NE and DA are catabolized by a mitochondrial enzyme, monoamine oxidase (MAO), which suggests that inhibition of this enzyme could help to correct a deficiency state. Inhibition of the MAO-A enzyme is an effective means of treating depression, one of the secondary features of AD, but MAO-A blockers require careful control of diet and sympathomimetic medications to avoid serious hypertensive complications, which greatly limits their usefulness in demented patients.[100] L-deprenyl, or selegiline, is an orally administered irreversible MAO-B inhibitor that penetrates the blood-brain barrier and is used therapeutically for the treatment of Parkinson disease. A few controlled trials with L-deprenyl have demonstrated a small but statistically significant cognitive benefit in AD.[101–103] While L-deprenyl does increase to a limited extent the availability of NE, DA, and serotonin, its major beneficial effects in neurodegenerative disease are most likely due to reduced production of free radicals. In clinically suspected Lewy-body variant patients, antiparkinsonian medications—L-dopa/carbidopa and DA receptor agonists such as bromocriptine or pergolide—are often tried, but they typically have little or no effect on either cognitive or motor symptoms.

Tricyclic antidepressants are commonly used to alleviate depression in AD, and it is thought that they may do so through a blockade of NE reuptake.[100,104] Selective serotonin reuptake inhibitors (SSRIs), particularly venlafaxine (Effexor), may also increase NE availability. Depression is more prominent early in AD, when patients still have some awareness of their cognitive losses. Depression can itself sometimes mimic dementia, and if it is manifested as an early symptom, should be treated to rule it out as a contributor to impaired cognition.[105]

Agitation, another common secondary symptom complex in AD, encompasses mood swings, insomnia, pacing, belligerence, and hallucinations and delusions. Neuroleptics, which block the DA receptor, are often used to treat these symptoms, but they can produce disabling side effects such as akathisia, tardive dyskinesia, and parkinsonism. The deficits in aminergic neurotransmitters may make AD patients more sensitive to the therapeutic effects and extrapyramidal side effects of neuroleptics. Newer "atypical" neuroleptics such as clozapine and risperidone, which have more selective receptor specificity than older agents, may be useful for controlling agitation in AD with a lesser risk of side effects. All such medications should be given in the lowest effective doses, and alternatives, such as behavioral management, should be considered before neuropsychiatric drugs are prescribed.

Indoleamines Neurons producing serotonin (5-HT) are concentrated in the dorsal raphe nuclei of the brainstem, and these neurons are commonly affected by the classical lesions of AD. The serotonergic system projects widely to the neocortex and hippocampus as well as to the striatum.[106] Given the major role of 5-HT in mood regulation, it has been speculated that disruption of the serotonergic system may contribute to the clinical depression and impaired cognition seen in neurodegenerative diseases.[107,108] Selective serotonin reuptake inhibitors such as fluoxetine, paroxetine, sertraline, or trazodone increase serotonin activity, which can ameliorate depression.[102] Dietary tryptophan, a serotonin precursor, may also provide some benefit.

Excitatory Amino Acids Glutamate and aspartate are amino acids that serve as excitatory neurotransmitters in the brain and stimulate *N*-methyl-D-aspartate (NMDA) receptors. The functioning of the hippocampus is highly dependent on NMDA receptor–mediated excitatory connec-

tions between neurons. Alzheimer disease lesions tend to cluster in hippocampal and neocortical regions that are most dependent on excitatory neurotransmitters; it has been proposed that overstimulation of receptors for glutamate and aspartate may cause neuronal compromise and even cell death.[109,110] Whatever the neuropathologic processes are that begin AD, once they are set in motion further activation of NMDA receptor-mediated pathways may promote neuronal hyperstimulation, leading to excess free radical production and cell death.[109,111] The NMDA receptor modulators, such as milacemide and D-cycloserine, have been administered to AD patients in clinical trials but failed to improve cognition.[112,113]

Somatostatin and Other Neuropeptides Somatostatin is a neuropeptide that is concentrated in large neurons of the cortex and hippocampus and, among other roles, modulates the activity of neurons whose primary neurotransmitters is the inhibitory gamma-aminobutyric acid (GABA), which is widely distributed in the brain.[114] Immunocytochemistry has demonstrated reactivity to somatostatin and other neuropeptides (neuropeptide Y, cholecystokinin, vasoactive intestinal peptide, corticotrophin releasing factor) in neuritic plaques. Levels of somatostatin and many neuropeptides are diminished overall in AD.[115] The neuropathologic and clinical implications of these changes are not well understood, and treatments aimed at correcting these deficiencies have not yet been developed. Benzodiazepines, which act as GABA agonists, are often prescribed for relief of secondary symptoms of insomnia and agitation in AD patients.

Possible Enhancement of Neuronal Metabolism with Nootropic Agents A heterogeneous group of substances called nootropics may affect neuronal metabolism. The best known of these is a combination of four ergoloid mesylates marketed as Hydergine.[116] A metaanalysis of the most methodologically sound 47 out of 151 clinical trials evaluating this drug concluded that Hydergine did produce a small though statistically significant improvement in dementia, but mainly for vascular (infarct-associated) dementia rather than AD and mostly at doses of 4.5 mg/day or greater.[117] Another nootropic currently undergoing testing is cerebrolysin, the product of an enzymatic breakdown of pig brain proteins, separated from their lipid fraction and made up of low-molecular-weight peptides and unspecified "free amino acids."[118] Hydergine and cerebrolysin are claimed to enhance neuronal metabolism. Brain scans using positron emission tomography (PET) or single-proton emission tomography (SPECT) technology have found evidence of regional hypometabolism in AD patients, even at an early stage of the disease course,[119,120] which could provide a pathophysiologic rationale for nootropic agents.

Therapies Aimed at Slowing Disease Progression or Delaying Disease Onset

Though fully effective therapies for AD are still at a developmental stage, there are several potential mechanisms specifically related to AD neuropathology that could be targeted so as to modify the appearance or progression of this disease. Other research efforts have focused on processes associated with but not specific for AD neuropathology and have suggested more immediately attainable therapeutic interventions. Table 43-2 lists these disease-specific and disease-associated strategies, the mechanisms that they aim to modulate, and their presumed targets.

Amyloid Precursor Protein and β-Amyloid

The β-amyloid protein, which is widely believed to be the leading candidate for a causative agent in AD, is cleaved from a much larger amyloid precursor protein (APD). Modulation of the secretases that make these cleavages would reduce the overall production of β-amyloid. A more refined approach would be to selectively inhibit the biochemical processes involved in producing the longer, more neurotoxic forms of β-amyloid. Alternatively, it might be possible to facilitate clearance of β-amyloid to reduce the potential for neurotoxicity.

Tau

The accumulation of neurofibrillary tangles within neurons is a likely cause of cell death in AD. Neurofibrillary tangles are made up of tau protein which, when highly phosphorylated at specific sites, is unable to bind as it normally would to microtubules. Unbound tau may then self-aggregate into paired helical filaments (PHF). The phosphorylation state of tau depends on a balance between kinase and phosphatase enzymes; inhibition of the former or enhancement of the latter could potentially diminish PHF formation.

Apolipoprotein E

Apolipoprotein E (ApoE) is a protein found both in the peripheral tissues and in the brain and functions as a cholesterol transporter. Its synthesis occurs mainly in the liver, peripherally, and centrally within brain astrocytes.[121] There are three major forms of ApoE ($\varepsilon2$, $\varepsilon3$, and $\varepsilon4$), each of which is specified by a slightly different version (allele) of the ApoE gene on chromosome 19. Since one allele is inherited from each parent, six combinations are possible in a given individual. Among Caucasians in the general population, the $\varepsilon3/\varepsilon3$ and $\varepsilon3/\varepsilon2$ combinations are most prevalent (72 percent); about 24 percent of people have one $\varepsilon4$ allele ($\varepsilon4/\varepsilon3$ or $\varepsilon4/\varepsilon2$), and only 3 percent are $\varepsilon4/\varepsilon4$ homozygotes; $\varepsilon2/\varepsilon2$ homozygotes are very rare.[122] In many studies of AD patients, by contrast, the $\varepsilon4$ allele has a greatly increased frequency of 40 to 65 percent; the samples included autopsy-confirmed cases, family studies, and clinical series.[123,124] There is a similarly elevated frequency of the $\varepsilon4$ allele among the Lewy-body variant subtype of AD.[125] The effect of the $\varepsilon4$ allele is to decrease the age of onset of AD. In the original study of families with late-onset AD, the mean age at onset was 68 for $\varepsilon4/\varepsilon4$ homozygotes, 76 for $\varepsilon4$ heterozygotes, and 86 for patients lacking an $\varepsilon4$ allele.[123] There are several ways in which ApoE could contribute to AD. For example, ApoE $\varepsilon4$ may bind β-amyloid more avidly than $\varepsilon3$ or $\varepsilon2$, which could affect fibril formation.[126] Alternatively or in addition, ApoE $\varepsilon3$ binds to the tau protein in a way that does not interfere with microtubule function but may protect the microtubules from phosphorylation and assembly into PHF. Apolipoprotein E $\varepsilon4$, it appears, does not bind to tau and so exerts no protective effect, which may leave the neuron vul-

Table 43-2

Biochemical mechanisms in Alzheimer disease that underlie disease onset and progression and that may be targets for therapy

Mechanism	Evidence for role in AD	Potential therapy
Specific for AD		
APP processing, resulting in Aβ deposition and/or neurotoxicity	APP mutations in familial AD; transgenic mouse model of AD; AD lesions seen in Down syndrome	Inhibition of secretases or of Aβ aggregation or clearance
Phosphorylation of tau epitopes, leading to NFT formation	Correlation of NFT frequency in multiple brain regions with severity of AD dementia	Inhibition of kinases or enhancement of phosphatases
Apolipoprotein E polymorphism	The ApoE ε4 allele is a potent genetic risk factor for AD	Inhibition of ApoE ε4 activity; enhancement of ApoE ε3 activity
Associated with AD Neurodegeneration		
Estrogen deficiency	Effects of estrogen replacement in case-control studies	Estrogen replacement in female AD patients
Neurotrophic factors	Trophic support is needed for neuronal maintenance and survival	Increase neurotrophic factor availability; e.g., NGF
Inflammation	Complement deposition in SP; microglial activation	NSAIDs, prednisone
Free radical toxicity	Aβ toxicity and lipid damage in AD via free radicals; mitochondrial damage in AD	MAO inhibition with L-deprenyl; antioxidant vitamins C, E, beta carotene
Calcium toxicity	Aβ toxicity via increased intracellular calcium	Calcium channel blockers

Abbreviations: Aβ = β-amyloids; APP = amyloid precursor protein; MAO = monoamine oxidase; NFT = neurofibrillary tangles; NGF = nerve growth factor; NSAIDs = nonsteroidal anti-inflammatory drugs.

nerable to neurofibrillary tangle formation.[127] Once the mechanisms by which ApoE ε4 contributes to AD pathology are better understood, this knowledge may facilitate the design of more effective disease-delaying interventions.

Estrogens Since the female nervous system has a lifelong exposure to estrogens and estrogens have profound effects on tissues outside the nervous system, these hormones are being assessed in relation to AD. Retrospective studies indicate that aged female AD patients who received estrogen replacement therapy may have a later onset of AD and milder cognitive impairment than do female patients who never received estrogen replacement.[128,129] Research with rodents has demonstrated a colocalization of receptors for estro-

gens and nerve growth factor (NGF) on basal forebrain ACh-producing neurons, including those in the nucleus basalis.[130] These data imply that estrogens could help to maintain the trophic support needed to preserve the functional integrity of these neurons, the decline of which is strongly associated with AD dementia. Estrogen is currently being studied in clinical trials that are monitoring its potential not only for symptomatic improvement in cognition but also for slowing disease progression.

Neurotrophic Factors The interest in nerve growth factor (NGF) in the treatment of AD is centered on its therapeutic potential to enhance the function of residual cholinergic neurons. Over the last decade, several animal models have been used to address NGF responsiveness in cholinergic basal forebrain neurons. These models include (1) cholinergic deafferentation of the hippocampus using fimbria-fornix transection in rodents and nonhuman primates, (2) cholinergic deafferentation of the cortex by lesioning the nucleus basalis in rodents and nonhuman primates, and (3) aging models in rodents and primates.

Intraventricular administration of NGF can partially reverse lesion and age-related behavioral, biochemical, and histologic deficits in all of these animal models. Treatment with NGF ameliorates memory and learning deficits in the Morris water maze task,[131,132] increases the activity of ChAT,[132] and increases cortical ACh synthesis.[133] Histologic reversal of cellular atrophy due to lesioning[134] or aging[131] of cholinergic basal forebrain neurons has also been demonstrated after intraventricular NGF administration.

Nevertheless, a number of caveats exist regarding the potential use of NGF for the treatment of humans. Nerve growth factor must be administered intraventricularly, a complex invasive procedure. Adverse events may occur, including an increase in APP expression,[135] an increase in sympathetic innervation of cerebral blood vessels,[136] the stimulation of neurite outgrowth from sensory neurons and dorsal root ganglia,[137] and stimulation of other central nervous system NGF-responsive neurons.[138]

Anti-Inflammatory Drugs The immune system is programmed to react against tissue pathology through generation of an inflammatory response. The brain is limited in the extent to which it can mount such a reaction, but indicators of production of complement proteins associated with the major histocompatibility complex are seen in the brains of AD patients, frequently in the same pyramidal neurons that are most vulnerable to neurofibrillary tangle formation.[139] There is evidence of major histocompatibility complex immunoreactivity of microglia (scavenger cells) adjacent to senile plaques in AD patients, and it has been speculated that microglial activation could contribute to neuron loss, synaptic remodeling, and amyloid formation.[140,141] In support of this evidence that inflammatory changes may contribute to AD, clinical

studies have found a possible therapeutic effect of anti-inflammatory agents. In one study of twins discordant for AD, the twin with prior exposure to either glucocorticoids or nonsteroidal anti-inflammatory drugs (NSAIDs) was less likely to become demented.[142] Further evidence comes from a study in which AD patients treated with indomethacin for 6 months appeared to have a slower rate of disease progression than those given placebo.[143] Prednisone is currently undergoing further study in clinical trials.

Free Radical Inhibitors Free radicals, such as peroxide and superoxide, are reactive species derived mainly from oxygen and lipids that are produced by oxidative metabolism. In general, cells with high levels of oxidative metabolism (e.g., neurons) carry a particularly high risk of free radical–induced damage.[144] These substances, particularly in combination with iron and ferritin, which are frequently deposited in the course of neurodegenerative disease, may overwhelm neuronal antioxidant defenses.[145] The defenses consist primarily of enzymes such as superoxide dismutase and glutathione peroxidase, reductase, and transferase, along with free radical acceptors (i.e., reducing agents) such as vitamins E and C, beta carotene, and membrane lipids. There are several lines of evidence implicating free radical mechanisms in AD, including promotion of free radical formation by β-amyloid toxicity or neurotransmitter catabolism, impairment of mitochondrial function, and lipid peroxidation. Parkinsonism can be exogenously induced in humans and primates by ingestion of 1-methyl-4-phenyl-1,2,3,6 tetrahydropyridine (MPTP) which, when metabolized to a free radical form by MAO-B, selectively injures monoaminergic neurons in the brain.[104] Even without such a toxic substrate being present, the normal catabolic activity of MAO generates potentially neurotoxic free radicals. The MAO-B inhibitor L-deprenyl has a small but significant ameliorative effect on AD dementia.[101–103] This effect may be mediated by a decrease in free radical production. These mechanisms provide a rationale for treatment of AD with antioxidants,[146,147] and trials of vitamin E and MAO-B inhibitors are in progress.

Calcium Channel Blockers Fibrillar β-amyloid may interfere with neuronal regulation of calcium influx, leading to excess intracellular calcium, vulnerability to excitotoxicity, and cell death.[22,23] These findings have prompted clinical trials of calcium channel blockers like nimodipine in AD patients.[148]

CONCLUSION

The great advances that have been made in our understanding of the neuropathology and neurochemistry of AD, though not yet offering a complete description of its causes and cure, have pointed the way toward two productive pathways for future investigation and therapy. First, we are more aware than before of the intricate relationship between neurotransmitter deficiencies and the cognitive and behavioral symptoms of AD. Cholinergic enhancement with tacrine improves cognition in AD, and this lead will be followed by the design of relatively selective drugs, analogous to the SSRIs that are used to treat depression with minimal side effects. Second, continued clarification of the complex biochemical cascade that ends with neurodegeneration in AD should eventually provide the data base needed for development of safe and effective disease-modifying agents. We anticipate that the efficacy of many potential therapeutic agents for AD will be examined in clinical trials over the next decade.

ACKNOWLEDGMENT

This work was supported by a VA Memorial Fellowship and by grants from the National Institutes of Health: AG 05131, AG 10483, and AG000353.

REFERENCES

1. Alzheimer A: Über eine eigenartige Erkrangkung der Hirnrinde. *All Z Psychiatr* 64:146–148, 1907.
2. Mirra SS, Hart MN, Terry RD: Making the diagnosis of Alzheimer's disease. *Arch Pathol Lab Med* 117:132–134, 1993.
3. Khachaturian Z: Diagnosis of Alzheimer's disease. *Arch Neurol* 42:1097–1104, 1985.
4. Robbins SL, Cotran RS, Kumar V: *Pathologic Basis of Disease,* 3d ed. Philadelphia: Saunders, 1984.
5. Glenner GG: Congophilic microangiopathy in the pathogenesis of Alzheimer's syndrome. *Med Hypoth* 5:1231–1236, 1979.
6. Kawai M, Kalaria RN, Harik SI, Perry G: The relationship of amyloid plaques to cerebral capillaries in Alzheimer's disease. *Am J Pathol* 137:1435–1446, 1990.
7. McKee AC, Kowall NW, Kosik KS: Microtubular reorganization and dendritic growth response in Alzheimer's disease. *Ann Neurol* 26:652–659, 1989.
8. Masters CL, Simms G, Weinman NA, et al: Amyloid core protein in Alzheimer disease and Down syndrome. *Proc Natl Acad Sci USA* 82:4245–4249, 1985.
9. Selkoe DJ: Alzheimer's disease: A central role for amyloid. *J Neuropathol Exp Neurol* 53:438–447, 1994.
10. Golde TE, Estrus S, Younkin LH, et al: Processing of the amyloid protein precursor to potentially amyloidogenic derivatives. *Science* 255:728–730, 1992.
11. Haas C, Koo EH, Mellon A, et al: Targeting of cell-surface β-amyloid precursor protein to lysosomes: Alternative processing into amyloid-bearing fragments. *Nature* 357:500–503, 1992.
12. Shoji M, Golde TE, Ghiso J, et al: Production of the amyloid β-peptide by normal proteolytic processing. *Science* 359:322–325, 1992.
13. Haas C, Schlossmacher MG, Hung AY, et al: Amyloid β-peptide is produced by cultured cells during normal metabolism. *Nature* 359:322–325, 1992.
14. Youngkin SG: Evidence that Aβ42 is the real culprit in Alzheimer's disease. *Ann Neurol* 37:287–288, 1995.
15. Kowall NW, McKee AC, Yankner BA, Beal MF: In vivo neurotoxicity of beta-amyloid [β(1-40)] and the β(25-25) fragment. *Neurobiol Aging* 13:537–542, 1992.
16. Games D, Khan KM, Soriano FG, et al: Lack of Alzheimer pathology after β-amyloid protein injections in the rat. *Aging* 13:569–576, 1992.
17. Stein-Behrens B, Adams K, Yeh M, Sapolsky R: Failure of beta amyloid protein fragment 25-35 to cause hippocampal damage in the rat. *Neurobiol Aging* 13:577–579, 1992.
18. Yankner BA: Commentary and perspective on

studies of beta amyloid neurotoxicity. *Neurobiol Aging* 13:615–616, 1992.

19. Busciglio J, Lorenzo A, Yeh J, Yankner BA: β-amyloid fibrils induce tau phosphorylation and loss of microtubule binding. *Neuron* 14:879–888, 1995.

20. Jarrett JT, Berger EP, Lansbury PT Jr: The C-terminus of the beta protein is critical in amyloidogenesis. *Ann NY Acad Sci* 695:144–148, 1993.

21. Jarrett JT, Berger EP, Lansbury PT Jr: The carboxy terminus of the beta amyloid protein is critical for the pathogenesis of Alzheimer's disease. *Biochemistry* 32:4693–4697, 1993.

22. Mattson MP, Cheng B, Davis D, et al: β-amyloid peptides destabilize calcium homeostasis and render human cortical neurons vulnerable to excitotoxicity. *J Neurosci* 12:376–389, 1990.

23. Cotman CW, Pike CJ, Capani A: β-amyloid neurotoxicity: A discussion of in vitro findings. *Neurobiol Aging* 13:617–621, 1992.

24. Mattson MP, Rydel RE: β-amyloid precursor protein and Alzheimer's disease: The peptide plot thickens. *Neurobiol Aging* 13:617–621, 1992.

25. Abraham CR, Selkoe DJ, Potter H: Immunochemical identification of the serine protease inhibitor α-1-antichymotrypsin in the brain amyloid deposits of Alzheimer's disease. *Cell* 52:487–501, 1988.

26. Snow AD, Mor H, Nochlin D, et al: The presence of heparan sulfate proteoglycans in the neuritic plaques and congophilic angiopathy in Alzheimer's disease. *Am J Pathol* 133:456–463, 1988.

27. Eikelenboom P, Hack CE, Rozemuler JM, Stam FC: Complement activation in amyloid plaques in Alzheimer's dementia. *Virchow's Arch [B]* 56:259–262, 1989.

28. Gomez-Pinilla F, Cummings BJ, Cotman CW: Induction of basic fibroblast growth factor in Alzheimer's disease and pathology. *Neurol Rep* 1:211–214, 1990.

29. Namba Y, Tomonaga M, Kawasaki H, et al: Apolipoprotein E immunoreactivity in cerebral amyloid deposits and neurofibrillary tangles in Alzheimer's disease and Kuru plaque amyloid in Creutzfeldt-Jakob disease. *Brain Res* 541:163–166, 1991.

30. Terry RD, Gonatas NK, Weiss M: Ultrastructural studies in Alzheimer's presenile dementia. *Am J Pathol* 44:269–297, 1964.

31. Cole GM, Masliah E, Shelton ER, et al: Accumulation of *N*-terminal sequence but not C-terminal sequence of beta-protein precursor in the neuritic component of Alzheimer disease senile plaques. *Neurobiol Aging* 12:85–91, 1991.

32. Joachim C, Games D, Morris J, et al: Antibodies to non-beta regions of the beta-amyloid precursor protein detect a subset of senile plaques. *Am J Pathol* 138:373–384, 1991.

33. Birecree E, Whetsell WO Jr, Soscheck C, et al: Immunoreactive epidermal growth factor receptors in neuritic plaques from patients with Alzheimer's disease. *J Neuropathol Exp Neurol* 47:549–560, 1988.

34. Masliah E, Mallory M, Hansen L, et al: Localization of amyloid precursor protein in GAP 43-immunoreactive aberrant sprouting neurites in Alzheimer's disease. *Brain Res* 574:312–316, 1992.

35. Perry G, Friedman R, Shaw G, Chau V: Ubiquitin is detected in neurofibrillary tangles and senile plaque neurites of Alzheimer's brain. *Proc Natl Acad Sci USA* 84:3033–3036, 1987.

36. Arai H, Lee VM, Otvos L Jr, et al: Defined neurofilament, tau, and beta-amyloid precursor protein epitopes distinguish Alzheimer from non-Alzheimer senile plaques. *Proc Natl Acad Sci USA* 87:2249–2253, 1990.

37. Armstrong DM, Benzing WC, Evans J, et al: Substance P and somatostatin coexist within neuritic plaques: Implication for the pathogenesis of Alzheimer's disease. *Neuroscience* 31:663–671, 1989.

38. Goate A, Chortier-Harlin M, Brown J, et al: Segregation of a missense mutation in the amyloid precursor protein gene with familial Alzheimer's disease. *Nature* 349:704–706, 1991.

39. Mullan M, Crawford F: Genetic and molecular advances in Alzheimer's disease. *Trends Neurosci* 16:398–403, 1993.

40. Mullan M, Crawford F, Houlden H, et al: A pathogenic mutation for probable Alzheimer's disease in the APP gene at the N-terminus of β-amyloid. *Nature Genet* 1:345–347, 1992.

41. Axelman K, Basun H, Winblad B, Lannfelt L: A large Swedish family with Alzheimer's disease with a codon 670/671 amyloid precursor protein. *Arch Neurol* 51:1193–1197, 1994.

42. Games D, Adams D, Alessandrini R, et al: Development of neuropathology similar to Alzheimer's disease in transgenic mice overexpressing the 717V—F β-amyloid precursor protein. *Nature* 373:523–527, 1995.

43. Glenner GG, Wong CW: Alzheimer disease and Down's syndrome: Sharing a unique cerebrovascular amyloid fibril protein. *Biochem Biophys Res Com* 122:1131–1135, 1984.

44. Hof PR, Bouras C, Perl DP, et al: Age-related

distribution of neuropathologic changes in the cerebral cortex of patients with Down's syndrome. *Arch Neurol* 52:379–391, 1995.

45. Iwatsubo MD, Mann DMH, Odaka O, et al: Amyloid β protein (Aβ) deposition: Aβ42(43) precedes Aβ40 in Down syndrome. *Ann Neurol* 37:294–299, 1995.

46. Rogers J, Morrison JH: Quantitative morphology and regional and laminar distributions of senile plaques in Alzheimer's disease. *J Neurosci* 5:2801–2808, 1985.

47. Terry RD, Hansen LA, DeTeresa R, Davies P: Senile dementia of the Alzheimer type without neocortical neurofibrillary tangles. *J Neuropathol Exp Neurol* 46:262–268, 1987.

48. Pearson RCA, Esiri MM, Hiorns RW, et al: Anatomical correlates of the distribution of the pathological change in the neocortex in Alzheimer's disease. *Proc Natl Acad Sci USA* 82:4531–4534, 1985.

49. Arriagada PV, Marzloff K, Hyman BT: Distribution of Alzheimer-type pathologic changes in nondemented elderly individuals matches the pattern in Alzheimer's disease. *Neurology* 42:1681–1688, 1992.

50. Berg, L, McKeel DW, Miller P, et al: Neuropathological indexes of Alzheimer's disease in demented and nondemented persons aged 80 years and older. *Arch Neurol* 50:349–358, 1993.

51. Lee V M-Y, Trojanowski JQ: The disordered neuronal cytoskeleton in Alzheimer's disease. *Curr Opin Neurobiol* 2:653–656, 1992.

52. Mori H, Kondo J, Ihara Y: Ubiquitin is a component of paired helical filaments in Alzheimer's disease. *Science* 235:1641–1644, 1987.

53. Hyman BT, Van Hoesen GW, Wolozin BL, et al: Alz-50 antibody recognizes Alzheimer-related neuronal changes. *Ann Neurol* 23:371–379, 1988.

54. Lee VM-Y, Balin BJ, Otvos L, Trojanowski JQ: A68: A major subunit of paired helical filaments and derivatized forms of normal tau. *Science* 251:675–677, 1991.

55. Braak E, Braak H, Mandelkow E-M: A sequence of cytoskeleton changes related to the formation of neurofibrillary tangles and neuropil threads. *Acta Neuropathol* 87:554–567, 1994.

56. Braak H, Braak E: Neuropathological staging of Alzheimer-related changes. *Acta Neuropathol* 82:239–259, 1991.

57. Terry RD: Neuropathological changes in Alzheimer's disease, in Svennerholm L, Asbury AK,

Reisfeld RA, et al (eds): *Progress in Brain Research.* Vol. 101. New York: Elsevier, 1994.

58. Samuel WS, Henderson VE, Miller CE: Severity of dementia in Alzheimer disease and neurofibrillary tangles in multiple brain regions. *Alz Dis Assoc Disord* 5:1–11, 1991.

59. Samuel W, Terry RD, DeTeresa R, et al: Clinical correlates of cortical and nucleus basalis pathology in Alzheimer dementia. *Arch Neurol* 51:772–778, 1994.

60. Terry RD, Masliah E, Salmon DP, et al: Physical basis of cognitive alterations in Alzheimer's disease: Synapse loss is the major correlate of cognitive impairment. *Ann Neurol* 30:572–580, 1991.

61. Samuel W, Masliah E, Hill LR, et al: Hippocampal connectivity and Alzheimer's dementia: Effects of synapse loss and tangle frequency in a two-component model. *Neurology* 44:2081–2088, 1994.

62. Bondareff W, Mountjoy CQ, Roth M, et al: Neuronal degeneration in locus ceruleus and cortical correlates of Alzheimer disease. *Alzheimer Dis Assoc Disord* 1:256–262, 1987.

63. Arriagada PV, Growdon JH, Hedley-White T, Hyman BT: Neurofibrillary tangles but not senile plaques parallel duration and severity in Alzheimer's disease. *Neurology* 42:631–639, 1992.

64. Bierer LM, Hof PR, Purohit DP, et al: Neocortical neurofibrillary tangles correlate with dementia severity in Alzheimer's disease. *Arch Neurol* 52:81–88, 1995.

65. Terry RD, Peck A, DeTeresa R, et al: Some morphometric aspects of the brain in senile dementia of the Alzheimer type. *Ann Neurol* 10:184–192, 1981.

66. Jobst KA, Smilth AD, Szatmari M, et al: Detection in life of confirmed Alzheimer's disease using a simple measurement of medial temporal lobe atrophy by computed tomography. *Lancet* 340:1179–1183, 1992.

67. Luxenberg J, Haxby J, Creasy H, et al: Rate of ventricular enlargement in dementia of the Alzheimer type correlates with rate of neuropsychological deterioration. *Neurology* 37:1135–1139, 1987.

68. Kesslak JP, Nalcioglu O, Cotman CW: Quantification of magnetic resonance scans for hippocampal and parahippocampal atrophy in Alzheimer's disease. *Neurology* 41:51–54, 1991.

69. Jack CR, Peterson RC, O'Brien PC, Tangalos EG: MR-based hippocampal volumetry in the diagnosis of Alzheimer's disease. *Neurology* 42:183–188, 1992.

70. Mann DMA, Marcyniuk B, Yates PO, et al: The

progression of the pathological changes of Alzheimer's disease in frontal and temporal neocortex examined both at biopsy and at autopsy. *Neuropathol Appli Neurobiol* 14:177–195, 1988.

71. Terry RD: Neuronal populations in normal and abnormal aging, in Goldstein AL (ed): *Biomedical Advances in Aging*. New York: Plenum Press, 1990, pp 435–440.

72. Ball MJ: Neuronal loss, neurofibrillary tangles, and granulovacuolar degeneration in the hippocampus with aging and dementia: A quantitative study. *Acta Neuropathol* 37:111–118, 1977.

73. Hyman BT, Van Hoesen GW, Damasio AR, Barnes CL: Alzheimer's disease: Cell-specific pathology isolates the hippocampal formation. *Science* 225:1168–1170, 1984.

74. Vogels OJM, Broere AJ, TerLaak HJ, et al: Cell loss and shrinkage in the nucleus basalis Meynert complex in Alzheimer's disease. *Neurobiol Aging* 11:3–13, 1990.

75. Bondareff W, Mountjoy CQ, Roth M: Loss of neurons of origin of the adrenergic projection to cerebral cortex (nucleus locus ceruleus) in senile dementia. *Neurology* 32:164–168, 1982.

76. Aletrino MA, Vogels OJM, Van Domburg PHMF, Ten Doneklaar HJ: Cell loss in the nucleus raphe dorsalis in Alzheimer's disease. *Neurobiol Aging* 13:461–468, 1990.

77. DeKosky ST, Scheff SW: Synapse loss in frontal cortex biopsies in Alzheimer's disease: Correlation with cognitive severity. *Ann Neurol* 27:428–437, 1990.

78. Scheff SW, De Kosky ST, Price DA: Quantitative assessment of cortical synaptic density in Alzheimer's disease. *Neurobiol Aging* 11:29–37, 1990.

79. Masliah E, Hansen L, Albright T, et al: Immunoelectron microscopic study of synaptic pathology in Alzheimer disease. *Acta Neuropathol* 81:428–433, 1991.

80. Scheff SW, Price DA: Synapse loss in the temporal lobe in Alzheimer's disease. *Ann Neurol* 33:190–199, 1993.

81. Masliah E, Terry RD, Alford M, DeTeresa R, et al: Cortical and subcortical patterns of synaptophysinlike immunoreactivity in Alzheimer's disease. *Am J Pathol* 138:235–246, 1991.

82. Terry RD, Hansen LA, DeTeresa R, et al: Senile dementia of the Alzheimer type without neocortical neurofibrillary tangles. *J Neuropathol Exp Neurol* 46:262–268, 1987.

83. Hansen LA, Masliah E, Galasko D, Terry RD: Plaque-only Alzheimer disease is usually the Lewy body variant, and vice versa. *J Neuropathol Exp Neurol* 52:648–654, 1993.

84. Hansen L, Salmon D, Galasko D, et al: The Lewy body variant of Alzheimer's disease: a clinical and pathologic entity. *Neurology* 40:1–8, 1990.

85. Lennox G, Lowe J, Landon M, et al: Diffuse Lewy body disease: Correlative neuropathology using anti-ubiquitin immunocytochemistry. *J Neurol Neurosurg Psychiatry* 52:1236–1247, 1989.

86. Samuel W, Galasko D, Masliah E, Hansen LA: Neocortical Lewy body counts correlate with dementia in the Lewy body variant of Alzheimer's disease. *J Neuropathol Exp Neurol* 55:44–52, 1996.

87. Mesulam M-M, Geula C: Nucleus basalis (Ch 4) and cortical cholinergic innervation in the human brain: Observations based on the distribution of acetylcholinesterase and choline acetyltransferase. *J Comp Neurol* 275:216–240, 1988.

88. Hansen LA, DeTeresa R, Davies P, Terry RD: Neocortical morphometry, lesion counts, and choline acetyltransferase levels in the age spectrum of Alzheimer's disease. *Neurology* 38:48–54, 1988.

89. Perry EK, Haroutunian V, Davis KL, et al: Neocortical cholinergic activities differentiate Lewy body dementia from classical Alzheimer's disease. *Neuroreport* 5:747–749, 1994.

90. Mountjoy CQ: Correlations between neuropathological changes and neurochemical changes. *Br Med Bull* 42:81–85, 1986.

91. Dekker JAM, Connor DJ, Thal LJ: The role of cholinergic projections from the nucleus basalis in memory. *Neurosci Behav Res* 15:299–317, 1991.

92. Saper CB, German DC, White CL: Neuronal pathology in the nucleus basalis and associated cell groups in senile dementia of the Alzheimer's type: Possible role in cell loss. *Neurology* 35:1089–1095, 1985.

93. Muir JL, Page KJ, Sirinathsinghji DJS, et al: Excitotoxic lesions of basal forebrain cholinergic neurons: Effects on learning, memory, and attention. *Behav Brain Res* 57:123–131, 1993.

94. Davis KL, Thal LJ, Gamzu ER, et al: A double-blind, placebo-controlled multicenter study of tacrine for Alzheimer's disease. *N Engl J Med* 327:1253–1259, 1992.

95. Farlow M, Gracon SI, Hershey LA, et al: A controlled trial of tacrine in Alzheimer's disease. *JAMA* 268:2523–2529, 1992.

96. Knapp MJ, Knopman DS, Solomon PR, et al: A 30-week randomized controlled trial of high-dose

tacrine in patients with Alzheimer's disease. *JAMA* 271:985–991, 1994.

97. Francis PT, Palmer AM, Sims NR: Neurochemical studies of early-onset Alzheimer's disease. *N Engl J Med* 313:7–11, 1985.

98. Langlais PJ, Thal L, Hansen L, et al: Neurotransmitters in basal ganglia and cortex of Alzheimer's disease with and without Lewy bodies. *Neurology* 43:1927–1934, 1993.

99. DeLong MR, Alexander GE, Miller WC, Crutcher MD: Anatomical and functional aspects of basal ganglia-thalamocortical circuits, in Franks AJ, Ironside JW, Mindham RHS (eds): *Function and Dysfunction in the Basal Ganglia*. New York: St. Martin's Press and Manchester University Press, 1990.

100. Bauer MS, Frazer A: Mood disorders, in Frazer A, Molinoff P, Winokur A (eds): *Biological Bases of Brain Function and Disease*. New York: Raven Press, 1994.

101. Burke WJ, Roccaforte WH, Wengel SP, et al: L-deprenyl in the treatment of mild dementia of the Alzheimer type: Results of a 15 month trial. *J Am Geriatr Soc* 41:1219–1225, 1993.

102. Finali G, Piccirilli M, Oliani C, Piccinin GL: Deprenyl therapy improves verbal memory in amnesic Alzheimer patients. *Clin Neuropharmacol* 14:523–536, 1991.

103. Mangoni A, Grassi MP, Frattola L, et al: Effects of a MAO-B inhibitor in the treatment of Alzheimer disease. *Eur Neurol* 31:101–107, 1991.

104. Edwards RH: Neural degeneration and the transport of neurotransmitters. *Ann Neurol* 34:638–645, 1993.

105. McDonald WM, Krishnan KRR: Pharmacologic management of the symptoms of dementia. *Am Fam Phys* 42:123–132, 1990.

106. Jellinger K: Changes in subcortical nuclei in Parkinson's disease, in Franks AJ, Ironside JW, Mindham RHS (eds): *Function and Dysfunction in the Basal Ganglia*. New York: St. Martin's Press and Manchester University Press, 1990.

107. Mayeux R, Stern V, Cote L, Williams JBW: Altered serotonin metabolism in depressed patients with Parkinson's disease. *Neurology* 34:642–646, 1984.

108. Birkmayer W, Riederer P: Biological aspects of depression in Parkinson's disease. *Psychopathology* 19(supp 2):58–61, 1986.

109. Greenamyre JT: Neuronal bioenergetic defects, excitotoxicity, and Alzheimer's disease: "Use it and lose it." *Neurobiol Aging* 12:334–336, 1991.

110. Miulli DE, Norwell DY, Schwartz FN: Plasma concentrations of glutamate and its metabolites in patients with Alzheimer's disease. *J Am Osteopath Assoc* 93:670–676, 1993.

111. Henneberry RC: The role of neuronal energy in the neurotoxicity of excitatory amino acids. *Neurobiol Aging* 10:611–613, 1989.

112. Dysken MW, Mendels J, LeWitt P, et al: Milacemide: A placebo-controlled study in senile dementia of the Alzheimer type. *J Am Geriatr Soc* 40:503–506, 1992.

113. Randolph C, Roberts JW, Tierney MC, et al: D-cycloserine treatment of Alzheimer disease. *Alz Dis Assoc Disord* 8:198–205, 1994.

114. Chan-Palay V: Somatostatin immunoreactive neurons in the human hippocampus and cortex shown by immunogold/silver intensification of vibratome section: Coexistence with neuropeptide Y neurons, and effects on Alzheimer-type dementia. *J Comp Neurol* 260:201–233, 1987.

115. Kowell NW, Flint-Beal M: Cortical somatostatin, neuropeptide Y, and NADPH diaphorase neurons: Normal anatomy and alterations in Alzheimer's disease. *Ann Neurol* 23:105–114, 1988.

116. Thompson TL, Filley CM, Mitchell WD, et al: Lack of efficacy of hydergine in patients with Alzheimer's disease. *N Engl J Med* 323:445–448, 1990.

117. Schneider LS, Olin JT: Overview of clinical trials of hydergine in dementia. *Arch Neurol* 51:787–798, 1994.

118. Ruther E, Ritter R, Apecechea M, et al: Efficacy of the peptidergic nootropic drug cerebrolysin in patients with senile dementia of the Alzheimer type (SDAT). *Pharmacopsychiatry* 27:32–40, 1994.

119. Smith GS, deLeon MJ, George AE, et al: Topography of cross-sectional and longitudinal glucose metabolic deficits in Alzheimer's disease. *Arch Neurol* 49:1142–1150, 1992.

120. Wolfe N, Reed BR, Everling JL, Jagust WJ: Temporal lobe perfusion on single photon emission computed tomography predicts the rate of cognitive decline in Alzheimer's disease. *Arch Neurol* 52:257–262, 1995.

121. Mahley RW: Apolipoprotein E: Cholesterol transport protein with expanding role in cell biology. *Science* 240:622–630, 1988.

122. Menzel H, Kladetzky RG, Assman G: Abetalipoprotein E polymorphism and coronary artery disease. *Arteriosclerosis* 3:310–315, 1983.

123. Corder EH, Saunders AM, Strittmatter WJ, et al: Gene dose of apolipoprotein E type 4 allele and the

risk of Alzheimer's disease in late onset families. *Science* 261:921–923, 1993.

124. Saunders AM, Strittmatter WJ, Schmechel D, et al: Association of apolipoprotein E ε4 with late-onset familial and sporadic Alzheimer's disease. *Neurology* 43:1467–1472, 1993.

125. Galasko D, Saitoh T, Xia Y, et al: The apolipoprotein E allele ε4 is over-represented in patients with the Lewy body variant of Alzheimer disease. *Neurology* 44:1950, 1994.

126. Strittmatter WJ, Saunders AM, Schmechel D, et al: Apolipoprotein E: High-avidity binding to β-amyloid and increased frequency of type 4 allele in late-onset familial Alzheimer disease. *Proc Natl Acad Sci USA* 90:1977–1981, 1993.

127. Strittmatter WJ, Weisgraber KH, Goedert M, et al: Hypothesis: Microtubule instability and paired helical filament formation in the Alzheimer's disease brain are related to apolipoprotein E genotype. *Exp Neurol* 125:163–171, 1994.

128. Henderson VW, Paganini-Hill A, Emanuel CK, et al: Estrogen replacement therapy in older women: Comparisons between Alzheimer's disease cases and nondemented control subjects. *Arch Neurol* 51:896–900, 1994.

129. Fillit H, Weinreb H, Cholst I, et al: Observations in a preliminary open trial of estradiol therapy for senile dementia: Alzheimer's type. *Psychoneuroendocrinology* 11:337–345, 1986.

130. Toran-Allerand D, Miranda RC, Bentham WDL, et al: Estrogen receptors colocalize with low-affinity nerve growth factor receptors in cholinergic neurons of the basal forebrain. *Proc Natl Acad Sci USA* 89:4668–4672, 1992.

131. Fischer W, Wictorin K, Bjorklund A, et al: Amelioration of cholinergic neuron atrophy and spatial memory impairment in aged rats by nerve growth factor. *Nature* 329:65–68, 1987.

132. Dekker AJ, Gage FH, Thal LJ: Delayed treatment with nerve growth factor improves acquisition of a spatial task in rats with lesions of the nucleus basalis magnocellularis: Evaluation of the involvement of different neurotransmitter systems. *Neuroscience* 48:111–119, 1992.

133. Dekker AJ, Langdon DJ, Gage FH, Thal LJ: NGF increases cortical acetylcholine release in rats with lesions of the nucleus basalis. *Neuroreport* 2:577–580, 1991.

134. Gage FH, Armstrong DM, Williams LR, Varon S: Morphological response of axotomized septal

neurons to nerve growth factor. *J Comp Neurol* 269:147–155, 1988.

135. Mobley WC, Neve RL, Prusiner SB, McKinley MP: Nerve growth factor increased mRNA levels for the prion protein and the β-amyloid protein precursor in developing hamster brain. *Proc Natl Acad Sci USA* 85:9811–9815, 1988.

136. Isaacson LG, Saffran BN, Crutcher KA: Intracerebral NGF infusion induces hyperinnervation of cerebral blood vessels. *Neurobiol Aging* 11:51–55, 1990.

137. Lewin GR, Ritter AM, Mendell LM: Nerve growth factor-induced hyperalgesia in the neonatal and adult rat. *J Neurosci* 13:2136–2148, 1993.

138. Williams L: Hypophagia is induced by intracerebroventricular administration of nerve growth factor. *Exp Neurol* 113:31–37, 1991.

139. Johnson SA, Lampert-Etchells M, Pasinetti GM, et al: Complement mRNA in the mammalian brain: Responses to Alzheimer's disease and experimental lesioning. *Neurobiol Aging* 13:641–648, 1992.

140. Dickson DW, Lee SC, Mattiace LA, et al: Microglia and cytokines in neurological disease, with special reference to AIDS and Alzheimer's disease. *Glia* 7:75–83, 1993.

141. Rogers J, Cooper NR, Webster S, et al: Complement activation by β-amyloid in Alzheimer disease. *Proc Natl Acad Sci USA* 89:10016–10020, 1992.

142. Breitner JCS, Gau BA, Welsh KA, et al: Inverse association of anti-inflammatory treatments and Alzheimer's disease: Initial results of a co-twin control study. *Neurology* 40:227, 1994.

143. Rogers J, Kirby LC, Hempelman SR, et al: Clinical trial of indomethacin in Alzheimer's disease. *Neurology* 43:1609–1611, 1993.

144. Jenner P: Oxidative damage in neurodegenerative disease. *Lancet* 344:796–798, 1994.

145. Connor JR, Snyder BS, Beardl JL, et al: Regional distribution of iron and iron-regulatory proteins in the brain in aging and Alzheimer's disease. *J Neurosci Res* 31:327–335, 1992.

146. Ames BN, Shigenaga MK, Hagen TM: Oxidants, antioxidants and the degenerative disease. *Proc Natl Acad Sci USA* 90:7915–7922, 1993.

147. Behl C, Davis JB, Lesley R, Schubert D: Hydrogen peroxide mediates amyloid beta protein toxicity. *Cell* 77:817–827, 1994.

148. Tollefson GD: Short-term effects of the calcium channel blocker nimodepine (Bay-e-9736) in the management of primary degenerative dementia. *Biol Psychiatry* 27:1133–1142, 1990.

Chapter 44

PICK DISEASE

Mario F. Mendez

In 1892 Arnold Pick described a patient with dementia and circumscribed atrophy of the left temporal lobe.[1] The disease that now bears his name consists of prominent lobar atrophy of gray and white matter and argentophilic intranuclear inclusions known as Pick bodies.[2] Although Pick disease cannot be diagnosed definitively without neuropathologic examination, it is suspected in the presence of a frontotemporal dementia and frontotemporal atrophy on neuroimaging (Fig. 44-1).[3–8]

EPIDEMIOLOGY

Clinicopathologic studies suggest that Pick disease represents 2 to 3 percent of all dementias and 20 to 25 percent of frontotemporal dementias.[7–9] The frontotemporal dementias are the second most common degenerative dementia after Alzheimer disease, especially when the age of onset is less than 65 years.[6,8] The age of onset of Pick disease averages about 56 to 58 years with a wide range, and the average duration of the disease is 8 to 11 years.[7,10] Males and females are equally affected. No specific gene has been implicated in the disease; however, 42 to 50 percent of patients with Pick disease have a first-degree relative with a frontotemporal dementia.[11–13]

CLINICAL FEATURES

In Pick disease and the frontotemporal dementias, personality changes usually precede or over-shadow cognitive disabilities (Table 44-1).[3,7] Common behaviors include apathy, decreased initiative, disinhibition, and impulsivity. Patients neglect their hygiene and behave in socially inappropriate ways—for example, making sexual or facetious comments, touching or kissing strangers, wandering unclothed, or urinating or defecating in public. Emotional changes occur, especially depression but also mania, lability, anger, and irritability.[3,7] In addition, Pick patients tend toward decreased verbal output, progressing to complete mutism, nonfluency, dysarthria, and reiterative speech such as echolalia, palilalia, and the repetition of stories, phrases, sounds.[14]

Bilateral temporal lobe involvement with damage to the amygdalar nuclei predisposes to the Klüver-Bucy syndrome.[7,15,16] This includes hypermetamorphosis, hyperorality, hypersexuality, visual agnosia, and blunted emotional reactivity. Hypermetamorphosis is the compulsion to attend to any visual stimuli. Patients are driven to explore and manipulate objects, particularly with their mouths. Hyperorality results in overeating and the eating of inedible items; it may require restraints to prevent suffocation. Hypersexuality is most often expressed as sexual overtures rather than increased sexual activity or drive. Visual object recognition is most commonly impaired, but difficulty with auditory and tactile recognition may occur. Finally, patients with the Klüver-Bucy syndrome lose their normal emotional reactivity and can become quite placid.

On neuropsychological testing, frontal-exec-

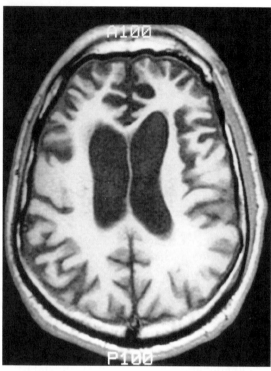

A

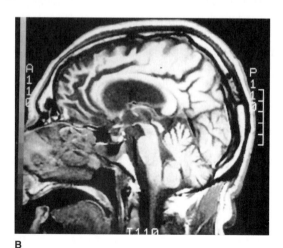

B

Figure 44-1

Magnetic resonance imaging scans of patient with frontotemporal dementia proven to be Pick disease on autopsy. T_1-weighted horizontal (A) and sagittal (B) images demonstrating frontotemporal atrophy. (Courtesy of Dr. Ronald Saul.)

Table 44-1

Core mental status features for frontotemporal dementia

Behavioral disorder
    Insidious onset and slow progression
    Early loss of personal awareness (neglect of personal hygiene)
    Early loss of social awareness (lack of social tact)
    Early signs of disinhibition (e.g., unrestrained sexuality)
    Mental rigidity and inflexibility
    Hyperorality (oral/dietary changes, overeating)
    Stereotyped and perseverative behavior (roaming, compulsions)
    Utilization behavior (unrestrained exploration)
    Distractibility, impulsivity, and impersistence
    Early loss of insight . . . pathologic change of own mental state

Affective symptoms
    Depression, anxiety, excessive sentimentality, suicidal and fixed ideation, delusion (early and evanescent)
    Hypochondriasis, bizarre somatic preoccupation (early, evanescent)
    Emotional unconcern (indifference, lack of empathy, apathy)
    Amimia (inertia, aspontaneity)

Speech disorder
    Progressive reduction of speech (economy of utterance)
    Stereotypy of speech (repetition of same words, phrases, themes)
    Echololalia and perseveration
    Late mutism

Spatial orientation and praxis preserved

Source: From the Lund and Manchester Groups,[6] with permission.

utive functions are compromised early, memory is less impaired, and occipitoparietal functions are relatively preserved.[17,18] Frontal-executive functions such as planning and follow-through, set-shifting and sequencing, and judgment are abnormal. Memory is eventually compromised, but there is relative preservation of recognition memory compared to free recall. This reflects a general retrieval deficit with difficulty retrieving established memories without a temporal gradient—that is, there is equal impairment across all life periods.[18] Lexical retrieval is also profoundly impaired. Visuospatial functions, however, remain intact in most patients.

A few additional clinical features suggest Pick disease or a frontotemporal dementia. Pick patients exhibit "roaming" behavior; they travel with the purpose of exploration.[7] Many have dietary changes, weight gain, and carbohydrate craving. Occasionally, frontotemporal dementia patients present with prominent compulsions or with assaultive behavior.[7,19] In some frontotemporal dementia patients, examination discloses the presence of apraxia, parkinsonism, primitive reflexes, or a history of urinary or fecal incontinence.

CLINICAL VARIANTS

In recent years, investigators have identified several variants of Pick disease.[19–26] In addition to the usual frontotemporal combination, there are patients with predominant frontal or predominant temporal Pick disease. The neuropathologic features can be asymmetrical, with predominant left-hemispheric or right-hemispheric Pick disease. Furthermore, there can be significant involvement of parietal lobes, basal ganglia and subcortical gray matter, and spinal motor neurons.[20]

Some patients with Pick disease lateralized to the left hemisphere present with an isolated "primary progressive aphasia" years before other clinical manifestations appear.[14,21,22] There is a progressive anomia (semantic variant) with word-finding difficulty or a nonfluent aphasia with hesitant, broken, dysarthric, and telegraphic speech. These patients have preserved awareness of the language deficit. An interesting variation occurs in Japanese when Pick disease affects the posterior temporal gyri in the dominant hemisphere. The reading of kanji, a primarily ideographic script, may be impaired, but not the reading of kana, a phonetic script.[23]

A right-hemispheric variant of Pick disease also exists. Investigators report a right-sided frontotemporal dementia associated with psychosis, bizarre or religious ideas, and hoarding behavior, with a flattened or nonempathetic affect.[24] The personalities of such patients appeared remote, and social interactions with them were uncomfortable. One of these patients subsequently proved to have Pick disease on autopsy (B. L. Miller, personal communication).

Pick disease may involve the parietal lobes, basal ganglia, thalamus, and substantia nigra. The combination of frontotemporal dementia with asymmetrical involvement of the parietal lobe and basal ganglia plus brainstem basophilic (corticobasal) inclusions may be identical with corticobasal-ganglionic degeneration. These patients have asymmetrical parkinsonism, myoclonus, ideomotor apraxia, and an "alien limb" that feels foreign and has involuntary, semipurposeful movements.[25,26] In addition, when the caudate nuclei are differentially affected in Pick disease, there may be prominent compulsions to the point of obsessive-compulsive disorder.[19] Compulsive behaviors among Pick patients commonly involve urination, bowel movements, oral behaviors, touching, roaming, and grabbing.[7,14,19]

DIFFERENTIAL DIAGNOSIS

Pick disease presents as a frontotemporal dementia often without cognitive deficits sufficient for dementia criteria and before evidence of lobar atrophy on neuroimaging scans.[4] Clinicians diagnose a frontotemporal dementia after excluding other conditions that can present as a frontal dementia, such as vascular dementia, normal pressure hydrocephalus, Huntington disease, progressive subcortical gliosis, and frontotemporal mass lesions. During life, Pick disease is most commonly confused with Alzheimer disease, but the two may be clinically distinguishable.[7] In addition to lobar atrophy on neuroimaging, 76 percent of Pick patients present with a personality change, as compared with 31 percent of Alzheimer disease patients; disinhibition, hyperorality, and roaming behavior are significantly more frequent among Pick patients than among Alzheimer disease patients.[7] The characteristic speech changes and the absence of severe amnesia further support the diagnosis of Pick disease.

NEUROIMAGING

There are no definitive tests for Pick disease, but neuroimaging can help confirm the presence of a frontotemporal dementia.[4,11] Although absent early, most frontotemporal dementia patients eventually show frontotemporal atrophy on computed tomography (CT) or magnetic resonance imaging (MRI) (see Fig. 44-1). Pick patients with obsessive-compulsive disorder may have MRI evidence of bilateral atrophy of the caudate nucleus.[19] Moreover, there is decreased regional cerebral blood flow in the frontal cortex,[27] and functional imaging scans with single photon emission tomography or positron emission tomography demonstrate asymmetrical frontotemporal hypometabolism (see Fig. 44-2, Plate 13).[3,28]

NEUROPATHOLOGIC FEATURES

Pick disease requires the presence of both frontotemporal dementia and Pick bodies (see Figs. 44-3

and 44-4).[2,8] The relationship between Pick disease and the other two frontotemporal dementias, nonspecific frontal lobe degeneration and frontotemporal dementia with motor neuron disease, is unclear.[5,8,29] All three frontotemporal dementias have neuronal cell loss, swollen "ballooned" neurons (Pick cells), astrogliosis, and spongiosis with minute cavities (microvacuolation), which are more marked in the outer, supragranular layers of the frontotemporal cortex. The diagnosis of Pick disease occurs when there are additional Pick bodies with or without more intense and widespread cortical gliosis.[6] Pick bodies are spherical, argentophilic intraneuronal inclusions consisting of straight 10- to 20-nm neurofilaments and constricted 160-nm fibrils, which are particularly concentrated in neocortical layers II–III and V–VI.[30] Pick bodies share antigenic determinants with neurofibrillary tangles, which occur in Pick disease as well as in Alzheimer disease. These pathologic changes of Pick disease occur in advance of overt clinical symptoms.[31]

In subcortical structures, pathologic changes frequently involve the basal ganglia, thalamus, amygdala, nucleus basalis of Meynert, substantia nigra, locus ceruleus, hippocampus, frontotem-

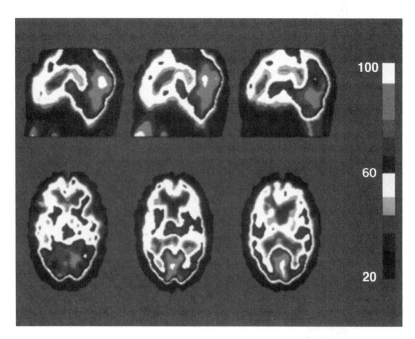

Figure 44-2

Tc99-HMPAO single-photon emission tomography scans (gray scale) *of a patient with Pick disease, demonstrating frontal and anterior temporal hypometabolism* (lighter anterior regions).

100
60
20

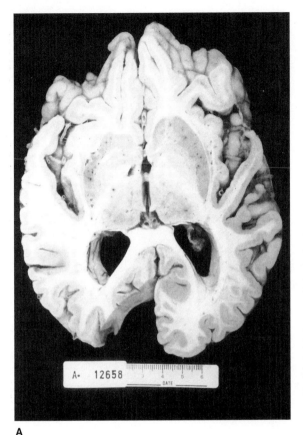

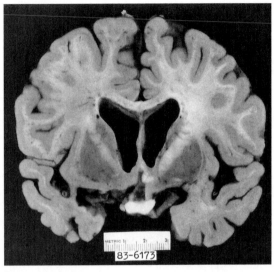

Figure 44-3
Gross neuropathologic features of Pick disease, demonstrating disproportionate atrophy of the frontal and temporal lobes. A is a horizontal cut; B, is a coronal cut. (Courtesy of Dr. Linda Chang and Dr. Bruce L. Miller.)

poral-pontine circuits, and other white matter tracts.[5,29] The hippocampal formation often has many Pick bodies, particularly in the granular layer of the dentate gyrus and in sector CA1.[30] Furthermore, other neurodegenerative disorders—such as striatonigral degeneration, olivopontocerebellar degeneration, and progressive supranuclear palsy—may overlap with the neuropathologic features of Pick disease.[32,33]

The neurotransmitter changes primarily involve serotonin. There are decreases in serotonin receptors and in postsynaptic serotonin.[31] On the other hand, choline acetyltransferase activity is comparable with that of normal controls, and

scopolamine infusion may not improve memory in Pick disease.[28,34] Finally, cerebrospinal fluid and brain tissue studies suggest that dopamine is relatively spared but somatostatin is decreased.[28,34]

CONCLUSIONS

Pick disease is suspected in the presence of a frontal personality change, elements of the Klüver-Bucy syndrome, and frontotemporal atrophy on neuroimaging. The clinical variants of Pick disease include progressive aphasia, psychosis with profound aprosodia, a corticobasal-

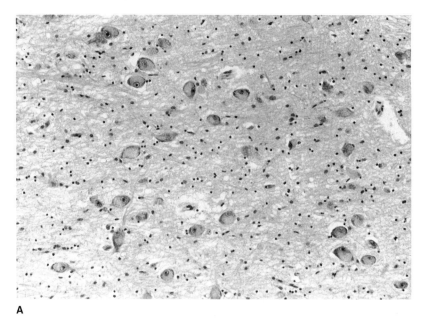

A

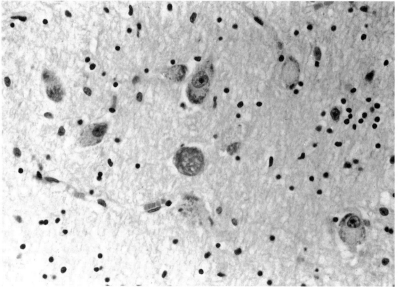

B

Figure 44-4
Microscopic neuropathologic features of Pick disease, demonstrating neocortical Pick bodies (large cells with inclusion bodies). A and B differ in magnification.

ganglionic degeneration-like picture, obsessive-compulsive disorder, and in association with amyotrophic lateral sclerosis. Although there is no specific treatment for Pick disease, many symptomatic therapies can be tried, such as carbamazepine for Klüver-Bucy symptoms and clomipramine and the selective serotonin reuptake inhibitors for compulsions. Much work remains to be done in the management of this disorder, in understanding the genetics of Pick disease, and in clarifying its relationship to other frontotemporal dementias.

REFERENCES

1. Pick A:. Über die Beziehungen der senilen Hirna-trophie zur Aphasie. *Prog Med Wochenshr* 17:165–167, 1892.

2. Baldwin B, Forstl H: "Pick's disease"—101 years on. Still there, but in need of reform. *Br J Psychiatry* 163:100–104, 1993.

3. Miller BL, Cummings JL, Villanueva-Meyer J, et al: Frontal lobe degeneration: Clinical, neuropsychological, and SPECT characteristics. *Neurology* 41:1374–1382, 1991.

4. Knopman DS, Christiansen KJ, Schut LJ, et al: The spectrum of imaging and neuropsychological findings in Pick's disease. *Neurology* 39:362–368, 1989.

5. Neary D, Snowden JS, Mann DMA: The clinical pathological correlates of lobar atrophy. *Dementia* 4:154–159, 1993.

6. The Lund and Manchester Groups: Clinical and neuropathological criteria for frontotemporal dementia. *J Neurol Neurosurg Psychiatry* 57:416–418, 1994.

7. Mendez MF, Selwood A, Mastri AR, Frey WH II: Pick's disease versus Alzheimer's disease: A comparison of clinical characteristics. *Neurology* 43:289–292, 1993.

8. Brun A: Frontal lobe degeneration of non-Alzheimer type: I. Neuropathology. *Arch Gerontol Geriatr* 6:193–208, 1987.

9. Gustafson L, Brun A, Risberg J: Frontal lobe dementia of non-Alzheimer type. *Adv Neurol* 51:65–71, 1990.

10. Heston LL, White JA, Mastri AR: Pick's disease: Clinical genetics and natural history. *Arch Gen Psychiatry* 44:409–411, 1987.

11. Groen JJ, Hekster REM: Computed tomography in Pick's disease: Findings in a family affected in three consecutive generations. *J Comput Assist Tomogr* 6:907–111, 1982.

12. Neary D, Snowden JS, Northen B, et al: Dementia of the frontal-lobe type. *J Neurol Neurosurg Psychiatry* 51:353–361, 1988.

13. Gustafson L: Frontal lobe degeneration of non-Alzheimer type: II. Clinical picture and differential diagnosis. *Arch Gerontol Geriatr* 6:209–233, 1987.

14. Snowden JS, Neary D, Mann MA, et al: Progressive language disorder due to lobar atrophy. *Ann Neurol* 21:174–183, 1992.

15. Cummings JL, Duchen LW: Klüver-Bucy syndrome in Pick's disease: Clinical and pathological correlations. *Neurology* 31:1415–1422, 1981.

16. Lilly R, Cummings JL, Benson DF, Frankel M: The human Klüver-Bucy syndrome. *Neurology* 33:1141–1145, 1983.

17. Johanson A, Hagberg B: Psychometric characteristics in patients with frontal lobe degeneration of non-Alzheimer type. *Arch Gerontol Geriatr* 8:129–137, 1989.

18. Hodges JR, Gurd JM: Remote memory and lexical retrieval in a case of frontal Pick's disease. *Arch Neurol* 51:821–827, 1994.

19. Tonkonogy JM, Smith TW, Barreira PJ: Obsessive-compulsive disorders in Pick's disease. *J Neuropsychiatry Clin Neurosci* 6:176–180, 1994.

20. Sam M, Butmann L, Schochet SS, Doshi H: Pick's disease: A case clinically resembling amyotrophic lateral sclerosis. *Neurology* 41:1831–1833, 1991.

21. Graff-Radford NR, Damasio AR, Hyman BT, et al: Progressive aphasia in a patient with Pick's disease: A neuropsychological, radiologic, and anatomic study. *Neurology* 40:620–626, 1991.

22. Kertesz A, Hudson L, Mackenzie IR, Munoz DG: The pathology and nosology of primary progressive aphasia. *Neurology* 44:2065–2072, 1994.

23. Jibiki I, Yamaguchi N: The Gogi (word-meaning) syndrome with impaired kanji processing: Alexia with agraphia. *Brain Lang* 45:61–69, 1993.

24. Miller BL, Chang L, Mena I, et al: Progressive right frontotemporal degeneration: Clinical, neuropsychological and SPECT characteristics. *Dementia* 4:204–213, 1933.

25. Jendroska K, Rossor MN, Mathias CJ, Daniel SE: Morphological overlap between corticobasal degeneration and Pick's disease: A clinicopathological report. *Mov Disord* 10:111–114, 1995.

26. Lang AE, Bergeron C, Pollanen MS, Ashby P: Parietal Pick's disease mimicking cortical-basal ganglionic degeneration. *Neurology* 44:1436–1440, 1994.

27. Alexander CE, Prohovnik I, Sackeim HA, et al: Cortical perfusion and gray matter weight in frontal lobe dementias. *J Neuropsychiatry Clin Neurosci* 7:188–196, 1995.

28. Friedland RP, Koss E, Lerner A, et al: Functional imaging, the frontal lobes, and dementia. *Dementia* 4:192–203, 1993.

29. Brun A: Frontal lobe dementia of the non-Alzheimer type revisited. *Dementia* 4:126–131, 1993.

30. Hof PR, Bouras C, Perl DP, Morrison JH: Quantitative neuropathologic analysis of Pick's disease cases: Cortical distribution of Pick bodies and coexistence with Alzheimer's disease. *Acta Neuropathol (Berl)* 87:115–124, 1994.

31. Sparks DL, Danner FW, Davis DG, et al: Neurochemical and histopathologic alterations characteristic of Pick's disease in a non-demented individual. *J Neuropathol Exp Neurol* 53:37–42, 1994.

32. Horoupian DS, Dickson DW: Striatonigral degeneration, olivopontocerebellar atrophy and atypical Pick disease. *Acta Neuropathol (Berl)* 81:287–295, 1991.

33. Arima K, Murayama S, Oyanagi S, et al: Presenile dementia with progressive supranuclear palsy tangles and Pick bodies: An unusual degenerative disorder involving the cerebral cortex, cerebral nuclei, and brain stem nuclei. *Acta Neuropathol (Berl)* 84:128–134, 1992.

34. Francis PT, Holmes C, Webster MT, et al: Preliminary neurochemical findings in non-Alzheimer dementia due to lobar atrophy. *Dementia* 4:172–177, 1993.

Chapter 45

DEMENTIA IN PARKINSON DISEASE, HUNTINGTON DISEASE, AND OTHER DEGENERATIVE CONDITIONS

Diane M. Jacobs
Yaakov Stern
Richard Mayeux

PARKINSON DISEASE

Epidemiology

The idiopathic form of Parkinson disease is one of the most common neurologic disorders, affecting between 80 to 200 people per 100,000.[1] The prevalence of Parkinson disease increases with advancing age. Although the average age of onset is approximately 65 years, more than 1 percent of persons in the United States over age 80 have Parkinson disease. The annual incidence is 1 per 10,000 people.

Estimates of the prevalence of dementia among Parkinson patients vary widely, depending upon the population studied and the criteria used to diagnose dementia. Rajput and colleagues[2] found that only 9 percent of their patients were demented on the basis of clinical examination, while Pirozzolo and colleagues[3] reported dementia in 93 percent of their Parkinson patients based upon performance on formal neuropsychological measures. Estimates of dementia prevalence ranging from 30 to 50 percent have frequently been reported.[1,4,5] In a community-based study, Mayeux and associates[1] found an overall prevalence rate of Parkinson disease with dementia of 41.1 per 100,000, with prevalence increasing with age from 0 below age 50 to 787.1 per 100,000 above age 79.

The risk of incident dementia among patients with Parkinson disease is far greater than that expected among individuals of the same age without Parkinson disease. Rajput and colleagues[6] found a significantly higher cumulative probability of developing dementia among Parkinson patients (21 percent) than among age-referenced controls (5.7 percent). Similarly, in a population-based community study, Marder and colleagues[7] reported that the risk of dementia in Parkinson patients was nearly twice that of healthy elderly matched in age and gender. The identification of dementia in patients with Parkinson disease is of clinical significance, as dementia is the single most important factor limiting standard pharmacotherapy of Parkinson disease.[8] Dementia also increases the mortality rate for Parkinson patients.[9]

Among Parkinson patients, risk factors for developing dementia include advancing age and older age at onset of Parkinson disease; severity of motor symptoms; depression; poor tolerance of levodopa or other standard treatment for Parkinson disease, including serious side effects such as hallucinations, delusions, and delirium; and facial masking as a presenting sign.[10,11]

Characteristics of Dementia

The dementia associated with Parkinson disease is generally characterized by predominant impairment of executive functions (e.g., initiating responses, planning, set shifting), visuospatial skills, free-recall memory, and verbal fluency. Language functions other than verbal fluency are relatively preserved, as are orientation, cued recall, and recognition memory. The neuropsychological profile of dementia in Parkinson disease is similar to the pattern of impaired and preserved cognitive abilities associated with damage to the frontal lobes, particularly the prefrontal cortex[12,13] (see Chaps. 30 and 31).

Impairment of executive functions in Parkinson dementia may be disproportionately severe relative to deficits in other cognitive domains. Executive functions commonly affected by Parkinson disease include response initiation, planning, set-shifting, and ability to benefit from feedback. The neuropsychological measure most frequently used to evaluate executive dysfunction in Parkinson disease is the Wisconsin Card Sorting Test (WCST), a task in which the patient is asked to sort a deck of cards based upon three categorical sorting rules.[14] Because successful performance on the WCST requires the ability to form concepts, shift set, monitor one's responses, and benefit from feedback provided by the examiner, it is highly sensitive to the pattern of executive dysfunction often observed in patients with Parkinson disease.

Bowen and colleagues[15] were the first to examine the performance of Parkinson disease patients on the WCST, and their results have been replicated numerous times. In their original investigation, Bowen et al. found that Parkinson patients were impaired in their ability to form concepts, and had an increased number of total and nonperseverative errors. Further, patients were able to verbalize the correct response but failed to use this information to modify their behavior appropriately. This dissociation between thought and action had been observed previously in patients with frontal-lobe lesions[16,17] and thereby lent further support to the notion that dementia in Parkinson disease was due, at least in part, to frontal-lobe dysfunction.

The extent to which the neuropsychological profile of dementia in Parkinson disease differs from that associated with Alzheimer disease is controversial. Several extensive reviews of comparative studies have been written.[18–20] While some investigators have concluded that the two

dementias differ in etiology and phenomenology,[21] others propose that the similarities between Parkinson and Alzheimer dementia far outweigh the differences.[19,22] Perhaps the most frequently replicated observed difference on neuropsychological testing between demented patients with Parkinson and Alzheimer disease is performance on delayed memory testing relative to immediate recall. In Alzheimer disease, delayed recall and recognition memory of recently learned information is severely impaired relative to normative data and to performance on immediate recall; that is, Alzheimer patients rapidly forget information that was recalled accurately on immediate memory testing.[23,24] In contrast, delayed recall and recognition memory in Parkinson disease may be impaired relative to normative data but often is commensurate with the level of recall on testing of immediate memory. Hence, Parkinson disease is associated with relatively good retention of newly acquired information over a delay interval. The memory impairment associated with Parkinson disease is considered primarily a retrieval deficit, while Alzheimer disease is characterized by deficient encoding or consolidation of information (Table 45-1).

Even in the absence of overt dementia, cognitive impairment occurs frequently in Parkinson disease. Common domains of relative impairment in nondemented Parkinson disease patients include attentional and executive functions, visuospatial skills, recall memory, and verbal fluency. Circumscribed cognitive impairments have been observed even in very high functioning Parkinson patients.[25] Nevertheless, the mild or relatively circumscribed cognitive dysfunction that is evident in many patients with Parkinson disease does not progress to frank dementia in all affected individuals. Jacobs and colleagues[26] found that the performance of nondemented patients with Parkinson disease on tests of letter and category fluency was a highly sensitive neuropsychological predictor of incident dementia. Stern and colleagues[23] concluded that although cognitive problems preceding dementia in Parkinson disease patients continue to worsen with the onset of dementia, there is also a qualitative shift in the pattern of cognitive

Table 45-1

Neuropsychological characteristics of dementia in Alzheimer, Parkinson, and Huntington diseases and progressive supranuclear palsy

	Alzheimer disease	Parkinson disease	Huntington disease	Progressive supranuclear palsy
Orientation	Impaired	Normal	Normal	Normal
Memory				
Immediate recall	Impaired	Impaired	Impaired	Normal–mildly impaired
Delayed recall	Severely impaired	Impaired	Impaired	Normal–mildly impaired
Delayed recognition	Severely impaired	Normal	Normal	Normal
Percent retained[a]	0–50	50–80+	50–80+	50–80+
Executive functions/ problem solving	Severely impaired	Severely impaired[b]	Severely impaired[b]	Severely impaired[b]
Language				
Naming	Severely impaired; anomia, para-phasia	Normal–mildly impaired; anomia	Normal; visual misperceptions	Normal; visual misperceptions
Verbal fluency	Impaired	Severely impaired	Severely impaired	Severely impaired
Visuospatial skills	Impaired	Impaired	Severely impaired	Impaired

[a]Percent retained = (immediate recall/delayed recall) × 100.

[b]Executive functions often are disproportionately impaired relative to other cognitive abilities.

deficits, with substantial broadening and worsening of memory dysfunction, as dementia emerges.

Depression is common in Parkinson disease, occurring in approximately 45 percent of patients.[27] The incidence rate of depression in Parkinson disease is 1.86 percent per year.[27] Depression has been found to coexist with dementia in some Parkinson patients[28] and has been identified as a risk factor for incident dementia in nondemented patients.[10,11]

Pathology

The pathologic hallmark of Parkinson disease is loss of pigmented cells in the substantia nigra and other pigmented nuclei. Lewy bodies are found within the neurons remaining in the affected areas.[29,30] The pattern of neuropsychologic deficit typical of dementia in Parkinson disease, including prominent impairment on "frontal lobe" or executive tasks, has been attributed to degeneration of the medial substantia nigra, with associated loss of nigral projections of dopamine to the limbic and frontal areas,[31] and to cholinergic deficiency,[32] although numerous other neurotransmitter systems also have been implicated.[30,33] Other pathologic entities that have been proposed as the neuropathologic basis for dementia in Parkinson disease include coincident Alzheimer disease[34,35] and cortical Lewy bodies.[36,37]

HUNTINGTON DISEASE

Epidemiology

Huntington disease is an autosomal dominant disorder with complete penetrance that is characterized by progressive involuntary choreiform movements, psychiatric features, and dementia. The genetic mutation has been identified as an unstable trinucleotide repeat (CAG) on the short arm of chromosome 4.[38] Prevalence estimates of Huntington disease range from 4 to 10 per 100,000.[39]

Dementia is a ubiquitous feature of Huntington disease; however, the severity of cognitive impairment does vary from patient to patient. The juvenile-onset form is associated with severe and rapidly progressive dementia, while cognitive dysfunction is relatively mild and slowly progressive in patients with onset of motor symptoms after age 50.[40] The dementia associated with midlife onset of Huntington disease, the most frequent presentation, is intermediate between the juvenile and late onset in terms of severity and rapidity of course. Degree of dementia is closely associated with severity of motor involvement.[41]

Characteristics of Dementia

The neuropsychological profile of dementia associated with Huntington disease is similar to that observed in patients with Parkinson disease and is characterized by lack of initiative, impaired attention and executive functions, poor memory and visuospatial skills, but relatively preserved language functions with the exception of verbal fluency. Impairment on tests of visuospatial function may be partly attributable to abnormalities in eye movement that are common in patients with Huntington disease. Errors made on tests of visual confrontation naming are often visual misperceptions of the test stimuli rather than paraphasic or anomic errors, again suggesting that eye-movement abnormalities may contribute to these errors. Nevertheless, specific impairments manipulating egocentric space (i.e., perceiving an object with reference to its distance and direction from the observer) in Huntington disease have been described.[42,43]

The memory impairment of Huntington disease, like that of Parkinson disease, is characterized by poor performance on all memory measures (e.g., immediate and delayed free recall, cued recall) relative to normative data. Rates of retention

from immediate to delayed testing, however, are relatively preserved,[24] and Huntington disease patients demonstrate significantly more improvement on testing of delayed recognition memory than do patients with Alzheimer disease.[44] As in Parkinson disease, the memory impairment of Huntington disease is characterized by severely impaired retrieval of stored information. Patients have difficulty initiating and organizing systematic retrieval strategies (see Table 45-1).

Personality changes and psychiatric disturbances are common and prominent features of Huntington disease, which may precede the onset of motor or cognitive symptoms by as much as 10 years.[45] Apathy, irritability, and poor impulse control are common. Major depression occurs at some time in nearly 40 percent of patients with Huntington disease.[46,47] Five to 10 percent of patients experience schizophrenia-like disorders, characterized by auditory and tactile hallucinations, paranoid delusions, and thought disorder.[48]

Pathology

The core pathologic feature of Huntington disease is atrophy of the caudate and putamen bilaterally. Bamford and colleagues[49] demonstrated that the cognitive impairment in 60 drug-free Huntington patients—including performance on tests of complex psychomotor skill, verbal memory, and visuospatial functioning—was closely linked to the extent of caudate atrophy as measured by computed tomography scan.

PROGRESSIVE SUPRANUCLEAR PALSY

Epidemiology

Clinical characteristics of progressive supranuclear palsy include supranuclear ophthalmoplegia primarily affecting vertical gaze, pseudobulbar palsy, dysarthria, and axial and nuchal rigidity.[50] The prevalence of progressive supranuclear palsy (PSP) has been estimated as 1.4 per 100,000, with an age-adjusted prevalence for the population over age 55 of 7 per 100,000.[51] It has, however, been suggested that the prevalence of progressive supranuclear palsy has been underestimated because it often is misdiagnosed as Parkinson disease.[52] The usual age of onset is between 60 and 70, but onset as early as the mid-40s has been reported.[51] Symptom onset is insidious, and the disease course is progressive, leading to death in 5 to 7 years. Dementia is a common although not ubiquitous feature of progressive supranuclear palsy. Cognitive or behavioral symptoms were reported in seven of the nine cases described by Steele and coworkers.[50] Subsequent estimates of the prevalence of dementia in progressive supranuclear palsy range from 20 to 60 percent.

Characteristics of Dementia

The neuropsychological profile of dementia in progressive supranuclear palsy is often considered prototypical of "subcortical" or "subcorticofrontal" dysfunction. Albert and colleagues[53] described forgetfulness, slowed thought processes, emotional or personality changes, and impaired ability to manipulate acquired knowledge as typical cognitive changes in progressive supranuclear palsy. Executive dysfunction is a prominent feature at all stages of the disease course.[54,55] Although performance on relatively simple attentional tasks may be normal, performance on more complex tasks—such as those requiring sequencing, mental flexibility, abstraction, and reasoning—is severely impaired. Slowness of information processing is pervasive and marked. Dubois and colleagues[56] found processing time in patients with progressive supranuclear palsy to be increased, even relative to patients with Parkinson disease. Albert and colleagues[53] reported that when patients were allowed additional time to respond (sometimes as long as 4 to 5 min for a single question), their performance improved by as much as 50 percent. Verbal fluency is generally very severely impaired; however, other language functions remain preserved. As in Huntington patients, erroneous responses on tests of visual confrontation naming are frequently visual misperceptions[57] and may be secondary to the oculomotor impairments that characterize this disorder. Anomic and paraphasic errors are uncommon. Although language is relatively preserved, severe dysarthria often impairs communicative ability.[57] The memory disorder of progressive supranuclear palsy is generally mild.[58] Although PSP patients may be impaired on memory tasks requiring free recall, they are able to benefit from retrieval cues and perform normally on tests of cued recall (see Table 45-1).[59]

The most commonly reported personality changes in progressive supranuclear palsy are apathy and inertia.[53,60] These symptoms likely reflect the mental slowing that is typical of this disorder. Irritability and depression are also common. Emotional disinhibition (i.e., either laughing or crying excessively with preserved affect) has also been described.

Pathology

Cell loss and pathology in progressive supranuclear palsy occur in various regions of the basal ganglia, brainstem, and cerebellum, including the pallidum, subthalamic nucleus, red nucleus, substantia nigra, superior colliculi, nuclei cuneiformis and subcuneiformis, periaqueductal gray matter, pontine tegmentum, and the dentate nucleus. Consistent with the clinical picture of dementia in progressive supranuclear palsy, functional brain imaging shows subfrontal glucose hypometabolism.[61] Pillon and colleagues[54] interpreted the clinicopathologic association in progressive supranuclear palsy as "frontal deafferentation."

CORTICAL-BASAL GANGLIONIC DEGENERATION

Epidemiology

Cortical-basal ganglionic degeneration (CBGD) is a relatively rare condition characterized by rigidity, focal dystonias or myoclonus, supranuclear gaze palsy, "alien-limb" phenomena, cortical sensory loss, postural-action tremor, postural instability, and severe apraxia.[62,63] Muscle strength is generally preserved. Signs and symptoms are often strikingly asymmetric. Although many of the signs of CBGD are similar to those found in Parkinson disease, the alien-limb phenomena and marked apraxia are distinguishing features. Alien-limb signs often observed in CBGD include levitation and posturing of the arm, particularly when attention is diverted or the eyes are closed.

Prevalence estimates for CBGD are unavailable, and there are no known risk factors. Onset is typically between age 60 and 70, and the average duration of disease from onset to death is 6 to 8 years. Although dementia was not described as a prominent feature in the initial report of this disorder,[62] subsequent reports have found dementia to be common and in some cases severe.[64]

Characteristics of Dementia

The neuropsychological profile of dementia associated with CBGD is characterized by a prominent dysexecutive syndrome, similar to that of patients with PSP; deficient dynamic motor control (e.g., bimanual coordination, temporal organization); asymmetric praxis disorders; and poor free recall but intact cued recall and recognition memory.[59] The most notable and frequently reported feature is the presence of ideational and ideomotor apraxia. Often patients can accurately describe an action (e.g., using a key to open a door) that they are completely unable to perform. Other reported neuropsychological characteristics include "decreased intellectual efficiency"[62] or slowing of thought processes, aphasia (anomia, paraphasia),[63,65] acalculia,[65] right-left confusion,[63] and perseveration.[63] Rediess and Satran[66] reported a patient who was tested serially with a comprehensive neuropsychological battery. One year after onset of motor and personality changes, this patient had impairments of psychomotor speed, verbal fluency, visuoperceptual ability, and nonverbal memory. Verbal memory was strikingly preserved. Four years after symptom onset, however, the patient's dementia was global and severe.

Changes in personality that have been reported in association with CBGD include irritability[66] and increased aggression.[63]

Pathology

Cortical basal ganglionic degeneration is associated with atrophy of frontal and parietal cortex.[62,67] Convolutional atrophy is often greater in the cerebral hemisphere contralateral to the side of the body with pronounced motor involvement. Cortical cell loss, gliosis, and Pick cells are observed, as are nerve cell loss and gliosis in the substantia nigra, locus ceruleus, thalamus, lentiform nucleus, subthalamic nucleus, red nucleus, and midbrain tegmentum.[67] Pathology is generally absent in the temporal and hippocampal regions.[67]

MULTIPLE-SYSTEM ATROPHY AND CEREBELLAR DEGENERATION

The term *multiple-system atrophy* has been applied to several disorders of the motor system sometimes referred to as Parkinson-plus syndromes. These disorders include striatonigral degeneration, sporadic olivopontocerebellar atrophy, and Shy-Drager syndrome. Each of these disorders is characterized by parkinsonian motor signs plus a unique feature that distinguishes it from idiopathic Parkinson disease.[68] Tremor is absent in striatonigral degeneration, and the response to levodopa is limited, as striatal neurons containing dopamine receptors are lost. Olivopontocerebellar atrophy is characterized by parkinsonism plus ataxia and other cerebellar signs. Familial olivopontocerebellar atrophy is a dominantly inherited disorder that presents as a cerebellar syndrome. Finally, Shy-Drager syndrome is characterized by parkinsonism plus autonomic dysfunction, particularly progressive, primary orthostatic hypotension. Although striatonigral degeneration, sporadic olivopontocerebellar atrophy, and Shy-Drager syndrome had previously been considered to be distinct and separate entities, they are now felt to represent different manifestations of a single disease process.[69]

Although motor signs are the prominent and distinguishing features of multiple-system atrophy, changes in cognition may also be present. The profile of cognitive impairment is generally one of relatively preserved overall intellectual functioning but with poor performance on tests of executive function, especially those requiring sequencing and set shifting.[70] Thought processes may be slowed. Performance on tests of language and visual perception generally is within normal limits with the possible exception of verbal fluency.

Cognitive impairment may also be associated with pure cerebellar atrophy.[71-75] As in patients with multiple-system atrophy, overall intelligence is generally preserved in patients with pure cerebellar atrophy; however, performance on tests of executive function may be impaired. Reported areas of cognitive deficit include planning on a complex problem-solving task, response initiation, shifting of attention, and verbal fluency. Appollonio and colleagues[74] found patients with cerebellar degeneration to be impaired relative to normal subjects on "effort-demanding" tests of memory, but the poor memory performance of these subjects was felt to be secondary to their executive dysfunction.

ACKNOWLEDGMENTS

This work was supported by Federal grants AG07232, AG08702, RR00645, and the Parkinson's Disease Foundation.

REFERENCES

1. Mayeux R, Denaro J, Hemenegildo N, et al: A population-based investigation of Parkinson's disease with and without dementia: Relationship to age and gender. *Arch Neurol* 49:492–497, 1992.
2. Rajput AH, Offord K, Beard CM, Kurland LT: Epidemiological survey of dementia in parkinsonism and control population, in Hassler RG, Christ JF (eds): *Advances in Neurology. Parkinson-Specific Motor and Mental Disorders.* New York: Raven Press, 1986, vol 40, pp 229–234.
3. Pirozzolo FJ, Hansch EC, Mortimer JA, et al: Dementia in Parkinson disease: A neuropsychological analysis. *Brain Cogn* 1:71–83, 1982.
4. Lieberman A, Dziatolowski M, Kupersmith M, et al: Dementia in Parkinson disease. *Ann Neurol* 6:355–359, 1979.
5. Celesia GG, Wanamaker WM: Psychiatric disturbances in Parkinson's disease. *Dis Nerv Syst* 33:577–583, 1972.
6. Rajput AH, Offord KP, Beard CM, Kurland LT: A case-control study of smoking habits, dementia, and other illnesses in idiopathic Parkinson's disease. *Neurology* 37:226–232, 1987.
7. Marder K, Tang M-X, Cote LJ, et al: Predictors of dementia in community-dwelling elderly patients with Parkinson's disease. *Neurology* 43:S115, 1993.
8. Mayeux R: A current analysis of behavioral problems in patients with idiopathic Parkinson's disease (review). *Move Dis* 4(suppl 1):S48–S56, 1989.
9. Marder K, Leung D, Tang M, et al: Are demented patients with Parkinson's disease accurately reflected in prevalence surveys? A survival analysis. *Neurology* 41:1240–1243, 1991.
10. Stern Y, Marder K, Tang MX, Mayeux R: Antecedent clinical features associated with dementia in Parkinson's disease. *Neurology* 43:1690–1692, 1993.
11. Marder K, Tang M-X, Cote L, et al: The frequency and associated risk factors for dementia in patients with Parkinson's disease. *Arch Neurol* 52:695–701, 1995.
12. Bondi MW, Kaszniak AW, Bayles KA, Vance KT: Contributions of frontal system dysfunction to memory and perceptual abilities in Parkinson's disease. *Neuropsychology* 7:89–102, 1993.
13. Taylor AE, Saint-Cyr JA, Lang AE, Kenny FF: Frontal lobe dysfunction in Parkinson's disease: The cortical focus of neostriatal outflow. *Brain* 109:845–883, 1986.
14. Berg EA: A simple objective test for measuring flexibility in thinking. *J Gen Psychol* 39:15–22, 1948.
15. Bowen FP: Behavioral alterations in patients with basal ganglia lesions, in Yahr MD (ed): *The Basal Ganglia.* New York: Raven Press, 1976, pp 169–180.
16. Milner B: Effects of different brain lesions on card sorting: The role of the frontal lobes. *Arch Neurol* 9:90, 1963.
17. Teuber HL: The frontal lobes and their functions: Further observations in carnivores, subhuman primates and man. *Int J Neurol* 5:282–300, 1966.
18. Dubois B, Boller F, Pillon B, Agid Y: Cognitive deficits in Parkinson's disease, in Boller F, Grafman J (eds): *Handbook of Neuropsychology.* Amsterdam: Elsevier, 1991, vol 5, pp 195–240.
19. Brown RG, Marsden CD: "Subcortical dementia": The neuropsychological evidence. *Neuroscience* 25:363–387, 1988.
20. Mahler ME, Cummings JL: Alzheimer's disease and

the dementia of PD: Comparative investigations. *Alz Dis Assoc Disord* 4:133–149, 1990.

21. Cummings JL: Subcortical dementia. Neuropsychology, neuropsychiatry and pathophysiology. *Br J Psychiatr* 149:682–697, 1986.

22. Whitehouse PJ: The concept of subcortical dementia: Another look. *Ann Neurol* 19:1–6, 1986.

23. Stern Y, Richards M, Sano M, Mayeux R: Comparison of cognitive changes in patients with Alzheimer's and Parkinson's disease. *Arch Neurol* 50:1040–1045, 1993.

24. Troster AI, Butters N, Salmon DP, et al: The diagnostic utility of savings scores: Differentiating Alzheimer's and Huntington's diseases with the Logical Memory and Visual Reproduction tests. *J Clin Exp Neuropsychol* 15:773–788, 1993.

25. Mohr E, Juncos J, Cox C, et al: Selective deficits in cognition and memory in high functioning Parkinson's patients. *J Neurol Neurosurg Psychiatr* 53:603–606, 1990.

26. Jacobs DM, Marder K, Cote LJ, et al: Neuropsychological characteristics of preclinical dementia in Parkinson's disease. *Neurology* 45:1691–1696, 1995.

27. Dooneief G, Mirabello E, Bell K, et al: An estimate of the incidence of depression in idiopathic Parkinson's disease. *Arch Neurol* 49:305–307, 1992.

28. Sano M, Stern Y, Williams J, et al: Coexisting dementia and depression in Parkinson's disease. *Arch Neurol* 46:1284–1286, 1989.

29. Gibb WRG, Scott T, Lees AJ: Neuronal inclusions of Parkinson's disease. *Move Disord* 6:2–11, 1991.

30. Jellinger K: New developments in the pathology of Parkinson's disease, in Streifler MB, Korczyn AD, Melamed E, Youdim MBH (eds): *Advances in Neurology: Parkinson's Disease: Anatomy, Pathology, and Therapy.* New York: Raven Press, 1991, vol 53, pp 1–16.

31. Rinne JO, Rummukainen J, Paljarvi L, Rinne UK: Dementia in Parkinson's disease is related to neuronal loss in the medial substantia nigra. *Ann Neurol* 26:47–50, 1989.

32. Dubois B, Pillon B, Lhermitte F, Agid Y: Cholinergic deficiency and frontal dysfunction in Parkinson's disease. *Ann Neurol* 28:117–121, 1990.

33. Hornykiewicz O: Movement disorders, in Marsden CD, Fanh S (eds): *Brain Neurotransmitter Changes in Parkinson's Disease.* London: Butterworth, 1982, pp 41–58.

34. Hakim AM, Mathieson G: Dementia in Parkinson's disease: A neuropathologic study. *Neurology* 29:1209–1214, 1979.

35. Paulus W, Jellinger K: The neuropathologic basis of different clinical subgroups of Parkinson's disease. *J Neuropathol Exp Neurol* 50:743–755, 1991.

36. Kosaka K, Tsuchiya K, Yoshimura M: Lewy body disease with and without dementia: A clinicopathological study of 35 cases. *Clin Neuropathol* 7:299–305, 1988.

37. Byrne EJ, Lennox GG, Godwin-Austin RB, et al: Dementia associated with cortical Lewy bodies: Proposed clinical diagnostic criteria. *Dementia* 2:283–284, 1991.

38. Huntington's Disease Collaborative Research Group: A novel gene containing a trinucleotide repeat that is expanded and unstable on Huntington's disease chromosomes. *Cell* 72:971–983, 1993.

39. Harper PS: The epidemiology of Huntington's disease. *Hum Genet* 89:365–376, 1992.

40. Bird ED: The brain in Huntington's chorea. *Psychol Med* 8:357–360, 1978.

41. Brandt J, Strauss ME, Larus J, et al: Clinical correlates of dementia and disability in Huntington's disease. *J Clin Neuropsychol* 6:401–412, 1984.

42. Potegal M: A note on spatial-motor deficits in patients with Huntington's disease: A test of hypothesis. *Neuropsychologia* 9:233–235, 1971.

43. Fedio P, Cox CS, Neophytides A, et al: Neuropsychological profile of Huntington's disease: Patients and those at risk, in Chase TN, Wexler NS, Barbeau A (eds): *Advances in Neurology.* New York: Raven Press, 1979, vol 23, 239–271.

44. Delis DC, Massman PJ, Butters N, et al: Profiles of demented and amnesic patients on the California Verbal Learning Test: Implications for the assessment of memory disorders. *Psychol Assess* 3:19–26, 1991.

45. Martin JB: Huntington's disease: New approaches to an old problem. *Neurology* 34:1059–1072, 1984.

46. Caine E, Shoulson I: Psychiatric syndromes in Huntington's disease. *Am J Psychiatry* 140:728–733, 1983.

47. Folstein SE: *Huntington's Disease.* Baltimore: Johns Hopkins University Press, 1989.

48. Shoulson I. Huntington's disease: Cognitive and psychiatric features. *Neuropsychiatry Neuropsychol Behav Neurol* 3:15–22, 1990.

49. Bamford KA, Caine ED, Kido DK, et al: Clinical-pathologic correlation in Huntington's disease: A neuropsychological and computed tomography study. *Neurology* 39:796–801, 1989.

50. Steele JC, Richardson JC, Olszewski J: Progressive supranuclear palsy. *Arch Neurol* 10:333–358, 1964.

51. Golbe LI, Davis PH, Schoenberg BS, Duvoisin RC: Prevalence and natural history of progressive supranuclear palsy. *Neurology* 38:1031–1034, 1988.

52. Lees AJ: Progressive supranuclear palsy (Steele-Richardson-Olszewski syndrome), in Cummings JL (ed): *Subcortical Dementia*. New York: Oxford University Press, 1990.

53. Albert ML, Feldman RG, Willis AL: The "subcortical dementia" of progressive supranuclear palsy. *J Neurol Neurosurg Psychiatry* 37:121–130, 1974.

54. Pillon B, Dubois B, Ploska A, Agid Y: Severity and specificity of cognitive impairment in Alzheimer's, Huntington's, and Parkinson's diseases and progressive supranuclear palsy. *Neurology* 41:634–643, 1991.

55. Litvan I: Cognitive disturbances in progressive supranuclear palsy. *J Neural Trans* 42:69–78, 1994.

56. Dubois B, Pillon B, Legault F, et al: Slowing of cognitive processing in progressive supranuclear palsy. *Arch Neurol* 45:1194–1199, 1988.

57. Podoll K, Schwarz M, Noth J: Language functions in progressive supranuclear palsy. *Brain* 114:1457–1472, 1991.

58. Milberg W, Albert M: Cognitive differences between patients with progressive supranuclear palsy and Alzheimer's disease. *J Clin Exp Neuropsychol* 11:605–614, 1989.

59. Pillon B, Blin J, Vidailhet M, et al: The neuropsychological pattern of corticobasal degeneration: comparison with progressive supranuclear palsy and Alzheimer's disease. *Neurology* 45:1477–1483, 1995.

60. Janati A, Appell AR: Psychiatric aspects of progressive supranuclear palsy. *J Nerv Ment Dis* 172:85–89, 1984.

61. Foster NL, Gilman S, Berent S, et al: Cerebral hypometabolism in progressive supranuclear palsy studied with positron emission tomography. *Ann Neurol* 24:399–406, 1988.

62. Rebeiz JJ, Kolodny EH, Richardson EP: Cortico-dentatonigral degeneration with neuronal achromasia. *Arch Neurol* 18:20–33, 1968.

63. Riley DE, Lang AE, Lewis A, et al: Cortical-basal ganglionic degeneration. *Neurology* 40:1203–1212, 1990.

64. Watts RL, Williams RS, Growdon JD, et al: Corticobasal ganglionic degeneration (abstr). *Neurology* 35(suppl 1):178, 1985.

65. Case records of the Massachusetts General Hospital. *N Engl J Med* 313:739–748, 1985.

66. Rediess S, Satran R: Corticobasal degeneration: Serial neuropsychological examination of a case (abstr). *J Int Neuropsychol Soc* 1:147, 1995.

67. Gibb RG, Luthert PJ, Marsden CD: Corticobasal degeneration. *Brain* 112:1171–1192, 1989.

68. Fahn S: Parkinsonism, in Rowland LP (ed): *Merritt's Textbook of Neurology,* 9th ed. Baltimore, MD: Williams & Wilkins, 1995, pp 713–730.

69. Penney JB: Multiple systems atrophy and nonfamilial olivopontocerebellar atrophy are the same disease. *Ann Neurol* 37:553–554, 1995.

70. Robbins TW, James M, Lange KW, et al: Cognitive performance in multiple system atrophy. *Brain* 115:271–291, 1992.

71. Grafman J, Litvan I, Massaquoi S, et al: Cognitive planning deficit in patients with cerebellar atrophy. *Neurology* 42:1493–1496, 1992.

72. Akshoomoff NA, Courchesne E, Press GA, Iragui V: Contribution of the cerebellum to neuropsychological functioning: Evidence from a case of cerebellar degenerative disorder. *Neuropsychologia* 30:315–328, 1992.

73. Fiez JA, Petersen SE, Cheney MK, Raichle ME: Impaired non-motor learning and error detection associated with cerebellar damage. *Brain* 115:155–178, 1992.

74. Appollonio IM, Grafman J, Schwartz V, et al: Memory in patients with cerebellar degeneration. *Neurology* 43:1536–1544, 1993.

75. Akshoomoff NA, Courchesne E: A new role for the cerebellum in cognitive operations. *Behav Neurosci* 106:731–738, 1992.

Chapter 46

VASCULAR DEMENTIA

John V. Bowler
Vladimir Hachinski

Over the past century, our concept of vascular dementia has evolved remarkably. It has developed from a poorly described condition, confused first with neurosyphilis and more recently with Alzheimer disease, to the position of being recognized as the second commonest cause of dementia. However, it has not yet reached clinical maturity, as fundamental disagreements about its nature remain. These center upon several observations; (1) that vascular dementia is not a single condition but has several etiologies, the clinical features and treatments of which may differ; (2) that the current definition is based on Alzheimer disease, requiring prominent memory loss, and may be inappropriate; (3) that the level of cognitive impairment required for "dementia" is too severe and will prevent identification of early cases; (4) the inclusion of major stroke; (5) the inclusion of intracerebral and subarachnoid hemorrhage; (6) the role of leukoaraiosis; and (7) the volumes and sites of infarction that are consistent with dementia. The lack of agreement profoundly limits the observations that can be made regarding its behavioral and psychological aspects, and interpretation of the data that do exist must be made in the context of these uncertainties, which are reviewed below.

CRITERIA FOR VASCULAR DEMENTIA

The recognition of Alzheimer disease as the commonest cause of dementia in western society resulted in the criteria used to define dementia[1,2]

being based on Alzheimer's disease. Thus prominent features of dementia have come to include early and prominent memory loss, progression, irreversibility, and a level of cognitive impairment sufficient to affect normal daily activities. Rather than using specific criteria for vascular dementia, it has been traditional to identify dementia according to Alzheimer-based criteria and then to separate Alzheimer disease from multi-infarct dementia using clinical features thought to reflect vascular risk factors, vascular events, and the manifestations of systemic and cerebral vascular disease. These elements are often operationalized using the ischemic score.[3-6] Thus, for historical reasons, the criteria for multi-infarct dementia have come to emphasize memory loss and the progression and irreversibility of cognitive decline. None of these necessarily accompany the cognitive decline due to cerebrovascular disease.[7,8] Furthermore, patients cannot be diagnosed as demented until they have developed impairment in normal day-to-day activities, a degree of severity that will prevent treatment until it is too late.

The available criteria for the diagnosis of vascular dementia fall into two groups. The first of these are the criteria contained in general diagnostic tools—i.e., the *Diagnostic and Statistical Manual of Mental Disorders,* 4th ed. (DSM-IV),[2] and the *International Classification of Diseases,* 10th rev. ed. (ICD-10).[1] Both are very general in nature and do not operationalize their criteria. The second group—the criteria of the State of California Alzheimer's Disease Diagnostic and

Treatment Centers,[9] the criteria of the National Institute of Neurological Disorders and Stroke, and those of the Association Internationale pour la Recherche at L'Enseignement en Neurosciences (NINDS-AIREN)[6]—are developments of the first two and attempt to operationalize the criteria.

The Criteria of the State of California Alzheimer's Disease Diagnostic and Treatment Centers

These criteria are given in Table 46-1.[9] Hemorrhagic and anoxic lesions are not included. The number and type of cognitive defects are deliberately not specified but are not confined to a single narrow category and memory loss is not emphasized. The severity should be sufficient to interfere with the conduct of the patient's customary affairs of life, and this judgment is to be made on clinical criteria, not by neuropsychological testing. Two or more ischemic strokes, by history and examination or imaging, are required, though rarely one stroke with a clear temporal relationship to the onset of dementia may be allowed. Unlike most of the other criteria, these criteria do not ask for a clear temporal relationship between infarcts and dementia except where a single infarct is the alleged cause of the dementia. The reason for this is that vascular cases may progress gradually, without a clear-cut association between events and cognitive decline, such that establishing a temporal relationship can be difficult. These points are valid but the criteria risk diagnosing all cases of dementia with two or more infarcts as cases of vascular dementia.

NINDS-AIREN Criteria

The NINDS-AIREN criteria[6] define dementia according to the ICD-10, requiring impaired functioning in daily living and a decline in memory and at least two other domains. The memory deficits may be less severe than in Alzheimer disease, and a diagnosis of vascular dementia is made uncertain or unlikely by the presence of early-onset memory deficit and progressive worsening of memory without corresponding focal lesions. A temporal association between stroke and dementia onset is required and is arbitrarily set at 3 months. An abrupt deterioration in cognition or a stepwise progression of dementia is acceptable if the 3-month criterion is not met. Neuroimaging is required, as the absence of a vascular lesion on magnetic resonance imaging (MRI) or computed tomography (CT) excludes the possibility of vascular dementia, but there are no criteria regarding lesion volume. A single lesion is acceptable. Specific recommendations regarding the sites of lesions and the minimum amount of white matter disease are given in Table 46-2. The recommendations regarding white matter changes should be treated with caution, as the correlation between white matter changes on MRI and cognition is extremely weak.[10] Correlation of the MRI or CT changes with the clinical picture is required on the grounds that there are no pathognomonic CT or MRI correlates of vascular dementia. Hemorrhagic lesions are permitted.

These elements are synthesized by requiring evidence of (1) dementia, (2) vascular disease, and (3) an association between the two without evidence of any other cause for a diagnosis of probable vascular dementia to be made. A diagnosis of possible vascular dementia is made if (1) there are no neuroimaging data but there is clinical evidence of cerebrovascular disease, (2) in the absence of a clear temporal relationship between dementia and stroke, or (3) in those with a subtle onset and variable course. Definite vascular dementia is diagnosed if probable dementia exists, it is accompanied by histopathologic evidence of cerebrovascular disease, and there is no histopathologic evidence of other possible causes of the cognitive loss. Mixed dementia is not recognized, but the coexistence of vascular dementia with Alzheimer disease is termed Alzheimer disease with cerebrovascular disease.

Limitations of the Current Definitions

While the criteria listed above are the only operational criteria available, it is important to realize that they are based on supposition and not on fact. The NINDS-AIREN criteria were also developed

Table 46-1

Criteria for Alzheimer disease from the State of California Alzheimer's Disease Diagnostic and Treatment Centers

1. Dementia

   Dementia is a deterioration from a known or estimated prior level of intellectual function sufficient to interfere broadly with the conduct of the patient's customary affairs of life, which is not isolated to a single narrow category of intellectual performance, and which is independent of level of consciousness.

   This deterioration should be supported by historical evidence and documented by either bedside mental status testing or ideally by more detailed neuropsychological examination, using tests that are quantifiable, reproducible, and for which normative data are available.

2. Probable IVD

   A. The criteria for the clinical diagnosis of PROBABLE IVD include ALL of the following:

      1. Dementia;

      2. Evidence of two or more ischemic strokes by history, neurologic signs, and/or neuroimaging studies (CT or T1-weighted MRI) or occurrence of a single stroke with a clearly documented temporal relationship to the onset of dementia;

      3. Evidence of at least one infarct outside the cerebellum by CT or T1-weighted MRI.

   B. The diagnosis of PROBABLE IVD is supported by

      1. Evidence of multiple infarcts in brain regions known to affect cognition;

      2. A history of multiple transient ischaemic attacks;

      3. History of vascular risk factors (e.g., hypertension, heart disease, diabetes mellitus);

      4. Elevated Hachinski Ischaemic Scale (original or modified version)

   C. Clinical features that are thought to be associated with IVD, but await further research, include

      1. Relatively early appearance of gait disturbance and urinary incontinence;

      2. Periventricular and deep white matter changes on T2-weighted MRI that are excessive for age;

      3. Focal changes in electrophysiological studies (e.g., EEG, evoked potentials) or physiologic neuroimaging studies (e.g., SPECT, PET, NMR, spectroscopy).

   D. Other clinical features that do not constitute strong evidence either for or against a diagnosis of PROBABLE IVD include

      1. Periods of slowly progressive symptoms;

      2. Illusions, psychosis, hallucinations, delusions;

      3. Seizures.

   E. Clinical features that cast doubt on a diagnosis of PROBABLE IVD include

1. Transcortical sensory aphasia in the absence of corresponding focal lesions on neuroimaging studies;

2. Absence of central neurologic symptoms/signs, other than cognitive disturbance.

3. Possible IVD

A clinical diagnosis of POSSIBLE IVD may be made when there is

1. Dementia;

   and one or more of the following:

2a. A history or evidence of a single stroke (but not multiple strokes) without a clearly documented temporal relationship to the onset of dementia;

   or

2b. Binswanger's syndrome (without multiple strokes) that includes all of the following:

   I. Early-onset urinary incontinence not explained by urologic disease, or gait disturbance (eg, parkinsonian, magnetic, apraxic, or "senile" gait) not explained by peripheral cause,

   II. Vascular risk factors, and

   III. Extensive white matter changes on neuroimaging.

   IV. Definite IVD
   A diagnosis of DEFINITE IVD requires histopathologic examination of the brain, as well as

   A. Clinical evidence of dementia;

   B. Pathologic confirmation of multiple infarcts, some outside the cerebellum.

Note: If there is evidence of Alzheimer's disease or some other pathologic disorder that is thought to have contributed to the dementia, a diagnosis of MIXED dementia should be made.

V. Mixed dementia

A diagnosis of MIXED dementia should be made in the presence of one or more other systemic or brain disorders that are thought to be causally related to the dementia.

The degree of confidence in the diagnosis of IVD should be specified as possible, probable, or definite, and the other disorder(s) contributing to the dementia should be listed. For example: mixed dementia due to probable IVD and possible Alzheimer's disease or mixed dementia due to definite IVD and hypothyroidism.

VI. Research classification

Classification of IVD for research purposes should specify features of the infarcts that may differentiate subtypes of the disorder, such as

Location: cortical, white matter, periventricular, basal ganglia, thalamus

Size: volume

Distribution: large, small or microvessel

Severity: chronic ischaemia versus infarction

Etiology: embolism, atherosclerosis, arteriosclerosis, cerebral amyloid angiopathy, hypoperfusion.

Source: From Chui et al.,[9] with permission.

Table 46-2
Radiologic features considered compatible with vascular dementia by the NINDS-AIREN criteria

1. Site
   A. Large-vessel strokes in the following territories:
      a. bilateral anterior cerebral artery
      b. posterior cerebral artery
      c. parietotemporal and temporo-occipital association areas
      d. the superior frontal and parietal watershed territories
   B. Small vessel disease:
      a. basal ganglia and frontal white matter lacunes
      b. extensive periventricular white matter lesions
      c. bilateral thalamic lesions
2. Severity
   A. Large-vessel lesions of the dominant hemisphere
   B. Bilateral large-vessel hemispheric strokes
   C. Leukoencephalopathy involving at least 25% of the total white matter

Source: From Roman et al.,[6] with permission.

with a view to epidemiologic convenience rather than to clinical accuracy. They are at fault in several respects, and the reader is encouraged to review them critically before applying them.

Involvement of Memory   The adoption of criteria from Alzheimer disease, in which the mesial temporal lobes are affected early and prominently, may be erroneous, as the mesial temporal lobes are not especially involved in cerebrovascular disease. The data that exist suggest that executive, subcortical, and frontal lobe functions are affected at least as prominently as memory.[11-26]

Severity of Dementia   The proposals define dementia on the basis of a clear loss of cognitive function. This will deny early cases the most appropriate opportunity for secondary preventive measures by failing to detect the disorder.[8,27-30] Early cases need to be identified.

Infarct Volume   That an infarct volume of 50 to 100 cm³ distinguished between vascular dementia and "senile dementia" was suggested in early work.[31] However, these data were based on highly selected cases, and dementia can exist with much smaller infarct volumes;[7,32-35] moreover, cognitive impairment short of dementia can be seen with very small infarct volumes.[24] Correlation between infarct volume and neuropsychological deficit is poor when all stroke types are studied together.[23,35,36] This is not surprising, as site is at least as important as size. It is therefore unlikely that there is a precise volume of infarction other than at meaninglessly large volumes that can reliably predict vascular dementia.

Infarct Site   Infarct site is crucial[37] but has never been formally investigated. Such evidence as exists is inconsistent because of variability in the study populations and protocols. The following sites are putatively important in the production of cognitive loss: bilateral,[32,34,38] left-sided,[22,34,35,39] thalamic,[38] anterior cerebral,[22] and frontal lesions.[40] Some work favors a special role for "lacunar" and other deep lesions over cortical lesions,[7,39,41-43] but other work does not.[22,33-35] Fisher felt that dementia in association with lacunes was rare,[44] but cognitive impairment in association with small numbers and volumes of subcortical infarcts is readily detectable.[24,45]

Multiple Types of Vascular Dementia   All of the current criteria largely treat vascular dementia as a single condition. This is an important error, since vascular lesions capable of causing cognitive loss arise from many different etiologies, and differing causes require different treatments. In addition, events falling short of stroke may be relevant. Episodes of hypotension, leukoaraiosis, and incomplete infarction are all associated with cognitive impairment and all have some vascular basis but do not necessarily cause or consist of infarcts.[19,25,26,46-55]

Leukoaraiosis   Leukoaraiosis seen on CT affects cognition.[45,48,52,55-57] Leukoaraiosis demonstrated on MRI has a weaker association with cognitive loss. Some studies have found a correlation between neuropsychological deficits and the extent of leukoaraiosis,[19,25,26,47,50,51,53,54] but in others the correlation becomes insignificant after correction for age.[58,59] Other studies have been negative,[60-63] but may have been negative for methodologic reasons, including the use of insensitive tests of cognition,[62] the summarizing of data from several neuropsychological tests together in a way that may mask changes in a few positive tests,[58] too little disease,[61] too few cases,[62] and the use of a simple dichotomy between demented and nondemented.[60,63] Overall, it seems the evidence shows that leukoaraiosis of relatively minor degree can affect cognition, but that the effects can be very subtle.

Inclusion of Major Stroke   Clinical medicine is usually concerned with unitary diseases with a single definition that do not overlap other conditions. The vascular dementias pose a problem in this regard as they overlap with stroke. Major cerebral infarction, identified by the production of substantial motor, sensory, visual, or language deficits, is a group of conditions for which the epidemiology, risk factors, primary and secondary preventative therapy, and prognoses are relatively well established. If the purpose of defining vascular dementia is to identify a group of conditions for which there may be special risk factors, perhaps different from stroke in general, for which patients may benefit from appropriate preventative therapy, then the inclusion of patients with major stroke is inappropriate. Alternatively, if the purpose is to describe the economic burden of cognitive decline due to stroke, a more inclusive approach is necessary. All of the current criteria implicitly or explicitly include major stroke.

OTHER PROPOSALS—VASCULAR COGNITIVE IMPAIRMENT

Progress in this field may best be served by moving away from vascular dementia toward a new concept, that of vascular cognitive impairment (VCI).[29] This broader concept includes cases now described as vascular dementia but would not include nonischemic cases and major stroke. In VCI, the term *vascular* refers to all causes of ischemic cerebrovascular disease, while *cognitive impairment* encompasses all levels of cognitive decline, from the earliest steps.

THE MECHANISM OF COGNITIVE IMPAIRMENT IN CEREBROVASCULAR DISEASE

Lesions interact synergistically in impairing cognition.[64,65] Neural nets may explain this as they provide scope for recovery after lesions, but as lesions' numbers increase, the scope for recovery decreases; the net sequelae of each successive lesion thus increase. Neural nets also give clues to the likely order of cognitive decline produced by multiple lesions, suggesting that frontal involvement may be the most prominent.[16,66] Evidence of prominent frontal system involvement following multiple lacunar infarction supports this.[16] Memory, which also depends on an extensive neural net,[66] may also be affected relatively early, but not most prominently. Where the basis of vascular dementia was a single lesion or a few large ones, this would not hold, and the pattern of cognitive loss would be closely linked to the site of the lesion. Even so, patients with right-sided lesions exhibit impairment in verbal IQ, and patients with left-sided lesions exhibit impairment in performance IQ,[18] clearly showing the importance of generalized cognitive processing, presumably based on neural nets, as opposed to the more traditional localization of function. Support for a role for neural nets in global cognitive decline after stroke comes from factorial analyses of neuropsychological deficits after stroke. These show that a relatively small number of factors,[36,67,68] distinct from the traditionally recognized cognitive domains, may form a mechanism by which dementia could occur based on multiple infarcts. These factors may reflect neural nets. Further support comes from emission tomography that shows extensive diaschisis, extending to the contralateral hemisphere, after a variety of lesions.[41,69-72] While there is doubt about whether these changes are causative or simply consequences,[73–75] they do reflect functional disconnection and so might indicate the more important projections of the affected neural nets.

GENERAL IMPAIRMENT OF COGNITION AFTER STROKE

The global cognitive changes after stroke, as distinct from the more traditionally considered focal effects, may be relevant in the description of the cognitive deficits seen in vascular dementia, as it is likely that they have many etiological aspects in common even if the presence of a major stroke is considered to be an exclusion from vascular dementia.

There is evidence that subcortical processes are commonly affected by stroke and that these processes may show a considerable degree of improvement,[23] an observation that would be consistent with disturbance of an underlying, complex, and flexible network[66] capable of rerouting to bypass damaged signal pathways. After multiple lacunar strokes, frontal deficits are common and subcortical involvement is also seen.[16] Attention may not be impaired with lacunar lesions alone, while a combination of lacunes and cortical infarcts may impair attention, language, visuospatial function, and motor programming.[17] While memory is not spared, memory deficits are not predominant over all other aspects of cognition after stroke.[22,23] Many domains may be involved, including orientation, language, and attention as well as memory, while abstract reasoning and visuospatial skills may be relatively spared.[22]

Over one-quarter of patients admitted with stroke become demented.[39] Importantly, further stroke, coexistent Alzheimer disease, and depression do not account for this.[20] Age, education, race, prior stroke, hemispheric stroke, lacunar stroke, left hemispheric lesions, and diabetes are all risk factors for dementia in this group, while hypertension, myocardial infarction, angina, congestive heart failure, atrial fibrillation, hypercholesterolemia, claudication, transient ischemic attacks alone, aspirin use, tobacco use, and alcohol use are

not risk factors. In the demented patients, visual neglect, hemiparesis, frontal release signs, urinary incontinence, and gait impairment were more common, whereas aphasia, hemianopia, and sensory loss were not.[39] A study with data on 71 patients seen after ischemic stroke that identified dementia in 40 had similar results. Age, duration of history of stroke, number of strokes, neurologic symptoms, and neurologic signs were similar in both groups, but in the demented patients, dominant hemisphere disease and bilateral symptoms were more common. Hypertension was more common in the demented patients, while heart disease, diabetes, blood viscosity, and fibrinogen were not different. Normal CT scans were more common in non-demented subjects, while bilateral infarcts and atrophy with infarcts were more common in the demented patients.[38]

NEUROPSYCHOLOGICAL DEFICITS IN VASCULAR DEMENTIA

Subcortical and Frontal Deficits in Vascular Dementia

The data that exist on the patterns of cognitive impairment seen in cerebrovascular disease suggest that impairment of subcortical and frontal lobe functions are the most common features.[11–26,40]

Binswanger Disease

Despite doubt as to the nosology, Binswanger's disease[76–78] may be considered to be a form of vascular dementia, and diagnostic criteria have been published.[79] The clinical picture is typically that of a patient slightly more often male than female in the sixth or seventh decade of life. A history of hypertension is present in 80 percent or more, and the hypertension is often poorly controlled. Other risk factors for vascular disease, especially diabetes, are often present.[77,80] Dementia is variable and not necessarily the presenting symptom. It evolves over 3 to 10 years and is intermittently progressive, but it may become gradually progressive without further clear-cut vascular events. Aphasia, amnestic intervals, and neglect are seen in some cases. Memory loss is not prominent.[81] Dysarthria, focal motor signs, and a gait disturbance, with features of spasticity, parkinsonism, and ataxia[82] evolve during the illness and may appear relatively early. Incontinence develops later but may occur while cognition is still at least grossly intact.[81,83] The dysarthria is part of a pseudobulbar palsy, and while both are variable in degree, they are nearly universally present.[81] Dizziness, faints, and—less commonly—epilepsy also occur.[76] A history of stroke at some stage is almost universal, but exceptions occur and, in rare instances, focal signs may be absent even late in the disease.[84] Behavioral changes are early and prominent and may be the presenting feature. Some patients exhibit an early manic phase, but in most progressively increasing abulia develops later in the illness.[81] Depression is common[79] and mood disturbances are seen.[83]

In light of numerous recent reports of "Binswanger disease" diagnosed by MRI, it is to be emphasized that Binswanger disease is a clinical syndrome and cannot be diagnosed by MRI alone. Extensive leukoaraiosis on MRI without clinical correlates is not Binswanger disease.

Neuropsychological Aspects of Vascular Dementia and Alzheimer Disease Contrasted

In comparing these two conditions, selection bias may affect data. Many studies report data from patients seen in memory clinics. In our memory clinic, cases of vascular dementia were rare, amounting to only 4.6 percent. Indeed, only 1 of 136 new cases seen by us in the memory clinic in the last 3 years had vascular dementia, while 43 percent had Alzheimer disease (Bowler and Hachinski, unpublished observations). Conversely, the Canadian Study of Health and Aging,[85] which is a population-based study, established that vascular dementia was responsible for 29 percent of all dementia. Furthermore, in 100 consecutive referrals to the vascular clinic, we found that 25 percent were cognitively impaired and 10 percent were

demented (Bowler and Hachinski, unpublished observations) according to Folstein's Mini-Mental State Examination,[86] using cutoffs of 26 and 24 respectively. These discrepancies suggest that cases of vascular dementia detected in memory clinics, as opposed to those detected in population surveys or vascular clinics, represent a subset of all cases of vascular dementia. We speculate that this is a subgroup in which the presentation mimics Alzheimer disease unusually closely.

Methodological differences also make comparisons of the two conditions difficult. Many studies identifying differences between Alzheimer disease and vascular dementia have not matched their cases for severity. In one series, language and orientation were worse in vascular dementia,[87] but the vascular dementia cases were globally worse than the Alzheimer disease cases. Other series[11–13] reported extensive neuropsychological differences between Alzheimer disease and vascular dementia, but in this work the Alzheimer patients were globally much more impaired than the vascular cases, which could explain all the differences. Greater difficulty in accessing the lexicon in Alzheimer disease cases compared to greater difficulty with syntax in vascular dementia cases has been reported,[88] but in this series the patients with vascular dementia were 10 years younger than those with Alzheimer disease, and there is no mention of or correction for education, occupation, or overall level of cognition.

In those studies in which the cases were matched for severity, differences between the Alzheimer disease and vascular dementia groups are typically sparse or nonexistent except that such work has often found aspects of memory to be more severely impaired in Alzheimer disease,[21,89–92] although others have found no difference.[93–97] Shuttleworth and Huber[94] found that only picture absurdities, which were worse in Alzheimer disease,[94] distinguished early Alzheimer disease and early vascular dementia, while visual memory, Raven matrices, geographic orientation, and copying of figures were not different. A study comparing aspects of visual function in Alzheimer's disease and vascular dementia found that the vascular cases did better on recognition memory for faces and on famous faces but found no difference in block design and line orientation.[98] Erkinjuntti and colleagues also found little neuropsychological difference between Alzheimer disease and vascular dementia.[95,96] In their series, motor functions, reading, and writing were worse in the vascular cases, while most cognitive functions, including memory, did not differ between the two groups. Fischer and coworkers also found no differences in semantic memory.[97] Several aspects of language may be relatively more impaired in Alzheimer disease,[92,99] including the understanding of temporal relationships and complex grammatical structures, repetition of sentences and stories, and word span,[92,99,100] while mechanical problems may be greater in vascular dementia.[100] Functions thought to have frontal or subcortical components—including motor performance, picture arrangement, writing, object assembly, and block design—are more severely affected in vascular dementia.[92] These findings are largely supported in other work, in which patients with Alzheimer disease did better on measures of attention, executive function, self-regulation, and fine motor control, while the patients with vascular dementia were better oriented and had better recall and language.[21]

BEHAVIORAL CHANGES IN VASCULAR DEMENTIA

The study of behavioral changes in vascular dementia has been impaired by the use of behavioral changes in some criteria used for vascular dementia. The International Classification of Diseases[1] specifically suggests that personality is relatively well preserved but allows that personality changes may occur in some cases with features of "apathy, disinhibition, or accentuation of previous traits such as egocentricity, paranoid attitudes, or irritability." The ischemia score,[4] which is often used to help identify vascular dementia, includes several behavioral items. The NINDS-AIREN criteria for vascular dementia[6] attach significance to incontinence, mood (particularly depression), and personality changes. Data obtained using any of these

criteria cannot properly be used to determine the behavioral changes seen in vascular dementia because of the selection of cases for the very features under investigation.

Only incontinence, among various behavioral changes, distinguished demented from nondemented stroke patients,[7] while in lacunar infarcts, behavioral changes may be more prominent than intellectual differences,[33] suggesting that behavioral changes may be important in identifying vascular dementia. Comparison of patients with lacunar infarcts with controls without infarcts suggests that depression, apathy, and perseveration[16] are associated with lacunar infarcts.

In a comparison of Alzheimer disease and vascular dementia, delusions were not more common in the former than in the latter,[101] occurring in about half of all cases in each condition. Hallucinations occur only rarely in both conditions. Severe depression occurs in about 25 percent of cases of vascular dementia, while depression of any severity occurs in about 60 percent of such cases; this is over four times that seen in Alzheimer disease.[101] A further comparative study of Alzheimer disease and vascular dementia, which used patients with dementia of moderate severity, found that distractability, perplexity, disorientation, speech defects, and long-term memory[102] were worse in the Alzheimer group, while on 10 other measures of behavioral disturbance, there were no differences between the two groups.

THE EPIDEMIOLOGY OF VASCULAR DEMENTIA

Dementia from all causes affects about 8 percent of the population over the age of 65; between 9 and 39 percent of these dementias are of vascular origin[103,104] and an additional 11 to 43 percent may be mixed dementia.[104] The prevalence of vascular dementia varies considerably, from 0 to 2 percent in the 60 to 69 age group and up to 16 percent for males aged 80 to 89, though more typical figures are between 3 and 6 percent.[105] As a proportion of cases of dementia, one study in men and women aged 60 to 79 suggested figures of 13.6 and 12 percent respectively, falling to 4.8 and 7 percent at age 80 to 89.[105] A more recent study suggested that vascular dementia accounted for 47 percent of cases of dementia in 85-year-olds and that the overall prevalence of vascular dementia was 14 percent at that age.[106] Males are more commonly affected than females in most but not all studies.[41,104,105,107] Vascular dementia may account for 56 percent of dementia in Japan.[108] After stroke, the incidence of dementia may be as high as 26 percent[20,39] though exclusion of possible preexisting cases of Alzheimer disease reduces this to 16.3 percent,[20,22] and blacks may be at greater risk than whites.[20] The risk increases with age, from 14.8 percent in those aged 60 to 69 to 52.3 percent for those over 80, but 36.4 percent of these individuals were felt to have both Alzheimer disease and the sequelae of stroke.[20]

RISK FACTORS FOR VASCULAR DEMENTIA

Little consistent information exists regarding risk factors, differences arising because of varying populations and definitions. It is not clear whether the risk factors for vascular dementia are the same as those for stroke or not. As vascular dementia may be more often due to small vessel disease than stroke in general, hypertension may be a disproportionate risk factor for vascular dementia but this remains an unproven hypothesis. One study identified hypertension, heart disease, diabetes, hyperlipidaemia, smoking, and carotid bruits but not alcohol consumption as risk factors for multi-infarct dementia compared to normal controls[41] suggesting much similarity with stroke. Other studies have identified hypertension, age, male sex, education, race, prior stroke, diabetes, cardiac disease, ECG changes, hematocrit, smoking, history of myocardial infarction, and proteinuria.[33,34,38,39,107,108] The same studies have often yielded negative results for many other common stroke risk factors,[39,107] including cardiac disease, increased viscosity, and fibrinogen in one[38] and obesity, cholesterol, alcohol, cigarettes, and glucose intolerance in another based in Japan.[108] In-

terestingly, a study comparing elderly blacks with and without multi-infarct dementia who had been hospitalized for cerebral infarction found that elevated systolic blood pressure and obesity were protective.[107] The authors suggest that protection by elevated systolic blood pressure may be a true finding because the suggestion that a window of systolic blood pressure exists, below which cognition declines.[109] However, the finding has not been replicated, is unexpected and contradicts such other evidence as is available.

DIFFERENTIAL DIAGNOSIS OF VASCULAR DEMENTIA

The principal differential diagnosis is from Alzheimer disease. In 90 percent of cases where multiple infarcts are responsible, there is also a history of stroke or of transient ischemic attacks. The use of the ischemia scale score, classifying those with a score of 4 or less as Alzheimer, will correctly diagnose dementia due to Alzheimer disease in 87 percent of cases on the clinical findings alone. Scores of over 7 suggest a vascular etiology, though distinguishing between vascular and mixed cases is unreliable using the ischemia score alone. The use of CT to identify infarcts increases diagnostic accuracy. Of at least equal importance to the identification of vascular dementia itself is identification of the cause of the vascular events, as it is upon these that the treatment and prognosis depend. Binswanger disease is a subtype of vascular dementia. The remainder of the differential diagnosis is that of dementia.

THE INVESTIGATION OF VASCULAR DEMENTIA

The clinical history and examination alone can identify dementia. The examination should include an assessment for depression, as depression is both a common cause of pseudodementia and treatable. Imaging is required to confirm the occurrence of infarction and to exclude structural causes. While MRI will better show leukoaraiosis and may be essential if certain conditions such as

CADASIL[110–112] are suspected, CT is sufficient in routine clinical practice. The presence of white matter lesions on CT (but not on MRI) may help to distinguish vascular dementia from Alzheimer disease.[113,114] Cortical sulcal atrophy and left ventricular enlargement are more severe in patients with multiple infarcts and dementia than in those with multiple infarcts without dementia,[34] but there is no evidence to suggest that this is sufficiently discriminating to be a useful part of the evaluation. Syphilis and human immunodeficiency virus (HIV) serology are necessary, and thyroid function, vitamin B_{12}, and red cell folic acid levels are needed to exclude abnormalities in these as possible causes of cognitive decline.

The vascular component of the investigations should be directed by clinical suspicion. Not all investigations are routinely required. However, a complete blood count, erythrocyte sedimentation rate, blood glucose test, and electrocardiogram should be obtained. Where appropriate, carotid duplex Doppler, chest x-ray, echocardiography, Holter monitoring, coagulation screen, lipid profile, lupus anticoagulant, anticardiolipin antibodies,[115] and autoantibody screen are justifiable. A glycosylated hemoglobin may detect unsuspected diabetes.[116] Cerebral angiography is indicated if carotid surgery is considered or to demonstrate beading of the smaller cerebral vessels if a cerebral vasculitis is suspected, but it is not a routine investigation. Examination of the cerebrospinal fluid may be required if an infectious or inflammatory etiology is suspected; also, rarely, may be dural or brain biopsy may be called for.

A number of investigations have been proposed as being useful in the diagnosis of multi-infarct dementia. Focal abnormalities on electroencephalography favor multi-infarct dementia[117,118] but are a poor discriminator. Intracranial hemodynamics may help distinguish multi-infarct dementia from Alzheimer disease and normal subjects,[119] but this has not been confirmed. Single photon emission computed tomography demonstrates more perfusion defects in Alzheimer disease than in multi-infarct dementia[120–122] but has not been assessed as a discriminatory test. These investigations are not recommended.

THE PREVENTION AND TREATMENT OF VASCULAR DEMENTIA

There is no good information regarding the prevention and treatment of vascular dementia as distinct from stroke. No satisfactory trials have been done. Aspirin has been proposed on the basis of a pilot study done without placebo,[123] and in a small uncontrolled, unblinded study, cessation of cigarette smoking was suggested along with lowering blood pressure to a window of 135 to 150 mmHg. Reductions below a systolic of 135 mmHg were detrimental.[109] Cessation of smoking[124] and control of blood pressure[125] increase cerebral blood flow, but the implications of these observations for therapy are unclear. At present, therefore, the medical management of vascular dementia is the management of stroke and risk factors for stroke, while the social, economic, and legal management is similar to that for Alzheimer disease.

THE PROGNOSIS OF VASCULAR DEMENTIA

Multi-infarct dementia shortens life expectancy[126] to about 50 percent of normal at 4 years from initial evaluation,[127,128] though females, those with higher education, and those who perform well on some neuropsychological tests do better.[127] In the very elderly, 3-year mortality may reach two-thirds, almost three times that of controls;[106] in one study, the 6-year survival was only 11.9 percent, about a quarter of that expected,[129] though many of these patients were elderly and severely demented at entry. About one-third die from complications of the dementia itself, one-third from cerebrovascular disease, 8 percent from other cardiovascular disease, and the rest from miscellaneous causes, including malignancy.[129]

CONCLUSION

Vascular disease is a common cause of dementia, but despite this, relatively little is known about it. The lack of knowledge is partially due to the use of inappropriate criteria for the diagnosis of vascular dementia, which has resulted in the selection and study of what it is likely to prove to be a subset of all the vascular dementias, selecting only more advanced cases and those in which memory loss is a prominent feature. The data that exist show frontal dysfunction and a subcortical pattern of dementia to be the most prominent characteristics of the cognitive deficits seen when vascular dementia is treated as a single entity. Memory is affected, but this is not a preeminent feature. Depression, apathy, perseveration, and incontinence have been identified as common behavioral changes in vascular dementia, but it must be borne in mind that the criteria used to diagnose vascular dementia specify similar deficits, and some part of the findings may ultimately prove to be tautological when cases of vascular dementia are studied in a more open fashion without the use of the current criteria, which are not supported by independent evidence.

REFERENCES

1. The World Health Organization: *The ICD-10 Classification of Mental and Behavioural Disorders. Diagnostic Criteria for Research.* Geneva: World Health Organization, 1993.

2. The American Psychiatric Association: *Diagnostic and Statistical Manual of Mental Disorders,* 4th ed. Washington, DC: American Psychiatric Association, 1994.

3. Hachinski VC, Lassen NA, Marshall J: Multi-infarct dementia: A cause of mental deterioration in the elderly. *Lancet* 2:207–209, 1974.

4. Hachinski VC, Iliff LD, Zilkha E, et al: Cerebral blood flow in dementia. *Arch Neurol* 32:632–637, 1975.

5. Wade JPH, Mirsen T, Hachinski VC, et al: The clinical diagnosis of Alzheimer's disease. *Arch Neurol* 44:24–29, 1987.

6. Roman GC, Tatemichi TK, Erkinjuntti T, et al: Vascular dementia: Diagnostic criteria for research studies. Report of the NINDS-AIREN international workshop. *Neurology* 43:250–260, 1993.

7. del Ser T, Bermejo F, Portera A, et al: Vascular dementia: A clinicopathological study. *J Neurol Sci* 96:1–17, 1990.

8. Hachinski VC: Preventable senility: A call for action against the vascular dementias. *Lancet* 340:645–647, 1992.

9. Chui HC, Victoroff JI, Margolin D, et al: Criteria for the diagnosis of ischemic vascular dementia proposed by the State of California Alzheimer's Disease Diagnostic and Treatment Centers. *Neurology* 42:473–480, 1992.

10. Kinkel WR, Jacobs L, Polachini I, et al: Subcortical arteriosclerotic encephalopathy (Binswanger's disease): Computed tomographic, nuclear magnetic resonance, and clinical correlations. *Arch Neurol* 42:951–959, 1985.

11. Perez FI, Gay JR, Taylor RL: WAIS performance of neurologically impaired aged. *Psychol Rep* 37:1043–1047, 1975.

12. Perez FI, Gay JR, Taylor RL, Rivera VM: Patterns of memory performance in the neurologically impaired aged. *Can J Neurol Sci* 2:347–355, 1975.

13. Perez FI, Rivera VM, Meyer JS, et al: Analysis of intellectual and cognitive performance in patients with multi-infarct dementia, vertebrobasilar insufficiency with dementia, and Alzheimer's disease. *J Neurol Neurosurg Psychiatry* 38:533–540, 1975.

14. Wade DT, Parker V, Langton Hewer R: Memory disturbance after stroke: Frequency and associated losses. *Int Rehabil Med* 8:60–64, 1986.

15. Wade DT, Wood VA, Hewer RL: Recovery of cognitive function soon after stroke: A study of visual neglect, attention span and verbal recall. *J Neurol Neurosurg Psychiatry* 51:10–13, 1988.

16. Wolfe N, Linn R, Babikian VL, et al: Frontal systems impairment following multiple lacunar infarcts. *Arch Neurol* 47:129–132, 1990.

17. Babikian VL, Wolfe N, Linn R, et al: Cognitive changes in patients with multiple cerebral infarcts. *Stroke* 21:1013–1018, 1990.

18. Hom J, Reitan RM: Generalized cognitive function after stroke. *J Clin Exp Neuropsychol* 12:644–654, 1990.

19. Pujol J, Junque C, Vendrell P, et al: Cognitive correlates of ventricular enlargement in vascular patients with leukoaraiosis. *Acta Neurol Scand* 84:237–242, 1991.

20. Tatemichi TK, Desmond DW, Mayeux R, et al: Dementia after stroke: Baseline frequency, risks, and clinical features in a hospitalized cohort. *Neurology* 42:1185–1193, 1992.

21. Villardita C: Alzheimer's disease compared with cerebrovascular dementia: Neuropsychological

similarities and differences. *Acta Neurol Scand* 87:299–308, 1993.

22. Tatemichi TK, Desmond DW, Stern Y, et al: Cognitive impairment after stroke: Frequency, patterns, and relationship to functional abilities. *J Neurol Neurosurg Psychiatry* 57:202–207, 1994.

23. Bowler JV, Hadar U, Wade JPH: Cognition in stroke. *Acta Neurol Scand* 90:424–429, 1994.

24. Corbett A, Bennett H, Kos S: Cognitive dysfunction following subcortical infarction. *Arch Neurol* 51:999–1007, 1994.

25. Breteler MM, van Amerongen NM, van Swieten JC, et al: Cognitive correlates of ventricular enlargement and cerebral white matter lesions on magnetic resonance imaging: The Rotterdam Study. *Stroke* 25:1109–1115, 1994.

26. Breteler MMB, van Swieten JC, Bots ML, et al: Cerebral white matter lesions, vascular risk factors, and cognitive function in a population-based study: The Rotterdam Study. *Neurology* 44:1246–1252, 1994.

27. Hachinski VC: The decline and resurgence of vascular dementia. *Can Med Assoc J* 142:107–111, 1990.

28. Hachinski VC: Multi-infarct dementia: A reappraisal. *Alzheimer Dis Assoc Disord* 5:64–68, 1991.

29. Hachinski VC, Bowler JV: Vascular dementia. *Neurology* 43:2159–2160, 1993.

30. Erkinjuntti T, Hachinski VC: Rethinking vascular dementia. *Cerebrovasc Dis* 3:3–23, 1993.

31. Tomlinson BE, Blessed G, Roth M: Observations on the brains of demented old people. *J Neurol Sci* 11:205–242, 1970.

32. Erkinjuntti T, Haltia M, Palo J, et al: Accuracy of the clinical diagnosis of vascular dementia: A prospective clinical and post-mortem neuropathological study. *J Neurol Neurosurg Psychiatry* 51:1037–1044, 1988.

33. Loeb C, Gandolfo C, Bino G: Intellectual impairment and cerebral lesions in multiple cerebral infarcts: A clinical-computed tomography study. *Stroke* 19:560–565, 1988.

34. Gorelick PB, Chatterjee A, Patel D, et al: Cranial computed tomographic observations in multi-infarct dementia: A controlled study. *Stroke* 23:804–811, 1992.

35. Liu CK, Miller BL, Cummings JL, et al: A quantitative MRI study of vascular dementia. *Neurology* 42:138–143, 1992.

36. Bowler JV: Cerebral infarction and ^{99}Tc^m HMPAO *SPECT,* MD Thesis. University of London, 1993.

37. Hijdra A: Vascular dementia, in Bradley WG, Daroff RB, Fenichel GM, Marsden CD (eds): *Neurology in Clinical Practice.* Boston: Butterworth-Heinemann, 1991, pp 1425–1435.

38. Ladurner G, Iliff LD, Lechner H: Clinical factors associated with dementia in ischaemic stroke. *J Neurol Neurosurg Psychiatry* 45:97–101, 1982.

39. Tatemichi TK, Desmond DW, Paik M, et al: Clinical determinants of dementia related to stroke. *Ann Neurol* 33:568–575, 1993.

40. Fukuda H, Kobayashi S, Okada K, Tsunematsu T: Frontal white matter lesions and dementia in lacunar infarction. *Stroke* 21:1143–1149, 1990.

41. Meyer JS, McClintic KL, Rogers RL, et al: Aetiological considerations and risk factors for multi-infarct dementia. *J Neurol Neurosurg Psychiatry* 51:1489–1497, 1988.

42. Meyer JS, Rogers RL, Mortel KF: Multi-infarct dementia: demography, risk factors and therapy, in Ginsberg MD, Dietrich WD (eds): *Cerebrovascular Diseases: Sixteenth Research (Princeton) Conference.* New York: Raven Press, 1989, pp 199–206.

43. Parnetti L, Mecocci P, Santucci C, et al: Is multi-infarct dementia representative of vascular dementias? A retrospective study. *Acta Neurol Scand* 81:484–487, 1990.

44. Fisher CM: Lacunes: Small, deep cerebral infarcts. *Neurology* 15:774–784, 1965.

45. Miyao S, Takano A, Teramoto J, Takahashi A: Leukoaraiosis in relation to prognosis for patients with lacunar infarction. *Stroke* 23:1434–1438, 1992.

46. Lassen NA: Incomplete cerebral infarction—Focal incomplete ischaemic tissue necrosis not leading to emollision. *Stroke* 13:522–523, 1982.

47. Cummings JL, Benson DF: Subcortical dementia: Review of an emerging concept. *Arch Neurol* 41:874–879, 1984.

48. Steingart A, Hachinski VC, Lau C, et al: Cognitive and neurologic findings in subjects with diffuse white matter lucencies on computed tomographic scan (leukoaraiosis). *Arch Neurol* 44:32–35, 1987.

49. Goto K, Ishii N, Fukasawa H: Diffuse white matter disease in the geriatric population: A clinical, neuropathological and CT study. *Radiology* 141:687–695, 1989.

50. Kertesz A, Polk M, Carr T: Cognition and white matter changes on magnetic resonance imaging in dementia. *Arch Neurol* 47:387–391, 1990.

51. Bowen BC, Barker WW, Loewenstein DA, et al:

MR signal abnormalities in memory disorder and dementia. *Am J Neuroradiol* 11:283–290, 1990.

52. Diaz JF, Merskey H, Hachinski VC, et al: Improved recognition of leukoaraiosis and cognitive impairment in Alzheimer's disease. *Arch Neurol* 48:1022–1025, 1991.

53. Wahlund LO, Andersson Lundman G, Julin P, et al: Quantitative estimation of brain white matter abnormalities in elderly subjects using magnetic resonance imaging. *Magn Reson Imaging* 10:859–865, 1992.

54. Almkvist O, Wahlund L, Andersson-Lundman G, et al: White-matter hyperintensity and neuropsychological functions in dementia and healthy aging. *Arch Neurol* 49:626–632, 1992.

55. Skoog I, Berg S, Johansson B, et al: The influence of white matter lesions on neuropsychological functioning in demented and non-demented 85 year olds, in Skoog I (ed): *Mental Disorders in the Elderly: A Population Study in 85-Year-Olds.* Göteborg: University of Göteborg, 1993.

56. Steingart A, Hachinski VC, Lau C, et al: Cognitive and neurologic findings in demented patients with diffuse white matter lucencies on computed tomographic scan (leukoaraiosis). *Arch Neurol* 44:36–39, 1987.

57. Skoog I, Palmertz B, Andreasson L: The prevalence of white matter lesions on computed tomography of the brain in demented and non-demented 85 year olds. *J Geriatr Psychiatry Neurol* 7:169–175, 1994.

58. Hunt AL, Orrison WW, Yeo RA, et al: Clinical significance of MRI white matter lesions in the elderly. *Neurology* 39:1470–1474, 1989.

59. Tupler LA, Coffey CE, Logue PE, et al: Neuropsychological importance of subcortical white matter hyperintensity. *Arch Neurol* 49:1248–1252, 1992.

60. Hershey LA, Modic MT, Greenough PG, Jaffe DF: Magnetic resonance imaging in vascular dementia. *Neurology* 37:29–36, 1987.

61. Rao SM, Mittenberg W, Bernardin L, Haughton V, Leo GJ: Neuropsychological test findings in subjects with leukoaraiosis. *Arch Neurol* 46:40–44, 1989.

62. Mirsen TR, Lee DH, Wong CJ, et al: Clinical correlates of white-matter changes on magnetic resonance imaging scans of the brain. *Arch Neurol* 48:1015–1021, 1991.

63. Erkinjuntti T, Gao F, Lee DH, et al: Lack of difference in brain hyperintensities between patients with early Alzheimer's disease and control subjects. *Arch Neurol* 51:260–268, 1994.

64. Hachinski VC: Multi-infarct dementia. *Neurol Clin* 1:27–36, 1983.

65. Wolfe N, Babikian VL, Linn RT, et al: Are multiple cerebral infarcts synergistic? *Arch Neurol* 51:211–215, 1994.

66. Mesulam M: Large-scale neurocognitive networks and distributed processing for attention, language and memory. *Ann Neurol* 28:597–613, 1990.

67. Fillenbaum GG, Heyman A, Wilkinson WE, Haynes CS: Comparison of two screening tests in Alzheimer's disease: The correlation and reliability of the mini-mental state examination and modified Blessed test. *Arch Neurol* 44:924–927, 1987.

68. Brandt J, Welsh KA, Breitner JCS, et al: Hereditary influences on cognitive functioning in older men: A study of 4000 twin pairs. *Arch Neurol* 50:599–603, 1993

69. D'Antona R, Baron JC, Pantano P, et al: Effects of thalamic lesions on cerebral cortex metabolism in humans. *J Cereb Blood Flow Metab* 5(suppl 1):S457–S458, 1985.

70. Dobkin JA, Levine RL, Lagreze HL, et al: Evidence for transhemispheric diaschisis in unilateral stroke. *Arch Neurol* 46:1333–1336, 1989.

71. Szelies B, Herholz K, Pawlik G, et al: Widespread functional effects of discrete thalamic infarction. *Arch Neurol* 48:178–182, 1991.

72. Baron JC, Levasseur M, Mazoyer B, et al: Thalamocortical diaschisis: Positron emission tomography in humans. *J Neurol Neurosurg Psychiatry* 55:935–942, 1992.

73. Bowler JV, Wade JPH: Ipsilateral cerebellar diaschisis following pontine infarction. *Cerebrovasc Dis* 1:58–60, 1991.

74. Bowler JV, Costa DC, Jones BE, et al: High resolution SPECT, small deep infarcts and diaschisis. *J R Soc Med* 85:142–146, 1992.

75. Bowler JV, Wade JPH, Jones BE, et al: The contribution of diaschisis to the clinical deficit in human cerebral infarction. *Stroke* 26:1000–1006, 1995.

76. Olszewski J: Subcortical arteriosclerotic encephalopathy: Review of the literature on the so-called Binswanger's disease and presentation of two cases. *World Neurol* 3:359–375, 1962.

77. Babikian V, Ropper AH: Binswanger's disease: A review. *Stroke* 18:2–12, 1987.

78. Hachinski VC, Potter P, Merskey H: Leuko-araiosis. *Arch Neurol* 44:21–23, 1987.

79. Bennett DA, Wilson RS, Gilley DW, Fox JH: Clin-

ical diagnosis of Binswanger's disease. *J Neurol Neurosurg Psychiatry* 53:961–965, 1990.

80. Loizou LA, Kendall BE, Marshall J: Subcortical arteriosclerotic encephalopathy: A clinical and radiological investigation. *J Neurol Neurosurg Psychiatry* 44:294–304, 1981.

81. Caplan LR, Schoene WC: Clinical features of subcortical arteriosclerotic encephalopathy (Binswanger disease). *Neurology* 28:1206–1215, 1978.

82. Thompson PD, Marsden CD: Gait disorder of subcortical arteriosclerotic encephalopathy: Binswanger's disease. *Move Disord* 2:1–8, 1987.

83. Delong GR, Kemper TL, Pogacar S, Lee HY: Clinical neuropathological conference. *Dis Nerv Syst* 35:286–291, 1974.

84. Burger PC, Burch JG, Kunze U: Subcortical arteriosclerotic encephalopathy (Binswanger's disease): A vascular etiology of dementia. *Stroke* 7:626–631, 1976.

85. The Canadian Study of Health and Aging Working Group: The Canadian study of health and aging: study methods and prevalence of dementia. *Can Med Assoc J* 150:899–913, 1994.

86. Folstein MF, Folstein SE, McHugh PR: "Mini-mental state": A practical method for grading the cognitive state of patients for the clinician. *J Psychiatr Res* 12:189–198, 1975.

87. Baldy-Moulinier M, Valmier J, Touchon J, et al: Clinical and neuropsychological rating scales for differential diagnosis of dementias. *Gerontology* 32(suppl 1):89–97, 1986.

88. Hier DB, Hagenlocker K, Shindler AG: Language disintegration in dementia: Effects of etiology and severity. *Brain Lang* 25:117–133, 1985.

89. Carlesimo GA, Fadda L, Bonci A, Caltagirone C: Differential rates of forgetting from long-term memory in Alzheimer's and multi-infarct dementia. *Int J Neurosci* 73:1–11, 1993.

90. Gainotti G, Parlato V, Monteleone D, Carlomagno S: Neuropsychological markers of dementia on visual-spatial tasks: A comparison between Alzheimer's type and vascular forms of dementia. *J Clin Exp Neuropsychol* 14:239–252, 1992.

91. Muramoto O: Selective reminding in normal and demented aged people: Auditory verbal versus visual spatial task. *Cortex* 20:461–478, 1984.

92. Kertesz A, Clydesdale S: Neuropsychological deficits in vascular dementia vs Alzheimer's disease. Frontal lobe deficits prominent in vascular dementia. *Arch Neurol* 51:1226–1231, 1994.

93. Almkvist O, Backman L, Basun H, Wahlund LO: Patterns of neuropsychological performance in Alzheimer's disease and vascular dementia. *Cortex* 29:661–673, 1993.

94. Shuttleworth EC, Huber SJ: The picture absurdities test in the evaluation of dementia. *Brain Cogn* 11:50–59, 1989.

95. Erkinjuntti T: Differential diagnosis between Alzheimer's disease and vascular dementia: Evaluation of common clinical methods. *Acta Neurol Scand* 76:433–442, 1987.

96. Erkinjuntti T, Laaksonen R, Sulkava R, et al: Neuropsychological differentiation between normal aging, Alzheimer's disease and vascular dementia. *Acta Neurol Scand* 74:393–403, 1986.

97. Fischer P, Gatterer G, Marterer A, Danielczyk W: Nonspecificity of semantic impairment in dementia of Alzheimer's type. *Arch Neurol* 45:1341–1343, 1988.

98. Ricker JH, Keenan PA, Jacobson MW: Visuoperceptual-spatial ability and visual memory in vascular dementia and dementia of the Alzheimer type. *Neuropsychologia* 32:1287–1296, 1994.

99. Kontiola P, Laaksonen R, Sulkava R, Erkinjuntti T: Pattern of language impairment is different in Alzheimer's disease and multi-infarct dementia. *Brain Lang* 38:364–383, 1990.

100. Powell AL, Cummings JL, Hill MA, Benson DF: Speech and language alterations in multi-infarct dementia. *Neurology* 38:717–719, 1988.

101. Cummings JL, Miller B, Hill MA, Neshkes R: Neuropsychiatric aspects of multi-infarct dementia and dementia of the Alzheimer type. *Arch Neurol* 44:389–393, 1987.

102. Bucht G, Adolfsson R: The Comprehensive Psychopathological Rating Scale in patients with dementia of Alzheimer type and multiinfarct dementia. *Psychiatr Scand* 68:263–270, 1983.

103. Kase CS, Wolf PA, Bachman DL, et al: Dementia and stroke: The Framingham study, in Ginsberg MD, Dietrich WD (eds): *Cerebrovascular Diseases: Sixteenth Research (Princeton) Conference.* New York: Raven Press, 1989, pp 193–197.

104. Kase CS: Epidemiology of multi-infarct dementia. *Alz Dis Assoc Disord* 5:71–76, 1991.

105. Rocca WA, Hofman A, Brayne C, et al: The prevalence of vascular dementia in Europe: Facts and fragments from 1980–1990 studies. EURODEM-Prevalence Research Group. *Ann Neurol* 30:817–824, 1991.

106. Skoog I, Nilsson L, Palmertz B, et al: A population-

based study of dementia in 85-year-olds. *N Engl J Med* 328:153–158, 1993.

107. Gorelick PB, Brody J, Cohen D, et al: Risk factors for dementia associated with multiple cerebral infarcts: A case-control analysis in predominantly African-American hospital-based patients. *Arch Neurol* 50:714–720, 1993.

108. Ueda K, Kawano H, Hasuo Y, Fujishima M: Prevalence and etiology of dementia in a Japanese community. *Stroke* 23:798–803, 1992.

109. Meyer JS, Judd BW, Tawaklna T, et al: Improved cognition after control of risk factors for multi-infarct dementia. *JAMA* 256:2203–2209, 1986.

110. Bousser MG, Lasserve ET: Summary of the proceedings of the first international workshop on CADASIL. *Stroke* 25:704–707, 1994.

111. Bowler JV, Hachinski VC: Progress in the genetics of cerebrovascular disease: Inherited subcortical arteriopathies. *Stroke* 25:1696–1698, 1994.

112. Tournier Lasserve E, Joutel A, et al: Cerebral autosomal dominant arteriopathy with subcortical infarcts and leukoencephalopathy maps to chromosome 19q12. *Nature Genet* 3:256–259, 1993.

113. Erkinjuntti T, Ketonen L, Sulkava R, et al: Do white matter changes on MRI and CT differentiate vascular dementia from Alzheimer's disease? *J Neurol Neurosurg Psychiatry* 50:37–42, 1987.

114. Erkinjuntti T, Ketonen L, Sulkava R, et al: CT in the differential diagnosis between Alzheimer's disease and vascular dementia. *Acta Neurol Scand* 75:262–270, 1987.

115. Coull BM, Bourdette DN, Goodnight SH Jr, et al: Multiple cerebral infarctions and dementia associated with anticardiolipin antibodies. *Stroke* 18:1107–1112, 1987.

116. Riddle MC, Hart J: Hyperglycemia, recognized and unrecognized, as a risk factor for stroke and transient ischemic attacks. *Stroke* 13:356–359, 1982.

117. Erkinjuntti T, Larsen T, Sulkava R, et al: EEG in the differential diagnosis between Alzheimer's disease and vascular dementia. *Acta Neurol Scand* 77:36–43, 1988.

118. Leuchter AF, Newton TF, Cook IA, et al: Changes in brain functional connectivity in Alzheimer-type and multi-infarct dementia. *Brain* 115:1543–1561, 1992.

119. Ries F, Horn R, Hillekamp J, et al: Differentiation of multi-infarct and Alzheimer dementia by intracranial hemodynamic parameters. *Stroke* 24:228–235, 1993.

120. Smith FW, Besson JA, Gemmell HG, Sharp PF: The use of technetium-99m-HM-PAO in the assessment of patients with dementia and other neuropsychiatric conditions. *J Cereb Blood Flow Metab* 8:S116–S122, 1988.

121. Neary D, Snowden JS, Shields RA, et al: Single photon emission tomography using 99mTc-HM-PAO in the investigation of dementia. *J Neurol Neurosurg Psychiatry* 50:1101–1109, 1987.

122. Launes J, Sulkava R, Erkinjuntti T, et al: 99Tcm-HMPAO SPECT in suspected dementia. *Nucl Med Comm* 12:757–765, 1991.

123. Meyer JS, Rogers RL, McClintic K, et al: Randomized clinical trial of daily aspirin therapy in multi-infarct dementia: A pilot study. *J Am Geriatr Soc* 37:549–555, 1989.

124. Rogers RL, Meyer JS, Judd BW, Mortel KF: Abstention from cigarette smoking improves cerebral perfusion among elderly chronic smokers. *JAMA* 253:2970–2974, 1985.

125. Meyer JS, Rogers RL, Mortel KF: Prospective analysis of long term control of mild hypertension on cerebral blood flow. *Stroke* 16:985–990, 1985.

126. Martin DC, Miller JK, Kapoor W, et al: A controlled study of survival with dementia. *Arch Neurol* 44:1122–1126, 1987.

127. Hier DB, Warach JD, Gorelick PB, Thomas J: Predictors of survival in clinically diagnosed Alzheimer's disease and multi-infarct dementia. *Arch Neurol* 46:1213–1216, 1989.

128. Barclay LL, Zemcov A, Blass JP, Sansone J: Survival in Alzheimer's disease and vascular dementias. *Neurology* 35:834–840, 1985.

129. Molsa PK, Marttila RJ, Rinne UK: Survival and cause of death in Alzheimer's disease and multi-infarct dementia. *Acta Neurol Scand* 74:103–107, 1986.

Chapter 47

INFECTIOUS CAUSES OF DEMENTIA INCLUDING HUMAN IMMUNODEFICIENCY VIRUS

John J. Sidtis
Richard W. Price

A consideration of the infectious causes of dementia, especially the dementia associated with the human immunodeficiency virus type 1 (HIV-1), provides an opportunity to address several issues—namely, the concept of dementia and pathophysiologic mechanisms at the cellular and metabolic levels.[1,2] The term *dementia* has widely become synonymous with Alzheimer disease; consequently, memory loss is often viewed as the most prominent feature of any dementia. The AIDS dementia complex (ADC) has provided a compelling reminder that the broader definition of dementia characterizes this condition as the sustained, chronic, progressive loss of acquired intellectual function. This broader definition is certainly better suited for the range of behavioral changes constituting the dementias that can accompany infectious processes. Although the pathophysiologic mechanisms underlying ADC are not yet understood, the possible factors suggest several processes that may produce a dementia in an infected brain. Finally, studies of cerebral metabolism in ADC illustrate a systems-level pathophysiology that is not likely to be unique to this condition.

PRESENTATION OF THE AIDS DEMENTIA COMPLEX

Although the dementia associated with advanced HIV infection has been referred to in various ways, the term *AIDS dementia complex* retains its value as a descriptor. The designation *AIDS* was chosen to represent association with a syndrome that occurs at the later stages of HIV-1 infection, when the dementia is most likely to occur. The term *dementia* was chosen to indicate the loss of intellectual function, and the term *complex* was included to convey the fact that the syndrome typically consists of generalized cognitive slowing, diminished motor control, and behavioral changes. Because of these features, ADC has often been classified among the subcortical dementias.[1] At the early stages, the ADC patient characteristically complains of lapses in concentration, increased difficulty in performing tasks that were once routine, forgetfulness, difficulty walking, diminished legibility in handwriting, loss of interest in daily activities, and social withdrawal. In contrast to the dementia of Alzheimer disease, early ADC does not present primarily as an amnestic disorder, and insight into personal capacity is generally well maintained. Further, cognitive and motor slowing commonly occur in tandem.

The AIDS dementia complex progresses to a state in which the patient has significant functional impairment in the activities of daily living as a result of intellectual impairment. Basic self-care can be maintained for a time, but this too is lost as the disease progresses. Motor function is similarly progressively affected. At the final stage, the ADC patient is nearly vegetative, with only rudimentary intellectual function.[3,4] The staging scheme for ADC is presented in Table 47-1.

Table 47-1

Staging scheme for the AIDS dementia complex (ADC)[a]

ADC stage	Characteristics
Stage 0 (normal)	Normal mental and motor function.
Stage 0.5 (equivocal/subclinical)	Either minimal or equivocal *symptoms* of cognitive or motor dysfunction characteristic of ADC or mild signs (snout response, slowed extremity movements) but *without impairment of work or capacity to perform activities of daily living* (ADL). Gait and strength are normal.
Stage 1 (mild)	Unequivocal evidence (symptoms, signs, neuropsychological test performance) of functional, intellectual, or motor impairment characteristic of ADC but able to perform *all but the more demanding aspects of work or ADL.* Can walk without assistance.
Stage 2 (moderate)	Cannot work or maintain the more demanding aspects of daily life but able to perform *basic activities of self-care.* Ambulatory but may require a single prop.
Stage 3 (severe)	*Major intellectual incapacity* (cannot follow news or personal events, cannot sustain complex conversation, considerable slowing of all output), *or motor disability* (cannot walk unassisted, requiring walker or personal support, usually with slowing and clumsiness of arms as well).
Stage 4 (end stage)	*Nearly vegetative.* Intellectual and social comprehension and responses are at a rudimentary level. Nearly or absolutely mute. Paraparetic or paraplegic with double incontinence.

[a]Stages 1 through 4 of the ADC are reserved for unequivocal abnormalities that impair the patient's functional capacity. Stage 0.5 is reserved for patients with minor symptoms or "soft" signs, for whom ADC must be considered subclinical or equivocal.[3,4]

NEUROPATHOGENESIS OF THE AIDS DEMENTIA COMPLEX

The neuropathogenesis of ADC is not fully understood, but it likely involves a temporally evolving, dynamic interaction among three components: the virus, the immune system, and the central nervous system.[2,4] In this model, the virus is the primary agonist and initiator of the pathologic process underlying ADC, while the immune system serves as both defender and secondary agonist through its capacity to produce immunopathology. The target of both primary and secondary pathologic processes is the central nervous system. The immune system is affected by HIV-1 through both immunosuppression and immune activation. The immune system affects HIV-1 infection by initially controlling viral replication and contributing to the selection of virus variants. Both HIV-1 and the immune system act on the central nervous system through infection, elaboration of virus-coded neurotoxins, and stimulation of cell-coded neurotoxins. Over time, the immune system loses control of viral replication and virus variants with altered cell tropism and virulence emerge.

PATHOPHYSIOLOGY OF THE AIDS DEMENTIA COMPLEX AT THE SYSTEMS LEVEL

The pathogenetic model outlined above can be placed in the context of systems-level pathology to better appreciate the processes involved in ADC. Immunohistochemical methods detect viral antigen in macrophages, microglia, and derivative multinucleated cells. Further, the distribution of infected cells preferentially involves deep brain structures, especially the basal ganglia and the central white matter.[5] Further insight into how infectious processes in deep gray nuclei and central white matter result in ADC is suggested by neuroimaging studies. Patterns of regional cerebral metabolism, as measured using positron emission tomography (PET), suggest a temporal evolution of metabolic pathology. At the earlier stages of ADC, cerebral metabolism is notable for relative subcortical hypermetabolism. The subcortical changes are associated with a broader pattern of altered metabolism involving multiple cortical regions as well. As the disease progresses to end stage, the metabolic pattern shifts to increasing global hypometabolism.[5,7]

At the systems level, then, ADC represents a situation in which infection largely restricted to subcortical areas has widespread and significant effects on cerebral metabolism. As in the model of pathogenesis at the cellular level, where the pathogenetic process is likely multifactorial, the systems-level changes in ADC appear to represent primary and secondary pathologic alterations.

INFECTION AND DEMENTIA DUE TO HUMAN IMMUNODEFICIENCY VIRUS TYPE 1

Although the above discussions represent only a brief sketch of the clinical and pathophysiologic features of ADC, they should serve to illustrate some of the general features that are likely to be relevant, in varying degrees, to other infectious processes resulting in dementia. Pathogenesis is likely to represent the effects of both infection and host response, and even localized areas of pathology are likely to produce secondary metabolic abnormalities in areas remote from the primary process. Both factors will contribute to the clinical syndrome.

OTHER VIRAL INFECTIOUS CAUSES OF DEMENTIA

Detailed reviews of other viral causes of dementia are beyond the scope of this chapter, but the major infectious processes that can result in a dementia are briefly reviewed. More detailed discussions of viral infections of the central nervous system can be found elsewhere.[8]

Herpes simplex encephalitis is a common form of viral infection of the central nervous system. There is a bimodal age predilection with heightened incidence in young adults and older individuals, but there is no gender preference in this infection. Patients typically experience headache and fever initially, with symptoms evolving over hours to days. Confusion and personality change progress to a focal encephalopathy with altered cognition and a decreasing level of consciousness. Findings include cerebral spinal fluid pleocytosis and proteinosis, abnormal electroencephalogram (EEG), and medial temporal lobe or orbital frontal lobe abnormalities on neuroimaging. The most definitive means of diagnosis is brain biopsy. After the acute phase, the patient can be left with global dementia or an amnestic syndrome.[9,10]

Progressive multifocal leukoencephalopathy (PML) is a disease that develops in immunocompromised patients. Apart from patients with AIDS, it tends to be a disease of later life. The evolution of neurologic symptoms occurs over days to weeks. The most common symptoms at onset relate to focal brain affliction, usually also accompanied by focal neurologic signs (hemiparesis, aphasia, visual field defects). The course is variable, but progression to death usually occurs within months. Magnetic resonance imaging reveals extensive lesions in the white matter.[11]

Subacute sclerosing panencephalitis is a rare disease of late childhood and adolescence. There is a male-to-female ratio of 2 or 3 to 1. The presentation is variable, occurring over weeks to years; initially, however, there is behavioral change and cognitive decline but no abnormal neurologic signs and a normal EEG. The next stage of progression is often marked by myoclonus taking the form of loss of posture followed by rapid recovery with jerking movements. This occurs without loss of consciousness. At this stage there are abnormal neurologic signs (ataxia, spasticity, involuntary movements, and dementia). Further progression leads to compromised level of consciousness, eventually resulting in stupor and coma. The final stage is a decerebrate state.[11,12]

Spongiform encephalopathies, including Creutzfeld-Jacob disease and its variants, result in a progressive dementia often associated with myoclonic jerks. It is a rare disease of later life that is usually sporadic but can also occur in families. In retrospect, nonspecific symptoms such as anorexia, insomnia, mood change, and malaise may be seen to have developed over weeks or months. The dementia can consist of changes in both cognition and behavior, and the ataxia may precede cognitive changes. The onset may be rapid or insidious and the EEG becomes abnormal as the symptoms emerge. Progression to a vegetative state and death typically occurs within 1 year.[11,13]

OTHER INFECTIOUS CAUSES OF DEMENTIA

Paretic neurosyphilis, another rare condition, is a late complication of syphilis occurring decades after the original infection. The pathologic characterization is that of a meningoencephalitis. Early symptoms include fatigue, irritability, personality changes, forgetfulness, and tremor. Symptoms at the late stage include impaired memory and judgment, confusion and disorientation, seizures, dysarthria, myoclonus, and poor motor control.[14]

SUMMARY

Dementia, broadly defined, can result from a number of infections of the central nervous system. With the exceptions of ADC and herpes simplex encephalitis, these conditions are uncommon and untreatable. As in the case of ADC, the cognitive changes associated with these infectious diseases are generally part of a symptom complex that includes changes in mood, personality, and behavior as well as impairments in motor function. The pathogenetic processes underlying the dementias in these conditions are not well understood, but they likely reflect pathogen-host interactions at

the cellular level as well as primary and secondary metabolic abnormalities at the systems level. For the most part, these conditions are progressive, leading to profound impairment and death.

REFERENCES

1. Price RW, Brew B, Sidtis JJ, et al: The brain in AIDS: Central nervous system HIV-1 infection and the AIDS dementia complex. *Science* 239:586, 1988.
2. Price RW: Understanding the AIDS dementia complex (ADC), in Price RW, Perry SW (eds): *HIV, AIDS and the Brain.* New York, Raven Press, 1994, pp 1–45.
3. Sidtis JJ, Price RW: Early HIV-1 infection and the AIDS dementia complex. *Neurology* 40:323, 1990.
4. Price RW: Management of AIDS dementia complex and HIV-1 infection of the nervous system. *AIDS* 9(suppl A):S221, 1995.
5. Brew BJ, Rosenblum M, Cronin K, Price RW: AIDS dementia complex and HIV-1 brain infection: Clinical-virological correlations. *Ann Neurol* 38:563, 1995.
6. Rottenberg DA, Moeller JR, Strother SC, et al: The metabolic pathology of the AIDS dementia complex. *Ann Neurol* 22:700, 1987.
7. Van Gorp WG, Mandelkern MA, Gee M, et al: Cerebral metabolic dysfunction in AIDS: Findings in a sample with and without dementia. *J Neuropsychiatry* 4:280, 1992.
8. Lambert HP (ed): *Infections of the Nervous System.* Philadelphia, Decker, 1991.
9. Whitley RJ: Viral encephalitis. *N Engl J Med* 323:242, 1990.
10. Goldsmith SM, Whitely RJ: Herpes simplex encephalitis, in Lambert HP (ed): *Infections of the Nervous System.* Philadelphia, Decker, 1991, pp 283–299.
11. Matthews WB: Slow viruses and the central nervous system, in Lambert HP (ed): *Infections of the Nervous System.* Philadelphia, Decker, 1991, pp 329–342.
12. Graves M: Subacute sclerosing panencephalitis. *Neurol Clin* 2:267, 1984.
13. Brown P, Cathala F, Castaigne P, et al: Creutzfeld-Jakob disease: Clinical analysis of a consecutive series of 230 neuropathologically verified cases. *Ann Neurol* 20:597, 1986.
14. Rowland LP: Spirochete infections: Neurosyphilis, in Rowland LP (ed): *Merritt's Textbook of Neurology.* Philadelphia, Lea & Febiger, 1989, pp 152–161.

Chapter 48

WERNICKE-KORSAKOFF AND RELATED NUTRITIONAL DISORDERS OF THE NERVOUS SYSTEM

Mieke Verfaellie
Laird S. Cermak

CLINICAL PRESENTATION

In 1881, Wernicke described a neurologic syndrome of acute onset characterized by ataxia, ophthalmoplegia, nystagmus, polyneuropathy in the arms and legs, and a global confusional state. Shortly thereafter, Korsakoff described the chronic changes in mental status and memory he observed in patients with disorders involving polyneuropathy.[1] Not until several years later[2] was it realized that the symptoms described by Wernicke and Korsakoff often occur sequentially in the same patients and represent a functional syndrome now generally referred to as Wernicke-Korsakoff syndrome (WKS). Although most commonly associated with chronic alcoholism, the syndrome is also seen in a number of other disorders leading to nutritional insufficiency, including prolonged vomiting, gastrointestinal carcinoma, dialysis, and acquired immunodeficiency syndrome (AIDS).

The onset of WKS is usually marked by an acute phase in which the patient is disoriented, confused and apathetic, and unable to maintain a coherent conversation. This confusional state is accompanied by ataxia and oculomotor problems, although there is considerable variability in the severity of these symptoms across patients.[3] Unless treated with thiamine, the patient is in danger of having fatal midbrain hemorrhages. Given appropriate treatment, however, the neurologic signs improve rapidly and markedly. Once the acute confusion clears, the patient is typically left with an enduring dense amnesia, characteristic of the Korsakoff stage of the disorder. Although some patients have been described to recover to a premorbid level of functioning, this is a rare occurrence.[4] Because of considerable variability in its presentation, Wernicke encephalopathy may at times go unrecognized until autopsy.[5] Indeed, some patients may evolve to the Korsakoff stage of the disorder without clinical evidence of an antecedent Wernicke encephalopathy.[4,6]

The hallmark of the chronic stage of WKS is the inability to retrieve recent memories and learn new information in the context of otherwise relatively preserved cognitive functioning. The selective and acute nature of the memory disorder sets it apart from alcoholic dementia, a syndrome characterized by more global impairments in intellectual functioning that evolve gradually over time.[7,8] Despite differences in clinical presentation between these two syndromes, controversy remains as to whether a nosologic distinction is justified on neuropathologic grounds.[9–11]

The incidence of WKS is rare, having been estimated in one study at approximately 10 per million of first psychiatric admissions.[12] Other statistics, based on hospital admissions as well as general population studies, estimate its occurrence at approximately 50 per million.[13,14] Notwithstanding its rare occurrence, the neuropsychological sequelae of WKS have been studied in extensive detail because patients with WKS provided one of the first opportunities to systematically examine

609

the information processing deficits underlying selective amnesia (e.g., Refs. 15 and 16).

NEUROPSYCHOLOGICAL PROFILE

General Cognitive Status

Despite severe amnesia, general intelligence is commonly well preserved in WKS.[15,16] Accordingly, many group studies of WKS patients report mean IQ scores as measured by the WAIS-R in the average range (see, e.g., Ref. 17). Table 48-1 illustrates the WAIS-R performance of a representative group of 10 patients followed at the Memory Disorders Research Center. As can be seen, these patients perform normally on all subtests of the WAIS-R with the exception of the Digit Symbol subtest, a measure of visuomotor performance. The same table also illustrates the severity of these

Table 48-1

Mean WAIS-R and WMS-R scores in a representative group of Korsakoff patients[a]

WAIS-R	
Full scale IQ	98.7
Verbal IQ	96.9
Information	9.3
Digit span	9.9
Vocabulary	9.2
Arithmetic	11.1
Comprehension	9.4
Similarities	9.8
Performance IQ	101.3
Picture completion	10.4
Picture arrangement	10.2
Block design	10
Object assembly	11.3
Digit symbol	8.5
WMS-R	
General memory	78.8
Verbal memory	81.2
Visual memory	86.3
Attention	98.5
Delayed memory	56.5

[a]WAIS-R subtest scores are age-scaled.

patients' memory deficit as indicated by performance on the Wechsler Memory Scale–Revised.[18] A discrepancy between IQ and Delayed Memory Quotient of almost three standard deviations (42 points in the current patient sample) is commonly observed.[19] Of note is the average Attentional Quotient, a finding indicative of the integrity of simple attentional functions in WKS. The difference between the Attentional and General Memory Quotient therefore provides a good indication of the severity of amnesia in this patient group.[19]

Despite their relatively well-preserved intellectual abilities, WKS patients do demonstrate deficits in a number of domains other than memory. Impairments in visuospatial and visuoperceptual functioning have been observed in a number of tasks. These include digit symbol and symbol digit substitution tests,[20–22] embedded figures tests,[15,20,21] and tests of figure-ground reversal.[15] Since early processing of visual information is intact,[23] these deficits have often been attributed to an impairment in the analysis of contour or configural information (see also Ref. 24).

Deficits in olfactory and gustatory functioning have also consistently been observed. Patients with WKS have difficulty in making qualitative discriminations between smells or tastes,[25,26] but whether these deficits are related to heightened sensory thresholds is still unclear.[26,27] Regardless of the exact level at which these processing deficits occur, they can be linked directly to atrophy of diencephalic structures associated with these sensory systems.

The extramemorial deficits most commonly noted in WKS are deficits in problem solving and concept formation,[28,29] deficits linked to impaired frontal executive control. Indeed, WKS patients typically perform poorly on clinical tests of frontal lobe functioning, such as the Wisconsin Card Sorting Test,[15,30] Verbal Fluency,[22,30,31] and Trails B.[22] Although perseveration and poor planning are frequently cited as underlying causes, executive deficits are likely to be multiply determined.[32]

An often cited clinical characteristic of WKS that may be linked to impaired executive control is patients' tendency to confabulate when faced with questions they cannot answer. This is by no means a central feature of the disorder, however, and occurs almost exclusively during the acute phase. Even then, confabulations are mostly provoked by the examiner's questioning and rarely occur spontaneously.

Anterograde Amnesia

The cardinal symptom of WKS is a profound inability to acquire new verbal and nonverbal information. Patients typically are unable to learn new names, faces, or facts, even in the face of multiple repetitions, and they forget events that happened just minutes before. These deficits are not due to impairments in the immediate registration of information, as patients are able to repeat information in the absence of any delay.[33–36] However, given distracting activity for as little as 9 s, performance can be markedly impaired.[16,34,37,38] Some information may be learned on an initial learning trial, but on subsequent trials marked deficits occur because of interference from information that was presented earlier. This increased sensitivity to interference is generally considered to be the most prominent feature of the anterograde amnesia. Some theorists[39,40] have suggested that interference occurs because the patient is unable to inhibit competition from irrelevant material at the time of *retrieval,* a hypothesis supported by the fact that retrieval cues that eliminate response competition improve performance.[41,42] Other investigators[16,37] have suggested that the learning deficits are due primarily to a failure to *encode* all the attributes of a stimulus. When left to their own devices, patients analyze the phonemic and associative features of stimuli, but they fail to analyze the semantic features of stimuli.[43–45] In the past, the relative contribution of encoding and retrieval deficits has been vigorously debated (for reviews, see Refs. 46 and 47), but there is now general agreement that a true understanding of the anterograde amnesia of WKS lies in the interaction between these factors.[48]

Although the anterograde amnesia of WKS is in many respects quite similar to that seen in patients with amnesias of other etiologies, the question arises as to whether frontal executive deficits influence the character of the memory disorder in this patient group. One feature that distinguishes WKS patients from amnesic patients of other etiologies is their increased propensity to commit prior-item intrusions, a finding that has been attributed to their superimposed frontal pathology.[49] Another feature of the memory disturbance in WKS that has been linked to frontal dysfunction is the failure of these patients to demonstrate release from proactive interference (PI).[30] However, more recent studies have suggested that frontal dysfunction is not in itself sufficient[50,51] or necessary[52] to cause impaired release from PI. Another feature that distinguishes WKS patients from other amnesic subgroups is their disproportionate impairment on tasks that tap memory for temporal information.[30,53–55] Since similar contextual deficits occur in patients with focal frontal lesions,[56] it has been suggested that these deficits in WKS may be secondary to superimposed frontal deficits.[30] The absence of reliable correlations between contextual memory performance and both structural and behavioral indices of frontal dysfunction, however, casts doubt on this view.[55,57] It appears that contextual memory deficits are an inseparable feature of WKS amnesia.

In addition to primary cognitive disturbances, motivational and arousal deficits may also contribute to patients' severe learning and memory problems. Patients with WKS generally display a profound apathy, passivity, and lack of initiative, features indicative of defective arousal and activation mechanisms. Several investigators have suggested that these deficits may interfere with the encoding and retrieval of information.[15,58] Partial support for this view comes from studies demonstrating that WKS patients show better learning when the information is emotionally salient or otherwise arousing.[59–61] These arousal effects appear to be transient, however, as no benefits are observed in the long-term retention of this information.[62,63]

Notwithstanding the severe impairments in new learning, several areas of preserved memory capacity should be mentioned briefly. These include the ability to acquire new motor[64,65] and perceptual skills[66,67] as well as preserved performance on a range of implicit memory tasks (see Chap. 36) in which memory is indicated by changes in speed, accuracy, or bias of processing a stimulus as a consequence of prior experience with that stimulus (for review, see Ref. 68).

Retrograde Amnesia

Patients with WKS have significant difficulty retrieving public as well as personal autobiographical events that occurred prior to the onset of their illness. This retrograde impairment is usually very extensive, but memories from childhood and early adulthood are typically remembered better than memories from the recent past. Such a temporal gradient has been observed in tests of autobiographical knowledge[57,69] as well as tests of public events and famous faces.[70–72a] Even when events from recent and remote time periods are carefully equated in terms of task difficulty,[72–74] this pattern remains, suggesting that it is not just an artifact of differential exposure and overlearning.

A popular explanation[72,73] for this temporal gradient posits that two factors may jointly contribute to the observed remote memory impairment in WKS: a gradually developing anterograde memory deficit that is related to patients' alcohol abuse and a general retrieval deficit that appears acutely during the Wernicke phase of the illness and affects all time periods equally. The gradual building of new learning deficits is thought to account for the presence of a temporal gradient, while the general retrieval deficit explains the fact that across all decades, remote memory is worse in WKS patients than in chronic alcoholics.

However, the contribution of new learning deficits to retrograde amnesia was called into question by the report of patient P.Z.,[75] a college professor who had written his autobiography 2 years prior to developing WKS. This patient demonstrated a temporally graded remote memory impairment for material mentioned in his autobiography. Clearly this could not be due to an inability to learn this material originally. Instead, Cermak and colleagues[75,76] explained the existence of a gradient in P.Z. by suggesting that information

from different time periods may tap qualitatively different forms of memory. Information from the recent past seems anchored in a temporal and spatial context, but information from the distant past often loses its contextual qualities through continued rehearsing and retelling. As a consequence, recent items may tap primarily episodic memory, whereas remote items may tap primarily semantic memory. According to this view, P.Z.'s performance may reflect the fact that episodic memories are more vulnerable to disruption than are semantic memories. Recent evidence, however, challenges this view. Memory for semantic information acquired prior to the onset of amnesia is also impaired in WKS and is characterized by a similar temporal gradient.[77] Thus, it appears that more recent memories, whether episodic or semantic, are more vulnerable to disruption than are remote memories. Even though P.Z. was able to describe recent events in his autobiography, these memories may have been less well established and less frequently rehearsed, hence their higher vulnerability.

Of note, several studies[57,77] have demonstrated that the extent of retrograde amnesia in WKS is correlated with performance on tests of frontal lobe functioning. A number of investigators (e.g., Refs. 78 and 79) have suggested that the frontal lobes play an important role in the planning and initiation of systematic memory search. Such deficits in strategic control may underlie the inability to retrieve premorbidly acquired information, regardless of its recency of occurrence.

ETIOLOGY OF WERNICKE-KORSAKOFF SYNDROME

It is now generally accepted that Wernicke encephalopathy is directly linked to severe avitaminosis and especially deficiency of thiamine (vitamin B_1). Autopsied brain samples of patients with WKS have been found to be severely and selectively deficient in thiamine-dependent enzymes.[80] Furthermore, in animals with induced thiamine deficiency, neurologic symptoms of Wernicke encephalopathy have been observed[81,82] as well as significant memory disorders.[83–85] This thiamine deficiency is due primarily to inadequate dietary intake of the vitamin, but impaired metabolism, possibly because of a genetic predisposition, is also thought to play a role.[86,87] Severe reductions in thiamine may trigger a series of metabolic events (see Ref. 84), leading to compromised energy metabolism and ultimately cell death.

In addition to thiamine deficiency, direct toxic effects of alcohol may also contribute to the neuropathology seen in patients with alcoholic WKS. There is now impressive evidence to suggest that patients with chronic alcohol abuse but without signs of WKS have signs of cognitive impairment and brain damage.[88–90] The similarity between the visuoperceptual and problem-solving deficits of WKS patients and those of chronic alcoholics has led to the suggestion that direct toxic effects of alcohol on association cortex may underlie these nonmnemonic deficits.[91] The link between frontal deficits and alcohol abuse per se remains controversial, however,[35] in part because frontal deficits have also been documented in patients with WKS of nonalcoholic origin.[92] It is likely, therefore, that multiple neuropathologic mechanisms contribute to the observed frontal deficits. Whether these deficits reflect direct structural damage to frontal cortex or a functional disconnection resulting from disruption of subcortical-frontal pathways also remains unclear.

NEUROPATHOLOGIC FINDINGS

The main pathology of WKS, described in detail by Victor and colleagues,[4] consists of symmetrically placed punctate lesions in the area of the third ventricle, fourth ventricle, and aqueduct, areas that are known to be very sensitive to thiamine deficiency. While it is generally agreed that lesions in the midbrain and cerebellum are responsible for the neurologic symptoms of the Wernicke stage,[93] diencephalic lesions are thought to play a critical role in amnesia. Although both the mammillary bodies of the hypothalamus and medial thalamic structures are commonly involved in WKS, controversy remains regarding the minimal critical lesion responsible for the severe amnesia. Victor and colleagues[4] report that of 43 brains in which the thalamus was systematically examined, 38 had extensive atrophy of the dorsomedial nucleus (DMN). The 5 patients without DMN damage were not amnesic, even though they showed severe atrophy of the mammillary bodies. Based on these findings, the authors concluded that involvement of DMN was essential in the causation of memory deficits. No case of WKS, however, has been reported with damage restricted to the DMN. Therefore, it remains possible that combined damage of DMN and the mammillary bodies is responsible for amnesia, a view consistent with the proposal that damage to both the amygdala and hippocampal circuits is necessary to produce severe amnesia.[94] The possibility that combined lesions of DMN and the mammillary bodies are responsible for the amnesia in WKS receives support from two neuropathologic studies of patients whose memory impairments were extensively documented during life.[95,96] Both studies report marked neuronal loss from the mammillary bodies as well as a thin band of gliosis between the wall of the third ventricle and the medial thalamus, in an area occupied by the paratenial nucleus. Whether in those cases the medial thalamic lesion extended into DMN itself, however, is difficult to ascertain. Figure 48-1 represents a section of a WKS brain studied at our center that demonstrates generally similar pathology. The figure illustrates lesions in the mammillary bodies and gray matter surrounding the third ventricle.

Other neuropathologic studies have questioned whether medial diencephalic damage is sufficient to account for the amnesia seen in WKS, raising the possibility that damage to the basal forebrain and hippocampus may also play a role.[4,96,97] Lesions in these latter areas, however, are not always present. Although they may contribute to the observed behavioral deficits, they do not appear to be mandatory.

Structural neuroimaging studies have confirmed the presence of diencephalic lesions in WKS[98–101] but have also focused attention on the presence of neocortical involvement, especially in the parietal and frontal lobes. Evidence for cortical

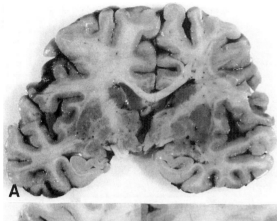

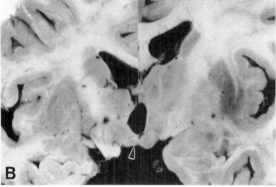

Figure 48-1

Coronal section of a Korsakoff brain (A) illustrating sulcal widening, loss of white matter, and enlarged ventricles. Significant atrophy of the mammillary bodies is highlighted by comparing the left hemisphere of the Korsakoff brain with the right hemisphere of an age-matched control (B).

atrophy comes from findings of enlargement of the lateral ventricles and widening of the sylvian and interhemispheric fissures, particularly between the frontal lobes. It should be noted, however, that the presence of frontal atrophy is characteristic of alcoholics both with and without WKS.[22,99,102]

To date, few studies have focused on quantitative measurements of cerebral blood flow and metabolism in WKS. In the acute phase, widespread depression of metabolism has been observed in both cortical and subcortical areas, but significant recovery has been noted following thiamine treatment.[103,104] In the chronic phase, decreased metabolism in diencephalic areas is the most noticeable feature.[104,105] Frontal metabolic deficits have been observed in one[106] but not in another study,[105] a finding that again points to the variability in the neuropathology of WKS.

In comparison to a wealth of structural neuroanatomic studies, relatively little research has addressed the biochemical deficiencies that may underlie the amnesia in WKS. One exception, however, is the work of McEntee and colleagues.[107,108] They have drawn attention to the fact that the areas in the midbrain and diencephalon that are typically compromised in WKS are the very areas in which the monoaminergic pathways are located. Consistent with a monoaminergic disruption, they found significant reductions in the concentration of MHPG, the primary metabolite of norepinephrine, in the CSF of WKS patients. Moreover, the magnitude of this reduction was correlated with the severity of the patients' memory impairment,[109] and administration of the norepinephrine agonist clonidine had a beneficial effect on patients' anterograde memory capabilities.[110] This latter effect, however, has been difficult to replicate.[111] Another neurotransmitter that deserves further scrutiny is acetylcholine. As a consequence of thiamine depletion, cholinergic deficiencies are present in the acute phase of WKS.[84] However, whether cholinergic systems are also involved in the chronic stage of the disorder remains to be determined.

ACKNOWLEDGMENTS

Preparation of this chapter was supported by NINDS grant NS26985 to Boston University School of Medicine.

REFERENCES

1. Victor M, Yakovlev PI: SS Korsakoff's psychic disorder in conjunction with peripheral neuritis: A translation of Korsakoff's original article with brief comments on the author and his contribution to clinical medicine. *Neurology* 5:394–406, 1955.

2. Gudden H: Klinische und anatomische Beitraege zur Kenntniss der multiplen Alkoholneuritis nebst Bemerkungen ueber die Regenerationsvorgaenge im peripheren Nervensystem. *Arch Psychiatr Nervenkrankh* 28:643–741, 1896.

3. Reuler JB, Girard DE, Cooney TG: Current concepts: Wernicke's encephalopathy. *N Engl J Med* 312:1035–1039, 1985.

4. Victor M, Adams RA, Collins GH: *The Wernicke-Korsakoff Syndrome and Related Neurologic Disorders due to Alcoholism and Malnutrition,* 2d ed. Philadelphia, Davis, 1989.

5. Harper CG, Giles M, Finlay-Jones R: Clinical signs in the Wernicke-Korsakoff complex: A retrospective analysis of 131 cases diagnosed at necropsy. *J Neurol Neurosurg Psychiatry* 49:341–345, 1986.

6. Blansjaar BA, Van Dijk JG: Korsakoff minus Wernicke syndrome. *Alcohol* 27:435–437, 1992.

7. Cutting J: The relationship between Korsakov's syndrome and alcoholic dementia. *Br J Psychiatry* 132:240–251, 1978.

8. Jacobson RR, Lishman WA: Selective memory loss and global intellectual deficits in alcoholic Korsakoff syndrome. *Psychol Med* 17:649–655, 1987.

9. Victor M, Adams RA: The alcoholic dementias, in Frederiks J (ed): *Handbook of Clinical Neurology.* Amsterdam, Elsevier, 1985, vol 2, pp 335–352.

10. Bowden SC: Separating cognitive impairment in neurologically asymptomatic alcoholism from Wernicke-Korsakoff syndrome: Is the neuropsychological distinction justified? *Psychol Bull* 107:355–366, 1990.

11. Joyce EM: Aetiology of alcoholic brain damage: Alcoholic neurotoxicity or thiamine malnutrition? *Br Med Bull* 50:99–114, 1994.

12. Centerwall BS, Criqui MH: Prevention of the Wernicke-Korsakoff syndrome: A cost-benefit analysis. *N Engl J Med* 299:285–289, 1978.

13. Blansjaar BA, Horjus MC, Nijhuis HG: Prevalence of the Korsakoff syndrome in the Hague, the Netherlands. *Acta Psychiatr Scand* 75:604–607, 1987.

14. Victor M, Laureno R: Neurologic complications of alcohol abuse: Epidemiologic aspects, in Schoenberg B (ed): *Advances in Neurology:* vol 19. *Neuroepidemiology.* New York, Raven Press, 1978, pp 603–617.

15. Talland G: *Deranged Memory: A Psychonomic Study of the Amnesic Syndrome.* New York: Academic Press, 1965.

16. Butters N, Cermak LS: *Alcoholic Korsakoff's Syndrome: An Information-Processing Approach to Amnesia.* London, Academic Press, 1980.

17. Parkin AJ, Leng NR: *Neuropsychology of the Amnesic Syndrome.* London, Erlbaum, 1993.

18. Wechsler D: *Wechsler Memory Scale-Revised.* New York, Psychological Corporation, 1987.

19. Butters N, Salmon DP, Cullum CM, et al: Differentiation of amnesic and demented patients with the Wechsler memory Scale-Revised. *Clin Neuropsychol* 2:133–148, 1988.

20. Glosser G, Butters N, Kaplan E: Visuoperceptual processes in brain-damaged patients on the digit-symbol substitution test. *Int J Neurosci* 7:59–66, 1977.

21. Kapur N, Butters N: Visuoperceptive deficits in long-term alcoholics with Korsakoff's psychosis. *J Studies Alcohol* 38:2025–2035, 1977.

22. Jacobson RR, Acker CF, Lishman WA: Patterns of neuropsychological deficit in alcoholic Korsakoff's syndrome. *Psychol Med* 20:321–334, 1990.

23. Deary IJ, Hunter R, Langan SJ, et al: Inspection time, psychometric intelligence and clinical estimates of cognitive ability in pre-senile Alzheimer's disease and Korsakoff's psychosis. *Brain* 114:2543–2554, 1991.

24. Dricker J, Butters N, Berman G, et al: Recognition and encoding of faces by alcoholic Korsakoff and right hemisphere patients. *Neuropsychologia* 16:683–695, 1978.

25. Jones BP, Moskowitz HR, Butters N: Olfactory discrimination in alcoholic Korsakoff patients. *Neuropsychologia* 13:173–179, 1975.

26. Jones BP, Butters N, Moskowitz HR, et al: Olfactory and gustatory capacities of alcoholic Korsakoff patients. *Neuropsychologia* 16:323–337, 1978.

27. Mair RG, Capra C, McEntee WL, et al: Odor discrimination and memory in Korsakoff's psychosis. *J Exp Psychol Hum Percept Perform* 6:445–448, 1980.

28. Oscar-Berman M: Hypothesis testing and focusing behavior during concept formation by amnesic Korsakoff patients. *Neuropsychologia* 11:191–198, 1973.

29. Becker JT, Butters N, Rivoira P, et al: Asking the right questions: Problem solving in male alcoholics and male alcoholics with Korsakoff's syndrome. *Alcoholism: Clin Exp Res* 10:641–646, 1986.

30. Squire LR: Comparisons between forms of amnesia: Some deficits are unique to Korsakoff's Syndrome. *J Exp Psychol Learn Mem Cog* 8:560–571, 1982.

31. Butters N, Granholm E, Salmon DP, et al: Episodic and semantic memory: A comparison of amnesic and demented patients. *J Clin Exp Neuropsychol* 9:479–497, 1987.

32. Delis DC, Squire LR, Bihrle A, et al: Componential analysis of problem-solving ability: Performance of patients with frontal lobe damage and amnesic patients on a new sorting test. *Neuropsychologia* 30:683–697, 1992.

33. Haxby JV, Lundgren SL, Morley GK: Short-term retention of verbal, visual shape and visuospatial location information in normal and amnesic subjects. *Neuropsychologia* 21:25–33, 1983.

34. Kopelman MD: Rates of forgetting in Alzheimer-type dementia and Korsakoff's syndrome. *Neuropsychologia* 23:623–638, 1985.

35. Joyce EM, Robbins TW: Frontal lobe function in Korsakoff and non-Korsakoff alcoholics: Planning and spatial working memory. *Neuropsychologia* 29:709–723, 1991.

36. Wiegersma S, De Jong E, Dieren MV: Subjective ordering and working memory in alcoholic Korsakoff patients. *J Clin Exp Neuropsychol* 13:847–853, 1991.

37. Kinsbourne M, Wood F: Short-term memory processes and the amnesic syndrome, in Deutsch DD, Deutsch JA (eds): *Short-Term Memory.* New York, Academic Press, 1975, pp 258–291.

38. Meudell PR, Butters N, Montgomery K: Role of rehearsal in the short-term memory performance of patients with Korsakoff's and Huntington's Disease. *Neuropsychologia* 16:507–510, 1978.

39. Warrington EK, Weiskrantz L: Amnesic syndrome: Consolidation or retrieval? *Nature* 228:628–630, 1970.

40. Warrington EK, Weiskrantz L: An analysis of short-term and long-term memory defects in man, in Deutsch J (ed): *The Physiological Basis of Memory.* New York, Academic Press, 1973, pp 365–395.

41. Warrington EK, Weiskrantz L: Organizational aspects of memory in amnesic patients. *Neuropsychologia* 9:67–73, 1971.

42. Warrington EK, Weiskrantz L: The effect of prior learning on subsequent retention in amnesic patients. *Neuropsychologia* 12:419–428, 1974.

43. Cermak LS, Reale L: Depth of processing and retention of words by alcoholic Korsakoff patients. *J Exp Psychol Hum Learn Mem* 4:165–174, 1978.

44. McDowall J: Effects of encoding instructions and retrieval cuing on recall in Korsakoff patients. *Mem Cog* 7:232–239, 1979.

45. Biber C, Butters N, Rosen J, et al: Encoding strategies and recognition of faces by alcoholic Korsakoff and other brain-damaged patients. *J Clin Neuropsychol* 3:315–330, 1981.

46. Cermak LS: Models of memory loss in Korsakoff and alcoholic patients, in Parsons O, Butters N, Nathan P (eds): *Neuropsychology of Alcoholism.* New York, Guilford Press, 1987, pp 207–226.

47. Butters N, Stuss DT: Diencephalic amnesia, in Squire LR (ed): *Handbook of Neuropsychology* (Boller F, Grafman J: volume editors). Amsterdam, Elsevier, 1991, vol 3, pp 107–148.

48. Verfaellie M, Cermak LS: Neuropsychological issues in amnesia, in Martinez J, Kesner R (eds): *Learning and Memory: A Biological View.* San Diego, CA, Academic Press, 1992, pp 467–497.

49. Kixmiller JS, Verfaellie M, Chase KA, Cermak LS: Comparison of figural intrusion errors in three amnesic subgroups. *J Int Neuropsychol Soc* 1:561–567, 1995.

50. Freedman M, Cermak LS: Semantic encoding deficits in frontal lobe disease and amnesia. *Brain Cog* 5:108–114, 1986.

51. Kopelman MD: Frontal dysfunction and memory deficits in the alcoholic Korsakoff syndrome and Alzheimer-type dementia. *Brain* 114:117–137, 1991.

52. Becker JT, Furman JM, Panisset M, et al: Characteristics of the memory loss of a patient with Wernicke-Korsakoff's syndrome without alcoholism. *Neuropsychologia* 28:171–179, 1990.

53. Parkin AJ, Leng NR, Hunkin NM: Differential sensitivity to context in diencephalic and temporal lobe amnesia. *Cortex* 26:373–380, 1990.

54. Shimamura AP, Janowski JS, Squire LR: Memory for the temporal order of events in patients with frontal lobe lesions and amnesic patients. *Neuropsychologia* 28:803–813, 1990.

55. Hunkin NM, Parkin AJ: Recency judgements in Wernicke-Korsakoff and post-encephalitic amnesia: Influences of proactive interference and retention interval. *Cortex* 29:485–499, 1993.

56. Milner B, Petrides M, Smith ML: Frontal lobes and the temporal organisation of memory. *Hum Neurobiol* 4:137–142, 1985.

57. Kopelman MD: Remote and autobiographical memory, temporal context memory and frontal at-

rophy in Korsakoff and Alzheimer patients. *Neuropsychologia* 27:437–460, 1989.

58. Oscar-Berman M: Neuropsychological consequences of long-term alcoholism. *Am Sci* 68:410–419, 1980.

59. Kovner R, Mattis S, Goldmeier E: A technique for promoting robust free recall in chronic organic amnesia. *J Clin Exp Neuropsychol* 5:65–71, 1983.

60. Kopelman MD: Recall of anomalous sentences in dementia and amnesia. *Brain Lang* 29:154–170, 1986.

61. Markowitsch HJ, Kessler J, Denzler P: Recognition memory and psychophysiological responses to stimuli with neutral or emotional content: A study of Korsakoff patients and recently detoxified and long-term abstinent alcoholics. *Int J Neurosci* 29:1–35, 1986.

62. Davidoff D, Butters N, Gerstman L, et al: Affective-motivational factors in the recall of prose passages by alcoholic Korsakoff patients. *Alcohol* 1:63–69, 1984.

63. Granholm E, Wolfe J, Butters N: Affective-arousal factors in the recall of thematic stories by amnesic and demented patients. *Dev Neuropsychol* 4:317–333, 1985.

64. Cermak LS, Lewis R, Butters N, et al: Role of verbal mediation in performance of motor tasks by Korsakoff patients. *Percept Motor Skills* 37:259–262, 1973.

65. Brooks DN, Baddeley AD: What can amnesic patients learn? *Neuropsychologia* 14:111–122, 1976.

66. Cohen NJ, Squire LR: Preserved learning and retention of pattern-analyzing skill in amnesia: Dissociation of knowing how and knowing that. *Science* 210:207–210, 1980.

67. Martone M, Butters N, Payne M, et al: Dissociations between skill learning and verbal recognition in amnesia and dementia. *Arch Neurol* 41:965–970, 1984.

68. Moscovitch M, Vriezen E, Gottstein J: Implicit tests of memory in patients with focal lesions or degenerative brain disorders, in Spinnler H, Boller F (eds): *Handbook of Neuropsychology* (Boller F, Grafman J: volume editors). Amsterdam, Elsevier, 1993, vol 8, pp 133–173.

69. Zola-Morgan S, Cohen NJ, Squire LR: Recall of remote episodic memory in amnesia. *Neuropsychologia* 21:487–500, 1983.

70. Seltzer B, Benson DF: The temporal pattern of retrograde amnesia in Korsakoff's disease. *Neurology* 24:527–530, 1974.

71. Marslen-Wilson ND, Teuber H-L: Memory for remote events in anterograde amnesia: Recognition of public figures from news photographs. *Neuropsychologia* 13:347–352, 1975.

72. Albert MS, Butters N, Levin J: Temporal gradients in the retrograde amnesia of patients with alcoholic Korsakoff's disease. *Arch Neurol* 36:211–216, 1979.

72a. Cohen NJ, Squire LR: Retrograde amnesia and remote memory impairment. *Neuropsychologia* 19:337–356, 1981.

73. Butters N, Albert MS: Processes underlying failures to recall remote events, in Cermak L (ed): *Human Memory and Amnesia.* Hillsdale, NJ, Erlbaum, 1982, pp 257–274.

74. Squire LR, Cohen NJ: Remote memory, retrograde amnesia and the neuropsychology of memory, in Cermak L (ed): *Human Memory and Amnesia.* Hillsdale, NJ, Erlbaum, 1982, pp 275–303.

75. Butters N, Cermak LS: A case study of the forgetting of autobiographical knowledge: Implications for the study of retrograde amnesia, in Rubin D (ed): *Autobiographical Memory.* New York, Cambridge University Press, 1986, pp 253–272.

76. Cermak LS: The episodic/semantic distinction in amnesia, in Squire LR, Butters N (eds): *The Neuropsychology of Memory.* New York, Guilford Press, 1984, pp 55–62.

77. Verfaellie M, Reiss L, Roth HL: Knowledge of new English vocabulary in amnesia: An examination of premorbidly acquired semantic memory. *J Int Neuropsychol Soc* 1:443–453, 1995.

78. Stuss DT, Benson DF: *The Frontal Lobes.* New York: Raven Press, 1986.

79. Dall'Ora P, Della Sala S, Spinnler H: Autobiographical memory: Its impairment in amnesic syndromes. *Cortex* 25:197–217, 1989.

80. Butterworth RF, Krill JK, Harper CG: Thiamine-dependent enzyme changes in the brains of alcoholics: Relationship to the Wernicke-Korsakoff syndrome. *Alcoholism Clin Exp Res* 17:1084–1088, 1993.

81. Dreyfus PM: Diseases of the nervous system in chronic alcoholics, in Kissin B, Begleiter H (eds): *The Biology of Alcoholism: Clinical Pathology.* New York, Plenum Press, 1974, vol 3, pp 265–291.

82. Mesulam M-M, Van Hoesen G, Butters N: Clinical

manifestations of chronic thiamine deficiency in the rhesus monkey. *Neurology* 27:239–245, 1977.

83. Markowitsch HJ, Pritzel M: The neuropathology of amnesia. *Prog Neurobiol* 25:189–287, 1985.

84. Witt ED: Neuroanatomical consequences of thiamine deficiency: A comparative analysis. *Alcohol Alcoholism* 20:202–221, 1985.

85. Mair RG, Knoth RL, Rabchenuk SA, et al: Impairment of olfactory, auditory, and spatial serial reversal learning in rats recovered from pyrithiamine-induced thiamine deficiency. *Behav Neurosci* 105:360–374, 1991.

86. Blass JP, Gibson GE: Abnormality of a thiamine-requiring enzyme in Wernicke-Korsakoff syndrome. *N Engl J Med* 297:1367–1370, 1977.

87. Martin PR, McCool BA, Singleton CK: Genetic sensitivity to thiamine deficiency and development of alcoholic organic brain disease. *Alcoholism Clin Exp Res* 17:31–37, 1993.

88. Ron MA, Acker W, Shaw GK, et al: Computerized tomography of the brain in chronic alcoholism. *Brain* 105:497–514, 1982.

89. Butters N, Brandt J: The continuity hypothesis: The relationship of long-term alcoholism to the Wernicke-Korsakoff syndrome, in Galanter M (ed): *Recent Developments in Alcoholism.* New York, Plenum Press, 1985, vol 3, pp 207–227.

90. Lishman WA, Jacobson RR, Acker C: Brain damage in alcoholism: Current concepts. *Acta Med Scand Suppl* 717:5–17, 1987.

91. Butters N: Alcoholic Korsakoff's syndrome: Some unresolved issues concerning etiology, neuropathology, and cognitive deficits. *J Clin Exp Neuropsychol* 7:181–210, 1985.

92. Parkin AJ, Blunden J, Rees JE, et al: Wernicke-Korsakoff syndrome of non-alcoholic origin. *Brain Cog* 15:69–82, 1991.

93. Brierly JB: Neuropathology of amnesic states, in Whitty C, Zangwill O (eds): *Amnesia,* 2d ed. Boston, Butterworth, 1977, pp 199–223.

94. Aggleton JP, Mishkin M: Visual recognition impairments following medial thalamic lesions in monkeys. *Neuropsychologia* 21:189–197, 1983.

95. Mair WG, Warrington EK, Weiskrantz L: Memory disorder in Korsakoff's psychosis: A neuropathological and neuropsychological investigation of two cases. *Brain* 102:749–783, 1979.

96. Mayes AR, Meudell PR, Mann D, et al: Location of lesions in Korsakoff's syndrome: Neuropsychological and neuropathological data on two patients. *Cortex* 24:367–388, 1988.

97. Arendt T, Bigl V, Arendt A, et al: Loss of neurons in the nucleus basalis of Meynert in Alzheimer's disease, paralysis agitans and Korsakoff's disease. *Acta Neuropathol* 61:101–108, 1983.

98. Charness ME, DeLaPaz RL: Mammillary body atrophy in Wernicke's encephalopathy: Antemortem identification using magnetic resonance imaging. *Ann Neurol* 22:595–600, 1987.

99. Shimamura AP, Jernigan TL, Squire LR: Korsakoff's syndrome: Radiological (CT) findings and neuropsychological correlates. *J Neurosci* 8:4400–4410, 1988.

100. Squire LR, Amaral D, Press G: Magnetic resonance imaging of the hippocampal formation and mammillary nuclei distinguish medial temporal lobe and diencephalic amnesia. *J Neurosci* 10:3106–3117, 1990.

101. Jernigan TL, Schafer K, Butters N, et al: Magnetic resonance imaging of alcoholic Korsakoff patients. *Neuropsychopharmacology* 4:175–186, 1991.

102. Jernigan TL, Butters N, DiTraglia G, et al: Reduced cerebral grey matter observed in alcoholics using magnetic resonance imaging. *Alcoholism Clin Exp Res* 15:418–427, 1991.

103. Hata T, Meyer JS, Tanahashi N, et al: Three-dimensional mapping of local cerebral perfusion in alcoholic encephalopathy with and without Wernicke-Korsakoff syndrome. *J Cereb Blood Flow Metab* 7:35–44, 1987.

104. Heiss W-D, Pawlik G, Holthoff V, et al: PET correlates of normal and impaired memory functions. *Cereb Brain Metab Rev* 4:1–27, 1992.

105. Perani D, Kartsounis LD, Costello A: Korsakoff's psychosis: A neuropsychological and positron emission tomography study of two cases, in Vallar G, Cappa SF, Wallesch C-W (eds): *Neuropsychological Disorders Associated with Subcortical Lesions.* Oxford, Oxford University Press, 1992, pp 169–180.

106. Hunter R, McLuskie J, Wyper D, et al: The pattern of function-related regional cerebral blood flow investigated by single photon emission tomography with 99mTc-HM-PAO in patients with presenile Alzheimer's disease and Korsakoff's psychosis. *Psychol Med* 19:847–855, 1989.

107. McEntee WJ, Mair RG, Langlais PJ: Neurochemical pathology in Korsakoff's psychosis; Implications for other cognitive disorders. *Neurology* 34:648–652, 1984.

108. McEntee WJ, Mair RG: The Korsakoff syndrome:

A neurochemical perspective. *Trends Neurosci* 13:340–344, 1990.

109. McEntee WJ, Mair RG: Memory impairments in Korsakoff's psychosis: A correlation with brain noradrenergic activity. *Science* 202:905–907, 1978.

110. McEntee WJ, Mair RG: Memory enhancement in Korsakoff's psychosis by clonidine: Further evidence for a noradrenergic deficit. *Ann Neurol* 7:466–470, 1980.

111. O'Carroll RE, Moffoot A, Ebmeier KP, et al: Korsakoff's syndrome, cognition and clonidine. *Psychol Med* 23:341–347, 1993.

Chapter 49

NEUROBEHAVIORAL ASPECTS OF VASCULITIS AND COLLAGEN VASCULAR SYNDROMES

Nancy N. Futrell
Clark H. Millikan

Collagen vascular and vasculitic diseases are overlapping categories of autoimmune diseases. Central nervous system (CNS) involvement with alterations in behavior may occur. Of these diseases systemic lupus erythematosus (SLE) is most frequently encountered in neurologic or psychiatric practice. It has the widest spectrum of behavioral changes, with multiple etiologies for the CNS involvement. The vasculitic diseases most likely to involve the CNS are those which produce stroke, either from CNS vasculitis or from systemic involvement, which predisposes to cardiogenic embolism or a hypercoagulable state.

SYSTEMIC LUPUS ERYTHEMATOSUS

Background

Systemic lupus erythematosus was first reported as an erythematous skin disorder by von Hebra in 1845, with systemic manifestations described by Kaposi in 1872.[1] Kaposi reported disturbed consciousness, including stupor and coma, although some of these cases were complicated by pulmonary infections, including tuberculosis.

The first report of focal brain dysfunction was made by Osler in 1904. After evaluating a lupus patient with repetitive episodes of right hemiparesis and aphasia, he postulated that vasculitis, similar to that seen in the skin, could produce focal neurologic abnormalities.[2] The first major neuropathologic autopsy study, done by Johnson and Richardson in 1968,[3] was remarkable for the

rarity of true vasculitis in the brain. Subsequent studies by Devinsky and Petito in 1988[4] and Hanly in 1990[5] strengthened the evidence that vasculitis in lupus is rare but that cerebral infarcts from cardioembolic sources are relatively common. None of the pathologic series have reported cerebritis other than that caused by infectious organisms.

A vast spectrum of neurologic involvement of both the central and peripheral nervous system has been described, including stroke,[6,7] seizure,[3] dementia,[8] psychosis,[9,10] coma,[11] peripheral neuropathy, and myositis.[12] This heterogeneous group of disorders is often referred to simply as "neuropsychiatric SLE."[13,14] Although this term persists, there is increasing recognition of the need to accurately classify the neurologic abnormalities in each patient and to recognize both direct and indirect mechanisms of SLE-related damage to the nervous system.[15,16] Clearly, "CNS-SLE" is not a single disease[17] but includes a spectrum of neurologic disorders, each with different potential etiologies.[18]

Stroke

Stroke in SLE patients presents with the same constellation of behavioral changes that occur in other stroke patients. The major difference is the great propensity for multiple strokes,[7] producing variable combinations of aphasias, agnosias, and apraxias in addition to motor, sensory, and visual abnormalities. These patients are often misdiagnosed with either confusion or primary psychiatric disease and are sometimes labeled "lupus cerebritis." If a neurologic evaluation is done, multifocal abnormalities are present clinically and on imaging studies (Fig. 49-1).

Figure 49-1

A 27-year-old woman with SLE and a history of five spontaneous abortions. The patient had a sudden onset of left hemiparesis and hemisensory deficit in her face, arm, and leg 5 months previously and was having episodic visual loss in the left eye of 5 to 30 min duration. The patient had a mild residual spastic hemiparesis with a Babinski sign on the left. The patient had been given a diagnosis of lupus cerebritis. A. Clock face drawn by the patient. B. Three-dimensional box, examiner's example on the left, patient's attempt on the right. Over the next 18 months, the patient continued to have repeated cerebral infarcts, presenting with unilateral and bilateral visual field defects, visual agnosia, cognitive dysfunction, and multifocal motor and sensory deficits. Anticoagulant was started following a pulmonary embolus. Although recurrent focal neurologic episodes stopped abruptly, the patient was already severely debilitated.

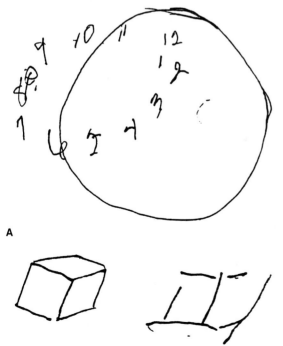

A

B

The cause of stroke in SLE is generally cardiogenic embolism or a hypercoagulable state.[7] Transesophageal echocardiography is used to detect potential cardiac sources of emboli. A hypercoagulable state in lupus may present as stroke, multiple spontaneous abortions, or venous thrombosis without predisposing events. This coagulopathy is often associated with the lupus anticoagulant (LA) or antiphospholipid antibodies (APL). Lupus anticoagulant is diagnosed by an elevated partial thromboplastin time (PTT) that is not corrected with fresh frozen plasma or, alternatively, a Russell's vipor venom time or a kaolin clotting time. Both LAs and APLs cause a hypercoagulable state by multiple mechanisms, including binding to endothelial cells[19] and inhibition of fibrinolysis.[20]

Patients with SLE face a very high risk of recurrent stroke, with over 50 percent of stroke patients having subsequent strokes. Preventive treatment with aggressive anticoagulant therapy is now generally accepted,[21,22] with an international normalized ratio (INR) of at least 3. Contraindications to anticoagulation—including thrombocytopenia, uncontrolled hypertension, history of GI bleeding, seizures, falls, dementia, and noncomplaince—are frequent in SLE patients and may limit preventive therapy. Steroids sometimes decrease APL titers[23] but do not reliably prevent strokes[21] and have serious long-term side effects. They can be used on a short-term basis in patients who have anticoagulant contraindications or who continue to have events on therapeutic anticoagulants.

Psychosis

Psychiatric disorders are common in SLE.[24] In our series of 91 patients located by consecutive hospital admissions, suicide attempts occurred in 6, generally during an acute psychotic outburst.[18] Diffuse atrophy is often seen on CT of the brain.[25] The EEG often shows diffuse slowing,[26] but this finding is nonspecific.

The etiology of psychosis in SLE is unknown. Reports of an association between psychosis and antiribosomal P antibodies have been variable.[9,27] A newly described antibody against a membrane protein in brain synaptic terminals has been associated with various CNS disorders in lupus, including psychosis, but the potential pathogenetic role of this protein has not been elucidated.[28]

The treatment includes standard antipsychotic medications. Although steroids and immunosuppressants are often given, this is controversial, as a direct immunologic etiology has never been proven for psychiatric disease in lupus.[13,29] Treatment is often guided by the activity of the systemic disease.

Encephalopathy

An acute or subacute diffuse encephalopathy of unknown etiology occurs in SLE. The clinical presentation is highly variable, with confusion, disorientation, and often decreased consciousness. Although the EEG frequently shows diffuse slowing and shifting asymmetry,[30] this is nonspecific, also occurring in psychotic patients with SLE.

Decreased consciousness is often a manifestation of advanced infections in patients with SLE, and the prognosis is grim if the infection is not identified and treated quickly.[18] Pneumonia, with organisms including bacteria, fungi, and acid-fast bacilli (both *Mycobacterium* and *Nocardia*), is the most frequent infection.[18] Patients with SLE may also present with abscesses, osteomyelitis, and CNS infections, including viral cerebritis and both fungal and bacterial meningitis.[31] Susceptibility to infection in SLE patients is increased;[32] however, the diagnosis may be delayed as the infections often mimic active SLE. Such delays lead to a high rate of sepsis, which will produce encephalopathy in 70 percent of patients.[33]

All SLE patients with encephalopathy should have a complete evaluation for infections, including lumbar puncture. Appropriate antimicrobial treatment is necessary. In patients without infection, steroids and immunosuppressive agents are often used, but their effectiveness has not been proven[34] and side effects can be serious.

Cognitive Decline

In addition to the acute and subacute processes listed above, there is an insidious, chronic cognitive decline in as many as 47 percent of patients with SLE.[13,35] Visuospatial abnormalities are prominent.[36] Memory deficits, both recent and remote, fluctuate with activity of the systemic disease.[37] Chronic "neurotic depression" is described but may not be more frequent than in patients with other chronic diseases such as rheumatoid arthritis.

The cause of this cognitive decline is unknown, but lymphocytotoxic antibodies are associated in several studies.[36,38,39] Other secondary factors, such as uremia, hypertension, and metabolic abnormalities related to the systemic disease, may be important.[40] There are no guidelines for treatment other than control of the systemic disease.

Figure 49-2

A T_2-weighted MRI done on a 26-year-old woman with SLE who presented with "confusion," which was actually mild aphasia, and mild gait apraxia. The radiographic diagnosis was vasculitis. Brain biopsy revealed areas of normal tissue, areas of edema, and two areas with subacute infarcts. There was no vasculitis.

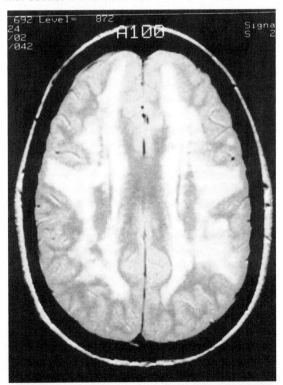

Table 49-1

Vasculitic diseases and treatment

Disorder	Systemic vasculitis	CNS vasculitis	Treatment
Systemic lupus erythematosus	+	−	S,AC
Primary antiphospholipid antibody syndrome	−	−	AC
Takayasu arteritis	++	+	S
Primary angiitis of the CNS	−	++	I
Rheumatoid arthritis	+	+	I
Periarteritis nodosa	++	+	I
Wegener granulomatosis	++	+	I
Scleroderma	±	−	S
Temporal arteritis, giant cell arteritis	++	+	S

Key: Presence of CNS vasculitis generally does not occur (−), occurs occasionally (+), occurs frequently (++); standard treatment with steroids (S), immunosuppressive agents (I), anticoagulants (AC).

Vasculitis

Although focal and diffuse neurologic abnormalities in SLE are often attributed to "CNS vasculitis," autopsy studies suggest that this is rare.[3,4] Radiographic features, including diffuse white matter hyperintensity on T_2-weighted magnetic resonance imaging[41] (Fig. 49-2) or "beading" on angiography, are nonspecific.[42] If CNS vasculitis is suspected in a lupus patient, a biopsy should be performed, as immunosuppressive therapy would be given for confirmed vasculitis.

OTHER VASCULITIC DISEASES

The other vasculitic and collagen vascular diseases are listed in Table 49-1, including the tendency for CNS vasculitis and the general category of treatment for CNS involvement.

The primary APL syndrome presents as multiple systemic or cerebral thrombotic events, multiple spontaneous abortions, or livedo reticularis, with a high titer of APLs.[43] This syndrome may be a *form fruste* of SLE.[43] Patients with the primary APL syndrome are much like the SLE patients, presenting frequently with multiple cerebral infarcts.[44] Biopsy, when done, reveals multiple thrombi rather than vasculitis.[45] Anticoagulation with coumadin with an INR of at least 3 is recommended.[46]

Patients with primary angiitis of the CNS may present with headache, dementia, or any combination of focal or multifocal neurologic abnormalities due to cerebral infarcts.[47–49] The diagnosis is suggested by pleocytosis in the CSF and beading or multiple vascular narrowings on angiography. In patients with suspected CNS vasculitis in association with primary angiitis of the CNS or SLE, biopsy should be obtained.[42] If CNS vasculitis is confirmed, immunosuppressive agents would be considered.[42] In systemic necrotizing vasculitides, such as periarteritis nodosa or Wegener granulomatosis, which require immunosuppressive agents to treat the systemic disease, biopsy confirmation of CNS vasculitis as the etiology of CNS symptoms is not necessary.

REFERENCES

1. Kaposi MK: Neue Beiträge zur Kenntniss des Lupus erythematosus. *Arch Derm Syph* 4:36–78, 1872.

2. Osler W: On the visceral manifestations of the erythema group of skin diseases. *Am J Med Sci* 127:1–23, 1904.

3. Johnson RT, Richardson EP: The neurological manifestations of systemic lupus erythematosus: A clinical-pathological study of 24 cases and review of the literature. *Medicine (Baltimore)* 47:337–369, 1968.

4. Devinsky O, Petito CK, Alonso DR: Clinical and neuropathological findings in systemic lupus erythematosus: The role of vasculitis, heart emboli and thrombotic thrombocytopenic purpura. *Ann Neurol* 23:380–384, 1988.

5. Hanly JG, Walsh NMG, Sangalang V: Brain pathology in systemic lupus erythematosus. *J Rheumatol* 71:416–422, 1991.

6. Derksen RHWM, Bouma BN, Kater L: The association between the lupus anticoagulant and cerebral infarction in systemic lupus erythematosus. *Scand J Rheumatol* 15:179–184, 1986.

7. Futrell N, Millikan C: Frequency, etiology, and prevention of stroke in patients with systemic lupus erythematosus. *Stroke* 20:583–591, 1989.

8. Asherson RA, Mercey D, Phillips G, et al: Recurrent stroke and multi-infarct dementia in systemic lupus erythematosus: Association with antiphospholipid antibodies. *Ann Rheum Dis* 46:605–611, 1987.

9. Bonfa E, Glombek SJ, Kaufman LD, et al: Association between lupus psychosis and anti-ribosomal P protein antibodies. *N Engl J Med* 317:265–271, 1987.

10. Sergent JS, Lockshin MD, Klempner MS, Lipsky BA: Central nervous system disease in systemic lupus erythematosus: Therapy and prognosis. *Am J Med* 58:644–654, 1975.

11. Bennahum DA, Messner RP: Recent observations on central nervous system lupus erythematosus. *Semin Arthritis Rheum* 4:253–266, 1975.

12. Omdal R, Mellgran SI, Husby G: Clinical neuropsychiatric and neuromuscular manifestations in systemic lupus erythematosus. *Scand J Rheumatol* 17:113–117, 1988.

13. Denburg JA, Temesvari P: The pathogenesis of neuropsychiatric lupus. *Can Med Assoc J* 128:257–260, 1983.

14. Singer J, Denburg JA, Ad Hoc Neuropsychiatric Lupus Workshop Group: Diagnostic criteria for neuropsychiatric systemic lupus erythematosus: The results of a consensus meeting. *J Rheumatol* 17:1397–1402, 1990.

15. O'Connor P: Diagnosis of central nervous system lupus. *Can J Neurol Sci* 15:257–260, 1988.

16. Robbins ML, Kornguth SE, Bell CL, et al: Antineurofilament antibody evaluation in neuropsychiatric systemic lupus erythematosus. *Arthritis Rheum* 31:623–631, 1988.

17. Kaell AT, Shetty M, Lee BCP, Lockshin MD: The diversity of neurologic events in systemic lupus erythematosus. *Arch Neurol* 43:273–276, 1986.

18. Futrell N, Schultz LR, Millikan C: Central nervous system disease in patients with systemic lupus erythematosus. *Neurology* 42:1649–1657, 1992.

19. Vismara A, Meroni PL, Tincani A, et al: Relationship between anti-cardiolipin and anti-endothelial cell antibodies in systemic lupus erythematosus. *Clin Exp Immunol* 74:247–253, 1988.

20. Nilsson TK, Lofvenberg E: Decreased fibrinolytic capacity and increased von Willebrand factor levels as indicators of endothelial cell dysfunction in patients with lupus anticoagulant. *Clin Rheumatol* 8:58–63, 1989.

21. Futrell N, Millikan CH: Prevention of recurrent stroke in patients with systemic lupus erythematosus or lupus anticoagulant. *J Stroke Cerebrovasc Dis* 1:9–20, 1991.

22. Levine SR, Welch KMA: Neurological manifestations associated with antiphospholipid antibodies. *Ann Neurol* 22:161, 1987.

23. Derksen RHWM, Beisma D, Bouma BN, et al: Discordant effects of prednisone on anticardiolipin antibodies and the lupus anticoagulant (letter). *Arthritis Rheum* 29:1295–1296, 1986.

24. Hay EM, Huddy A, Black D, et al: A prospective study of psychiatric disorder and cognitive function in systemic lupus erythematosus. *Ann Rheum Dis* 53:298–303, 1994.

25. Gonzalez-Scarano F, Lisak RP, Bilaniuk LT, et al: Cranial computed tomography in the diagnosis of systemic lupus erythematosus. *Ann Neurol* 5:158–165, 1979.

26. Matsukawa Y, Sawada S, Hayama T, et al: Suicide in patients with systemic lupus erythematosus: A clinical analysis of seven suicidal patients. *Lupus* 3:31–35, 1994.

27. Teh LS, Hay EM, Amos N, et al: Anti-P antibodies are associated with psychiatric and focal cerebral disorders in patients with systemic lupus erythematosus. *Br J Rheumatol* 32:287–290, 1993.

28. Hanson VG, Horowitz M, Rosenbluth D, et al: Systemic lupus erythematosus patients with central nervous system involvement show autoantibodies to a 50-kD neuronal membrane protein. *J Exp Med* 176:565–573, 1992.

29. Derksen RHWM, van Dam AP, Meyling FHJG, et al: A prospective study on antiribosomal P proteins

in two cases of familial lupus and recurrent psychosis. *Ann Rheum Dis* 49:779–782, 1990.

30. Ritchlin CT, Chabot RJ, Alper K, et al: Quantitative electroencephalography. *Arthritis Rheum* 35:1330–1342, 1992.

31. Al-Rasheed SA, Al-Fawaz IM: Cryptococcal meningitis in a child with systemic lupus erythematosus. *Ann Trop Paediatr* 10:323–326, 1990.

32. Yu CL, Chang KL, Chiu CC, et al: Defective phagocytosis, decreased tumour necrosis factor-alpha production, and lymphocyte hyporesponsiveness predispose patients with systemic lupus erythematosus to infections. *Scand J Rheumatol* 18:97–105, 1989.

33. Bolton CF, Young GB, Zochodne DW: The neurological complications of sepsis. *Ann Neurol* 33:94–100, 1993.

34. Sibley JT, Olszynski WP, Decoteau WE, Sundaram MB: The incidence and prognosis of central nervous system disease in systemic lupus erythematosus. *J Rheumatol* 19:47–52, 1992.

35. Edwards KK, Lindsley HB, Lai C, VanVeldhuizen PJ: Takayasu arteritis presenting as retinal and vertebrobasilar ischemia. *Rheumatology* 16:1000–1002, 1989.

36. Denburg SD, Behmann SA, Carbotte RM, Denburg JA: Lymphocyte antigens in neuropsychiatric systemic lupus erythematosus. *Arthritis Rheum* 37:369–375, 1994.

37. Martinez X, Tintore M, Montalban J, et al: Antibodies against gangliosides in patients with SLE and neurological manifestations. *Lupus* 1:299–302, 1992.

38. Denburg SD, Carbotte RM, Long AA, Denburg JA: Neuropsychological correlates of serum lymphocytotoxic antibodies in systemic lupus erythematosus. *Brain Behav Immun* 2:222–234, 1994.

39. Denburg JA, Behmann SA: Lymphocyte and neuronal antigens in neuropsychiatric lupus: Presence of an elutable, immunoprecipitable lymphocyte/neuronal 52 kd reactivity. *Ann Rheum Dis* 53:304–308, 1994.

40. Putterman C, Naparstek Y: Neuropsychiatric involvement in systemic lupus erythematosus. *Isr J Med Sci* 28:458–460, 1992.

41. Shintani S, Ono K, Hinoshita H, et al: Unusual neuroradiological findings in systemic lupus erythematosus. *Eur Neurol* 33:13–16, 1993.

42. Moore PM: Diagnosis and management of isolated angiitis of the central nervous system. *Neurology* 39:167–173, 1989.

43. Asherson RA, Khamashta MA, Ordi-Ros J, et al: The "primary" antiphospholipid syndrome: Major clinical and serological features. *Medicine* 68:366–374, 1989.

44. Asherson RA, Merry P, Acheson JF, et al: Antiphospholipid antibodies: A risk factor for occlusive ocular vascular disease in systemic lupus erythematosus and the "primary" antiphospholipid syndrome. *Ann Rheum Dis* 48:358–361, 1989.

45. Westerman EM, Miles JM, Backonja M, Sundstrom WR: Neuropathologic findings in multi-infarct dementia associated with anticardiolipin antibody. *Arthritis Rheum* 35:1038–1041, 1992.

46. Khamashta MA, Cuadrado MJ, Mujic F, et al: The management of thrombosis in the antiphospholipid-antibody syndrome. *N Engl J Med* 332:993–1027, 1995.

Chapter 50

SYMPTOMATIC OR NORMAL PRESSURE HYDROCEPHALUS IN THE ELDERLY

Neill R. Graff-Radford

Patients with possible symptomatic hydrocephalus (also termed normal pressure hydrocephalus, or NPH) are often encountered in clinical practice and comprise up to 6 percent of patients in some dementia studies.[1] To the neurologist, the commonly asked question is, "Which patients with the clinical triad of dementia, gait abnormality, and incontinence of urine—together with the radiologic finding of hydrocephalus—should be recommended for shunt surgery?" The motivation for this question is that only half the individuals with this constellation of findings improve with surgery;[2,3] moreover, shunt surgery has about a 30 percent long-term complication rate.[4,5] An important corollary question is why half the patients with the clinical triad and hydrocephalus fail to improve with surgery. One of the answers to this is that each of the clinical findings associated with symptomatic hydrocephalus are common in the elderly and may have multiple causes. Severe dementia may occur in up to 5 percent of people over 65 years of age and a milder form may be present in many more.[6] Incontinence occurs in 15 percent of women and 10 percent of men over age 70.[7] Gait abnormality is also common in the elderly and has been shown to have multiple etiologies.[8] The cerebral ventricles increase in size with age,[9] and ventriculomegaly is a common accompaniment of Alzheimer disease.[10] Since none of its cardinal findings is specific to symptomatic hydrocephalus, it is not surprising that a patient can exhibit the typical clinical triad plus hydrocephalus on computed tomography (CT) and yet not re-

spond to surgery. How can the neurologist best make the decision regarding recommendation for surgery? The first section of this chapter deals with the useful information already in the literature.

USEFUL INFORMATION IN DECIDING WHOM TO RECOMMEND FOR SHUNT SURGERY

History

Several important questions should be asked in taking a history from these patients and their families:

How long has the patient been demented? If this is more than 2 years, it is less likely that the patient will respond to surgery.[5,11] Note that the question is not how long the patient has had gait abnormality but how long the patient has been demented. Please refer to Table 50-1 to see how reliable this information was in predicting surgical outcome in our series.[11]

Which started first, gait abnormality or dementia? If the gait abnormality began before or at the same time as dementia, then there is a better chance for successful surgery. Whereas if dementia started before gait abnormality, shunting is less likely to help[11,12,19] (Table 50-1).

Is there a history of alcohol abuse? Alcohol abuse is a poor prognostic indicator.[13]

Is there a secondary cause of hydrocephalus? Examples are subarachnoid hemorrhage, meningi-

Table 50-1

Variables predicting surgical outcome in symptomatic hydrocephalus

Variable	No. of patients	Odds ratio	p value[a]	95% confidence interval for odds ratio[b]	Correct classification	
					Unimproved	Improved
Age	30	1.031	0.59	0.919–1.157		
Education	30	0.906	0.41	0.716–1.146		
Sex	30	4.615	0.215[c]	0.423–233.0		
Gait abnormality (years)	30	1.133	0.51	0.789–1.626		
Incontinence (years)	30	1.441	0.402	0.614–3.408		
Dementia (years)	30	9.002	<0.001	1.542–52.56	5/7	21/23
Order of onset (gait versus dementia)	30	0	0.009[c]	0–0.425	3/7	23/23
Percent time B-waves present	28	0.969	0.04	0.937–1.001	2/6	22/22
Percent time pressure >15 mmHg	28	0.968	0.055	0.930–1.006	0/6	22/22
Percent time pressure >20 mmHg	28	0.979	0.23	0.940–1.020		
Visual naming test	25	0.941	0.093	0.875–1.013	2/7	17/18
Visual naming, pass/fail	25	8.750	0.058[c]	0.887–113.3	5/7	14/18
Cerebral blood flow (anterior/posterior ratio slice 4)	30	1.120	<0.001	1.026–1.224	5/7	22/23
CSF conductance	23	0.254	0.956	0–infinity		
CSF conductance, 0.08 as cutoff value	23	1.071	1.00[c]	0.065–67.354		

[a]*p* value based on likelihood ratio test.

[b]Based on Wald test (which is slightly different from likelihood ratio test) and on Fisher exact test when this test was used.

[c]*p* value based on Fisher exact test.

Source: From Graff-Radford and Godersky,[18] with permission.

tis, previous brain surgery, and head injury. If any of these are present, the chances of improvement with surgery are better.[5,14,15]

Examination

On examination, the following issues should be addressed:

Measure the head circumference. If greater than 59 cm in males or 57.5 cm in females (i.e., greater than the 98th percentile for head circumference) the patient could have congenital hydrocephalus that has become symptomatic in later life.[16,17]

Exclude diseases that may mimic symptom- *atic hydrocephalus,* such as Parkinson disease, cervical spondylosis with spinal cord compression, progressive supranuclear palsy, multisystem degenerative disorder, phenothiazine use, Alzheimer disease with extrapyramidal features, and multiple subcortical infarctions. This is sometimes easier said than done, but keeping this differential diagnosis in mind during the examination is helpful.

Neuropsychology

Look for evidence of aphasia. If there is evidence of aphasia (e.g., anomia), this is a poor prognostic indicator for surgical success[11,13,18] (see Table 50-1).

Cerebrospinal Fluid Drainage Procedures

If the patient's gait improves after a large quantity of cerebrospinal fluid (CSF) *has been removed by lumbar puncture* (30 to 50 mL, and this can be repeated daily), he or she would be a good candidate for shunt surgery.[20,21] A modification of this technique, *continuous CSF drainage,* has also been reported and is executed via a catheter placed in the lumbar CSF space.[22,23] To do this, a thin subarachnoid catheter is placed in the lumbar CSF space and led into a drainage bag. The height of the drainage bag is adjusted to allow drainage of 5 to 10 mL/h and yet avoid CSF hypotensive symptoms of headache. This is a closed system and allows an average of 150 mL drainage per day. The closed system helps prevent infection and the thin tube prevents rapid CSF drainage, cutting down the risk of subdural hemorrhage. There are other methods of doing this. Hanley and coworkers,[23] for example, use a larger (16-gauge) catheter through which CSF pressure can also be monitored. They pay attention to the level of the drainage bag, aiming to drain 240 mL/day. To minimize infection, the drainage system is kept in for 2 to 5 days. If symptoms of headache and nausea develop, one should be concerned that too much CSF is being drained.

There are shortcomings to these diagnostic tests. We have seen patients who eventually responded to shunt surgery but had no obvious improvement for the first postsurgical week. The drainage test could have given a falsely negative result in these patients. When this test is being done, the patient may appear improved for the duration of the test (the placebo effect) but fail to maintain the response, thus producing a false-positive result. In addition, meningitis and subdural hematoma are possible complications of the continuous CSF drainage procedures.

COMPUTED TOMOGRAPHY AND MAGNETIC RESONANCE IMAGING

Computed Tomography

Since the advent of computed tomography (CT), the documentation of ventriculomegaly has become easier. This has had both advantages and disadvantages. There is a clear advantage to not having to subject patients to the uncomfortable procedure of air encephalography to diagnose hydrocephalus; however, physicians are often held responsible for knowing that a patient has ventriculomegaly when the scan may have been ordered for an unrelated indication.

A patient has ventriculomegaly (above the 95th percentile) when the modified Evans ratio is greater than 3.2.[24] The Evans ratio can be calculated on the axial CT slice where the frontal horns are largest. One measures the maximal diameter of the frontal horns and the inner table of the skull at the same level and then calculates the two measures as a ratio, the inner table of the skull in relation to the maximal diameter of the frontal horns. The ventricles normally enlarge with age,[25] a point that should be taken into account in diagnosing hydrocephalus. There is slow ventricular enlargement to age 60 years and then the rate of enlargement increases. In Barron's study,[25] the mean ventricular size was 5.2 percent (percent of intracranial area) in the decade from 50 to 59 years, 6.4 percent from 60 to 69 years, 11.5 percent from 70 to 79 years, and 14.1 percent from 80 to 89 years. If a patient has hydrocephalus without sulcal enlargement, this is a favorable factor in surgical prognosis; however, if there is sulcal enlargement and hydrocephalus, patients can still improve with surgery. Borgesen and Gjerris[15] measured the largest sulcus in the high frontal or parietal region and found that if the cortical sulci were less than 1.9 mm, 17 of 17 patients shunted improved; if the sulci were 1.9 to 5 mm, 17 of 20 shunted patients improved; and if the sulci were 5 mm or more, 15 of 27 patients shunted improved. Figure 50-1 shows a pre- and postoperative CT in a patient with symptomatic hydrocephalus.

Magnetic Resonance Imaging

Magnetic resonance imaging (MRI) is an excellent method for evaluating patients with possible symptomatic hydrocephalus. It has the advantage of being able to visualize structures in the posterior fossa that may be related to the patient's problem, such as the cerebral aqueduct, the level of the

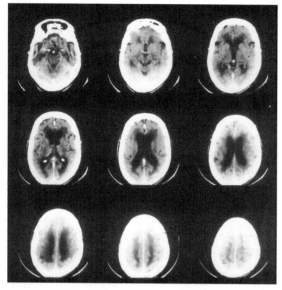

A

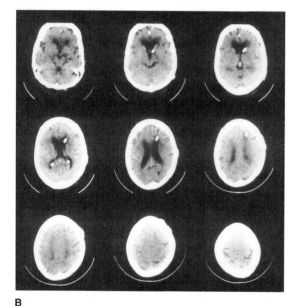

B

Figure 50-1

A. *Preoperative CT of patient with symptomatic hydro-cephalus.* B. *Postoperative CT of the same patient. This patient improved with surgery. Note that the ventricles are smaller after surgery. Sometimes this decrease in ventricular size is not as obvious, even in patients who improve.*

cerebellar tonsils, and infarctions in the brainstem. Further, MRI can be used to obtain volumetric measures of medial temporal lobe structures, a technique that has been shown to be useful in separating patients with Alzheimer disease from normal elderly controls.[26] About 10 percent of elderly patients with symptomatic hydrocephalus may have congenital hydrocephalus that becomes symptomatic in later years.[16] The clinical clue to this is that the patient has a head circumference above the 98th percentile. On MRI, the ventricular enlargement shows no or little associated periventricular increased signal on T_2-weighted imaging, indicating a chronic process. In addition, a cause for the congenital hydrocephalus may be found, such as an Arnold Chiari malformation.

Deep white matter changes on MRI have many possible causes and may also be seen on CT as "transependymal flow." Some report that the presence of transependymal flow may be related to a good surgical prognosis. In the study of Borgesen and Gjerris,[15] 16 of 16 with periventricular hypodensity on CT improved with surgery, whereas in the study of Bradley and colleagues,[27] MRI images were rated for deep white matter changes, and the presence or extent of these did not correlate with outcome. Jack and colleagues[28] retrospectively reviewed the charts in 57 patients, 17 with NPH, 8 with obstructive hydrocephalus, 8 with Alzheimer disease, and 21 with non-Alzheimer dementia. They looked at increased periventricular signal and white matter signal on T_2-weighted images, CSF flow void in the aqueduct, and corpus callosum thinning. Increased periventricular signal, increased white matter signal, and corpus callosum thinning were not useful in distinguishing among the four groups. All 17 NPH patients underwent shunt surgery, and a better response was noted in patients without increased white matter signal but with increase in periventricular signal. In a postmortem MRI study of fixed brains and the histologic analysis of the same brains, Munoz and coworkers[29] found the white matter changes seen on MRI are correlated with decreased density of axons and myelinated fibers, diffuse vacuolation of white matter (so called spongiosis), and decreased density of glia. Infarctions were not common in these areas. While this study does not necessarily apply to the white matter changes seen in hydrocephalic patients, it does indicate that white matter MRI findings do not necessarily indicate irreversible periventricular infarctions, making shunt surgery unlikely to be effective.

We have seen numerous patients improve with or without white matter changes on MRI. In more acute hydrocephalus, as might occur after subarachnoid hemorrhage, breakdown of the ependyma and CSF migration at the frontal horn angle occurs.[30,31] Thus Borgesen and Gjerris's observation[15] that transependymal flow is a good prognostic indicator may be more applicable to patients with secondary hydrocephalus because their series was heavily weighted with such patients. However, patients with chronic hydrocephalus characteristically have little transependymal flow, and these patients often improve with surgery.[16]

Another area where MRI has the potential to be helpful prognostically is in volumetric measurements of certain structures in the temporal lobe. Jack and colleagues[26] developed a technique for measuring the volumes of structures in the anterior temporal lobe and hippocampal formation. The volume of the hippocampal formation has also been shown to correlate with relevant cognitive variables. Occasionally when patients are shunted for symptomatic hydrocephalus and do not respond, they are ultimately found to have Alzheimer disease. This procedure is being evaluated for its predictive value in this clinical situation. Magnetic resonance imaging has advanced our knowledge regarding hydrocephalus and, in our opinion, is the imaging method of choice in these patients.

Detection of Cerebrospinal Fluid Flow through the Aqueduct by Magnetic Resonance Imaging

In 1991 Bradley and coworkers[32] retrospectively reviewed the MRI scans of 20 patients who had undergone ventriculoperitoneal shunt surgery for NPH. The investigators rated initial surgical outcome as excellent, good, or poor and correlated this with the extent of flow void in the cerebral aqueduct. They found a significant correlation between extent of increased aqueductal flow void and initial surgical outcome. More specifically, 8 out of 10 with increased CSF flow void scores had an excellent or good response to surgery, whereas only 1 out of 9 who normal flow void scores improved with surgery. The investigators speculate that the increased flow in the aqueduct in hydrocephalus is based on the following mechanism. A major cause of CSF motion is systolic expansion of the cerebral hemispheres and choroid plexus.[33] Systolic enlargement of the hemispheres normally results in outward expansion (with venting of cortical blood) and expansion inwardly with venting of CSF. However, in hydrocephalus, the brain is tighter against the skull, allowing less outward expansion during systole and resulting in more inward expansion and increased CSF venting. Again, we believe that this is a promising method for predicting surgical prognosis in symptomatic hydrocephalus. Future studies should be prospective, have better quantitation of flow through the aqueduct, and have more objective measures of surgical outcome.

Summary of Factors to be Addressed on Imaging

Hydrocephalus must be present. The modified Evans ratio (maximum width of the frontal horns/measure of the inner table at the same place) should be greater than 3.1.[15]

Is cortical atrophy prominent? If there is extensive cortical atrophy, this reduces but does not eliminate the chance of improvement with surgery.[5,15,34]

The pattern of atrophy may be useful diagnostically e.g., does it involve the medial temporal lobes, as is seen in Alzheimer disease? Although data on this point are lacking, it may be that prominent medial temporal cortical atrophy decreases the chances for surgical improvement because these patients may have Alzheimer disease.[35–37]

Is there evidence of congenital hydrocephalus? For example is there aqueductal stenosis or an Arnold-Chiari malformation?[16,17]

Newer MRI techniques such as cine-MRI involving the analysis of a CSF flow void in the aqueduct of Sylvius may be helpful in predicting who will respond to a shunt.[27,32,33,38]

REGIONAL CEREBRAL BLOOD FLOW

It has been reported that regional cerebral blood flow (rCBF) is decreased in the frontal areas in hydrocephalus[39] and in the parietotemporal areas in Alzheimer disease.[40] On the presumption that many of the nonimproved group have Alzheimer disease (which we have confirmed in two who came to autopsy), we tried to differentiate those who will respond to shunt surgery from those who will not on the basis of the pattern of preoperative rCBF.[41] To do this, we calculated the ratio of frontal over posterior regional blood flow, expecting a lower frontal posterior ratio in true symptomatic hydrocephalus and a higher ratio in pseudosymptomatic hydrocephalus patients with Alzheimer disease. In fact, this has been a good method in predicting surgical outcome: the ratio predicted 5 of 7 unimproved and 22 of 23 improved patients in our series[11] (see Table 50-1).

CISTERNOGRAPHY

Our experience with cisternography is limited, but the literature suggests that there are numerous patients with a positive test (radioisotope seen within the ventricles 48 to 72 h after being injected in the lumbar area) who do not improve with surgery and patients with equivocal or negative tests who do improve. Further, the test itself may be difficult to interpret. Black and colleagues, in a review of their experience with this test, suggest that a positive test is helpful but an equivocal or negative test is not.[14] A recent study by Vanneste and associates[42] reported that "cisternography did not improve the accuracy of combined clinical and computerized tomography in patients with presumed normal-pressure hydrocephalus." We do not use cisternography.

MONITORING OF CEREBROSPINAL FLUID PRESSURE

There have been reports of a significant relationship between measures of intracranial cerebrospinal fluid pressure monitoring and surgical outcome for symptomatic hydrocephalus—e.g., in the Borgesen and Gjerris study[15] and in our study,[11] the greater the percentage of time B waves were present, the greater the chance of a good outcome. Also in our series, the longer the pressure was more than 15 mmHg, the better the chance of successful surgery (see Table 50-1). This implies that increased pressure may be pathogenetic in symptomatic hydrocephalus.

These data raise the issue of what is meant by NPH. Does it mean normal pressure at one spinal tap or does it imply that the pressure remains normal all the time? We do not know what 24-h recordings of CSF pressure in normal people would show. It follows that we do not know whether the pressure is normal or abnormal in those who respond to surgery but have CSF pressures greater than 15 mmHg some of the time. For this reason, at present, we prefer the term *symptomatic hydrocephalus* over *normal pressure hydrocephalus.*

A continuous printout over 24 to 72 h with a paper speed between 50 and 150 mm/h is needed to assess the overall intracranial pressure (ICP) and presence of B waves. Sedation may be helpful at night to reduce the frequency of artifact in the recording.

INFUSION TESTS

Borgesen and Gjerris[15] described the *CSF conductance test,* in which CSF absorption is measured at different CSF pressures. They reported in their series a greater than 90 percent accuracy in predicting short-term prognosis following shunt surgery and about an 85 percent accuracy in predicting long-term prognosis. They concluded that the greater the pressure needed to obtain an amount of absorption, the better the chances of that patient improving with shunt surgery. In our study,[11] we found no significant correlation between CSF conductance and improvement (see Table 50-1). However, we chose our patients on the basis of conductance result, so this was not an independent variable. In addition, most of our patients had idiopathic hydrocephalus, whereas many of Borgenson and Gerris's patients had secondary hydrocephalus. The conductance test, which relates to CSF absorption, may be a better predictor of outcome in secondary hydrocephalus, in which an absorption defect may be causative.

SHUNT COMPLICATIONS

Shunt complications, both major and minor, unfortunately occur in about 30 percent of patients.[4,5] These include intraoperative complications related to general anesthesia in an elderly population, intracranial hemorrhage from ventricular catheter placement, intraabdominal injury (rare), and arrhythmias from incorrect ventriculoatrial distal catheter placement. Perioperative complications include infection (3 to 8 percent of cases), CSF hypotensive headaches, and the development of subdural effusions or hematomas. This last problem is more likely to occur in those with marked reduction in ventricular size postshunting and is more common when low-pressure valves are utilized to treat these effusions. Depending on symptoms, conservative or surgical therapy may be indicated. Long-term complications are primarily related to shunt occlusion or catheter breakage. Infection after the first 2 months is unusual.

HOW TO ASSESS PATIENT IMPROVEMENT

Traditionally, patient improvement has been assessed on a five-point rating scale.[4,15] This may be problematic, because levels on the scale overlap and it is a subjective judgment into which level the patient falls. We have tried to develop more objective measures and use the following:

Serial Videotaping of the Patient's Gait

Preoperatively and 2 and 6 months postoperatively, we videotape the patient's neurologic exam-

ination, including walking. Scales have been developed and published to both qualitatively and quantitatively measure the patient's gait performance.[11,19]

Katz Index of Activities of Daily Living[43]

This scale rates the patient on six items: bathing, dressing, toileting, transferring, continence, and feeding. The worst score for each item is 3 and the best is 1. Thus the worst obtainable score is 18 and the best is 6. There is a written description for each score in each item. We regard a change of 2 or more in this index as significant. This allows measurements of small but functionally important changes. An example of a 2-point improvement on this index might be as follows: a change from "occasional urinary accidents" to "controls urination and bowel movements completely by self" (1-point improvement) plus "moves in and out of bed or chair with assistance" to "moves in and out of bed as well as chair without assistance" (1-point improvement).

Neuropsychological Testing

Our patients receive a battery of neuropsychological tests before surgery and then 2 and 6 months postoperatively.[11] These tests sample orientation, intelligence, verbal and visual memory, language, visuospatial functioning, and executive control. We judge the patient neuropsychologically improved when there has been a significant increase in the test scores in two or more neuropsychological areas evaluated, provided that there is no decline in another area. Only about 50 percent of those responding to shunt surgery improve cognitively by the above criteria.

HOW TO DECIDE WHOM TO RECOMMEND FOR SURGERY

Bearing the above information in mind, we recommend the following. Take a careful history from the patient and family. Try to establish time of onset of dementia and gait abnormality by asking questions such as, "How did the patient walk last

Christmas or on her last birthday?'' Noting the differential diagnoses mentioned above, ask appropriate questions to find other causes of the constellation of findings. For example, has the patient had cervical spondylosis or a previous neck injury? Has the patient been a heavy drinker? Is there another cause for urinary difficulty, such as prostatism or the birth of multiple children? What medications does the patient take? Are there symptoms of autonomic dysfunction such as postural hypotension? Is there a secondary cause for hydrocephalus, such as a head injury, meningitis, or subarrachnoid hemorrhage? Has the patient had a large head since childhood? Does the patient have symptoms of Parkinson disease involving the hands, such as micrographia or tremor? On examination, measure the head size, measure the postural blood pressure, look for signs of Parkinson disease involving the arms, (making parkinsonism more likely), vertical-gaze paresis (unusual in symptomatic hydrocephalus in the elderly), and upper motor neuron signs in the legs and or lower motor neuron signs in the arms (raising suspicion of cervical spondylosis). Do formal psychometric testing looking for evidence of aphasia (especially anomia). Let the patient have a head CT and/or MRI and analyze this, keeping in mind the points mentioned above in the discussion of CT and MRI. If necessary, order a cervical MRI. Make a videotape of the patient walking about 20 yd, turning and walking back. At this time you may be able to make your decision about surgery. If you are still uncertain, perform daily serial lumbar punctures for 3 to 5 days, videotaping the patient before and after. If the patient improves, surgery is likely to help, but if there is no improvement, the patient could still improve and therefore should still be followed. Before recommending surgery, be sure to point out that complications occur in about 30 percent of patients undergoing shunt surgery. Also tell the patient and family that even if the patient improves, it is likely that he or she will not return to normal. In those that respond favorably, gait and incontinence usually improve, but cognition improves in only 50 percent. These are important improvements and may prevent a patient's placement in a nursing home, but the patient and family should have realistic expectations. If at this stage you are still unsure of what to do, you can defer the decision and let the patient return in 3 months, repeating the videotape at that time. Longitudinal information documenting whether the problem is stable or progressive may factor into your decision. Alternative diagnostic tests such as rCBF, CSF pressure monitoring, infusion studies, and continuous CSF drainage studies are not universally available but can be used as adjunctive information in centers that use these tests.

THE RELATIONSHIP OF IDIOPATHIC SYMPTOMATIC HYDROCEPHALUS AND SYSTEMIC HYPERTENSION

Several lines of evidence in the literature now point to a relationship between hydrocephalus and systemic hypertension. A number of postmortem examinations of NPH patients have found associated hypertensive cerebrovascular changes.[44–46] In our own series,[47] a significantly higher prevalence of systemic hypertension was found in patients with idiopathic NPH than in matched, demented controls and in the U.S. population, of the same age.

Another line of evidence showing that systemic hypertension and hydrocephalus may be related comes from the Cooperative Aneurysm Study.[48] In over 3000 patients with subarachnoid hemorrhage, it was found that a preoperative history of hypertension, the admission blood pressure, measurement and sustained hypertension during hospitalization after surgery were all significantly related to the patients' development of hydrocephalus. Greitz and coworkers[49] found a high prevalence of hypertension in patients with hydrocephalus from aqueductal stenosis.

The observation of the association of hypertension and hydrocephalus is corroborated by reports in the animal literature.[50–53] Thus, a body of information is accumulating that systemic hypertension and hydrocephalus are probably associated. If this proves to be so, it remains to be shown whether hypertension causes hydrocephalus, hydrocephalus causes hypertension, or both.

FACTORS ASSOCIATED WITH THE PATHOGENESIS OF HYDROCEPHALUS IN THE ELDERLY

Regarding the etiology and pathogenesis of symptomatic hydrocephalus in the elderly the following are some of the important factors: (1) *Congenital hydrocephalus* that becomes symptomatic in the elderly (this made up about 10 percent of our series[16,19]). (2) *Impaired CSF absorption.* There are many lines of evidence supporting this factor. For example, in the cooperative subarachnoid hemorrhage study,[48] items associated with the development of hydrocephalus were intraventricular hemorrhage, diffuse subarachnoid blood, and thick focal accumulation of blood; thin accumulation of blood and intracerebral hematoma were not associated with hydrocephalus. Patients with posterior circulation aneurysms (near the foramina of Luschka and Magendie and thus interfering with CSF egress from the fourth ventricle) have a significantly higher incidence of hydrocephalus, while patients with middle cerebral aneurysms have a significantly lower incidence of hydrocephalus. (3) *Increasing age.* The evidence in favor of this factor is that this is a disease of older individuals. Further, in the cooperative subarachnoid aneurysm study, increasing age was significantly associated with the development of hydrocephalus.[48] (4) *Systemic hypertension.* See discussion of this subject above.

ACKNOWLEDGMENTS

This work was supported in part by NIA grant AG08031-06S1 and the State of Florida Alzheimer's Disease Initiative.

REFERENCES

1. Wells CE: Diagnosis of dementia. *Psychosomatics* 20:517–522, 1979.
2. Katzman R: Normal pressure hydrocephalus, in Katzman R, Terry R, Bick KC (eds): *Alzheimer's Disease: Senile Dementia and Related Disorders (Aging).* New York: Raven Press, 1978, pp 115–124.
3. Hughes CP, Siegal BA, Coxe WS, et al: Adult idiopathic communicating hydrocephalus with and without shunting. *J Neurol Neurosurg Psychiatry* 41:961–971, 1978.
4. Black PMcL: Idiopathic normal pressure hydrocephalus. *Neurosurgery* 52:371–377, 1980.
5. Peterson RC, Mokri B, Laws ER: Surgical treatment of idiopathic hydrocephalus in elderly patients. *Neurology* 35:307–311, 1985.
6. Mortimer JA, Shuman LM, French LR: Epidemiology of dementing illness, in Mortimer JA, Shuman LM (eds): *The Epidemiology of Dementia.* New York: Oxford University Press, 1981.
7. Yarnell JW, St Leger AS: The prevalence, severity, and factors associated with urinary incontinence in a random sample of the elderly. *Age Ageing* 8:81–85, 1979.
8. Sudarsky L, Ronthal M: Gait disorders among elderly patients: A survey of 50 patients. *Arch Neurol* 40:740–743, 1983.
9. Barron SA, Jacobs L, Kinkel W: Changes in size of normal lateral ventricles during aging determined by computerized topography. *Neurology* 26:1011–1013, 1976.
10. Damasio H, Eslinger P, Damasio AR, et al: Quantitative computed tomographic analysis in the diagnosis of dementia. *Arch Neurol* 40:715–719, 1983.
11. Graff-Radford NR, Godersky JC, Jones MP: Variables predicting outcome in symptomatic hydrocephalus in the elderly. *Neurology* 39:1601–1604, 1989.
12. Fisher CM: The clinical picture in occult hydrocephalus. *Clin Neurosurg* 24:270–315, 1977.
13. DeMol J: Facteurs pronostiques du resultat therapeutique dans l'hydrocephalie a pression normale. *Acta Neurol Belg* 85:13–29, 1985.
14. Black PMcL, Ojemann RG, Tzouras A: CSF shunts for dementia, incontinence, and gait disturbance. *Clin Neurosurg* 32:632–656, 1985.
15. Borgesen SE, Gjerris F: The predictive value of conductance to outflow of CSF in NPH. *Brain* 105:65–86, 1982.
16. Graff-Radford NR, Godersky JC: Symptomatic congenital hydrocephalus in the elderly simulating normal pressure hydrocephalus. *Neurology* 39:1596–1600, 1989.
17. McHugh PR: Occult hydrocephalus. *Q J Med* 130:297–308, 1964.
18. Graff-Radford NR, Godersky JC, Tranel D, et al: Neuropsychological testing in normal pressure hy-

drocephalus, in Hoff JT, Betz AL (eds): *Intracranial Pressure.* Berlin: Springer-Verlag, 1989, vol VII, pp 422–424.

19. Graff-Radford NR, Godersky JC: Normal pressure hydrocephalus: Onset of gait abnormality before dementia predicts a good surgical outcome. *Arch Neurol* 43:940–942, 1986.

20. Wikkelso C, Andersson C, Blomstrand C, et al: The clinical effect of lumbar puncture in NPH. *J Neurol Neurosurg Psychiatry* 45:64–69, 1982.

21. Wikkelsö C, Anderson H, Blomstrand C, et al: Normal pressure hydrocephalus: Predictive value of the cerebrospinal fluid tap-test. *Acta Neurol Scand* 73:566–573, 1986.

22. Haan J, Thormeer RTWM: Predictive value of temporary external lumbar drainage in normal pressure hydrocephalus. *Neurosurgery* 22:388–391, 1988.

23. Hanley DF, Borel CO, Herdman S: Normal-pressure hydrocephalus, in Johnson RT (ed): *Current Therapy in Neurological Disease,* 3d ed. Philadelphia: Decker, 1990, pp 305–309.

24. Gyldensted C: Measurements of the normal ventricular system and hemispheric sulci of 100 adults with computed tomography. *Neuroradiology* 14:183–192, 1977.

25. Barron SA, Jacobs L, Kinkel W: Changes in size of normal lateral ventricles during aging determined by computerized tomography. *Neurology* 26:183–192, 1976.

26. Jack CR, Petersen RC, O'Brien PC, Tangalos EG: MR-based hippocampal volumetry in the diagnosis of Alzheimer's disease. *Neurology* 42:183–188, 1992.

27. Bradley WG, Kortman KE, Burgoyne B: Flowing cerebrospinal fluid in normal and hydrocephalic states: Appearance on MR images. *Radiology* 159:611–616, 1986.

28. Jack CR, Mokri B, Laws ER, et al: MR findings in normal-pressure hydrocephalus: Significance and comparison with other forms of dementia. *J Comput Assist Tomogr* 11:923–931, 1987.

29. Munoz DG, Hasak SM, Harper B, et al: Pathological correlates of increased signals of the centrum ovale on magnetic resonance imaging. *Arch Neurol* 50:492–497, 1993.

30. Di Chiro G, Arimitau T, Brooks RA, et al: Computed tomography profiles of periventricular hypodensity in hydrocephalus and leukencephalopathy. *Radiology* 130:661–666, 1979.

31. Mori K, Honda H, Murata T, Nahano Y: Periven-

tricular lucency in computed tomography of hydrocephalus and cerebral atrophy. *J Comput Assist Tomogr* 4:204–209, 1980.

32. Bradley WG, Whittemore AR, Kortman KE, et al: Marked cerebrospinal fluid void: Indicator of successful shunt in patients with suspected normal-pressure hydrocephalus. *Radiology* 178:459–466, 1991.

33. Feinberg DA, Mark AS: Human brain motion and cerebrospinal fluid circulation demonstrated with MR velocity imaging. *Radiology* 163:793–799, 1987.

34. Huckman MS: Normal pressure hydrocephalus: Evaluation of diagnosis and prognostic tests. *AJNR* 2:385–395, 1981.

35. George AE, De Leon MJ, Miller J, et al: CT diagnostic features of Alzheimer's disease: Importance of the choroidal/hippocampal fissure complex. *AJNR* 11:101–107, 1990.

36. Kido DK, Caine ED, LeMay M, et al: Temporal lobe atrophy in patients with Alzheimer's disease: A CT study. *AJNR* 10:551–555, 1989.

37. Sandor T, Albert M, Stafford J, Harpley S: Use of computerized analysis to discriminate between Alzheimer patients and normal control subjects. *AJNR* 9:1181–1187, 1988.

38. Enzmann DR, Pelc NJ: Normal flow patterns of intracranial and spinal cerebrospinal fluid defined with phase-contrast CINE-MRI imaging. *Radiology* 178:467–474, 1991.

39. Foster NL, Chase TN, Fedio P, et al: Alzheimer's disease: Focal cortical changes shown by positron emission tomography. *Neurology* 33:961–965, 1983.

40. Jagust WJ, Friedland RP, Budinger TF: Positron emission tomography with (^{18}F)-fluodeoxyyglucose differentiates normal pressure hydrocephalus from Alzheimer-type dementia. *J Neurol Neurosurg Psychiatry* 48:1091–1096, 1985.

41. Graff-Radford NR, Rezai K, Godersky JC, et al: Regional cerebral blood flow in normal pressure hydrocephalus. *J Neurol Neurosurg Psychiatry* 50:1589–1596, 1987.

42. Vanneste J, Augustijn P, Davies GAG, et al: Normal-pressure hydrocephalus. *Arch Neurol* 49:366–370, 1992.

43. Kane RA, Kane RL: *Assessing the Elderly: A Practice Guide to Measurements.* Lexington, MA: Lexington Books, 1981.

44. Koto A, Rosenberg G, Zingesser LH, et al: Syndrome of normal pressure hydrocephalus: Possible relation to hypertensive arteriosclerotic vasculo-

pathy. *J Neurol Neurosurg Psychiatry* 40:73–79, 1977.

45. Earnest MP, Fahn S, Karp JH, Rowland LP: Normal pressure hydrocephalus and hypertensive cerebrovascular disease. *Arch Neurol* 31:262–266, 1974.

46. Coblentz JM, Mattis S, Zingesser LH, et al: Presenile dementia. *Arch Neurol* 29:299–308, 1973.

47. Graff-Radford NR, Godersky JC: Idiopathic normal pressure hydrocephalus and systemic hypertension. *Neurology* 37:868–871, 1987.

48. Graff-Radford NR, Torner J, Adams HP, Kassell NF: Factors associated with hydrocephalus after subarachnoid hemorrhage: A report of the Cooperative Aneurysm Study. *Arch Neurol* 46:744–752, 1989.

49. Greitz T, Levander BE, Lopez J: High blood pressure and epilepsy in hydrocephalus due to stenosis of the aqueduct of Sylvius. *Acta Neurochir (Wien)* 24:201–206, 1971.

50. Ritter S, Dinh TT: Progressive postnatal dilatation of brain ventricles in spontaneously hypertensive rats. *Brain Res* 370:327–332, 1986.

51. Portnoy HD, Chopp M, Branch C: Hydraulic model of myogenic autoregulation and the cerebrovascular bed: The effects of altering systemic arterial pressure. *Neurosurgery* 13:482–498, 1983.

52. Peltarossi VE, Di Rocci C, Mancinelli R, et al: Communicating hydrocephalus induced by mechanically increased amplitude of the intraventricular cerebrospinal fluid pulse pressure: Rationale and method. *Exp Neurol* 59:30–39, 1978.

53. Bering RA Jr, Salibi B: Production of hydrocephalus by increased cephalic-venous pressure. *Arch Neurol Psychiatry* 81:693–698, 1959.

Part 7

EPILEPSY AND RELATED ISSUES

Chapter 51

NEUROBEHAVIORAL ASPECTS OF EPILEPSY

Joel Paraiso
Orrin Devinsky

Epilepsy is associated with behavioral changes that can occur in the peri-ictal, ictal, and interictal states. The diversity of these behavioral changes reflects the anatomic foci, patterns of spread, and biological and psychological differences among patients.[21,24,51,55,114] Although interictal cognitive and behavioral changes in epilepsy have clearly been established (see Table 51-1), defining the relation between behavior and the direct effects of epilepsy is difficult. Coexisting factors alter behavior. These include structural lesions, anti-epilepsy drugs, and existing psychosocial problems. The interictal period is dynamic, and the behavioral changes noted in this state may be paroxysmal (e.g., fear) or fairly continuous (e.g., viscosity).

The association of behavior and epilepsy has been recognized since the dawn of recorded history and was noted by Hippocrates in *The Sacred Disease.*[69] Although severe stigma and misperception dominated lay and medical communities for most of the past two millennia, the late 1800s saw the dawn of a new era. Reynolds[123] in 1861 observed that while epilepsy is often accompanied by behavioral and cognitive changes, it does not necessarily involve any personality change. Gowers[52] in 1885 reported that many patients have normal intellect and personality but that interictal behavioral changes in epilepsy are multifactorial, with epilepsy a prominent factor in most cases. Wilson[171] suggested that psychosocial factors are important in the pathogenesis of interictal behavior.

The association of temporal lobe epilepsy (TLE) and psychopathology began with the finding of Gibbs and coworkers[48] that abnormal behavior was more frequent in patients with psychomotor epilepsy when compared to those with other focal or generalized seizures. Slater and Beard[144] reported a significantly increased incidence of psychosis among epilepsy patients, supporting a widely held clinical impression that TLE predisposes toward psychosis. Waxman and Geshwind[164] defined an interictal behavior syndrome in TLE characterized by deepened emotion, altered religious and sexual concerns, and hypergraphia. They stressed behavioral changes rather than behavioral disorder, emphasizing that behaviors are not necessarily maladaptive or negative. Notably, epilepsy has been associated with positive traits, including military genius, artistic creativity, philosophical and religious insights, and profound deepening of emotions.[15]

Despite intensive study on the association of epilepsy and behavioral changes, our understanding remains fragmentary. The controversies surrounding behavior and epilepsy arise from three basic problems: (1) conflicting and nonstandardized research methods to measure personality and psychopathology, (2) disparate epilepsy and comparison group populations because of changes in the classification of epilepsy, and (3) the humanistic concern to avoid increasing the social stigma of epilepsy by associating it with abnormal behavior.

Table 51-1

Interictal behavioral changes associated with epilepsy

Aggression	Hypermoralism
Altered sexual interest	Hypomoralism
Dissociative disorders	Increased emotionality
Circumstantiality	Irritability
Decreased emotionality	Obsessionalism
Dependence, passivity	Paranoia
Elation, euphoria	Philosophical interest
Emotional lability	Religiosity
Guilt	Sadness
Humorlessness, sobriety	Sense of personal destiny
Hypergraphia	Viscosity

PERSONALITY CHANGES

Certain personality traits have been reported as being more common in epilepsy patients. These traits (Table 51-1) were identified from anecdotal observations as well as studies utilizing inventories [Bear and Fedio Temporal Lobe Epilepsy Inventory (BF-TLEI), Minnesota Multiphasic Personality Inventory (MMPI)] administered to epilepsy patients and control groups. The results are conflicting, although few experts doubt that among some epilepsy patients, personality can change or differ from that of individuals without chronic disabilities and other brain disorders. Much of the conflict concerns control groups. For example, in the large study performed by Guerrant and colleagues,[54] the control and TLE groups each had an approximately 80 percent incidence of behavioral disorder. However, the frequency of psychotic traits was much higher in the TLE group, although the authors concluded that there were no significant differences.

In Bear and Fedio's study,[5] TLE patients showed significant difference from normal and neuromuscular control groups regarding all 18 traits surveyed, with the most prominent changes in humorlessness, circumstantiality, dependence, and sense of personal destiny. Differences in per-

sonality traits between patients with right and left TLE were also found. Patients with right-sided TLE displayed more emotional traits and exhibited "denial" or "polished" their images, whereas those with left temporal lobe foci exhibited more ideational traits and "tarnished" their self-images. A recent study of epilepsy patients with personality changes found an association between auras and the development of personality disorders, particularly if the auras are not followed by secondary generalized seizure activity.[97]

Studies comparing trait differences between patients with TLE and primary generalized epilepsy failed to show any significant differences.[60,129] However, the critical issue may be the specific features of behavior, not the absolute percentage with a behavioral disorder. These studies and case reports led to further study on specific personality traits, both positive and negative. Several are considered below.

Altered Sexual Interest

Altered sexuality has been observed during the interictal, ictal, and postictal periods (Table 51-2). Interictal hyposexuality is most common and presents with impotence and decreased libido.[41,68,142] However, these complaints are often not perceived as a problem by the patient but more often by the spouse. Hyposexuality occurs in various types of epilepsy, affecting approximately

Table 51-2

Sexual behavioral changes seen in temporal lobe and frontal lobe epilepsy

Ictal	Interictal
Genital sensations	Hyposexuality
Sexual thoughts/arousal	Impotence
Pelvic thrusting	Hypersexuality
Masturbation	Altered sexual
Erection	preference
Orgasm	Exhibitionism
Undressing	Fetishism
Postictal	Transvestism
Undressing	Transsexualism
Erection	

half of TLE patients regardless of sex. In some cases hyposexuality resolves with good seizure control.[117] Barbiturates are an important cause of impotence that resolves when the medication is withdrawn.

Deviant sexual behavior interictally—including exhibitionism, transvestism, transsexualism, and fetishism—has been reported in isolated TLE.[71,130] Interictal hypersexuality, although rare, can occur and may respond to antiepileptic medications.[46,142] Hypersexuality rarely follows successful epilepsy surgery.

Ictal sexual phenomena can occur. Somatosensory sensations in the genitalia have been reported by patients with parietal and temporal lobe seizure foci.[18,44,122] Automatic genital manipulation, pelvic thrusting, and the uttering of obscenities can occur during frontal lobe seizures.

Postictal sexual arousal, erection, and undressing have all been observed following complex partial and generalized tonic-clonic seizures.

Hypergraphia

Hypergraphia, a tendency toward extensive and in some cases compulsive writing with striking preoccupation to details, is associated with epilepsy, occurring in approximately 8 percent of TLE patients.[64,65,132,164] These patients tend to define, redefine, underline, and use parentheses to make word meanings absolutely clear with a preponderance of focus on moral and religious concerns. These observations were interpreted as an extension of the interictal behavioral changes, especially deepening of emotions and viscosity.[164]

Religiosity

Various forms of religious experiences, mysticism, or conversions are associated with epilepsy. While Hippocrates attempted to refute the prevailing belief that epilepsy was a curse from the gods or that epileptics possessed prophetic powers,[69] religious and magical treatments of epilepsy predominated during the next two thousand years.[157] In the nineteenth century, the religiosity of epileptics was stressed by physicians such as Esquirol,[34] Morel,[105,106] and Maudsley.[92]

Dostoyevsky[33] eloquently described his personal epilepsy-related religious experience:

> *The air was filled with a big noise, and I thought that it had engulfed me. I have really touched God. He came into me myself, yes, God exists, I cried, and I don't remember anything else. You all, healthy people, he said, can't imagine the happiness which we epileptics feel during the second before our attack. I don't know if this felicity lasted for seconds, hours, or months, but believe me, for all the joys that life may bring, I would not exchange this one. . . . Such instants were characterized by a fulguration of the consciousness and by a supreme exaltation of emotional subjectivity.*

Religious aura or premonitory periods that may last for hours or days were reported by 53 of 1325 patients with epilepsy.[146] A temporal relationship between sudden religious conversion and first seizure or an increase in seizure frequency has been reported. Less often, there is a significant decrease in seizures before conversion.[29] Epileptiform activities have been documented during a religious ecstatic seizure.[16]

Religiosity is not a common interictal personality feature among patients with epilepsy. Two studies utilizing detailed religion questionnaires failed to reveal any significant differences between patients with right versus left TLE, TLE versus generalized epilepsy, or between epilepsy subjects and controls.[160,170]

Viscosity

Viscosity is an interpersonal style characterized by cohesive and "sticky" behavior favoring prolonged verbal contacts. Speech is often repetitive and circumstantial. This has been associated with TLE and appears to be more common with left-sided seizure foci. Viscosity is also more common among patients with primary generalized epilepsy as compared with normal controls.[11,70]

Viscosity may result from a combination of language impairment, mental slowness, psychological dependence, and a tendency for social cohesion. A direct correlation between left temporal seizure foci and impaired naming and circumstantiality suggests that in some cases viscosity is an interictal language impairment rather than a distinct personality trait.[93] The emotional need of some patients for interpersonal closeness may contribute to viscosity. This aspect is difficult to quantify but may have a biological basis, since animals with septal lesions tend to remain in greater contact with each other.[100]

Genius

A remarkable number of historical figures in politics, religion, and the fields of arts, sciences, and literature allegedly had epilepsy.[28] The question of whether epilepsy contributes to genius, extraordinary ambitions, and successes or whether this association is just coincidental remains unanswered. Some other attributes associated with epilepsy, such as deepened emotion, religiosity, hypergraphia, obsessiveness, and a personal sense of destiny, may provide the motivation that underlies extraordinary accomplishments among some individuals with epilepsy.

PSYCHOPATHOLOGY

Patients with epilepsy have a significantly increased incidence of mental pathology compared to a normal population.[77,168] However, the incidence of psychopathology among patients with epilepsy is only slightly increased (most often for psychoses, depression, and anxiety)[54,147] or the same[75,91,152] as compared with the incidence in patients with chronic medical or neurologic illnesses. Higher rates of psychiatric hospitalization among patients with epilepsy as compared with those with other chronic illnesses largely reflect the increased incidence of psychoses in epilepsy.[168] Various studies report psychopathology in 29 to 88 percent of epilepsy populations.[54,77,149,152] The interictal psychopathologic disorders reported among epilepsy patients are listed in Table 51-3.

Comparisons of TLE and non-TLE groups

Table 51-3
Reported interictal psychopathologic disorders

Mood disorder
    Depression
        Major depression
        Dysthymia
    Mania

Psychosis
    Schizophrenialike but with preserved emotions
    Forced normalization

Anxiety disorders
    Panic disorder
    Generalized anxiety disorder
    Phobias

Personality disorders
    Obsessive-compulsive disorder
    Paranoid disorder
    Dissociative disorders
        Depersonalization
        Poriomania
        Multiple personality
    Disorder of impulse control
        Intermittent explosive disorder
        Conduct disorder

(generalized epilepsy or focal, nontemporal epilepsy) have not revealed consistent findings. Studies utilizing MMPI and other psychopathology scales and psychiatric diagnoses do not demonstrate significant intergroup differences.[50,61,81,102,145,149] In a nonselected adult epilepsy population, psychological problems occurred in 29 percent (51 percent of TLE subgroup), and 7 percent had been hospitalized for psychiatric illness (21 percent in the TLE subgroup).[119]

Several variables may increase psychopathology among epilepsy patients. These include seizure phenomenology, brain pathology, antiepileptic drugs, and psychosocial factors (Table 51-4), e.g., early seizure onset,[61,72,139,166] multiple seizure types,[59,128] total lifetime number of seizures,[31,86] mesial-limbic temporal (in contrast to neocortical-lateral) foci,[110,166] left temporal foci,[2,42,96,116,137,140,151,156] right temporal foci,[42] bilateral temporal foci,[59,128] male sex,[129,155] female sex,[156] focal atrophic lesion on head computed

Table 51-4
Factors associated with psychopathology in epilepsy

Genetic predisposition	Brain pathology
Gender	Known cause
Epilepsy-related	Diffuse brain dysfunction
Anatomic focus	Early brain injury
Lateralization	Temporal lobe pathology
Temporal	Lateralized cerebral injury
Frontal	Cognitive impairment
Multifocal	Antiepilepsy drugs
Seizure type	Polytherapy
Simple partial	Withdrawal
Complex partial	Acute or chronic toxicity
Generalized tonic-clonic	Psychosocial factors
Myoclonic	Low socioeconomic status
Prolonged seizures	Low educational level
Status epilepticus	Vocational problems
Low seizure frequency	Premorbid personality
Seizure cluster/increased frequency	Stigmatization
Age of onset	Discrimination
	Fear of seizures
	Deprivation

tomography or magnetic resonance imaging,[120] and ictal fear.[55,59,67]

Depression

Depression can occur during the prodromal, ictal, interictal, and postictal periods. Depression is a common affective prodrome, occurring hours to days prior to a seizure,[9] and the second most common ictal affect next to fear-anxiety.[23,169] Feelings of sadness can persist for days after a seizure.[169] Prolonged depressive affect can occur with simple partial status.[167]

Depression is the most common interictal psychiatric disorder in patients with epilepsy, occurring in approximately one-third of patients. This prevalence is significantly higher as compared with prevalence in a comparatively disabled population.[104] When directly questioned, up to 80 percent of epilepsy patients report depression.[96,104,147] Endogenous depression occurs in up to 40 percent of patients with epilepsy.[124] The rate of suicide attempts and gestures among epilepsy patients has

been reported to be 30 percent as compared to 7 percent in a comparatively disabled control group.[96] These observations suggest that the higher incidence of depression among epilepsy patients is not simply a reaction to chronic illness; biological factors also contribute. Biological factors include a family history of depression, left-sided seizure focus, and antiepileptic medications (especially, barbiturates).[2,110,116,124] Notably, greater depressive reactions are observed in left hemispheric lesions and left-sided amobarbital injections as compared to right-sided ones.[125,126,158] Bilateral inferior frontal hypometabolism has been correlated with depression in epilepsy patients.[12]

Psychosocial problems accompanying epilepsy can contribute to depression. These include (1) neurologic impairment in patients with structural pathology or frequent seizures; (2) social bias and stigma, leading to restrictions on employment, living situations, and companionship; and (3) disturbed family relations (e.g., dependency, overprotection, rejection, negative self-image), which all act to reduce an individual's capacity to enjoy life and grow.[66,90,130,163]

Depression can be devastating to a patient with epilepsy. Given the high prevalence and associated morbidity and mortality, recognition and treatment of depression in patients with epilepsy should be a prime concern for neurologists. Effective treatments are available. Epilepsy is not an absolute contraindication for the use of antidepressants. Although these medications can lower the seizure threshold, most patients tolerate them without increased seizure frequency.[111]

Psychoses

The relationship between epilepsy and psychosis is controversial. Studies have shown a positive correlation between psychosis and epilepsy, particularly among patients with TLE.[13,115,121,144] However, there are no controlled epidemiologic studies of prevalence rates for psychosis in epilepsy.[150] Both retrospective and prospective studies show that the prevalence rate of psychosis is increased among patients with epilepsy as compared with prevalence in the general population and in patients with other medical or neurologic illnesses.[87,115,144,168] This observation, together with the finding that psychosis typically occurs after the onset of epilepsy in most patients with both disorders, suggests that the association is more than coincidental.

Ictal Psychosis   Ictal psychosis is rare, but recognition is essential for prompt treatment. Absence status—which causes confusion, impaired responsiveness, and subtle facial myoclonus—can be confused with psychosis.[85] Similar clinical presentations occur in other forms of atypical generalized nonconvulsive status, which rarely present in the elderly as the first manifestation of epilepsy.[84,108] Rarely, partial complex status epilepticus can cause psychosis.[134] Between discrete partial complex seizures, there may be clouding of consciousness with automatisms or agitation.

Simple partial status may be associated with different forms of psychopathology, including hallucinations, depersonalization, or derealization.[174]

These patients usually retain some insight into the perceived ictal phenomena.[135]

Postictal Psychosis   Postictal psychosis accounts for at least 25 percent of psychoses among epilepsy patients.[135] The psychosis usually follows a series of primary or secondary generalized tonic-clonic and complex partial seizures.[21,32,89] Typically, psychosis emerges after a lucid interval of 6 to 48 h following an increase in seizure frequency.[21] The duration of psychosis varies from hours to months. Prominent mood changes are common. Spontaneous recovery is usual, but lorazepam and molindone for 1 to 4 days has been our treatment of choice. Patients at high risk include those with bilateral independent seizure foci or a history of encephalitis or prior psychiatric hospitalization.[21]

Peri-ictal delirium must be distinguished from psychosis. Delirium is transient and causes a global deterioration of cognitive functions with impaired attention, orientation, autonomic activity, and sleep.[88] In contrast, in postictal psychosis, attention is relatively preserved. The hallucinations or delusions associated with postictal psychosis are more systematized and structured than the fragments of delirium.[57,89]

Interictal Psychosis   Interictal psychosis is more common in patients with epilepsy, especially those with TLE.[47,144] There are differences between schizophrenia and the schizophrenialike psychoses of epilepsy. The latter are characterized by a relatively preserved warm affect and personality, with a predominance of visual rather than auditory hallucinations.[94,144] Formal thought disorder, incoherent thought, emotional withdrawal, catatonia, and negative symptoms are less common in epileptic psychosis.[13,49,79] Outcome is more favorable among patients with epilepsy, with less need for neuroleptics or institutionalization.[141] Despite these clinical differences, extensive symptomatic overlap exists.[80] Also, epilepsy and schizophrenia may coexist.

Possible risk factors for psychosis in patients

Table 51-5
Possible risk factors for interictal psychosis

Genetic predisposition

Female sex

Epilepsy variables
    Onset before 20 years of age
    Duration of greater than 10 years
    History of complex partial seizures
    Left-sided seizure focus
    ? Temporal > frontal lobe seizure focus

Brain pathology
    Glial tumors
    Hamartomas

Pharmacologic factors
    Polytherapy
    High-dose antiepileptic drug therapy

Psychosocial factors
    Social deterioration
    Life events

with epilepsy are listed in Table 51-5. Identification of these risk factors may allow effective preventive therapies for high-risk epilepsy patients. New behavioral complaints and social or functional deterioration warrant a careful assessment.

Forced normalization (paradoxical normalization) was first described by Landolt[82] in 1953; the term refers to acute psychosis occurring after achievement of good clinical seizure control or resolution of interictal epileptiform discharges. This phenomenon appears more commonly with generalized epilepsies.[172] While generally considered rare, this phenomenon may account for as much as 8 percent of all psychoses associated with epilepsy.[173] Forced normalization is clinically more pleomorphic than most other forms of interictal psychosis.[113] Most patients are successfully treated with antipsychotic medications.

Anxiety Disorder

Anxiety and related feelings of fear and paranoia can occur in epilepsy patients as (1) simple partial seizures, (2) psychological reaction to other symptoms that alert a patient that a seizure is imminent, (3) postictal states, (4) interictal behavioral changes related to epilepsy, or (5) anxiety or panic disorders which are unrelated to epilepsy.[56,103,109,130,165] The boundaries between these mechanisms are usually clear but may overlap and blur.[56,130,165] Other causes of anxiety must be considered, including mitral valve prolapse, hyperthyroidism, hypoglycemia, pheochromocytoma, Cushing syndrome, alcohol or sedative drug withdrawal, and central nervous system stimulants.

Ictal Fear Fear and anxiety account for 10 to 15 percent of simple partial seizure symptoms[74,143,153] and are the most common affective symptoms in spontaneous and electrically induced partial seizures.[8,23,51,55,169] Spontaneous fear and anxiety are associated with anteromedial temporal[26,51,53] and less often cingulate seizure foci.[101] The quality and intensity of ictal anxiety-fear vary tremendously. As with other simple partial seizure symptoms, the onset of ictal fear is paroxysmal, usually lasting 30 to 120 s.[27] In contrast, panic attacks often build up gradually and last over 5 or 10 min.[58,95]

Ictal fear is associated with an increased frequency of psychopathology in some patients,[22,55,59,67] including psychiatric hospitalization, interictal anxiety, and increased MMPI scores for psychopathic deviancy, paranoia, schizophrenia, and social introversion. It is unknown whether behavioral effects of recurrent ictal fear or pathophysiologic changes associated with a specific anatomy contribute to psychopathy.

Differentiation between spontaneous ictal and reactive ictal fear can be difficult. Spontaneous fear is a sudden emotion unprovoked by a frightening thought or stimulus, while reactive fear is a patient's response to the realization that a seizure may occur.

Postictal Fear Some patients develop postictal fear or anxiety that can last hours or days, like depressive affect. These patients often have fear or anxiety as their aura, and postictal anxiety frequently follows a cluster of complex partial seizures. Ictal and postictal anxiety are treated with antiepileptic drugs.

Interictal Fear and Anxiety   Interictal anxiety symptoms are common in patients with epilepsy, occurring in as many as 66 percent of patients with limbic epilepsy.[56,103,107] There may also be an increased rate of these disorders among patients with juvenile myoclonic epilepsy.[162] In epilepsy patients with generalized anxiety or panic disorders, behavioral or pharmacologic treatment is indicated.

Dissociative Disorder

Dissociative disorders are characterized by a sudden or gradual alteration in the integrative functions of identity, memory, or consciousness. The transient or chronic disturbances of self include loss of memory for self-referential information (psychogenic amnesia), elaboration of secondary identities (e.g., psychogenic fugue, multiple personalities), or depersonalization (loss of personal reality; feeling detached from one's mind, like an automaton). Memory disturbances usually consist of amnesia for recall of events during a dissociative state which may be complete or partial. Ictal dissociative phenomena include depersonalization, derealization, autoscopy, and, rarely, personality changes. In a study of patients with partial epilepsy, 15 percent had depersonalization, 18 percent had derealization, and 6 percent had autoscopy.[23] Cases of dual or multiple personality states temporarily associated with seizures are rare[7,99,133] and are often psychogenic.[25]

Poriomania is a prolonged period of confusion in which an epilepsy patient may travel and subsequently be amnesic for events during this period (i.e., fugue state). The pathophysiology remains undefined. These rare cases are not well documented and probably represent postictal delirium or psychosis.

Aggression

Aggression is the most controversial behavior associated with epilepsy. Aggression and epilepsy remain inappropriately linked in medical and lay perceptions.[40] This association, based largely on inaccurate data and anecdotal reports, has significantly advanced the stigma of epilepsy. Aggression and epilepsy are common among patients with brain insults (see Chap. 57). However, the contribution of epilepsy to the aggressive behavior in patients with brain lesions is difficult to assess. In some cases, aggression has been linked to the seizures, occurring before, during, and most commonly after seizures. Nonspecific psychological changes—such as irritability, verbal aggression, anxiety, or depression—can occur hours or days before (i.e., prodromal) a seizure.[78,127]

Ictal Aggression   Although rare, aggression can occur during a seizure. Only 19 of 5400 patients whose seizures were studied on video-EEG monitoring displayed aggressive behavior.[19] These acts were unprovoked and, although they appeared highly coordinated, were associated with confusion and were inappropriate to the situation. The aggressive acts were usually verbal or physical and nondirected or directed toward inanimate objects. This behavior could be the first manifestation of a seizure or could occur as the seizure progressed. The behavior often consisted of pushing and shoving, although there have been reports of directed violence during a seizure.[37,38,39,159]

The violent repetitive rapid movements that can occur during frontal lobe complex partial seizures can be misinterpreted as aggression. Aggression, which is confusional, can result from continuous temporal lobe seizure activity. This behavior rapidly responds to diazepam, which temporarily interrupts the seizure activity.[36]

Postictal Aggression   The most common and best documented form of aggressive behavior in epilepsy occurs after a generalized tonic-clonic seizure and less often a complex partial seizure. Verbal or physical aggression can occur during the recovery period, when the subject is still confused. In this setting, physical restraint can provoke aggression, which almost always stops when the restraint is withdrawn.[40,129] Aggression may also be a prominent feature of postictal psychoses, particularly in patients with paranoid delusions and threatening hallucinations.

Interictal Aggression   Interictal aggressive behavior has been reported in patients with epilepsy, especially TLE, but a direct association remains controversial. There are no conclusive prospective or controlled studies of aggression in the general epilepsy population. Reported rates of interictal behavioral aggression vary from 5 to 50 percent.[17,45,112,129] In one prospective study of 100 consecutive children with TLE, 36 percent had rage episodes.[87] In another study, 30 percent of patients with partial or generalized seizures admitted to experiencing interictal intense episodic irritability or moodiness, as compared with 2 percent in normal or neurologic controls.[23]

Several studies failed to demonstrate an increased incidence of interictal behavioral aggression between patients with TLE and those with other forms of epilepsy, neurologic disorders, or psychiatric disturbances.[63] Interictal violence has a greater correlation with psychopathology and mental retardation than with epileptiform activity.[98] Most studies demonstrate an increased incidence of aggression in all groups over the expected rate in the general population. This pattern can be explained by the presence of identified risk factors for aggression coexisting with epilepsy. These factors include exposure to violence as a child, violent behavior as a child, male sex, left-handedness, low socioeconomic status, focal or diffuse neurologic lesions, cognitive impairment, and medications such as barbiturates.[112,148,155] In contrast, consecutive but highly selected neurosurgical series reported pathologic aggression in 27 to 36 percent of patients.[139,155] Despite the selection bias, reduced aggression in more than 35 percent of these violent patients after temporal lobectomy suggests that the dysfunctional temporal lobe contributed to aggressive behavior.[35] Interictal aggression can occur after development of a limbic epileptic focus in patients without developmental or sociologic risk factors for aggression.[22] Experimental temporal lobe seizure foci in animals increase aggressive behavior.[1,14,53,118,138] Reduced

aggressive behavior follows temporolimbic resection in humans and animals.[76,161] Together, these findings suggest that, in selected cases and situations, epilepsy can be associated with aggressive behavior.

PATHOGENESIS

The wide spectrum of behavioral changes associated with epilepsy results from a dynamic and complex interplay of many variables. These include biological and social as well as iatrogenic factors. Dissecting the etiologic factors of behavior in epilepsy is limited by the lack of consensus as to the definition of the behavioral changes, their prevalence, and in which group they occur. Potential biological mechanisms involved in epilepsy-related behavioral changes include changes in neuronal connections, excitation, or inhibition.

Gastaut and coworkers[45] recognized that many behavioral changes associated with TLE (e.g., decreased sexual appetite, hypoactivity, and increased level of aggression) are opposite to the behavioral changes of the Kluver-Bucy syndrome.[76] A model of sensory-limbic hyperconnection or enhanced affective association was proposed by Bear to explain the behavioral changes in TLE.[6] Interictal frontotemporal hypometabolism, well documented in patients with complex partial seizures, suggests that functional hypoactivity may contribute to some behavioral changes in these patients. Other interictal behaviors, however, such as hyposexuality and deepened emotions, are not consistent with functional hypoactivity. These behaviors suggest functional hyperactivity of limbic areas, perhaps resulting from selective impairment of inhibitory neurons. Scans with single-proton emission computed tomography of two patients with left TLE and psychosis showed hypoperfusion during the interictal period and normal or hyperperfusion of the amygdala or left temporal lobe during psychosis.[73]

The organic pathology causing epilepsy may be static, but at a functional level, the process is dynamic and can cause a sustained alteration of behavior. This is the basis of Sir Charles Symonds's[154] hypothesis of the epileptogenic disorder of function:

> If then neither the fits nor the temporal lobe damage can be held directly responsible for the psychosis, what is the link? . . . Epileptic seizures and epileptiform discharges in the EEG are epiphenomena. They may be regarded as occasional expressions of a fundamental and continuous disorder of neuronal function. The essence of this disorder is loss of the normal balance between excitation and inhibition at the synaptic junctions. From moment to moment there may be excess either of excitation or inhibition—or even both at the same time in different parts of the same neuronal system. The epileptogenic disorder of function may be assumed to be present continuously but with peaks at which seizures are likely to occur.

Antiepileptic drugs can alter behavior and cognition. Decreased concentration, depression, and irritability are common complaints of patients, particularly those who are on barbiturates.[20,30] Antiepileptic medications can cause lethargy and decreased cognitive functions and initiative.[10] Individual sensitivity to drugs may explain prominent manifestations with low serum levels. While most behaviorial effects of antiepileptic drugs are secondary to changes in normal brain activity, some changes may result from suppression of epileptogenic activity. Patients may complain of irritability, tension, depression, and poor attention span after prolonged seizure-free interval. In such patients, suppression of seizures with antiepileptic drugs can enhance undesirable interictal behaviors. This process may be akin to forced normalization, where improvement in the electroencephalogram or seizure control produced by antiepileptic medications is associated with behavioral deterioration.[83]

Social factors influence and affect the interictal behavior of epilepsy patients, as do intrapersonal factors. These include the feeling of shame, perceived stigma and discrimination, feeling of helplessness, and lack of control over their lives because of epilepsy.[3,4,131] Extrapersonal factors play a significant role in the behavior of epilepsy patients as well. The social stigma and discrimination against epilepsy are widely recognized. Epilepsy patients have been unfairly denied employment[43] and socially excluded and devalued as people.[136] Learned helplessness may contribute to interictal behavioral changes such as depression.[62,63]

SUMMARY

Epilepsy is associated with alterations in cognition, affect, personality, and other elements of behavior. These changes manifest in the peri-ictal, ictal, and interictal stages. Negative traits (i.e., depression, apathy, anxiety, and altered sexual behavior) as well as positive traits (i.e., genius and creativity) have been reported. Multiple factors—including neurobiological, social, and iatrogenic factors—have been proposed as causes. Studies of the behavioral changes associated with epilepsy point to diversity as a unifying theme, and a single "epileptic constitution or personality complex" does not exist. However, certain behavioral traits, such as hyposexuality and viscosity, are more common among patients with epilepsy. In caring for epilepsy patients, physicians must remain vigilant to detect early behavioral changes that herald deterioration.

REFERENCES

1. Adamec RE, Starl-Adamec C: Limbic control of aggression in the cat. *Prog Neuro-psychopharmacol Biol Psychiatry* 7:505–512, 1983.
2. Altschuler LL, Devinsky O, Post RM, Theodore WH: Depression, anxiety, and temporal lobe epilepsy: Laterality of focus and symptomatology. *Arch Neurol* 47:284–288, 1990.
3. Arnston P, Droge D, Norton R, Murray E: The perceived psychosocial consequences of having epilepsy, in Whitman S, Hermann BP (eds): *Psychopathology in Epilepsy: Social Dimensions.* New York: Oxford University Press, 1986, pp 143–161.

4. Bagley C: Social prejudice and the adjustment of people with epilepsy. *Epilepsia* 13:33–45, 1972.

5. Bear DM, Fedio P: Quantiative analysis of interictal behavior in temporal lobe epilepsy *Arch Neurol* 34:454–467, 1977.

6. Bear DM: Temporal lobe epilepsy—A syndrome of sensory-limbic hyperconnection. *Cortex* 15:357–384, 1979.

7. Benson DF, Miller BL, Signer SF: Dual personality associated with epilepsy. *Arch Neurol* 43:471–474, 1986.

8. Bingley T: Mental symptoms in temporal lobe epilepsy and temporal lobe gliomas. *Acta Psychiatr Neurol Scand* 33(suppl):1–151, 1958.

9. Blanchet P, Fomment GP: Mood changing preceding epileptic seizures. *J Nerv Ment Dis* 174:471–476, 1986.

10. Bourgeois B: Natriumvalproat und kognitive Funktionen. *Schweiz Rundschau Med Praxis* 83:1122–1225, 1994.

11. Brandt J, Seidman LJ, Kohl D: Personality characteristics of epileptic patients: A controlled study of generalized and temporal lobe cases. *J Clin Exp Neuropsychol* 7:25–38, 1985.

12. Broomfield EB, Altshuler L, Leiderman DB, et al: Cerebral metabolism and depression in patients with complex partial seizures. *Epilepsia* 31:625–626, 1990.

13. Bruens JH: Psychoses in epilepsy. *Psychiatry Neurol Neurochir* 74:175–192, 1971.

14. Brutus M, Shaikh MB, Edinger H, Siegal A: Effects of experimental temporal lobe seizures upon hypothalamically elicited aggressive behavior in the cat. *Brain Res* 366:53–63, 1986.

15. Bryant JE: *Genius and Epilepsy.* Concord, MA: Ye Old Depot Press, 1953.

16. Cirignotta F, Todesco CV, Lugaresi E: Temporal lobe epilepsy with ecstatic seizures (so-called Dostoyevsky epilepsy). *Epilepsia* 21:705–710, 1980.

17. Currie S, Healthfield KWG, Henson RA, Scott DF: Clinical course and prognosis of temporal lobe epilepsy: A survey of 666 patients. *Brain* 94:173–190, 1971.

18. Currier RD, Little SC, Suess JF, Andy OJ: Sexual seizures. *Arch Neurol* 25:260–264, 1971.

19. Delgado-Escueta AV, Mattson RH, King L, et al: The nature of aggression during epileptic seizures. *N Engl J Med* 305:711, 1981.

20. Devinsky O: Cognitive and behavioral effects of antiepileptic drugs. *Epilepsia* 36(suppl 2):S46–65, 1995.

21. Devinsky O, Abramson H, Alper K, et al: Post ictal psychosis: A case control series of 20 patients and 150 controls. *Epilepsy Res* 20:247–253, 1995.

22. Devinsky O, Bear D: Varieties of aggressive behavior in temporal lobe epilepsy. *Am J Psychiatry* 141:651–656, 1984.

23. Devinsky O, Feldman E, Emoto S, et al: Structured interview for partial seizures: Clinical phenomenology and diagnosis. *J Epilepsy* 3:107–116, 1991.

24. Devinsky O, Kelley K, Yacubian EM, et al: Postictal behavior: A clinical and subdural electroencephalographic study. *Arch Neurol* 51:254–259, 1994.

25. Devinsky O, Putnam F, Grafman J, et al: Dissociative states and epilepsy. *Neurology* 39:835–840, 1989.

26. Devinsky O, Sato S, Theodore WH, Porter RJ: Fear episodes due to limbic seizures with normal scalp EEG: A subdural electrographic study. *J Clin Psychiatry* 50:28–30, 1989.

27. Devinsky O: Fear and epilepsy, in Canger R, Saccheti E, Perini GI, Canevini MP (eds): *Carbamazepine: A Bridge between Epilepsy and Psychiatric Disorders.* Origio, Italy: Ciba-Geigy Edizioni, 1990, pp 41–48.

28. Devinsky O: Interictal behavioral changes in epilepsy, in Devinsky O, Theodore WH (eds): *Epilepsy and Behavior.* New York: Wiley-Liss, 1991, pp 1–21.

29. Dewhurst K, Beard AW: Sudden religious conversions in temporal lobe epilepsy. *Br J Psychiatry* 117:497–507, 1970.

30. Dodrill CB: Effects of antiepileptic drugs on abilities. *J Clin Psychiatry* 49:31–34, 1988.

31. Dodrill CB: Correlates of generalized tonic seizures with intellectual, neuropsychological, emotional, and social function in patients with epilepsy. *Epilepsia* 27:399–411, 1986.

32. Dongier S: Statistical study of clinical and electroencephalographic manifestations of 536 psychotic episodes occurring in 516 epileptics between clinical seizures. *Epilepsia* 1:117–142, 1959/60.

33. Dostoyevsky FM: *The Idiot.* Magarshack D (transl). London: Penguin Books, 1955.

34. Esquirol E: *Mental Maladies: A Treatise on Insanity.* Hunt EK (transl). Philadelphia: Lea & Blanchard, 1845.

35. Falconer MA: Reversibility by temporal lobe resection of the behavioral abnormalities of temporal lobe epilepsy. *N Engl J Med* 289:451–455, 1973.

36. Fenwick P: Precipitation and inhibition of seizures,

in Reynolds E, Trimble M (eds): *Epilepsy and Psychiatry*. Edinburgh: Churchill Livingstone, 1981, pp 306–321.

37. Fenwick P: Aggression and epilepsy, in Bolwig H, Trimble M (eds): *Aspects of Epilepsy and Psychiatry*. Chichester, England: Wiley, 1986, pp 62–98.

38. Fenwick P: Is dyscontrol epilepsy? in Trimble M, Reynolds E (eds): *What Is Epilepsy?* Edinburgh: Churchill Livingstone, 1986, pp 161–182.

39. Fenwick P: Dyscontrol, in Reynolds E, Trimble M (eds): *The Bridge between Neurology and Psychiatry* Edinburgh: Churchill Livingstone, 1989, pp 263–287.

40. Fenwick P: Aggression and epilepsy, in Devinsky O, Theodore WH (eds): *Epilepsy and Behavior*. New York: Liss, 1991, pp 85–96.

41. Fenwick PBC, Toone BK, Wheeler MJ, et al: Sexual behavior in a centre for epilepsy. *Acta Neurol Scand* 71:428–435, 1985.

42. Flor-Henry P: Psychosis and temporal lobe epilepsy: A controlled investigation. *Epilepsia* 10:363–395, 1969.

43. Fraser RT, Clemmons DC: Vocational and psychosocial interventions for youth with seizure disorders, in Hermann BP, Seidenberg M (eds): *The Childhood Epilepsies: Neuropsychological, Psychosocial, and Intervention Aspects*. Chichester, England: Wiley, 1989, pp 201–219.

44. Freemon FR, Nevis AH: Temporal lobe sexual seizures. *Neurology* 19:87–90, 1969.

45. Gastaut H, Morin G, Leserve N: Etude du comportement des epileptiques psychomoteurs dans l'intervalle de leurs crises. *Ann Med Psychol* 113:1–27, 1955.

46. Geshwind N, Shader RI, Bear D, et al: Behavioral changes with temporal lobe epilepsy: Assessment and treatment. *J Clin Psychiatry* 41:89–95, 1980.

47. Gibbs FA: Ictal and non-ictal psychiatric disorders in temporal lobe epilepsy. *J Nerv Ment Dis* 113:522–528, 1951.

48. Gibbs FA, Gibbs EL, Fuster B: Psychomotor epilepsy. *Arch Neurol Psychiatry* 60:331–339, 1948.

49. Glaser GH: The problem of psychosis in psychomotor temporal lobe epilepsy. *Epilepsia* 5:271–278, 1964.

50. Glass DH, Mattson RJ: Psychopathology and emotional precipitation of seizures in temporal lobe and nontemporal lobe epileptics. Proceedings of the 81st Annual Convention of the American Psychological Association, 1973, pp 425–426.

51. Gloor P, Olivier A, Quensney LF, et al: The role of the limbic system in experimental phenomena in temporal lobe epilepsy. *Ann Neurol* 12:129–144, 1982.

52. Gowers WR: *Epilepsy and Other Chronic Convulsive Disorders*. New York: William Wood, 1985, p 101.

53. Griffith N, Engel J, Bandler R: Ictal and enduring interictal disturbances in emotional behavior in an animal model of temporal lobe epilepsy. *Brain Res* 400:360–364, 1987.

54. Guerrant J, Anderson WW, Fischer A, et al: *Personality in Epilepsy*. Springfield, IL: Charles C Thomas, 1962.

55. Halgren E, Walter RD, Cherlow DG, Crandall PH: Mental phenomena evoked by electrical stimulation of the human hippocampal formation and amygdala. *Brain* 101:83–117, 1978.

56. Harper M, Roth M: Temporal lobe epilepsy and the phobic anxiety-depersonalization syndrome: Part I. A comparative study. *Compr Psychiatry* 3:129–151, 1962.

57. Hauser P, Devinsky O, De Bellis M, et al: Benzodiazepine withdrawal delirium with catatonic features. *Arch Neurol* 46:696–699, 1989.

58. Henricksen GF: Status epileticus partialis with fear as clinical expression. *Epilepsia* 14:39–46, 1973.

59. Hermann BP, Dikmen S, Schwartz MS, Karnes WE: Psychopathology in TLE patients with ictal fear: A quantitative investigation. *Neurology* 32:7–11, 1982.

60. Hermann BP, Reil P: Interictal personality and behavioral traits in temporal lobe and generalized epilepsy. *Cortex* 17:125–128, 1981.

61. Hermann BP, Schwartz MS, Karnes WE, Vahdat P: Psychopathology in epilepsy: Relationship to seizure type to age at onset. *Epilepsia* 21:15–23, 1980.

62. Hermann BP, Stone JL: A historical review of the epilepsy surgery program at the University of Illinois Medical Center: The contributions of Bailey, Gibbs, and collaborators to the refinement of anterior temporal lobectomy. *J Epilepsy* 2:155–163, 1989.

63. Hermann BP, Whitman S: Behavioral and personality correlates of epilepsy: A review, methodological critique, and conceptual model. *Psychol Bull* 95:451–497, 1984.

64. Hermann BP, Whitman S, Arnston P: Hypergraphia in epilepsy: Is there a specificity to temporal lobe epilepsy? *Cortex* 17:125–128, 1981.

65. Hermann BP, Whitman S, Wyler AR, et al: The

neurological, psychosocial and demographic corre-lates of hypergraphia in patients with epilepsy. *J Neurol Neurosurg Psychiatry* 51:203–208, 1988.

66. Hermann BP, Whitman S: Psychosocial predictors of interictal depression. *J Epilepsy* 2:231–237, 1989.

67. Hermann BP, Chhabria S: Interictal psychopathol-ogy in patients with ictal fear: Examples of sensory-limbic hyperconnection. *Arch Neurol* 37:667–668, 1981.

68. Hierons R, Saunders M: Impotence in patients with temporal lobe lesions. *Lancet* 2:761–763, 1966.

69. Hippocrates: The Sacred Disease, in *The Genuine Works of Hippocrates.* London: Sydenham Society, 1846, pp 843–858.

70. Hoeppner JB, Garron DC, Wilson RS, Koch-Wesser MP: Epilepsy and verbosity. *Epilepsia* 28:35–40, 1987.

71. Hooshmand H, Brawley BW: Temporal lobe sei-zures and exhibitionism. *Neurology* 19:1119–1124, 1969.

72. Jensen I, Larsen JK: Mental aspects of temporal lobe epilepsy. *J Neurol Neurosurg Psychiatry* 42:256–265, 1979.

73. Jibiki I, Maeda T, Kubota T, Yamaguchi N: ^{123}I-IMP SPECT brain imaging in epileptic psychosis: A study of two cases of temporal lobe epilepsy with schizophrenia-like syndrome. *Neuropsycho-biology* 28:207–211, 1993.

74. King DW, Marsan CA: Clinical features and ictal patterns in epileptic patients with temporal lobe foci. *Neurology* 2:138–147, 1977.

75. Klove H, Doehring H: MMPI in epileptic groups with different etiology. *J Clin Psychol* 18:149–153, 1962.

76. Kluver H, Bucy PC: Preliminary analysis of func-tions of the temporal lobe in monkeys. *Arch Neurol Psychiatry* 42:979–1002, 1939.

77. Kogeorgos J, Fonagy P, Scott DF: Psychiatric symptom profiles of chronic epileptics attending a neurologic clinic: A controlled investigation. *Br J Psychiatry* 140:236–243, 1982.

78. Kolb B, Nonneman AJ: Frontolimbic lesions and social behavior in the rat. *Physiol Behav* 13:637–643, 1974.

79. Koreniowski L: Les problemes diagnostiques corncernant les psychoses paranoiaques schizo-phreniformes en epilepsie. *Ann Med Psychol* 123:35–42, 1965.

80. Kraft AM, Price TRP, Peltier D: Complex partial seizures and schizophrenia. *Compr Psychiatry* 25:113–124, 1984.

81. Lachar D, Lewis R, Kupke T: MMPI in differentia-tion of temporal lobe and nontemporal lobe epi-lepsy: Investigation of three levels of test perfor-mance. *J Consult Clin Psychol* 47:186–188, 1979.

82. Landolt H: Serial electroencephalographic investi-gations during psychotic episodes in epileptic pa-tients and during schizophrenic attacks, in Lorentz de Haas AM (ed): *Lectures on Epilepsy.* Amster-dam: Elsevier, 1953, pp 99–133.

83. Landolt H: Serial encephalographic investigations during psychotic episodes in epileptic patients and during schizophrenic attacks, in de Hass L (ed): *Lectures on Epilepsy.* Amsterdam: Elsevier, 1958, pp 91–133.

84. Lee SI: Nonconclusive status of epilepticus. *Arch Neurol* 42:778–781, 1985.

85. Lennox WG: The treatment of epilepsy. *Med Clin North Am* 29:1114–1128, 1945.

86. Lennox WG: *Epilepsy and Related Disorders.* Bos-ton: Little, Brown, 1960, vols 1 and 2.

87. Lindsay J, Ounstead C, Richards P: Long-term outcome in children with temporal lobe seizures: III. Psychiatric aspects in childhood and adult life. *Dev Med Child Neurol* 21:630–636, 1979.

88. Lipowski ZJ: *Delirium: Acute Brain Failure in Man.* Springfield, IL: Charles C Thomas, 1980.

89. Logsdail SJ, Toone BK: Post-ictal psychoses. *Br J Psychiatry* 152:246–252, 1988.

90. Long CG, Moore JL: Parental expectations for their epileptic child. *J Child Psychol Psychiatry* 20:299–312, 1979.

91. Matthews CG, Klove H: MMPI performance in major motor, psychomotor, and mixed seizure clas-sifications of known and unknown etiology. *Epilep-sia* 9:43–53, 1968.

92. Maudsley H: *The Pathology of Mind.* London: Macmillan, 1879, p 446.

93. Mayeux R, Brandt J, Rosen J, Benson DF: Interic-tal memory and language impairment in temporal lobe epilepsy. *Neurology* 30:120–125, 1980.

94. McKenna PJ, Kane JM, Parrish K: Psychotic symp-toms in epilepsy. *Am J Psychiatry* 142:895–904, 1985.

95. McLachlan RS, Blume WT: Isolated fear in com-plex partial status epilepticus. *Ann Neurol* 8:639–641, 1980.

96. Mendez MF, Cummings JL, Benson DF: Depres-sion in epilepsy. *Arch Neurol* 38:176–181, 1986.

97. Mendez MF, Doss RC, Taylor JL: Interictal vio-lence in epilepsy: Relationship to behavior and

seizure variable. *J Nerv Ment Dis* 181:566–569, 1993.

98. Mendez MF, Doss RC, Taylor JL, Arguello R: Relationship of seizure variables to personality disorders in epilepsy. *J Neuropsychiatry Clin Neurosci* 5:283–286, 1993.

99. Mesulam MM: Dissociative states with abnormal temporal lobe EEG. *Arch Neurol* 38:176–181, 1981.

100. Meyer DR, Ruth RA, Lavond DG: The septal social cohesiveness effect: Its robustness and main determinants. *Physiol Behav* 21:1027–1029, 1978.

101. Meyer G, McElhaney M, Martin W, McGraw CP: Stereotactic cingulotomy with results of acute stimulation and serial psychological testing, in Laitinen LV, Livingston KE (eds): *Surgical Approaches in Psychiatry.* Baltimore: University Park Press, 1973, pp 39–58.

102. Mignone RJ, Donnelly EF, Sadowsky D: Psychological and neurological comparisons of psychomotor and nonpsychomotor epileptic patients. *Epilepsia* 11:345–359, 1970.

103. Mittan RJ, Locke GE: Fear of seizures: Epilepsy's forgotten problem. *Urban Health* Jan/Feb:38–39, 1982.

104. Mittan RJ, Locke GE: The other half of epilepsy: Psychosocial problems. *Urban Health* Jan/Feb:38–39, 1982.

105. Morel BA: *Traite des maladies mentales.* Paris: Masson, 1960.

106. Morel BA: D'une forme de delire, suite d'une surexcitation nerveuse se rattachant a une variete non encore decrite d'epilepsie (Epilepsie larvee). *Gaz Hebdom Med Chir* 7:773–775, 819–821, 836–841, 1860.

107. Mulder DW, Daly D: Psychiatric symptoms associated with lesions of temporal lobe. *JAMA* 150:173–176, 1952.

108. Nakane Y: Absence status: With special reference to the psychiatric symptoms directly related to the occurrence of seizure activity. *Folia Psychiatry Neurol Jpn* 37:227–238, 1983.

109. Nickell PV, Uhde TW: Anxiety disorders and epilepsy, in Devinsky O, Theodore WH (eds): *Epilepsy and Behavior.* New York: Wiley-Liss, 1991, pp 67–84.

110. Nielsen H, Kristensen O: Personality correlates of sphenoidal EEG foci in temporal lobe epilepsy. *Acta Neurol Scand* 64:289–300, 1981.

111. Ojemann LM, Baugh-Bookman C, Dudley DL: Effect of psychotropic medications on seizure control in patients with epilepsy. *Neurology* 37:1525–1527, 1987.

112. Ounstead C: Aggression and epilepsy: Rage in children with temporal lobe epilepsy. *J Psychosom Res* 13:237–242, 1969.

113. Pakalnis A, Drake ME, John K, Kellum BJ: Forced normalization: Acute psychosis after seizure control in seven patients. *Arch Neurol* 44:289–292, 1987.

114. Penfiled W, Jasper H: *Epilepsy and the Functional Anatomy of the Human Brain.* Boston: Little, Brown, 1954.

115. Perez MM, Trimble MR: Epileptic psychosis—Diagnostic comparison with process schizophrenia. *Br J Psychiatry* 137:245–249, 1980.

116. Perini GL, Mendius R: Depression and anxiety in complex partial seizures. *J Nerv Ment Dis* 172:287–290, 1984.

117. Peters UH: Sexualstorungen bei psychomotorischer Epilepsie. *J Neurovis Relat* (suppl 10):491–497, 1971.

118. Pinel JPJ, Treit D, Rovner LI: Temporal lobe aggression in rats. *Science* 197:1088–1089, 1977.

119. Pond DA, Bidwell BH: A survey of epilepsy in fourteen general practices: II. Social and psychological aspects. *Epilepsia* 1:285–299, 1959/60.

120. Provinchiali L, Franciolini B, del Pesce M, et al: Influence of neurological factors on the personality profile of patients with temporal lobe epilepsy. *J Epilepsy* 2:239–244, 1989.

121. Ramani V, Gumnit RJ: Intensive monitoring of interictal psychosis in epilepsy. *Ann Neurol* 11:613–622, 1981.

122. Remillard GM, Andermann F, Testa GR, et al: Sexual ictal manifestations predominate in women with temporal lobe epilepsy: A finding suggesting sexual dimorphism in the human brain. *Neurology* 33:323–330, 1983.

123. Reynolds JR: *Epilepsy: Its Symptoms, Treatment and Relation to Other Chronic Convulsive Disorders.* London: John Churchill, 1861, pp 39–77.

124. Robertson MM, Trimble MR, Townsend HRA: The phenomenology of depression in epilepsy. *Epilepsia* 28:364–372, 1987.

125. Robinson RG, Kubus KL, Starr LB, et al: Mood disorders in stroke patients: Importance of location of lesion. *Brain* 42:441–447, 1984.

126. Robinson RH, Szetela B: Mood changes following left hemispheric brain injury. *Ann Neurol* 9:447–453, 1981.

127. Rodin E, Schmaltz S: The Bear-Fedio personality

inventory and temporal lobe epilepsy. *Neurology* 34:591–596, 1984.

128. Rodin EA, Katz M, Lennox D: Differences between patients with temporal lobe seizures and those with other forms of epileptic attacks. *Epilepsia* 17:313–320, 1976.

129. Rodin EA: Psychomotor epilepsy and aggressive behavior. *Arch Gen Psychiatry* 28:210–213, 1973.

130. Roth M, Harper M: Temporal lobe epilepsy and the phobic anxiety-depersonalization syndrome: Part II. Practical and theoretical considerations. *Compr Psychiatry* 3:215–226, 1962.

131. Ryan R, Kempner K, Emlen AC: The stigma of epilepsy as a self-concept. *Epilepsia* 21:433–444, 1980.

132. Sachdev HS, Waxman SG: Frequency of hypergraphia in temporal lobe epilepsy: An index of interictal behavior syndrome. *J Neurol Neurosurg Psychiatry* 44:358–360, 1981.

133. Schenk L, Bear D: Multiple personality and related dissociative phenomena in patients with temporal lobe epilepsy. *Am J Psychiatry* 138:1131–1316, 1981.

134. Schmitz B: Psychosen bei Epilepsia: Eine epidemiologische Untersuchung (thesis). Berlin: Free University, 1988.

135. Schmitz B, Wolf P: Psychoses in epilepsy, in Devinsky O, Theodore WH (eds): *Epilepsy and Behavior.* New York: Wiley-Liss, 1991, pp 97–128.

136. Schneider JW, Conrad P: In the closet with epilepsy: Epilepsy stigma potential and information control. *Soc Probl* 28:32–44, 1980.

137. Seidman L: Lateralized cerebral dysfunction, personality, and cognition in temporal lobe epilepsy (thesis). Ann Arbor, MI: University Microfilms International, 1980.

138. Seigel A, Brutus M, Shaikh MB, Edinger H: Effects of temporal lobe epileptiform activity upon aggressive behavior in the cat. *Int J Neurol* 19,20:59–73, 1985/86.

139. Serafetinides EA: Aggressiveness in temporal lobe epileptics and its relation to cerebral dysfunction and environmental factors. *Epilepsia* 6:33–42, 1965.

140. Sherwin I: Differential psychiatric features in epilepsy: Relation to lesion laterality. *Acta Psychiatr Scand* 69(suppl 313):92–103, 1984.

141. Sherwin I: Psychosis associated with epilepsy: Significance of the laterality of the epileptogenic lesion. *J Neurol Neurosurg Psychiatry* 44:83–85, 1981.

142. Shulka GD, Hrivastava ON, Katiyar BC: Sexual disturbances in temporal lobe epilepsy: A controlled study. *Br J Psychiatry* 134:288–292, 1979.

143. Silberman EK, Post RM, Nurenberger J, et al: Transient sensory, cognitive and affective phenomena in affective illness: A comparison with partial epilepsy. *Br J Psychiatry* 146:81–89, 1985.

144. Slater E, Beard AW: The schizophrenic like psychoses of epilepsy. *Br J Psychiatry* 109:95–150, 1968.

145. Small JG, Milstein V, Stevens JR: Are psychomotor epileptics different? A controlled study. *Arch Neurol* 7:187–194, 1962.

146. Spratling WP: *Epilepsy and Its Treatment.* Philadelphia: Saunders, 1904, pp 473–474.

147. Standage KF, Fenton GW: Psychiatric symptom profiles of patients with epilepsy: A controlled investigation. *Psychol Med* 5:152–160, 1975.

148. Stevens JR, Hermann B: Temporal lobe epilepsy, psychopathology and violence: The state of the evidence. *Neurology* 31:1127–1132, 1981.

149. Stevens JR, Milstein V, Goldstein S: Psychometric test performance in relation to the psychopathology of epilepsy. *Arch Gen Psychiatry* 26:532–538, 1972.

150. Stevens JR: Interictal manifestions of complex partial seizures, in Penry JK, Daly DD (eds): *Advances in Neurology.* New York: Raven Press, 1975, vol 11.

151. Stores G: School children with epilepsy at risk for learning and behavior problems. *Dev Med Child Neurol* 20:502–508, 1978.

152. Strauss E, Risser A, Jones MN: Fear responses in patients with epilepsy. *Arch Neurol* 39:626–630, 1982.

153. Strobos RJ: Mechanisms in temporal lobe seizures. *Arch Neurol* 5:48–57, 1961.

154. Symonds C: Discussion. *Proc R Soc Med* 55:314–315, 1962.

155. Taylor D: Aggression and epilepsy. *J Psychosom Res* 13:229–236, 1969.

156. Taylor DC: Factors influencing the occurrence of schizophrenia-like psychosis in patients with temporal lobe epilepsy. *Psychol Med* 5:249–254, 1975.

157. Temkin O: *The Falling Sickness,* 2d ed. Baltimore: Johns Hopkins University Press, 1971.

158. Terzian H: Behavioral and EEG effects of intracarotid sodium amyal injection. *Acta Neurochir* 12:230–239, 1964.

159. Trieman D, Delgado-Escueta AV: Violence and epilepsy: A critical review. In Pedley T, Meldrum

B (eds): *Recent Advances in Epilepsy 1.* Edinburgh: Churchill Livingstone, 179–209, 1983.

160. Tucker DM, Novelly RA, Walker PJ: Hyperreligiosity in temporal lobe epilepsy: Redefining the relationship. *J Nerv Ment Dis* 175:181–184, 1987.

161. Vaernet K, Madsen A: Stereotaxic amygdalatomy and basofrontal tractotomy in psychotics with aggressive behavior. *J Neurol Neurosurg Psychiatry* 33:858–863, 1970.

162. Vasquez B, Devinsky O, Luciano D, et al: Juvenile myoclonic epilepsy: Clinical features and factors related to misdiagnosis. *J Epilepsy* 6:233–238, 1993.

163. Ward F, Bower BD: A study of certain social aspects of epilepsy in childhood. *Dev Med Child Neurol* 39(suppl):1–50, 1978.

164. Waxman SG, Geschwind N: Hypergraphia in temporal lobe epilepsy. *Neurology* 24:629–631, 1974.

165. Weilberg JP, Bear DM, Sachs G: Three patients with concomitant panic attacks and seizure disorder: Possible clues to the neurology of anxiety. *Am J Psychiatry* 144:1053–1056, 1983.

166. Weiser HG: Selective amygdalohippocampectomy: Indications, investigative technique and results. *Adv Tech Stand Neurosurg* 13:39–133, 1986.

167. Wells CE: Transient postictal psychosis. *Arch Gen Psychiatry* 32:1201–1203, 1975.

168. Whitman S, Hermann BP, Gordon A: Psychopathology in temporal lobe epilepsy: How great is the risk? *Biol Psychiatry* 19:213–236, 1984.

169. Williams D: The structure of emotions relected in epileptic experiences. *Brain* 79:29–67, 1956.

170. Willmore LJ, Heilman KM, Fennell E, Pinnas RM: Effect of chronic seizures on religiosity. *Trans Am Neurol Assoc* 105:85–87, 1980.

171. Wilson SAK: *Neurology.* Baltimore: Williams & Wilkins, 1940, p 1486.

172. Wolf P: The clinical syndromes of forced normalization. *Folia Psychiatr Neurol Jpn* 38:187–192, 1984.

173. Wolf P: Discussion, in Trimble MR, Bolwig TG (eds): *Aspects of Epilepsy and Psychiatry.* Chichester, England: Wiley, 1986, p 162.

174. Wolf P: Status epilepticus and psychosis, in Akimoto H, Kazamatsuri H, Semo M, Ward A (eds): *Advances in Epileptology: XIIIth Epilepsy International Symposium.* New York: Raven Press, 1982, pp 211–217.

Chapter 52

NEUROPSYCHOLOGICAL ASSESSMENT FOR EPILEPSY SURGERY

David W. Loring
Kimford J. Meador

Neuropsychological assessment and Wada testing are performed to document seizure onset laterality, identify patients who are at risk for significant memory decline following surgery, and establish the laterality of cerebral language and memory dominance. As in patients with other neurologic disorders, neuropsychological assessment in epilepsy surgery candidates also assists in identifying psychiatric disorders and directing vocational rehabilitation.

Neuropsychological testing and the Wada procedure provide important confirmatory evidence of seizure onset laterality in patients with complex partial seizures whose seizures originate in temporal lobes.[1,2] These behavioral measures may be sensitive to small structural changes that are difficult to detect radiologically and may also reflect functional (as opposed to structural) abnormalities resulting from epilepsy. Consequently, neurobehavioral evaluation of seizure surgery candidates is an important aspect of the evaluation of epilepsy surgery patients. This chapter focuses on temporal lobe seizure patients undergoing anterior temporal lobectomy (ATL), since this is the most common type of ablative epilepsy surgery. Corpus callosotomy is discussed elsewhere in this volume (Chap. 32).

PREOPERATIVE NEUROPSYCHOLOGICAL ASSESSMENT

Cognitive Abilities

Neuropsychological testing is employed during the preoperative evaluation for epilepsy surgery to measure functional deficits associated with the seizure focus. The baseline neuropsychological evaluation varies among epilepsy centers but includes a combination of tests designed to assess intelligence, memory, language, visual-spatial ability, attention, sensory and motor function, and applied problem-solving strategies.

Patients with generalized or multifocal areas of dysfunction have poorer postoperative seizure control, although mixed results have been reported.[3] Full-scale IQ reflects, in part, general cerebral impairment and may be considered in determining candidacy for ATL, since low IQs are consistent with generalized impairment in which focal resection is less likely to be beneficial. Although comparison of verbal IQ with performance IQ may reflect lateralized cerebral impairment in other neurologic populations, the use of these measures in epilepsy surgery candidates does not help in the lateralization of unilateral temporal lobe seizures.[4] Although nonlateralized neuropsychological findings occur more frequently in groups with poor seizure outcomes,[5] the concordance of the side of seizure onset and laterality of neuropsychological findings is not necessarily related to outcome.[6]

Because medial temporal lobe structures are crucial for acquisition of new material into memory, memory assessment is central in the neuropsychological evaluation for ATL. Although some functional reorganization may occur when hippocampal tissue is dysfunctional, compensation is rarely complete, and recent memory is typically impaired.[7] In addition, ongoing seizure activity and repetitive interictal discharges may also impair memory.[8] When seizure onset is unilateral, the associated memory deficits may be material-specific. Verbal memory deficits associated with left temporal lobe seizure onset is a robust finding and has been shown across surgery centers and with a variety of verbal memory tests.[2,9–13] Visuospatial memory deficits are associated with right temporal seizure onset; however, this relationship is much less robust and reliable than the association of verbal memory impairment and left temporal seizure onset.[14]

Material-specific memory impairment associated with the temporal lobe contralateral to a seizure focus (i.e., verbal memory impairment in right temporal lobe epilepsy (TLE) or visuospatial memory impairment in left TLE) may indicate a higher risk for postoperative memory change because it raises the possibility of contralateral temporal lobe impairment. Thus, the reliability of visuospatial memory impairment is an important issue. Because replication attempts have been unable to reliably reproduce selective visuospatial memory impairments in right TLE and because poor visuospatial memory impairments may be present in left TLE patients and normal in right TLE patients, visuospatial memory performance alone does not typically play a prominent role in assessing risk for postoperative memory decline.

Many complex partial seizure patients undergoing evaluation for ablative surgery have seizures that arise in lateral, orbital, or medial frontal regions. Neuropsychological deficits associated with frontal seizure onset are not only less well lateralized compared with memory deficits in TLE but also less well localized to the frontal lobes. For example, a common measure used to assess frontal lobe function is the Wisconsin Card Sorting Test (WCST). However, WCST performance may be decreased in patients with postcentral lesions and may be normal in certain cases of confirmed frontal lobe pathology.[15] Further, poor WCST scores may be present both in patients with temporal lobe seizure onset and in patients with frontal seizure onset.[16] Generative fluency tasks are also commonly used as measures of frontal lobe function, and preliminary evidence has been presented to suggest the utility of comparing word generation to figure generation in discriminating left from right lobe impairment.[17] However, its prospective application for individual patient prediction is not universally agreed upon.[18] Neuropsychological testing in other nontemporal seizure patients is used primarily to establish whether anticipated cognitive deficits in those areas are present and is not typically employed for prognostic purposes.

Personality and Psychosocial Function

Neuropsychological testing of epilepsy surgery candidates also includes assessment of personality and psychosocial status. In some centers, the presence of serious psychopathology—such as severe psychosis or severe depression, personality disorders, or frequently nonepileptic seizures—is considered contraindicative to surgery.[19] This is based on the perceived risk for postoperative psychiatric deterioration, difficulty in patient management during evaluation and treatment, and the potential need for extensive resources and intervention during postoperative rehabilitation. However, other centers do not consider there to be any psychiatric contraindication. This disparity in views may be due to the absence of well-controlled, large-scale studies of psychiatric morbidity.

Psychosocial status, including mood and the patient's perception of his or her quality of life, is increasingly considered in the evolution for epilepsy surgery. Although cognitive abilities and psychological adjustment interact, with poorer adjustment present in patients with greater cognitive impairments, there is still a large area of independence between cognition and quality of life. Fraser reported that 40 percent of job failures in epilepsy were due to emotional/attitudinal problems. The most commonly employed measure of personality is the Minnesota Multiphasic Personality Inventory (MMPI). Examples of psychosocial and quality-of-life measures include the Washington Psychosocial Seizure Inventory[20] and the Quality-of-Life in Epilepsy Inventory.[21,22]

THE WADA TEST

The Wada procedure is employed to lateralize language function and assess memory preoperatively.[23,24] The procedure pharmacologically inactivates the distribution of the ipsilateral anterior and middle cerebral arteries for several minutes, during which time the patient is presented with multiple cognitive tasks. The three main goals of Wada testing for epilepsy surgery evaluation are (1) establishing cerebral language representation, (2) predicting patients who are at risk for developing a postsurgical amnestic syndrome, and (3) identifying lateralized dysfunction to help confirm seizure onset laterality. However, the goals and the procedure itself vary among centers. Variations in the procedure include differences in drug administration (e.g., dosage, concentration, and injection rate) and method of behavioral assessment (e.g., type and timing of stimuli).

Language

Language information derived from the Wada procedure may be used to determine the need for preoperative grid studies or intraoperative cortical mapping (see Chap. 53) and may be considered in planning the extent of surgical resection. Most epilepsy surgery centers (93 percent) employ naming as a criterion for establishing speech lateralization for the dominant hemisphere, as well as unspecified aphasic signs (78 percent), counting ability (80 percent), familiar word/phrase repetition (61 percent), and unfamiliar word/phrase repetition (65 percent).[24] In contrast, more heterogeneous criteria are used to infer the presence of speech representation in the nondominant hemisphere, including mouthing appropriately, groaning, singing, object naming, partial phoneme vocalization, serial rote speech, and expression of familiar words. Thus, it should not be surprising that some centers never observed bilateral language representation, whereas others reported bilateral language in as many as 60 percent of cases. We consider positive paraphasic responses as the strongest single evidence of language representation in the hemisphere being studied. Confidence is further enhanced if evidence of deficits across multiple language domains is induced.

Test sensitivity is particularly important in inferring exclusive right-hemispheric language representation. Speech arrest, for example, may be present following right cerebral injection but may be unrelated to language representation.[23,26] In addition, patients with "right cerebral language dominance" by Wada testing have developed transient aphasia following left-hemispheric surgery, showing some left-hemispheric language representation.[27] Similarly, other "right cerebral language"–dominant patients by Wada testing have had left-hemispheric language areas identified during cortical stimulation mapping using subdural electrodes.[28] Thus, many patients considered right cerebral language dominant may have some left-hemispheric language representation as well. Our experience is that most patients who are not left cerebral language dominant have varying degrees of bihemispheric language representation, with exclusive right-hemispheric language representation rarely being observed.[29] Right-hemispheric language may also be observed without a corresponding shift in handedness and may be present in some dextral patients with either left[30] or right temporal seizure onset.[31,32]

Atypical language representation alters the confidence with which inferences from neuropsychological findings are made. For example, in a patient with bilateral language representation (R > L) and a right temporal lobe seizure focus, both pre- and postoperative neuropsychological studies revealed impaired visuospatial memory and normal verbal memory.[32] Further, memory testing during electrical hippocampal stimulation via depth electrodes indicated reliance on left-hemispheric medial temporal lobe structures for verbal memory. Thus, the patient presented with verbal memory more lateralized to the left hemisphere and visuospatial memory more lateralized the right hemisphere, despite greater right-hemispheric language representation. Cerebral dominance for language and verbal memory are not necessarily linked.

Memory

Wada memory testing is employed partly to assess whether the hemisphere contralateral to a unilateral seizure focus can sustain memory function following temporal lobectomy.[33] In contrast to the formal neuropsychological evaluation in which material-specific measures of verbal and visuospatial memory are obtained, Wada memory testing frequently employs memory stimuli that are encodable in a variety of ways, since one primary goal is to identify risk for amnesia. In addition, the use of material-specific memory stimuli will be confounded by the amobarbital-induced generalized hemispheric dysfunction.[34] For example, impaired recall of written words following language-dominant injection may reflect aphasia during stimulus presentation rather than the inability of the temporal lobe to acquire new information.

Wada memory performance is related to both hippocampal cell counts[35] and to hippocampal volumes as gauged by magnetic resonance imaging (MRI).[36] Although the posterior hippocampus is not directly supplied by the distribution of the internal carotid artery, depth record electroencephalographic (EEG) slowing occurs in this region following intracarotid amobarbital administration.[37] Thus, both a structural and functional relationship exists between Wada memory and the hippocampus.

Despite the above findings, Wada memory testing should not be employed as an absolute measure of hippocampal function. Patients failing the Wada memory component may successfully undergo surgery if other evidence suggests a low likelihood of risk to recent memory, such as structural evidence (tumor or hippocampal atrophy) or a consistent unilateral seizure onset. Several reports describe patients who have failed the Wada memory test but did not develop postoperative amnesia or who failed an initial Wada test and subsequently passed a repeat study.[38–40] However, marked Wada memory asymmetries that are inconsistent with an established seizure focus suggest caution. For example, if a patient with a right temporal lobe focus recognizes all the memory items following left-hemispheric injection but recognizes none of the memory items following right-hemispheric injection, the patient would be considered at increased risk for both poor memory and a poor seizure outcome.[41]

Wada Prediction of Lateralized Dysfunction

Wada memory asymmetries may be helpful in identifying functional impairments associated with the primary seizure focus.[40,42,43] Even when the test is applied on an individual basis, a significant relationship exists between the side of seizure onset and asymmetries in ipsilateral/contralateral Wada memory performance.[44,45] Strong Wada memory asymmetries may help in documenting seizure onset laterality in patients whose seizure workups have been suggestive but inconclusive. In these cases, a definite Wada memory asymmetry may eliminate the need for invasive monitoring before surgery.

Patients are more likely to have poor memory performance following injection contralateral to a seizure focus if significant hippocampal sclerosis exists.[43,46,47] This relationship is presumably due to the degree of bilateral temporal lobe dysfunction created by the injection. Minimal functional hippocampal capacity is present with severe hippocampal sclerosis; consequently, contralateral amobarbital perfusion creates greater bilateral temporal lobe dysfunction with a concomitant increase in the likelihood of greater Wada memory asymmetry, since the ipsilateral injection would be less likely to impair memory. In contrast, patients with mild sclerosis perform better following contralateral injection. In this case, the contralateral side is significantly impaired due to the disruptive effects of amobarbital, but the epileptogenic hippocampus with only minimal sclerosis has residual functional capacity and can contribute to new memory acquisition.[48] However, patients with mild sclerosis still do worse following the contralateral rather than ipsilateral injections.

Wada Seizure Outcome Prediction

Evidence of well-lateralized temporal lobe dysfunction increases the likelihood of a good surgical outcome. Patients with significant volumetric MRI hippocampal asymmetries are more likely to have a good outcome following ATL.[49] Since the presence of hippocampal atrophy is related to postoperative seizure frequency and because Wada memory asymmetries are related to MRI hippocampal volume asymmetries,[36] an association between Wada memory and seizure outcome would be anticipated. In one report, 89 percent of patients with Wada memory asymmetries were seizure-free. In contrast, only 63 percent of the patients without asymmetries were seizure-free.[50] Wada memory asymmetries contribute unique information to outcome prediction, beyond the information provided by other clinical factors such as presence of tumor or earliest age of possible brain abnormality.[51]

POSTOPERATIVE NEUROPSYCHOLOGICAL OUTCOME

Postoperative Memory Change

One of the most famous patients in neuropsychology is H.M., who, on September 1, 1953, underwent bilateral temporal lobectomy for seizure control. William B. Scoville was the neurosurgeon and reported the changes in H.M.'s memory at the Harvey Cushing Society Meeting: "[B]ilateral resection . . . has resulted in no marked physiologic or behavioral changes with the exception of a very grave, recent memory loss, so severe as to prevent the patient from remembering the locations of the rooms in which he lives, the names of his close associates, or even the way to toilet and urinal. . . ."[52] Two patients in addition to H.M. with significant recent memory impairment following bilateral temporal lobectomy were presented in the original report. Describing the first patient, Scoville and Milner[53] comment: "At the examiner's request he drew a dog and an elephant, yet half an hour later did not even recognize them as his own drawings." The second additional case displayed a profound retrograde amnesia such that "her immediate recall of stories and drawings was inaccurate and fragmentary, and delayed recall was impossible for her even with prompting; when the material was presented again she failed to recognize it."

In addition to postoperative amnesia following bilateral temporal lobe resection, memory impairment was also noted in some early cases following unilateral temporal lobectomy. Although not as severe as in the bilateral cases, it was sufficiently severe to prevent the patients from returning to their previous jobs and to interfere with activities of daily living. The memory impairment was postulated to result from the effects of the surgery in conjunction with preexisting contralateral damage.[54] This hypothesis was subsequently confirmed in one patient who was shown to have a pale and shrunken right hippocampus at autopsy[55] and provided the rationale for Milner to include memory testing as part of the Wada procedure,[56] which, until that time, was used exclusively to determine language laterality. Subsequently developments in neuroimaging, invasive EEG monitoring, and Wada testing have all contributed to a decline in the incidence of amnesia after temporal lobectomy. Nevertheless, recent reports show that amnesia continues to be a risk associated with ATL.[41]

The development of global amnesia is a rare event. Patients undergoing epilepsy surgery are at risk for experiencing significant decline in material-specific verbal memory following left ATL or decline in visuospatial memory following right ATL. Although not as devastating as global amnesia, a significant decline in verbal memory may interfere with quality of life, including occupational function.[14] Verbal memory decline following dominant-hemispheric temporal lobectomy is more frequently described by patients than changes in nonverbal memory following right ATL. Not only is the relationship between verbal memory impairment and left TLE easier to demonstrate neuropsychologically prior to surgery but the material-specific memory decline is more apparent following left ATL.

Despite the risk of postoperative memory decline, not all patients will have poorer memory at their follow-up neuropsychological examination. Eliminating the disruptive effects of the seizure focus and decreasing or eliminating antiepileptic medications may increase general cognitive abilities, including memory. These factors contribute to greater improvement in material-specific memory performance for measures contralateral to the seizure focus (i.e., improved visual memory following left temporal lobectomy and improved verbal memory performance following right temporal lobectomy). In both cases, the material-specific memory typically associated with the side of seizure onset remains constant or declines after surgery.

Predictors of Postoperative Verbal Memory Decline

Greater risk of memory decline is associated with resection of relatively nonsclerotic hippocampus and, by extension, one that has greater residual functional capacity. Larger memory declines following left ATL are observed in patients with minimal left hippocampal sclerosis.[57,58] Similarly, poorer memory outcome is seen following resection of relatively nonatrophic left hippocampus as reflected by MRI volumetry.[7] These studies suggest that patients without evidence of hippocampal pathology are more likely to experience decline in verbal memory following left ATL, since functional tissue is included in the mesial temporal lobe resection.

Wada memory performance is also related to postoperative verbal memory function. Patients declining on verbal memory tasks (at least one standard deviation) following left ATL have more symmetrical Wada memory scores.[59] In contrast, patients with Wada memory asymmetries suggesting left unilateral temporal impairment tend to show no decline in verbal memory following left ATL. Good memory performance following amobarbital perfusion contralateral to the seizure focus has been associated with verbal memory decline following left ATL.[48] As with other studies of right ATL effects employing visuospatial memory stimuli, no consistent relationship with changes in visuospatial memory following right ATL has been found.

Baseline memory assessment itself also provides a measure of risk to memory change following temporal lobectomy. Patients with normal verbal memory are less likely to have left hippocampal atrophy, and higher preoperative memory is associated with greater decline following left ATL.[9,60] In contrast, no similar relationship is present for visuospatial memory change following right ATL, a consistent theme throughout the temporal lobectomy literature.

Risk for significant postoperative memory decline depends partly on the level of preoperative memory impairment and two other factors: (1) memory must be sufficiently intact in order to have the potential for decline following surgery, and (2) even when declines occur that are noticeable to the family, there must be sufficient sensitivity of the neuropsychological instruments employed to measure a decline and avoid what is referred to as "floor effect" of the neuropsychological measures. High-functioning patients with intact verbal memory show the greatest verbal memory declines postoperatively, and this decline is not explained solely by statistical regression to the mean. Chelune and coworkers[9] reported that patients with Wechsler Memory Scale—Revised Verbal Memory Index scores that were in the average range or greater (i.e., scores ≥90) had a 75 percent change of experiencing a 10 percent decline in verbal memory at their 6-month follow-up.

Patients who are not seizure-free following surgery are also more likely to show greater verbal memory impairments than those without postoperative seizures, although verbal memory impairment may be present in seizure-free patients.[12,61] In addition, patients older than 40 years of age may be at increased risk for greater postoperative memory decline.[62]

The length of the follow-up interval produces some effect on memory results. After the initial acute effects, there are very mild improvements in certain aspects of memory over the first postoperative year, although this is a surprisingly small effect.[63] However, over longer intervals ranging from 5 to 10 years and beyond, there continues to be mild improvement on neuropsychological memory tasks.[64]

Postoperative Language Change

Decline in language function provides the rationale for functional cortical speech mapping during surgery. Although acute language deficits are common following temporal lobectomy, they largely resolve over longer intervals.[65] Hermann and co-workers[66] demonstrated no statistical group decline in language in patients who underwent stimulation mapping during surgery. However, when examined on an individual basis, several individuals showed significant language declines, although the factors that might be related to the language decline could not be identified. These same authors compared postoperative language in patients who received mapping to those who did not in a consecutive patient series at the same epilepsy center.[67] The only pre- to postoperative change in patients undergoing left ATL who were not mapped was on a confrontation task and was roughly one-half standard deviation. This study suggests that mapping provides some benefit in avoiding mild anomia following surgery.

Patients who undergo surgery encroaching on primarily language areas, of course, may experience greater language decline. In cases in which seizures arise near primarily language regions, mapping is thought to decrease the magnitude of language decline, although good postoperative data do not exist. Multiple subpial transection decreases but does not eliminate postoperative language effect for epilepsy surgery involving language cortex.[68]

Postoperative Psychosocial Function/Quality of Life

Quality of life and improvement in psychosocial status appears to be greatest in patients who become seizure-free following surgery.[69] However, preoperative psychosocial status is more closely related to postoperative psychosocial status than is seizure outcome.[3,70] Additional determinants of psychosocial status following epilepsy surgery need to be more clearly delineated.

SUMMARY AND FUTURE DIRECTIONS

Neuropsychological testing and Wada evaluation will continue to play a prominent role in the evaluation of epilepsy surgery patients. In many patients, they not only measure functional deficits with known cerebral lesions but also contribute to establishing laterality of seizure onset and provide some estimate of the risk to memory following ATL. With both approaches, however, there will continue to be procedural refinement based upon correlations with MRI volumetry, fMRI, and MRI spectroscopy and also correlations with long-term cognitive, vocational, and seizure outcome. New noninvasive measures of brain function, including fMRI, are likely, eventually, to provide much of the same information as that derived from Wada testing. However, it remains to be established if a procedure that relies on activation of cognitive functions can provide data comparable to those of the Wada test, which as an inactivation procedure, and thus more directly models the effects of surgery on cognition. Nevertheless, there continues to be an important need for further refinement in the ability to predict and avoid significant postoperative cognitive deficits. Greater understanding of the interaction between cognitive, psychiatric, and quality-of-life variables and how these factors contribute to the overall outcome of epilepsy surgery will provide a richer description of postsurgical results than simply reporting postoperative seizure frequency. Delineation of these issues will contribute to improved care of patients undergoing epilepsy surgery.

REFERENCES

1. Engel J, Rausch R, Leib J, Kuhl DE, Crandall PH: Correlation of criteria used for localizing epileptic foci in patients considered for surgical therapy in epilepsy. *Ann Neurol* 19:215–224, 1981.
2. Milner B: Psychological aspects of focal epilepsy and its neurosurgical management, in Purpura D, Penry J, Walter R (eds): *Advances in Neurology: vol 8. Neurosurgical Management of the Epilepsies.* New York: Raven Press, 1975, pp 299–321.
3. Dodrill CB, Hermann BP, Rausch R, et al: Neuropsychological testing for assessing prognosis following surgery for epilepsy, in Engel J (ed): *Surgical Treatment of the Epilepsies.* New York: Raven Press, 1993, vol 2, pp 263–271.
4. Hermann BP, Gold J, Pusakulich R, et al: Wechsler Adult Intelligence Scale—Revised, in the evaluation of anterior temporal lobectomy candidates. *Epilepsia* 36:480–487, 1995.
5. Bengzon ARA, Rasmussen T, Gloor P, et al: Prognostic factors in the surgical treatment of temporal lobe epileptics. *Neurology* 18:717–731, 1968.
6. Dodrill CB, Wilkus RJ, Ojemann GA, et al: Multidisciplinary prediction of seizure relief from cortical resection surgery. *Ann Neurol* 20:2–12, 1986.
7. Trenerry MR, Jack Jr CR, Ivnik RJ, et al: MRI hippocampal volumes and memory function before and after temporal lobectomy. *Neurology* 43:1800–1805, 1993.
8. Solomon PR, Solomon SD, Schaaf EV, Perry HE: Altered activity in the hippocampus is more detrimental to classical conditioning than removing the structure. *Science* 220:329–331, 1983.
9. Chelune GJ, Naugle RI, Lüders H, Awad IA: Prediction of cognitive change as a function of preoperative ability status among temporal lobectomy patients seen at 6-month follow-up. *Neurology* 41:399–404, 1991.
10. Hermann BP, Wyler AR, Richey ET, Rea JM: Memory function and verbal learning ability in patients with complex partial seizures of temporal lobe origin. *Epilepsia* 28:547–554, 1987.
11. Loring DW, Lee GP, Martin RC, Meador KJ: Material-specific learning in patients with partial complex seizures of temporal lobe origin: convergent validation of memory constructs. *J Epilepsy* 1:53–59, 1988.
12. Novelly RA, Augustine EA, Mattson RH, et al: Selective memory improvement and impairment in temporal lobectomy for epilepsy. *Ann Neurol* 15:64–67, 1984.

13. Rausch R: Psychological evaluation, in Engel J Jr (ed): *Surgical Treatment of the Epilepsies.* New York: Raven Press, 1987, pp 181–195.
14. Ivnik RJ, Sharbrough FW, Laws ER: Anterior temporal lobectomy for the control of partial complex seizures: Information for counseling patients. *Mayo Clinic Proc* 63:783–793, 1988.
15. Anderson SW, Damasio H, Jones RD, Tranel D: Wisconsin card sorting test performance as a measure of frontal lobe damage. *J Clin Exp Neuropsychol* 13:821–830, 1991.
16. Hermann BP, Wyler AR, Richey ET: Wisconsin card sorting test performance in patients with complex partial seizures of temporal-lobe origin. *J Clin Exp Neuropsychol* 10:467–576, 1988.
17. Jones-Gotman M, Milner B: Design fluency: The invention of nonsense drawings after focal cortical lesions. *Neuropsychologia* 15:653–674, 1977.
18. Jones-Gotman M, Smith ML, Zatorre RJ: Neuropsychological testing for localizing and lateralizing the epileptogenic region, in Engel J (ed): *Surgical Treatment of the Epilepsies.* New York: Raven Press, 1993, vol 2, pp 245–261.
19. Fenwick PCB, Blumer DP, Caplan R, et al: Presurgical psychiatric assessment, in Engel J (ed): *Surgical Treatment of the Epilepsies.* New York: Raven Press, 1993, vol 2, pp 273–290.
20. Dodrill C, Batzel LW, Queisser HR, Tempkin NR: An objective method for the assessment of psychological and social problems among epileptics. *Epilepsia* 21:123–135, 1980.
21. Perrine KR: A new quality-of-life inventory for epilepsy patients: Interim results. *Epilepsia* 34(suppl 4):S28–S33, 1993.
22. Vickrey BG: A procedure for developing a quality-of-life measure for epilepsy surgery patients. *Epilepsia* 34(suppl 4):S22–S37, 1993.
23. Loring DW, Meador KJ, Lee GP, King DW: *Amobarbital Effects and Lateralized Brain Function: The Wada Test.* New York: Springer-Verlag, 1992.
24. Rausch R, Silvenius H, Wieser H-G, et al: Current practices of intra-arterial amobarbital procedures, in Engel J (ed): *Surgical Treatment of the Epilepsies.* New York: Raven Press, 1993, vol 2, pp 341–357.
25. Snyder PJ, Novelly RA, Harris LJ: Mixed speech dominance in the intracarotid sodium Amytal procedure: Validity and criteria issues. *J Clin Exp Neuropsychol* 12:629–643, 1992.
26. Oxbury SM, Oxbury JM: Intracarotid amytal test in the assessment of language dominance, in FC Rose (ed): *Advances in Neurology. Progress in*

Aphasiology. New York: Raven Press, 1984, vol 42, pp 115–123.

27. Branch C, Milner B, Rasmussen T: Intracarotid sodium amytal for the lateralization of cerebral speech dominance: Observations in 123 patients. *J Neurosurg* 21:399–405, 1964.

28. Wyllie E, Lüders H, Murphy D, et al: Intracarotid amobarbital (Wada) test for language dominance: Correlation with results of cortical stimulation. *Epilepsia* 31:156–161, 1990.

29. Loring DW, Meador KJ, Lee GP, et al: Cerebral language lateralization: Evidence from intracarotid amobarbital testing. *Neuropsychologia* 28:831–838, 1990.

30. Rausch R, Walsh G: Right-hemisphere language dominance in right-handed epileptic patients. *Arch Neurol* 41:1077–1080, 1984.

31. Rosenbaum T, DeToledo J, Smith DB, et al: Preoperative assessment of language laterality is necessary in all epilepsy surgery candidates: A case report (abstr). *Epilepsia* 30:712, 1989.

32. Loring DW, Meador KJ, Lee GP, et al: Crossed aphasia in a patient with complex partial seizures: Evidence from intracarotid amobarbital testing functional cortical mapping and neuropsychological assessment. *J Clin Exp Neuropsychol* 12:340–354, 1990.

33. Jones-Gotman MJ: Commentary: Psychological evaluation: Testing hippocampal function, in Engel J (ed): *Surgical Treatment of the Epilepsies.* New York: Raven Press, 1987, pp 203–211.

34. Perrine K, Gershengorn J, Brown ER, et al: Material-specific memory in the intracarotid amobarbital procedures. *Neurology* 43:706–711, 1993.

35. Sass KJ, Lencz T, Westerveld M, et al: The neural substrate of memory impairment demonstrated by the intracarotid amobarbital procedure. *Arch Neurol* 48:48–52, 1991.

36. Loring DW, Murro AM, Meador KJ, et al: Wada memory testing and hippocampal volume measurements in the evaluation for temporal lobectomy. *Neurology* 43:1789–1793, 1993.

37. Gotman J, Bouwer MS, Jones-Gotman M: Intracranial EEG study of brain structures affected by internal carotid injection of amobarbital. *Neurology* 42:2136–2143, 1992.

38. Girvin JP, McGlone J, McLachlan RS, Blume WT: Validity of the sodium amobarbital test for memory in selected patients (abstr). *Epilepsia* 28:636, 1987.

39. Novelly RA, Williamson PD: Incidence of false-positive memory impairment in the intracarotid Amytal procedure (abstr). *Epilepsia* 30:711, 1989.

40. Loring DW, Lee GP, Meador KJ, et al: The intracarotid amobarbital procedure as a predictor of memory failure following unilateral temporal lobectomy. *Neurology* 40:605–610, 1990.

41. Loring DW, Hermann BP, Meador KJ, et al: Amnesia following unilateral temporal lobectomy: A case report. *Epilepsia* 35:757–763, 1994.

42. Lesser RP, Dinner DS, Lüders H, Morris HH: Memory for objects presented soon after intracarotid amobarbital sodium injections in patients with medically intractable complex partial seizures. *Neurology* 36:895–899, 1986.

43. Rausch R, Babb TL, Engel J Jr, Crandall PH: Memory following intracarotid amobarbital injection contralateral to hippocampal damage. *Arch Neurol* 46:783–788, 1989.

44. Wyllie E, Naugle R, Chelune G, et al: Intracarotid amobarbital procedure: II. Lateralizing value in evaluation for temporal lobectomy. *Epilepsia* 32:865–869, 1991.

45. Loring DW, Meador KJ, Lee GP, et al: Stimulus timing effects on Wada memory testing. *Arch Neurol* 51:806–810, 1994.

46. Sass KJ, Lencz T, Westerveld M, et al: The neural substrate of memory impairment demonstrated by the intracarotid Amytal procedure. *Arch Neurol* 48:48–52, 1991.

47. O'Rourke DM, Saykin AJ, Gilhool JJ, et al: Unilateral hemispheric memory and hippocampal neuronal density in temporal lobe epilepsy. *Neurosurgery* 32:547–581, 1993.

48. Kneebone AC, Chelune GJ, Dinner D, et al: Intracarotid amobarbital procedure as a predictor of material-specific memory change after anterior temporal lobectomy. *Epilepsia* 36:857–865, 1995.

49. Jack CR Jr, Sharborough FW, Cascino GD, et al: Magnetic resonance based imaging-based hippocampal volumetry: Correlation with outcome after temporal lobectomy. *Ann Neurol* 31:138–146, 1992.

50. Loring DW, Meador KJ, Lee GP, et al: Wada memory performance predicts seizure outcome following anterior temporal lobectomy. *Neurology* 44:2322–2324, 1994.

51. Sperling MR, Saykin AJ, Glosser G, et al: Predictors of outcome after anterior temporal lobectomy: The intracarotid amobarbital test. *Neurology* 44;2325–2330, 1994.

52. Scoville WB: The limbic lobe in man. *J Neurosurg* 11:64–66, 1954.

53. Scoville W, Milner B: Loss of recent memory after bilateral hippocampal lesions. *J Neurol Neurosurg Psychiatry* 20:11–21, 1957.

54. Penfield W, Milner B: Memory deficit produced by bilateral lesions in the hippocampal zone. *Arch Neurol Psychiatry* 79:475–497, 1958.

55. Penfield W, Mathieson G: Memory: Autopsy findings and comments on the role of the hippocampus in experimental recall. *Arch Neurol* 3:1145–1154, 1974.

56. Milner B, Branch CL, Rasmussen T: Study of short-term memory after intracarotid injection of sodium Amytal. *Trans Am Neurol Assoc* 87:224–226, 1962.

57. Hermann BP, Wyler AR, Somes G, et al: Pathological status of the mesial temporal lobe predicts memory outcome from left anterior temporal lobectomy. *Neurosurgery* 31:652–657, 1992.

58. Hermann BP, Wyler AR, Somes G, et al: Declarative memory following anterior temporal lobectomy in humans. *Behav Neurosci* 108:3–10, 1993.

59. Loring DW, Meador KJ, Lee GP, et al: Wada memory asymmetries predict verbal memory decline following anterior temporal lobectomy. *Neurology* 45:1329–1333, 1995.

60. Rausch R, Babb TL, Ary C, Crandall PH: Memory changes following unilateral temporal lobectomy reflect preoperative integrity of the temporal lobe. Paper presented at the annual meeting of the International Neuropsychological Society, Houston, 1984.

61. Rausch R, Crandall PH: Psychological status related to surgical control of temporal lobe seizures. *Epilepsia* 23:191–202, 1982.

62. Loring DW, Lee GP, Meador KJ, et al: Age effects on verbal and visual-spatial memory following temporal lobectomy. *Epilepsia* 34:72, 1993.

63. Loring DW, Trenerry MR, Naugle RI, et al: Time effects on post-temporal lobectomy memory: A multicenter cooperative report. *Clin Neuropsychol* 6:350, 1992.

64. Blakemore CB, Falconer MA: Long-term effects of anterior temporal lobectomy on certain cognitive function. *J Neurol Neurosurg Psychiatry* 30:364–367, 1967.

65. Loring DW, Meador KJ, Lee GP: Effects of temporal lobectomy on generative fluency and other language functions. *Arch Clin Neuropsychol* 9:229–238, 1994.

66. Hermann BP, Wyler AR: Effects of anterior temporal lobectomy on language function: A controlled study. *Ann Neurol* 23:585–588, 1988.

67. Hermann BP, Wyler AR, Sommes G: Language function following anterior temporal lobectomy. *J Neurosurg* 74:560–566, 1991.

68. Devinsky O, Perrine K, Vazquez B, et al: Multiple subpial transections in the language cortex. *Brain* 117:255–265, 1994.

69. Vickrey BG, Hays RD, Graber J, et al: A health related quality of life instrument of patients evaluated for epilepsy surgery. *Med Care* 330:299–319, 1992.

70. Hermann BP, Wyler AR, Somes G: Preoperative psychological adjustment and surgical outcome are determinants of psychosocial status after anterior temporal lobectomy. *J Neurol Neurosurg Psychiatry* 55:491–496, 1992.

Chapter 53

CORTICAL STIMULATION (INTERFERENCE) DURING BEHAVIOR

Barry Gordon
John Hart, Jr.
Dana Boatman
Ronald P. Lesser

There are three major approaches that can be taken to understanding behavior and its underlying neural mechanisms. The first is purely *behavioral*, whereby parameters of a behavior are varied and the consequences observed. This is the traditional approach in experimental psychology. The second is *observational* or correlational. A behavior is performed while neural activity is measured, without otherwise perturbing the neural activity. Studies using measures of regional cerebral metabolism, cerebral blood flow, and regional electrical activity fall into this category. The third general method is *lesional*. Changes in a behavior are observed (or inferred) after brain tissue is lesioned or disturbed in some way. While lesional methods have a long history in neuroscience, rigorous, prospective lesional studies have usually been confined to animals. Until recently, the bulk of evidence from lesional studies in humans had to rely on accidental lesions produced by illness or trauma. Now, however, with increasing frequency, techniques that produce temporary, relatively focal neuronal dysfunction have been applied in humans to serve clinical as well as research purposes. These techniques include such methods as transcranial magnetic or electrical stimulation[1] and direct cortical electrical stimulation.

Direct cortical electrical stimulation appears to have two major types of effects: (1) *Positive effects,* which are the elicitation of motor movements, sensations, or at times behaviors. Positive motor effects have been attributed to stimulation of subcortical white matter.[2,3] (2) *"Negative" or lesional effects,* which appear to involve temporary disruption of an ongoing behavior. Electrical current applied directly to the surface of the brain has been shown both by simulations[4] and empirical studies to induce strong electrical fields in the subjacent neuronal tissue. These cause both direct neuronal effects and, perhaps, indirect vascular effects[5] (but see Ref. 6).

In terms of the direct neuronal effects, suprathreshold stimulation, such as the method we use, would be expected to (1) depolarize most neurons into inactivity;[2] (2) stimulate intracortical and subcortical axons;[2,3] and therefore (3) have transsynaptic effects on some neurons in the vicinity[2] and perhaps (4) on other, more distant neurons connected by intracortical U fibers and/or callosal pathways.[2] In animals, transcallosal effects appear to be mostly inhibitory (hyperpolarizing),[2] perhaps explaining why stimulation of the nondominant hemisphere does not seem to induce dysfunction of roughly homologous regions of the dominant hemisphere (Lesser, Gordon et al., unpublished observations). Collectively, these negative effects cause a temporary functional "lesion." Simulation studies[4] and functional analyses[7,8] suggest that the functional lesion produced under these circumstances is fairly small, on the order of 1.0 cm^2 or less. Moreover, under the usual conditions of interference (0.3-ms pulses of alternating polarity applied at a rate of 50 pulses per second at currents of up to 17 mA), these functional lesions appear to have nearly immediate onset as well as nearly immediate offset.

Direct cortical electrical interference applied in the operating room has a long history, dating back at least to Cushing in 1909. While intraoperative direct cortical electrical stimulation continues to be used for clinical and research purposes, the last decade has seen the increasing use of indwelling electrode strips and grids. These provide longer access to the cortical surface (days instead of hours), with greater patient comfort. A number of investigators have now used indwelling strips and arrays to map language and other functions for clinical and research purposes (e.g., Refs. 9 to 12). The method used at our institution evolved from procedures used by Lüders, Lesser, and their colleagues at the Cleveland Clinic.[13] This chapter summarizes our use of the technique of direct cortical electrical interference to dissect behavior. However, we must note that we employ all three investigative approaches—behavioral, correlational, and the "functional lesion" afforded by direct cortical electrical interference—if at all possible in both our clinical and research work. Used together, they help us obtain the least biased understanding of the underlying behavioral abilities and their neural substrates.

GENERAL METHODS

Patients/Subjects

Candidates for implantation of indwelling electrode arrays are patients for whom focal cerebral resections are being strongly considered to treat such conditions as epilepsy of focal origin, arteriovenous malformations,[14] and tumors.[15] The implantations serve to permit (1) recording of the ictal electroencephalographic (EEG) pattern associated with seizures in order to identify the seizure focus prior to resection or (2) cortical electrical interference mapping of language and other functions in order to identify cortical regions relevant for performing these functions. This information, in turn, helps us to plan the surgical resection.

Electrodes

Subdural electrode grids consist of arrays of electrodes embedded in medical-grade Silastic (Wyler

type, Adtech Medical Instrument Co., Racine, WI). The electrodes are platinum-iridium. They consist of 3-mm disks (with 2.3-mm-diameter areas exposed), embedded in square arrays with 1.0-cm center to center. Standard arrays consist of varieties such as 8×8 and 8×2 electrode arrangements. These are cut as necessary for the particular placements planned.

Placement

Placement is tailored to the particular clinical needs of each patient, guided by the dual requirements of best localizing ictal seizure activity (if epilepsy is the issue) and functional mapping for the anticipated surgical resection. Hence, preimplantation intracarotid amobarital injection[16,17] is used in essentially all patients to help determine language laterality and to identify patient with possibly aberrant language laterality. Because of the need for more detailed functional mapping of language, most grids are implanted on the left (dominant) side. The electrode arrays usually cover the temporal lobe, parts of the inferior temporal region, posterior perisylvian region, and often the inferior post- and precentral gyri. However, grids have also been placed interhemispherically (both frontally and occipitally), over the dorsolateral frontal lobe, over the lateral occipital lobe, and bilaterally. An effort is made to align the rows of electrodes with the gyri on the temporal lobe.

Up to 174 electrodes have been implanted at a time. A few patients have had additional arrays implanted while the first set was still in place, to map regions not initially appreciated (typically, the borders of epileptogenic zones). A few have also had array implantations on two separate occasions. Surgical aspects of array implantation are discussed by Uematsu and coworkers.[18] The electrode arrays are typically left in for 10 to 14 days for localization of ictal foci and for interference mapping, but shorter periods have also proven adequate in some patients.

Electrode Localization

Volumetric magnetic resonance images (MRIs) are obtained preimplantation, and three-dimensional (3D) computed tomography (CT) scans of the electrodes are obtained in the middle of the postimplantation period. In some cases, volumetric MRI scans are also obtained postimplantation. In addition, plain skull films are obtained postimplantation. Intraoperative photographs are also taken preimplantation, immediately after implantation, and upon reoperation, when the grid is about to be removed and the brain resected. The available data confirm that in most cases there is no appreciable shift of cerebral tissues after implantation of the electrode array(s). Therefore, a 3D reconstruction of the preimplantation MRI is fused with a 3D reconstruction of the electrodes from the CT scan to obtain the most accurate localization of the electrodes with respect to that individual's sulci and gyri. This is checked against the intraoperative photographs and the plain skull films. Recently, in some cases, the intraoperative location of the electrode has also been checked using a wand to mark the stereotactic coordinates of selected electrodes.

Testing Procedures

The approach we use has been described; see, for example, Refs. 10 and 17 for further details.

For clinical purposes, horizontally adjacent pairs of electrodes on the grid are treated as potential sites for "functional lesioning," and every such "site" is stimulated in initial screening. If clinical needs warrant, the region is tested in more anatomic detail using appropriate combinations of electrodes. Electrode assignment for research purposes generally covers the anatomic region of interest with all possible combinations of adjacent electrodes. Our current anatomic strategy is to use adjacent electrodes for interference testing because, for both empirical[19] and theoretical[4,8] reasons, these produce the smallest functional lesions and the most precise functional-anatomic correlations. When longer interelectrode distances have been used (e.g., Ref. 20) somewhat different patterns of deficits are found than typically produced by stimulating adjacent electrodes.

The usual functional lesion for both clinical

and research purposes is the most complete interference that can be produced at a site. This is achieved by applying the maximal allowable current, which is determined at a given site as follows: Initial current application of 1.0 mA is increased in 1.0-mA increments. With each increment in current, the patient is observed for motor activity, asked about subjective sensations, and the EEG is monitored for signs of afterdischarges or seizures. Incrementing continues until reaching either the maximal current the stimulator can deliver (15 to 16.7 mA, depending upon the stimulator model, the most common reason; development of unavoidable afterdischarges, the next most common reason; or the occurrence of pain from stimulation of dural afferents.[13]

When peak current is achieved, testing for the consequences of the functional lesioning proceeds. Testing requires at least two people: one to present stimuli or monitor psychological stimulus presentation and patient response and other to control or monitor the cortical electrical stimulation itself. Testing itself is always semi-double blind (in that the tester presents stimuli and/or records results without prior knowledge of whether cortical stimulation is being applied, and the patient does not know stimulation is being applied unless he or she has a subjective experience or appreciates errors). Cortical electrical stimulation is applied in two ways: (1) on a trial-by-trial basis, wherein it is pseudorandomly intermixed with nonstimulated trials; or in short blocks, with stimulation applied through two to three psychological trials, which are then mixed pseudorandomly with unstimulated blocks of trials. The latter method is used more for screening purposes or when time is limited.

At the current time, in most cases, the direct presentation of stimuli and the recording of electrical and response parameters is handled through a computer operated by the second individual described above, while the first individual monitors the subject directly face to face so as to be sensitive to nuances of expression and responsiveness while scoring responses.

The functions tested at each site are partly determined by prior experience and expectations, partly by the specific needs of the individual patient. Language functions are usually tested at all sites. If time permits, seven functions are tested: spontaneous speech (about the patient's favorite topics); auditory comprehension (with a shortened version of the Token test),[22] auditory repetition of single words, reading of single words and passages, visual confrontation naming, and naming to description. If time is short, several modifications to the language testing are possible: a smaller set of tasks (visual confrontation naming, spontaneous speech or reading passages, and auditory comprehension). To assess visual processing, tasks such as object color identification, visual object decision (real/unreal object), and other functions have been tested.[18]

Stimuli for each subject and for each session are drawn from a set kept constant across all subjects. Where possible, the same stimuli are used for all the tasks. All subjects are pretested with the stimuli; stimuli causing errors because of lack of familiarity are not presented again after this screening.

When presented via computer, visual stimuli are typically either words in an enlarged, serif typeface or 2D black-and-white line drawings, although color pictures can also be shown. They are shown on a monitor placed a comfortable distance in front of the patient. Auditory stimuli presented via the computer are segments of natural speech, recorded in a sound studio by a trained male native speaker of American English, and digitized at 44 kHz with 16-bit resolution. Auditory stimuli are presented via calibrated insert earphones. All sessions are videotaped with a high-quality audio soundtrack recorded by boom microphone.

The computer records response times (via voice key or button press); response correctness is entered immediately (by the second tester) and later checked against a videotape of the session. Responses are recorded as errors if the subject makes no response, the response is abnormally delayed, or the response is erroneous (e.g., a paraphasia). Correct responses made after the offset of stimulation when no response was possible during stimulation (not a rare event) are also counted as errors. However, codes are kept for each trial indicating the nature of the error that occurred.

Statistical Analysis

Statistical significance is assessed in several ways. The most basic method is sitewise, comparing, for each task, responses with interference at a site to all responses when interference was not applied during that test session (a test session is defined as a continuous 2- to 3-h block of testing, usually either in the morning or the midafternoon). Because baseline (nonstimulated) performance is usually at ceiling and performance measures are discrete (e.g., percent correct), statistical comparisons are made using methods such as distribution-free McNemar's tests, direct calculation of odds ratios, and Mantel-Hanszel Chi-Square tests (the latter because it is based on conditional likelihood functions and therefore is less sensitive to small sample sizes). Examples of such analyses applied to research data are given in Refs. 20 and 23.

The sitewise method, while perhaps the most traditional, has the potential problem of ignoring a priori probabilities and interregional correlations. Therefore both Bayesian and geographic inference models have been investigated.

Data are kept in two forms: as a functional map overlaid on each individual's anatomic map and as a functional map overlaid on a normalized brain atlas. The normalization is based on the Talairach bilinear transformation[24,25] into a single two-dimensional lateral reference figure. Electrode locations are placed on this normalized atlas to respect in particular (1) the sylvian fissure and (2) their anterior-posterior distance in relation to electrodes along the superior temporal gyrus. Assignment of electrode locations is done by an individual who is not part of the testing team and who is blind to the results of that particular patient. Electrode locations are determined by consensus data from plain lateral skull films, pre- and postimplantation MRI and x-ray CT, intraoperative photographs, and maps drawn by the neurosurgeon or epileptologist at the time of electrode implantation.

For clinical purposes, experience has shown

that even a single erroneous response is *statistically* significant by many different statistical approaches. The *clinical* significance of any deficits found by cortical interference mapping—as opposed to the strict statistical significance—is determined by additional considerations, such as whether and what other functions are impaired at a site; the presence of any impairments at adjacent sites; expectations based on individual history, handedness, and intracarotid amobarbital injection; data from prior patients; and consideration of both immediate and long-term risk-benefit ratios. These considerations are taken up in parallel with consideration of the resection planned for the treatment of the epilepsy or other primary condition. This joint process usually takes place almost simultaneously, culminating in a meeting of all concerned the evening before the planned resection. The medical recommendation (or recommendations) is (are) then presented to the patient and family for consideration. As a result, the clinical interpretation of the cortical inference mapping also takes the patient's individual concerns, goals, and cognitive abilities into account.

CONCLUSIONS

Direct cortical electrical interference behaves like a hyperacute, anatomically limited, totally reversible "lesion" for most of the functions, regions, and individuals that we have tested. Probably as a result, the deficits found with direct cortical electrical interference tend to be more behaviorally limited and more profound than those found in the more chronic state, after much larger cerebral lesions. For example, stimulation of some sites can cause profound deficits in visual confrontation naming without affecting other language functions; detailed investigations of some of these instances has shown that the underlying functional deficit appears to be limited to semantic-to-phonologic processing.[21] Direct cortical electrical interference therefore allows a method of probing human mental functions and their neuronal substrate that is not necessarily possible by other methods, either by traditional studies of normal subjects or

of fixed brain lesions or by newer techniques such as regional cerebral blood flow. It is likely that multiple methods will have to be used to develop the best picture of behavioral-brain relationships apart from the distortions introduced by each particular technique.

ACKNOWLEDGMENTS

This research was supported in part by grants from The National Institute on Deafness and Other Communication Disorders (R03-DC01881 and K08-DC00099), The National Institute of Neurological Disorders and Stroke (R01-NS26553 and R01-29973), and by the Seaver Foundation, the Whittier Foundation, and the McDonnell-Pew Program in Cognitive Neuroscience. Pamela Schwerdt, Barbara Cyszk, and Mary Bare were directly involved in testing and in perfecting testing techniques; Jeffery Sieracki with developing the cognitive testing computer and its interfaces. We wish to thank Drs. Karen Bandeen-Roche and Charles Hall for statistical advice and support, Dr. Ola Selnes for general advice on language-brain relationships, and Jennifer Hopp, Valencia Booth, and Frank Hajamadi for technical assistance. Dr. Nitish Thakor, Surendar Nathan, Veena Agarwal, and S. R. Sirha developed the simulation of direct cortical electrical stimulation. Dr. Sumio Uematsu (deceased) was the neurosurgeon who initially implemented the indwelling electrode technique at Johns Hopkins; his efforts are gratefully acknowledged. Finally, this technique and our interpretation of its results have benefited immensely from numerous conversations over the years with our colleagues in neurolinguistics, cognitive science, behavioral neurology, biomedical engineering, and other fields.

REFERENCES

1. Mills KR, Murray NM, Hess CW: Magnetic and electrical transcranial brain stimulation: Physiological mechanisms and clinical applications. *Neurosurgery* 20:164–168, 1987.
2. Li C-H, Chou SN: Cortical intracellular synaptic

potentials and direct cortical stimulation. *J Cell Comp Physiol* 60:1–16, 1962.

3. Landau WM, Bishop GH, Clare MH: Site of excitation in stimulation of the motor cortex. *J Neurophysiol* 28:1206–1222, 1965.

4. Nathan SS, Sinha SR, Gordon B, et al: Determination of current density distributions generated by electrical stimulation of the human cerebral cortex. *Electrocephalogr Clin Neurophysiol* 86:183–192, 1993.

5. Pudenz RH, Bullara LA, Dru D, Tallala A: Electrical stimulation of the brain II: Effects on the blood-brain barrier. *Surg Neurol* 4, 265–270, 1975.

6. Agnew WF, McCreery DB, Bullara LA, Yuen TGH: Development of safe techniques for selective activation of neurons (NINCDS Contract #N01-NS-62397). *Quarterly Progress Report #1,* January 1, 1987.

7. Ojemann GA: Common cortical and thalamic mechanisms for language and motor functions. *Am J Physiol* 246:R901–R903, 1984.

8. Agarwal, V: Modelling electrical stimulation of the human cerebral cortex. Masters Thesis, Johns Hopkins University, 1994.

9. Andy OJ, Bhatnagar SC: Right-hemispheric language: Evidence from cortical stimulation. *Brain Lang* 23:159–166, 1984.

10. Lesser IM, Mena I, Boone KB, et al: Reduction of cerebral blood flow in older depressed patients. *Arch Gen Psychiatry* 51:677–686, 1994.

11. Perrine K, Devinsky O, Uysal S, et al: Left temporal neocortex mediation of verbal memory: Evidence from functional mapping with cortical stimulation. *Neurology* 44:1845–1850, 1994.

12. Risinger MW, Sutherling WW, Wilson CL, et al: Comprehension deficits with electrical stimulation of Wernicke's area. *Neurology* 38(suppl 1):185, 1988.

13. Lesser RP, Lueders H, Klem G, et al: Extraoperative cortical functional localization in patients with epilepsy. *J Clin Neurophysiol* 4:27–53, 1987.

14. Lesser RP, Lueders H, Dinner DS, et al: The location of speech and writing functions in the frontal

language area: Results of extraoperative cortical stimulation. *Brain* 107:275–291, 1984.

15. Burchiel KJ, Clarke H, Ojemann GA, et al: Use of stimulation mapping and corticography in the excision of arteriovenous malformations in sensorimotor and language-related neocortex. *Neurosurgery* 24:322–327, 1989.

16. Morris HH, Luders H, Hahn JF, et al: Neurophysiological techniques as an aid to surgical treatment of primary brain tumors. *Ann Neurol* 19:559–567, 1986.

17. Milner B: Psychological aspects of focal epilepsy and its neurosurgical management, in Purpura DP, Penry JK, Walter RD (eds): *Advances in Neurology, 8.* New York: Raven Press, 1975.

18. Hart J Jr, Lesser RP, Gordon B: Selective interference with the representation of size in the human by direct cortical electrical stimulation. *J Cog Neurosci* 4:337–344, 1992.

19. Uematsu S, Lesser RP, Fisher RS, et al: Tailored resection of epileptogenic cerebral tissue with aid of a subdural grid-electrode. Second International Cleveland Clinic Symposium, Cleveland, June 1990.

20. Boatman DF, Lesser RP, Hall CB, Gordon B: Auditory perception of segmental features: A functional-neuroanatomic study. *J Neuroling* 8:225–234, 1994.

21. Gordon B, Hart J, Lesser RP, et al: Dissociations in mixed transcortical aphasia produced by direct cortical electrical stimulation. Paper presented to the Academy of Aphasia, Montreal, October 1988.

22. Selnes OA, Knopman DS, Niccum N, et al: Computed tomographic scan correlates of auditory comprehension deficits in aphasia: A prospective recovery study. *Ann Neurol* 13:558–566, 1983.

23. Boatman DF, Lesser RP, Gordon B: Auditory speech processing in the left temporal lobe: An electrical interference study. *Brain Lang* 51:269–290, 1995.

24. Talairach J, Szikla G: *Atlas of Stereotaxic Anatomy of the Telencephalon: Anatomo-Radiological Studies.* Paris: Masson, 1967.

25. Talairach J, Tournoux P: *Co-Planar Stereotactic Atlas of the Human Brain.* New York: Thieme, 1988.

Part 8
EMOTIONAL DISORDERS

Chapter 54

EMOTION AND THE BRAIN: AN OVERVIEW

Kevin S. LaBar
Joseph E. LeDoux

The psychological and neuroscientific investigation of the nature of emotion has a long and varied history. While fundamental questions regarding the concept of emotion continue to be debated,[1] a resurgent interest in examining emotion and the brain has emerged in recent years. Significant progress has already been made in identifying brain regions involved in certain domains of emotional behavior, particularly fear. Most of this advance in knowledge has evolved from animal models of emotion, although extensions of this work into human populations have begun to be established. The purpose of this chapter is to provide an overview of research aimed at understanding the neural basis of emotion. We begin with a review of early pioneering studies linking emotion and the brain. We then present current conceptualizations of emotional information processing networks and propose directions for future research. Because of the vast nature of this topic, certain aspects of emotional processing will undoubtedly be underemphasized; the reader is referred to other recent reviews in this area.[2–14]

HISTORICAL PERSPECTIVE

William James[15] was among the leading late-nineteenth-century thinkers to postulate a specific relationship between brain-body function and emotional states. His feedback hypothesis stated that peripheral physiologic changes in the body determined emotional experience by their influence on

sensory and motor areas in the neocortex. This view, shared to a large extent by Lange,[16] suggested that emotion can be differentiated on the basis of internal monitoring of autonomic and somatic changes and that a specialized brain network regulating emotion need not exist.

The James-Lange theory was soon challenged by physiologists examining autonomic function and brain localization of emotion. Studies in decorticate animals showed that transection of the cerebral cortex left intact mechanisms of emotional expression, particularly elicitation of "sham rage,"[17] but that midbrain transection eliminated integrated emotional reactions.[18,19] Thus, emotional expression appeared to be mediated by diencephalic structures, including the thalamus and hypothalamus, located below the cortex but above the midbrain.[20,21] In addition, the diffuse sympathetic arousal in the periphery seemed to be too undifferentiated to determine distinct emotional states.[22] According to the Cannon-Bard formulation, sensory input reaching the diencephalon simultaneously produced emotional expression, by projections to peripheral organs, and emotional experience, by projections to the neocortex. In contrast to the James-Lange theory, this hypothesis suggested that structures specialized in emotional processing were present in the brain and that bodily feedback was not required to produce emotional feeling.

Papez[23] incorporated the notions of Cannon and Bard into an anatomic framework. His emotional circuit consisted of the hypothalamus, ante-

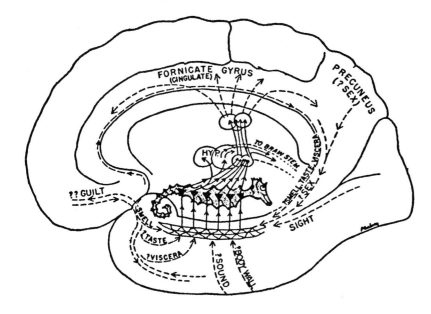

Figure 54-1
MacLean's visceral brain, the foundation of the limbic system theory of emotion. According to this conception, the hippocampus, or "sea horse," played a central role in emotional experience. (From MacLean,[26] with permission.)

rior thalamus, cingulate gyrus, and hippocampal formation. Papez viewed the cingulate gyrus as the cortical area for emotional experience, while the hypothalamus imbued incoming sensory signals with affective coloration. At the same time, Klüver and Bucy[24,25] reported a behavioral deficit in monkeys with bilateral temporal lobe lesions. The syndrome they reported consisted of an emotional tameness or hypoemotionality, increased oral tendencies, visual agnosia ("psychic blindness"), and altered feeding habits and sexual behavior. The constellation of behaviors observed in these animals indicated that they lacked the ability to evaluate the affective significance of objects in their environment, which Klüver and Bucy attributed to the destruction of the hippocampus, the medial temporal lobe component of Papez's model.

The Papez circuit was subsequently reconceived by MacLean[26,27] in what has become an influential *limbic system* theory of emotion. MacLean expanded upon Papez's neuroanatomic model by incorporating such areas as the amygdala, orbitofrontal cortex, septum, and portions of the basal ganglia to form a "visceral brain" engaged in emotion and survival functions (see Fig. 54-1). The centerpiece of this conceptualization

was the hippocampal formation, which he viewed as playing a key evaluative role in combining external stimuli and internal states into conscious emotional experience. In this view, the hippocampus, rather than the cingulate gyrus, was the cortical seat of emotional feeling.

CONTEMPORARY CHALLENGES TO THE LIMBIC SYSTEM CONCEPT

The limbic system concept was an important and persuasive development toward understanding the neural correlates of emotional processing. At the time of its development, very little was known about the anatomy and physiology of the structures contained within the limbic forebrain, and subsequent research on emotion was inspired and guided by this conceptual framework. Recently, however, the limbic system theory has been challenged on both anatomic[28,29] and functional[30–32] grounds. Anatomically, a consistent set of inclusion criteria for the classification of structures into this system has not been substantiated. In addition, it is now clear that some of the regions originally contained within this system primarily subserve functions other than those related to emotion. In particular, the hippocampus, the cornerstone of the limbic system concept, has been primarily linked to cognitive functions, such as declarative memory,[33] spatial cognition,[34,35] and contextual/configural/relational processes.[36–38] Importantly, selective lesions of the amygdala, and not the hippocampus, produce the emotional disturbances constituting the Klüver-Bucy syndrome in monkeys.[39] Subsequent work has consistently implicated the amygdala in emotional processing.[40] Thus, the inclusion of the amygdala by MacLean may explain the long-standing survival of the limbic system concept as a model for emotional processing in the brain.

EMOTION AND BRAIN: A REFORMULATION

Recent advances in understanding brain function have greatly benefited by the decomposition of global behavioral constructs into component parts or subdomains. This approach has led to the discovery of parallel processing streams in vision[41] and to the development of multiple memory systems in the brain.[42–44] We believe that the application of this strategy holds great promise for identifying neural systems involved in emotion and that a renewed neuropsychological theory of emotion can emerge from this line of inquiry. Methodologic examination of the neural bases of specific instances of emotional behavior can provide an architectural foundation upon which more comprehensive conjectures regarding emotion can be structured. Insights gained from brain studies derived in this manner will complement psychological investigation into the nature of emotion and may help guide or constrain current debates, such as the influence of peripheral feedback on emotional states[45,46] and the relation between emotion and cognition.[47–51] Progress in this direction has already been made for some emotions, most notably fear. Next, we review the functional anatomy of fear as revealed by animal studies and consider the role of these brain regions in other aspects of emotional processing in animals and in the generation of human emotion.

FEAR CONDITIONING: A MODEL SYSTEMS APPROACH

Background and Definitions

Threatening stimuli produce a variety of species-typical defensive responses, such as changes in autonomic activity (e.g., heart rate, arterial pressure, skin conductance, pupillary dilation), endocrine function ("stress"), behavioral reactions (cessation of movement, or "freezing"), reflex modulation (fear-potentiated startle), and pain sensitivity. This repertoire of fear reactivity is largely biologically innate; however, through learning, novel stimuli can come to control these responses through their association with threatening stimuli.[52] One way in which emotional learning can be achieved in the laboratory is through classical conditioning procedures.[53,54] In classical fear conditioning, an emotionally neutral stimulus, such as a tone, is presented in association with an aversive event, such as the presentation of a mild electric shock. The tone is called a conditioned stimulus (CS), and the shock is called an unconditioned stimulus (US). The US elicits a set of unconditioned defensive responses (URs), and over several CS-US pairings, conditioned fear responses (CRs) develop in reaction to the CS itself.[55]

By this arrangement of stimulus contingencies, fear-conditioning paradigms provide an experimentally controlled method to investigate how emotional significance is attached to novel stimuli. The initially neutral tone acquires aversive signaling properties through its predictive affiliation with the shock; as the animal learns the relationship between these stimuli, the set of defensive responses the animal exhibits to the US come under the control of the CS. Conditioned fear responses develop very quickly (within one trial if the US is sufficiently intense[56]) and are long-lasting.[57] Because the set of stimuli and responses involved in fear conditioning is relatively simple and well defined, it has been possible to track the neural pathways mediating this type of emotional memory formation. More complex aspects of emotional processing have also been assessed within this model, such as the establishment and retention

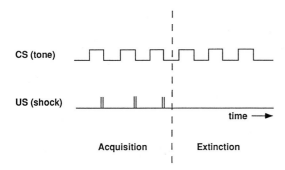

Figure 54-2

Schematic diagram of a typical fear-conditioning experiment. CS = conditioned stimulus, US = unconditioned stimulus. During the acquisition phase, the CS (e.g., a tone) is presented several times in association with a noxious US (e.g., a mild electric shock). During the extinction phase, the CS is repeatedly presented alone.

of emotional reactions to contextual cues[58–60] and control of emotional responses involving higher-order interactions of the CS-US contingency.[61,62] Finally, extinction of emotional learning has been examined by studies in which the CS is repeatedly presented alone after a CR has been acquired.[63] A schematic depiction of the experimental parameters in a typical fear-conditioning procedure is given in Fig. 54-2.

Animal Studies Reveal the Neural Circuitry

Using modern neuroanatomic, behavioral, and electrophysiologic recording techniques, research-

ers have begun to uncover the neural circuits involved in emotional learning and memory as measured by fear conditioning. Across several species and experimental paradigms, the amygdala has emerged as a brain region critical for the learning and/or expression of conditioned fear associations.[10,64–68] Lesions of the amygdala disrupt the development of CRs on a variety of fear indices, some of which are illustrated in Fig. 54-3. In addition, the firing patterns of neuronal subpopulations within this region[69–71] (as well as the sensory neocortex[14]) change during conditioning, although the functional implications of these findings require further investigation. Finally, a number of pharmacologic agents with anxiolytic properties used in the treatment of human anxiety disorders reduce conditioned fear in both humans[72,73] and animals.[66,74] Some of these drug effects have been localized to action sites within the amygdala.[66,75–77]

The pathways by which sensory information reaches the amygdala for emotional evaluation in fear conditioning have also been detailed, particularly in the auditory domain. Auditory CS transmission to the amygdala occurs by both a direct thalamoamygdala projection and an indirect thalamocorticoamygdala loop.[10,65,78] The direct route is faster than the indirect route, but it provides cruder information regarding stimulus features. The direct pathway may function to prime the amygdala to respond quickly to danger, leaving more intricate analysis of the incoming signal for the cortical pathway. This neurobiological warning signal can grant organisms an evolutionary advan-

Figure 54-3

Some examples of the effects of amygdala lesions on indices of conditioned fear. A. Ibotenic acid lesions of the central nucleus (ACE) block differential heart rate conditioned responses (HR CR), measured as a difference in HR changes over baseline to one tone paired with a periorbital shock (CS+) and another tone presented alone (CS−). (From McCabe et al.,[100] with permission.) B. Electrolytic lesions of the lateral nucleus (L AMYG) disrupt both conditioned arterial pressure responses and conditioned freezing duration. (From LeDoux et al.,[81] with permission.) C. NMDA lesions of the lateral/basolateral nuclei block fear-potentiated startle, measured as a difference in startle amplitude evoked by the auditory startle stimulus presented alone and the startle stimulus presented in the presence of a visual conditioned stimulus. (From Sananes and Davis,[68] with permission.)

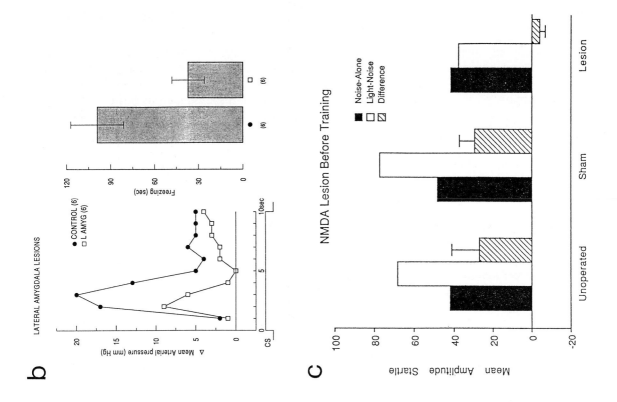

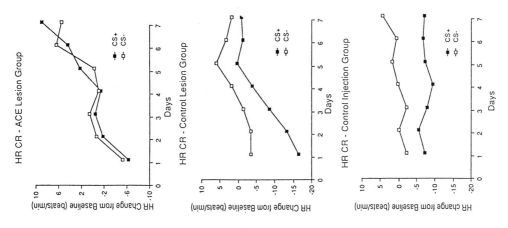

tage by rapidly communicating the existence of potentially threatening environmental stimuli. Either of these transmission routes is sufficient to mediate conditioned fear to single auditory cues,[79] but the cortical pathway may be necessary for appropriate responses to tones that must be discriminated from one another.[80]

These parallel input pathways converge in the lateral nucleus of the amygdala, which serves as a sensory interface to the region.[81] Neurons in the lateral nucleus that respond to acoustic input are also sensitive to somatosensory stimulation.[82] The lateral nucleus may thus function as a site of CS-US integration, a place where emotional associations can be formed and directed to output pathways regulating emotional responses. Synaptic plasticity through the induction of long-term potentiation (LTP) has been observed in the thalamoamygdala pathway,[83,84] the corticoamygdala pathway,[85] and in the acoustic thalamus itself.[86] Although the relationship between LTP and learning and memory processes remains tenuous,[87–90] LTP in the lateral amygdala is accompanied by concurrent enhancement of auditory evoked responses,[84] providing a link between LTP mechanisms and natural sensory transmission.

Once incoming sensory information is processed by the lateral nucleus, it is relayed by intra-amygdala connections[91–93] to the central nucleus, the main output station of the amygdala. Target zones of central nucleus innervation in the brainstem and diencephalon are critical for the generation of emotional responses, although these efferent structures exert specialized control over particular facets of emotional expression. For example, central nucleus projections to the dorsal motor nucleus of the vagus nerve mediate parasympathetic responses;[64] projections to the lateral hypothalamus have been implicated in sympathetic regulation;[94,95] projections to the central gray region are crucial for conditioned freezing responses and conditioned analgesia;[67,95] and projections to the pons are important for fear-potentiated startle.[66] Lesions to these efferent target sites disrupt the generation of individual conditioned emotional responses, leaving others intact;[95] however, ablation of the central nucleus itself produces

global deficits in CR production regardless of response modality.[96–100] The central nucleus of the amygdala therefore serves to coordinate divergent emotional response output during aversive fear conditioning, and there is also evidence that it may direct attentional orienting systems during appetitive conditioning tasks.[101,102]

Contribution of Other Brain Structures

While it is clear that the amygdala plays a central role in the computation of emotional stimulus value, there is recent evidence that other brain regions make contributions to aspects of emotional processing within a fear-conditioning framework. The integrity of the hippocampus, for example, is not essential for conditioning to simple phasic cues but is critical for conditioning to contextual stimuli.[58–60] The effect of hippocampal lesions on the retention of contextual fear is shown in Fig. 54-4. These findings are consistent with cognitive theories regarding the role of the hippocampus in complex stimulus processing.[35–38] This contextual information may be important in al-

Figure 54-4

Effect of electrolytic hippocampal lesions on retention of contextual fear. Lesions were made either 1, 7, 14, or 28 days after training. The hippocampus appears to have an important but time-limited role in conditioned fear memories elicited by contextual stimuli, as measured by the percentage of time spent freezing to the context following training. ○ = *control;* ● = *hippocampal lesions;* ■ = *cortex lesions. (From Kim and Fanselow,[58] with permission.)*

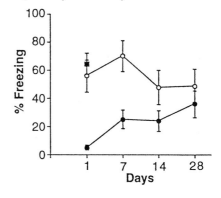

lowing organisms to learn and remember the environmental subtexts in which threatening stimuli occur. The hippocampus may be exerting its influence via anatomic interactions with the amygdala. These connections provide a neural passageway by which higher-order cognitive and mnemonic processes can trigger and shape emotional experience, and vice versa.

In addition, lesions of the ventromedial prefrontal cortex selectively interfere with the extinction of emotional learning in fear conditioning studies.[63,103] This result extends the long-observed perseveration phenomena following prefrontal cortex damage[104,105] into the emotional domain. The extinction process appears to involve active brain processing,[106] which may be regulated by prefrontal-amygdala projections.[107] The neural traces laid down in amygdala neurons during emotional learning are relatively indelible, and their suppression requires neocortical input.[13,108] If extended into human populations, these results may have clinical relevance for neurologic patients with persistent affective disorders (see "Fear Conditioning in Humans," below).

Fear Conditioning in Humans

Figure 54-5 summarizes a current model of the neural circuitry involved in the emotional processing of conditioned fear. As this model becomes refined through animal studies, the question of whether these structures perform similar functions in humans arises. Human subjects do exhibit reliable conditioned fear responses,[109–111] although these responses may be influenced somewhat by certain personality characteristics[112,113] and cognitive processes.[114] Despite its success in animal research, fear conditioning has not been widely used in the neuropsychological assessment of human brain function, where little is known about the neural basis of emotion. Fear conditioning was once attempted in H.M., a well-studied amnesic patient with extensive bilateral medial temporal lobe excision for the surgical treatment of medically refractory epilepsy.[115,116] However, H.M. did not show skin conductance responses to electric shock, even at high intensity levels, so the fear

conditioning experiment was terminated.[116] Recently, we examined fear conditioning in human epileptic patients with unilateral medial temporal lobe resection, including the amygdala.[117] These patients exhibited intact skin conductance responses to a loud white-noise US but showed impaired CR acquisition during discriminative conditioning tasks (see Fig. 54-6). This result suggests that, as in other species, the integrity of the medial temporal lobe is important for conditioned emotional learning in humans, although assessment of the relative contributions of particular structures within this region must await future investigation in patients with more restricted damage and functional imaging studies in healthy adults.

Fear conditioning paradigms have also been proposed as a model system for studying emotional processing in clinical populations with affective and traumatic memory disorders.[118,119] The clinical symptomatology of human anxiety shares many markers with measures of conditioned fear in animals,[66] and, in general, anxious patients show elevated electrodermal activity during fear-conditioning tasks.[120–122] Schizophrenic patients, in contrast, tend to show decreased skin conductance responses on conditioning tasks,[123,124] although these patients must be divided into subpopulations based on overall electrodermal reactivity.[125] Moreover, a line of research growing out of biological preparedness theory[126] has demonstrated that fear conditioning with phobic material produces greater resistance to extinction than does conditioning with neutral stimuli.[127] Behavioral therapies based on conditioning principles have been largely successful in the treatment of phobic disorders,[128] although remission is sometimes observed after systematic desensitization or counterconditioning. Spontaneous remission and renewal processes are currently being viewed in terms of contextual effects in animal models of fear conditioning,[57] which may have important implications for work in clinical settings.[129] Finally, conditioning interpretations have been postulated to account for initial attack episodes in patients with panic disorder, although the maintenance of panic disorder once it has developed may be guided by other factors.[130] Cognitive appraisal mechanisms,

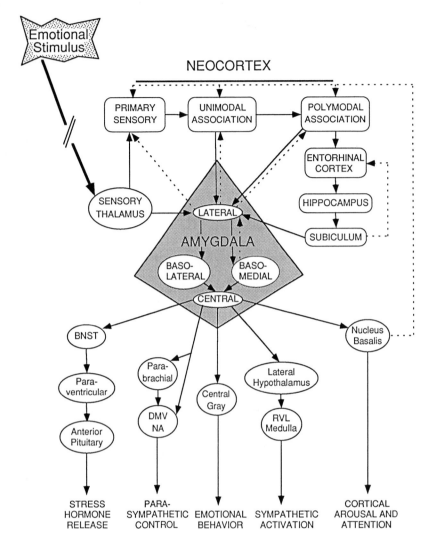

Figure 54-5
An emotional processing network based on studies of conditioned fear. Increasingly complex information transmitted by parallel afferent projections to the lateral nucleus of the amygdala is integrated and sent via intraamygdala connections to the central nucleus of the amygdala, which functions to coordinate diverse effector systems to produce appropriate emotional responses. Feedforward projections are indicated by solid lines, while feedback projections are indicated by dashed lines. Additional outputs of the central nucleus are not shown. BNST = bed nucleus of the stria terminalis, DMV = dorsal motor nucleus of the vagus, NA = nucleus ambiguus, RVL medulla = rostral ventrolateral nuclei of the medulla.

vicarious learning, and coping strategies are also crucial to the development and maintenance of other fear-related disorders.[131] In this regard, behavioral therapies have evolved to incorporate contemporary theories of conditioning, instrumental learning, and cognition.[132]

TOWARD AN INTEGRATIVE VIEW OF THE EMOTIONAL BRAIN

Fear-conditioning paradigms have immensely guided our current understanding of how emotion-

ally significant events are learned and remembered. The model systems approach, as outlined above, is beginning to bridge the gap in emotion research aimed at various levels of nervous system organization, from molecular/genetic studies[133,134] to behavioral/computational models.[135] This is a major step toward the integration of disparate research domains across experimental techniques and species. In addition, though, it is important to consider the extent to which the brain regions mediating conditioned fear more generally govern the processing of fear and other emotions. Although an extensive review of the literature is be-

Figure 54-6

Impaired simple discrimination acquisition in human epileptic patients with unilateral anteromedial temporal lobe resection, including the amygdala. Data from each experimental phase are collapsed across trials. Difference skin conductance responses (SCR) above zero reflect intact discrimination performance during the acquisition phase, with relatively greater conditioning to a tone paired with a loud noise unconditioned stimulus compared to another tone presented alone. μS = microsiemens. (From LaBar et al.,[117] with permission.)

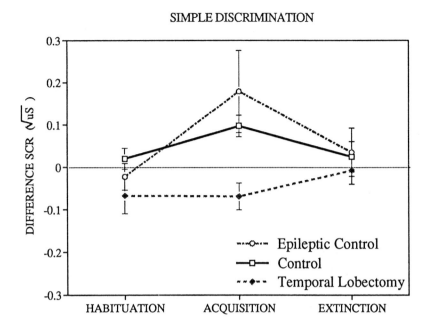

SIMPLE DISCRIMINATION

yond the scope of this overview, we will briefly mention several points regarding the role of particular limbic forebrain structures in emotional processing beyond conditioning.

First, the amygdala has been implicated in other aspects of fear regulation in both human[136–140] and nonhuman[141–143] studies. The amygdala also appears to be involved in stimulus-reward learning[13,144,145] and may contribute to dysfunction characterized by other disorders of affect and dementia.[7,137,146–148] Second, Gray[8,149,150] has incorporated the septohippocampal system into a behavioral inhibition model of anxiety and stress, with an emphasis on its role in cognitive monitoring and coping strategies. This conception reflects how cognitive influences enter into emotional networks and complements the investigation of the role of the hippocampus in more complex aspects of conditioned fear. Third, the integrity of the orbitofrontal cortex is critical for the appropriate adjustment of behavioral responses to changing reinforcement contingencies, which may account for some of the emotional deficits following frontal lobe damage.[13] The orbitofrontal cortex may also function as a link be-

tween internal somatic states and social perceptions in the guidance of behavior,[151] and prefrontal-cingulate-amygdala connectivity with effector structures seems to be particularly important for mediating socioemotional interactions.[5,152] Thus, particular structures of the limbic forebrain appear to play distinct roles in affective processing, some of which can be understood as relating to more general functions of these regions outside of the emotional domain. Of the structures comprising MacLean's limbic system hypothesis, the amygdala has been most consistently linked with emotional stimulus evaluation, a function originally attributed to the hypothalamus by previous theorists (see "Historical Perspective" above). The generality of these findings and the amygdala's contribution to other sensoricognitive areas, however, remain to be elucidated.

To conclude, the greatest advances in affective neuroscience to date have been made in discrete domains of emotional behavior tested through experimentally controlled and well-defined models, as exemplified by the discussion of fear conditioning in the present chapter. These kinds of studies have yielded an emerging view of the emotional brain with much greater specificity than has previously been possible. Most of this precision has been achieved from animal models of emotion, but with the advent of more refined neuroimaging techniques, human research will become more informative in terms of both structural localization in lesion analysis and in the development of functional brain mapping. This advance will be particularly useful in assessing the contribution of the neocortex and its interaction with limbic and brainstem control of affect and arousal. Finally, future research will need to expand upon the breadth of existing behavioral paradigms, particularly for affiliative emotions, in order to provide a more complete account of the range, complexity, and subtlety of emotional experience. The result of these efforts will provide the foundation for a more integrative view of emotional processing in the brain.

REFERENCES

1. Ekman P, Davidson RJ: *The Nature of Emotion.* New York: Oxford University Press, 1994.
2. Heilman KM, Bowers D, Valenstein E: Emotional disorders associated with neurological diseases, in Heilman KM, Valenstein E (eds): *Clinical Neuropsychology,* 3d ed. New York: Oxford University Press, 1993, pp 461–498.
3. Damasio AR: *Descartes' Error: Emotion, Reason, and the Human Brain.* New York: Putnam, 1994.
4. Bloom FE: Cellular mechanisms active in emotion, in Gazzaniga M (ed): *The Cognitive Neurosciences.* Cambridge, MA: MIT Press, 1995, pp 1063–1070.
5. Brothers L: Neurophysiology of the perception of intentions by primates, in Gazzaniga M (ed): *The Cognitive Neurosciences.* Cambridge, MA: MIT Press, 1995, pp 1107–1116.
6. Davidson RJ: Cerebral asymmetry, emotion, and affective style, in Davidson RJ, Hugdahl K (eds): *Brain Asymmetry.* Cambridge, MA: MIT Press, 1995, pp 361–388.
7. Drevets WC, Raichle ME: Positron emission tomographic imaging studies of human emotional disorders, in Gazzaniga M (ed): *The Cognitive Neurosciences.* Cambridge, MA: MIT Press, 1995, pp 1153–1164.
8. Gray JA: A model of the limbic system and basal ganglia: Applications to anxiety and schizophrenia, in Gazzaniga M (ed): *The Cognitive Neurosciences.* Cambridge, MA: MIT Press, 1995, pp 1165–1180.
9. Halgren E, Marinkovic K: Neurophysiological networks integrating human emotions, in Gazzaniga M (ed): *The Cognitive Neurosciences.* Cambridge, MA: MIT Press, 1995, pp 1137–1152.
10. LeDoux JE: In search of an emotional system in the brain: Leaping from fear to emotion and consciousness, in Gazzaniga M (ed): *The Cognitive Neurosciences.* Cambridge, MA: MIT Press, 1995, pp 1049–1062.
11. Liotti M, Tucker DM: Emotion in asymmetric corticolimbic networks, in Davidson RJ, Hugdahl K (eds): *Brain Asymmetry.* Cambridge, MA: MIT Press, 1995, pp 389–424.
12. McEwen BS: Stressful experience, brain, and emotions: Developmental, genetic, and hormonal influences, in Gazzaniga M (ed): *The Cognitive Neurosciences.* Cambridge, MA: MIT Press, 1995, pp 1117–1136.
13. Rolls ET: A theory of emotion and consciousness, and its application to understanding the neural basis of emotion, in Gazzaniga M (ed): *The Cognitive Neurosciences.* Cambridge, MA: MIT Press, 1995, pp 1091–1106.
14. Weinberger NM: Retuning the brain by fear conditioning, in Gazzaniga M (ed): *The Cognitive Neurosciences.* Cambridge, MA: MIT Press, 1995, pp 1071–1090.
15. James W: What is an emotion? *Mind* 9:188–205, 1884.
16. Lange CG: *Über Gemüthsbewegungen.* Leipzig: Thomas, 1887.
17. Cannon WB, Britton SW: Pseudoaffective medulliadrenal secretion. *Am J Physiol* 72:283–294, 1925.
18. Woodworth RS, Sherrington CS: A pseudoaffective reflex and its spinal path. *J Physiol Lond* 31:234–243, 1904.
19. Bazett HC, Penfield WG: A study of the Sherrington decerebrate animal in the chronic as well as the acute condition. *Brain* 45:185–265, 1922.
20. Cannon WB: The James-Lange theory of emotions: A critical examination and an alternative theory. *Am J Psychol* 39:106–124, 1927.
21. Bard P: A diencephalic mechanism for the expression of rage with special reference to the sympathetic nervous system. *Am J Physiol* 84:490–515, 1928.
22. Cannon WB: *Bodily Changes in Pain, Hunger, Fear, and Rage.* 2d ed. New York: Appleton, 1929.

23. Papez JW: A proposed mechanism of emotion. *Arch Neurol Psychiatry* 79:217–224, 1937.

24. Klüver H, Bucy PC: "Psychic blindness" and other symptoms following bilateral temporal lobectomy in rhesus monkeys. *Am J Physiol* 119:352–353, 1937.

25. Klüver H, Bucy PC: Preliminary analysis of functions of the temporal lobes in monkeys. *Arch Neurol Psychiatry* 42:979–1000, 1939.

26. MacLean PD: Psychosomatic disease and the visceral brain: Recent developments bearing on the Papez theory of emotion. *Psychosom Med* 11:338–353, 1949.

27. MacLean PD: Some psychiatric implications of physiological studies on frontotemporal portion of limbic system (visceral brain). *Electroencephalogr Clin Neurophysiol* 4:407–418, 1952.

28. Brodal A: *Neurological Anatomy.* New York: Oxford University Press, 1982.

29. Swanson LW: The hippocampus and the concept of the limbic system, in Seifert W (ed): *Neurobiology of the Hippocampus.* London: Academic Press, 1983, pp 3–19.

30. Kotter R, Meyer N: The limbic system: A review of its empirical foundation. *Behav Brain Res* 52:105–127, 1992.

31. LeDoux JE: Emotion, in Plum F (ed): *Handbook of Physiology:* I. *The Nervous System. Higher Functions of the Brain.* Bethesda, MD: American Physiological Society 1987, vol 5, pp 419–460.

32. LeDoux JE: Emotion and the limbic system concept. *Concepts Neurosci* 2:169–199, 1991.

33. Squire LR: Mechanisms of memory. *Science* 232:1612–1619, 1987.

34. O'Keefe J, Nadel L: *The Hippocampus as a Cognitive Map.* Oxford, England: Clarendon, 1978.

35. Nadel L: Hippocampus and space revisited. *Hippocampus* 1:221–229, 1991.

36. Hirsh R: The hippocampus and contextual retrieval of information from memory: A theory. *Behav Biol* 12:421–444, 1974.

37. Sutherland RJ, Rudy JW: Configural association theory: The role of the hippocampal formation in learning, memory, and amnesia. *Psychobiology* 17:129–144, 1989.

38. Cohen NJ, Eichenbaum H: *Memory, Amnesia, and the Hippocampal System.* Cambridge, MA: MIT Press, 1993.

39. Weiskrantz L: Behavioral changes associated with ablation of the amygdaloid complex in monkeys. *J Comp Physiol* 49:381–391, 1956.

40. LeDoux JE: Emotion and the amygdala, in Aggleton JP (ed): *The Amygdala: Neurobiological Aspects of Emotion, Memory, and Mental Dysfunction.* New York: Wiley-Liss, 1992, pp 339–352.

41. Ungerleider LG, Mishkin M: Two cortical visual systems, in Ingle DJ, Goodale MA, Mansfield RJW (eds): *Analysis of Visual Behavior.* Cambridge, MA: MIT Press, 1982.

42. Tulving E, Schacter DL: Priming and human memory systems. *Science* 247:301–306, 1990.

43. Weiskrantz L: Problems of learning and memory: One or multiple memory systems? *Phil Trans R Soc Lond B* 329:99–108, 1990.

44. Squire LR, Knowlton B, Musen G: The structure and organization of memory. *Annu Rev Psychol* 44:453–495, 1993.

45. Levenson RW: Emotion and the autonomic nervous system: A prospectus for research on autonomic specificity, in Wagner H (ed): *Social Psychophysiology and Emotion: Theory and Clinical Applications.* London: Wiley, 1988, pp 17–42.

46. Izard CE: *The Psychology of Emotions.* New York: Plenum, 1991.

47. Schacter S, Singer JE: Cognitive, social, and physiological determinants of emotional state. *Psychol Rev* 69:379–399, 1962.

48. Lazarus RS: On the primacy of cognition. *Am Psychol* 39:124–129, 1984.

49. Zajonc RB: On the primacy of affect. *Am Psychol* 39:117–123, 1984.

50. Leventhal H, Scherer K: The relationship of emotion to cognition: A functional approach to a semantic controversy. *Cogn Emot* 1:3–28, 1987.

51. LeDoux JE: Cognitive-emotional interactions in the brain. *Cogn Emot* 3:267–289, 1989.

52. Blanchard DC, Blanchard RJ: Innate and conditioned reactions to threat in rats with amygdaloid lesions. *J Comp Physiol Psychol* 81:281–290, 1972.

53. Pavlov IP: *Conditioned Reflexes.* New York: Dover, 1927.

54. Estes WK, Skinner BF: Some quantitative properties of anxiety. *J Exp Psychol* 29:390–400, 1941.

55. McAllister WR, McAllister DE: Behavioral measurement of conditioned fear, in Brush FR (ed): *Aversive Conditioning and Learning.* New York: Academic Press, 1971, pp 105–179.

56. Fanselow MS: Conditional and unconditional components of postshock freezing. *Pavlov J Biol Sci* 15:177–182, 1980.

57. Bouton ME: Context, ambiguity, and classical conditioning. *Curr Dir Psychol Sci* 3:49–53, 1994.

58. Kim JJ, Fanselow MS: Modality-specific retrograde amnesia of fear. *Science* 256:675–677, 1992.

59. Phillips RG, LeDoux JE: Differential contribution of amygdala and hippocampus to cued and contextual fear conditioning. *Behav Neurosci* 106:274–285, 1992.

60. Phillips RG, LeDoux JE: Lesions of the dorsal hippocampal formation interfere with background but not foreground contextual fear conditioning. *Learn Mem* 1:34–44, 1994.

61. Rickert EJ, Bennett TL, Lane PL, French J: Hippocampectomy and the attenuation of blocking. *Behav Biol* 22:147–160, 1978.

62. Kaye H, Pearce JM: Hippocampal lesions attenuate latent inhibition of a CS and of a neutral stimulus. *Psychobiology* 15:293–299, 1987.

63. Morgan MA, Romanski LM, LeDoux JE: Extinction of emotional learning: Contribution of medial prefrontal cortex. *Neurosci Lett* 163:109–113, 1993.

64. Kapp BS, Wilson A, Pascoe J, et al: A neuroanatomical systems analysis of conditioned bradycardia in the rabbit, in Gabriel M, Moore J (eds): *Learning and Computational Neuroscience: Foundations of Adaptive Networks.* Cambridge, MA: MIT Press, 1990, pp 53–90.

65. LeDoux JE: Information flow from sensation to emotion: Plasticity in the neural computation of stimulus value, in Gabriel M, Moore J (eds): *Learning and Computational Neuroscience: Foundations of Adaptive Networks.* Cambridge, MA: MIT Press, 1990, pp 3–52.

66. Davis M: The role of the amygdala in conditioned fear, in Aggleton JP (ed): *The Amygdala: Neurobiological Aspects of Emotion, Memory, and Mental Dysfunction.* New York: Wiley-Liss, 1992, pp 255–306.

67. Fanselow MS: Neural organization of the defensive behavior system responsible for fear. *Psychonom Bull Rev* 1:429–438, 1994.

68. Sananes CB, Davis M: *N*-Methyl-D-aspartate lesions of the lateral and basolateral nuclei of the amygdala block fear-potentiated startle and shock sensitization of startle. *Behav Neurosci* 106:72–80, 1992.

69. Applegate CD, Frysinger RC, Kapp BS, Gallagher M: Multiple unit activity recorded from amygdala central nucleus during Pavlovian heart rate conditioning in the rabbit. *Brain Res* 238:457–462, 1982.

70. Pascoe JP, Kapp BS: Electrophysiological characteristics of amygdaloid central nucleus neurons

during Pavlovian fear conditioning in the rabbit. *Behav Brain Res* 16:117–133, 1985.

71. Quirk GJ, Tao P, Repa JC, LeDoux JE: Simultaneously recorded neurons in the lateral amygdala of freely moving rats during fear conditioning. *Soc Neurosci Abstr* 20:1007, 1994.

72. Molander L: Effect of melperone, chlorpromazine, haloperidol, and diazepam on experimental anxiety in normal subjects. *Psychopharmacology* 77:109–113, 1982.

73. Hensman R, Guimarães FS, Wang M, Deakin JFW: Effects of ritanserin on aversive classical conditioning in humans. *Psychopharmacology* 104:220–224, 1991.

74. Fanselow MS, Helmstetter FJ: Conditional analgesia, defensive freezing, and benzodiazepines. *Behav Neurosci* 102:233–243, 1988.

75. Davis M: Pharmacological and anatomical analysis of fear conditioning. *NIDA Research Monograph* 97:126–162, 1990.

76. Gallagher M, Kapp BS, McNall CL, Pascoe JP: Opiate effects in the amygdala central nucleus on heart rate conditioning in rabbits. *Pharmacol Biochem Behav* 14:497–505, 1981.

77. Gallagher M, Kapp BS, Pascoe JP: Enkephalin analogue effects in the amygdala central nucleus on conditioned heart rate. *Pharmacol Biochem Behav* 17:217–222, 1982.

78. LeDoux JE: Sensory systems and emotion. *Integr Psychiatry* 4:237–248, 1986.

79. Romanski LM, LeDoux JE: Equipotentiality of thalamo-amygdala and thalamo-cortico-amygdala projections as auditory conditioned stimulus pathways. *J Neurosci* 12:4501–4509, 1992.

80. Jarrell TW, Gentile CG, Romanski LM, et al: Involvement of cortical and thalamic auditory regions in retention of differential bradycardia conditioning to acoustic conditioned stimuli in rabbits. *Brain Res* 412:285–294, 1987.

81. LeDoux JE, Cicchetti P, Xagoraris A, Romanski LM: The lateral amygdaloid nucleus: Sensory interface of the amygdala in fear conditioning. *J Neurosci* 10:1062–1069, 1990.

82. Romanski LM, Clugnet MC, Bordi F, LeDoux JE: Somatosensory and auditory convergence in the lateral nucleus of the amygdala. *Behav Neurosci* 107:444–450, 1993.

83. Clugnet MC, LeDoux JE: Synaptic plasticity in fear conditioning circuits: Induction of LTP in the lateral nucleus of the amygdala by stimulation of

the medial geniculate body. *J Neurosci* 10:2818–2824, 1990.

84. Rogan MT, LeDoux JE: LTP is accompanied by commensurate enhancement of auditory-evoked responses in a fear conditioning circuit. *Neuron* 15:1–20, 1995.

85. Chapman PF, Kairiss EW, Keenan CL, Brown TH: Long-term synaptic potentiation in the amygdala. *Synapse* 6:271–278, 1990.

86. Gerren RA, Weinberger NM: Long term potentiation in the magnocellular medial geniculate nucleus of the anesthetized cat. *Brain Res* 265:138–142, 1983.

87. McNaughton BL, Barnes CA: From cooperative synaptic enhancement to associative memory: Bridging the abyss. *Semin Neurosci* 2:403–416, 1990.

88. Laroche S, Doyère V, Rédini-Del Negro C: What role for long-term potentiation in learning and the maintenance of memories? in Baudry M, Davis JL (eds): *Long-Term Potentiation: A Debate of Current Issues.* Cambridge, MA: MIT Press, 1991, pp 301–316.

89. Morris RGM: Is there overlap between the characteristics of learning and the physiological properties of LTP? in Squire LR (ed): *The Encyclopedia of Learning and Memory.* New York: Macmillan, 1992, pp 369–372.

90. Gallistel CR: Is long-term potentiation a plausible basis for memory? in McGaugh JL, Weinberger NM, Lynch G (eds): *Brain and Memory.* New York: Oxford University Press, 1995, pp 328–337.

91. McDonald AJ: Cell types and intrinsic connections of the amygdala, in Aggleton JP (ed): *The Amygdala: Neurobiological Aspects of Emotion, Memory, and Mental Dysfunction.* New York: Wiley-Liss, 1992, pp 67–96.

92. Pitkänen A, Stefanacci L, Farb CR, et al: Intrinsic connections of the rat amygdaloid complex: Projections originating in the lateral nucleus. *J Comp Neurol* 356:288–310, 1995.

93. Savander V, Go C-G, LeDoux JE, Pitkänen A: Intrinsic connections of the rat amygdaloid complex: Projections originating in the basal nucleus. *J Comp Neurol* 361:345–368, 1995.

94. Smith OA, Astley CA, Devito JL, et al: Functional analysis of hypothalamic control of the cardiovascular responses accompanying emotional behavior. *Fed Proc* 39:2487–2494, 1980.

95. LeDoux JE, Iwata J, Cicchetti P, Reis DJ: Different projections of the central amygdaloid nucleus mediate autonomic and behavioral correlates of conditioned fear. *J Neurosci* 8:2517–2529, 1988.

96. Kapp BS, Frysinger RC, Gallagher M, Haselton J: Amygdala central nucleus lesions: Effect on heart rate conditioning in the rabbit. *Physiol Behav* 23:1109–1117, 1979.

97. Gentile CG, Jarrell TW, Teich A, et al: The role of amygdaloid central nucleus in the retention of differential Pavlovian conditioning of bradycardia in rabbits. *Behav Brain Res* 20:263–273, 1986.

98. Hitchcock J, Davis M: Lesions of the amygdala but not of the cerebellum or red nucleus block conditioned fear as measured with the potentiated startle paradigm. *Behav Neurosci* 100:11–22, 1986.

99. Iwata J, LeDoux JE, Meeley MP, et al: Intrinsic neurons in the amygdaloid field projected to by the medial geniculate body mediate emotional responses conditioned to acoustic stimuli. *Brain Res* 383:195–214, 1986.

100. McCabe PW, Gentile CG, Markgraf CG, et al: Ibotenic acid lesions in the amygdaloid central nucleus but not in the lateral subthalamic area prevent the acquisition of differential Pavlovian conditioning of bradycardia in rabbits. *Brain Res* 580:155–163, 1992.

101. Gallagher M, Holland PC: Understanding the function of the central nucleus: Is simple conditioning enough? in Aggleton JP (ed): *The Amygdala: Neurobiological Aspects of Emotion, Memory, and Mental Dysfunction.* New York: Wiley-Liss, 1992, pp 307–321.

102. Gallagher M, Holland PC: The amygdala complex: Multiple roles in associative learning and attention. *Proc Natl Acad Sci USA* 91:11771–11776, 1994.

103. Morgan MA, LeDoux JE: Differential contribution of dorsal and ventral medial prefrontal cortex to the acquisition and extinction of conditioned fear in rats. *Behav Neurosci* 109:681–688, 1995.

104. Fuster JM: *The Prefrontal Cortex: Anatomy, Physiology, and Neuropsychology of the Frontal Lobe,* 2d ed. New York: Raven Press, 1989.

105. Janowsky JS, Shimamura AP, Kritchevsky M, Squire LR: Cognitive impairment following frontal lobe damage and its relevance to human amnesia. *Behav Neurosci* 103:548–560, 1989.

106. Falls WA, Miserendino MJD, Davis M: Extinction of fear-potentiated startle: Blockade by infusion of an NMDA antagonist into the amygdala. *J Neurosci* 12:854–863, 1992.

107. Amaral DG, Price JL, Pitkänen A, Carmichael ST: Anatomical organization of the primate amygda-

loid complex, in Aggleton JP (ed): *The Amygdala: Neurobiological Aspects of Emotion, Memory, and Mental Dysfunction.* New York: Wiley-Liss, 1992, pp 1–66.

108. LeDoux JE, Romanski LM, Xagoraris AE: Indelibility of subcortical emotional memories. *J Cogn Neurosci* 1:238–243, 1989.

109. Hodes RL, Cook EW, Lang PJ: Individual differences in autonomic response: Conditioned association or conditioned fear? *Psychophysiology* 22:545–560, 1985.

110. Grillon C, Ameli R, Woods SW, et al: Fear-potentiated startle in humans: Effects of anticipatory anxiety on the acoustic blink reflex. *Psychophysiology* 28:588–595, 1991.

111. Fredrickson M, Annas P, Georgiades A, et al: Internal consistency and temporal stability of classically conditioned skin conductance responses. *Biol Psychol* 35:153–163, 1993.

112. Eysenck HJ: The conditioning model of neurosis. *Behav Brain Sci* 2:155–199, 1979.

113. Guimarães FS, Hellewell J, Hensman R, et al: Characterization of a psychophysiological model of classical fear conditioning in healthy volunteers: Influence of gender, instruction, personality and placebo. *Psychopharmacology* 104:231–236, 1990.

114. Davey G (ed): *Cognitive Processes and Pavlovian Conditioning in Humans.* Chichester, England: Wiley, 1987.

115. Scoville WB, Milner B: Loss of recent memory after bilateral hippocampal lesions. *J Neurol Neurosurg Psychiatry* 20:11–21, 1957.

116. Milner B, Corkin S, Teuber H-L: Further analysis of the hippocampal amnesic syndrome: 14-year follow-up study of H.M. *Neuropsychologia* 6:215–234, 1968.

117. LaBar KS, LeDoux JE, Spencer DD, Phelps EA: Impaired fear conditioning following unilateral temporal lobectomy in humans. *J Neurosci* 15:6846–6855, 1995.

118. Öhman A: Fear-relevance, autonomic conditioning, and phobias: A laboratory model. in Sjödén PO, Bates S, Dockens WS (eds): *Trends in Behavior Therapy.* New York: Academic Press, 1979, pp 107–133.

119. Charney DS, Deutch AY, Krystal JH, et al: Psychobiologic mechanisms of posttraumatic stress disorder. *Arch Gen Psychiatry* 50:294–305, 1993.

120. Ashcroft K, Guimarães FS, Wang M, Deakin JFW: Evaluation of a psychophysiological model of clas-

sical fear conditioning in anxious patients. *Psychopharmacology* 104:215–219, 1991.

121. Pitman RK, Orr SP: Test of the conditioning model of neurosis: Differential aversive conditioning of angry and neutral facial expressions in anxiety disorder patients. *J Abnorm Psychol* 95:208–213, 1986.

122. Howe ES: GSR conditioning in anxiety states, normals, and chronic functional psychotic subjects. *J Abnorm Soc Psychol* 56:183–189, 1958.

123. Ax AF, Banford JL, Beckett PGS, et al: Autonomic conditioning in chronic schizophrenia. *J Abnorm Psychol* 76:140–154, 1970.

124. Gorham IC, Novelly RA, Ax A, Frohman CE: Classically conditioned autonomic discrimination and tryptophan uptake in chronic schizophrenia. *Psychophysiology* 15:158–164, 1978.

125. Öhman A: Electrodermal activity and vulnerability to schizophrenia: A review. *Biol Psychol* 12:87–145, 1981.

126. Seligman MEP: Phobias and preparedness. *Behav Ther* 2:307–320, 1971.

127. Marks I, Tobena A: Learning and unlearning fear: A clinical and evolutionary perspective. *Neurosci Biobehav Rev* 14:365–384, 1989.

128. Masters JC, Burish TG, Hollon SD, Rimm DC: *Behavior Therapy: Techniques and Empirical Findings.* 3d ed. New York: Harcourt Brace Jovanovich, 1987.

129. Bouton ME, Schwartzentruber D: Sources of relapse after extinction in Pavlovian and instrumental learning. *Clin Psychol Rev* 11:123–140, 1991.

130. Wolpe J, Rowan VC: Panic disorder: A product of classical conditioning. *Behav Res Ther* 26:441–450, 1988.

131. Carr AT: The psychopathology of fear, in Sluckin W (ed): *Fear in Animals and Man.* New York: Van Nostrand Reinhold, 1979, pp 199–235.

132. Thorpe GL, Olson SL: *Behavior Therapy: Concepts, Procedures, and Applications.* Boston: Allyn & Bacon, 1990.

133. Chen C, Rainnie DG, Greene RW, Tonegawa S: Abnormal fear response and aggressive behavior in mutant mice deficient for α-calcium-calmodulin kinase II. *Science* 266:291–294, 1994.

134. Tully T, Preat T, Boynton SC, Del Vecchio M: Genetic dissection of consolidated memory in *Drosophila. Cell* 79:35–47, 1994.

135. Armony JL, Servan-Schreiber D, Cohen JD, LeDoux JE: An anatomically constrained neural

network model of fear conditioning. *Behav Neurosci* 109:1–12, 1995.

136. Adolphs R, Tranel D, Damasio H, Damasio AR: Impaired recognition of emotion in facial expressions following bilateral damage to the human amygdala. *Nature* 372:669–672, 1994.

137. Aggleton JP: The functional effects of amygdala lesions in humans: A comparison with findings from monkeys, in Aggleton JP (ed): *The Amygdala: Neurobiological Aspects of Emotion, Memory, and Mental Dysfunction.* New York: Wiley-Liss, 1992, pp 485–504.

138. Gloor P: Role of the amygdala in temporal lobe epilepsy, in Aggleton JP (ed): *The Amygdala: Neurobiological Aspects of Emotion, Memory, and Mental Dysfunction.* New York: Wiley-Liss, 1992, pp 505–538.

139. Halgren E: Emotional neurophysiology of the amygdala within the context of human cognition, in Aggleton JP (ed): *The Amygdala: Neurobiological Aspects of Emotion, Memory, and Mental Dysfunction.* New York: Wiley-Liss, 1992, pp 191–228.

140. Raichle ME: Exploring the mind with dynamic imaging. *Semin Neurosci* 2:307–315, 1990.

141. Fernandez de Molina A, Hunsperger RW: Central representation of affective reactions in forebrain and brain stem: Electrical stimulation of amygdala, stria terminalis, and adjacent structures. *J Physiol* 145:251–265, 1959.

142. Shibata K, Kataoka Y, Yamashita K, Ueki S: An important role of the central amygdaloid nucleus and mammillary body in the mediation of conflict behavior in rats. *Brain Res* 372:159–162, 1986.

143. Slotnick BM: Fear behavior and passive avoidance deficits in mice with amygdala lesions. *Physiol Behav* 11:717–720, 1973.

144. Gaffan D: Amygdala and the memory of reward, in Aggleton JP (ed): *The Amygdala: Neurobiological Aspects of Emotion, Memory, and Mental Dysfunction.* New York: Wiley-Liss, 1992, pp 471–484.

145. Everitt BJ, Robbins TW: Amygdala-ventral striatal interactions and reward-related processes, in Aggleton JP (ed): *The Amygdala: Neurobiological Aspects of Emotion, Memory, and Mental Dysfunction.* New York: Wiley-Liss, 1992, pp 401–430.

146. Cummings JL, Duchen LW: Klüver-Bucy syndrome in Pick's disease: Clinical and pathological correlations. *Neurology* 31:1415–1422, 1981.

147. Mann DMA: The neuropathology of the amygdala in ageing and in dementia, in Aggleton JP (ed): *The Amygdala: Neurobiological Aspects of Emotion, Memory, and Mental Dysfunction.* New York: Wiley-Liss, 1992, pp 575–594.

148. Reynolds GP: The amygdala and the neurochemistry of schizophrenia, in Aggleton JP (ed): *The Amygdala: Neurobiological Aspects of Emotion, Memory, and Mental Dysfunction.* New York: Wiley-Liss, 1992, pp 561–574.

149. Gray JA: *The Psychology of Fear and Stress.* 2d ed. Cambridge, England: Cambridge University Press, 1987.

150. Gray JA, McNaughton N: Comparison between the behavioural effects of septal and hippocampal lesions: A review. *Neurosci Biobehav Rev* 5:109–132, 1983.

151. Damasio A, Tranel D, Damasio H: Somatic markers and the guidance of behavior: Theory and preliminary testing, in Levin H, Eisenberg H, Benton A (eds): *Frontal Lobe Function and Dysfunction.* New York: Oxford University Press, 1991, pp 217–229.

152. Damasio H, Grabowski T, Frank R, et al: The return of Phineas Gage: Clues about the brain from the skull of a famous patient. *Science* 264:1102–1105, 1994.

Chapter 55

EMOTIONAL DISORDERS IN RELATION TO UNILATERAL BRAIN DAMAGE

Guido Gainotti

The hypothesis of hemispheric specialization for psychological phenomena other than language and cognitive functions, such as emotions and affect, is a recent one in the history of neuropsychology. Thus, only 30 years ago, and a century after the discovery of left hemispheric dominance for language,[1,2] the classic viewpoint on this subject was summarized in these words by Hécaen:[3] "When there is a disturbance of the activities of synthesis (such as personality disturbances derived from cerebral lesions) no difference can be found between left and right lesions." About the same time, however, the problem of a possible hemispheric asymmetry in the regulation of emotions was raised by some clinical observations, independently made during pharmacologic inactivation of the right and left hemispheres[4-6] and during observation of the emotional behavior of unilaterally brain-damaged patients.[7,8] The interest of these early clinical studies does not reside only in the fact that they called the attention of neuropsychologists to a problem that had been previously substantially neglected. It also stems from the fact that the theoretical models proposed by those who made these clinical observations later served to orient most of the experimental studies devised to clarify the links between emotions and hemispheric specialization.

THE FIRST CLINICAL STUDIES

Those who observed the emotional behavior of patients submitted to the Wada test found that a "depressive-catastrophic" reaction is often noted after the injection of sodium amytal into the left carotid artery, whereas a "euphoric-maniacal" reaction is observed after pharmacologic inactivation of the right hemisphere. Taking implicitly as a reference point the biological model of the bipolar maniac-depressive psychosis, these authors considered the depressive-catastrophic reaction to be a form of endogenous depression, resulting from inactivation of a "center for positive emotions" located in the left hemisphere. Analogously, they considered the euphoric-maniacal reaction to be a hypomanic state resulting from inactivation of a "center for negative emotions" located in the right hemisphere.

The clinical observations made by Gainotti[7,8] while studying the emotional behavior of right- and left-brain-damaged patients were at first similar to those made by previous authors during the Wada test. Patients with left brain damage typically showed a "catastrophic reaction" (i.e., increasing signs of anxiety and/or sudden bursts of tears) in the face of their difficulties of verbal communication, whereas those with right brain damage showed a strange "indifference reaction" toward failures and disabilities. However, clinical considerations concerning the typical context of catastrophic reactions and the qualitative features of indifference reactions led Gainotti[8-10] to reject the interpretation linking the former to an endogenous depression and the latter to a manic state. Gainotti noticed that catastrophic reactions were usually triggered by frustrating, repeated attempts at verbal expression. He therefore suggested that catastrophic reactions should be considered a dramatic but psychologically appropriate form of reaction to a catastrophic event rather than a biologically based form of depression. He also noticed that, from the qualitative point of view, the indifference reactions of right-brain-damaged patients did not show the features of excitement and euphoric mood typical of a manic state but rather consisted of a heterogeneous and rather paradoxical set of emotional abnormalities. A first set of features, which could properly be grouped under the heading of indifference, included overt expressions of unawareness or of minimization of the disease, an obvious lack of concern for the disability, and an attitude of indifference toward failures met during the neuropsychological examination. A second pattern of behavior, which could be labeled verbal disinhibition, consisted of a tendency to joke in a fatuous, ironic, or sarcastic manner, which sometimes gave an impression of childish euphoria but at other times that of black humor. A last set of behavioral patterns seemed to suggest an implicit attitude of denial of illness and of rejection of the paralyzed limbs. This set included delusions about the paralyzed limbs (somatoparaphrenia), which were felt as unattached to the patient's body and were attributed to someone else;[11,12] confabulations of denial,[13] consisting of a marked tendency to tell stories which, although not explicitly concerning the paralyzed limbs, were clearly inconsistent with the patient's disease; expressions of hatred toward the paralyzed limbs (misoplegia), usually couched in grotesque, exaggerated, or sarcastic language.[14] (See Chaps. 22 and 28.) All these patterns of behavior are reported here in some detail because they are surprising and paradoxical and represent the emotional disturbances more frequently observed in patients with right brain damage. Gainotti noticed that they are, in any case, much more abnormal and less psychologically appropriate than the catastrophic reactions of left-brain-damaged patients. He therefore proposed that the difference between the emotional behavior of left- and right-brain-damaged patients could be better explained by the contrast between "appropriate" and "inap-

propriate" forms of emotional reaction than by the opposition between depression and euphoria. According to this interpretation, the right hemisphere might play a critical role in emotions and affects. When this hemisphere is intact (as in left-brain-damaged patients), the emotional reaction may be dramatic but psychologically appropriate. When, on the contrary, the lesion impinges upon right hemispheric structures crucially involved in emotional behavior, a composite set of abnormal emotional responses (grouped for the sake of simplicity under the heading of indifference reactions) would usually ensue.

COMPREHENSION AND EXPRESSION OF EMOTIONS IN RIGHT- AND LEFT-BRAIN-DAMAGED PATIENTS

Since the exact nature of the emotional modifications observed after right and left brain injury remained controversial, a large series of investigations were undertaken to clarify this issue by means of experiments with both normal subjects and patients with unilateral hemispheric damage. Although these investigations have explored various aspects of the emotional behavior, the attention of neuropsychologists has been focused mainly on the most cognitive components of emotions, namely the comprehension of emotional stimuli and the (facial or vocal) expression of emotions. This was partly due to the assumption that the type of information processing typical of the right hemisphere (and characterized by a syncretic and holistic rather than by a sequential and analytical style) may be particularly suited to the treatment of emotional information.[15] Since a critical review of investigations conducted in normal subjects obviously exceeds the scopes of this chapter, it will be limited to giving some details about studies conducted on patients with unilateral brain injury and to summarizing results of research conducted on normal subjects.

The methodology of investigations conducted on patients with focal brain injury has consisted in matching the capacity of right- and left-brain-damaged patients to comprehend and/or express emotions at the facial level or through the tone of voice. Following this research strategy, several authors have shown that right-brain-damaged patients are consistently impaired in recognizing emotions expressed through tone of voice,[16–21] in the identification of facial emotional expressions,[19,22–25] and in the ability to express emotions through facial movements[25–27] or with the prosodic contours of speech.[17,19,28] On the other hand, investigations conducted on normal subjects have allowed a better control of the hypothesis, assuming a different specialization of the right and left hemispheres for negative and positive emotions, respectively. Even if some studies have supported the hypothesis of an interaction between hemisphere and positive or negative emotional valence, most have failed to confirm it (see Refs. 9, 10, and 29 for surveys). On the contrary, the great majority of these investigations have substantially confirmed the hypothesis of a general superiority of the right hemisphere for functions of emotional comprehension and expression.

This fact has led some authors to hypothesize that right hemispheric dominance for emotions may mainly concern the communicative aspects of emotional behavior rather than other, more basic components of emotions. This line of thought has been developed in particular by Ross (Refs. 18, 28, and Chap. 56 in this volume), who has suggested that disorders of nonverbal communication might be the primary defect of right-brain-damaged patients and that emotional disturbances usually observed in these patients may simply be a consequence of their basic inability to comprehend and express emotions. According to this viewpoint, the indifference reaction of right-brain-damaged patients should not be considered as an inappropriate form of emotional behavior but simply the consequence of a basic inability to correctly evaluate emotional signals and to express an otherwise intact emotional experience. Three main objections can be addressed to this interpretation of the indifference reaction of right-brain-damaged patients. The first refers to the heterogeneity of the patterns of behavior grouped under the general heading of "indifference reaction." As we have seen in discussing the clinical aspects of the emo-

tional behavior of right- and left-brain-damaged patients, different behavioral patterns are grouped under this heading. Some of them, namely those considered as indifference proper, could more easily be interpreted as a consequence of a reduced ability to communicate an otherwise intact emotional experience. Other behavioral patterns, however—namely, those considered as manifestations of a verbal disinhibition and, even more, those suggesting an attitude of denial of the disability and of rejection of the paralyzed limbs—are inconsistent with this interpretation and point to a deeper emotional disorder. The second objection refers to the fact that several investigations have failed to confirm a significant difference between right- and left-brain-damaged patients in the capacity to express and comprehend emotional signals. Thus, in research conducted at the expressive level, no difference has been found between right- and left-brain-damaged patients in the facial expressions elicited by positive, neutral, and strongly negative emotional movies;[30] in the ability to produce posed rather than spontaneous facial emotional expressions;[31,32] or in the capacity to express emotions through emotional contours of speech.[33,34]

Analogously, in studies conducted at the receptive level, no difference between right- and left-brain-damaged patients has been found on tasks requiring the identification of facial emotional expressions[10,35] or the recognition of the emotion expressed through the prosodic components of speech.[33,34] All these data suggest that right hemispheric dominance for functions of emotional communication has probably been overemphasized in previous studies and that the emotional indifference of right-brain-damaged patients cannot simply be considered the consequence of a defect of emotional communication.

AUTONOMIC COMPONENTS AND EXPERIENCE OF EMOTIONS IN PATIENTS WITH RIGHT HEMISPHERIC DAMAGE

The third objection that can be raised to the hypothesis considering as apparent the emotional indifference of right-brain-damaged patients consists in the fact that this hypothesis is at variance with results obtained in studies that have investigated the autonomic components of emotions in right- and left-brain-damaged patients. As a matter of fact, if one accepts that the autonomic components of emotion play an important role in the generation (or, in any case, in determining the intensity and duration) of the emotional experience,[36–38] then these components of emotions should be intact in right-brain-damaged patients if their apparent indifference is basically due to an inability to express an otherwise intact emotional experience. This prediction, however, is at variance with results of investigations that have studied the electrodermal responses (or other indices of autonomic activation) in right- and left-brain-damaged patients submitted to presentation of emotional stimuli. Thus several authors have observed in right- but not in left-brain-damaged patients a flattened galvanic skin response to painful stimuli applied to the hand ipsilateral to the damaged hemisphere,[39] to emotion-provoking slides,[40,41] and to emotionally arousing movies.[42] Other authors have observed that right-brain-damaged patients fail to show the normal cardiac deceleration in response to emotional stimuli[42] and during an attention-demanding task.[43] Taken together, these data suggest that the emotional indifference of right-brain-damaged patients is real and might at least in part be due to a reduced capacity to react to emotionally laden stimuli with an appropriate autonomic response. This claim is also supported by an unexpected observation made by Mammucari and coworkers[30] while studying, in right- and left-brain-damaged patients, the facial expression of emotions elicited by the presentation of emotional movies.

These authors noticed that during the presentation of a very unpleasant emotional film, normal subjects and left-brain-damaged patients tended to divert the gaze from the screen, whereas similar avoidance eye movements were not shown by right-brain-damaged patients. The investigators argued that normal subjects and left-brain-damaged patients diverted their gaze from the screen because they were emotionally distressed by the crude scenes of the film, whereas right-brain-damaged patients did not look away from the screen because they were much less emotionally involved. This interpretation is supported by experimental data obtained by Caltagirone and associates[44] studying, in the same subjects, the relationships between modifications of heart rate and presence of the avoidance eye movements. In normal subjects and in left-brain-damaged patients, heart rate deceleration was much greater in subjects who watched the entire film sequence than in those who displayed avoidance eye movements, whereas in right-brain-damaged patients, heart rate changes were very mild, regardless of the presence or absence of avoidance eye movements.

In conclusion, results of investigations conducted in right- and left-brain-damaged patients seem to show that right hemispheric damage disrupts not only the communicative aspects of emotions but also the generation of the autonomic components of the emotional response and therefore the inner experience of emotions. Data consistent with the hypothesis of a leading role of the right hemisphere in the generation of the autonomic components of emotions and of the concomitant emotional experience have also recently been obtained by Wittling and Roscmann[45,46] during lateralized presentation of emotionally laden films to normal subjects. These authors found that both the increase of diastolic and systolic blood pressure and the subjective rating of the intensity of the emotional experience were higher during presentation of the film to the right rather than to the left hemisphere.

THE RELATIONSHIP BETWEEN POSTSTROKE DEPRESSION AND LESION OF LEFT FRONTAL CORTEX

We have seen above that investigations of the communicative aspects of emotions have failed to support the hypothesis of a different specialization of the right and left hemispheres for negative and positive emotions, respectively. In order to circumvent these negative results, some authors have tried to reformulate the original theory in slightly different terms. In particular, Davidson and To-marken[47–49] have proposed that the specialization of the left hemisphere for positive emotions and of the right hemisphere for negative emotions may account only for the expressive but not for the evaluative aspects of emotions. Even if the experimental evidence supporting this theory consists mostly of data obtained with psychophysiologic procedures in normal subjects (see Refs. 49 and 50 for contrasting viewpoints on this subject), a series of anatomoclinical studies conducted by Robinson and coworkers[51–54] on patients with poststroke depression seems consistent with the Davidson's hypothesis. These studies are discussed here in some detail, since they are more relevant to the scope of the present volume. In their papers, Robinson and coworkers have distinguished, on the basis of DMS-III[55] diagnostic criteria, two different types of poststroke depression: a major form, considered as an endogenous (psychotic) depression, and a minor form, considered as a dysthymic (neurotic or reactive) depression. According to these authors, the former is thought to result from interruption of the monoaminergic pathways linking the brainstem to the cerebral cortex and is usually due to left frontal lesions, whereas the latter is thought to be caused by less specific (psychological) mechanisms and shows no relationship with a specific locus of lesion. Now, even if the neurochemical mechanism proposed by Robinson and coworkers cannot be easily reconciled with the hypothesis of a "center for positive emotions" located in the left frontal cortex, the observation that a form of major depression results from injury to the left frontal lobe could be consistent with Davidson's theory.

During the last few years, however, some methodologic and empiric objections have been addressed to the claim that a form of "major" depression is specifically caused by left frontal lesions. From the methodologic point of view, it has been argued that the criteria suggested by DSM-III to make a diagnosis of "major" depression cannot be valid for patients with an organic form of depression. According to this manual, in fact, a diagnosis of major depression can be made if, in addition to a depressed mood, the patient pre-

sents at least five symptoms out of a series of eight that include, among others, sleep disorders, loss of weight and/or appetite, fatigue, apathy, and concentration disorders. The objection that, in a stroke patient, some of these symptoms may be due to the brain injury per se has been tested in a recent study[56] in which the main symptoms of patients classified (on the basis of DSM-III diagnostic criteria) as major depression of vascular and functional origin have been compared. In patients classified as having major poststroke depression, part of the symptomatology seemed due either to the direct effect of the brain damage or to the psychological reaction of the patient to the disabilities and handicaps provoked by the lesion. Furthermore, from the empiric point of view, the assumption of a strong link between left frontal lesions and major poststroke depression has been only partly confirmed by further investigations. In particular, some studies[56–58] have found that patients with anterior lesions are more depressed than those with posterior lesions but also that this is true irrespectively of the hemispheric side of injury. These findings can, perhaps, be reconciled with Robinson's hypothesis, assuming that the poststroke depression may be due to a disruption of pathways providing the monoaminergic input to the neocortex. They are, however, clearly inconsistent with Davidson's theory, assuming a different lateralization of structures subserving the expression of positive and negative emotions at the level of the left and right frontal lobes.

Also inconsistent with this theory are the results of studies, in right- and left-brain-damaged patients, of expressive facial responses to positive and negative emotional stimuli. In these experiments, some authors (e.g., Refs. 25, 26, and 27) have found that right-brain-damaged patients are significantly less expressive than left-brain-damaged patients or normal controls. Other authors (e.g., Ref. 30) have failed to observe significant differences between the two groups in the tendency to produce a facial expression congruent with the emotional stimulus. In no case, however, was there an interaction between hemispheric side of lesion and tendency to produce a particular emotional response. Furthermore, a trend in the direction opposite to the theory was found in a study in which a difference was observed between right- and left-brain-damaged patients in the expression of various kinds of emotions. In this study,[27] right-brain-damaged patients produced significantly less smiles and laughs and nonsignificantly more cries than patients with a left hemispheric injury.

CONCLUDING REMARKS

Taken together, results of investigations conducted in patients with unilateral brain damage and in normal subjects seem more consistent with the hypothesis assuming a general dominance of the right hemisphere for various aspects of emotional behavior than with the alternative hypothesis assuming a different specialization of the right and left hemispheres for opposite aspects of the mood. It is also possible that the difference between the right and left hemispheres in the regulation of emotions may be qualitative rather than simply quantitative and that the two sides of the brain may play complementary roles in emotional behavior. The author has, in fact, hypothesized elsewhere[50] that the right hemisphere might be involved mainly in the more basic and automatic aspects of emotions (namely in the generation of the autonomic components of the emotional response, in the correlative subjective experience, and in the spontaneous expression of emotions), whereas the left hemisphere might play a more important role in control functions, particularly in the intentional control of the emotional expressive apparatus.

Obviously, this is not the place to dwell upon this rather speculative issue. However, it is worthwhile to stress the fact that emotions are based on a highly complex and articulated system, which can be fractionated according to different criteria. Two of these criteria, namely the emotional valence (i.e., the positive or negative polarity of the emotional experience) and the functional subcomponents of the emotional system (i.e., communicative aspects, autonomic response, and subjective experience of emotions) have been taken into ac-

count in the present survey. Other criteria, however—such as, for example, the automatic or controlled level of the emotional behavior—could be relevant to the problem of the relationships between emotions and hemispheric specialization.

REFERENCES

1. Broca P: Sur la faculté du langage articulé. *Bull Soc Antropol* 6:377–393, 1865.
2. Dax M: Lésions de la moité gauche de l'encéphale coincidant avec l'oubli des signes de la pensée. *Gaz Hebd Med Chir* 2:259–260, 1865.
3. Hécaen H: Clinical symptomatology in right and left hemisphere lesions, in Mountcastle VB (ed): *Interhemispheric Relations and Cerebral Dominance.* Baltimore: Johns Hopkins Press, 1962, pp 215–243.
4. Terzian H, Cecotto C: Determinazione e studio della dominanza emisferica mediante iniezione intracarotide di Amytal sodico nell'uomo: I. Modificazioni cliniche. *Boll Soc Ital Biol Sper* 35:1623–1626, 1959.
5. Alema G, Donini G: Sulle modificazioni cliniche ed elettroencefalografiche da introduzione intracarotidea di isoetil-barbiturato di sodio nell'uomo. *Boll Soc Ital Biol Sper* 36:900–904, 1960.
6. Perria L, Rosadini G, Rossi GF: Determination of side of cerebral dominance with amoarbital. *Arch Neurol* 4:173–181, 1961.
7. Gainotti G: Réaction "catastrophiques" et manifestations d'indifférence au cours des atteintes cérébrales. *Neuropsychologia* 7:195–204, 1969.
8. Gainotti G: Emotional behavior and hemispheric side of the lesion. *Cortex* 8:41–55, 1972.
9. Gainotti G: Disorders of emotional behavior and of autonomic arousal resulting from unilateral brain damage, in Ottoson D (ed): *The Dual Brain.* London: Macmillan, 1987, pp 161–179.
10. Gainotti G: The meaning of emotional disturbances resulting from unilateral brain injury, in Gainotti G, Caltagirone C (eds): *Emotions and the Dual Brain.* Heidelberg: Springer-Verlag, 1989, pp 147–167.
11. Gestmann J: Problem of imperception of disease and of impaired body territories with organic lesions: Relation to body scheme and its disorders. *Arch Neurol Psychiatry* 48:890–913, 1942.
12. Nathanson M, Bergman PS, Gordon GG: Denial of illness: Its occurrence in one hundred consecutive

cases of hemiplegia. *Arch Neurol Psychiatry* 68:380–387, 1952.

13. Gainotti G: Confabulations of denial in senile dementia. *Psychiatr Clin* 8:99–108, 1975.

14. Critchley M: Personification of paralysed limbs in hemiplegics. *Br Med J* 30:284–286, 1955.

15. Tucker DM: Neural substrates of thought and affective disorders, in Gainotti G, Caltagirone C (eds): *Emotions and the Dual Brain.* Heidelberg: Springer-Verlag, 1989, pp 225–234.

16. Heilman KM, Scholes R, Watson RT: Auditory affective agnosia. *J Neurol Neurosurg Psychiatry* 38:69–72, 1975.

17. Tucker DM, Watson RT, Heilman KM: Discrimination and evocation of affectively intoned speech in patients with right parietal disease. *Neurology* 27:947–950, 1977.

18. Ross ED: The aprosodias. *Arch Neurol* 38:561–569, 1981.

19. Benowitz LI, Bear DM, Rosenthal R, et al: Hemispheric specialization in nonverbal communication. *Cortex* 19:5–11, 1983.

20. Heilman KM, Bowers D, Speedie L, Coslett HB: Comprehension of affective and nonaffective prosody. *Neurology* 34:917–921, 1984.

21. Blonder LX, Bowers D, Heilman KM: The role of the right hemisphere in emotional communication. *Brain* 114:1115–1127, 1991.

22. Cicone M, Wapner W, Gardner H: Sensitivity to emotional expressions and situations in organic patients. *Cortex* 16:145–158, 1980.

23. DeKosky S, Heilman KM, Bowers D, Valenstein E: Recognition and discrimination of emotional faces and pictures. *Brain Lang* 9:206–214, 1980.

24. Bowers D, Bauer RM, Coslett HB, Heilman KM: Processing of faces by patients with unilateral hemisphere lesions: Dissociation between judgments of facial affect and facial identity. *Brain Cogn* 4:258–272, 1985.

25. Borod JC, Koff E, Perlman-Lorch M, Nicholas M: The expression and perception of facial emotion in brain-damaged patients. *Neuropsychologia* 24:169–180, 1986.

26. Buck R, Duffy RJ: Nonverbal communication of affect in brain-damaged patients. *Cortex* 16:351–362, 1980.

27. Blonder LX, Burns A, Bowers D, et al: Right hemisphere facial expressivity during natural conversation. *Brain Cogn* 21:44–56, 1993.

28. Ross ED: Right hemisphere's role in language, affective behavior, and emotion. *Trends Neurosci* 7:342–346, 1984.

29. Etcoff NL: Recognition of emotions in patients with unilateral brain damage, in Gainotti G, Caltagirone C (eds): *Emotions and the Dual Brain.* Heidelberg: Springer-Verlag, 1989, pp 168–186.

30. Mammucari A, Caltagirone C, Ekman P, et al: Spontaneous facial expression of emotions in brain-damaged patients. *Cortex* 24:521–533, 1988.

31. Caltagirone C, Ekman P, Friesen W, et al: Posed emotional expression in unilateral brain damaged patients. *Cortex* 25:653–663, 1989.

32. Weddel RA, Miller DJ, Trevarthen C: Voluntary emotional facial expression in patients with focal cerebral lesions. *Neuropsychologia* 28:43–60, 1990.

33. Bradvik B, Dravins C, Holtas S, et al: Do single right hemisphere infarcts or transient ischemic attacks result in aprosody? *Acta Neurol Scand* 81:61–70, 1990.

34. Cancelliere AEB, Kertesz A: Lesion localization in acquired deficits of emotional expression and comprehension. *Brain Cogn* 13:133–147, 1990.

35. Weddel RA: Recognition memory for emotional facial expressions in patients with focal cerebral lesions. *Brain Cogn* 11:1–17, 1989.

36. Hohmann G: Some effects of spinal cord lesions on experimental emotional feelings. *Psychophysiology* 3:143–156, 1966.

37. Schachter S: Cognition and peripheralist-centralist controversies in motivation and emotion, in Gazzaniga MS, Blakmore C (eds): *Handbook of Psychobiology.* New York: Academic Press, pp 529–564, 1975.

38. Le Doux JE: Cognitive-emotional interactions in brain. *Cogn Emotion* 3:267–289, 1989.

39. Heilman KM, Schwartz H, Watson RT: Hypoarousal in patients with the neglect syndrome and emotional indifference. *Neurology* 28:229–232, 1978.

40. Morrow L, Vrtunsky PB, Kim Y, Boller F: Arousal responses to emotional stimuli and laterality of lesion. *Neuropsychologia* 20:77–81, 1982.

41. Zoccolotti P, Scabini D, Violani V: Electrodermal responses in patients with unilateral brain damage. *J Clin Neuropsychol* 4:143–150, 1982.

42. Zoccolotti P, Caltagirone C, Benedetti N, Gainotti G: Perturbation des réponses végétatives aux stimuli émotionnels au cours des lésions hémisphériques unilatérales. *Encéphale* 12:263–268, 1986.

43. Yokoyama K, Jennings R, Ackles P, et al: Lack of heart rate changes during an attention demanding

task after right hemisphere lesions. *Neurology* 37:624–630, 1987.

44. Caltagirone C, Zoccolotti P, Originale G, et al: Autonomic reactivity and facial expression of emotions in brain-damaged patients, in Gainotti G, Caltagirone C (eds): *Emotions and the Dual Brain.* Heidelberg: Springer-Verlag, 1989, pp 204–221.

45. Wittling W: Psychophysiological correlates of human brain asymmetry: Blood pressure changes during lateralized presentation of an emotionally laden film. *Neuropsychologia* 28:457–470, 1990.

46. Wittling W, Roscmann R: Emotion-related hemisphere asymmetry: Subjective emotional response to laterally presented films. *Cortex* 29:431–448, 1993.

47. Davidson RJ: Hemispheric specialization for cognition and affect, in Gale A, Edwards J (eds): *Physiological Correlates of Human Behavior.* London: Academic Press, 1985.

48. Davidson RJ, Tomarken AJ: Laterality and emotions: An electrophysiological approach, in Boller F, Grafman J (eds): *Handbook of Neuropsychology.* North Holland: Elsevier, 1989, vol 3, pp 419–441.

49. Davidson RJ: Cerebral asymmetry and emotion: Conceptual and methodological conundrums. *Cogn Emotion* 7:115–138, 1993.

50. Gainotti G, Caltagirone C, Zoccolotti P: Left/right and cortical/subcortical dichotomies in the neuropsychological study of human emotions. *Cogn Emotion* 7:71–93, 1993.

51. Robinson RG, Kubos KL, Starr LB, et al: Mood changes in stroke patients: Relationship to lesion location. *Comp Psychiatry* 24:555–566, 1983.

52. Robinson RG, Kubos KL, Starr LB, et al: Mood disorders in stroke patients: Importance of location of lesion. *Brain* 107:81–93, 1984.

53. Starkstein SE, Robinson RG, Price TR: Comparison of patients with and without poststroke major depression matched for size and location of lesion. *Arch Gen Psychiatry* 45:247–252, 1988.

54. Starkstein SE, Robinson RG: Affective disorders and cerebrovascular disease. *Br J Psychiatry* 154:170–182, 1989.

55. American Psychiatric Association: *Diagnostic and Statistical Manual of Mental Disorders,* 3d ed (DSM-III). Washington, DC: American Psychiatric Press, 1980.

56. Gainotti G, Azzoni A, Lanzillotta M, et al: Some preliminary findings on a new scale for the assessment of depression and related symptoms in stroke patients. *Ital J Neurol Sci* 16:439–451, 1995.

57. Sinyor D, Jacques P, Kaloupek DG, et al: Poststroke depression and lesion location: An attempted replication. *Brain* 109:537–546, 1986.

58. House A, Dennis M, Warlow C, et al: Mood disorders after stroke and their relation to lesion location. *Brain* 113:1113–1129, 1990.

Chapter 56

THE APROSODIAS

Elliott D. Ross

As a result of the fundamental discoveries of Broca[1] and Wernicke[2] that focal lesions in the left hemisphere cause spectacular deficits in the verbal aspects of language, clinical studies of human communication have, for the most part, focused on the aphasias. These studies have led to the widely held belief that language is a dominant function of the left hemisphere, with the right hemisphere being relegated to a "minor" or "nondominant" role in language and behavior.[3,4] Over the last two decades, however, considerable evidence has accrued to support the thesis that communication functions are distributed between the hemispheres.[5—33] The left is primarily concerned with processing the verbal, syntactic, and other language-related functions such as pantomime, pragmatics, denotation, and the linguistic and dialectal aspects of prosody, while the right is primarily concerned with processing affective prosody, gestures, and certain word-related functions such as connotation, thematic inference, and comprehension of nonliteral phrases and complex linguistic relations. In addition, both focal cerebral blood flow[34] and positron emission tomography (PET)[7,35,36] scanning studies have established an active role for the right hemisphere in language, even though three of the four studies were designed primarily to assess linguistic processes. The most intensively analyzed right hemispheric function has been affective prosody and gestures.

ELEMENTS OF LANGUAGE AND COMMUNICATION

Language and communication are characterized by four major constituents: the lexicon (vocabulary), syntax (grammar), prosody, and kinesics. The segment is the smallest articulated feature of a language, which, in nontechnical terms, is most closely allied with the syllable.[37,38] Segments, therefore, might be thought of as the primary building blocks for creating the words that form the lexicon. Words, in turn, are concatenated into grammatical relationships to form phrases, sentences, and discourse. It is the segmentally related or verbal-propositional features of language that are primarily disrupted by focal left-brain injury, thus causing aphasic syndromes.

Prosody is a nonverbal or suprasegmental feature of language that conveys various levels of information to the listener, including linguistic, affective (attitudinal and emotional), dialectical, and idiosyncratic data.[27,38–41] The acoustical features underlying prosody include pitch, intonation, melody, cadence, loudness, timbre, tempo, stress, accent, and pauses. Although the preeminence of the propositional aspects of language is well accepted, developmental studies have established that the earliest building blocks of language are prosodic-intonational rather than verbal-segmental features.[42,43] As children acquire the verbal-segmental features of language, prosodic phenomena eventually become embedded and carried by the articulatory line.

Kinesics refers to the limb, body, and facial movements associated with language and communication.[44] Movements that are used for semiotic purposes, such as the "V for victory" sign, are classified as pantomime, since they convey specific semantic information, whereas movements used to color, emphasize, and embellish speech are classified as gestures.[44,45] Most spontaneous kinesic activity associated with discourse usually blends gestures and pantomime into a single movement.

Neurology of Prosody

The first in-depth inquiry into the neurology of prosody was initiated by Monrad-Krohn.[40,46] During World War II, he cared for a native Norwegian woman who sustained a shrapnel wound to the left frontal area, causing an acute Broca aphasia. The woman made an excellent recovery except for a lingering accent, which caused her great emotional distress during the Nazi occupation, since she was consistently mistaken for being German and was, consequently, socially ostracized. Her speech was reported to have preserved melody, as evidenced by her ability to sing, intone, and emote. The acquired foreign accent was due to inappropriate application of stresses and pauses to the articulatory line.

On the basis of this patient and others, Monrad-Krohn[40] divided prosody into four basic components, as indicated by the italicized words. *Intrinsic* (linguistic) prosody provides the means for using nonverbal features to enhance the linguistic functions of a language, for example, raising the intonation at the end of a statement to indicate a question, changing the stress and timing on certain segments of a phrase to clarify meaning—i.e., "the *red*coats (British regulars) are coming" versus "the red coats (red-colored coats) are coming"—or changing the stress on certain words and altering the pause structure to clarify potentially ambiguous syntax—i.e., "The *man* . . . and woman dressed in black . . . came to visit" (only the woman was dressed in black) versus "The man and woman dressed in *black* . . . came to visit"

(both were dressed in black).[27,39,41] Dialectal and idiosyncratic prosody are also to some degree subsumed by the term *intrinsic prosody,* since they involve regional and individual differences in speech quality. *Intellectual* prosody imparts attitudinal information to discourse that may drastically alter meaning. For example, if the sentence "He is clever" is emphatically stressed on *is,* it becomes a resounding acknowledgment of the person's ability, whereas if the emphatic stress resides on *clever* with a terminal rise in intonation, sarcasm becomes apparent. *Emotional* prosody injects primary types of emotions into speech, such as happiness, sadness, fear, and anger. The term *affective prosody* refers to the combination of attitudinal and emotional prosody. *Inarticulate* prosody is the use of certain paralinguistic nonverbal elements, such as grunts and sighs, to embellish discourse.

Monrad-Krohn[40] also described various clinical disorders of prosody. *Dysprosody* is a change in voice quality that gives rise to a foreign-accent syndrome. Since it is encountered primarily in patients with fairly good recovery from motor types of aphasia, it is associated with left hemispheric lesions that alter the patient's dialectal and idiosyncratic aspects of prosody. *Aprosody* is the general lack of prosody encountered in Parkinson disease as part of the akinesia, masked facies, and soft monotone voice. *Hyperprosody* refers to the excessive use of prosody observed in mania or in patients with Broca aphasia who have very few words at their disposal but use them to their utmost to convey attitudes and emotions. Although Monrad-Krohn did not describe prosodic disorders from focal right brain damage, he did predict that disorders of prosodic comprehension should also be encountered in brain-damaged patients.

Recent clinical studies have shown that focal right brain damage may seriously impair, in various combinations, the production, comprehension, and repetition of the affective-prosodic elements of language without disrupting its propositional elements (see below).[4–6,8,9,12,13,15,18–21,23–26,31,33] These affective-prosodic components, coupled with gestures, impart a vitality to discourse that, in many instances, makes them far more important than the verbal-linguistic message. Various studies have shown that if a statement contains an affective-prosodic message that is at variance with its verbal-linguistic meaning, then the prosodic message normally takes precedence in adults and to a lesser degree in children.[8,47-49] For example, if the sentence "I had a really great day" is spoken using irony, it will be understood as communicating a meaning that is actually opposite to its linguistic content.

Neurology of Kinesics

Disturbances in the production and comprehension of pantomimal kinesics have been firmly linked to left brain damage.[50,51] Goodglass and Kaplan[52] proposed that pantomimal disorders in aphasics with significant comprehension deficits can be attributed to their general inability to comprehend symbols, whereas pantomimal disorders in aphasics without significant comprehension deficits can be attributed to ideomotor apraxia. Other investigators, however, have not shown such tight correlation of a specific pantomimal disturbance with a specific linguistic disturbance,[53-55] although all studies to date have found that disorders of pantomime are almost always due to left hemispheric damage resulting in aphasic disturbances.[52-56]

Gestural kinesics, on the other hand, has not been well studied neurologically, although occasionally clinical researchers have mentioned that gestural activity may be preserved in aphasic patients.[44,45] The first paper to specifically address the possible relationship of gestures to right brain damage and loss of affective prosody was published in 1979 by Ross and Mesulam.[4] They observed that lesions of the right frontal operculum may cause complete loss of spontaneous gestural activity in the nonparalyzed right face and limbs without any disturbance in praxis. The suggestion was made, therefore, that the gestural behavior as opposed to pantomime was a dominant function of the right hemisphere. Since then a number of studies have lent further support to this hypothesis by showing that the right hemisphere is specialized not only for producing gestures but also for comprehending their meaning.[5,18,23,57-60]

THE APROSODIAS

Although Hughlings-Jackson[45] suggested over a hundred years ago that the right hemisphere may have a dominant role in emotional communication, the first clinical study of affective prosody was published in 1975 by Heilman and coworkers.[20] They assessed the ability of patients with right and left hemispheric strokes in the posterior sylvian distribution to recognize the affective content of verbally neutral statements that were spoken with various emotional intonations. Right-brain-damaged patients were markedly impaired on the task as compared with normals and mildly aphasic left-brain-damaged patients. In a follow-up study, Tucker and colleagues[26] found that right-but not left-brain-damaged patients also had great difficulty in inserting affective variation into verbally neutral sentences on request and on a repetition task.

In 1979, Ross and Mesulam[4] described two patients with infarctions of the right anterior suprasylvian region verified by computed tomography (CT). Neither patient was aphasic or apraxic, but both complained bitterly of their almost total inability to insert affective variation into their speech and gestural behavior. Neither patient seemed to have difficulty in perceiving affective displays in others, and both insisted that they could feel and experience emotions inwardly. Based on these patients and the previous publications by Heilman and associates,[20,26] it was hypothesized that (1) the right hemisphere was dominant for organizing the affective-prosodic components of language and gestural behavior and (2) the functional/anatomic organization of affective language in the right hemisphere was analogous to the organization of propositional language in the left hemisphere. An issue not resolved in the paper, however, was whether the prosodic deficits from right brain damage also involved the linguistic aspects of prosody. Subsequent studies by Weintraub and colleagues,[31] Heilman and coworkers,[19] and Danly and associates[61-62] have looked more carefully at this issue in both right- and left-brain-damaged patients. The composite data indicate that the linguistic features of prosody may be impaired by either right or left brain damage but that the affective components seem to be disrupted exclusively by right brain damage.

In 1981, Ross[23] approached the issue of whether the anatomic organization of affective language in the right hemisphere was, in fact, similar to the organization of propositional language in the left hemisphere. Ten patients with focal right brain damage, localized by CT scan, underwent a bedside assessment, similar to that utilized for propositional language, of their ability to modulate affective prosody and gestures. Thus, the patients were examined qualitatively for (1) spontaneous use of affective prosody and gesturing during conversation, (2) ability to repeat verbally neutral sentences with affective variation, (3) abil-

ity to auditorily comprehend affective prosody, and (4) ability to visually comprehend gestures. All patients who had lesions bordering the right sylvian fissure had some disorder of affective language. Because specific combinations of affective-prosodic deficits occurred following circumscribed lesions in the right hemisphere that were analogous to the functional-anatomic clustering of aphasic deficits observed after focal left brain damage,[3] these particular syndromes were called *aprosodias,* and the same modifiers were applied for classification purposes as those used in the aphasias (Fig. 56-1, Table 56-1).[23] In a follow-up study, using blinded evaluations of affective language, Gorelick and Ross[18] corroborated that patients with focal right brain lesions display various deficits

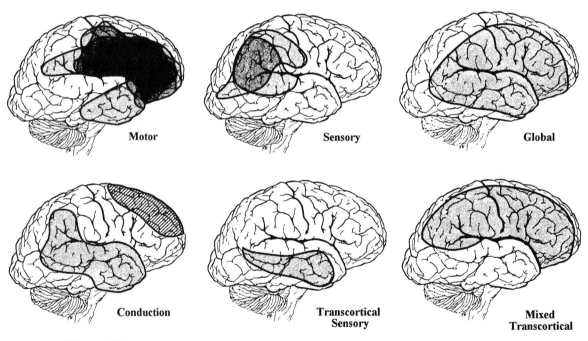

Figure 56-1

Composite cortical distribution of published CT scan lesions associated with various aprosodias[18,23] projected onto a lateral template of the right hemisphere. Stippled areas represent ischemic infarctions except for the patient with transcortical sensory aprosodia, who had a discrete hemorrhage without edema. Although the stippled lesion should have produced sensory rather than conduction aprosodia, an analogous lesion in the left hemisphere may occasionally cause conduction rather than Wernicke (sensory) aphasia.[3,94,95] The patient represented by the hatched-marked lesion had a mild conduction aprosodia that evolved from an initial motor-type aprosodia.[23]

Table 56-1

The aprosodias

Type of aprosodia[a]	Spontaneous affective prosody and gesturing	Affective prosodic repetition	Affective prosodic comprehension	Comprehension of emotional gesturing
Motor	Poor	Poor	Good	Good
Sensory	Good	Poor	Poor	Poor
Global	Poor	Poor	Poor	Poor
Conduction	Good	Poor	Good	Good
Transcortical motor	Poor	Good	Good	Good
Transcortical sensory	Good	Good	Poor	Poor
Mixed transcortical	Poor	Good	Poor	Poor
"Agestic"[a]	(Good)	(Good)	(Good)	(Poor)

[a]"Agestic" aprosodia (agnosia for gestures with otherwise intact processing of affective prosody), akin to anomic aphasia[3] (anomia accompanied by alexia and agraphia), has not yet been described in the literature; however, a patient reported by Bowers and Heilman[93] may have had this syndrome; motor, sensory, global, and transcortical sensory aprosodias have good anatomic correlation with lesions in the left hemisphere known to cause analogous aphasias (see Fig. 56-1).

in affective language that corresponded with the aprosodic classifications and localizations published previously. They also reported that the prevalence of aprosodia following right brain damage was equal to the prevalence of aphasia following left brain damage, thus underscoring that the aprosodias are common rather than esoteric syndromes.

Quantitative acoustic and neuropsychological testing paradigms exist for assessing affective prosody and communication;[22,24,25] however, with some practice and familiarization, clinicians can readily incorporated an assessment of aprosodia into their bedside neurologic examination, similar to the techniques used to assess patients for aphasia.

Spontaneous Affective Prosody and Gesturing During the interview, observations are made as to whether the patient gestures and imparts affect into his or her spontaneous conversation, especially when asked emotionally loaded questions about the current illness or about past emotional experiences. Overall loudness or softness of speech should be ignored, with attention paid to intonational variation in voice and gesturing to

determine whether emotional information appropriate to the situation under discussion is incorporated into the patient's discourse.

Repetition of Affective Prosody A declarative sentence, void of emotional words, is used to test affective repetition. After producing a token sentence—using, for example, a happy, sad, tearful, disinterested, angry, or surprised tone of voice—the examiner immediately asks the patient to repeat the sentence. Repetition should be judged on how well the patient imitates the affective prosody of the examiner; if the patient raises or lowers the overall loudness of voice, slightly raises the voice at the end of a statement to indicate a question rather than surprise, or produces an incorrect emotion, the response should not be considered correct.

Comprehension of Affective Prosody A declarative statement, void of emotional words, is used. The examiner injects the sentence with different affects and asks the patient either to identify the emotion verbally or choose the correct answer from a verbal list of five choices. By standing behind the patient during this assessment, the examiner avoids giving the patient visual clues through gestural behaviors.

Comprehension of Gestures This is accomplished by standing in front of the patient and conveying a particular affective state using only gestural activity involving the face and limbs. As with affective-prosodic comprehension, the patient is requested either to identify the emotion verbally or, if necessary, choose the correct answer from a verbal list of five choices.

Using the bedside evaluation outlined above, aprosodias may be identified and subtyped as shown in Table 56-1. Computed tomography correlates of aprosodias involving a predominantly corticosubcortical distribution are presented in Fig. 56-1. For detailed clinical descriptions of the aprosodias, Refs. 18, 23, and 33 should be consulted.

To date, the aprosodias appear to have a functional-anatomic organization in the right hemisphere analogous to the aphasias in the left hemisphere. In addition, some of the recovery patterns observed in patients with aprosodia[23] are similar to those described with aphasias,[3,63] and subcortical lesions in the right hemisphere may produce aprosodias,[18,23,33,64] just as subcortical lesions in the left hemisphere may produce aphasias.[65–67] There have also been case reports of crossed aprosodia, in which a strongly right-handed patient becomes aprosodic but not aphasic following a left hemispheric stroke, similar to cases of crossed aphasia in which a strongly right-handed patient becomes aphasic following a right hemispheric stroke.[68] Last, acquired aprosodias in children[69] and developmental disorders of affective prosody associated with aberrant psychosocial development resulting from early right brain damage[70–72] have been reported that are comparable with the syndromes of acquired aphasia in children and developmental dyslexia.

Hemispheric Lateralization of Affective Prosody

The terms *dominant* and *lateralized* brain function are used interchangeably in the literature, even though they have overlapping but somewhat different neurologic implications. A brain function is considered dominant if a unilateral lesion produces a behavioral deficit that subtends both sides of space.[73,74] a criterion easily met by the various aphasic and aprosodic syndromes. For a function to be strongly lateralized, however, it must also be shown that the behavioral deficit does not occur following lesions of the opposite hemisphere. In this regard, it is of historic interest that, soon after his initial discovery that damage to the foot of the left third frontal convolution caused loss of articulate speech,[1] Broca[75] reported that right hemispheric lesions did not result in the loss of articulate speech, thus establishing that articulation was both a dominant and highly lateralized function of the left hemisphere.[76] Unlike the aphasias, however, the degree of lateralization of affective prosody has not been established, since various publications have documented affective-prosodic disturbances in aphasic patients with left hemispheric strokes (see Chap. 55). In some instances, authors have assumed incorrectly that all prosodic systems—intrinsic, affective, idiolectal, and dialectal—rather than just affective prosody, are modulated by the right hemisphere.[77,78] Nevertheless, certain publications[79–82] have reported considerable disturbances in the production and comprehension of affective prosody in left-brain-damaged patients with severe aphasias, suggesting that affective prosody may not be strongly lateralized to the right hemisphere even though it appears to be a dominant function of the right hemisphere.

De Bleser and Poeck[79] examined prosodic intonation in severe global aphasics whose speech output was restricted to one or two recurring syllables. Their intonations tended to be very stereotypic, bringing into question the original observations by Hughlings-Jackson[45] that severely aphasic patients are able to communicate through emotional channels. Schlanger and coworkers[80] reported affective-prosodic comprehension deficits in aphasics in opposition to the original studies by Heilman and associates.[20] A review of the data published by both groups suggests that the discrepancy is most likely attributable to the distribution and severity of aphasic deficits; Heilman and associates[20] used patients with relatively preserved comprehension, whereas Schlanger and coworkers[80] used patients with significant deficits in verbal comprehension. More importantly, however, when Schlanger and colleagues[80] sorted their patients into "low-verbal" and "high-verbal" groups, the low-verbal aphasics were significantly more impaired on the emotional comprehension task than the high-verbal aphasics. Similarly, Seron and coworkers[81] have also reported a significant positive correlation between scores of affective performance and verbal comprehension in aphasic patients. This would suggest, therefore, that verbal impairments per se rather than a primary defect in affective processing underlie deficient performance on affective comprehension tasks in aphasic patients.

To address this issue further, Ross and colleagues[82] assessed affective prosody in a series of right-brain-damaged and left-brain-damaged patients using a quantitative testing paradigm in which the verbal-articulatory demands were progressively reduced by using token sentences in which various emotions are carried by words, a repeated monosyllable ("ba ba ba ba ba ba"), and an asyllabic articulation ("aaaaaahhhhhhh"). In the left-brain-damaged patients, reducing the verbal-articulatory load caused statistically robust improvement in their ability to comprehend and produce affective prosody on a repetition task, whereas no improvement occurred in the right-brain-damaged patients. Interestingly, the performance of left-brain-damaged patients was not correlated to the presence, severity, or type of aphasic deficit(s). Based on functional-anatomic correlations for both spontaneous affective prosody and affective-prosodic repetition, deep white matter lesions located below the supplementary motor area that disrupt interhemispheric connections coursing through the mid-rostral corpus callosum seem to contribute to affective-prosodic deficits that are both additive and independent of any aphasic deficits. These findings, therefore, sustain the hypothesis that affective prosody is both a dominant and a lateralized function of the right hemisphere and lend strong support to research

by Blonder and coworkers[6] and Bowers and associates[8,9] suggesting loss of affective-communicative representations caused by right brain damage as the theoretical basis for the aprosodias, similar to loss of verbal-syntactic representations caused by left brain damage as the theoretical basis for the aphasias.[82]

Neurology of Emotions

The aprosodias represent disturbances of graded emotional behavior encompassing both affective prosody and gestures. These behaviors are organized predominantly at the level of the neocortex as part of the language-related systems of communication. Since the experiential and display aspects of emotions are available to patients with aprosodia,[23,83,84] seemingly paradoxical behaviors may occur during clinical and social interactions. The most dramatic examples reported to date are patients with motor types of aprosodia who are also experiencing severe depression. Because of their aprosodia, they exhibit a flat affective demeanor even when they are discussing highly emotional issues, such as suicide.[83,84] Consequently, their verbal reports of emotional distress can easily be discounted by both clinicians and family. Other patients may verbally deny depression but have vegetative indicators of melancholia that respond readily to antidepressant treatment. Current evidence has implicated the temporal limbic system, in particular the amygdala, as the nodal point of a neuroanatomic network for experiencing emotions and related phenomena.[85–89] Patients with motor or global aprosodia may also be observed to display extremes of emotion during very sad, happy, or angry situations despite their otherwise affectively flat demeanor.[18,23,83,84] The displays tend to be all or none, uncontrollable, and socially embarrassing, giving them the quality of pathologic regulation of affect, similar to behaviors encountered in patients with pseudobulbar palsy.[3,90,91] Thus, the organization of emotional displays must also be modulated by areas outside the right neocortical motor system. The critical areas seem to reside in the temporal limbic system and basal forebrain, which have descending connections to alpha motor neurons through the hypothalamus, periaqueductal gray, locus ceruleus, subceruleus, and the median raphe,[84,92] since lesions and epileptic discharges in these regions are known to induce sham emotional displays that usually take the form of pathologic regulation of affect.[90] For a more complete review of the neurology of emotions, the reader is referred to Chap. 54 by LaBar and LeDoux and Chap. 55 by Gainotti in this book and a recent article by Ross and coworkers[88] addressing the differential hemispheric lateralization of emotions and related behaviors based on the concept that emotions may be classified as having either primary or social properties.

ACKNOWLEDGMENTS

This work was supported in part by grants from the Neuropsychiatric Research Institute, Fargo, ND; the Merit Review Board, Department of Veterans Affairs, Washington, DC; and the EJLB Foundation, Montreal, Canada.

REFERENCES

1. Broca P: Remarques sur le siege de la faculte du langage articule, suives d'une observation d'aphemie. *Bull Soc Anthropol Paris* 6:330–337, 1861.
2. Wernicke C: *Der aphasische Symptomencomplex: Eine psychologische Studie auf anatomischer Basis.* Breslau: Cohn & Weigert, 1874. (Translated in Eggert GH: *Wernicke's Works on Aphasia: Sourcebook and Review.* The Hague: Mouton, 1977.)
3. Benson DF: *Aphasia, Alexia and Agraphia.* Edinburgh: Churchill Livingstone, 1979.
4. Ross ED, Mesulam MM: Dominant language functions of the right hemisphere? Prosody and emotional gesturing. *Arch Neurol* 36:144–148, 1979.
5. Benowitz LI, Bear DM, Rosenthal R, et al: Hemispheric specialization in nonverbal communication. *Cortex* 19:5–14, 1983.
6. Blonder LX, Bowers D, Heilman KM: The role of the right hemisphere in emotional communication. *Brain* 114:1115–1127, 1991.
7. Bottini G, Corcoran R, Sterzi R, et al: The role of the right hemisphere in the interpretation of figurative aspects of language: A positron emission tomography activation study. *Brain* 117:1241–1253, 1994.
8. Bowers D, Coslett HB, Bauer RM, et al: Comprehension of emotional prosody following unilateral hemispheric lesions: Processing defect versus distraction defect. *Neuropsychologia* 25:317–328, 1987.
9. Bowers D, Bauer RM, Heilman KM: The nonverbal affect lexicon: Theoretical perspectives from neuropsychological studies of affect perception. *Neuropsychology* 7:433–444, 1993.
10. Brownell HH, Potter HH, Bihrle A: Inference deficits in right brain-damaged patients. *Brain Lang* 29:310–321, 1986.
11. Brownell HH, Potter HH, Michelow D, Gardner H: Sensitivity to lexical denotation and connotation in brain-damaged patients: A double dissociation? *Brain Lang* 22:253–265, 1984.
12. Darby DG: Sensory aprosodia: A clinical clue to lesions of the inferior division of the right middle cerebral artery? *Neurology* 34:567–572, 1993.
13. Denes G, Caldognetto EM, Semenza C, et al: Discrimination and identification of emotions in human voice by brain damaged subjects. *Acta Neurol Scand* 69:154–162, 1984.
14. Edmondson JA, Ross ED, Chan JL, Seibert GB: The effect of right-brain damage on acoustical measures of affective prosody in Taiwanese patients. *J Phonet* 15:219–233, 1987.
15. Ehlers L, Dalby M: Appreciation of emotional expressions in the visual and auditory modality in normal and brain-damaged patients. *Acta Neurol Scand* 76:251–256, 1987.
16. Emmorey K: The neurologic substrates for the prosodic aspects of speech. *Brain Lang* 30:305–320, 1987.
17. Foldi NC: Appreciation of pragmatic interpretations of indirect commands: Comparison of right and left brain-damaged patients. *Brain Lang* 31:88–108, 1987.
18. Gorelick PB, Ross ED: The aprosodias: Further functional-anatomic evidence for the organization of affective language in the right hemisphere. *J Neurol Neurosurg Psychiatry* 50:553–560, 1987.
19. Heilman KM, Bowers D, Speedie L, Coslett HB: Comprehension of affective and nonaffective speech. *Neurology* 34:917–921, 1984.
20. Heilman KM, Scholes R, Watson RT: Auditory affective agnosia: Disturbed comprehension of affective speech. *J Neurol Neurosurg Psychiatry* 38:69–72, 1975.
21. Hughes CP, Chan JL, Su MS: Aprosodia in Chinese

patients with right cerebral hemisphere lesions. *Arch Neurol* 40:732–736, 1983.

22. Kent RD, Rosenbeck JC: Prosodic disturbances and neurologic lesion. *Brain Lang* 15:259–291, 1982.

23. Ross ED: The aprosodias: Functional-anatomic organization of the affective components of language in the right hemisphere. *Arch Neurol* 38:561–569, 1981.

24. Ross ED, Edmondson JA, Seibert GB, Homan RW: Acoustic analysis of affective prosody during right-sided Wada test: A within-subjects verification of the right hemisphere's role in language. *Brain Lang* 33:128–145, 1987.

25. Shapiro B, Danly M: The role of the right hemisphere in the control of speech prosody in propositional and affective contexts. *Brain Lang* 25:19–36, 1985.

26. Tucker DM, Watson RT, Heilman KM: Discrimination and evocation of affectively intoned speech in patients with right parietal disease. *Neurology* 27:947–950, 1977.

27. Van Lancker D: Cerebral lateralization of pitch cues in the linguistic signal. *Int J Hum Commun* 13:201–277, 1980.

28. Van Lancker D: The neurology of proverbs. *Behav Neurol* 3:169–187, 1990.

29. Van Lancker D, Kempler D: Comprehension of familiar phrases by left- but not right-hemisphere damaged patients. *Brain Lang* 32:256–277, 1987.

30. Wapner W, Hamby S, Gardner H: The role of the right hemisphere in the apprehension of complex linguistic materials. *Brain Lang* 14:15–33, 1981.

31. Weintraub S, Mesulam MM, Kramer L: Disturbances in prosody. *Arch Neurol* 38:742–744, 1981.

32. Winner E, Gardner H: The comprehension of metaphor in brain-damaged patients. *Brain* 100:717–729, 1977.

33. Wolfe GI, Ross ED: Sensory aprosodia with left hemiparesis from subcortical infarction: Right hemisphere analogue of sensory-type aphasia with right hemiparesis? *Arch Neurol* 44:661–671, 1987.

34. Larsen B, Skinhoj E, Lassen NA: Variations in regional cortical blood flow in the right and left hemispheres during automatic speech. *Brain* 101:193–209, 1978.

35. Paulesu E, Firth CD, Frackowiak RSJ: The neural correlates of the verbal component of working memory. *Nature* 363:583–584, 1993.

36. Wise R, Chollet F, Hadar U, et al: Distribution of cortical neural networks involved in word compre-

hension and word retrieval. *Brain* 114:1803–1817, 1991.

37. Ladefoged P: *A Course in Phonetics.* New York: Harcourt Brace Jovanovich, 1975.

38. Kent RD, Read C: *The Acoustic Analysis of Speech.* San Diego, CA: Singular Publishing, 1992.

39. Crystal D: *The English Tone of Voice.* New York: St. Martin's, 1975.

40. Monrad-Krohn GH: The third element of speech: Prosody and its disorders, in Halpern L (ed): *Problems in Dynamic Neurology.* Jerusalem: Hebrew University Press, 1963, pp 101–118.

41. Van Lancker D, Canter GJ, Terbeek D: Disambiguation of ditropic sentences: Acoustic and phonetic cues. *J Speech Hearing Res* 24:330–335, 1981.

42. Crystal D: Non-segmental phonology in language acquisition: Review of the issues. *Lingua* 32:1–45, 1973.

43. Lewis A: *Infant Speech: A Study of the Beginnings of Language.* New York: Harcourt Brace, 1936.

44. Critchley M: *The Language of Gesture.* London: Edward Arnold, 1939.

45. Hughlings-Jackson J: On affections of speech from diseases of the brain. *Brain* 38:106–174, 1915.

46. Monrad-Krohn GH: Dysprosody or altered "melody of language." *Brain* 70:405–415, 1948.

47. Ackerman BP: Form and function in children's understanding of ironic utterances. *J Exp Child Psychol* 35:487–508, 1983.

48. Bolinger D (ed): *Intonation.* Hardmondsworth, England: Penguin Press, 1972.

49. De Groot A: Structural linguistics and syntactic laws. *Word* 5:1–12, 1949.

50. De Renzi E, Motti F, Nichelli P: Imitating gestures: A quantitative approach to ideomotor apraxia. *Arch Neurol* 37:6–10, 1980.

51. Gainotti G, Lemmo M: Comprehension of symbolic gestures in aphasia. *Brain Lang* 3:451–460, 1976.

52. Goodglass H, Kaplan E: Disturbance of gesture and pantomime in aphasia. *Brain* 86:703–720, 1963.

53. Cicone M, Wapner W, Foldi N, et al: The relationship between gesture and language in aphasic communication. *Brain Lang* 8:324–349, 1979.

54. Delis D, Foldi NS, Hambe S, et al: A note on temporal relations between language and gestures. *Brain Lang* 8:350–354, 1979.

55. Feyereisen P, Seron X: Nonverbal communication and aphasia: A review (in 2 parts: I. Comprehension, II. Expression). *Brain Lang* 16:191–212, 213–236, 1982.

56. Seron X, Van der Kaa MA, Remitz A, Van der

Linden M: Pantomime interpretation and aphasia. *Neuropsychologia* 17:661–668, 1979.

57. Borod JC, Koff E, Lorch MP, Nicholas M: Channels of emotional communication in patients with unilateral brain damage. *Arch Neurol* 42:345–348, 1985.

58. Borod JC, Koff E, Perlman M, et al: The expression and perception of facial emotion on focal lesion patients. *Neuropsychologia* 24:169–180, 1986.

59. Cicone M, Wapner W, Gardner H: Sensitivity to emotional expressions and situations in organic patients. *Cortex* 16:145–158, 1980.

60. DeKosky ST, Heilman KM, Bowers D, Valenstein E: Recognition and discrimination of emotional faces and pictures. *Brain Lang* 9:206–214, 1980.

61. Danly M, Cooper WE, Shapiro B: Fundamental frequency, language processing, and linguistic structure in Wernicke's aphasia. *Brain Lang* 19:1–24, 1983.

62. Danly M, Shapiro B: Speech prosody in Broca's aphasia. *Brain Lang* 16:171–190, 1982.

63. Kertesz A: *Aphasia and Associated Disorders.* New York: Grune & Stratton, 1979.

64. Ross ED, Harney JH, de Lacoste C, Purdy P: How the brain, integrates affective and propositional language into a unified brain function: Hypotheses based on clinicopathological correlations. *Arch Neurol* 38:745–748, 1981.

65. Ross ED, Anderson B, Morgan-Fisher A: Crossed aprosodia in strongly dextral patients. *Arch Neurol* 46:206–209, 1989.

66. Alexander MP, LoVerme SR: Aphasia after left hemispheric intracerebral hemorrhage. *Neurology* 30:1193–1202, 1980.

67. Damasio AR, Damasio H, Rizzo M, et al: Aphasia with nonhemorrhagic lesions in the basal ganglia and internal capsule. *Arch Neurol* 39:15–20, 1982.

68. Naeser MA, Alexander MP, Helm-Estabrooks N, et al: Aphasia with predominantly subcortical lesion sites: Description of three capsular/putaminal aphasia syndromes. *Arch Neurol* 39:2–14, 1982.

69. Bell WL, Davis DL, Morgan-Fisher A, Ross ED: Acquired aprosodias in children. *J Child Neurol* 5:19–26, 1989.

70. Weintraub S, Mesulam MM: Developmental learning disabilities of the right hemisphere: Emotional, interpersonal, and cognitive components. *Arch Neurol* 40:463–468, 1983.

71. Manaoch DS, Sandson TA, Weintraub S: The developmental social-emotional processing disorder is associated with right hemisphere abnormalities. *Neu-*

ropsychiatr Neuropsychol Behav Neurol 8:99–105, 1995.

72. Voeller KKS: Right hemisphere deficit syndrome in children. *Am J Psychol* 143:1004–1009, 1986.

73. Denny-Brown D, Banker BQ: Amorphosynthesis from left parietal lesion. *Arch Neurol Psychiatry* 71:302–313, 1954.

74. Denny-Brown D, Meyer JS, Horenstein S: The significance of perceptual rivalry resulting from parietal lesion. *Brain* 75:433–471, 1952.

75. Broca P: Du siege de la faculte du langage articule. *Bull Soc Anthropol Paris* 6:337–393, 1865.

76. Lecours AR, Lhermitte F: Historical review: From Franz Gall to Pierre Marie, in Lecours AR, Lhermitte F, Bryans B (eds): *Aphasiology.* London: Bailliere Tindall, 1983, pp 12–14.

77. Ryalls J: Concerning right-hemisphere dominance for affective language. *Arch Neurol* 45:337–338, 1988.

78. Ross ED: Prosody and brain lateralization: Fact vs fancy or is it all just semantics? *Arch Neurol* 45:338–339, 1988.

79. de Bleser R, Poeck K: Analysis of prosody in the spontaneous speech of patients with CV-recurring utterances. *Cortex* 21:405–416, 1985.

80. Schlanger BB, Schlanger P, Gerstmann LJ: The perception of emotionally toned sentences by right hemisphere-damaged and aphasic subjects. *Brain Lang* 3:396–403, 1976.

81. Seron X, van der Kaa MA, van der Linden M, et al: Decoding paralinguistic signals: Effect of semantic and prosodic cues on aphasic comprehension. *J Commun Disord* 15:223–231, 1982.

82. Ross ED, Stark RD, Yenkosky JP: Lateralization of affective prosody in brain and the callosal integration of hemispheric language functions. *Brain Lang.* In press.

83. Ross ED, Rush AJ: Diagnosis and neuroanatomical correlates of depression in brain-damaged patients: Implications for a neurology of depression. *Arch Gen Psychiatry* 38:1344–1354, 1981.

84. Ross ED, Stewart R: Pathological display of affect in patients with depression and right focal brain damage: An alternative mechanism. *J Nerv Ment Dis* 175:165–172, 1978.

85. Gloor P: Experiential phenomena of temporal lobe epilepsy: Facts and hypothesis. *Brain* 113:1673–1694, 1990.

86. Gloor P, Olivier A, Quesney LF, et al: The role of the limbic system in experiential phenomena of

temporal lobe epilepsy. *Ann Neurol* 12:129–144, 1982.

87. LeDoux JE: Emotion and the amygdala, in Aggleton JP (ed): *The Amygdala: Neurobiological Aspects of Emotion, Memory, and Mental Dysfunction.* New York: Wiley-Liss, 1992, pp 339–351.

88. Ross ED, Homan RW, Buck R: Differential hemispheric lateralization of primary and social emotions: Implications for developing a comprehensive neurology for emotion, repression, and the subconscious. *Neuropsychiatr Neuropsychol Behav Neurol* 7:1–19, 1994.

89. Zola-Morgan S, Squire LR, Alvarez-Royo P, Clower RP: Independence of memory functions and emotional behavior: Separate contributions of the hippocampal formation and the amygdala. *Hippocampus* 1:207–220, 1991.

90. Poeck K: Pathophysiology of emotional disorders associated with brain damage, in Vinken PJ, Bruyn GW (eds): *Handbook of Clinical Neurology.* Amsterdam: North-Holland, 1969, vol 3, pp 343–367.

91. Wilson SAK: Some problems in neurology: II. Pathological laughing and crying. *J Neurol Psychopathol* 4:299–333, 1924.

92. Kuypers HGJM: A new look at the organization of the motor system. *Prog Brain Res* 57:381–403, 1982.

93. Bowers D, Heilman KM: Dissociation between the processing of affective and nonaffective faces: A case study. *J Clin Neuropsychol* 6:367–379, 1984.

94. Benson DF, Sheremata WA, Bouchard R, et al: Conduction aphasia: A clinicopathologic study. *Arch Neurol* 28:339–346, 1973.

95. Damasio H, Damasio AR: The anatomical basis of conduction aphasia. *Brain* 103:337–350, 1980.

Chapter 57

VIOLENCE AND THE BRAIN

Jonathan M. Silver
Stuart C. Yudofsky

EPIDEMIOLOGY OF VIOLENCE IN ORGANIC BRAIN DISORDERS

Explosive and violent behavior has long been associated with neuropsychiatric disorders. These episodes range in severity from irritability to outbursts that result in damage to property or assaults on others. A full discussion of the neuropsychiatry of violent behavior and the assessment and treatment of aggression is beyond the scope of this chapter (see Refs. 1 to 3). In this chapter, the authors review several of the major neuropsychiatric conditions associated with aggressive and violent behavior, summarize the major neurobiologic findings, and outline treatment procedures.

Among a sample of outpatients with senile dementia of the Alzheimer type (SDAT), Reisberg and coworkers[4] reported that 48 percent exhibited agitation, 30 percent violent behavior, and 24 percent verbal outbursts, which together accounted for the most common of all behavioral problems in this population.

Aggression is highly prevalent in both the acute and chronic recovery stages from traumatic brain injury. In the acute recovery period, 35 to 96 percent of patients are reported to have exhibited agitated behavior. After the acute recovery phase, irritability or bad temper is common. In follow-up periods ranging from 1 to 15 years after injury, these behaviors occur in 31 to 71 percent of patients who have experienced severe traumatic brain injury.[1]

Studies of the emotional and psychiatric syn-

dromes associated with epilepsy have documented an increase in hostility, irritability, and aggression interictally.[5] In a retrospective survey of aggressive and nonaggressive patients with temporal lobe epilepsy, Herzberg and Fenwick[6] found that aggressive behavior was associated with early onset of seizures, a long duration of behavioral problems, and male gender.

Those patients who have mental retardation and require institutionalization frequently exhibit aggressive behaviors. In a group of severely or profoundly mentally retarded individuals, approximately 33 percent were irritable and 20 percent were injurious to themselves.[7] In a survey of patients in community residences or institutions for the mentally retarded, 30 to 40 percent of the residents showed either disruptive behaviors or injury to self, others, or property.[8]

EVALUATION

Aggressive outbursts that result from organic brain dysfunction have typical characteristics.[9] These features include the reactive, nonreflective, nonpurposeful nature of the outbursts that are explosive and periodic. The diagnostic category in the fourth edition of the APA's *Diagnostic and Statistical Manual* (DSM-IV) is "Personality Change Due to a General Medical Condition."[10] Patients with aggressive behavior would be specified as "Aggressive Type."

Patients who exhibit aggressive behavior require a thorough assessment. It is important to assess systematically the presence of concurrent neuropsychiatric disorders, since this may guide subsequent treatment. Thus, the clinician must diagnose psychosis, depression, mania, mood lability, anxiety, seizure disorders, and other concurrent neurologic conditions, including central nervous system neoplasms, head trauma, cerebrovascular disease, Huntington disease, epilepsy, infectious conditions with central nervous system involvement (e.g., human immunodeficiency virus), endocrine conditions (e.g., hypothyroidism, hypo- and hyperadrenalcorticalism), and autoimmune conditions with central nervous system involvement (e.g., systemic lupus erythematosus).[2,10]

Drug effects and side effects commonly result in disinhibition or irritability.[1,2] By far the most common drug associated with aggression is alcohol, during both intoxication and withdrawal. Stimulating drugs, such as cocaine and amphetamines, as well as the stimulating antidepressants commonly produce severe anxiety and agitation in patients with or without brain lesions. Antipsychotic medications often increase agitation through anticholinergic side effects, and agitation and irritability usually accompany severe akathisia. Many other drugs may produce confusional states, especially anticholinergic medications that cause agitated delirium.[11]

Psychosocial factors are important in the expression of aggressive behavior. Certain brain-injured patients become aggressive only in specific circumstances, as in the presence of particular family members. This suggests that the patient maintains some level of control over aggressive behaviors and that the level of control may be modified by behavioral therapeutic techniques. Most families require professional support to adjust to the impulsive behavior of a violent relative with organic dyscontrol of aggression.

BIOLOGY OF AGGRESSION

Neuroanatomy

Many areas of the brain are involved in the production and mediation of aggressive behavior, and lesions at different levels of neuronal organization can elicit specific types of aggressive behavior.[12,13] The regulation of the neuroendocrine and autonomic response is controlled by the hypothalamus, which is involved in "flight or fight" reactions. Investigations in animals have shown that lesions in the ventromedial hypothalamus result in nondirected rage with stereotypic behavior (i.e., scratching, biting, etc.).[14]

The limbic system, especially the amygdala, is responsible for mediating impulses from the prefrontal cortex and hypothalamus; it adds emotional content to cognition and associates biological drives with specific stimuli (i.e., searching for food when hungry).[15] Activation of the amygdala, which can occur in seizurelike states or in kindling, may result in enhanced emotional reactions, such as outrage at personal slights. Damage to the amygdaloid area has resulted in violent behavior.[16] Injury to the anterior temporal lobe, which is a common site for contusions, has been associated with the "dyscontrol syndrome." Some patients with temporal lobe epilepsy exhibit emotional lability, impairment of impulse control, and suspiciousness.[17]

The most recent region of the brain to evolve, the neocortex, coordinates timing and observation of social cues, often prior to the expression of associated emotions. Lesions in this area give rise to disinhibited anger after minimal provocation, characterized by an individual showing little regard for the consequences of the affect or behavior. Patients with violent behavior have been found to have a high frequency of frontal lobe lesions.[18] Frontal lesions may result in the sudden discharge of limbic and/or amygdala-generated affects, which are no longer modulated, processed, or inhibited by the frontal lobe. In this condition, the patient overresponds with rage and/or aggression upon thoughts or feelings that would ordinarily have been modulated, inhibited, or suppressed. In summary, prefrontal damage may cause aggression by a secondary process involving lack of inhibition of the limbic areas.

Neurochemistry

Many neurotransmitters are involved in the mediation of aggression; this area has been reviewed in detail by Eichelman.[19] Among the neurotransmitter systems, serotonin, norepinephrine (NE), dopamine, acetylcholine, and the gamma aminobutyric acid (GABA) systems have prominent roles in influencing aggressive behavior.

Animal studies suggest that NE enhances aggressive behavior, including sham rage, affective aggression, and shock-induced fighting.[19] Higley and coworkers[20] found an association between aggression in free-ranging rhesus monkeys and cerebrospinal fluid (CSF) norepinephrine. Humans who exhibit aggressive or impulsive behavior have been shown to have increased levels of the NE metabolite 5-hydroxy-3 methyoxypheneleneglycol (5-MHPG).[21] Stimulation of the amygdala produces sham rage and is associated with decrease in brainstem levels of NE (indicative of NE release).[22] The major NE tracts in the brain start in the locus ceruleus and the lateral tegmental system and courses to the forebrain, and are, thus, vulnerable to traumatic injury.[23] Beta$_1$-adrenergic receptors are located in the limbic forebrain and cerebral cortex, areas known to be involved in the mediation of aggressive behavior.[24]

Lowered levels of serotonergic activity have been associated with increased aggression in a number of studies, including studies of predatory aggression and shock-induced fighting in rats[19] and in a study of free-ranging rhesus monkeys.[20] Clinical studies have confirmed the role of decreased serotonin in the expression of aggressiveness and impulsivity in humans[25,26]—particularly as it applies to self-destructive acts. A link between the gene for tryptophan hydroxylase and levels of CSF 5-hydroxyindoleacetic acid (5-HIAA) in impulsive aggressive individuals has been reported.[27] Olivier and colleagues[28] suggest that serotonin-specific drugs with putative antiaggressive properties bind to the 5-HT-1B subtype of the serotonin receptor, which can be found in the neocortex and hypothalamus, among other brain regions. Interestingly, 5-HT-2 receptor antagonists, including antipsychotic drugs, have antiaggressive properties.[29] It has been reported that deleting the 5-HT-1B gene increases aggression.[30]

Increases in dopamine may lead to aggression in several animal models,[19] and agitation is a common symptom in schizophrenia, often treated with antidopaminergic medications. Acetylcholine has been reported to increase aggressive behaviors.[19] Increasing GABA, via benzodiazepines, results in reduced aggressive behavior in animals,[19] and GABA agonists such as the benzodiazepines have been reported to be associated with paradoxical rage attacks.[31]

Neurophysiology of Aggression

Aggressive behavior may result from neuronal excitability of limbic system structures. For example, subconvulsive stimulation (i.e., kindling) of the amygdala leads to permanent changes in neuronal excitability.[32] Epileptogenic lesions in the hippocampus in cats, induced by the injection of the excitotoxic substance kainic acid, result in interictal defensive rage reactions.[33] When the cat experiences partial seizures, it exhibits heightened emotional reactivity and lability. In addition, defensive reactions can be elicited by excitatory injections to the midbrain periaqueductal gray region. Hypothalamus-induced rage reactions can be modulated by amygdaloid kindling.[34]

TREATMENT

Aggressive and agitated behaviors may be treated in a variety of settings, including the acute brain injury unit in a general hospital, a "neurobehavioral" unit in a rehabilitation facility, a nursing home, a residential facility for mentally retarded individuals, an outpatient environment, and the home setting. A multifactorial, multidisciplinary, collaborative approach to treatment is necessary in most cases. The continuation of family treatments as well as psychopharmacologic interventions, and insight-oriented psychotherapeutic approaches are often required. We have reviewed the treatment of aggressive behavior in detail elsewhere.[1,2] Therefore, the important general principles of treatment are reviewed here.

Documentation of Aggressive Episodes

Before therapeutic intervention to treat violent behavior is initiated, the clinician should document the baseline frequency of these behaviors.[35,36] It is essential that the clinician establish a treatment plan that utilizes objective documentation of aggressive episodes to monitor the efficacy of interventions and to designate specific time frames for the initiation and discontinuation of pharmacotherapy of acute episodes as well as the initiation of pharmacotherapy for chronic aggressive behavior.

The Overt Aggression Scale (OAS) is an operationalized instrument of proven reliability and validity that can be used to rate, easily and effectively, aggressive behavior in patients with a wide range of disorders.[35,37] The OAS comprises items that assess verbal aggression, physical aggression against objects, physical aggression against self, and physical aggression against others. Aggressive behavior can be monitored by staff or family members utilizing this instrument.

Treatment

Pharmacotherapy Although no drug is approved by the FDA specifically for the management of acute or chronic aggression, medications are widely used (and commonly misused) for this purpose. After diagnosis and treatment of underlying causes of aggression and evaluation and doc-

umentation of aggressive behaviors, the use of pharmacologic interventions can be considered in two categories: (1) The use of the sedating effects of medications, as required in acute situations, so that the patient does not harm self or others, and (2) The use of nonsedating antiaggressive medications to treat for chronic aggression when necessary. The clinician must be aware that patients may not respond to just one medication but may require combination treatment, as is done in the pharmacotherapy of refractory depression.

Acute Aggression and Agitation In the treatment of agitation and for treating acute episodes of aggressive behavior, medications that are sedating, such as antipsychotic drugs or benzodiazepines, may be indicated. However, as these drugs are not specific in their ability to inhibit aggressive behaviors, there may be detrimental effects on arousal and cognitive function. In addition, due to the potential for interference with respiration and temperature regulation, these drugs should be administered only under careful medical supervision. Therefore, the use of sedation-producing medications must be time-limited to avoid the emergence of seriously disabling side effects ranging from oversedation to tardive dyskinesia.

Table 57-1
Psychopharmacologic treatment of chronic aggression

Agent	Indications	Special clinical considerations
Antipsychotics and benzodiazepines	Psychotic and anxiety symptoms	Over sedation, multiple side effects, paradoxical rage

Anticonvulsants
    Carbamazepine (CB2)
    Valproic acid (VPA)
	Seizure disorder	Bone marrow suppression (CBZ) and hepatoxicity (CBZ and VPA)

Lithium	Manic excitement or bipolar disorder	Neurotoxicity and confusion
Buspirone	Persistent, underlying anxiety and/or depression	Delayed onset of action
Propanolol (and other beta blockers)	Chronic or recurrent aggression	Latency of 4 to 6 weeks
Serotonergic antidepressants	Depression or mood lability with irritability	May require usual clinical doses

Source: From Yudofsky et al.,[9] with permission.

Chronic Aggression If a patient continues to exhibit periods of agitation or aggression beyond several weeks, the use of specific antiaggressive medications should be initiated to prevent these episodes from occurring. The choice of medication may be guided by the underlying hypothesized mechanism of action (i.e., effects on serotonin system, adrenergic system, kindling, etc.), or in consideration of the predominant clinical features. Since no medication has been approved by the FDA for the treatment of aggression, the clinician must use medications that may be antiaggressive but that have been approved for other uses (i.e., for seizure disorders, depression, hypertension, etc).

Table 57-1 summarizes our recommendations for the utilization of various classes of drugs in the treatment of aggressive disorders. In treating aggression, the clinician, where possible, should diagnose and treat underlying disorders, and utilize, where possible, antiaggressive agents specific for those disorders. When there is a partial response after a therapeutic trial with a specific medication, adjunctive treatment with a medication with a different mechanism of action should be instituted. For example, a patient with a partial response to beta blockers may show further improvement with the addition of an anticonvulsant or a serotonergic antidepressant.

Behavioral Treatment It is clear that aggression can be caused and influenced by a combination of environmental and biological factors. Because of the dangerous and unpredictable nature of aggression, caretakers, both in institutions and at home, have intense and sometimes unjudicious reactions to aggression when it occurs. Behavioral treatments have been shown to be highly effective in treating patients with organic aggression and may be useful when combined with pharmacotherapy. Behavioral strategies—including a token economy, aggression replacement strategies, and decelerative techniques—may reduce aggression in the inpatient setting and can be combined effectively with pharmacologic treatment. A review of this subject is found in Ref. 38.

CONCLUSION

Aggressive behavior in the presence of brain damage is common and can be highly disabling. Neuroanatomic, neurochemical, and neurophysiologic factors may have an etiologic or mediating role in the production of violence. After appropriate evaluation and assessment of possible etiologies, treatment begins with the documentation of the aggressive episodes. Psychopharmacologic strategies may be divided into those intended to treat acute aggression and those intended to prevent episodes in the patient with chronic aggression. While the treatment of acute aggression involves the judicious use of sedation, the treatment of chronic aggression is guided by underlying diagnoses and symptomatologies. Behavioral strategies remain an important component in the comprehensive treatment of aggression.

REFERENCES

1. Silver JM, Yudofsky SC: Aggressive disorders, in Silver JM, Yudofsky SC, Hales RE (eds): *Neuropsychiatry of Traumatic Brain Injury.* Washington, DC: American Psychiatric Press, 1994.
2. Yudofsky SC, Silver JM, Hales RE: Treatment of aggressive disorders, in Schatzberg A, Nemeroff C (eds): *American Psychiatric Press Textbook of Psychopharmacology.* Washington, DC: American Psychiatric Press, 1995, pp 735–751.
3. Volavka J: *Neurobiology of Violence.* Washington, DC: American Psychiatric Press, 1995.
4. Reisberg B, Borenstein J, Salob SP, et al: Behavioral symptoms in Alzheimer's disease: Phenomenology and treatment. *J Clin Psychiatry* 48(5, suppl):9–15, 1987.
5. Robertson MM, Trimble MR, Townsend HRA: Phenomenology of depression in epilepsy. *Epilepsia* 28:364–372, 1987.
6. Herzberg JL, Fenwick PBC: The aetiology of aggression in temporal-lobe epilepsy. *Br J Psychiatry* 153:50–55, 1988.
7. Reid AH, Ballinger BR, Heather BB, et al: The natural history of behavioral symptoms among severely and profoundly mentally retarded patients. *Br J Psychiatry* 145:289–293, 1984.
8. Hill BK, Balow EA, Bruininks RH: A national study

of prescribed drugs in institutions and community residential facilities for mentally retarded people. *Psychopharmacol Bull* 21:279–284, 1985.

9. Yudofsky SC, Silver JM, Hales RE: Pharmacologic management of aggression in the elderly. *J Clin Psychiatry* 51(10, suppl):22–28, 1990.

10. American Psychiatric Association: *Diagnostic and Statistical Manual of Mental Disorders,* 4th ed. Washington, DC: American Psychiatric Association, 1994.

11. Beresin E: Delirium in the elderly. *J Geriatr Psychiatry Neurol* 1:127–143, 1988.

12. Ovsiew F, Yudofsky SC: Aggression: A neuropsychiatric perspective, in Roose S, Glick RD (eds): *Rage, Power, and Aggression.* New Haven, CT: Yale University Press, 1993.

13. Garza-Trevino E: Neurobiological factors in aggressive behavior. *Hosp Commun Psychiatry* 45:690–699, 1994.

14. Valzelli L: *Psychobiology of Aggression and Violence.* New York: Raven Press, 1981.

15. Halgren E: Emotional neurophysiology of the amygdala within the context of human cognition, in Aggleton JP (ed): *The Amygdala: Neurobiological Aspects of Emotion, Memory, and Mental Dysfunction.* New York: Wiley-Liss, 1992, pp 191–228.

16. Tonkonogy TM: Violence and temporal lobes lesion: Head CT and MRI data. *J Neuropsychiatry Clin Neurosci* 3:189–196, 1991.

17. Garyfallos G, Manos N, Adamopoulou A: Psychopathology and personality characteristics of epileptic patients: Epilepsy, psychopathology and personality. *Acta Psychiatr Scand* 78:87–95, 1988.

18. Heinrichs RW: Frontal cerebral lesions and violent incidents in chronic neuropsychiatric patients. *Biol Psychiatry* 25:174–178, 1989.

19. Eichelman B: Neurochemical and psychopharmacologic aspects of aggressive behavior, in Meltzer HY (ed): *Psychopharmacology: The Third Generation of Progress.* New York: Raven Press, 1987, pp 697–704.

20. Higley JD, Mehlman PT, Taum DM, et al: Cerebrospinal fluid monoamine and adrenal correlates of aggression in free-ranging rhesus monkeys. *Arch Gen Psychiatry* 49:436–441, 1992.

21. Brown GL, Goodwin FK, Ballenger JC, et al: Aggression in humans correlates with cerebrospinal fluid amine metabolites. *Psychiatry Res* 1:131–139, 1979.

22. Reis DJ: The relationship between brain norepinephrine and aggressive behavior. *Res Publ Assoc Res Nerv Ment Dis* 50:266–297, 1972.

23. Cooper JR, Bloom FE, Roth RH: *The Biochemical Basis of Neuropharmacology,* 6th ed. New York: Oxford University Press, 1991.

24. Alexander RW, Davis JN, Lefkowitz RJ: Direct identification and characterization of β-adrenergic receptors in rat brain. *Nature* 258:437–440, 1979.

25. Kruesi MJP, Hibbs ED, Zahn TP, et al: A 2-year prospective follow-up study of children and adolescents with disruptive behavior disorders: Prediction by cerebrospinal fluid 5-hydroxyindoleacetic acid, homovanillic acid, and autonomic measures? *Arch Gen Psychiatry* 49:429–435, 1992.

26. Linnoila VMI, Virkkunen M: Aggression, suicidality, and serotonin. *J Clin Psychiatry* 53(10, suppl):46–51, 1992.

27. Nielsen DA, Goldman D, Virkkunen M, et al: Suicidality and 5-hydroxyindoleacetic acid concentration associated with a tryptophan hydroxylase polymorphism. *Arch Gen Psychiatry* 51:34–38, 1994.

28. Olivier B, Mos J, Rasmussen DL: Behavioural pharmacology of the serenic, eltoprazine. *Drug Metab Drug Interact* 8:31–38, 1990.

29. Mann JJ: Violence and aggression, in Bloom FE, Kupfer DJ (eds): *Psychopharmacology: The Fourth Generation of Progress.* New York: Raven Press, 1995, pp 1919–1928.

30. Hen R, Boschert U, Lemeur M, et al: 5-HT-1B receptor "knock out": Pharmacological and behavioral consequences (abstr). Society for Neuroscience 23d Annual Meeting, Washington, DC, 19:632, 1993.

31. Salzman C, Kochansky GE, Shader RI, et al: Chloridazepoxide-induced hostility in a small group setting. *Arch Gen Psychiatry* 31:401–405, 1974.

32. Post RM, Uhde TW, Putnam FE, et al: Kindling and carbamazepine in affective illness. *J Nerv Ment Dis* 170:717–731, 1982.

33. Engel J Jr, Bandler R, Griffith NC, et al: Neurobiological evidence for epilepsy-induced interictal disturbances, in Smith D, Treiman D, Trimble M (eds): *Advances in Neurology:* Vol 55. *Neurobehavioral Problems in Epilepsy.* New York: Raven Press, 1991.

34. Adamec RE, Stark-Adamec C: Kindling and interictal behavior: An animal model of personality change. *Psychiatr J U Ottawa* 10:220–230, 1985.

35. Silver JM, Yudofsky SC: Documentation of aggression in the assessment of the violent patient. *Psychiatr Ann* 17:375–384, 1987.

36. Silver JM, Yudofsky SC: The Overt Aggression Scale: Overview and clinical guidelines. *J Neuropsychiatry Clin Neurosci* 3:S22–S29, 1991.

37. Yudofsky SC, Silver JM, Jackson W, et al: The Overt Aggression Scale for the objective rating of verbal and physical aggression. *Am J Psychiatry* 143:35–39, 1986.

38. Corrigan PW, Yudofsky SC, Silver JM: Pharmacological and behavioral treatments for aggressive psychiatric inpatients. *Hosp Commun Psychiatry* 44:125–133, 1993.

Part 9

NEUROBEHAVIORAL DISORDERS IN CHILDREN

Chapter 58

THE NEUROBEHAVIORAL EXAMINATION IN CHILDREN

Martha Bridge Denckla*

The first large difference between mental status examination in adult acquired and child/developmental contexts is that, in the latter, one must

---

*The title of this chapter could as well be "The Mental Status Examination in a Developmental Context," with the added qualification, "with Special Emphasis on the Interface between Motor Functions and Cognition." The reader of this chapter will benefit from the knowledge that the author thereof was, in the beginning, a behavioral neurologist trained to examine adults with aphasia or dementia; construction of a neurobehavioral examination for children (and adults with disorders of development) was approached by this author in apprenticeship to pediatric neurologists and developmental neuropsychologists. Through the didactic generosity of the pediatric neurologists then (1968–1976) at the Neurological Institute (Columbia University's College of Physicians and Surgeons) and the late Rita G. Rudel, to all of whom this author is deeply indebted, this chapter was made possible. Through a subsequent brief but intense growth period experienced in Boston (with the authors of the chapter that follows) this chapter was further facilitated. The author makes no clear line of demarcation other than that dictated by custom or convenience between the "neurobehavioral" and "neuropsychological" examination of children; neuropsychologists may use the timed motor exam and behavioral neurologists use digit span. Long ago, Rita G. Rudel came to the conclusion that these were the boundaries; neuropsychologists could not use the neurologist's reflex hammer or other physical examination instruments, while neurologists could not trepass upon the subtests used to compute IQ.

memorize or carry around for reference normative data arranged according to age expectations. This author was inspired to construct and norm a developmental neuromotor examination by the experience of having, in a weekly clinic, to ask a pediatric neurologist such questions as, "Should a 4-year-old child be able to hop on her nonpreferred foot?" Although the evolution of research on aging and dementia has increased awareness in all behavioral neurologists that all adults do not, decade by decade, perform across tasks at a uniform level of expectation, those who see children must have an annualized normative frame of reference and a sense of when each neurodevelopmental domain spurts steeply and then enters a plateau (temporary or ultimate). Thus, with minor exceptions, the developmental neurobehavioral examination relies on tests or tasks with norms, requires scoring, and demands additional "behind the scenes" time for looking up age-referenced expectations for performance before a profile can be described and/or diagnostic decisions reached.

Apart from such tests or tasks themselves, for each of which there is a rationale, there is an aspect of evaluation that goes beyond the term *examination* and is indispensable to developmental "mental status"; this is the history and description of the patient by parents and teachers. Of course, this is shared with all of behavioral neurology, since the literal confines of *examination* cannot sample complex social, vocational, and communal behaviors relevant to any patient's mental status. For the developmental clinic, however, the need to collect and interpret parent- and teacher-derived data relates with urgency to decisions about certain diagnostic "entities" that are shared by professional colleagues in psychiatry and education. Whatever our neurologically based intellectual qualms about some of these "diagnoses," service to the patients demands that data considered to be the basis of these "entities" be included in the neurobehavioral assessment (see Table 58-1).

Above and beyond these "formal" diagnosis-oriented obligations, there is a genuine need for the developmental neurobehavioral assessment to include descriptions and illustrative anecdotes of how the patient functions in the home, the family, the classroom, and in extracurricular activities. These situations of environmental complexity and social dynamics reveal aspects of "mental status" that no clinical "examination" can approximate. The historical perspective is particularly important, because the record of when skills and

Table 58-1

Rating scales and questionnaires for use in conjunction with history

---

Broad-band mental health dimensional screening (externalizing, internalizing, somaticizing, socializing)
    Sources: Parent
                   Child/adolescent
                   Teacher

ADHD-oriented checklists and rating scales
    1. For hyperactivity/impulsivity
    2. For inattention/disorganization
    Sources: Parent
                   Teacher(s)
                   Self (if adolescent or adult)
                   "Significant other" (if adult)

Autistic spectrum questionnaires
    1. For communication level
    2. For socialization level
    3. For range of activities (versus restricted repertoire)
    4. For unusual sensory responsivity (hyper- or hypoactivity)
    Sources: Parent
                   Teacher(s)

---

capacities became evident is itself part of the diagnostic formulation; for example, disproportionate delay in speech/language "milestones" (compared with normal or precocious emergence of motor skills) would fit with and convergently validate an examination data set in which the same profile is apparent. Yet it is even more urgent to fill in the "social mental status" and the "self-regulatory" or broader "executive function" mental status from history taking alone; we are at the mercy of the history to assess the capacity to delay gratification, to accept limits set by parents and teachers, to attend to and process nonverbal social/interpersonal cues from others (particularly peers), and to organize space/plan time. It is naive to expect to sample or elicit such naturally occurring behaviors in a clinic. In examining an individual patient in the one-on-one clinical setting, the developmental behavioral neurologist typically provides an adult authoritative structure that, while facilitating collection of data about many domains of importance in the mental status examination, effectively bypasses the self-regulatory, the social, and the executive. Many are the adorably compliant examinees whose history of oppositional-defiant behaviors comes as a shock to clinicians or physician-assistant colleagues (see below) who test "blind" to history.

A "parallel assessment" format evolved for the most pragmatic of reasons—this author's goals of (1) no child sitting alone in a waiting area and (2) two visits per family, only one of which involves the child and the second of which is a parent informing/interpreting/advising session. In addition, because schools are the major settings for the "treatment" of most developmental disorders (and even of the less numerous referrals for chronic states following closed head injury or brain tumor survival), an educator (preferably a special educator) was the chosen professional for a specialized physician-assistant colleague who (blind to history) directly tests/examines in parallel during the time that the neurologist looks over the questionnaires, rating scales, and report cards and does the formal history-oriented interview of the parent(s) or (as more adults are being evaluated) of the adult patient's "significant other." The special educator/neuropsychological colleague is trained to write down qualitative observations and impressions and then score (from raw to age-referenced norms) as much as possible during the second half of the evaluation visit, during which the neurologist (who is not blind to history but at this point blind to whatever aspects of the direct examination were done by the assistant) examines the patient. In the week usually intervening between the evaluation visit and the conference visit, the neurologist meets with his or her colleague; together, they generate a profile, a diagnostic formulation, and a set of recommendations. Most of the time, the assistant (whose unique contribution is the educator's perspective) joins the conference, which itself serves as another opportunity for expanding and refining the history, because frequently the other parent (or some professional already involved with the patient) attends the conference. The conference also serves as a dress rehearsal for report preparation. Reports have to serve many purposes; it takes quite a bit of experience and art to produce *one* report that addresses referring physicians, parents, teachers, and sometimes other agencies, in language appropriate for diverse "subcultures."

As is the case with the ultimate report, what is included in the evaluation is multidetermined. To be unkind, one could call the "menu" of what is included a "hodgepodge"; to be generous, one could call it eclectic and pragmatic. It is not a fixed battery; it changes with conceptual and data-driven shifts in the current relevant literatures. For example, as there emerged convergent consensus that phonologic coding skills are the basis for reading acquisition, the inclusion of direct norm-referenced measures of phoneme segmentation, phonologic memory, and reading (decoding) nonsense words became standard in the "learning disability"–oriented workup. Depending on the chief complaint, which varies somewhat from patient to patient and age group to age group, only a "core" is invariant; but a certain set of mental status constructs is assessed flexibly, on an individualized basis. As Rita G. Rudel so aptly warned, "Don't assault (patients) with your battery."

It will be perfectly obvious and recognizable to any professional trained to engage in the mental status examination that the developmentalist surveys language, attention, memory, visual perception, and (emphatically) motor skills. In the approach that this author has adopted, only the history (of all domains) and motor skills are exclusively the responsibility of the neurologist. The other domains are divided up between the neurologist and the colleague (the person with a neuropsychoeducational background). At the beginning of the partnership, it is best to allocate to the colleague (assuming at least minimal neuropsychological training in his or her background) those aspects of the neuropsychological tests requiring the least qualitative appraisal; specifically, multiple-choice tests of "perception" or recognition memory can be done while, simultaneously, the neurologist is interviewing parents and taking the history. Even at the beginning, however, the colleague should be exhorted to write down observations of every aspect of *how* the patient does the multiple-choice task. Impulsive or perseverative choices, wandering eyes (off task), and an obbligato of chatter are extremely useful clinical data. The neurologist will assess those tasks requiring spoken or graphomotor output, because the nature of errors and quality of responses will have major implications well beyond the quantitative level of performance. As the colleague in clinical practice becomes more sophisticated (usually because he or she participates in the informing/interpreting sessions), the colleague and the neurologist may decide to alter the pattern of "who does what" so as to avoid habituation or downright boredom. Table 58-2 lists a proposed division of labor for a $2\frac{1}{2}$-h visit; the reader is cautioned against taking this 1995 "menu" as "carved in stone."

It should also be taken into consideration that this system of evaluation is based upon the assumption that IQ and academic testing are carried out elsewhere, with the results made available for integration with the neurobehavioral examination. It should also be noted that, were the author of this chapter working in a setting alongside the authors of the next chapter, the neurobehavioral visit would be shortened and reshaped to take into consideration the particularly enriched offerings

Table 58-2
A model for the developmental neurobehavioral examination

Neurologist	Colleague (EdD, PhD)
History/interview	Multiple-choice tests
Questionnaires	Visual "what" perception
Rating scales	Visual "where" perception
Review other reports	Visual recognition memory (what, where)
	Design copying
	Target search
	Simple/choice reaction time
	Go/no go with reaction time
	Receptive language (sentence level)
	Word fluency
	Basic reading
	Nonsense
	Real words
	Basic calculations
Confrontation naming	
Complex design copying	
Word-list learning	
Neurodevelopmental motor[a]	
Praxis	

[a]Described in Table 55-3.

of that environment. Similarly, pragmatic constraints may alter the format; scheduling and reimbursement strictures may rule out the luxury of a $2\frac{1}{2}$-h initial evaluation visit followed by a $1\frac{1}{2}$-h visit informing, interpreting, and advising patients and/ or families. There is no universal "usual and customary" format, just as there is no "battery" of tests.

The most "neurologic" core of the developmental mental status examination is located at the interface where motor control is adjacent to cognitive control. An eye-movement examination would, in fact, be the most elegant instance of such assessment; in fact, getting the equipment and neuroopthalmologic training to do a "saccade battery" is a good plan for the future. At present, however, the neurodevelopmental general motor examination is the most practical and relevant one to emphasize.

The reader may be puzzled by the lack of emphasis on "higher cortical sensory" portions of the neurobehavioral examination. Certainly, it goes without saying that vision and hearing should have been elsewhere assessed and, if need be, corrected. Basic pain, temperature, vibration, and touch sensations are not considered part of the mental status examination or often enough relevant to chief complaints to warrant time spent on examining them. Problems with the intuitively relevant "higher-order" sensory functions are that (1) task demands, such as keeping eyes closed and responding with good attention to each stimulus, are frequently not met, due to deficits in the youngsters being evaluated, and (2) the significance of "finger agnosia" or "graphesthesia" failures is even less clear in a developmental context than in adult acquired cases, as attachment of some name, numbering, or "mapping" system to a sensory input is not necessarily "sensory" in any meaningful way. Little is known about firmness of association between mental image or visual memory of a letter, the name of the letter, and the dynamic-tactile experience of "graphesthesia," especially in children. To put it bluntly, one may waste a lot of time on "higher cortical sensation" and come up with little meaningful nonredundant data about the patient.

By contrast, the motor examination—even as it transcends the basics of strength, tone, and reflexes—gives the neurologist information that is both directly and indirectly relevant. For greater detail about the motor function examination, the reader is referred to Denckla and Roeltgen (Table 58-3).[1]

The directly relevant items most often bear upon "excuse slips" for gym or, more commonly, for handwriting. Sometimes a child's balance—hopping, tandem, and tone—are so much below age expectation that playground and athletic accommodations are advisable. Far more commonly, the examination elicits characteristics that lead to a recommendation that handwriting be minimized and, where unavoidable, be deemphasized in the teacher's attitude or grading/marking responses. The two most common handwriting-relevant findings are, in order of frequency, (1) choreiform movements and (2) slowness of finger sequencing (successive tapping against thumb of index, middle, ring, and little fingers). Choreiform movements are elicited by instructing the patient to stand with eyes closed, holding arms extended in front and all fingers extended and abducted. Rather than describe these as "involuntary movements," it is useful to describe them to parents and teachers as lapses in postural stability. Indeed, one can see the consequences of choreiform lapses, as recorded on design-copying tasks, in wobbly line quality and excessive pressure. Thus, there is cross-validation of choreiform postural instability between the neurologic manuever for elicitation and the design-copying elicitation of the abnormality. The patient's unconscious compensatory maneuver of excessive pen/pencil pressure, while somewhat corrective of the irregular jerks and jiggles caused by the choreiform syndrome, leads to fatigue during handwriting and gradual aversive conditioning toward tasks involving handwriting.

Slow finger sequencing correlates with poor handwriting;[3] in that sense it is not as direct a causal link to poor handwriting as is the choreiform syndrome, because it is by the adjacent neural substrate for sequence-of-pencil-moves (graphomotor praxis) that slow/poor finger sequencing bears directly on handwriting. In the original normative studies of timed motor coordination,[4,5] 5 percent of boys in kindergarten could not even perform finger sequencing; subsequent clinical experience has shown that illegible "dyspraxic" handwriting correlates with such nonperformance. Drawing unconstrained, self-generated pictures does not correlate with finger sequencing, while precise copying of designs does serve as a "surrogate" for handwriting in 5- and 6-year-olds.

The timed motor coordination examination [revised and itself a part of the revision of the National Institute of Mental Health–initiated Physical and Neurological Examination for Subtle (Soft) Signs][2] is a source of evidence of finger slowing. Motor speeds may also reveal or unmask subtle left/right differences of "classic" lateralizing significance. As youngsters are followed over

Table 58-3

Motor function: Neurodevelopmental examination

Observations
    Hand and eye (gaze) preference
    Pencil grasp
    Choreiform movements
    Extraneous overflow movements

Semiquantified tasks[a]
    Heel, toe, outside-of foot gaits (10 steps)
    Tandem gait (10 steps forward, 10 steps backward—if age > 10)
    Unipedal balance (to limit 30 s)
    Tandem balance (to limit 20 s)
    Hop (to limit 50 times)

Quantified "time to do 20 movements"
    Tongue wiggles
    Finger repetitive, finger sequential taps
    Hand pats, hand pronation-supination
    Foot taps, foot heel-toe alternations

[a]Physical and Neurological Examination for Subtle Signs (PANESS).

Source: From Denckla,[2] with permission.

years, changes in motor speed can be used to track their age-expected development or, in the shorter run, medication effects (for better or for worse) of stimulants, psychotropics, or anticonvulsants.

Of indirect relevance, as markers of the development of control processes in whose brain neighborhood they reside, are those aspects of the neurodevelopmental examination with which child neurologists are most familiar; these are the extraneous or overflow movements normally seen early in development and expected to disappear in an orderly, "milestone"-like fashion.[6] It is presumed that this disappearance reflects the maturation of inhibitory pathways. When bilaterally symmetrical, such extraneous movements as "feet-to-hands overflow" are markers of developmental failure to meet milestones; had the child been younger, the "imitative"-looking (but actually uninhibited) hand postures accompanying heel walking or outsides-of-feet walking would have been expected. When unilateral or asymmetrical, extraneous overflow movements may have subtle classic lateralizing significance. In children less than 10 years old with recovering congenital hemiparesis, mirror movements of the intact hand are elicited by the formerly hemiplegic hand's performance of a unimanual task. In these same children, when they are older than 10 years, the intact hand's mirroring decreases but a mild degree of mirroring is seen bilaterally in such tasks as finger sequencing that normally (up to age 13 years) elicit subtle mirror overflow. (For an in-depth explanation and discussion, the reader is referred to Nass.[7]) The meaning of the prominence and distribution of extraneous overflow must be derived from an integrated history and examination. As "archaeology" of the brain's anterior control systems, this part of the examination can make a surprising contribution to the assessment of adults presenting with questions about having residual signs and symptoms of attention deficit hyperactivity disorder. The deficit in age-appropriate motor inhibition can be quite striking and diagnostically helpful when the clinical problem concerns the origin of disinhibited adult behavior. To quote Norman Geschwind's clinical teaching maxim, "where we are so ignorant, we cannot afford to throw out information." Findings that implicate motor control/inhibition deficits in adults are like "laboratory data" that help to confirm the neurodevelopmental origins of certain persistent cognitive problems, especially when (as is far from uncommon) there are comorbid depressive or anxious states.

Pencil grasp is another observable motor characteristic of interest. Each grasp reflects the degree to which there is deviation from the ideal mature pencil control, that which allows movements from the distal phalanges of thumb and forefinger. Stability (not movement or pressure) is contributed by the middle finger and the ulnar "cushion" of the hand. Common deviations are depicted in Fig. 58-1 as (1) "one plus," (2) "two plus," and (3) "three plus" inefficient, reflecting movement (respectively) from (1) proximal portions of fingers, (2) too many fingers, and (3) hand muscles. Not depicted (because so rarely seen) is the truly primitive ulnar (also called simian) grasp that reflects forearm movement.

Interpretation of pencil grasp is not as straightforward as is noting its practical effect on handwriting, in terms of lack of ease or frank fatigue. A pencil grasp, like a regional accent, is a hard-to-change early-acquired motor habit; some individuals may show inefficient pencil grasps as residual indicators of the state of maturation of their motor system at the time they began to use a pencil. Sometimes it is far from easy to obtain this history of the chronological age at which pencil use began. Hence, pencil grasp does not clearly "stigmatize" the patient's *current* motor repertoire but may be like an old snapshot of past status during the period of motor skill learning.

Hand and eye preference (the latter actually a surrogate for "gaze" preference) are standard neurologic observations; rarely are they in any way diagnostic or clinically applicable. However, as research data someday to be proven relevant to understanding variations in underlying brain organization patterns of motor preference, these observations may well prove their worth, as Geschwind taught. There is one clinical situation in which the neurologist can use the observation of left-handedness or right-hand/left-"eye" preference (although "eye" is really gaze preference):

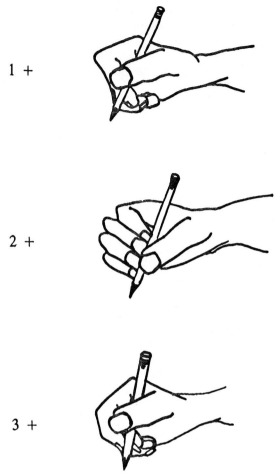

Figure 58-1
Pencil grasp as an indicator of motor control. "One plus" reflects movement from proximal portions of fingers, "two plus" from too many fingers, and "three plus" from hand muscles—all common deviations from normal.

this is to reassure parents whose 5- or 6-year-olds "mirror-write." This is easily corrected by explicit teaching and is not a predictor of any kind of reading or learning disability unless other risk factors coexist.

Finally, the neurodevelopmental motor examination must be integrated with other mental status findings. As is true in all behavioral neurology, certain clusters occur in a way that confirms the existence of recognizable syndromes (conver-

gent validity). These do not conform well to official educational, legal, and mental health syndromes but do at least overlap with the constructs of "reading disability," "nonverbal learning disability," and the subtypes (preponderantly inattentive and/or preponderantly hyperactive-impulsive) of attention deficit hyperactivity disorder (ADHD). For example, the prototypical case of "reading disability" (RD), while not conforming exactly to the neurologic construct of "developmental dyslexia," will show phonologic coding deficits, with confrontation naming and word memory recall being deficits that occur outside of the reading task per se; and on the timed motor exam, the "dyslexic" person often shows slow tongue wiggling and finger sequencing. Significant "negatives" for the pure RD patient are executive control tasks of search and choice, visuospatial and visual memory, and nongraphomotor visuoconstructive skills.

By contrast, the pure ADHD case (more likely to visit a neurologist if ADHD is of the preponderantly inattentive type) usually shows variability or some discrepantly low scores *within* the verbal or visuospatial domain in proportion to the executive control demands of such tasks (e.g., poor letter/word fluency despite excellent confrontation naming and reasonably average semantic word fluency), looks worst in terms of speed and consistency of reaction time, disorganized on target search tasks (the simpler the worse!) and shows much "young-for-age" motor overflow and incoordination. Visual-motor design-copying tasks are also poorly done by most patients with ADHD, and qualitatively the appearance of the copy products differs from that of the patient with RD. Copying standard designs is thus a very sensitive but, unless evaluated qualitatively, nonspecific screening test for those "at risk" developmentally.

Beyond attempts to document "syndromes" that overlap entities recognizable to the schools and clinics where treatment is carried out, the neurobehavioral examination is free to describe the strengths and weaknesses of each patient. Rarely is "localization" or classic brain-behavior correlation the purpose of the evaluations. Explanation of the cluster of deficits or the profile, consistent with established knowledge of brain organization, helps to legitimize educational approaches or accommodations. Sometimes brain-based explanations even serve to clarify prognosis. At the very least, brain-based explanations usually help to avoid irrational or harmful treatments and, for those patients mature enough to attempt to understand themselves, self-knowledge and insight are the not inconsiderable benefits.

ACKNOWLEDGMENTS

This work was supported by grant #P50 HD25806 from the National Institutes of Health. The author wishes to acknowledge Pamula D. Yerby for her help in the preparation of this manuscript.

REFERENCES

1. Denckla MB, Roeltgen DP: Disorders of motor function and control, in Rapin I, Segalowitz SJ (vol eds). Boller F, Grafman J (series eds): *Handbook of Neuropsychology:* vol 6. *Child Neuropsychology.* Amsterdam: Elsevier, 1992, pp 455–476.

2. Denckla MB: Revised neurological examination for subtle signs. *Psychopharm Bull* 21:773–779, 1985.

3. Berninger VW, Rutberg J: Relationship of finger function to beginning writing: Application to diagnosis of writing disabilities. *Dev Med Child Neurol* 34:198–215, 1992.

4. Denckla MB: Development of speed in repetitive and successive finger movements in normal children. *Dev Med Child Neurol* 15:635–645, 1973.

5. Denckla MB: Development of motor coordination in normal children. *Dev Med Child Neurol* 16:729–741, 1974.

6. Wolff PH, Gunnoe CE, Cohen C: Associated movements as a measure of developmental age. *Dev Med Child Neurol* 25:417–429, 1983.

7. Nass R: Mirror movement asymmetries in congenital hemiparesis: The inhibition hypothesis revisited. *Neurology* 35:1059–1062, 1985.

BIBLIOGRAPHY

Pennington BF: *Diagnosing Learning Disorders: A Neuropsychological Framework.* New York: Guilford, 1991, pp vii–x, 32–34.

Touwen BCL: Examination of the child with minor neurological dysfunction, in *Clinical Developmental Medicine,* No. 71, 2d ed. London: MacKeith, 1979.

Chapter 59

PEDIATRIC NEUROPSYCHOLOGICAL ASSESSMENT

Jane Holmes Bernstein
Deborah P. Waber

In contemporary practice, neuropsychological assessment of children, like that of adults, is undertaken within one of two broad frameworks. "Fixed battery" approaches are highly regimented and consist of menus of well-normed psychological tests and associated statistical procedures that provide the basis for assigning a diagnosis.[1-4] In contrast, "flexible" approaches can be more eclectic in terms of the actual test instruments used and can respond more flexibly to variation from child to child.[5-9] Assessments may be primarily function-oriented or primarily centered on the child. A flexible strategy, as applied in the pediatric setting, is rarely child-centered in the Lurian tradition;[10] it typically involves—but to varying degrees—both a consistent set of measures that is routinely administered to all patients and selected tasks that address specific referral questions, findings elicited by the core measures, symptoms characteristic of given disorders, and/or potential models of intervention. How these are integrated depends on the theoretical framework brought to bear by the assessor. While there may be no a priori algorithm for arriving at a diagnosis, as is the case for the "fixed" approaches, there should be principles that guide the diagnostic formulation.[5,11-16] The choice of a particular model is best based on considerations such as the setting in which it is applied, the qualifications of the examiner, the fit between the examiner's preferred style of assessment and the format of different approaches, and the demands of the clinical practice in which the method is applied.

Each of the approaches has obvious advantages and disadvantages. Fixed approaches are sturdy in a variety of settings. Because reliability and validity are well established (assuming that the tests are administered in the prescribed fashion), they are not vulnerable to variations in the training or the biases of the examiner, to variations in the manner of administration of tests, or to subtle social variables that may impinge on the test situation. Disadvantages are primarily related to the clinical utility of such approaches. They are structured primarily to provide for group discrimination (e.g., normal versus abnormal) but cannot provide the more descriptive information that is most valuable for intervention (e.g., learning style, social/personality variables, developmental context).

The more flexible approaches have the obvious disadvantage of limited reliability and validity. These latter approaches can be far more dependent on the skill of "experts" who may or may not provide useful diagnostic information, depending on their training, experience, and theoretical sophistication.[4] Advantages, however, include the ability to assimilate a broad range of information (including but not limited to test scores), to provide extensive descriptive information that is valuable in intervention, and to draw conclusions and make predictions that are based on a developmental context.

In the present chapter, we review specific considerations entailed in the neuropsychological assessment of children; these should inform any approach that is employed. We then provide a conceptual description of our own "systemic" approach, which integrates developmental principles more formally into the assessment process. Each of these discussions would obviously be worthy of much lengthier treatment. In the present format, significant issues are outlined relatively briefly in order to provide an overview of the major issues involved.

CONSIDERATIONS IN THE NEUROPSYCHOLOGICAL ASSESSMENT OF CHILDREN

In many ways, pediatric neuropsychology has been defined by contrast with that of adults. Early attempts at assessing children were derived largely from adult models. In a defining paper, Fletcher and Taylor[12] set forth four inferential fallacies that characterized many of those efforts (Table 59-1). Their critique led to a reexamination of practices and especially data interpretation. However, the points they raised are often not accorded adequate consideration, and other issues have emerged as developmental neuropsychology has evolved in the years since their critique and particularly as our understanding of brain-behavior relationships

Table 59-1
Fletcher and Taylor's four inferential fallacies

Fallacy	Error
Differential sensitivity	Brain-behavior relationships in adults with brain lesions will predict such relationships in childhood neuropathology
Similar skills	Tests developed and normed on adults will measure the same abilities in children
Special sign	Specific pathognomonic signs in adults imply the same CNS pathology in children
Brain-behavior isomorphism	Behavioral deficit equals brain dysfunction

Source: Adapted from Fletcher and Taylor,[12] with permission.

in general has advanced. A summary of relevant considerations is presented here.

Focal versus Nonfocal Neural Substrates

Modern perspectives on brain-behavior relationships in humans derive primarily from clinicoanatomic correlative studies of brain lesions in adults. These form a basis for notions such as hemispheric specialization, the differential functions of prefrontal and frontal cortex, substrates for motor coordination, and so forth. More recent analyses of the neural substrates for behavioral functions have highlighted the importance of functional networks,[17] work that has been increasingly elaborated with advances in neuroimaging techniques, particularly functional imaging techniques—e.g., positron emission tomography (PET) and functional magnetic resonance imaging (fMRI). Nonetheless, studies of individuals with focal lesions or specific forms of neuropathology continue to occupy a central position in adult neuropsychology.

Focal lesions, however, are rare in children; the most prevalent forms of childhood neuropathology that are the basis for correlative studies tend to be more disseminated (e.g., periventricular lesions associated with prematurity, structural correlates of neurogenetic disorders and malformations, effects of lead intoxication and other environmental hazards). In this developmental context, the functional network becomes a far more salient concept than that of the focally organized deficit. Furthermore, a substantial subset of children who present for neuropsychological assessment are assumed to have a developmental disorder (e.g., learning disability, developmental delay) with as yet no known neural correlates. These types of disorders, for which the focal lesion model has limited relevance, must also be conceptualized within the assessment process.

Modularity versus Nonmodularity

A related issue is the architecture of cognition. In the adult, specific cognitive functions, it can be argued, assume a modular structure.[18] That is, cognition can be understood to be "packaged" in modules, and (focal) brain injury can thus manifest itself by alteration of such a module, with relative sparing of other functions.

In the child, cognition is not yet organized in such discrete packages but assumes a more global, dynamic, and systemically integrated architecture. Indeed, one of the hallmarks of cognitive development is progressive differentiation of functions (and possibly associated limitations in terms of plasticity and recovery of function). Hence, even when brain injury does occur in a child, it will not necessarily result in a disorder of a specific cognitive function but can have more wide-ranging effects in terms of the broader organization of cognition.

Stability versus Developmental Change

While changes in neurobehavioral structure clearly occur throughout the life span,[19] such changes are far more dramatic in children. Relatively speaking, therefore, brain injury or pathologic changes in the adult can be understood in the context of a stable cognitive profile. In children, pathologic changes and normative developmental differences are equally rooted in the ontogenetic course of cognition in childhood.[20] Although such changes can manifest themselves empirically on psychological tests as an apparently linear accretion of knowledge or skill, developmental psychology has consistently demonstrated that these apparent changes actually represent sequential organization and reorganization of cognitive functions, presumably reflecting underlying maturational changes in interaction with experiential influences. Thus, the developmental context, while superficially linear, is in fact nonlinear.[21] Functional differences will thus be transformed as a function of these developmental mandates, leading to recovery or compensation in some instances, or emergence of seemingly new problems in others. Diagnosis and, in particular, prediction must therefore be cognizant of the developmental context and its significance.

Pathognomonic Signs versus Developmental Normality

One of the most fascinating challenges for pediatric neuropsychologists is the extent to which signs or behaviors that are clearly pathologic in adults may be either normative (at certain ages), of equivalent pathologic significance, or pathognomonic—but of different systems—in children. It is important to recognize not only that such signs may not be indicative of pathology in the child but also that the underlying substrate may well be different. In any event, a firm grounding in normal development is an essential prerequisite to effective neuropsychological assessment of difference or disorder.

Neurobehavioral Deficits versus Environmental Expectations

In adult neuropsychology, the complaint that brings an individual to evaluation is most frequently apparent or suspected loss of function, most likely referable to some underlying pathologic process. For children, the issues are quite different. Many of the so-called acquired lesions of childhood occur in the pre- or perinatal period. In the context of neurobehavioral assessment of the child, the consequence of these early insults is that the impairment itself becomes a part of the broader developmental process. Most typically, the presenting problem is functional and there is no identifiable neural substrate. The issue, then, is not that someone has lost a previously acquired function but that the child is not able to meet normative expectations for adaptation and achievement comfortably. The nature of the failure to meet such expectations reflects the impact of developmental change on emerging neurobehavioral functions.[22] The task of the pediatric assessment, then, is not primarily (or optimally) to identify impairments (as in the adult) but to analyze the child's complement of skills and the environmental demands in a developmental context, with the aim of improving the "fit" between the two. We have referred to this elsewhere as the child-world system.[5]

THE SYSTEMIC APPROACH TO PEDIATRIC NEUROPSYCHOLOGICAL ASSESSMENT

The foregoing discussion highlights the importance of integrating developmental principles in a comprehensive approach to brain-behavior relationships in children. In the research context, current investigations include detailed analyses of brain-behavior relations in children,[23–25] growth-curve analysis,[26] alternative assessment strategies,[27] and age-referenced normative studies of neuropsychological tests for which brain-behavior relationships have been defined in the adult (to date, primarily tests of purported frontal system function).[28–31] Developmental principles, however, must also be integrated into the clinical assessment process.

Developmental theorists have long recognized the centrality of the interaction between the organism and the environment.[21,32] In this vein, the systemic approach derives from the developmental systemic tradition of Luria and Vygotsky.[33] It assumes as its focus not the child and specification of deficits, as has been typical in clinical pediatric neuropsychology, but the child-world system (see Bernstein and Waber[5] for a more detailed presentation). The neuropsychological component of this approach lies in the organization and interpretation of observations of the child in interaction with the environment in the context of brain function and its development. The relevant data derive from the developmental history, rigorous behavioral observation, and psychological testing.

The fundamental premise, much like that of structuralist psychology (e.g., Piaget), is that there is an essential and evolving neuropsychological diagnostic profile. This profile is framed in neuroanatomic terms (at minimum at a heuristic level) and organizes behavioral adaptation across functional domains. The goal of the assessment is to describe that profile, to analyze how it fits or does not fit environmental demands and expectations, to thus determine the child's "risk," and to recommend ways to reorganize the system so as to minimize that risk.

The Assessment: Diagnostic Method

Using this approach, the diagnostic process integrates models from medicine and behavioral neurology with those of neuropsychology. The clinician seeks to identify a diagnostic cluster of converging and discriminating behaviors on the basis of a review of (neuro)behavioral systems. These are manifest in the context of specific systemic interactions in the natural and testing environments and are referenced to the developmental status of the child. As noted above, the relevant data come from the family and developmental history, from detailed observation of the child's behavioral repertoire in a variety of contexts, and from performance on selected psychological tests.

Although it is well recognized that any behavioral datum is "neuropsychological" to the extent that it is used systematically by a trained clinician to make inferences about the central nervous system (CNS),[34,35] historic and observational data have most frequently been conceptualized as moderator variables, which influence the diagnostic inferences drawn from test performance but do not themselves contribute directly to the diagnosis. In contrast, the systemic approach assigns equivalent weight to historic, observation, and test-based sources of data. Indeed, we have demonstrated empirically that it is possible, largely on the basis of historic and observational aspects of the assessment, to derive biologically relevant behavioral profiles that are invisible to numeric test scores.[36]

Rigorously employed, psychometrically sound psychological tests are equally an essential component of the systemically based assessment. Tests should be administered in the standard fashion so that valid, norm-referenced scores can be generated. Testing of limits—that is, determining what modifications need to be made to facilitate a successful performance—can provide invaluable data for diagnostic formulation and intervention. Nevertheless, such testing must be done in a way that preserves the integrity of the test itself and allows for standardized use. In addition, assembling test protocols that are used on a relatively routine basis, with some allowance for flexibility to evaluate specific issues as needed, provides for consistency across children and enhances observational analyses as it becomes possible to build an experiential base of knowledge about the range of responses that children will demonstrate given the same set of challenges.

Forecasting the Future

The pediatric neuropsychological assessment is typically expected not only to evaluate current status but to render predictions about the future. These predictions do not derive from a test and a specific function that it is presumed to measure (e.g., visuomotor skill) but from the neuropsychological diagnostic profile, its developmental context, and environmental expectations. Very often, a child will manifest difficulties in one skill area at a specific developmental stage and in a different area later on. Such "time-reference symptoms"[37,38] are as much a function of academic and curricular demands as of the child. For example, a language-impaired child may struggle to decode the grapheme-phoneme code at the first-grade level, read at grade level by fifth grade, but be overwhelmed again in the face of junior high school written language expectations. Intervention requires education of family and teaching staff about the relationship between oral and written language and the persisting risk for difficulty in the face of (any) increase in curricular language demands throughout the school experience.

Similarly, the mathematical skills that have heretofore been a consistent strength for this child may suddenly pose major difficulty. Strict adherence to test findings would not have predicted this latter problem, since a strong score on a mathematics achievement test typically predicts for subsequent success. Closer examination reveals, however, that the difficulty has emerged in response to a change in the language demands of the mathematics curriculum. While underlying conceptual strengths may continue to be present, production and achievement can falter as the child struggles to manage the more complex verbal demands of a particular topic or indeed of a whole curriculum. In the systemic formulation, this would have been predicted directly—as a result of the child's neuro-

psychological diagnostic profile interacting with environmental demand as this responds to developmental change. In this instance, the recommendation would not be to institute math support but to emphasize specific elements of the curriculum over others or to modify the language demands of the existing curriculum.

Formulating an Intervention Strategy

Intervention should be aimed at achieving a better fit between the child's complement of skills and the demands of the environment. The approach is twofold. On the one hand, specific remediation can be employed to facilitate development in skill areas, management techniques can be instituted in the classroom to facilitate performance, or social skills instruction or psychotherapy may be undertaken to address social and emotional issues. On the other hand, it is important to acknowledge that the ultimate goal is not to normalize every child to the same level of performance but to maximize a particular child's progress and adaptation, given an underlying cognitive profile that is most likely going to be relatively stable (albeit through various developmental transformations). To this end, analysis and modification of environmental demands so that they are more appropriate for the child's neuropsychological profile must be central to any management plan.

Reporting the Findings

The feedback session(s) and the written report form the basis for the informing process, the latter also constituting a record of the assessment itself. While formal communication of findings is an essential component of any psychological assessment, its importance is heightened in the pediatric setting. Children come to the evaluation at the behest of adults and are dependent on parents and teachers for support of their development. Given that the goal of the assessment is not simply to evaluate the child but also to institute a process of change in a system that is not functioning optimally, education of parents and teachers to better understand the child and the risk posed for that child by demands is an essential component of modifying the system. Thus, the feedback session(s) and the report of the evaluation should not be a simple statement of findings and list of recommendations but should be viewed as a crucial opportunity to reframe models of attribution, to assign responsibility more appropriately, and to provide all involved with a working model of the child. For this to be maximally effective for the well-being and adjustment of the child, engaging parents and teachers in face-to-face dialogue is crucial. While specific recommendations are always helpful, in the systemic context the primary goal of both the feedback and the report is to help key adults not only to understand the diagnostic formulation of the child but also to assimilate it so that they can respond more effectively to the child on an on-line basis.

For example, reframing an apparent attentional problem in terms of a basic, underlying language processing problem can have a profound influence on the child-world system. Instead of viewing inattention as a "deficit" worthy of remediation, teachers can be encouraged to view the attentional failure as a signal that the child has not effectively processed the language and is, as a consequence, confused and distracted. The appropriate intervention in this context is to facilitate comprehension and ensure that the child is engaged with the classroom discussion or activity.

CONCLUSION

Pediatric neuropsychology is a rapidly evolving discipline in the furtherance of which clinicians and researchers are engaged in a dialogue to elucidate the nature of brain-behavior relationships in the child. Clinicians contribute to this dialogue via the practice of assessment. Assessment is not a set of techniques, learned once and for all by clinicians in training. It is itself a developmental process that uses psychometric tools and techniques in the context of a theoretical perspective informed by a changing knowledge base in the service of the child. It is an integral component of the search for new knowledge, a process that must be constantly reviewed in the light of additional information.

Differences in approach to the neuropsychological assessment of children reflect differences in populations, in types of neuropathology or behavioral disorders, in the goals of intervention and management, and in the training and expertise of clinicians. Differing approaches to assessment are not, however, exclusive; each contributes in complementary ways to extend our understanding of neurobehavioral development.

REFERENCES

1. Golden CJ: The Luria-Nebraska Children's Battery: Theory and formulation, in Hynd GW, Obrzut JE (eds): *Neuropsychological Assessment and the School-Age Child*. New York, Grune & Stratton, 1981, pp 277–302.
2. Reed HB, Reitan RM, Klove H: Influence of cerebral lesions on psychological test performances of older children. *J Consult Psychol* 29:247–251, 1965.
3. Reitan RM: Psychological effects of cerebral lesions on children of early school age, in Reitan RM, Davison LA (eds): *Clinical Neuropsychology: Current Status and Applications*. Washington, DC: Hemisphere, 1974, pp 53–89.
4. Rourke BP, Fisk J, Strang JD: *Neuropsychological Assessment of Children*. New York, Guilford Press, 1986.
5. Bernstein JH, Waber DP: Developmental neuropsychological assessment: The systemic approach, in Boulton AA, Baker GB, Hiscock M (eds): *Neuromethods: vol 17. Neuropsychology*. Clifton, NJ, Humana Press, 1990, pp 311–371.
6. Taylor HG, Fletcher JM: Neuropsychological assessment of children, in Goldstein G, Hersen M (eds): *Handbook of Psychological Assessment*, 2d ed. New York, Pergamon, 1990, pp 228–255.
7. Hartlage LC, Telzrow C: *Neuropsychological Assessment and Intervention with Children and Adolescents*. Sarasota, FL, Professional Resource Exchange, 1986.
8. Pennington BF: *Diagnosing Learning Disorders*. New York, Guilford Press, 1991.
9. Wilson BC: The neuropsychological assessment of the preschool child: A branching model, in Rapin I, Segalowitz SJ (eds): *Handbook of Neuropsychology: vol 6. Child Neuropsychology*. Amsterdam, Elsevier, 1992, pp 377–394.

10. Christensen AL: *Luria's Neuropsychological Investigation.* New York, Spectrum, 1975.

11. Fennell EB, Bauer RM: Modes of inference in evaluating brain-behavior relationships in children, in: Reynolds CR, Fletcher-Janzen E (eds): *Handbook of Clinical Child Neuropsychology.* New York, Plenum Press, 1989, pp 167–177.

12. Fletcher JM, Taylor HG: Neuropsychological approaches to children: Towards a developmental neuropsychology. *J Clin Neuropsychol* 6:39–56, 1984.

13. Morris RD, Fletcher JM, Francis DJ: Conceptual and psychometric issues in the neuropsychologic assessment of children: Measurement of ability discrepancy and change, in Rapin I, Segalowitz SJ (eds): *Handbook of Neuropsychology:* vol 6. *Child Neuropsychology.* Amsterdam, Elsevier, 1992, pp 341–352.

14. Rourke BP: Brain-behavior relationships in children with learning disabilities: A research program. *Am Psychol* 30:911–920, 1975.

15. Waber DP: Rate and state: A critique of models underlying the assessment of learning disabled children, in Zelazo PR, Barr RG (eds): *Challenges to Developmental Paradigms: Implications for Theory, Assessment and Treatment.* Hillsdale, NJ, Erlbraum, 1988, pp 29–41.

16. Wilson BC, Finucci DA: A model for clinical-quantitative classification: Application to language-disordered preschool children. *Brain Lang* 27:282–309, 1986.

17. Mesulam M-M: Large scale neurocognitive networks and distributed processing for attention, language and memory. *Ann Neurol* 28:597–613, 1990.

18. Fodor J: *Modularity of Mind.* Cambridge, MA, MIT Press, 1983.

19. Benes FM, Turtle M, Khan Y, et al: Myelination of a key relay zone in the hippocampal formation occurs in the human brain during childhood, adolescence, and adulthood. *Arch Gen Psychiatry* 51:477–484, 1994.

20. Segalowitz SJ, Hiscock M: The emergence of a neuropsychology of normal development: Rapprochement between neuroscience and developmental neuropsychology, in Rapin I, Segalowitz SJ (eds): *Handbook of Neuropsychology:* vol 6. *Child Neuropsychology.* Amsterdam, Elsevier, 1992, pp 45–71.

21. Sameroff AJ: Developmental systems: Contexts and evolution, in Mussen PH (series ed), Kessen W (ed): *Handbook of child psychology,* 4th ed: vol 1. *History, Theory, and Methods.* New York, Wiley, 1983, pp 237–294.

22. Dennis M: Assessing the neuropsychological abilities of children and adolescents for personal injury litigation. *Clin Neuropsychol* 3:203–229, 1989.

23. Diamond A: Neuropsychological insights into the meaning of object concept development, in Carey S, Gelman R (eds): *The Epigenesis of Mind: Essays on Biology and Knowledge.* Hillsdale, NJ, Erlbaum, 1993, pp 208–247.

24. Molfese DL, Morse PA, Peters CJ: Auditory evoked responses to names for different objects: Cross modal processing as a basis for infant language processing. *Dev Psychol* 26:780–795, 1990.

25. Fox NA: If it's not left, it's right: Electroencephalograph asymmetry and the development of emotion. *Am Psychol* 46:863–872, 1991.

26. Francis DJ, Fletcher JM, Stueberg KK, et al: Analysis of change: Modeling individual growth. *J Consult Clin Psychol* 59:27–37, 1991.

27. Naglieri JA, Das JP: Planning, attention, simultaneous and successive (PASS) cognitive processes as a model for intelligence. *J Psychoed Assess* 8:303–337, 1990.

28. Chelune GJ, Baer RA: Developmental norms for the Wisconsin Card Sorting Test. *J Clin Exp Neuropsychol* 8:219–228, 1986.

29. Levin HS, Culhane KA, Hart J, et al: Developmental changes in performance on tests of purported frontal lobe functioning. *Dev Neuropsychol* 7:377–395, 1991.

30. Passler MA, Isaac W, Hynd GW: Neuropsychological development of behavior attributed to frontal lobe functioning in children. *Dev Neuropsychol* 1:349–370, 1985.

31. Welsh MC, Pennington BF: Assessing frontal lobe functioning in children: Views from developmental psychology. *Dev Neuropsychol* 4:199–230, 1988.

32. Gottlieb G: Experiential canalization of behavioral development: Theory. *Dev Psychol* 27:4–13, 1991.

33. Luria AR: *The Working Brain.* New York, Basic Books, 1973.

34. Mattis S: Neuropsychological assessment of school-aged children, in Rapin I, Segalowitz SJ (eds): *Handbook of Neuropsychology:* vol 6. *Child Neuropsychology.* Amsterdam, Elsevier, 1992, pp 395–415.

35. Taylor HG: Neuropsychological testing: Relevance of assessing children's learning disabilities. *J Consult Clin Psychol* 56:795–800, 1988.

36. Waber DP, Bernstein JH, Kammerer BL, et al: Neuropsychological diagnostic profiles of children who received CNS treatment for acute lymphoblastic leukemia: Neurodevelopmental implications. *Dev Neuropsychol* 8:1–28, 1992.

37. Holmes JM: Natural histories in learning disabilities: Neuropsychological difference/environmental demand, in Ceci SJ (ed): *Handbook of Cognitive, Social and Neuropsychological Aspects of Learning Disabilities.* Hillsdale, NJ, Erlbaum, 1987, vol 2, pp 303–319.

38. Rudel RG: Residual effects of childhood reading disabilities. *Bull Orton Soc* 31:89–102, 1981.

Chapter 60

ACQUIRED DISORDERS OF LANGUAGE IN CHILDREN

Maureen Dennis

Childhood-acquired language disorder, or *childhood-acquired aphasia,* refers to language impairment that is evident after a period of normal language acquisition and that is precipitated by a demonstrable form of brain insult. It may be differentiated from language acquisition disorders without clearly established brain pathology as well as from language deficits that emerge during initial language acquisition or afterwards in children with neurodevelopmental brain disorders evident at birth (see Chaps. 61, 62, 66, and 67).

EARLIER (BEFORE 1980) VERSUS RECENT (AFTER 1980) VIEWS OF CHILDHOOD-ACQUIRED APHASIA

The earlier era of research highlighted the apparent differences between adults and children with acquired aphasia. The reference point for judging whether a child was aphasic was adult aphasia syndromes rather than age-inappropriate language development. Childhood-acquired aphasia was largely defined by negative features, aphasic symptoms that were classically present in the aphasic adult but not evident in the aphasic child.

Using adult aphasia as the reference point, the earlier view[1,2] was that childhood-acquired aphasia involved nonfluent and transient language defects that arose from nonfocal and poorly lateralized brain mechanisms. In this perspective, childhood and adult-acquired aphasias differed with respect to language symptoms, rate of language recovery, lesion localization, and lesion laterality. More important, these differences between aphasic children and aphasic adults were attributed to the differing ages at onset of aphasia.

The recent view of childhood-acquired aphasia is different from the earlier view, and a variety of influences have shaped it, among them the burgeoning number of empirical studies since 1980, the publication of better benchmarks and assessment instruments for normal language development, and the increased availability and accessibility of brain imaging techniques for identifying side and site of aphasia-causing lesions. All of this has occurred in the context of emerging evidence about the sometimes greater cognitive morbidity in younger rather than older children as a result of brain tumors and head injury, which has led to a less sanguine view about the protective function for cognition of a young age at brain injury.[3]

In the earlier view, the child with acquired aphasia was advantaged over the adult aphasic by virtue of an earlier age at aphasia onset. It now appears that the advantage, if any, is short-lived and concerns the faster abatement of acute-stage aphasic symptoms. With respect to long-term language function, children with acquired aphasia often fare poorly. Age at aphasia-producing brain injury has proved to be less predictive of aphasic symptoms but more relevant to long-term language function than was previously thought. Given a similar brain injury, children and adults exhibit similar aphasic symptoms in the acute stage of acquired aphasia; however, while children show a

737

faster resolution of aphasic symptoms than adults, their long-term language function may sometimes be poorer. These conclusions have emerged from studies conducted over the last 15 years, which have called into question all of the features once considered to define childhood-acquired aphasia.

Nonfluent Nature of Childhood-Acquired Aphasia

Historically, childhood-acquired aphasia was characterized by nonfluent and impoverished spontaneous speech,[4–6] ranging in severity from mutism to articulatory difficulties as well as by nonfluent language, often with simplified syntax, telegraphic speech, and word-finding difficulties (see Chap. 9 for a discussion of these aphasic signs). A period of mutism immediately postonset resolving to a nonfluent aphasia has long been reported in samples of childhood-acquired aphasia.[7–9] Even now, speech and language dysfluency is characteristic of many forms of childhood-acquired aphasia.[10]

One corollary of the traditional view of a primarily expressive deficit in childhood-acquired aphasia was that symptoms of adult fluent aphasia (logorrhea, verbal stereotypies, perseverations, neologisms, jargon, and paraphasias; see Chap. 9) would be absent in children with acquired language disorders.[8] More recent studies have shown that aphasic children do indeed exhibit fluent aphasia[11] that includes phonemic jargon, neologisms, and paraphasias.[12] In fact, there appear to be a large number of aphasic symptoms in children, more varied than previously thought.[13] Moreover, many adult aphasic syndromes have been described in children: jargon aphasia;[12,14] Wernicke's aphasia and transcortical sensory aphasia;[15] conduction aphasia;[16] transcortical sensory aphasia;[11,17] anomic aphasia;[18] and alexia without agraphia.[19 20] In short, most adult aphasic syndromes can be observed in children, albeit with different base frequencies.[21]

Many of the classic adult aphasic syndromes involve comprehension deficits, and these have also proved to be central to childhood-acquired aphasia. From its first description in 1957, the Landau-Kleffner syndrome (LKS),[22] whose defining feature is a severe and long-lasting verbal auditory agnosia for words and for sounds, became the paradigm of childhood-acquired aphasia.[23] Comprehension deficits are features of the long-term language function in several other childhood-acquired aphasic conditions and may even be more pronounced than in adults; for example, global aphasia from a childhood left middle cerebral artery infarct may resolve to a transcortical sensory aphasia characterized by poorer language comprehension than in comparable adult cases.[24] Thus, recent research has not confirmed the traditional idea that comprehension, especially auditory comprehension, is invariably preserved in childhood-acquired aphasia.

Transient Nature of Childhood-Acquired Aphasia

Recovery of aphasic symptoms in cases of childhood-acquired aphasia is often rapid,[25] although some 25 to 50 percent of cases still show aphasia 1 year postonset. More important is the observation that recovery of speech cannot be equated with recovery of language.[8]

Recent long-term follow-up studies have focused on recovery of language function rather than on abatement of aphasic symptoms. Considered in this manner, the consequences of childhood-acquired aphasia appear to be long-lasting and extend in time far beyond the disappearance of aphasic symptoms.[23] Although clinical signs of aphasia somewhat similar to those in the adult occur in the acute phase of childhood-acquired aphasia, long-term language outcome may still be poor after aphasic symptoms have resolved.[26] Even when clinical signs of aphasia abate, full and functional pragmatic language will not necessarily be acquired or restored.[27,28] And academic achievement in school-age children continues to be poor after clinical recovery from aphasic symptoms.[29–31] School difficulties—involving failure to accrue new learning[17]—may even become more pronounced with time, perhaps because of the escalating demands of academic work in the higher grades.[32]

Nonfocal Brain Bases of Childhood-Acquired Aphasia

The idea that childhood-acquired aphasia was based in nonfocal brain mechanisms arose for several reasons, among them the fact that early study groups of children with acquired aphasia had an overrepresentation of traumatic and infectious etiologies[7] and included patients with pathologic processes that appeared to be lateralized (on the basis of evidence of gross neurologic status, such as hemiplegia) but which actually affected functions bilaterally.[14] In addition, the early studies that shaped the traditional view of childhood-acquired aphasia could not include neuroimaging of the aphasia-producing lesions, resulting in inperfect information about lesion localization and extent.

In recent studies there has been increased recognition of the fact that child and adult aphasia-producing lesions may have different long-term effects on the brain. Some early lesions may leave little focal residual change,[33] with the result that the brain does not show characteristic gliotic changes but rather tissue shrinkage; thus, even with an initially focal insult, brain lesions in childhood may involve decreased brain volume.[34] This invalidates any simple comparison between children and adults at the point in time that aphasic symptoms are most florid.

Nonlateralized Brain Bases of Childhood-Acquired Aphasia

In the earlier view, language lateralization developed over the first decade of life in a gradual and linear manner. The question of whether cerebral dominance for language develops gradually or is innate, once considered so central to understanding childhood-acquired aphasia,[35] has in recent years come to seem less burning.[21] Perhaps more important, particular entailments of the view of a slowly-developing lateralization of language have been proven wrong, such as the idea that aphasia after right-sided lesions is more common in children than in adults.[14] If the left hemisphere has been damaged, the risk of acquired aphasia is approximately the same in right-handed children and right-handed adults;[25,36,37] evidently, childhood

aphasia is no more uncommon than adult aphasia, given a unilateral lesion to the dominant hemisphere.[38] Further, left-sided lesions to the classic posterior language areas in childhood produce a fluent aphasia with many neologisms and paraphasias[39] of the sort observed in adults with similar brain lesions. And finally, recovery from childhood-acquired aphasia depends on the integrity of the left posterior language areas,[30] which suggests that a lateralized and focal language representation is well established by middle childhood and also that recovery from childhood-acquired aphasia depends on the intact areas of the left hemisphere rather than on a language shift to the nondominant hemisphere.[40]

Age-Related versus Etiologic Differences in Adult and Childhood-Acquired Aphasia

In the traditional view, the apparent better recovery from aphasia in the childhood aphasic versus the adult was attributed to the younger age of the child (and to the putative plasticity of the brain for which the younger age was a marker). Early research selected study groups on the basis of aphasia and combined heterogeneous pathologies in assessing outcome.[7] If subjects are accrued to a study because they show aphasic symptoms, any group of children will have an overrepresentation of traumatic and convulsive etiologies and an underrepresentation of vascular disorders in relation to an adult group. Differences in age at aphasia onset are thereby correlated with differences in etiology.

The consequences of the correlation between age and etiology have not been trivial for views of childhood-acquired aphasia. Because theories about acquired aphasia tend to be based on data from the most frequently described etiologies for any age group, the nature of adult-acquired aphasia has been shaped from arteritic stroke while that for childhood-acquired aphasia has been understood from head injury and convulsive disorders.

Childhood- and adulthood-acquired aphasias typically differ in both age and etiology,[31] and, indeed, recovery is different according to etiologic categories.[26] Perhaps the most important recent advance in understanding childhood-acquired aphasia has involved the specification of etiology to a greater extent than in an earlier research era, together with the increased recognition of the diversity of short- and long-term outcome as a function of etiology. One consequence of this recognition has been the increased attention in recent publications to the question of etiologic differences in childhood-acquired aphasia.[2,41] The analysis of childhood-acquired aphasia according to both etiology and age has challenged the assumption that language differences between childhood and adulthood aphasias are due to differences in age at onset of the aphasia.

PRINCIPAL ETIOLOGIES OF CHILDHOOD-ACQUIRED APHASIA

This section reviews the characteristics of the principal etiologies of childhood-acquired aphasia. For each etiology, some general issues are discussed, and, where sufficient evidence is available, cross-etiology comparisons are facilitated by Tables 60-1 through 60-4.

Seizure and Seizure-Related Disorders: The Landau-Kleffner Syndrome

Seizure disorders affect language function, and language symptoms have been observed both as part of clinical seizures[42] and as part of ictal speech automatisms. In addition, recurrent generalized seizures and medication may have diffuse effects that can confound the interpretation of otherwise focal lesions. The most studied aphasia-producing seizure disorder, however, is the LKS,[22] the characteristics of which are reviewed in Table 60-1.

Vascular Disorders

Vascular disorders involve interruptions to the blood supply within the brain as a result of occlusion (ischemic stroke) or rupture (hemorrhagic stroke). Most vascular diseases observed in the adult also occur in children, albeit with different

base frequencies. Degenerative disorders like atherosclerosis are common in the middle-aged and elderly but rare in children, while vascular disorders associated with congenital heart disease occur principally in childhood[68] and may produce strokes by an embolism from the heart, from complications of heart surgery, or from hypoperfusion from prolonged hypotension. The characteristics of childhood-acquired aphasia from vascular diseases are reviewed in Table 60-2.

Traumatic Disorders

Traumatic head injury is a principal cause of childhood-acquired aphasia. Children exhibit a variety of aphasic symptoms and language disturbances after head injury.[76] The characteristics of childhood-acquired aphasia from traumatic disorders are reviewed in Table 60-3.

Brain Tumors

Brain tumors in children are not uncommonly associated with language disturbances.[11,79,95] For tumors above the tentorium, there are few data available on the type and localization of aphasia-producing lesions. Posterior fossa tumors occur with a high frequency in children relative to adults, with the result that this tumor type has provided the principal source of information about childhood brain tumors and language.[96] The characteristics of childhood-acquired aphasia from posterior fossa tumors are reviewed in Table 60-4.

Cancer Treatments

Radiotherapy and chemotherapy are often part of the treatment for such childhood cancers as acute lymphoblastic leukemia. Central nervous system (CNS) prophylaxis is known to cause structural and functional damage to the brain.[106,107] Children treated for cancer show a variety of deficits in speech and language,[108] including mutism, expressive aphasia, anomia, and problems with academic tasks. Much about these speech and language deficits remains to be understood, however, including the relation between degree of language impairment and prophylactic dose, the specificity of the language disorders within particular conditions, and the correlation between language function and neuropathology.

Infectious Conditions

Infectious diseases of the brain may involve viral, bacterial, spirochetal, and other microorganisms that infect the meninges (meningitis) and/or the brain (encephalitis). Infectious conditions are reported to produce childhood-acquired aphasia,[109] either as a primary effect of CNS involvement in conditions like herpes simplex encephalitis or as a secondary effect of sensorineural hearing loss in conditions such as bacterial meningitis or toxoplasmosis.

Studies of the effects of meningitis on language function have not provided clear information. While some studies have suggested that deficits in communication are an effect of meningitis, others have not.[109] Differences in research methods and assessment procedures for language may be responsible for the apparent inconsistency in results in studies of meningitis and language.

Commonly, aphasia is part of the morbidity of herpes simplex encephalitis,[15,29,40,110] even though antiviral medication in recent years has reduced the mortality associated with this condition. In the acute stage of encephalitis, there is a severe defect of comprehension similar to that seen in global aphasia following an initial period of mutism. The comprehension deficit involves a fluent aphasia with neologisms, semantic and phonemic paraphasias, stereotypies, and perseverations.[15,29,111] That a fluent form of aphasia is associated with herpes simplex encephalitis appears consistent with the fact that the herpesvirus has a tropism for the temporal lobes.[2]

Recovery from aphasia is especially poor after herpes simplex encephalitis.[109] Children with aphasia from this infection continue to show paraphasias and severe comprehension deficits in the recovery period as well as long-term difficulties in word finding.[15,29] The poor outcome may be related to the fact that, while some infections are unilateral, most have bilateral effects on the brain,[33] and also that the herpesvirus causes ne-

crotic brain lesions and significant neurologic sequelae.[112]

Hypoxic Disorders

Anoxia is a state in which the oxygen levels in the body fall below physiologic levels because oxygen supply is deficient or absent. Anoxia can come about from various causes—including severe hypotension, cardiac arrest, carbon monoxide poisoning, near-drowning, and suffocation—that involve a drop in the level of cerebral blood flow or the oxygen content of the blood. In turn, this results in cerebral anoxia, a prolonged period of which will produce permanent brain damage or anoxic encephalopathy, which is associated with a range of neurologic disorders, including language deficits.[113]

In children, anoxic encephalopathy produces short- and long-term language deficits. An initial mutism resolves into a variety of forms of language disorder, ranging from dysarthria, increased speech rate, problems initiating speech movements, and anomia.[29,114] Children who suffer a near-drowning episode show speech and language disorders that appear to recover in the longer term,[115,116] although that subset of children who initially present as comatose after a near-drowning episode may continue to be at risk for language disorders.[113]

The neuropathology of cerebral anoxia is fairly well known, although there have been few research studies in children that correlate language status and patterns of anoxic brain damage. In one study, subcortical lesions resulting from anoxic encephalopathy in adolescence have been related to motor speech disorders involving a progression from mutism to dysarthria.[114]

Metabolic Disorders

Systemic metabolic disorders that result in the accumulation of metabolites in the bloodstream cause structural alterations in the brain that may result in speech and language deficits. Some of the inborn errors of metabolism that have been shown to affect speech and language[117] include phenylke-

Table 60-1

Childhood-acquired aphasia and the Landau-Kleffner syndrome

Definition

- Landau-Kleffner syndrome (LKS) involves acquired aphasia with convulsive disorder[22] occurring in normal children who acutely or progressively lose previously acquired language ability.
- A variety of typologies have been proposed.[43]
- It was originally claimed that pregnancy, birth, and early development were normal in LKS,[44] and, classically, LKS occurs after some period of normal language development. More recently, however, it has been found that a history of language pathology may precede the onset of language deterioration and loss,[45] with some 75 percent of cases exhibiting language disturbance before the aphasia.[46]
- Loss of language is associated with either clinical seizures (generalized, partial, partial complex, or absence) or with an electroencephalogram (EEG) showing unilateral or paroxysmal activity, sometimes more prominent in slow-wave sleep.[47]
- It has been argued that LKS overlaps with other epileptic conditions: rolandic epilepsy, electrical status epilepticus during sleep (ESES), and autistic regression and disintegrative disorder associated with unilateral or bilateral centrotemporal spike/spike-wave discharges.[21]

Core Features

- A severe comprehension defect[48] occurs, characteristically with severe verbal auditory agnosia, which may involve both common sounds (such as a dog barking, or a doorbell ringing) and words.[2,49]
- Epileptic seizures occur in 70 to 75 percent of cases.[50]
- Severe behavior disturbances occur in 75 percent of cases.[50] Long-term (>7 years) follow-up studies have reported mild behavior disturbance (hyperactivity, impulsivity, and oppositional behavior) that is chronologically linked with the language disturbances and follows their fluctuations.[51]
- Oral expression is typically poorer than written expression,[52,53] although severe impairment of written language and mathematical skills has been reported.[48]
- Neurologic examination is reported to be normal.[54]
- Nonverbal intelligence appears to be well preserved.[55]
- Half the published cases present first with comprehension disorder, the other half with seizures.[50]
- Most LKS patients have a mild form of epilepsy that responds to drug therapy.[56]
- There is a correlation between the aphasia and the seizure disorder, although both may fluctuate out of phase,[56] so that the relation is not obvious.[57]

Epidemiology, Demography, and Risk Factors

- Some 200 cases have been reported from 1957 to 1995.[50]
- The male:female ratio is 2:1.[50]
- There are currently no epidemiologic data in regard to geography, infectious disease, toxins, nutrition, or environmental exposures.[58]

Age-Related Factors

- Onset occurs from 3 to 8 years in 50 percent of cases.[50]
- Onset is rare after 8 years, although several cases have been reported with loss of language after age 9. Later-onset cases are more likely to have a primarily expressive aphasia with dysfluency and word-finding difficulties.[59]
- An age-prognosis relationship has been proposed, such that the younger the child, the poorer the recovery from the acquired aphasia, the reasoning being that newly acquired language skills are particularly vulnerable to bilateral brain pathology.[44] However, age-prognosis effects, such as the claim that recovery is worse with a diagnosis before age 5,[60] have not been replicated with more clearly defined case selection criteria.[51]

Table 60-1 (Continued)

Time-Related Factors

- Language impairments in LKS persist for months or even years.[49]

- Long-term language outcome is often poor. When studied 10 to 28 years after onset of acquired aphasia, more than half of an LKS sample continued to show language disorder.[47] In a long-term follow-up of at least 7 years—into the adolescent years—no individual with LKS fully recovered language.[51]

- Typically, seizures remit before adulthood and the aphasia subsides, although not necessarily in parallel.[44]

- The long-term outcome of the aphasia has been considered to be unpredictable with respect to medical history features,[47] despite the fact that both epilepsy and EEG abnormalities improve.[61] There is an unpredictable prognosis on an individual case basis, with a fluctuating course of remissions and exacerbations for both aphasia and EEG abnormalities.

- In a long-term (2- to 15-year) follow-up of LKS cases, it was found that, even when the EEG normalized in the long term, few individuals achieved normal language, and, further, that no individual with persisting EEG abnormalities recovered normal or near normal language.[46] Thus, persisting EEG abnormalities appear to be a risk factor for continuing aphasia.

Neuropathologic Substrate

- Initially, it was unclear whether the language disturbances in LKS was functional or due to an identifiable brain lesion. Proposals for the brain basis of LKS have ranged widely.

- It has been suggested that LKS might involve focal subclinical epileptogenic discharges involving the language areas. In this view, aphasic symptoms arise because persistent epileptic discharges cause functional ablation of the primary cortical language areas.[62]

- Because the course of the aphasia in LKS may be linked to the appearance and disappearance of ESES,[61] LKS has been considered related to ESES. However, few children with ESES have specific language disorders, and the characteristic EEG of ESES is infrequently found in LKS.[56]

- The mild to moderate elevation of cerebrospinal fluid proteins in some LKS cases[47,63] has been used to suggest a low-grade focal inflammation of the brain as the mechanism of LKS aphasia.[64]

- Cortical biopsies in some LKS cases have shown changes indicative of a slow virus infection, implying that a subacute viral encephalitis might produce both aphasia and seizures, either from a low-grade selective encephalitis[55] or a subchronic viral encephalitis affecting both hemispheres.[44]

- The finding of a positive autoimmune reaction to myelin during clinical deterioration of language in LKS patients has been used to suggest a disorder of myelin metabolism and to account for the positive effect of corticosteroids as immunosuppressive therapy.[65]

- Computed tomography and structural magnetic resonance imaging are typically normal.[64]

- Angiography has shown isolated arteritis of some branches of the carotid arteries, which implies that focal cerebral vasculitis may be involved in the pathogenesis of LKS.[64]

- Positron emission tomography has shown abnormal glucose utilization during sleep, with lower metabolic rates in subcortical than in cortical areas.[66]

Treatment

- There is no convincing evidence of empirically effective therapy.[58]

- Various drug treatments (antiepileptics, corticosteroids) have been tried, with success on an individual case basis.

- Under the view that focal vasculitis is responsible for LKS, calcium channel blockers have been proposed as a possible therapy.[64]

- Subpial resection has been proposed as therapy in some cases of LKS.

- Speech and language therapy has long been used in the rehabilitation of individuals with LKS, but there has been controversy about whether therapy should involve enhancing the residue of oral language; intensive training in the visual domain (gestures, communication boards, signing, computers); brief training in the visual domain with rapid transfer to oral language; or a more pragmatic, multimodal approach. A recent review[67] suggests that no single therapy program will work, that LKS patients are not like deaf individuals, and that any therapy will likely take several years to be effective.

Table 60-2
Language disturbances from vascular etiologies

Definition

- Acquired aphasia may be precipitated by a vascular brain lesion, occurring in children who acutely or progressively lose previously acquired language skills.
- Brain localization depends on the pathophysiology of the stroke. In children, most strokes are secondary to intracranial occlusive disease and are localized in the basal ganglia;[69] however, cortical vascular lesions in the left temporoparietal lobe that produce aphasia have been reported to occur from cerebral arteritis[39] and ruptured arteriovenous malformations.[70]

Core Features

- The type of aphasia depends on the localization of the lesion. Aphasia is fluent in form with lesions to the posterior left hemisphere cortical language areas[71] but nonfluent with predominantly subcortical pathology.[72,73]
- In the fluent form of aphasia, anomia, word finding deficits, paraphasias, and circumlocutions occur.[39,70]
- Reading and spelling may be relatively preserved with cortical lesions in the left-hemispheric posterior language areas, despite anomia,[39,70] which suggests poor phonologic representation of target words.
- Reading and writing disorders are common in both the acute and chronic stages of subcortical vascular lesions.[73]

Epidemiology, Demography, and Risk Factors

- Few cases have been reported.[71]

Age-Related Factors

- Onset at any point throughout childhood.

Time-Related Factors

- There is significant recovery from aphasic symptoms after vascular lesions,[73] although naming and word-finding problems persist into the chronic stage of recovery.[39,70]

Neuropathologic Substrate

- The laterality and localization of cortical lesions are similar to those of anomic aphasia in adults; damage occurs to the posterior left hemisphere cortical language areas.[39,70]
- Most subcortical vascular aphasias of childhood also appear to accord with the clinical-radiologic correlation observed in adults with subcortical aphasias.[72,73]
- Lesion laterality may be related to the pattern of impaired language comprehension. In a mixed group of brain-injured children—many with acquired lesions from vascular etiologies—children with left-sided lesions were unable to integrate pragmatic knowledge with syntactic constraints,[74] whereas those with right-sided lesions showed impairments in lexical-semantic and pragmatic knowledge.[74,75]

Treatment

- None specific.

Table 60-3

Language disturbances from head injury

Definition

- Acquired aphasia may occur after a head injury, typically a closed head injury.
- The aphasia is precipitated by injury to the brain, which includes both immediate impact injury (contusions, diffuse axonal damage) and secondary brain damage involving intracranial events (hematomas, brain swelling, infections, subarachnoid hemorrhages, hydrocephalus) and extracranial factors (hypoxia, hypotension).
- Focal brain contusions are common in the frontal and temporal lobes after head injury, whether or not the head has been struck in these particular regions.[77]

Core Features

- Children with acquired aphasia from head injury show a variety of aphasic symptoms in the acute stage.[7,78,79]
- Frank aphasia and adultlike aphasic syndromes occur infrequently.[76]
- Mutism or reduced verbal output and anomia are common in the short term after head injury.[76,80,81]

Epidemiology, Demography, and Risk Factors

- Head injury is the leading cause of childhood death in North America,[82] with an incidence of 200 per 10,000 per year.[83] Eighty percent of survivors of severe childhood head injury have learning difficulties, including problems in language-related skills.[84]

Age-Related Factors

- Onset occurs at any point throughout childhood.
- A younger age at onset may be associated with more deficits in expressive language in the recovery phase, around 8 months postinjury.[85]
- Injury before age 7 versus injury at an older age is associated with more long-term difficulties in understanding the linguistic-symbolic nature of facial expressions, in metalinguistic awareness, and in comprehension monitoring.[86,87]

Time-Related Factors

- Aphasic symptoms resolve over time in children with acquired aphasia from head injury.[7,78,79]
- Anomia and reduced verbal fluency are consistent deficits after childhood head injury, even 18 months postinjury.[37,88–90]
- One group of persisting problems for children after head injury involve what have been termed nonaphasic language disorders with nonliteral language, discourse, and inferencing.[91] In the long term, head-injured children show a variety of discourse deficits, not so much in the gross aspects of communication[92,93] as in telling a story,[27] using and understanding idiomatic or ambiguous statements, making knowledge-based inferences in social scripts, and producing speech acts appropriate to particular contexts.[28]
- In the long term, children with head injury have difficulty in comprehension–monitoring tasks requiring them to evaluate statements that violate semantic selection rules, grammatical structures, or pragmatic constraints.[86]
- In the long term, children who have had a head injury at a younger rather than an older age are poor at referential communication tasks requiring them to judge the relevance of an instruction, suggesting poor metacognitive function.[86]
- Children with head injury have long-term difficulties in understanding how language is used to serve social-communicative goals that include emotional deception. These children have difficulty understanding the linguistic-symbolic nature of facial displays, such as those involved in the deceptive expression of emotion (e.g., they have difficulty selecting a neutral or happy expression when told that a story character is feeling sad but has a reason for hiding that feeling from another character).[87]
- Academic abilities in language-related areas are poor in the long-term after childhood head injury.[80,81]
- Vocabulary tests may deteriorate with increasing time, because head-injured children are unable to acquire new language-based knowledge at an age-appropriate rate.[29]

Neuropathologic Substrate

- The degree of residual language impairment appears to be related to the severity of the head injury,[5,81] and children with mild head injury recover functional language faster than do children with more severe injuries.[90]
- The clinical-pathologic correlation of language disorders in childhood head injury is poorly understood, particularly as it concerns contusional damage to the frontal and temporal lobes. However, it is known that frontal contusions and left-sided contusions in children and adolescents with head injury are variously associated with problems in understanding the linguistic-symbolic nature of facial expressions, in metalinguistic awareness, and in oral comprehension monitoring.[86,87]
- Early frontal lobe injury particularly affects nonaphasic discourse disorders in the long term after a childhood head injury,[86,87] which is consistent with the importance of an intact frontal lobe system for the development of social awareness and social cognition.[94]

Treatment

- None specific.

Table 60-4

Language disturbances after posterior fossa brain tumors

Definition

- Acquired aphasia occurs secondary to astrocytomas, medulloblastomas, and ependymomas of the cerebellum, fourth ventricle, and/or brainstem, occurring in children who acutely or progressively lose previously acquired language skills.

Core Features

- Mutism occurs commonly in acute-stage cerebellar lesions of childhood.[97,98]
- The mutism is not tumor-specific in that it involves various tumor pathologies.[97]
- A syndrome of mutism and subsequent dysarthria (MSD) has been identified,[99] not obviously related to cerebellar ataxia but characterized by a complete but transient loss of speech resolving into dysarthria.
- Analysis of the dysarthria of posterior fossa tumors in children suggests that it shares some of the features of adult dysarthria—namely, imprecise consonants, articulatory breakdowns, prolonged phonemes, prolonged intervals, slow rate of speech, lack of volume control, harsh voice, pitch breaks, variable pitch, and explosive onsets.[100]
- There appears to be no adultlike pattern of fluent or nonfluent aphasia in children treated for posterior fossa tumors.[100] However, children with treated posterior fossa tumors, including medulloblastomas, show mild language impairments in oral expression and auditory comprehension.[101]

Epidemiology, Demography, and Risk Factors

- As of 1994, a total of 36 cases of MSD have been reported.[99]
- In children with posterior fossa tumors, risk factors for the development of MSD are hydrocephalus at the time of tumor presentation, ventricular localization of the tumor, and postsurgical edema of the pontine tegmentum.[99]

Age-Related Factors

- Some 90 percent of MSD patients are less than 10 years of age, and the condition has been described in children as young as age 2.[99]

Time-Related Factors

- In cases of MSD, recovery of dysarthria to normal speech seems to be related to the recovery of complex movements of the mouth and tongue.[99]
- A range of short- and long-term intellectual, neuropsychological, and academic difficulties have been identified in children with posterior fossa tumors,[102] including language-related difficulties. Academic failure occurs frequently in survivors of posterior fossa tumors, and the rate is higher in survivors of medulloblastoma than in survivors of cerebellar astrocytomas.[103,104]

Neuropathologic Substrate

- Mutism may occur with a midline location of the tumor combined with postoperative complications that involve destruction of the midline roof structures and penetration of the peduncles and/or lateral wall or ventricular floor parenchyma.[97]
- Mutism occurs particularly with posterior fossa tumors located in the midline or vermis of the cerebellum, and with tumors invading both cerebellar hemispheres or the deep nuclei of the cerebellum.[97,98]
- Isolated lesions in cerebellar structures are not sufficient to produce MSD. An additional ventricular location of the tumor and adherence to the dorsal brainstem are necessary, an idea supported by the frequent occurrence of pyramidal and eye-movement signs in children with MSD.[99]
- Localization of the brainstem dysfunction in MSD appears to be rostral to the medulla oblongata and caudal to the mesencephalon.[99]
- It has been proposed that the mutism of MSD is related to bilateral involvement of the dentate nuclei and that the subsequent dysarthric speech represents a recovering cerebellar mechanism.[105]

Treatment

- None specific to the language disorders, only the appropriate course of tumor treatment.

tonuria (an absence of the liver enzyme phenylala-nine), galactosemia (an inability to utilize the sugars galactose and lactose because of disordered carbohydrate metabolism), and Wilson disease (a progressive degenerative disorder of the brain and liver resulting from inability to process dietary copper). Congenital hypothyroidism also affects intellectual functions, including language.[117] In addition to these relatively direct metabolic effects on the brain, other hereditary metabolic diseases such as homocystinuria, a disorder of amino acid metabolism, may cause vascular occlusive disease when enzyme deficiencies damage blood vessels, leading to thrombosis and ischemic stroke.[68] The specificity of speech and language disorders and the relation between language and neuropathology are poorly understood in these various metabolic conditions.

CONCLUSIONS AND FUTURE DIRECTIONS

In studies conducted over the last 15 years, separation of the principal etiologic subgroups, together with fuller descriptions of the language profiles associated with these etiologies, has significantly advanced our understanding of childhood-acquired aphasia. Descriptive studies of etiologies have provided the basis of more systematic knowledge about childhood-acquired aphasia: specifically, about the language symptoms and type of aphasia, the demographic and incidence factors, and the course of recovery or resolution of language symptoms as evidenced by longitudinal evaluations. A better information base has made it possible to consider some core issues about childhood-acquired aphasia, including its symptom spectrum, its similarities and differences with adult-acquired aphasia, its neuropathologic substrate, and the factors that promote or retard abatement of aphasic symptoms and recovery of language function.

Children show a wide range of language symptoms after brain damage that precipitates acquired aphasia, and there is no single profile of language loss in the acquired aphasic conditions of childhood. Various profiles of language loss are associated with different etiologies of childhood-acquired aphasias, ranging from the mutism of extensive cerebellar lesions through nonaphasic language disorders, pragmatic and social discourse impairments commonly observed in the long term after traumatic lesions.

While the types of symptoms manifest in the acute phase of childhood-acquired aphasia often differ according to etiology, it is also the case that some acquired aphasic symptoms are common to a range of etiologies while others occur in a more limited number of conditions. Many types of childhood-acquired aphasia, indeed, many types of brain injury in children,[118] resolve to anomic and word-finding deficits. The severe auditory agnosia commonly associated with LKS, however, has not been reported in other conditions.

Age-Related Issues: Similarities and Differences between Children of Different Ages and between Children and Adults

One age-related issue concerns the difference among children with acquired aphasia in relation to age at onset of language disorder. Language disturbances involving the use and understanding of mental states and social discourse are more common with an earlier rather than a later age at head injury.[86,87]

A second age-related issue concerns the consequences for language-related skills of the developmental timing of brain injury. If the onset of epilepsy coincides with beginning to read and write, it will impair the acquisition of written language.[42] In comparison with later prophylaxis, earlier treatment for acute lymphoblastic leukemia in childhood results in less utilization of phonemically based spelling strategies and, by inference, poorer phonemic awareness.[119] From data such as these, it has been proposed that the skills that are in a period of active development but not yet consolidated are more vulnerable to disruption than either less or more consolidated skills.

Aphasic mutism is of interest under the above model of heightened vulnerability for skills that are in the course of acquisition but not yet automatized. Mutism occurs more commonly in children than in adults, variously from a range of etiologies that include the acute phase of vascular, epileptogenic, traumatic, tumorigenic, and infectious conditions. The ubiquity of aphasic mutism in childhood-acquired aphasia over the age range of childhood suggests that the initiation of speech is a volatile language function during childhood, one that is easily disrupted by a range of aphasia-precipitating forms of brain damage; it suggests further that the initiation of speech is imperfectly automatized throughout much of childhood.

An important age-related issue concerns similarities and differences between childhood- and adulthood-acquired aphasia. Children and adults show more similarities in aphasic patterns than was earlier recognized. This is not to argue, however, that the aphasic symptoms and patterns are identical in children and adults; for one reason, the base frequencies of symptoms like mutism are higher in children than in adults, whereas the base frequencies of symptoms like neologisms are lower in children than in adults.

The neuroanatomy of childhood-acquired aphasia is both similar to and different from that of adulthood-acquired aphasia.[17] Only by comparing the same etiologies in childhood and in adulthood can the effect of age itself be evaluated; when the same etiology is compared in childhood and in adulthood, many language deficits prove to be similar. In children as well as in adults, a lesion in the left-hemispheric posterior cortical language areas produces a fluent aphasia and impaired comprehension;[95] specifically, the correlation between lesion site on computed tomography (CT) and aphasia in children duplicates the anatomic-clinical correlation in adults.[17] In accordance with these results, age does not predict recovery from aphasic symptoms when etiology is constant.[30]

To be sure, aphasic symptoms are not identical in children and adults with the same brain damage. Unlike adults, for example, children do not suffer speech disturbances from damage to the superior paravermal cortical regions associated with posterior fossa tumors.[99] It is also possible that differences in base rate and frequency of aphasic symptoms involve different underlying

neuropathologic substrates in children and adults. The neuroanatomy of superficially similar symptoms may prove to be different in children and adults in important ways.

The differences between acquired aphasia in children and in adults, once thought to concern short-term aphasic symptoms, now appear to relate more to long-term language function. With increasing time since aphasia, adult language improves, albeit at variable rates. Time does not always improve language function after childhood-acquired aphasia. Aphasic children may show an increasing inability to accrue a new verbal knowledge base, which results in chronic problems in reading and vocabulary development.[29,73]

Time-Related Issues and Their Importance for Theoretical Accounts and Taxonomies of Childhood-Acquired Aphasia

What seems to discriminate among the different etiologies of childhood-acquired aphasia is the time course of aphasic symptoms and recovery of language function. Aphasic symptoms arising from head injury resolve more quickly than do symptoms from infectious and vascular etiologies. Granted that abatement of symptoms varies according to etiology,[26] a continuing task in understanding childhood-acquired aphasia is to specify the time course of symptoms within conditions.

A better understanding of the time course and pattern of preserved and disrupted language skills is essential to establishing a more theoretically grounded account of the childhood-acquired aphasias. This is also relevant to the question of a taxonomy of childhood-acquired aphasic conditions.

At present, there are few plausible theories of the language disturbances underlying the principal forms of childhood-acquired aphasia. Certainly, no single theory is likely to be adequate to cover all the different etiologic manifestations of childhood aphasia. Even within a particular etiology, any theory must account for the vagaries of symptoms throughout the time course of the aphasia. For example, central receptive deficits have been proposed to be primary in LKS,[60] but a closer analysis of the time course in LKS cases with more slowly developing symptoms reveals a predominantly motor aphasia evident during a language deterioration phase,[45] which seems inconsistent with the idea of an exclusively receptive disorder at the core of this condition. Only by understanding patterns of language deficits that change over time is it possible to provide a theoretically motivated account of what distinguishes impaired from preserved language skills in childhood-acquired aphasia.

The neuroanatomy of symptom patterns over time is likely to provide important clues to the underlying mechanisms of language loss and hence to be part of any theory of acquired aphasia. It has been claimed that subcortical lesions in children may have similar long-term effects to cortical lesions; for example, one interpretation of the mutism from subcortical vascular lesions is that it arises from a transient frontal diaschisis secondary to subcortical damage.[73] Correlations between language and neuroimaging to allow a detailed comparison of cortical and subcortical lesions producing acquired aphasia have not yet been reported.

At present, the working hypothesis must be that the same acquired aphasic symptom may be produced by more than one neural mechanism. In support of this, the time course of resolution of aphasic mutism appears to be different with supratentorial and subtentorial lesions. In the case of posterior fossa tumors, the mutism resolves to dysarthria; with vascular subcortical lesions, however, the resolution of the mutism does not appear to include dysarthric symptoms.[72] This suggests a role for the cerebellum in the initiation and programming of speech, perhaps in keeping with recent concepts of its broader role in higher cognitive functions, including the timing of nonautomatized language operations.[120]

Without a theory of language disruption grounded in the time course of symptoms and long-term language function, there can be no workable taxonomy for childhood-acquired aphasia and its symptom patterns. For the most part, the loose descriptive taxonomy that exists among etiologies is based simply on frequency of reporting and aphasic symptoms for particular etiologies, with a condition like LKS somewhat over-represented in publications on childhood-acquired aphasia in relation to its frequency of occurrence.[2]

At present, neither the classic adult taxonomy of aphasia nor existing childhood language classification systems are adequate for describing childhood-acquired aphasia. When childhood-acquired aphasia cases are coded according to a taxonomy of adult aphasia,[121] some 30 to 50 percent of cases cannot be classified.[16,20,122,123] In fact, the majority of children with acquired aphasia cannot be classified in either the Goodglass adult taxonomy or a taxonomy devised for pediatric conditions.[124]

Existing taxonomies of childhood-acquired aphasia still seem to rely largely on models of adult aphasia rather than on cognitive-developmental paradigms of normal language development. Perhaps a productive approach to the issue of taxonomy would be one that used theory-driven paradigms of normal language development rather than a priori taxonomies. In recent reviews of childhood-acquired aphasia, there has been a more explicit awareness of the need for paradigms of normal language development.[54] At the same time, it has become apparent that any such paradigms must be complex and expressed as patterns of acquisition over very long time spans, because there are wide individual differences in the rate, strategy, and style of language acquisition in normally developing children, and brain damage affects language acquisition patterns in a number of different ways.[125]

Neuropathology of Language Disorders

One reason for the dearth of workable taxonomies of childhood-acquired aphasic conditions must be the limited number of clinical-pathologic correlations that would allow comparisons of patterns of neuropathology underlying language disorders. An important objective in studies of childhood-acquired aphasia has been to contrast the pathologic processes that produce acquired aphasia with those that do not.[33] Only noninvasive forms of neuroimaging make possible this endeavor; in recent years, structural and functional neuroimaging has provided information about the temporal and spatial extent of brain pathology, and hence information about the neuropathologic substrates of childhood-acquired aphasia. Of direct relevance are findings from functional neuroimaging studies suggesting what had long been suspected, that areas of brain dysfunction are much larger than the areas of structural lesion in some forms of aphasia-producing childhood vascular lesions.[126]

Studies that correlate language status with neuroimaging are able to identify the factors that produce poor recovery of language. Three such factors have been suggested: an infectious etiology, poor verbal comprehension, and involvement of Wernicke's area.[30] As a larger data base of such studies is accrued, it will become easier to understand the mechanism of recovery in cases of childhood-acquired aphasia.[10]

Because detailed structural and functional neuroimaging studies are of relatively recent origin, their potential value in shaping a taxonomy of childhood-acquired aphasia has not yet been exploited. It seems likely that the clinicopathologic correlation between language and neuroimaging will ground any taxonomy of childhood-acquired aphasic conditions.

ACKNOWLEDGMENTS

The author's research described in this paper was supported by project grants from the Ontario Mental Health Foundation and the Physicians' Services Incorporated Foundation. I thank Marcia Barnes for her critical comments on the text and Tamara Bashirullah-Abousleman for assistance with preparation of the manuscript.

REFERENCES

1. Collignon R, Hécaen H, Angelergues R: A propos de 12 cas d'aphasie acquise de l'enfant. *Acta Neurol Belg* 68:245–277, 1968.
2. Paquier P, Van Dongen HR: Current trends in acquired childhood aphasia: An introduction. *Aphasiology* 7:421–440, 1993.
3. Dennis M, Barnes MA: Developmental aspects of neuropsychology: Childhood, in Zaidel D (ed): *Handbook of Perception and Cognition: Neuropsychology.* New York: Academic Press, 1994, pp 219–246.
4. Freud S: Infantile cerebral paralysis (trans by LA Russin, 1968). Coral Gables, FL: University of Miami, 1897.
5. Assal G, Campiche R: Aphasie et troubles du langage chez l'enfant apres contusion cerebrale. *Neurochirurgie* 19(suppl 4):399–406, 1973.
6. Byers RK, McLean WT: Etiology and course of certain hemiplegias with aphasia in childhood. *Pediatrics* 29:376–383, 1962.
7. Guttmann E: Aphasia in children. *Brain* 65:205–219, 1942.
8. Alajouanine TH, Lhermitte F: Acquired aphasia in children. *Brain* 88:653–662, 1965.
9. Hécaen H: Acquired aphasia in children and the ontogenesis of hemispheric functional specialization. *Brain Lang* 3:114–134, 1976.
10. Satz P: Symptom pattern and recovery outcome in childhood aphasia: A methodological and theoretical critique, in Martins IP, Castro-Caldas A, Van Dongen HR, Van Hout A (eds): *Acquired Aphasia in Children.* Dordrecht, The Netherlands: Kluwer Academic, 1991, pp 95–114.
11. Van Dongen HR, Paquier P: Fluent aphasia in children, in Martins IP, Castro-Caldas A, Van Dongen HR, Van Hout A (eds): *Acquired Aphasia in Children.* Dordrecht, The Netherlands: Kluwer Academic, 1991, pp 125–141.
12. Visch-Brink EG, Van de Sandt-Koenderman M: The occurrence of paraphasias in the spontaneous speech of children with an acquired aphasia. *Brain Lang* 23:258–271, 1984.
13. Van Hout A: Characteristics of language in acquired aphasia in children, in Martins IP, Castro-Caldas A, Van Dongen HR, Van Hout A (eds): *Acquired Aphasia in Children.* Dordrecht, The Netherlands: Kluwer Academic, 1991, pp 117–124.
14. Woods BT, Teuber HL: Changing patterns of childhood aphasia. *Ann Neurol* 3:273–280, 1978.
15. Van Hout A, Evrard P, Lyon G: On the positive semiology of acquired aphasia in children. *Dev Med Child Neurol* 27:231–241, 1985.
16. Van Dongen HR, Loonen MCB, Van Dongen KJ: Anatomical basis for acquired fluent aphasia in children. *Ann Neurol* 17:306–309, 1985.
17. Cranberg LD, Filley CM, Hart EJ, Alexander MP: Acquired aphasia in childhood: Clinical and CT investigations. *Neurology* 37:1165–1172, 1987.
18. Hynd GW, Semrud-Clikeman M, Lorys AR, et al: Brain morphology in developmental dyslexia and

attention deficit disorder/hyperactivity. *Arch Neurol* 47:919–926, 1990.

19. Makino A, Soga T, Obayashi M, et al: Cortical blindness caused by acute general cerebral swelling. *Surg Neurol* 29:393–400, 1988.

20. Paquier P, Saerens J, Parizel PM, et al: Acquired reading disorder similar to pure alexia in a child with ruptured arteriovenous malformation. *Aphasiology* 3:667–676, 1989.

21. Rapin I: Acquired aphasia in children. *J Child Neurol* 10:267–270, 1995.

22. Landau WM, Kleffner FR: Syndrome of acquired aphasia with convulsive disorder in children. *Neurology* 7:523–530, 1957.

23. Paquier P, Van Dongen HR: Acquired childhood aphasia: A rarity? *Aphasiology* 7(suppl 5):417–419, 1993.

24. Ikeda M, Tanabe H, Yamada K, et al: A case of acquired childhood aphasia with evolution of global aphasia into transcortical sensory aphasia. *Aphasiology* 7(suppl 5):497–502, 1993.

25. Satz P, Bullard-Bates C: Acquired aphasia in children, in Sarno MT (ed): *Acquired Aphasia.* San Diego, CA: Academic Press, 1981, pp 399–426.

26. Loonen MCB, Van Dongen HR: Acquired childhood aphasia: Outcome one year after onset, in Martins IP, Castro-Caldas A, Van Dongen HR, Van Hout A (eds): *Acquired Aphasia in Children.* Dordrecht, The Netherlands: Kluwer Academic, 1991, pp 185–200.

27. Chapman SB, Culhane KA, Levin HS, et al: Narrative discourse after closed head injury in children and adolescents. *Brain Lang* 43:42–65, 1992.

28. Dennis M, Barnes MA: Knowing the meaning, getting the point, bridging the gap, and carrying the message: Aspects of discourse following closed head injury in childhood and adolescence. *Brain Lang* 3:203–229, 1990.

29. Cooper JA, Flowers CR: Children with a history of acquired aphasia: Residual language and academic impairments. *J Speech Hear Disord* 52:251–262, 1987.

30. Martins IP, Ferro JM: Recovery of acquired aphasia in children. *Aphasiology* 6(suppl 4):431–438, 1992.

31. Van Hout A: Outcome of acquired aphasia in childhood: Prognosis factors, in Martins IP, Castro-Caldas A, Van Dongen HR, Van Hout A (eds): *Acquired Aphasia in Children.* Dordrecht, The Netherlands: Kluwer Academic, 1991, pp 163–169.

32. Cross JA, Ozanne AE: Acquired childhood aphasia: Assessment and treatment, in Murdoch BE (ed): *Acquired Neurological Speech/Language Disorders in Childhood.* London: Taylor & Francis, 1990, pp 66–123.

33. Woods BT: Patient selection in studies of aphasia acquired in childhood, in Martins IP, Castro-Caldas A, Van Dongen HR, Van Hout A (eds): *Acquired Aphasia in Children.* Dordrecht, The Netherlands: Kluwer Academic, 1991, pp 27–34.

34. Taveras JM, Wood EH: *Diagnostic Neuroradiology,* 2d ed. Baltimore: Williams & Wilkins, 1976, vol 1.

35. Seron X: L'aphasie de l'enfant. *Enfance* 24:249–270, 1977.

36. Carter RL, Hohenegger MK, Satz P: Aphasia and speech organization in children. *Science* 218:797–799, 1982.

37. Hécaen H: Acquired aphasia in children: Revisited. *Neuropsychologia* 21:581–587, 1983.

38. Satz P, Lewis R: Acquired aphasia in children, in Blanken G, Dittmann J, Grimm H, Marshall JC, Wallesch C-W (eds): *Linguistic Disorders and Pathologies: An International Handbook.* Berlin: Walter de Gruyter, 1993, pp 646–659.

39. Dennis M: Strokes in childhood: I. Communicative intent, expression, and comprehension after left hemisphere arteriopathy in a right-handed nine-year-old, in Rieber R (ed): *Language Development and Aphasia in Children.* New York: Academic Press, 1980, pp 45–67.

40. Martins IP, Ferro JM: Recovery from aphasia and lesion size in the temporal lobe, in Martins IP, Castro-Caldas A, Van Dongen HR, Van Hout A (eds): *Acquired Aphasia in Children.* Dordrecht, The Netherlands: Kluwer Academic, 1991, pp 171–184.

41. Murdoch BE: *Acquired Speech and Language Disorders: A Neuroanatomical and Functional Neurological Approach.* London: Chapman & Hall, 1990.

42. Deonna T, Davidoff V, Roulet E: Isolated disturbance of written language acquisition as an initial symptom of epileptic aphasia in a 7-year old child: A 3-year follow-up study. *Aphasiology* 7(suppl 5):441–450, 1993.

43. Deonna T, Beaumanoir A, Gaillard F, Assal G: Acquired aphasia in childhood with seizure disorder: A heterogeneous syndrome. *Neuropadiatrie* 8:263–273, 1977.

44. Lou HC, Brandt S, Bruhn P: Aphasia and epilepsy in childhood. *Acta Neurol Scand* 56:46–54, 1977.

45. Marien P, Saerens J, Verslegers W, et al: Some

controversies about type and nature of aphasic symptomatology in Landau-Kleffner's syndrome: A case study. *Acta Neurol Belg* 93:183–203, 1993.

46. Soprano AM, Garcia EF, Caraballo R, Fejerman N: Acquired epileptic aphasia: Neuropsychologic follow-up of 12 patients. *Pediatr Neurol* 11(suppl 3):230–235, 1994.

47. MantoVani JF, Landau WM: Acquired aphasia with convulsive disorder. *Neurology* 30:524–529, 1980.

48. Papagno C, Basso A: Impairment of written language and mathematical skills in a case of Landau-Kleffner syndrome. *Aphasiology* 7:451–461, 1993.

49. Cooper JA, Ferry PC: Acquired auditory verbal agnosia and seizures in childhood. *J Speech Hear Disord* 43:176–184, 1978.

50. Appleton RE: The Landau-Kleffner syndrome. *Arch Dis Child* 72:386–387, 1995.

51. Dugas M, Gerard CL, Franc S, Sagar D: Natural history, course and prognosis of the Landau and Kleffner syndrome, in Martins IP, Castro-Caldas A, Van Dongen HR, Van Hout A (eds): *Acquired Aphasia in Children.* Dordrecht, The Netherlands: Kluwer Academic, 1991, pp 263–277.

52. Aicardi J: Syndrome of acquired aphasia with seizure disorder: Epileptic aphasia, Landau-Kleffner syndrome, and verbal auditory agnosia with convulsive disorder, in Aicardi J (ed): *Epilepsy in Children.* New York: Raven Press, 1986, pp 176–182.

53. Dugas M, Masson M, Le Heuzey MF, Regnier N: Aphasie "acquise" de l'enfant avec epilepsie (syndrome de Landau et Kleffner): Douze observations personnelles. *Rev Neurol* 138:755–780, 1982.

54. Martins IP: Introduction, in Martins IP, Castro-Caldas A, Van Dongen HR, Van Hout A (eds): *Acquired Aphasia in Children.* Dordrecht, The Netherlands: Kluwer Academic, 1991, pp 3–12.

55. Worster-Drought C: An unusual form of acquired aphasia in children. *Dev Med Child Neurol* 13:563–571, 1971.

56. Genton P, Guerrini R: The Landau-Kleffner syndrome or acquired aphasia with convulsive disorder. *Arch Neurol* 50:1009, 1993.

57. Van Dongen HR, De Wijngaert E, Wennekes MJ: The Landau-Kleffner syndrome: Diagnostic considerations, in Martins IP, Castro-Caldas A, Van Dongen HR, Van Hout A (eds): *Acquired Aphasia in Children.* Dordrecht, The Netherlands: Kluwer Academic, 1991, pp 253–261.

58. Landau WM: Landau-Kleffner syndrome. *Arch Neurol* 49:353, 1992.

59. Gerard C-L, Dugas M, Valdois S, Franc S, Lecendreux M: Landau-Kleffner syndrome diagnosed after 9 years of age: Another Landau-Kleffner syndrome? *Aphasiology* 7:463–473, 1993.

60. Bishop DVM: Age of onset and outcome in "acquired aphasia with convulsive disorder." *Dev Med Child Neurol* 27:705–712, 1985.

61. Paquier PF, Van Dongen HR, Loonen CB: The Landau-Kleffner syndrome or "acquired aphasia with convulsive disorder." *Arch Neurol* 49:354–359, 1992.

62. Shoumaker RD, Bennett DR, Bray PF, Curless RG: Clinical and EEG manifestations of an unusual aphasic syndrome in children. *Neurology* 24:10–16, 1974.

63. McKinney W, McGreal DA: An aphasic syndrome in children. *Can Med Assoc J* 110:637–639, 1974.

64. Pascual-Castroviejo I, Lopez Martin VL, Martinez Bermejo AM, Perez Higueras AP: Is cerebral arteritis the cause of the Landau-Kleffner syndrome? Four cases in childhood with angiographic study. *Can J Neurol Sci* 19:46–52, 1992.

65. Nevsimalova S, Tauberova A, Doutlik S, et al: A role of autoimmunity in the etiopathogenesis of Landau-Kleffner syndrome? *Brain Dev* 14:342–345, 1992.

66. Maquet P, Hirsch E, Dive D, et al: Cerebral glucose utilization during sleep in Landau-Kleffner syndrome: A PET study. *Epilepsia* 31:778–783, 1990.

67. De Wijngaert E, Gommers K: Language rehabilitation in the Landau-Kleffner syndrome: Considerations and approaches. *Aphasiology* 7(suppl 5):475–480, 1993.

68. Ozanne AE, Murdoch BE: Acquired childhood aphasia: Neuropathology, linguistic characteristics and prognosis, in Murdoch BE (ed): *Acquired Neurological Speech/Language Disorders in Childhood.* London: Taylor & Francis, 1990, pp 1–65.

69. Zimmerman RA, Bilaniuk LT, Packer RJ, et al: Computed tomographic-arteriographic correlates in acute basal ganglionic infarction in childhood. *Neuroradiology* 24:241–248, 1983.

70. Hynd GW, Leathem J, Semrud-Clikeman M, et al: Anomic aphasia in childhood. *J Child Neurol* 10:189–293, 1995.

71. Klein SK, Masur D, Farber K, et al: Fluent aphasia in children: Definition and natural history. *J Child Neurol* 7:50–59, 1992.

72. Aram DM, Rose DF, Rekate HI, Whitaker HA:

Acquired capsular/striatal aphasia in childhood. *Arch Neurol* 40:614–617, 1983.

73. Martins IP, Ferro JM: Acquired childhood aphasia: A clinicoradiological study of 11 stroke patients. *Aphasiology* 7(suppl 5):489–495, 1993.

74. Eisele JA: Selective deficits in language comprehension following early left and right hemisphere damage, in Martins IP, Castro-Caldas A, Van Dongen HR, Van Hout A (eds): *Acquired Aphasia in Children.* Dordrecht, The Netherlands: Kluwer, 1991, pp 225–238.

75. Eisele JA, Aram DM: Differential effects of early hemisphere damage on lexical comprehension and production. *Aphasiology* 7:513–523, 1993.

76. Jordan FM: Speech and language disorders following childhood closed head injury, in Murdoch BE (ed): *Acquired Neurological Speech/Language Disorders in Childhood.* London: Taylor & Francis, 1990, pp 124–147.

77. Ommaya AK, Grubb RL, Naumann RA: Coup and contrecoup injury: Observations on the mechanics of visible brain injuries in the rhesus monkey. *J Neurosurg* 35:503–516, 1971.

78. Van Dongen HR, Loonen MCB: Factors related to prognosis of acquired aphasia in children. *Cortex* 13:131–136, 1977.

79. Loonen MCB, Van Dongen HR: Acquired childhood aphasia: Outcome one year after onset. *Arch Neurol* 47:1324–1328, 1990.

80. Ewing-Cobbs L, Fletcher JM, Landry SH, Levin HS: Language disorders after pediatric head injury, in Darby JK (ed): *Speech and Language Evaluation in Neurology: Childhood Disorders.* San Diego, CA: Grune & Stratton, 1985, pp 97–111.

81. Ewing-Cobbs L, Fletcher JM, Levin HS, Eisenberg HM: Language functions following closed head injury in children and adolescents. *J Clin Exp Neuropsychol* 5:575–592, 1987.

82. Goldstein FC, Levin HS: Epidemiology of pediatric closed head injury: Incidence, clinical characteristics, and risk factors. *J Learn Disabil* 20:518–525, 1987.

83. Annegers JF: The epidemiology of head trauma in children, in Shapiro K (ed): *Pediatric Head Trauma.* Mt. Kisco, NY: Futura, 1983, pp 1–10.

84. Ewing-Cobbs L, Iovino I, Fletcher JM, et al: Academic achievement following traumatic brain injury in children and adolescents (abstr). *J Clin Exp Neuropsychol* 13:93, 1991.

85. Ewing-Cobbs L, Miner ME, Fletcher JM, Levin HS: Intellectual, motor, and language sequelae fol-lowing closed head injury in infants and preschoolers. *J Pediatr Psychol* 14:531–547, 1989.

86. Dennis M, Barnes MA, Donnelly RE, et al: Appraising and managing knowledge: Metacognitive skills after childhood head injury. *Dev Neuropsychol* 12:77–103, 1996.

87. Dennis M, Wilkinson M, Humphreys RP: How children with head injury represent real and deceptive emotion in short narratives. *Brain Lang* 1996. In press.

88. Jordan FM, Ozanne AE, Murdoch BE: Long-term speech and language disorders subsequent to closed head injury in children. *Brain Inj* 2:179–185, 1988.

89. Jordan FM, Ozanne AE, Murdoch BE: Performance of closed head injury children on a naming task. *Brain Inj* 4:27–32, 1990.

90. Jordan FM, Murdoch BE: A prospective study of the linguistic skills of children with closed-head injuries. *Aphasiology* 7:503–512, 1993.

91. McDonald S: Viewing the brain sideways? Frontal versus right hemisphere explanations of nonaphasic language disorders. *Aphasiology* 7:535–549, 1993.

92. Campbell TF, Dollaghan CA: Expressive language recovery in severely brain-injured children and adolescents. *J Speech Hear Disord* 55:567–586, 1990.

93. Jordan FM, Murdoch BE: Linguistic status following closed head injury in children: A follow-up study. *Brain Inj* 4:147–154, 1990.

94. Grattan LM, Eslinger PJ: Frontal lobe damage in children and adults: A comparative review. *Dev Neuropsychol* 7:283–326, 1991.

95. Martins IP, Ferro JM: Type of aphasia and lesions' localization, in Martins IP, Castro-Caldas A, Van Dongen HR, Van Hout A (eds): *Acquired Aphasia in Children.* Dordrecht, The Netherlands: Kluwer Academic, 1991, pp 143–159.

96. Hudson LJ: Speech and language disorders in childhood brain tumours, in Murdoch BE (ed): *Acquired Neurological Speech/Language Disorders in Childhood.* London: Taylor & Francis, 1990, pp 245–268.

97. Humphreys RP: Mutism after posterior fossa tumor surgery. *Concepts Pediatr Neurosurg* 9:57–64, 1989.

98. Rekate HL, Grubb RL, Aram DL, et al: Muteness of cerebellar origin. *Arch Neurol* 42:697–698, 1985.

99. Van Dongen HR, Catsman-Berrevoets CE, Van Mourik M: The syndrome of "cerebellar" mutism

and subsequent dysarthria. *Neurology* 44:2040–2046, 1994.

100. Hudson LJ, Murdoch BE, Ozanne AE: Posterior fossa tumours in childhood: Associated speech and language disorders post-surgery. *Aphasiology* 3:1–18, 1989.

101. Hudson LJ, Murdoch BE: Language recovery following surgery and CNS prophylaxis for the treatment of childhood medulloblastoma: A prospective study of three cases. *Aphasiology* 6:17–28, 1992.

102. Dennis M, Spiegler BJ, Hetherington CR, Greenberg ML: Neuropsychological sequelae of the treatment of children with medulloblastoma. *J Neurooncol* 1996. In press.

103. Hirsch JF, Reiner D, Czernichow P, et al: Medulloblastoma in childhood: Survival and functional results. *Acta Neurochir* 48:1–15, 1979.

104. Johnson DL, McCabe MA, Nicholson HS, et al: Quality of long-term survival in young children with medulloblastoma. *J Neurosurg* 80:1004–1010, 1994.

105. Ammirati M, Mirzai S, Samii M: Transient mutism following removal of a cerebellar tumour: A case report and review of the literature. *Childs Nerv Syst* 5:12–14, 1989.

106. Withers HR: Biological basis of radiation therapy for cancer. *Lancet* 339:156–159, 1992.

107. Dropcho EJ: Central nervous system injury by therapeutic irradiation. *Neurol Clin* 9:969–988, 1991.

108. Hudson LJ, Buttsworth DL, Murdoch BE: Effect of CNS prophylaxis on speech and language function in children, in Murdoch BE (ed): *Acquired Neurological Speech/Language Disorders in Childhood.* London: Taylor & Francis, 1990, pp 269–307.

109. Smyth V, Ozanne AE, Woodhouse LM: Communicative disorders in childhood infectious diseases, in Murdoch BE (ed): *Acquired Neurological Speech/Language Disorders in Childhood.* London: Taylor & Francis, 1990, pp 148–176.

110. Paquier P, Van Dongen HR: Two contrasting cases of fluent aphasia in children. *Aphasiology* 5:235–245, 1991.

111. Van Hout A, Lyon G: Wernicke's aphasia in a 10-year-old boy. *Brain Lang* 29:268–285, 1986.

112. Kleiman MB, Carver DH: Central nervous system infections, in Black P (ed): *Brain Dysfunction in Children: Etiology, Diagnosis, and Management.* New York: Raven Press, 1981, pp 79–107.

113. Murdoch BE, Ozanne AE: Linguistic status following acute cerebral anoxia in children, in Murdoch BE (ed): *Acquired Neurological Speech/Language Disorders in Childhood.* London: Taylor & Francis, 1990, pp 177–198.

114. Murdoch BE, Chenery HJ, Kennedy M: Aphemia associated with bilateral striato-capsular lesions subsequent to cerebral anoxia. *Brain Inj* 3:41–49, 1989.

115. Pearn JM, DeBuse P, Mohay M, Golden M: Sequential intellectual recovery after near-drowning. *Med J Aust* 1:463–464, 1979.

116. Reilly K, Ozanne AE, Murdoch BE, Pitt WR: Linguistic status subsequent to childhood immersion injury. *Med J Aust* 149:225–228, 1988.

117. Ozanne AE, Murdoch BE, Krimmer HL: Linguistic problems associated with childhood metabolic disorders, in Murdoch BE (ed): *Acquired Neurological Speech/Language Disorders in Childhood.* London: Taylor & Francis, 1990, pp 199–215.

118. Dennis M: Word finding after brain-injury in children and adolescents. *Top Lang Disord* 13:66–82, 1992.

119. Kleinman SN, Waber DP: Neurodevelopmental bases of spelling acquisition in children treated for acute lymphoblastic leukemia. *Cog Neuropsychol* 9:403–425, 1992.

120. Schmahmann JD: An emerging concept: The cerebellar contribution to higher function. *Arch Neurol* 48:1178–1186, 1991.

121. Goodglass H, Kaplan E: *The Assessment of Aphasia and Related Disorders.* Philadelphia: Lea & Febiger, 1972.

122. Marshall JC: The description and interpretation of aphasic language disorder. *Neuropsychologia* 24:5–24, 1986.

123. Martins IP, Ferro JM: Acquired conduction aphasia in a child. *Dev Med Child Neurol* 29:529–540, 1987.

124. Lees JA: Differentiating language disorder subtypes in acquired childhood aphasia. *Aphasiology* 7(suppl 5):481–488, 1993.

125. Bates E, Thal D, Janowsky JS: Early language development and its neural correlates, in Boller F, Grafman J (eds): *Handbook of Neuropsychology.* Amsterdam: Elsevier Science, 1992, vol 7, pp 69–110.

126. Shahar E, Gilday DL, Hwang PA, et al: Pediatric cerebrovascular disease: Alterations of regional cerebral blood flow detected by TC 99m–HMPAO SPECT. *Arch Neurol* 47:578–584, 1990.

Chapter 61

SPECIFIC LANGUAGE IMPAIRMENTS

Karin Stromswold

DEFINITION AND DIAGNOSIS OF SPECIFIC LANGUAGE IMPAIRMENTS

Without any formal instruction, essentially all normal children who are exposed to it acquire language in a remarkably uniform, rapid, and essentially error-free manner.[1,2] Over the years, researchers have reported that some apparently normal children inexplicably have difficulty acquiring language. These children have been said to suffer from childhood aphasia, congenital aphasia, congenital auditory imperception, congenital word deafness, developmental aphasia, developmental dysphasia, developmental language disorders, dyslogia, or idioglosia.[3] Today, *specific language impairments* (SLI) is the generally accepted term for developmental disorders characterized by severe deficits in the production and/or comprehension of language that cannot be explained by hearing loss, mental retardation, motor deficits, neurologic or psychiatric disorders, or lack of exposure to language. In order to receive the diagnosis of SLI, a child must meet inclusionary and exclusionary criteria such as those given in Table 61-1.[4–10] Special care must be taken to distinguish between developmental and acquired language disorders (see Chap. 60). Thus, in order to receive the diagnosis of SLI, a child cannot have risk factors associated with acquired brain injury (e.g., meningitis, head injuries resulting in loss of consciousness, etc.) or a clinical history consistent with acquired language disorders (e.g., cessation or regression of language skills). Last, children with SLI who are

unable to speak must be distinguished from those who choose not to speak (i.e., children with elective mutism).

TYPES OF SPECIFIC LANGUAGE IMPAIRMENT

Because SLI is a diagnosis of exclusion, SLI children are a very heterogeneous group. They vary in the degree to which expressive and/or receptive language skills are impaired and also in the degree to which the different subcomponents of language (i.e., syntax, semantics, morphology, phonology, pragmatics, and the lexicon) are affected. This heterogeneity can and does affect the outcome of behavioral and neurologic studies, with different studies frequently reporting different results, depending on how SLI subjects were selected. The heterogeneity of SLI is problematic not just for basic researchers who seek to discover the nature and etiology of SLI and for applied researchers who attempt to evaluate the efficacy of different types of therapeutic interventions but also for clinicians who must diagnose, evaluate, refer, and make prognoses about SLI children.

Researchers and clinicians have attempted to address this diversity by proposing classification systems for developmental language impairments (see Table 61-2). Developmental language disorders have been classified according to etiology,[11] language function (i.e., repetition, comprehension, production, etc.),[12–14] neuropsychological or neu-

Table 61-1

Diagnostic criteria for specific language impairments

1. Severe language disorder (e.g., performance on standardized language tests at least 6 to 12 months below chronological or mental age)

2. Normal hearing (hearing threshholds below 25 dB between 250 and 6000 Hz)

3. Normal nonverbal intelligence (performance IQ no more than 1 SD below the mean)

4. No "hard" neurologic signs ("soft" neurologic signs allowed)

5. No disorders, diseases, or injuries affecting the central nervous system (e.g., Down syndrome, cerebral palsy, familial dysautonomia, meningitis, severe head injury)

6. Articulation skills commensurate with expressive language skills (i.e., articulation no more than 6 months behind expressive language skills)

7. No obvious structural or functional peripheral oral-motor abnormalities

8. No evidence of a frank psychiatric, emotional, or behavioral disorder (e.g., no severe behavioral or adjustment problems noted by parents or teachers)

9. No history of neglect or abuse

10. Adequate exposure to language

11. No evidence of acquired language disorder (i.e., no cessation or regression of language)

Source: Adapted from Stark and Tallal,[10] with permission.

rolinguistic profile,[15–17] linguistic profile,[18,19] or some combination of the above.[20] Some of these classification systems are based on language-impaired children's patterns of performance on batteries of language tests,[13,15–17] and others are based on patterns of impairments clinically observed in language-impaired children.[12,19,20] However, none of these classification system has gained widespread acceptance in either clinical or research settings. Aram and colleagues[5] advocate that, given the lack of a widely accepted classification system and the varying degree of congruence between and among SLI populations identified by poor performance on standardized tests and those identified by clinical judgment, it is of paramount

importance that clinicians and researchers describe in detail how SLI children are identified.

THE ETIOLOGY OF SPECIFIC LANGUAGE IMPAIRMENTS: WHAT IS THE UNDERLYING DEFICIT?

Until recently, most studies of SLI have been concerned with the etiology or risk factors associated with SLI (see Table 61-3). Despite this, the etiology of SLI remains uncertain.[21] Researchers have proposed that SLI children suffer from impoverished or deviant linguistic input,[22,23] transient, fluctuating hearing loss,[24–27] impairment in short-term auditory memory,[28–30] impairment in auditory sequencing,[31,32] impairment in rapid auditory processing,[33–35] general impairment in sequencing,[36] general impairment in rapid sensory processing,[37] general impairment in representational or symbolic reasoning,[38–40] general impairment in hierarchical planning,[41] impairments in language perception or processing (e.g., the inability to acquire aspects of language that are not phonologically salient[42–44]), impairments in underlying grammar (e.g., the lack of linguistic features such as tense and number,[45–48] the inability to use government to analyze certain types of syntactic relations,[49] the inability to form certain types of agreement relations,[50–52] etc.), or some combination of the above. Some researchers have even suggested that SLI is not a distinct clinical entity, and that SLI children just represent the low end of the normal continuum in linguistic ability.[8,53]

None of the proposed etiologies of SLI have received unambiguous empirical support. A problem for theories that propose relatively general impairments as the basis of SLI[36–41] is that, although such general impairments might well cause secondary linguistic deficits, they should also cause more pervasive behavioral deficits. Another major difficulty in ascertaining the underlying impairment in SLI is distinguishing whether the impairment under investigation is the *cause* of the linguistic deficit or the *result* of the linguistic deficit. For example, although results of several studies suggest that parents may speak differently to SLI children than to normal children,[22,23,54] there are no convincing data to suggest that differences in parental input *cause* SLI.[55] Parents may speak differently to SLI children because they are compensating for their children's language impairments. In other words, SLI children's linguistic impairments may cause the differences in parental input, rather than vice versa. Results of a number of studies[26,56–59] indicate that, although there does seem to be a relationship between language delay and chronic otitis media, language delays tend to resolve once hearing impairments resolve and there is no convincing evidence that transient episodes of otitis media result in persistent language impairment (but see Ref. 27). Tallal and Piercy[33–35] have argued that SLI children's language disorders result from their general difficulty in processing auditory information that changes rapidly. They have shown, for example, that SLI children do not categorically perceive stop consonants (e.g., /b/ and /p/) in the same way that normal children do.[33–35] Although the inability to perceive consonants categorically could be the result of a disorder in rapid auditory processing, it is also possible that by virtue of their linguistic deficits, SLI children do not have normal exposure to the phonemes of their language. If this is the case, then it may be that SLI children do not perceive phonemes categorically for the same reason that adult Japanese speakers have difficulty perceiving /l/ and /r/ categorically:[60–62] neither SLI children nor Japanese adults have had enough exposure to the linguistic stimuli necessary to permit categorical perception of these speech sounds.

In many studies of SLI children's nonverbal abilities, SLI children must understand verbal instructions or respond verbally. For example, one of the studies most frequently cited as evidence that SLI children have a general representational deficit is a mental rotation study.[38] In this study, SLI and normal children had to decide whether pairs of geometric figures rotated 45, 90, and 135° were the same or were mirror images. In order to do this, the SLI children had to understand complex verbal instructions and they had to make subtle left/right judgments—two tasks that language-impaired children frequently have difficulty with.

Despite this, SLI children were just as accurate as normal children and differed only in the amount of time it took them to do the task. Even in studies that do not require verbal responses, having linguistic labels may be useful in performing the task.[41]

In summary, *the* cause of SLI is not known. Given the heterogeneity in the children diagnosed with SLI, it is extremely unlikely that all children with SLI suffer from the same underlying impairment. Furthermore, it is likely that in many cases, whether a child will have a clinically evident language impairment depends on multiple, interacting factors. For example, whereas transient, fluctuating hearing loss might have no noticeable effect on the linguistic development of children who are not at risk for SLI, it might have a devastating effect on the linguistic development of children who are at risk for SLI.[57] Similarly, whereas most children appear to be able to acquire language within a wide range of linguistic environments, children who are at risk for developing SLI might require an optimal linguistic environment in order to acquire normal language.

THE NEURAL BASIS OF SPECIFIC LANGUAGE IMPAIRMENTS

At the neural level, the cause of SLI is also uncertain. Prior to the advent of modern neuroimaging techniques, it was theorized that children with SLI had bilateral damage to the perisylvian cortical regions that subserve language in adults.[63] Contrary to the bilateral-damage theory, computed tomography (CT) and magnetic resonance imaging (MRI) scans of SLI children have failed to reveal the types of gross perisylvian lesions typically found in patients with acquired aphasia.[64–66] However, CT and MRI scans have revealed that the brains of SLI children often do not have the normal pattern of the left temporal plane being larger than the right temporal plane.[64–66] Results from dichotic listening[67–71] and auditory evoked response potential (AEP) experiments[72] suggest that at least some SLI children have aberrant functional lateralization for language, with language

Table 61-2

Classification systems for developmental language disorders

Aram and Nation (1975)[13]

Repetition strength
Nonspecific formulation-repetition deficit
Generalized low performance
Phonologic comprehension-formulation-repetition deficit
Comprehension deficit
Formulation-repetition deficit

Bishop and Rosenbloom (1987)[18]

Type of language disorder			Examples
Phonology			
	Expressive	Immature	Cluster reduction, final consonant deletion, fronting (e.g., "k" pronounced as "t")
		Deviant	Initial consonant deletion
	Receptive	Immature	?
		Deviant	?
Grammar			
	Expressive	Immature	Simple, telegraphic sentences lacking grammatical markers (e.g., "me want cookie")
			Grammatical overregularization ("goed" for "went")
		Deviant	Restricted use of a single sentence frame
			Bizarre syntax (e.g., "me buy go sweets")
	Receptive	Immature	Tendency to ignore inflectional endings
		Deviant	Systematic misunderstanding of some structures
Semantics			
	Expressive	Immature	Overextension of word meanings
		Deviant	Frequent failure to produce words that are known
	Receptive	Immature	Weak vocabulary
		Deviant	Confused if one word has different meanings
Pragmatic			
	Expressive	Immature	Failure to use polite forms
		Deviant	Use of inappropriately stilted language
	Receptive	Immature	Failure to recognize sarcasm
		Deviant	Tendency to respond to utterances literally

Bloom and Lahey (1978)[19]

Impairment in form (i.e., syntax, morphology, and phonology)
Impairment in content (i.e., semantics and the lexicon)
Impairment in use (i.e., pragmatics and discourse)

Curtiss and Tallal (1988)[14]

Expressive language disorder
Receptive language disorder
Mixed language disorder

Denckla (1981)[15]

Anomic disorder (impaired naming with intact comprehension and repetition)

Table 61-2

Classification systems for developmental language disorders (Continued)

Denckla (1981)[15]

Anomic disorder with repetition deficits
Dysphonemic sequencing disorder (phonemic substitutions and missequencing)
Verbal memory disorder
Mixed language disorder (impaired repetition, comprehension, and production)
Right hemisyndrome with mixed language disorder

DSM-IV (1994)[12]

Expressive language disorder
Mixed expressive/receptive language disorder
Phonologic disorder (developmental articulation disorder in DMS-IIIR)

Ingram (1969)[11]

Disorders of voicing (dysphonia)
Disorders of respiratory coordination (dysrhythmia)
Disorders of speech sound production (dysarthria)
Disorders of speech sound production secondary to other diseases or adverse environmental factors (e.g., mental retardation, deafness, psychiatric disorder, acquired dysphasias)
Developmental speech disorders—developmental expressive and receptive dysphasia

Korkman and Hakkinen-Rihu (1994)[16]

Specific dyspraxia subtype
Specific comprehension subtype
Specific dysnomia subtype
Global subtype

Rapin and Allen (1983)[20]

Phonologic syntactic syndrome (with or without oromotor dysfunction)
Severe expressive syndrome with good comprehension
Verbal auditory agnosia (phonetic decoding deficit)
Syntactic-pragmatic syndrome
Semantic-pragmatic syndrome without autism ("cocktail party" speech)
Mute autistic syndrome
Autistic syndrome with echolalia

Wilson and Risucci (1986)[17]

Auditory semantic comprehension disorder
Auditory and visual semantic comprehension disorder
Auditory semantic comprehension and auditory and visual short-term memory disorder
Expressive and/or receptive disorder
Global disorder
Auditory memory and retrieval disorder
Expressive disorder
No deficits

Table 61-3

Proposed etiologies and underlying impairments in specific language impairments

Disorders affecting adequate input
    Hearing loss
    Impoverished linguistic input

Disorders affecting adequate output
    Subtle structural or functional oral-motor disorders (e.g., oral motor dyspraxia)

Disorders affecting auditory processing
    Auditory short-term memory
    Auditory sequencing
    Rapid auditory processing

Non-modality-specific disorders
    Impairment in short-term memory/storage
    Impairment in sequencing
    Impairment in rapid sensory processing
    Impairment in representation/symbolic reasoning
    Impairment in hierarchical planning

Linguistic disorders
    Disorders of performance
    Disorders of competence

No disorder (SLI children represent the low end of normal continuum)

Multifactorial

either present bilaterally or predominantly in the right hemisphere. Single photon emission computed tomography (SPECT) studies of normal and language-impaired children have revealed hypoperfusion in the inferior frontal convolution of the left hemisphere (including Broca's area) in two children with isolated expressive language impairment,[73] hypoperfusion of the left temporoparietal region and the upper and middle regions of the right frontal lobe in 9 of 12 children with expressive and receptive language impairment,[73] and hypoperfusion in the left temporofrontal region of language-impaired children's brains.[74]

Because SLI is not a fatal disorder and people with SLI have normal life spans, only one brain of a possible SLI child has come to autopsy to date. Postmortem examination of this brain revealed atypical symmetry of the temporal planes and a dysplastic microgyrus on the inferior surface of the left frontal cortex along the inferior surface of the sylvian fissure,[75] findings similar to those reported for dyslexic brains.[76–80] Although it is tempting to use the results of this autopsy to argue—as Geschwind and Galaburda[79] have for dyslexia—that SLI is the result of subtle anomalies in the left perisylvian cortex, the child whose brain was autopsied had a performance IQ of only 74 (verbal IQ 70); hence, the anomalies noted on autopsy may be related to the child's general cognitive impairment rather than to her language impairment.

GENETIC STUDIES OF SPECIFIC LANGUAGE IMPAIRMENTS

Genetic studies of SLI are important for several reasons. If SLI is genetically transmitted, family history can aid in diagnosis. Genetically homogeneous groups are also advantageous for both basic and applied research. Last, if SLI is heritable, this suggests that it is not caused by impoverished linguistic environments or other environmental insults. Table 61-4 summarizes the results of 12 epidemiologic studies of familial aggregation of developmental spoken language disorders.[81–92] All 12 studies found that a higher percentage of language-impaired children had a positive family history of language impairment (between 30 and 70 percent) than did normal (control) children (between 11 to 46 percent).[81–92] In all but one of the 12 studies,[92] the difference was significant. All 12 studies also revealed that a higher percentage of the relatives of language-impaired children were language-impaired (between 9 to 42 percent) than were the relatives of the control children (between 2 and 18 percent).[81–92] In all but one of the 12 studies,[92] the difference was significant. Although it is possible that children who have language-impaired parents or siblings are more likely to be linguistically impaired themselves because they are exposed to deviant language, the deviant linguistic environment (DLE) account is unlikely for a number of reasons. First, research on language acquisition reveals that within a fairly wide range, linguistic environment has little or no effect on

Table 61-4

Family aggregation studies of language disorders

Authors	Sample size	Proband diagnosis	Other diagnoses counted for plus family history	Presence of positive family history in probands and controls	Frequency of impairment in relatives of probands and controls
Ingram (1959)	75 probands	Developmental speech and language disorders	None	24% positive parental history 32% positive sibling history	N.A.
Luchsinger (1970)	127 probands	Developmental speech retardation	None	36% probands	N.A.
Byrne, Willerman, and Ashmore (1974)	18 severely impaired, 20 moderately impaired	Delayed speech	None	17% "severe" probands 55% "moderate" probands[b]	N.A.
Neils and Aram (1986)	74 probands, 36 controls	Developmental language disorders	Dyslexia, stuttering, articulation	46% first-degree proband relatives 8% first-degree control relatives[d]	20% all proband relatives 3% all control relatives[c]
Lewis, Ekelman, and Aram (1989)	20 probands, 20 controls	Phonologic disorder	Dyslexia, stuttering, LD	N.A.	*LI:* 9% all proband relatives vs. 1% all control relatives[d] *All disorders:* 12% all proband relatives vs. 2% all control relatives[d]
Tallal, Ross, and Curtiss (1989)	62 probands, 50 controls	Specific language impairment	Dyslexia, LD, school problem	77% first-degree proband relatives 46% first-degree control relatives[c]	42% first-degree proband relatives vs. 19% first-degree control relatives[c]
Tomblin (1989)	51 probands, 136 controls	Receiving speech or language therapy	Stuttering, articulation	53% first-degree proband relatives Controls: N.A.	23% first-degree proband relatives vs. 3% first-degree control relatives[d]
Haynes and Naido (1991)	156 probands	Specific language impairment	None	54% all proband relatives 41% first-degree proband relatives	28% proband parents affected, 18% proband sibs affected
Tomblin, Hardy, and Hein (1991)	55 probands, 607 normal	Lowest 10th percentile on test (50) or clinical history (5)	+FH = 1 first-degree or >1 extended family member	35% of low language 17% of normals[c]	N.A.
Whitehurst et al. (1991)	62 probands, 55 controls	Isolated expressive language delay	Late talker, speech problem, school problem	N.A.	*Late-talker:* 12% first-degree proband vs. 7% first-degree control relatives, NS *Speech:* 12% first-degree proband relative vs. 8% first-degree control relatives, NS
Beitchman, Hood, and Inglis (1992)	136 probands, 138 controls	Speech, language, or voicing disorder or stuttering	Dyslexia, LD, articulation	47% all proband relatives vs. 28% all control relatives[c] 34% first-degree proband relatives vs. 11% first-degree control relative[d]	N.A.
Lewis (1992)	87 probands, 79 controls	Phonologic disorder	Dyslexia, LD, stuttering, hearing loss	N.A.	*LI:* 14% all proband relatives vs. 2% all control relatives[d] (26% vs 4% for first-degree[d]) Significant differences for dyslexia and LD but not stuttering or hearing loss.

Key: Statistical significance (one-tailed test): [a]$p < .05$, [b]$p < .01$, [c]$p < .001$, [d]$p < .0001$; FH = family history; LD = unspecified learning disability; LI = language impairment; NA = not available; NS = not significant.

Source: Adapted from Stromswold,[95] with permission.

language acquisition by normal children.[1,2,93,94] In addition, the DLE makes a number of predictions that were not borne out in these studies.[95] For example, contrary to the DLE, the more severely impaired children did not systematically have families with higher incidence of language impairment, and parents with a history of spoken language impairment who were no longer impaired were significantly more likely to have SLI children than were parents with no such history.

Monozygotic (MZ) twins and dizygotic (DZ) twins share essentially the same pre- and postnatal environment, whereas MZ twins share 100 percent of their genetic material and, on average, DZ twins share only 50 percent of their genetic material.[96] Therefore if, for a particular trait, MZ twins are more similar to one another than are DZ twins, this suggests that genetic factors play a role in the expression of that trait. Table 61-5 summarizes the results of five twin studies of spoken and written language disorders.[97–101] In all four studies that investigated the concordance rates for language disorders in twins.[97–99,101] the concordance rates were significantly greater for MZ twins (between 51 and 84 percent) than for DZ twins (between

20 and 32 percent), indicating that genetic factors play a role in written and spoken language disorders. DeFries and Gillis[98] also performed a multiple regression analysis on their twins' scores on standardized reading tests. This analysis revealed that 50 percent of their subjects' reading deficits were attributable to heritable factors.[98] In a different type of study, Locke and Mather[100] compared the articulation errors of MZ and DZ twins and found that MZ twins were significantly more likely to mispronounce the same target words than were DZ twins. However, MZ twins were no more likely to mispronounce a word in exactly the same way than were DZ twins.[100]

Stromswold[95] reviewed nine twin studies of spoken and written language disorders and found that in all nine studies, the pairwise and probandwise concordancy rates were greater for MZ than DZ twin pairs. Overall, the nine studies included 400 MZ twin pairs and 293 DZ twin pairs. The overall pairwise concordancy rates were 66.0 percent for MZ twins and 29.7 percent for DZ twins (chi square(1) = 89.19, $p < .0000005$).[95] The overall probandwise concordancy rates were 79.5 percent for MZ twins and 45.8 percent for DZ twins

Table 61-5

Twin studies of language

Study	MZ twins	DZ twins	Proband selection	MZ pairwise concordance rate	DZ pairwise concordance rate
Bakwin[97]	31 (19 male, 12 female)	31 (19 male, 12 female)	History of dyslexia	Overall, 84% Male, 84% Female, 83%	Overall, 29%[d] Male, 42%[b] Female, 8%[c]
Matheny, Dolan, and Wilson[101]	17 (sex N.A.)	10 (sex N.A.)	History of dyslexia or academic problems	76% concordant	20% concordant[b]
Locke and Mather[100]	13 (5 male, 8 female)	13 (5 male, 8 female)	Poor performance on TD articulation test (>15% errors)	82% of errors shared	56% of errors shared[a]
Lewis and Thompson[99]	32 (24 male, 8 female)	25 (18 male, 7 female)	History of spoken or written language disorder	Any disorder, 67% Articulation, 95% Learning disorder, 53% Delayed speech, 71%	Any disorder, 32%[c] Articulation, 22%[d] Learning disorder, 33% Delayed speech, 0%
DeFries and Gillis[98]	133 (58 male, 75 female)	98 (57 male, 41 female)	History of dyslexia *and* poor performance on word recognition, spelling, and comprehension PIAT	51% concordant	28% concordant[c]

Key: Statistical significance (one-tailed test): [a]$p < .05$, [b]$p < .01$, [c]$p < .001$, [d]$p < .0001$; MZ = monozygotic; DZ = dizygotic; PIAT = Peabody Individual Achievement Tests; TD articulation = Templin-Darley Screening Test of Articulation.

Source: Adapted from Stromswold,[95] with permission.

$(z = 8.77, p < .00000005)$. If spoken language disorders and written language disorders are distinct entities, including twins with both types of disorders in one analysis would be inappropriate and could either hide a significant difference or create a spuriously significant difference. Of the nine twin studies Stromswold[95] reviewed, five investigated written language disorders and four investigated spoken language disorders. Stromswold's[95] metaanalyses included 212 MZ and 199 DZ twins pairs in which at least one member of the twin pair had a written language disorder. For written language disorders, the overall pairwise concordance rates were 59.9 percent for MZ twins and 27.1 percent for DZ twins (chi square(1) = 44.73, $p < .0000005$), and the overall probandwise concordance rates were 74.9 percent for MZ twins and 42.7 percent for DZ twins $(z = 6.53, p < .00000005)$.[95] Stromswold[95] metaanalysis included 188 MZ and 94 DZ twin pairs in which at least one member of the twin pair had a spoken language disorder. For spoken language disorders, the overall pairwise concordance rates were 72.9 percent for MZ twins and 35.1 percent for DZ twins (chi square(1) = 37.330, $p < .0000005$), and the probandwise concordance rates were 84.3 percent for MZ twins and 52.0 percent for DZ twins $(z = 5.14, p < .00000025)$.[95]

If pedigree studies of large, multigeneration families reveal that the pattern of family members who are language-impaired and not language-impaired is consistent with particular modes of genetic transmission, this supports the notion that SLI is a genetic disorder. Pedigree analyses involve evaluating models of genetic transmission by *rejecting* possible modes of transmission based on which family members in a pedigree are affected.[102] Researchers have reported a number of kindreds with extremely large numbers of severely affected family members in which transmission seems to be autosomal dominant with variable expressivity and penetrance.[46–48,103–106] Samples and Lane[107] analyzed a family in which six of six siblings had a severe developmental language disorder and concluded that the mode of transmission in that family was a single autosomal recessive gene. Stromswold[108] analyzed a family with severe

verbal dyspraxia in which transmission appears to be either autosomal recessive or multifactorial. To date, only one published segregation study exists for probands with spoken language disorders other than stuttering.[109] In this study, pedigrees of 45 probands with a history of a moderate to severe speech or language disorder were analyzed and the results were most consistent with multifactorial transmission.[109] In summary, the results of genetic studies indicate that there is a strong genetic component to developmental language disorders and that SLI is probably a genetically heterogeneous disorder.

ARE THESE CHILDREN DEVIANT OR ARE THEY MERELY DELAYED?

One of the central questions in SLI research is whether the major (perhaps only) difference between SLI children and normal children is the rate of language acquisition or whether the course of language acquisition by SLI children is deviant.[9,40,46–48,110–116] Even within the restricted domain of inflectional morphology where researchers generally agree that many SLI children exhibit particular difficulty (having difficulty using inflectional morphemes such as the past tense morpheme -*ed*), there is debate about whether SLI children's morphologic impairments reflect deviant underlying grammars,[45–52,117–121] limitations in language processing,[42,43,122–124] limitations in sensory processing,[33–35,37] or protracted (though essentially normal) acquisition of language.[113,125]

LONGITUDINAL COURSE AND PROGNOSIS IN SPECIFIC LANGUAGE IMPAIRMENTS

Follow-up studies of children diagnosed as having a spoken language disorder in preschool generally indicate that 40 to 60 percent of these children continue to have difficulties in later years (e.g., see Refs. 126–128). Most of these children had difficulties with written language or academic subjects, but many continued to have trouble with spoken language. One study found that 50 percent of children who had both comprehension and production deficits at age 3 still had deficits at age 5, whereas only 13 percent of children who only had production deficits at age 3 still had language deficits at age 5 and only 4 percent of children who only had comprehension deficits at age 3 still had deficits at age 5.[129] A follow-up study of the same children at age 11 revealed that children diagnosed with a language delay at age 3 were more likely to have lower verbal and full-scale IQs and reading scores than were children who were not diagnosed as language-delayed at age 3.[130] At age 11, there were no significant differences in IQ for children who had isolated production or comprehension deficits at age 3, but children diagnosed with global language deficits at age 3 had significantly lower IQs than either group.[130] At age 11, children with isolated expressive or isolated receptive delays had reading levels 2 years behind children who were not language-delayed at 3, and children with global language delays had reading levels more than 2.5 years behind normal children.[130] A 10-year follow-up study of children diagnosed with a specific language impairment in preschool revealed that preschool scores on the nonverbal Leiter IQ test[131] were the best predictor of adolescent scores on standardized tests of spoken language, reading achievement, and placement in a regular classroom.[132] Preschool scores on the expressive section of the Northwest Syntax Screening Test[133] were also a strong predictor of adolescent language scores.[132]

RELATIONSHIP BETWEEN SPECIFIC LANGUAGE IMPAIRMENTS AND DYSLEXIA

There is a growing consensus that many reading disabilities are language-based in origin.[130,134–144] Prospective studies of kindergarten and preschool-age children who were later diagnosed as dyslexic have revealed that such children exhibit weaknesses in phonemic awareness,[140,145–149] phonologic production,[140,150] receptive and expressive vocabulary,[140,147,148,151] syntactic comprehension

and production,[140,147,152] and syntactic awareness.[153] Follow-up studies have generally shown that many children who had spoken language impairments when they were of preschool age later exhibit signs of written language disorders.[126–128,130,132] In one 10-year follow-up study, over 90 percent of children who had spoken language disorders in preschool later exhibited evidence of learning difficulties or disorders in reading, spelling, or mathematics.[132] In retrospective studies, parents report that dyslexic children were more likely to have had spoken language impairments than were children without dyslexia.[154,155] Results from genetic studies also suggest that dyslexia and SLI are related. For example, as part of a twin study, Johnston and coworkers[156] found that preschool language skill was the best predictor of reading ability, accounting for 33 percent of the variance in reading-age discrepancy. In a different twin study, phonologic coding deficits were revealed to be highly heritable and accounted for most of the heritable variance in word recognition, whereas orthographic coding deficits were not significantly heritable and accounted for much of the environmental variance in word recognition.[157] Last, studies suggest that children with developmental phonologic disorders have significantly more nuclear and extended family members with dyslexia than do control children.[85,86]

IMPLICATIONS OF SPECIFIC LANGUAGE IMPAIRMENTS FOR COGNITIVE SCIENCE AND LINGUISTICS

If language acquisition involves the development of specialized, modular structures and operations that have no counterparts in nonlinguistic domains, then it should be possible for a child to be cognitively intact and linguistically impaired. If, on the other hand, language acquisition involves the development of the same general symbolic structures and operations used in other cognitive domains, then dissociation of language and general cognitive development should not be possible. Thus, the existence of children with SLI supports the position that language is cognitively and neurally distinct (or modular) from general intellectual abilities. Genetic studies which show that SLI is heritable provide further support for the acquisition of language being the result of innate, linguistically specific structures and not the result of instruction and general cognitive and neural structures. To the extent that SLI children's language is markedly different from that of normal children, this is consistent with the cognitive and neural processes that SLI children use to generate language being qualitatively different from those used by normal children.

In many modern linguistic theories, the subcomponents of language (e.g., syntax, semantics, morphology, phonology, and the lexicon) are believed to be functionally distinct or modular from one another.[158] The existence of SLI children whose linguistic impairments preferentially involve the acquisition of some subcomponents of language but not others (e.g., the acquisition of morphology, but not the acquisition of lexical items) is consistent with modular linguistic theories. Modern linguistic theories (particularly generative theories of grammar) also frequently make a distinction between a person's knowledge of the rules of language (competence) and a person's actual use of language in real situations (performance).[158,159] Some researchers have argued that SLI children's impairments or limitations are at the level of competence,[46–49,51,119,121] whereas other researchers have argued that SLI children's limitations are at the level of performance.[42,122–124]

Just as analyses of adult aphasics' deficits have been used to test specific linguistic and psycholinguistic theories,[160–163] careful investigations of SLI children's linguistic deficits may be useful in testing specific linguistic and psycholinguistic theories. A number of researchers have argued that the patterns of impairment in SLI children's language are consistent with SLI children having very specific linguistic impairments. For example, van der Lely[49] has suggested that SLI children's linguistic impairments reflect their inability to use government to analyze certain types of syntactic relations. Clahsen[51] has argued that, within a parametric theory of language (in which all languages share a number of universal properties, but differ

in the settings chosen for certain parameters), SLI children's linguistic deficits could be the result of them having miss-set or missing parametric setting(s). Another possibility within a learning theoretic-parametric framework is that the *threshold* at which SLI children reset parameters is aberrant. If SLI children's parameter-setting thresholds are too high, this could result in SLI children staying in the normal stages of language acquisition for prolonged periods of time. If Rice and Wexler[121] are correct and SLI children have an extended optional infinitive stage, this could be the result of SLI children having abnormally high thresholds for setting parameters.

To get a sense of the types of specific linguistic and psycholinguistic accounts that have been proposed to explain SLI children's language impairments, consider the accounts recently offered for why SLI children have particular difficulty with certain aspects of morphology, such as tense, number, and case. Leonard[42,43,123,164] has proposed that SLI children have difficulty perceiving and processing brief, unstressed linguistic elements and that this directly affects their ability to build the morphologic paradigms that Pinker[165] proposes are a key component of normal language acquisition. As support for the phonological salience theory, Leonard and colleagues report that SLI children who are acquiring English and Italian have specific difficulty learning grammatical morphemes that are expressed as word final consonants, even though the syntactic and semantic functions of these grammatical morphemes frequently differ in the two languages.[42,43,123,164] Gopnik and colleagues have argued that children with SLI make frequent morphologic errors because they are missing certain abstract syntactic-semantic features such as number, tense, animacy, and aspect.[45–48] A number of researchers have proposed that SLI children's morphological errors result from a specific deficit or delay in the acquisition of functional categories.[117,119,120] Clahsen has proposed that SLI children have difficulty forming subject-verb agreement relationships and this causes them to make certain types of morphologic errors.[50,51] Recently, Rice and colleagues have suggested that SLI children's morphologic errors may be caused by specific difficulties with specifier-head agreement relations[52] or by SLI children remaining in the optional infinitive stage of language acquisition for an abnormally long period of time.[121]

SUMMARY

Despite decades of intensive and productive research on specific language impairments in children, the answers to a number of fundamental questions about SLI remain uncertain. Although clinicians and researchers generally agree that considerable diversity exists in the behavioral profiles and manifestations of children diagnosed with SLI and that it is important to distinguish between various subtypes of SLI, no system for classifying the different behavioral subtypes of SLI is generally accepted. Researchers disagree about the etiology or underlying impairment in SLI, and offer proposals ranging from a specific impairment in a circumscribed aspect of abstract linguistics to general cognitive/processing impairments to environmental causes. Researchers disagree about the nature of the linguistic manifestations of SLI (be they primary or secondary to some underlying cause). Researchers disagree whether language acquisition in SLI is deviant or merely a prolonged version of the normal course of language acquisition. Researchers also disagree about whether SLI represents an impairment in the underlying grammar (competence) or the use of that grammar (performance). Even among researchers who believe that SLI is an impairment of linguistic competence, there is disagreement about what aspect of the underlying grammar is impaired.

Structural and functional neuroimaging studies suggest that children with SLI may not have the pattern of left-right asymmetry that normally developing children and adults have, but this research is somewhat preliminary and it is possible that SLI children's aberrant asymmetries reflect their linguistic impairments rather than cause them. Although the vast majority of the genetic studies of developmental language impairments indicate that there is a heritable component to

written and spoken language disorders, we know relatively little about the mode(s) of transmission and gene(s) responsible for spoken language disorders. Studies generally show that many SLI children continue to exhibit language and learning difficulties, particularly with written language. However, estimates of the prevalence of later language and learning disabilities in preschool children diagnosed with SLI vary considerably and not all children with a history of spoken language impairments have difficulty learning to read.

ACKNOWLEDGMENTS

Preparation of this chapter was supported by grants to the author from the John Merck Foundation on the Biology of Developmental Disorders and the Johnson and Johnson Foundation.

REFERENCES

1. Pinker S: *The Language Instinct: How the Mind Creates Language.* New York: William Morrow, 1994.
2. Stromswold K: The cognitive and neural bases of language acquisition, in Gazzaniga M (ed): *The Cognitive Neurosciences.* Cambridge, MA: MIT Press, 1995, pp 855–870.
3. Myklebust HR: Childhood aphasia: An evolving concept, in Travis LE (ed): *Handbook of Speech Pathology and Audiology.* New York: Appleton-Century-Crofts, 1971, pp 1181–1202.
4. Aram DM: Comments on specific language impairment as a clinical category. *Lang Speech Hear Serv Schools* 22:84–87, 1991.
5. Aram DM, Morris R, Hall NE: Clinical and research congruence in identifying children with specific language impairment. *J Speech Hear Res* 36:580–591, 1993.
6. Dale PS, Cole KN: What's normal? Specific language impairment in an individual differences perspective. *Lang Speech Hear Serv Schools* 22:80–83, 1991.
7. Lahey M: Who shall be called language disordered? Some reflections and one perspective. *J Speech Hear Dis* 55:612–620, 1990.
8. Leonard L: Specific language impairment as a clini-

cal category. *Lang Speech Hear Serv Schools* 22:66–68, 1991.

9. Leonard LB: Language impairment in children. *Merrill-Palmer Q* 25:205–232, 1979.

10. Stark RE, Tallal P: Selection of children with specific language deficits. *J Speech Hear Dis* 46:114–122, 1981.

11. Ingram TTS: Disorders of speech development in childhood. *Br J Hosp Med* 4:1608–1625, 1969.

12. American Psychiatric Association: *Diagnostic and Statistical Manual of Mental Disorders,* 4th ed. Washington, DC: American Psychiatric Association, 1994.

13. Aram DM, Nation JE: Patterns of language behavior in children with developmental language disorders. *J Speech Hear Res* 18:229–241, 1975.

14. Curtiss S, Tallal P: Neurolinguistic correlates of specific developmental language impairment. *J Clin Exp Neuropsychol* 10:18–19, 1988.

15. Denkla MB: Minimal brain dysfunction and dyslexia: Beyond diagnosis by exclusion, in Blair ME, Rapin I, Kinsbourne M (eds): *Child Neurology.* New York: Spectrum, 1981.

16. Korkman M, Hakkinen-Rihu P: A new classification of developmental language disorders (DLD). *Brain Lang* 47:96–116, 1994.

17. Wilson B, Risucci D: A model for clinical-quantitative classification: Generation I: Application to language-disordered preschool children. *Brain Lang* 27:281–309, 1986.

18. Bishop D, Rosenbloom L: Childhood language disorders: Classification and overview, in Yule W, Rutter M (eds): *Language Development and Disorders.* Philadelphia: Lippincott, 1987, pp 16–41.

19. Bloom L, Lahey M: *Language Development and Language Disorder.* New York: Wiley, 1978.

20. Rapin I, Allen DA: Developmental language disorders: Nosological considerations, in Kirk U (ed): *Neuropsychology of Language, Reading, and Spelling.* New York: Academic Press, 1983, pp 155–183.

21. Bishop DVM: The underlying nature of specific language impairment. *J Child Psychol Psychiatry Allied Disc* 33:3–66, 1992.

22. Cramblit N, Siegel G: The verbal environment of a language-impaired child. *J Speech Hearing Dis* 42:474–482, 1977.

23. Lasky E, Klopp K: Parent-child interactions in normal and language-disordered children. *J Speech Hear Dis* 47:7–18, 1982.

24. Bishop DVM, Edmundson A: Is otitis media a major cause of specific developmental language disorders? *Br J Disord Commun* 21:321–338, 1986.

25. Gordon AG: Some comments on Bishop's annotation "Developmental dysphasia and otitis media." *J Child Psychol Psychiatry* 29:361–363, 1988.

26. Gravel JS, Wallace IF: Listening and language at 4 years of age: Effects of early otitis media. *J Speech Hear Res* 35:588–595, 1992.

27. Teele DW, Klein JO, Chase C, et al: Otitis media in infancy and intellectual ability, school achievement, speech, and language at age 7 years. *J Infect Dis* 162:685–694, 1990.

28. Graham NC: Response strategies in the partial comprehension of sentences. *Lang Speech* 17:205–221, 1974.

29. Graham NC: Short-term memory and syntactic structure in educationally subnormal children. *Lang Speech* 11:209–219, 1968.

30. Rapin I, Wilson BC: Children with developmental language disability: Neuropsychological aspects and assessment, in Wyke MA (ed): *Developmental Dysphasia.* London: Academic Press, 1978, pp 13–41.

31. Efron R: Temporal perception, aphasia and deja vu. *Brain* 86:403–424, 1963.

32. Monsee EK: Aphasia in children. *J Speech Hear Disord* 26:83–86, 1961.

33. Tallal P, Piercy M: Defects of non-verbal auditory perception in children with developmental dysphasia. *Nature* 241:468–469, 1973.

34. Tallal P, Piercy M: Developmental aphasia: Impaired rate of non-verbal processing as a function of sensory modality. *Neuropsychologia* 11:389–398, 1973.

35. Tallal P, Piercy M: Developmental aphasia: Rate of auditory processing as a selective impairment of consonant perception. *Neuropsychologia* 12:83–93, 1974.

36. Poppen R, Stark J, Eisenson J, et al: Visual sequencing performance of aphasic children. *J Speech Hear Res* 12:288–300, 1969.

37. Tallal P: Fine-grained discrimination deficits in language-learning impaired children are specific neither to the auditory modality nor to speech perception. *J Speech Hear Res* 33:616–621, 1990.

38. Johnston J, Weismer S: Mental rotation abilities in language-disordered children. *J Speech Hear Res* 26:397–403, 1983.

39. Kahmi A: Nonlinguistic symbolic and conceptual abilities in language-impaired and normally devel-

oping children. *J Speech Hear Res* 24:446–453, 1981.

40. Morehead D, Ingram D: The development of base syntax in normal and linguistically deviant children. *J Speech Hear Res* 16:330–352, 1973.

41. Cromer R: Hierarchical planning disability in the drawings and constructions of a special group of severely aphasic children. *Brain Cogn* 2:144–164, 1983.

42. Leonard LB: Language learnability and specific language impairment in children. *Appl Psycholing* 10:179–202, 1989.

43. Leonard LB: Some problems facing accounts of morphological deficits in children with specific language impairments, in Watkins RV, Rice ML (eds): *Specific Language Impairments in Children.* Baltimore: Brookes, 1994, pp 91–106.

44. Leonard LB, McGregor KK, Allen GD: Grammatical morphology and speech perception in children with specific language impairment. *J Speech Hear Res* 35:1076–1085, 1992.

45. Crago MB, Gopnik M: From families to phenotypes: Theoretical and clinical implications of research into the genetic basis of specific language impairment, in Watkins RV, Rice ML (eds): *Specific Language Impairments in Children.* Baltimore: Brookes, 1994, pp 35–52.

46. Gopnik M: Feature blindness: A case study. *Lang Acquis* 1:139–164, 1990.

47. Gopnik M: Feature-blind grammar and dysphasia. *Nature* 344:715, 1990.

48. Gopnik M, Crago MB: Familial aggregation of a developmental language disorder. *Cognition* 39:1–50, 1991.

49. van der Lely HKJ: Canonical linking rules: Forward versus reverse linking in normally developing and specifically language-impaired children. *Cognition* 51:29–72, 1994.

50. Clahsen H: *Child Language and Developmental Dysphasia: Linguistic Studies of the Acquisition of German.* Philadelphia: Benjamins, 1991.

51. Clahsen H: The grammatical characterization of developmental dysphasia. *Linguistics* 27:897–920, 1989.

52. Rice ML: Grammatical categories of children with specific language impairments, in Watkins RV, Rice ML (eds): *Specific Language Impairments in Children.* Baltimore: Brookes, 1994, pp 69–90.

53. Johnston JR: The continuing relevance of cause: A reply to Leonard's "Specific language impairment as a clinical category." *Lang Speech Hear Serv Schools* 22:75–79, 1991.

54. Conti-Ramsden G, Dykins J: Mother-child interactions with language-impaired children and their siblings. *Br J Disord Commun* 26:337–354, 1991.

55. Leonard L: Is specific language impairment a useful construct? in Rosenberg S (ed): *Advances in Applied Psycholinguistics: Disorders of First Language Development.* New York: Cambridge University Press, 1987, pp 1–39.

56. Friel-Patti S, Finitzo T: Language learning in a prospective study of otitis media with effusion in the first two years of life. *J Speech Hear Res* 33:188–194, 1990.

57. Hall DMB, Hill P: Does secretory otitis media affect language development? *Arch Dis Child* 61:42–47, 1986.

58. Paradise JL: Otitis media during early life: How hazardous to development? A critical review of the evidence. *Pediatrics* 68:869–873, 1981.

59. Paul R, Lynn T, Lohr-Flanders M: History of middle ear involvement and speech/language development in late talkers. *J Speech Hear Res* 36:1055–1062, 1993.

60. MacKain K, Best C, Strange W: Categorical perception of English /r/ and /l/ by Japanese bilinguals. *Appl Psycholing* 2:369–390, 1981.

61. Strange W, Dittman S: Effects of discrimination training on the perception of /r-l/ by Japanese adults learning English. *Percept Psychophys* 36:131–145, 1984.

62. Strange W, Jenkins JJ: Role of linguistic experience in the perception of speech, in Walk D, Pick Jr HJ (eds): *Perception and Experience.* New York: Plenum, 1978, pp 125–169.

63. Bishop DVM: The causes of specific developmental language disorder ("developmental dysphasia"). *J Child Psychol Psychiatry* 28:1–8, 1987.

64. Jernigan TL, Hesselink JR, Sowell E, Tallal PA: Cerebral structure on magnetic resonance imaging in language impaired and learning-impaired children. *Arch Neurol* 48:539–545, 1991.

65. Plante E, Swisher L, Vance R: Anatomical correlates of normal and impaired language in a set of dizygotic twins. *Brain Lang* 37:643–655, 1989.

66. Plante E, Swisher L, Vance R, Rapsak S: MRI findings in boys with specifically language impairment. *Brain Lang* 41:52–66, 1991.

67. Arnold G, Schwartz S: Hemispheric lateralization of language in autistic and aphasic children. *J Autism Dev Disord* 13:129–139, 1983.

68. Boliek CA, Bryden MP, Obrzut JE: Focused attention and the perception of voicing and place of articulation contrasts with control and learning-disabled children. The 16th Annual Meeting of the International Neuropsychological Society. New Orleans, LA, January 1988.

69. Cohen H, Gelinas C, Lassonde M, Geoffroy G: Auditory lateralization for speech in language-impaired children. *Brain Lang* 41:395–401, 1991.

70. Obrzut JE, Conrad PF, Boliek CA: Verbal and nonverbal auditory processing among left- and right-handed good readers and reading disabled children. 16th Annual Meeting of the International Neuropsychological Society. New Orleans, LA, 1988.

71. Obrzut JE, Conrad PF, Bryden MP, Boliek CA: Cued dichotic listening with right-handed, left-handed, bilingual and learning-disabled children. *Neuropsychologia* 26:119–131, 1988.

72. Dawson G, Finley C, Phillips S, Lewy A: A comparison of hemispheric asymmetries in speech-related brain potentials of autistic and dysphasic children. *Brain Lang* 37:26–41, 1989.

73. Denays R, Tondeur M, Foulon M, et al: Regional brain blood flow in congenital dysphasia studies with technetium-99m HM-PAO SPECT. *J Nuc Med* 30:1825–1829, 1989.

74. Lou HD, Henriksen L, Bruhn P: Focal cerebral dysfunction in developmental learning disabilities. *Lancet* 335:8–11, 1990.

75. Cohen M, Campbell R, Yaghmai F: Neuropathological abnormalities in developmental dysphasia. *Ann Neurol* 25:567–570, 1989.

76. Galaburda A: Neuropathologic correlates of learning disabilities. *Semin Neurol* 11:20–27, 1991.

77. Galaburda AM: Developmental dyslexia and animal studies: At the inferface between cognition and neurology. *Cognition* 50:133–149, 1994.

78. Geschwind N, Galaburda A: Cerebral lateralization: Biological mechanisms, associations, and pathology: I. *Arch Neurol* 42:428–459, 1985.

79. Geschwind N, Galaburda AM: *Cerebral Lateralization: Biological Mechanisms, Associations, and Pathology.* Cambridge, MA: MIT Press, 1987.

80. Livingstone MS, Rosen GD, Drislane FW, Galaburda AM: Physiological and anatomical evidence for a magnocellular defect in developmental dyslexia. *Proc Natl Acad Sci USA* 88:7943–7947, 1991.

81. Beitchman JH, Hood J, Inglis A: Familial transmission of speech and language impairment: A preliminary investigation. *Can J Psychiatry* 37:151–156, 1992.

82. Byrne BM, Willerman L, Ashmore LL: Severe and moderate language impairment: Evidence for distinctive etiologies. *Behav Genet* 4:331–345, 1974.

83. Haynes C, Naidoo S: *Children with Specific Speech and Language Impairment.* London: MacKeith Press, 1991.

84. Ingram TTS: Specific developmental disorders of speech in childhood. *Brain* 82:450–467, 1959.

85. Lewis BA: Pedigree analysis of children with phonology disorders. *J Learn Disabil* 25:586–597, 1992.

86. Lewis BA, Ekelman BL, Aram DM: A familial study of severe phonological disorders. *J Speech Hear Res* 32:713–724, 1989.

87. Luchsinger R: Inheritance of speech deficits. *Fol Phoniatr* 22:216–230, 1970.

88. Neils J, Aram DM: Family history of children with developmental language disorders. *Percept Motor Skills* 63:655–658, 1986.

89. Tallal P, Ross R, Curtiss S: Familial aggregation in specific language impairment. *J Speech Hear Disord* 54:167–173, 1989.

90. Tomblin JB: Familial concentrations of developmental language impairment. *J Speech Hear Dis* 54:287–295, 1989.

91. Tomblin JB, Hardy JC, Hein HA: Predicting poor-communication status in preschool children using risk factors present at birth. *J Speech Hear Res* 34:1096–1105, 1991.

92. Whitehurst GJ, Arnold DS, Smith M, et al: Family history in developmental expressive language delay. *J Speech Hear Res* 34:1150–1157, 1991.

93. Heath SB: *Ways with Words: Language, Life and Work in Communities and Classrooms.* New York: Cambridge University Press, 1983.

94. Singleton JL, Morford JP, Goldin-Meadow S: Once is not enough: Standards of well-formedness in manual communication created over three different timespans. *Language* 69:683–715, 1993.

95. Stromswold K: The genetic basis of language acquisition, in Stringfellow A, Cahana-Amitay D, Hughes E, Zukowski A (eds): *Proceedings of the 20th Annual Boston University Conference on Language Development.* Somerville, MA: Cascadilla Press, 1996, vol 2, pp 736–747.

96. Falconer DS: *Introduction to Quantitative Genetics.* New York: Ronald Press, 1960.

97. Bakwin H: Reading disabilities in twins. *Dev Medic Child Neurol* 15:184–187, 1973.

98. DeFries JC, Gillis JJ: Genetics of reading disability,

in Plomin R, McClearn GE (eds): *Nature, Nurture, and Psychology.* Washington, DC: American Psychological Association, 1993, pp 121–145.

99. Lewis BA, Thompson LA: A study of developmental speech and language disorders in twins. *J Speech Hear Res* 35:1086–1094, 1992.

100. Locke JL, Mather PL: Genetic factors in the ontogeny of spoken language: Evidence from monozygotic and dizygotic twins. *J Child Lang* 16:553–559, 1989.

101. Matheny AP, Dolan AB, Wilson RS: Twins with academic learning problems: Antecedent characteristics. *Am J Orthopsychiatr* 46:464–469, 1976.

102. Pauls DL: Genetic analysis of family pedigree data: A review of methodology, in Ludlow CL, Cooper JA (eds): *Genetic Aspects of Speech and Language Disorders.* New York: Academic Press, 1983, pp 139–147.

103. Arnold GE: The genetic background of developmental language disorders. *Fol Phoniatr* 13:246–254, 1961.

104. Hurst JA, Baraitser M, Auger E, et al: An extended family with a dominantly inherited speech disorder. *Dev Med Child Neurol* 32:347–355, 1990.

105. Lenneberg EH: *Biological Foundations of Language.* New York: Wiley, 1967.

106. Lewis BA: Familial phonological disorders: Four pedigrees. *J Speech Hear Disord* 55:160–170, 1990.

107. Samples J, Lane V: Genetic possibilities in six siblings with specific language learning disorders. *Am Speech Lang Hear Assoc* 27:27–32, 1985.

108. Stromswold K: Language comprehension without language production: Implications for theories of language acquisition. Boston University Conference on Language Development. Boston, January 1994.

109. Lewis BA, Cox NJ, Byard PJ: Segregation analysis of speech and language disorders. *Behav Genet* 23:291–297, 1993.

110. Benedict H: Early lexical development: Comprehension and production. *J Child Lang* 6:183–200, 1979.

111. Bishop DV, Edmundson A: Specific language impairment as a maturational lag: Evidence from longitudinal data on language and motor development. *Dev Med Child Neurol* 29:442–459, 1987.

112. Camarata S, Gandour J: Rule invention in the acquisition of morphology by a language-impaired child. *J Speech Hear Dis* 50:4–45, 1985.

113. Curtiss S, Katz W, Tallal P: Delay versus deviance

in the language acquisition of language-impaired children. *J Speech Hear Res* 35:373–383, 1992.

114. Gibson D, Ingram D: The onset of comprehension and production in a language delayed child. *Appl Psycholing* 4:359–375, 1983.

115. Grimm H, Weinert S: Is the syntax development of dysphasic children deviant and why? New findings to an old question. *J Speech Hear Res* 33:220–228, 1990.

116. Kahmi A: Metalinguistic abilities in language impaired children. *Topics Lang Disord* 7:1–12, 1987.

117. Guilfoyle E, Allen S, Moss S: Specific language impairment and the maturation of functional categories. BU Conference of Language Development. Boston, Oct 19, 1991.

118. Oetting JB, Rice ML: Plural acquisition in children with specific language impairment. *J Speech Hear Res* 36:1236–1248, 1993.

119. Rice ML, Oetting JB: Morphological deficits of children with SLI: Evaluation of number marking and agreement. *J Speech Hear Res* 36:1249–1257, 1993.

120. Rice ML, Oetting JB: Morphological deficits of SLI children: A matter of missing functional categories? BU Conference on Language Development. Boston, October 1991.

121. Rice ML, Wexler K: Extended optional infinitive (EIO) account of specific language impairment, in MacLaughlin D, McEwen S (eds): *19th Annual Boston University Conference on Language Development.* Boston: Cascadilla Press, 1995, pp 451–462.

122. Bishop DVM: Grammatical errors in specific language impairment: Competence or performance limitations. *Appl Psycholing* 15:507–550, 1994.

123. Leonard LB, Bortolini U, Caselli MC, et al: Morphological deficits in children with specific language impairment: The status of features in the underlying grammar. *Lang Acquis* 2:151–179, 1992.

124. Leonard LB, Sabbadini L, Volterra V, Leonard JS: Some influences on the grammar of English- and Italian-speaking children with specific language impairment. *Appl Psycholing* 9:39–57, 1988.

125. Lahey M, Liebergott J, Chesnick M, et al: Variability in children's use of grammatical morphemes. *Appl Psycholing* 13:373–398, 1992.

126. Aram DM, Nation JE: Preschool language disorders and subsequent language and academic difficulties. *J Commun Disord* 13:159–170, 1980.

127. Hall P, Tombin J: A follow-up study of children

with articulation and language disorders. *J Speech Hear Disord* 43:227–241, 1978.

128. King RR, Jones C, Lasky E: In retrospect: A fifteen-year follow-up report of speech-language disordered children. *Lang Speech Hear Serv School* 13:24–32, 1982.

129. Silva PA: The prevalence, stability, and significance of developmental language delay in preschool children. *Dev Med Child Neurol* 22:768–777, 1980.

130. Silva PA, Williams S, McGee R: A longitudinal study of children with developmental language delay at age three: Later intelligence, reading and behavior problems. *Dev Med Child Neurol* 29:630–640, 1987.

131. Arthur G: *The Arthur Adaptation of the Leiter International Performance Scale.* Washington, DC: Psychological Service Center Press, 1952.

132. Aram DM, Eklelman BL, Nation JE: Preschoolers with language disorders: 10 years later. *J Speech Hear Res* 27:232–244, 1984.

133. Lee LL: The developmental sentence scoring (DSS) reweighted scores, in Lee LLA (ed): *Developmental Sentence Analysis.* Evanston, IL: Northwestern University Press, 1974, pp 6–7.

134. Bowey JA, Patel RK: Metalinguistic ability and early reading achievement. *Appl Psycholing* 9:367–383, 1988.

135. Catts HW, Hu C-F, Larrivee L, Swank L: Early identification of reading disabilities in children with speech-language impairments, in Watkins RV, Rice ML (eds): *Specific Language Impairments in Children.* Baltimore: Brookes, 1994, pp 145–160.

136. Kahmi AG: Causes and consequences of reading disabilities, in Kahmi AG, Catts HW (eds): *Reading Disability: A Developmental Language Perspective.* Boston: Little, Brown, 1989, pp 67–99.

137. Kahmi AG, Catts HW: *Reading Disabilities: A Developmental Language Perspective.* Boston: Little, Brown, 1989.

138. Kavanagh JF, Yeni-Komshian G: *Developmental Dyslexia and Related Reading Disorders.* Bethesda, MD: National Institute of Child Health and Human Development, 1985.

139. Perfetti CA: *Reading Ability.* New York: Oxford University Press, 1985.

140. Scarborough HS: Very early language deficits in dyslexic children. *Child Dev* 61:1728–1743, 1990.

141. Scarborough HS, Dobrich W: Development of children with early language delay. *J Speech Hear Res* 33:70–83, 1990.

142. Snyder LS, Downey DM: The language-reading relationship in normal and reading-disabled children. *J Speech Hear Res* 34:129–140, 1991.

143. Stanovich KE: The right and wrong places to look for the cognitive locus of reading disability. *Ann Dyslexia* 38:154–177, 1988.

144. Vellutino FR: *Dyslexia: Theory and Research.* Cambridge, MA: MIT Press, 1979.

145. Bryant PE, Bradley L, Maclean M, Crossland J: Nursery rhymes, phonological skills, and reading. *J Child Lang* 16:407–428, 1989.

146. Mann VA, Ditunno P: Phonological deficiencies: Effective predictors of future reading problems, in Pavlides G (ed): *Perspectives on Dyslexia.* New York: Wiley, 1990, pp 105–131.

147. Share DL, Jorm AF, Maclean R, Matthews R: Sources of individual differences in reading acquisition. *J Educ Psychol* 76:1309–1324, 1984.

148. Stanovich KE, Cunningham AE, Cramer BB: Assessing phonological awareness in kindergarten children: Issues of task comparability. *J Exp Child Psychol* 38:175–190, 1984.

149. Stuart M, Coltheart M: Does reading develop in a sequence of stages? *Cognition* 30:139–181, 1988.

150. Silva PA, McGee R, Williams W: Some characteristics of 9-year-old boys with general reading backwardness or specific reading retardation. *J Child Psychol Psychiatry* 26:407–421, 1985.

151. Wolf M, Goodglass H: Dyslexia, dysnomia, and lexical retrieval: A longitudinal study. *Brain Lang* 28:154–168, 1986.

152. Butler SR, Marsh HW, Sheppard MJ, Sheppard JL: Seven-year longitudinal study of the early prediction of reading achievement. *J Educ Psychol* 77:349–361, 1985.

153. Tunmer WE, Herriman ML, Nesdale AR: Metalinguistic abilities and beginning reading. *Read Res Q* 23:134–158, 1988.

154. Ingram TTS, Mason AW, Blackburn I: A retrospective study of 82 children with reading disability. *Dev Med Child Neurol* 12:271–281, 1970.

155. Rutter M, Yule W: The concept of specific reading retardation. *J Child Psychol Psychiatry* 16:181–197, 1975.

156. Johnston C, Prior M, Hay D: Prediction of reading disability in twin boys. *Dev Med Child Neurol* 26:588–595, 1984.

157. Olson RK, Wise B, Conners F, et al: Specific deficits in component reading and language skills: Ge-

netic and environmental influences. *J Learn Disabil* 22(6):339–348, 1989.

158. Chomsky N: *Knowledge of Language: Its Nature, Origin, and Use.* New York: Praeger, 1986.

159. Chomsky N: *Syntactic Structures.* The Hague: Mouton, 1957.

160. Caramazza A, Laudanna A, Romani C: Lexical access and inflectional morphology. *Cognition* 28:297–332, 1988.

161. Garrett MF: Production of speech: Observations from normal and pathological language use, in Ellis A (ed): *Normality and Pathology in Cognitive Functions.* London: Academic Press, 1982.

162. Grodzinsky Y: *Theoretical Perspectives on Language Deficits.* Cambridge, MA: MIT Press, 1990.

163. Zurif E, Swinney D, Prather P, et al: An on-line analysis of syntactic processing in Broca's and Wernicke's aphasia. *Brain Lang* 45:448–464, 1993.

164. Leonard LB, Sabbadini L, Leonard JS, Volterra V: Specific language impairment in children: A cross-linguistic study. *Brain Lang* 32:233–252, 1987.

165. Pinker S: *Language Learnability and Language Development.* Cambridge, MA: Harvard University Press, 1984.

Chapter 62

DEVELOPMENTAL READING DISORDERS

Maureen W. Lovett

For more than a century, it has been recognized that a sizable minority of otherwise intelligent, healthy children unexpectedly fail to learn to read. In 1895, Hinshelwood[1,2] described specific reading problems as *visual word blindness* and hypothesized that such difficulties were caused by damage to a visual memory center for words localized to the left angular gyrus. Early recognition of developmental learning disorders was influenced strongly by case studies of brain-damaged adults with acquired cognitive disorders.[3] In 1896, Morgan[4] suggested a parallel between cases of acquired and developmental reading disorder and drew attention to the fact that a congenital form of word blindness could exist in children with otherwise normal development. The most influential early student of reading disability was Samuel Orton,[5,6] who described a condition he labeled *strephosymbolia,* which he attributed to incomplete or delayed cerebral dominance. Orton suggested that developmental delay in specialization of the left hemisphere for language could cause the condition. Orton's work formed the basis for a number of early educational therapies for the disorder,[7,8] some of which remain popular today.[9]

Over 25 years ago, the World Federation of Neurology defined *specific developmental dyslexia* by exclusionary criteria as "a disorder manifested by difficulty in learning to read despite conventional instruction, adequate intelligence, and sociocultural opportunity." The disorder was attributed to "fundamental cognitive disabilities which are frequently of constitutional origin."[10] Some authors attributed dyslexia to a "well defined defect in any one of several specific higher cortical functions,"[11] drawing attention to the heterogeneous presentation of the accompanying cognitive deficits. Other authors observed that the majority of dyslexic children have accompanying, potentially precursive, speech and language concomitants to their reading disorder: In 1979, Denckla[12] described dyslexia as the "index symptom of a developmental language disorder too subtle to lead to referral of the child in preschool life" (p. 550), a view reiterated by other authors over the past decade.[13–16] Developmental dyslexia occurs relatively frequently, with prevalence rates conservatively estimated at 3 to 6 percent.[17–19]

Exclusionary definitions of dyslexia fostered diagnostic approaches based on defining a discrepancy between reading achievement and intellectual potential as measured by standardized psychometric tests. Regression formulas are used to classify as dyslexic those children who are reading significantly below IQ-based expectations. A discrepancy-based definition of dyslexia or developmental reading disability has dominated clinical practice and research for decades and has been legislated into eligibility requirements for special education services in parts of the United States and Canada.[20–23]

At the heart of the discrepancy-based approach is the assumption that aptitude-achievement discrepancies yield a more homogeneous—and more specific—diagnostic profile than that provided by definitions based on low achievement criteria alone. It was assumed that higher-IQ disabled readers experienced a more specific form of dyslexia characterized by a unique deviant pattern of development in reading-related cognitive processes, while low-IQ disabled readers were handicapped by developmental lags in many reading-related *and* -unrelated cognitive processes.[16,23] Some authors considered the discrepancy group more "purely" dyslexic and of potentially different (biologically driven?) etiology than the no-discrepancy group of "garden-variety" poor readers.[24]

Recent research has demonstrated, however, that disabled readers with and without aptitude-achievement discrepancies do not differ on the information processing subskills (phonologic and orthographic coding) that underlie word recognition. Word recognition deficiencies define the index symptom of reading disability; and all of the differences between these two groups of disabled readers lay outside the word-recognition module.[23] Similarly, recent epidemiologic evidence provides no support for specificity of cognitive deficits in relation to IQ-based discrepancies.[25] This evidence confirms that the principal correlate of reading disability is linguistic, with the most reliable predictors found in the phonologic processing domain. An assessment of intellectual potential, while useful in practice, is not essential to the definition of developmental reading disorders. Therefore the definition of dyslexia, or *developmental reading disability* (often used synonymously), is based on indications of severe difficulties in reading acquisition despite access to instructional, linguistic, and environmental opportunities.

CURRENT DEFINITIONS OF DEVELOPMENTAL READING DISABILITY

Current research defines the most reliable indicator of reading disability as a failure to acquire rapid, context-free word-identification skill.[16,19,24,26–30] Although disabled readers experience problems with decoding accuracy, reading rate, and comprehension when reading connected text, the index symptom of their disability involves severe developmental failures of word-recognition learning and deficiencies in component processes within the word-identification domain.

Reading disability is often accompanied by associated deficits in some aspect of speech and language development, although this is not invariably true. In the past 15 years, there has been converging evidence that the core linguistic deficit characterizing developmental reading disability is deficient phonologic awareness. Phonologic awareness can be defined as "the ability to reflect explicitly on the sound structure of spoken words,"[31] a multifaceted ability with different levels of analysis developing at different rates.[32] A certain degree of phonologic awareness and an ability to segment and blend individual speech sounds are considered prerequisites to learning grapheme-phoneme (letter-sound) correspondences and acquiring an alphabetic code.[33–35] Many aspects of phonologic awareness and phonologic processing skills have been reported deficient in dyslexic individuals, including difficulties segmenting individual sounds within words, blending individual speech sounds to produce a word, and using phonologic codes to facilitate working memory processes.[16,28,36–38] Phonologic processing abilities measured in kindergarten have been demonstrated to be the best predictors of reading ability and disability at the end of second grade.[39,40] Phonologic processing deficits have been demonstrated to persist into adulthood even when individuals with childhood diagnoses of dyslexia were shown to attain reasonable standards of literacy.[41]

Children with reading disability also have problems rapidly retrieving and accessing names for visually presented material.[42–48] The deficit in visual naming speed characterizes disabled readers from kindergarten[47] through adulthood,[49–51] has been documented in dyslexics of other languages,[52–54] and has been suggested to be causally implicated in failures to acquire rapid, context-free word-identification skill.[44,46]

Developmental reading disability, therefore, appears characterized by two highly specific deficits in separate aspects of speech, language, and visible language development: (1) problems in the ability to represent and access individual speech sounds in words and (2) difficulty in rapidly accessing and retrieving names for visual symbols. Both deficits interfere with language and visible language processing at the lexical level and are compatible with evidence that the defining feature of the dyslexic reading disability is a failure to acquire rapid, context-free word-identification skill.[55–57]

GENETIC AND NEUROBIOLOGICAL BASES OF DEVELOPMENTAL READING DISORDERS

The Genetics of Dyslexia

The biological bases of developmental reading disorders have attracted considerable scientific interest. Evidence of the familiality of the disorder was suggested in several early case reports and in a few early family and twin studies.[58–60] In 1970, an influential epidemiologic study on the Isle of Wight reported that dyslexia was identified with a frequency of 34 percent among the parents and siblings of reading-disabled children but was identified in only 9 percent of the families of control children.[61] Later comparison of results from four different family studies reported similar findings and strong evidence of the familiality of dyslexia: the median increase in the risk of dyslexia to a child having a dyslexic parent was approximately eight times the population prevalence figure of 5 percent, with sibling recurrence estimated at a rate between 38 and 43 percent.[62–65] Twin studies using multiple regression techniques to estimate heritable and common environmental contributions supported early speculation that familial aggregation is at least partly based on genetic transmission.[66] DeFries and his colleagues in the Colorado Family Reading Study estimated that approximately 30 percent of the cognitive phenotype in developmental dyslexia could be attributed to heritable factors; later heritability estimates for reading (44 percent), spelling (62 percent), and nonword reading (75 percent) were even higher.[63,66–68] Precise

mechanisms of transmission for dyslexia, however, are not suggested from these data.

In recent years, two major findings have been reported from large-scale genetic studies of developmental dyslexia. To evaluate mode of transmission, segregation analyses were conducted on four independently ascertained family samples (1698 individuals from 204 families): Pennington and colleagues found evidence of major gene transmission (dominant or additive) with sex-dependent penetrance (estimated as complete in males, incomplete in females) in three samples, and the suggestion of multifactorial-polygenic transmission in the fourth sample.[69] The investigators are careful to note, however, that genetic heterogeneity existed even in families selected for apparent dominant transmission. These segregation findings are interpreted as strong evidence for sex-influenced, major locus transmission in a large proportion of dyslexic families.[63]

Other investigators using segregation and linkage analysis techniques have concluded that their results indicate genetic heterogeneity in the transmission of dyslexia.[70,71] Earlier work in the 1980s had suggested evidence for linkage between dyslexia and chromosome 15 heteromorphisms in a minority of families with apparent autosomal dominant transmission.[72] Although at least one study failed to confirm linkage between dyslexia and chromosome 15 heteromorphisms,[73] further work by the Colorado group estimated that dyslexia may be linked to chromosome 15 in a minority (<20 percent) of families.[65]

The second critical recent finding is a report of a major dyslexia locus on chromosome 6 in the majority of affected families not linked to chromosome 15. Investigators have reported what is described as "compelling evidence" for a quantitative trait locus for reading disability on chromosome 6 within the human leukocyte antigen region.[74] Derived from interval mapping of genetic data from two independent samples of sibling pairs, this quantitative trait locus is suggested to have either a recessive or dominant mode of expression. The search was targeted to this region of chromosome 6 because of the association observed by some investigators between dyslexia and immune disorders,[75,76] and knowledge that specific fragments of chromosome 6 had been identified as containing genes that contribute to disorders like hay fever, migraine headaches, asthma, thyroid disease, and allergies. Many behavioral geneticists consider this finding confirmatory evidence that a majority of cases of dyslexia will be linked to a small specific part of the human genome, and that a gene for dyslexia may be found.

Although recent findings are the most provocative yet reported on the behavioral genetics of reading disability, the notion that a specific gene for dyslexia will be identified remains controversial. Pennington[63] cautions that behavioral genetics may not identify a single locus for the dyslexic disorder itself but rather a major locus effect relevant to the transmission of reading ability and disability. The familiality, heritability, and transmission results for normal variability in reading ability parallel those found for reading disability,[77] leading to speculation that a small number of quantitative trait loci may contribute to the transmission of both normal reading skill and dyslexia.[63] Dyslexics may have more unfavorable alleles at these loci and/or greater environmental risk: Pennington suggests that the locus or loci, therefore, are better described as "susceptibility" loci for reading disorders.

Plomin[78] is even more cautious, warning that applications of molecular biology to the study of behavior may be unproductive if it is assumed that one or two major genes will prove largely responsible for genetic variation: Plomin contends that there is generally scant evidence to suggest that genetic influence on behavior can be attributed to a few major genes. He recommends an alternative approach that allows the identification of multiple genes that account for small amounts of variance, with recognition of the fact that genetic variance typically does not account for half of observed behavioral variance and that nongenetic sources of variance are equally significant.

The Neurobiology of Dyslexia

Interest in defining the neuroanatomic substrates of developmental reading disability has been strong since Hinshelwood's localization of visual word memory to the left angular gyrus at the beginning of this century. Two types of investigations have been reported in the search for what is different in the brain morphology and brain function of dyslexic individuals. These include neuroimaging studies of dyslexic and matched control samples and postmortem studies of dyslexic and control brains. Until relatively recently, evidence from these two empiric approaches appeared to converge, suggesting a tentative model of structural differences in the brain development of dyslexic children that appeared grossly compatible with behavioral observations of core symptoms. Recent results appear far more divergent, however: both inconsistent findings and growing awareness of methodologic limitations suggest our current understanding of the neurobiologic correlates of dyslexia to be quite tentative.[79]

Because reading involves processing language in visible form and because of the speech-based concomitants of dyslexia, many attempts to study the neuroanatomy of dyslexia focused on brain systems believed to subserve language function, particularly those in the perisylvian association cortex of the left hemisphere.[80,81] Particular attention has been directed to bilateral measurement of the planum temporale (PT), a neuroanatomical landmark on the upper surface of the temporal lobe that contains several subdivisions of auditory cortex, has been implicated by left-sided lesions causing Wernicke's aphasia, and is thought to subserve auditory perception and association in the left hemisphere.[82–85] Early computed tomography (CT) and magnetic resonance imaging (MRI) studies reported increased symmetry for dyslexics in the regions of the planum temporale and the parietal-occipital cortex,[86,87] findings consistent with those from the first postmortem studies on dyslexia.[88] Most of these early neuroimaging studies were criticized on methodologic grounds by Hynd and Semrud-Clikeman,[89] however, for reliance on questionable criteria in the diagnosis of dyslexia and for their failure to include comparison groups with other diagnosed developmental and neurocognitive disorders. Although directed at studies conducted in the early 1980s, these methodologic concerns remain relevant to many current neuroimaging studies. Hynd and Semrud-Clikeman contended that without other well-defined clinical control groups, any differences between dyslexic and normal controls could not be considered evidence of neuroanatomic involvement specific to dyslexia.

In the past few years, greater access to MRI technologies has encouraged further research on brain morphology and dyslexia. Hynd and Semrud-Clikeman conducted an MRI study in an attempt to define syndrome-specific patterns of brain involvement in two different (although frequently comorbid) developmental disorders, dyslexia and attention deficit hyperactivity disorder (ADHD). They found that 70 percent of normal and ADHD children exhibited the expected pattern of left > right plana asymmetry, but only 10 percent of the dyslexic children did.[90] Both clinical groups had smaller right anterior width measurements than the normal controls, but these investigators concluded the significant increase in the incidence of plana symmetry or reversed asymmetry to be unique to dyslexia and they postulated a relationship to deviant patterns of corticogenesis.

Larsen and coworkers[91] reported somewhat similar MRI results, noting that among dyslexics with documented phonologic deficits none exhibited expected patterns of plana asymmetry. These investigators suggested asymmetry of the plana may be a prerequisite for normal language development in the phonological domain. The Larsen and colleagues[91] and Hynd and coworkers[90] results were not similar, however, at another level of analysis. Larsen's results indicated a reversal of the expected left asymmetry in the report of a *greater right* planum temporale length in dyslexic subjects. Rather than a greater right planum, Hynd and associates reported a *smaller left* planum compared to the right and a smaller insular region bilaterally.

These discrepancies are frequent among different neuroimaging results reported on dyslexia, a fact that Schultz and associates[81] and Filipek[79] attribute to both (1) wide variations in (and lack of attention to) subjects' age, sex, handedness, and diagnostic criteria validity in different studies and (2) inherent difficulties in accurately and reliably measuring structures like the planum temporale. In an attempt to replicate previous MRI results on dyslexia, Schultz and colleagues[81] found initial evidence of smaller left hemispheric structures in dyslexic brains: when analyses were conducted controlling for age and overall brain size, however, no reliable differences between dyslexics and normal controls were found on a range of measures including those of surface area and symmetry of the planum temporale. Sex, age, and overall brain size were all found to significantly influence specific morphometric measures of the brain, especially the surface area of the planum temporale. After reviewing all of the recent MRI studies on developmental dyslexia, Filipek[79] concluded that none of the planum temporale measurements in these studies were comparable, and that definition of the plana temporale remains one of the most difficult challenges for MRI-based work. Filipek concludes that, at present, no consistent morphologic correlates of developmental reading disorders can be identified from neuroimaging studies.

The second line of neuroanatomic evidence on dyslexia is provided through postmortem studies of dyslexic brains. The first autopsy study was reported by Drake,[92] detailing postmortem findings on a 12-year-old boy with multiple learning disabilities and a family history of dyslexia who died of a massive cerebellar hemorrhage. Several neurodevelopmental abnormalities were found that could not be attributed to brain damage, including an abnormal convolutional pattern bilaterally in the parietal lobes, a thinned corpus callosum, and ectopic neurons deep in the white matter. These findings suggested deviations in cellular migration during gestation.[93]

Subsequent studies by Galaburda and colleagues confirmed the presence of minor cortical malformations in four male dyslexic brains and alterations in the expected patterns of brain asymmetry in the language areas, particularly the planum temporale.[88] In all four autopsies, neurodevelopmental abnormalities were found primarily in the left frontal and left perisylvian region. Postmortem studies of three female dyslexic brains again revealed symmetry of the planum temporale and cortical abnormalities identical to those reported for the male brains.[94] The malformations were suggested to occur in the second trimester of pregnancy.[82]

Supported by experimental studies with animal models,[95–97] Galaburda speculates that a genetic defect may result in a tendency to small cerebral vascular accidents (CVAs) in fetal life, and that the sequelae of these events is abnormal neuronal migration and the establishment of abnormal neuronal circuits in brain areas typically devoted to language functions: the dyslexic brain is suggested to have too many neurons in the posterior language areas, particularly in the right hemisphere, rather than too few.[83] Based on Behan and Geschwind's[98] theory about the interrelationships between immune deficiencies and deviations in neuronal migration, Galaburda[99] speculates that the focal brain injury may even be mediated through allergic mechanisms.

Although not emphasized in the report, the focal ectopias and dysplasias revealed in the Galaburda and coworkers[88] work were bilateral in nature and involved both left and right frontal regions. As Hynd and Semrud-Clikeman[89] note, the bilateral involvement of the anterior cortex is very relevant behaviorally, and may support speculation that the language disturbances associated with developmental dyslexia may extend beyond left anterior-central structures to include right hemispheric systems.

Additional evidence on the neurobiology of dyslexia is found in combined neurophysiologic and neuroanatomic studies. In a controversial report, Lovegrove and colleagues[100] had identified a specific visual abnormality associated with dyslexia, abnormally slow flicker fusion rates (i.e., the fastest rate at which a contrast reversal of a stimulus can be seen) observed only at low spatial frequencies and at low contrasts. In evoked potentials studies, Livingstone and coworkers,[101] and Lehmkuhle and colleagues[102] found that the parvocellular pathway (the slow, more contrast-insensitive, and color-selective visual pathway) seemed to be functioning normally in a dyslexic sample, but that the visual pathway handling fast, low-contrast stimuli appeared abnormally slow. Fast stimuli are handled by the magnocellular pathway,

the two pathways being differentiated in the retina and separate through the lateral geniculate nucleus (LGN), the primary visual cortex, and higher order visual cortices.[82] Livingstone and colleagues[101] compared the magnocellular and parvocellular layers of the LGN in five dyslexic and five control brains and found that the magnocellular cells were smaller in the dyslexic brains but the parvocellular cells were not. In subsequent work, Galaburda and coworkers[103] reported abnormal asymmetry in the medial geniculate nuclei (MGN) of five dyslexic brains; unlike control brains which were symmetrical, left MGN neurons were smaller than right MGN neurons in dyslexic brains. This finding implicated parallel difficulties in the auditory system, and was hypothesized relevant to behavioral observations of left hemisphere–based phonologic processing deficits. Livingstone and colleagues speculate that other cortical systems may be subdivided into fast and slow subsystems and that dyslexics may prove selectively deficient in fast subsystem functions across modalities.[82,101,103,104]*

---

*The reports of slowed visual function, related to the magnocellular pathway, are controversial in the dyslexia literature for several reasons: First, these results have not been consistently replicated in independent studies (e.g., see Ref. 102 versus Refs. 105 and 106); second, the methodology has been criticized for vulnerability to artifactual effects;[107] and third, the results appear to contradict the bulk of evidence on phonological core deficits as characteristic of dyslexia.[23,108] The relevance of detailed examination of rapid temporal processing functions in visual, auditory, and motor domains is suggested, however, by existing evidence of auditory temporal processing deficits in language impaired children,[109,110] visual naming speed deficits in dyslexic children,[46,47] and impaired temporal resolution in bimanual motor coordination in dyslexic children.[111] Wolff[111] cautions against any simplistic attribution of the temporal resolution deficit of dyslexics to a single temporal behavioral variable or to specific regions of the central nervous system neuroanatomically: Wolff[111] suggests instead that some of the core dyslexic deficits may relate to problems assembling components of behavior into "temporally ordered larger ensembles," problems which may be associated with developmental difficulty in motor, language, and reading domains.

Postmortem observations on developmental dyslexia are necessarily limited by small sample sizes, significant heterogeneity in the individual histories of the cases, and retrospective and variable diagnostic and behavioral data. Despite the obvious methodologic shortcomings, the neuroanatomic data provided through both the postmortem and animal research studies of Galaburda and colleagues have provided evidence on potential biological etiologies for reading disability and yielded a rich source of neurobiological hypotheses. With the expanding technologies available for functional neuroimaging and new awareness of critical design controls in neuroimaging studies with pediatric and adult samples,[79,81,112] the next decade should witness significant advances in our understanding of the structural and functional bases of dyslexic disorders in the developing brain.

THE TREATMENT OF DEVELOPMENTAL READING DISORDERS

Many approaches to treating reading disorders have been advocated. Some methods aim to remediate the nonreading deficit or set of deficits presumed causal to the reading disability, and a great diversity of interventions have been attempted in this tradition. These include perceptual and perceptual-motor training programs of the 1960s and 1970s (e.g., Refs. 113 and 114), pharmacologic interventions of the 1980s and 1990s,[115,116] and mechanical devices like the "electronic ear," which remain popular.[117] None of these methods has proven effective in the remediation of reading disability despite controlled research on their efficacy.[118–122] The second type of treatment intervention for reading disorders attempts to remediate the deficient reading process directly and address the primary symptoms leading to referral. Consideration of this approach to treatment and what we learn of the core disorder through a systematic study of treatment response constitutes the remainder of this chapter.

Before the mid 1980s, there existed no reliable or credible evidence from well-controlled studies of the relative merit of any one intervention approach over another.[26,123–125] This dearth of evidence led to inevitable questions about the amenability of the disorder to treatment. In the past decade, however, different investigators have reported positive findings from controlled intervention or training studies with samples of disabled readers.[33–35,126–134] Because the core deficit in phonologic awareness had been demonstrated to be a lifelong symptom, even with the attainment of some standard of literacy in adulthood,[41,135] reports of positive findings were particularly encouraging in demonstrating that children with developmental reading disability *are* able to benefit from some forms of literacy training.

The most recent treatment outcome data reveal the importance of addressing the core deficits defining the developmental reading disorder[127] rather than circumventing processing deficits and teaching to the child's "strengths." The best results appear with effective, well-directed treatment that remediates the basic phonologic and word-identification learning deficits. Both treatment successes and treatment failures from our intervention studies at the Hospital for Sick Children in Toronto have provided a window on the core acquisition deficits of children with developmental reading disability. Children with severe reading disabilities appear to have enormous difficulty abstracting grapheme-phoneme (letter-sound) pattern invariance. In one study, they failed to show significant transfer to uninstructed reading words even in situations where training on very similar instructed words had been clearly effective.[33] Despite their success on the training words, *line* and *mark,* for instance, dyslexic subjects were not reliably better after treatment in identifying *fine* and *dark.* In these studies, dyslexic subjects responded to intensive training by doubling their estimated reading vocabularies, yet they seemed to be acquiring specific lexical knowledge rather than systematic letter-sound knowledge that could facilitate their decoding of new, unknown words.

Transfer-of-Learning Issues

This pattern of dyslexic reading acquisition reflects basic difficulties in transfer of learning during the course of training. We have described these transfer-of-learning problems in the word-identification module and attributed them to difficulties in parsing syllables into subsyllabic units, a failure that limits dyslexic readers' acquisition of word recognition skill by preventing both large-unit (rime—i.e., the vowel and what comes after: the *ain* in *rain*) and smaller-unit (letter-sound, letter-cluster-sound) extraction of spelling-to-sound patterns when a new word is learned. We have attributed this difficulty to the phonemic awareness deficits known to characterize the most prevalent forms of developmental reading disability.[26,34] It has also been suggested that such difficulties may stem from the nature and/or accessibility of the lexical representations laid down in memory (e.g., Refs. 136 and 137) during learning.

Transfer-of-learning failures in reading acquisition are also exacerbated, however, by more general difficulties that many reading-disabled children experience in the metacognitive domain. The ability to identify new unknown words depends on age-appropriate phonologic processing skills, consolidated letter-sound knowledge, and also on effective and flexible strategies for identifying words and the child's ability to exert some metacognitive control over the decoding process. Children with reading disorders have been characterized as deficient and inefficient in the use of cognitive strategies.[138–142] Despite limitations in their phonemic awareness and letter-sound knowledge, disabled readers do not reliably use what they *do* know to help them decode what they do not.[127,143] Children with learning disorders have been characterized as lacking self-regulatory strategies, failing to self-monitor and self-correct the product of their efforts,[144–146] observations some authors have found suggestive of frontal lobe dysfunction.[147] Strategy acquisition, application, and monitoring is essential to any learning that extends beyond that which has been specifically taught; and strategy use and metacognitive knowledge are critical to achieving transfer of learning in many domains of functioning.[127,144,148]

Treating Transfer-of-Learning Failures

In a recent treatment outcome study, we have addressed two of the core deficits underlying developmental dyslexia and attempted to ameliorate transfer-of-learning difficulties in word-identification learning. Children with severe developmental reading disability were randomly assigned to two forms of word-identification training, both designed to promote transfer of learning, or to a study skills control program. One program addressed phonologic awareness and subsyllabic segmentation deficits through direct, intensive phonological training and direct instruction of letter-sound correspondences (PHAB/DI for Phonological Analysis and Blending/Direct Instruction).* The other program provided a metacognitive focus, training disabled readers in the acquisition, use, and monitoring of four metacognitive decoding strategies (WIST for Word Identification Strategy Training).† The two programs addressed subsyllabic segmentation with different-sized units, the phonologic program training the smallest units of spelling-to-sound mapping (letter-sound) and the metacognitive program dealing with larger spelling-to-sound units (i.e., the rime).

Results provided positive evidence of transfer of learning in the treatment of developmental reading disability.[127] Both intervention programs were associated with large positive effects, transfer attained on several different measures, and generalized achievement gains on standardized measures. Children who before training stumbled over high-frequency one-syllable words like *way, left,* and *put* were able (albeit slowly) after training to decode multisyllabic words like *unintelligible, mistakenly,* and *disengaged.* A critical finding of this research was the demonstration that the deficient phonologic processing skills of dyslexic children *are* amenable to treatment and that

---

*The PHAB/DI Program used direct instructional materials developed by Engelmann and colleagues at the University of Oregon[149–151] to train phonologic analysis, phonologic blending, and letter-sound association skills.

†The WIST Program was developed in our laboratory classrooms at the Hospital For Sick Children. This program is based in part on the Benchmark School Word Identification/Vocabulary Development Program developed by Gaskins and coworkers.[152]

phonologic segmentation, blending, and letter-sound learning abilities can be improved with effective and focused intervention methods. Both speech- and print-based phonologic skills of this impaired sample, although not normalized after 35 h of training, were significantly improved and closer to age-appropriate expectations. Different patterns of transfer were observed following the two different interventions, the phonologic program resulting in greater transfer across the phonologic domain, and the metacognitive program resulting in broader-based transfer for real English words (i.e., regular and exception words).

The success of both programs suggests that different routes of subsyllabic segmentation are possible in the remediation of reading disability: both the letter-sound (PHAB/DI) and the letter cluster-sound (WIST) approaches were associated with improved word identification and decoding skills. Some level of segmentation within the syllable, however, is essential to allow transfer from a just-learned word to a similarly spelled word: without subsyllabic segmentation that is explicitly trained and practiced, disabled readers will fail to transfer new word learning and be prevented from becoming independent readers.

In this study, both metacognitive and phonologically based training proved to be of merit in the remediation of developmental reading disability. These results are interpreted as evidence that only systematic deficit-directed remediation will allow severely disabled readers to overcome transfer-of-learning failures in the course of reading acquisition. Effective remediation of children with reading disabilities must address the problem of transfer of learning in every remedial lesson, and provide intensive remediation of the core processing deficits contributing to reading acquisition failure.[127]

SUMMARY COMMENTS

Developmental reading disability has been recognized as a specific developmental disorder for over a century. The term is usually reserved for those 3 to 6 percent of otherwise normally developing children who experience significant, often unexpected, difficulties in acquiring basic literacy skills. Once considered only to describe children reading below IQ-based predictions (i.e., those with higher IQs and lower reading achievement), the disorder is now recognized to affect children with a range of intellectual abilities and to be attributable to the same core processing deficits irrespective of a child's estimated intellectual potential.

Reading disorders are often accompanied by two highly specific deficits in separate aspects of speech and language development: (1) problems in the ability to represent and rapidly access individual speech sounds in words and (2) difficulty rapidly accessing and retrieving names for visual symbols. Both deficits have been found to persist into adulthood. Many reading-disabled children also appear generally deficient and inefficient in the use and monitoring of cognitive strategies, a tendency that exacerbates the difficulties attributable to their core processing deficits and makes it particularly hard for them to profit from remedial instruction. Our recent treatment results described severely reading-disabled children as experiencing basic problems with transfer of learning during the course of word-identification learning. Taught to read the words *rain* and *car,* these children could not reliably identify *pain* or *far,* a transfer failure we attribute to phonologically based difficulties in subsyllabic segmentation and a lack of effective decoding strategies.

The most recent treatment results with reading-disabled samples are encouraging in demonstrating that two of the above core deficits are amenable to treatment with systematic, intensive, and focused remediation: two different remedial teaching approaches were identified which allowed severely dyslexic children to improve their word identification and nonword decoding skills and demonstrate significant transfer of learning to a variety of words, nonwords, and reading tasks. While not completely ameliorated, the pervasive and persistent phonologic processing deficits of these children were significantly improved following intensive phonologic training. Similarly, children who stumbled over one-syllable words before treatment acquired the ability to decode difficult multisyllabic words following a metacognitive approach to literacy training. These results demonstrate that systematic deficit-directed remediation will allow severely dyslexic children to overcome transfer-of-learning problems: Effective remedial techniques are available to address the deficits contributing to reading acquisition failure in these children.

There are a number of neurobiological explanations advanced in research on the potential etiology of dyslexia. The possible heritability of dyslexia was recognized decades ago, with recognition that the disorder tended to familial aggregation. Although evidence for genetic heterogeneity is strong even for specially selected family samples, there is very recent evidence of a possible dyslexia locus on a specific region of chromosome 6. The search for neuroanatomic and neurophysiologic substrates of dyslexia has implicated areas of the left hemisphere specialized for language function but has also demonstrated evidence of bilateral frontal ectopias and other abnormalities in dyslexic brains. It has been speculated that deviations in neuronal pruning and neuronal migration in the second trimester of pregnancy result in too many neurons in the posterior language areas rather than too few, particularly in the right hemisphere. These deviations in fetal brain development have been attributed by different authors to possible viral infection in the mother,[153] small cerebrovascular accidents mediated through allergic mechanisms, or to conditions mediated by genetic predisposition.

Significant advances have been made in the definition, diagnosis, and treatment of developmental reading disabilities. At the same time, technical capabilities for functional neuroimaging research have expanded, and there is increasing commitment to methodologic rigor in the pursuit of a neurobiological perspective on reading, language, and their developmental disorders. With the wealth of interdisciplinary data now available, and the potential for new conceptualizations of developing brain and behavioral systems and their interrelationships, developmental dyslexia may become a model for examining development and developmental variability in this decade of the brain.

REFERENCES

1. Hinshelwood J: Word blindness and visual memories. *Lancet* 2:1566–1570, 1895.
2. Hinshelwood J: *Congenital Word Blindness.* London: Lewis, 1917.
3. Spreen O, Tupper D, Risser A, et al: *Human Developmental Neuropsychology.* New York: Oxford University Press, 1984.
4. Morgan WP: A case of congenital word-blindness. *Br Med J* 2:1378, 1896.
5. Orton ST: "Word-blindness" in school children. *Arch Neurol Psychiatry* 14:581–615, 1925.
6. Orton ST: Specific reading disability—Strephosymbolia. *J Am Med Assoc* 90:1095–1099, 1928.
7. Gillingham A, Stillman BW: *Remedial Training for Children with Specific Disability in Reading, Spelling, and Penmanship.* Cambridge, MA: Educators Publishing Service, 1960.
8. Orton ST: *Reading, Writing, and Speech in Children.* New York: Norton, 1937.
9. Ansara A: The Orton-Gillingham approach to remediation, in Malatesha RN, Aaron PG (eds): *Reading Disorders: Varieties and Treatment.* New York: Academic Press, 1982, pp 409–433.
10. Critchley M: *The Dyslexic Child.* Springfield, IL: Charles C Thomas, 1970.
11. Mattis S: Dyslexia syndromes: A working hypothesis that works, in Benton AL, Pearl D (eds): *Dyslexia: An Appraisal of Current Knowledge.* New York: Oxford University Press, 1978.
12. Denckla MB: Childhood learning disabilities, in Heilman KM, Valenstein E (eds): *Clinical Neuropsychology.* New York: Oxford University Press, 1979.
13. Bishop DVM, Adams C: A prospective study of the relationship between specific language impairment, phonological disorders and reading retardation. *J Child Psychol Psychiatry* 31:1027–1050, 1990.
14. Gathercole SE, Baddeley AD: The processes underlying segmental analysis. *Eur Bull Cogn Psychol* 7:462–464, 1987.
15. Scarborough HS: Very early language deficits in dyslexic children. *Child Devel* 61:1728–1743, 1990.
16. Stanovich KE: Annotation: Does dyslexia exist? *J Child Psychol Psychiatry* 55:579–595, 1994.

17. Hynd GW, Cohen M: *Dyslexia: Neuropsychological Theory, Research, and Clinical Differentiation.* New York: Grune & Stratton, 1983.

18. Rutter M: Prevalence and types of dyslexia, in Benton A, Pearl D (eds): *Dyslexia: An Appraisal of Current Knowledge.* New York: Oxford University Press, 1978.

19. Stanovich KE: Matthew effects in reading: Some consequences of individual differences in the acquisition of literacy. *Read Res Q* 21:360–407, 1986.

20. Frankenberger W, Fronzaglio K: A review of state's criteria and procedures for identifying children with learning disabilities. *J Learn Disabil* 24:495–500, 1991.

21. Frankenberger W, Harper J: State's criteria and procedures for identifying learning disabled children: A comparison of 1981/82 and 1985/86 guidelines. *J Learn Disabil* 20:118–121, 1987.

22. Satz P, Fletcher J: Minimal brain dysfunctions: An appraisal of research, concepts, and methods, in Rie HE, Rie ED (eds): *Handbook of Minimal Brain Dysfunctions: A Critical Review.* New York: Wiley, 1980, pp 669–714.

23. Stanovich KE, Siegel LS: Phenotypic performance profile of children with reading disabilities: A regression-based test of the phonological-core variable-difference model. *J Educ Psychol* 86:24–53, 1994.

24. Gough PB, Tunmer WE: Decoding, reading, and reading disability. *Remed Special Educ* 7:6–10, 1986.

25. Fletcher JM, Shaywitz SE, Shankweiler DP, et al: Cognitive profiles of reading disability: Comparisons of discrepancy and low achievement definitions. *J Educ Psychol* 86:6–23, 1994.

26. Lovett MW: Developmental dyslexia, in Rapin I, Segalowitz SJ (eds): *Handbook of Neuropsychology.* Amsterdam: Elsevier Science, 1992, pp 163–185.

27. Perfetti CA: *Reading Ability.* New York: Oxford University Press, 1985.

28. Stanovich KE: Changing models of reading and reading acquisition, in Rieben L, Perfetti CA (eds): *Learning to Read: Basic Research and Its Implications.* Hillsdale, NJ: Erlbaum, 1991, pp 19–31.

29. Vellutino FR: *Dyslexia: Theory and Research.* Cambridge, MA: MIT Press, 1979.

30. Wolf M, Vellutino F: A psycholinguistic account of the reading process, in Berko-Gleason J, Bernstein-Ratner N (eds): *Psycholinguistics.* New York: Macmillan, 1993, pp 352–391.

31. Snowling M, Hulme C: Developmental dyslexia and language disorders, in Blanken G, Dittmann J, Grimm H, et al (eds): *Linguistic Disorders and Pathologies: An International Handbook.* New York: Walter de Gruyter, 1993, pp 724–732.

32. Goswami U, Bryant PE: *Phonological Skills and Learning to Read.* Hillsdale, NJ: Erlbaum, 1990.

33. Lovett MW, Warren-Chaplin PM, Ransby MJ, Borden SL: Training the word recognition skills of reading disabled children: Treatment and transfer effects. *J Educ Psychol* 82:769–780, 1990.

34. Lovett MW: Reading, writing, and remediation: Perspectives on the dyslexic learning disability from remedial outcome data. *Learn Indiv Diff* 3:295–305, 1991.

35. Vellutino FR, Scanlon DM: Phonological coding, phonological awareness, and reading ability: Evidence from a longitudinal and experimental study. *Merrill-Palmer Q* 33:321–363, 1987.

36. Liberman IY, Shankweiler D: Phonology and the problems of learning to read and write. *Remed Spec Educ* 6:8–17, 1985.

37. Mann V: Why some children encounter reading problems, in: Torgesen J, Wong B (eds): *Psychological and Educational Perspectives on Learning Disabilities.* New York: Academic Press, 1986, pp 133–159.

38. Wagner RK, Torgesen JK: The nature of phonological processing and its causal role in the acquisition of reading skills. *Psychol Bull* 101:192–212, 1987.

39. Wagner RK, Torgesen JK, Laughon P, et al: Development of young readers' phonological processing abilities. *J Educ Psychol* 85:83–103, 1993.

40. Wagner RK, Torgesen JK, Rashotte CA: Development of reading-related phonological processing abilities: New evidence of bidirectional causality from a latent variable longitudinal study. *Dev Psychol* 30:73–87, 1994.

41. Bruck M: Persistence of dyslexics' phonological awareness deficits. *Dev Psychol* 28:874–886, 1992.

42. Bowers PG, Steffy RA, Tate E: Comparison of the effects of IQ control methods on memory and naming speed predictors of reading disability. *Read Res Q* 23:204–319, 1988.

43. Bowers PG, Swanson LB: Naming speed deficits in reading disability: Multiple measures of a singular process. *J Exp Child Psychol* 51:195–219, 1991.

44. Bowers PG, Wolf M: Theoretical links between naming speed, precise mechanisms, and ortho-

graphic skill in dyslexia. *Reading Writing* 5:69–85, 1993.

45. Wolf M: The word retrieval process and reading in children and aphasics, in Nelson K (ed): *Children's Language.* Hillsdale, NJ: Erlbaum, 1982, pp 473–493.

46. Wolf M: Naming speed and reading: The contribution of the cognitive neurosciences. *Read Res Q* 26:123–141, 1991.

47. Wolf M, Bally H, Morris R: Automaticity, retrieval processes, and reading: A longitudinal study in average and impaired readers. *Child Dev* 57:988–1000, 1986.

48. Wolf M, Obregon M: Early naming deficits, developmental dyslexia, and a specific deficit hypothesis. *Brain Lang* 42:219–247, 1992.

49. Felton RH, Brown IS: Phonological processes as predictors of specific reading skills in children at risk for reading failure. *Reading Writing* 2:39–59, 1990.

50. Wolff P, Michel G, Ovrut M: Rate variables and automatized naming in developmental dyslexia. *Brain Lang* 39:556–575, 1990.

51. Wolff P, Michel G, Ovrut M, Drake C: Rate and timing precision of motor coordination in developmental dyslexia. *Dev Psychol* 26:349–359, 1990.

52. Novoa L: *Word Retrieval Process and Reading Acquisition and Development in Bilingual and Monolingual Children.* Cambridge, MA: Harvard University Press, 1988.

53. Wolf M, Pfeil C, Lotz R, Biddle K: Towards a more universal understanding of the developmental dyslexias: The contribution of orthographic factors, in Berninger VW (ed): *The Varieties of Orthographic Knowledge, I.* Dordrecht: Kluwer, 1994, pp 137–171.

54. Yap R, Van der Liej A: Word processing in dyslexia: An automatic coding deficit? *Reading Writing* 5:261–279, 1993.

55. Bowers PG: Re-examining selected reading research from the viewpoint of the double-deficit-hypothesis. Society for Research in Child Development. Indianapolis, April 1995.

56. Lovett MW: Remediating dyslexic children's word identification deficits: Are the core deficits of developmental dyslexia amenable to treatment? Society for Research in Child Development. Indianapolis, April 1995.

57. Wolf M: The double deficit hypothesis for developmental reading disorders. Society for Research in Child Development. Indianapolis, April 1995.

58. Hinshelwood J: Four cases of congenital word-blindness occurring in the same family. *Br Med J* 2:1229–1232, 1907.

59. Hinshelwood J: Two cases of hereditary word-blindness. *Br Med J* 1:608–609, 1911.

60. Stephenson S: Six cases of congenital word-blindness affecting three generations of one family. *Ophthalmoscope* 5:482–484, 1907.

61. Rutter M, Tizard J, Whitmore K: *Education, Health, and Behavior.* New York: Krieger, 1970.

62. Gilger JW, Pennington BF, DeFries JC: Risk for reading disabilities as a function of parental history of learning problems: Data from three samples of families demonstrating genetic transmission. *Reading Writing* 3:205–217, 1991.

63. Pennington BF: Genetics of learning disabilities. *J Child Neurol* 10:S69–S77, 1995.

64. Vogler GP, DeFries JC, Decker SN: Family history as an indicator of risk for reading disability. *J Learn Disabil* 18:419–421, 1985.

65. Pennington BF: The genetics of dyslexia. *J Child Psychol Psychiatry* 31:193–201, 1990.

66. DeFries JC, Fulker DW, LaBuda MC: Reading disability in twins: Evidence for a genetic etiology. *Nature* 329:537–539, 1987.

67. DeFries JC, Stevenson J, Gillis JJ, Wadsworth SJ: Genetic etiology of spelling deficits in the Colorado and London twin studies of reading disability. *Reading Writing* 3:271–283, 1991.

68. Olson RK, Gillis JJ, Rack JP, et al: Confirmatory factor analysis of word recognition and process measures in the Colorado reading project. *Reading Writing* 3:235–248, 1991.

69. Pennington BF, Gilger JW, Pauls D, et al: Evidence for major gene transmission of developmental dyslexia. *JAMA* 26:1527–1534, 1991.

70. Lewitter FI, DeFries JC, Elston RC: Genetic models of reading disability. *Behav Genet* 10:9–30, 1980.

71. Smith SD, Pennington BF, Kimberling WJ, Ing PS: Familial dyslexia: Use of genetic linkage analysis to define subtypes. *J Am Acad Child Psychiatry* 29:204, 1990.

72. Smith SD, Kimberling WJ, Pennington BF, Lubs MA: Specific reading disability: Identification of an inherited form through linkage analysis. *Science* 219:1345–1347, 1983.

73. Bisgaard ML, Eiberg H, Moller N, Niebuhr E, et al: Dyslexia and chromosome 15 heteromorphism: Negative lod score in a Danish material. *Clin Genet* 32:118–119, 1987.

74. Cardon LR, Smith SD, Fulker FW, et al: Quantitative trait locus for reading disability on chromosome 6. *Science* 266:276–279, 1994.

75. Geschwind N, Behan P: Left-handedness: Association with immune disease, migraine, and developmental learning disorder. *Proc Natl Acad Sci USA* 79:5097–5100, 1982.

76. Pennington BF, Smith SR, Kimberling WJ, et al: Left-handedness and immune disorders in familial dyslexics. *Arch Neurol* 44:634–639, 1987.

77. Harris EL: The contribution of twin research to the study of the etiology of reading disability, in Smith SD (ed): *Genetics and Learning Disabilities*. San Diego, CA: College Hill Press, 1986, pp 3–19.

78. Plomin R: The role of inheritance in behavior. *Science* 248:183–188, 1990.

79. Filipek PA: Neurobiologic correlates of developmental dyslexia: How do dyslexics' brains differ from those of normal readers? *J Child Neurol* 10:S62–S69, 1995.

80. Caplan D: *Language: Structure, Processing, and Disorders*. Cambridge, MA: MIT Press, 1992.

81. Schultz RT, Cho NK, Staib LH, et al: Brain morphology in normal and dyslexic children: The influence of sex and age. *Ann Neurol* 35:732–742, 1994.

82. Galaburda AM: Neurology of developmental dyslexia. *Curr Opin Neurol Neurosurg* 5:71–76, 1992.

83. Galaburda AM: Neuroanatomic basis of developmental dyslexia. *Neurol Clin* 11:161–173, 1993.

84. Galaburda AM, Sanides F: Cytoarchitectonic organization of the human auditory cortex. *J Comput Neurol* 190:597–610, 1980.

85. Luria AR: *Higher Cortical Functions in Man*. New York: Basic Books, 1980.

86. Haslam RH, Dalby JT, Johns RD, Rademaker AW: Cerebral asymmetry in developmental dyslexia. *Arch Neurol* 38:679–682, 1981.

87. Rumsey JM, Dorwart R, Vermess M, et al: Magnetic resonance imaging of brain anatomy in severe developmental dyslexia. *Arch Neurol* 43:1045–1046, 1986.

88. Galaburda AM, Sherman GF, Rosen GD, et al: Developmental dyslexia: Four consecutive patients with cortical anomalies. *Ann Neurol* 18:222–233, 1985.

89. Hynd GW, Semrud-Clikeman M: Dyslexia and brain morphology. *Psychol Bull* 106:447–482, 1989.

90. Hynd GW, Semrud-Clikeman M, Lorys AR, et al: Brain morphology in developmental dyslexia and attention deficit disorder/hyperactivity. *Arch Neurol* 47:919–926, 1990.

91. Larsen JP, Hoien T, Lundberg I, Odegaard H: MRI evaluation of the size and symmetry of the planum temporale in adolescents with developmental dyslexia. *Brain Lang* 39:289–301, 1990.

92. Drake WE: Clinical and pathological findings in a child with a developmental learning disability. *J Learn Disabil* 1:486–502, 1968.

93. Hynd GW, Semrud-Clikeman M: Dyslexia and neurodevelopmental pathology: Relationships to cognition, intelligence, and reading skill acquisition. *J Learn Disabil* 22:204–220, 1989.

94. Humphreys P, Kaufmann WE, Galaburda AM: Developmental dyslexia in women: Neuropathological findings in three cases. *Ann Neurol* 28:727–738, 1990.

95. Humphreys P, Rosen BD, Press DM, et al: Freezing lesions of the developing rat brain: A model for cerebrocortical microgyria. *Neuropathol Exp Neurol* 50:145–160, 1991.

96. Sherman GF, Galaburda AM, Geschwind N: Cortical anomalies in brains of New Zealand mice: A neuropathologic model of dyslexia? *Proc Natl Acad Sci USA* 82:8072–8074, 1985.

97. Sherman GF, Galaburda AM, Behan PO, Rosen GD: Neuroanatomical anomalies in autoimmune mice. *Acta Neuropathol* 74:239–242, 1987.

98. Behan PO, Geschwind N: Dyslexia, congenital anomalies, and immune disorders: The role of the fetal environment. *Ann NY Acad Sci* 457:13–18, 1985.

99. Galaburda AM: Developmental dyslexia. *Buffalo Branch Orton Dyslexia Soc News* 5–11, 1993.

100. Lovegrove WJ, Garzia RP, Nicholson SB: Experimental evidence for a transient system deficit in specific reading disability. *J Am Optom Assoc* 61:137–146, 1990.

101. Livingstone MS, Rosen GD, Drislane FW, Galaburda AM: Physiological and anatomical evidence for a magnocellular defect in developmental dyslexia. *Proc Natl Acad Sci USA* 88:7943–7947, 1991.

102. Lehmkuhle S, Garzia RP, Turner BS, et al: A defective visual pathway in children with reading disability. *N Engl J Med* 328:989–996, 1993.

103. Galaburda AM, Menard MT, Rosen GD: Evidence for aberrant auditory anatomy in developmental dyslexia. *Proc Natl Acad Sci USA* 91:8010–8013, 1994.

104. Galaburda AM, Livingstone M: Evidence for a

magnocellular defect in developmental dyslexia. *Ann NY Acad Sci* 68:70–82, 1993.

105. Hayduk S, Bruck M, Cavanagh P: Low level processing skills of adults and children with dyslexia: A critical evaluation. *Cogn Neuropsychol.* In press.

106. Smith A, Early F, Grogan S: Flicker masking and developmental dyslexia. *Perception* 15:473–482, 1986.

107. Badcock D, Sevdalis E: Masking by uniform field flicker: Some practical problems. *Perception* 16:641–647, 1987.

108. Hulme C: The implausibility of low-level visual deficits as a cause of children's reading difficulties. *Cogn Neuropsychol* 5:369–374, 1988.

109. Tallal P, Stark RE, Mellits D: The relationship between auditory temporal analysis and receptive language development: Evidence from studies of developmental language disorder. *Neuropsychologia* 23:527–534, 1985.

110. Tallal P, Stark RE, Mellits D: Identification of language-impaired children on the basis of rapid perception and production skills. *Brain Lang* 25:314–322, 1985.

111. Wolff PH: Impaired temporal resolution in developmental dyslexia. *Ann NY Acad Sci* 682:87–103, 1993.

112. Shaywitz BA, Shaywitz SE, Pugh KR, et al: Sex differences in the functional organization of the brain for language. *Nature* 373:607–609, 1995.

113. Delacato CH: *Neurological Organization and Reading.* Springfield, IL: Charles C Thomas, 1966.

114. Frostig M: *Move, Grow, Learn.* Chicago, IL: Follet, 1969.

115. Wilsher CR, Bennett D, Chase CH, et al: Piracetam and dyslexia: Effects on reading tests. *J Clin Psychopharmacol* 7:230–237, 1987.

116. Levinson HN: *A Solution to the Riddle Dyslexia.* New York: Springer-Verlag, 1980.

117. Tomatis A: *Education and Dyslexia.* France-Quebec: Les Editions, 1978.

118. Di Ianni M, Wilsher C, Blank MS, et al: The effects of piracetam in children with dyslexia. *J Clin Psychopharmacology* 5:272–278, 1985.

119. Gittelman R, Feingold I: Children with reading disorders: I. Efficacy of reading remediation. *J Child Psychol Psychiatry* 24:167–191, 1983.

120. Kershner JR, Cummings RL, Clarke KA, et al: Evaluation of the Tomatis Listening Training Program with learning disabled children. *Can J Special Educ* 2:1–32, 1986.

121. Kershner JR, Cummings RL, Clarke KA, et al: Two-year evaluation of the Tomatis Listening Training Program with learning disabled children. *Learn Disabil Q* 13:43–53, 1990.

122. Robinson HM: Visual and auditory modalities related to methods for beginning readers. *Reading Res Q* 8:7–39, 1972.

123. Gittelman R: Treatment of reading disorders, in Rutter M (ed): *Developmental Neuropsychiatry.* New York: Guilford Press, 1983, pp 520–541.

124. Hewison J: The current status of remedial intervention for children with reading problems. *Dev Med Child Neurol* 24:183–186, 1982.

125. Johnson DL: Remedial approaches to dyslexia, in Benton AL, Pearl D (eds): *Dyslexia: An Appraisal of Current Knowledge.* New York: Oxford University Press, 1978, pp 397–421.

126. Lovett MW, Barron RW, Forbes JE, et al: Computer speech-based training of literacy skills in neurologically-impaired children: A controlled evaluation. *Brain Lang* 47:117–154, 1994.

127. Lovett MW, Borden SL, DeLuca T, et al: Treating the core deficits of developmental dyslexia: Evidence of transfer-of-learning following phonologically- and strategy-based reading training programs. *Dev Psychol* 30:805–822, 1994.

128. Lovett MW, Ransby MJ, Barron RW: Treatment, subtype, and word type effects in dyslexic children's response to remediation. *Brain Lang* 34:328–349, 1988.

129. Lovett MW, Ransby MJ, Hardwick N, et al: Can dyslexia be treated? Treatment-specific and generalized treatment effects in dyslexic children's response to remediation. *Brain Lang* 37:90–121, 1989.

130. Olson RK, Wise BW: Reading on the computer with orthographic and speech feedback. *Reading Writing* 4:107–144, 1992.

131. Olson RK, Wise B, Conners F, Rack J: Organization, heritability, and remediation of component word recognition and language skills in disabled readers, in Carr T, Levy BA (eds): *Reading and Its Development: Component Skills Approaches.* San Diego, CA: Academic Press, 1990, pp 261–322.

132. Roth SF, Beck IL: Theoretical and instructional implications of the assessment of two microcomputer word recognition programs. *Reading Res Q* 22:197–218, 1987.

133. Wise BW, Olson R, Anstett M, et al: Implementing a long-term computerized remedial reading program with synthetic speech feedback: Hardware,

software, and real world issues. *Behav Res Meth Instr Comput* 21:173–180, 1989.

134. Wise BW, Olson RK: Remediating reading disabilities, in Obrzut JE, Hynd GW (eds): *Neuropsychological Foundations of Learning Disabilities: A Handbook of Issues, Methods, and Practice.* San Diego, CA: Academic Press, 1991, pp 631–658.

135. Bruck M: The adult functioning of children with specific learning disabilities: A follow-up study, in Siegel IE (ed): *Advances in Applied Developmental Psychology.* Norwood, NJ: Ablex, 1985, pp 91–129.

136. Lemoine HE, Levy BA, Hutchinson A: Increasing the naming speed of poor readers: Representations formed across repetitions. *J Exp Child Psychol* 55:297–328, 1993.

137. Perfetti CA: Representations and awareness in the acquisition of reading competence, in Rieben L, Perfetti CA (eds): *Learning to Read: Basic Research and Its Implications.* Hillsdale, NJ: Erlbaum, 1991, pp 33–44.

138. Borkowski JG, Estrada MT, Milstead M, Hale CA: General problem-solving skills: Relations between metacognition and strategic processing. *Learn Disabil Q* 12:57–70, 1989.

139. Gaskins IW, Elliot TT: *Implementing Cognitive Strategy Training Across the School: The Benchmark Manual for Teachers.* Cambridge, MA: Brookline Books, 1991.

140. Kavale KA: The reasoning abilities of normal and learning disabled readers on measures of reading comprehension. *Learn Disabil Q* 3:34–45, 1980.

141. Meltzer L: Problem-solving strategies and academic performance in learning-disabled students: Do subtypes exist? in Feagans LV, Short EJ, Meltzer LJ (eds): *Subtypes of Learning Disabilities: Theoretical Perspectives and Research.* Hillsdale, NJ: Erlbaum, 1991, pp 163–188.

142. Paris SG, Oka ER: Strategies for comprehending text and coping with reading difficulties. *Learn Disabil Q* 12:32–42, 1989.

143. Gaskins IW, Downer MA, Anderson RC, et al: A metacognitive approach to phonics: Using what

you know to decode what you don't know. *Remed Special Educ* 9:36–41, 66, 1988.

144. Meltzer LJ: Assessment of learning disabilities: The challenge of evaluating the cognitive strategies and processes underlying learning, in Lyon GR (ed): *Frames of Reference for the Assessment of Learning Disabilities: New Views on Measurement Issues.* Baltimore: Brookes, 1994, pp 571–606.

145. Pressley M: Can learning-disabled children become good information processors? How can we find out? in Feagans LV, Short EJ, Meltzer LJ (eds): *Subtypes of Learning Disabilities: Theoretical Perspectives and Research.* Hillsdale, NJ: Erlbaum, 1991, pp 137–161.

146. Pressley M, Harris KR, Marks B: But good strategy instructors are constructivists! *Educ Psychol Rev* 4:3–33, 1992.

147. Levin BE: Organizational deficits in dyslexia: Possible frontal lobe dysfunction. *Dev Neuropsychol* 6:95–110, 1990.

148. Harris KR, Graham S, Pressley M: Cognitive-behavioral approaches in reading and written language: Developing self-regulated learners, in Singh NN, Beale IL (eds): *Learning Disabilities: Nature, Theory, and Treatment.* New York: Springer-Verlag, 1992, pp 415–451.

149. Engelmann S, Bruner EC: *Reading Mastery I/II Fast Cycle: Teacher's Guide.* Chicago: Science Research Associates, 1988.

150. Engelmann S, Carnine L, Johnson G: *Corrective Reading, Word Attack Basics, Decoding A.* Chicago: Science Research Associates, 1988.

151. Engelmann S, Johnson G, Carnine L, et al: *Corrective Reading: Decoding Strategies, Decoding B1.* Chicago: Science Research Associates, 1988.

152. Gaskins IW, Downer MA, Gaskins RW: *Introduction to the Benchmark School Word Identification/ Vocabulary Development Program.* Media, PA: Benchmark School, 1986.

153. Livingston R, Adam BS, Bracha HS: Season of birth and neurodevelopmental disorders: Summer birth is associated with dyslexia. *J Am Acad Child Adolesc Psychiatry* 32:612–616, 1993.

Chapter 63

NONVERBAL LEARNING DISABILITY

Marcel Kinsbourne

A learning disability designates isolated substandard achievement (and, by inference, ability) in one cognitive domain in an otherwise normally achieving child. Actually, the cognitive underpinnings of the learning disability do not appear to be the same whether or not the child otherwise learns normally.[1] So learning disability is tantamount to selective mental retardation. Extraneous cognitive strengths may offer "bypass" opportunities: the child learns within the affected curriculum, but by capitalizing on intact "channels" (teaching to strength,[2] e.g., in nonverbal learning disability). Nevertheless, the core and usually unavoidable teaching to weakness is unaffected by irrelevant strengths (except as useful morale boosters).

Outside the verbal domain, learning disability is nonverbal learning disability, notably in arithmetic learning disability, which is as prevalent as the higher-profile dyslexias.[3] It has been underinvestigated, perhaps because a fourth-grade level of functioning suffices for purposes of everyday living.[4] Art, design, and musical achievement are arbitrarily dismissed as not of "core" importance. Social learning disability[5] is considered in Chap. 64.

THE SPECTRUM OF LEARNING DISABILITIES

By definition, learning disability is selective, whereas mental retardation implicates all domains of mental function. In reality, learning disability and mental retardation are not discontinuous. Learning disability varies greatly, not only in severity within its primary domain (reading, writing, calculation, etc.), but also in its extension across domains. Most reading disabilities involve writing as well, and many also involve calculation (a nominally nonverbal activity). Additionally, persons with learning disability, sampled by discrepancy between performance on a target ability and a normative reference score, usually an IQ test, typically perform less well than a matched control group on most other mental tests. The more severe the learning disability, the more of the cognitive spectrum it involves.[7] "Pure" deficits are uncommon and perhaps confined to certain pedigrees. The construct of a syndrome, a constellation of deficits that co-occur beyond chance frequency, is equally problematic in learning disability, in which putative "components," such as dyscalculia and visuospatial deficit, are themselves ill-defined and probably hybrid disabilities, involving variable and extensive cerebral circuitry. These reflections argue against the concept of a handful of highly selective learning disabilities—dyslexia, dysgraphia, dyscalculia—and in favor of learning disability as a spectrum of overlapping deficits.

HEMISPHERE ASCRIPTIONS IN LEARNING DISABILITY

Various learning disability phenotypes have been ascribed to right hemisphere (RH) dysfunction and sometimes packaged together as RH learning disability, often based on a simplistic equation of left hemisphere (LH) with verbal and RH with nonverbal functioning. Conversely, the RH has been credited with specific roles in some ostensibly LH-based verbal learning disabilities.[6] These attributions are speculative. By definition, learning disability excludes underlying structural brain damage. Therefore, external validation by means of a consistently localized lesion site is not available. Neuropsychological analysis may point to underlying structural brain damage. Therefore, external validation by means of a consistently localized site is not available. Neuropsychological analysis may point to an underlying processing deficit of known localizing significance. But even if one ventures to equate the localizing values of comparable acquired and developmental deficits, there remains little demonstrated correspondence between the functional specializations of the hemispheres and patterns of academic achievement. Cerebral cortex is not organized by curricular entity. One has either to show deficiency in a specific lateralized mental operation or refer the components of the learning disability syndrome to corresponding mental operations localized in adjacent (neighboring) parts of the brain. The former concept assumes that a specific cognitive module fails to develop normally (e.g., for reasons of flawed genetic control). The latter concept ascribes learning disability to early brain damage, which does not respect the boundaries of any one cognitive module but does impact some limited area of brain. In practice, a child's learning disability is rarely clear-cut but rather occupies some point in a spectrum space.

WHAT DEFICITS MIGHT ARISE FROM RIGHT-HEMISPHERE UNDERDEVELOPMENT?

A host of functions have been attributed to what is, after all, half the cerebrum—from route-finding to face perception to number estimation and from awareness of internal states to discrepancy alerting to imagery. But the most straightforward answer

to the question is "None of the above." Hemispherectomy studies have demonstrated the prodigious ability of each hemisphere to compensate for loss of the other. For a hemisphere-specific deficit to appear in development, there has to be some reason why the other hemisphere does not take over its role in cognition—bilateral involvement or some inhibitory influence from the damaged hemisphere that prohibits compensation by the one that remains intact. To this extent, the idea of a right-hemisphere learning disability is undermined from the start. The topic of nonverbal learning disability is better addressed from the vantage point of its most important component, arithmetic learning disability.

ARITHMETIC LEARNING DISABILITY

Arithmetic learning disability may be selective or coincide with delayed language[8] or reading disability.[9] Several theorists have offered taxonomies of arithmetic learning disability, according to their understanding of the cognitive prerequisites for arithmetic acquisition.[3,10,11] Some of these problem types are rare; number concept is hardly ever lacking except in mental retardation, and inability to learn how to read and write numbers rarely occurs in isolation from comparable problems with letters and words.[12] The usual difficulties are (1) in acquiring fluency with number facts (i.e., in automatization),[13] (2) with place value when calculating with multidigit numbers, (3) in rule-governed computing,[14] and (4) in mathematical reasoning. Although these are not mutually exclusive, Temple[15] has reported double dissociation between number fact and computing skill.

Failure to automatize is sometimes found in attention deficit hyperactivity disorder (ADHD).[16] Place-value problems are often associated with similar (order) difficulties in spelling, in right-left orientation, and in finger identification,[17] analogous to the Gerstmann syndrome of left parietal injury (see also Ref. 18). Along similar lines, Siegel and Heaven[19] stress the relationship between arithmetic learning disability and difficulty with written work. Mathematical reasoning problems are associated with comparable problems in verbal syntax and semantics.

Both intuition and correlative studies[20] nominate spatial skill as a prerequisite for learning at least geometry and perhaps all of mathematics. This would then implicate the right hemisphere. Indeed, in a cerebral-palsied sample, arithmetic competence correlated significantly with the integrity of the right hemisphere.[21] However, neuropsychological case studies have demonstrated "acalculia" both with left- and with right-hemisphere lesions (see Chap. 15). Shalev and coworkers[22] grouped dyscalculic children with respect to associated signs of left- versus right-hemisphere dysfunction. They found both types to be similarly disabled, but the left-hemisphere group more severely so. One can only conclude that lesions of either hemisphere can impair arithmetic acquisition and that if different subskills are implicated by RH and LH lesions, these have yet to be identified. The mere presence of arithmetic learning disability is not evidence of RH dysfunction.

Both reading disability and arithmetic learning disability are deficient in short-term memory. Persons with arithmetic learning disability are less handicapped by auditory presentation and linguistic content.[9,23] Adolescents and adults grouped into reading disability, arithmetic learning disability, and reading and arithmetic learning disability differed similarly, with arithmetic learning disability and reading and arithmetic learning disability distinguished by low scores on a spatial task.[24]

The usual predominance of males in learning disability does not apply to arithmetic learning disability,[25] which occurs frequently in female carriers of fragile-X syndrome[26] and in Turner syndrome.[27] It is also seen in neurofibromatosis and in treated phenylketonuria.[28] It is the most frequent learning disability in epilepsy.[29]

RIGHT-HEMISPHERE LEARNING DISABILITY

Children manifest nonverbal learning disability[3] or specifically RH learning disability when they exhibit arithmetic, visuospatial, and social impairments, with or without left-sided neurologic signs, hard or soft.[31-33] Voeller[34] and Grace and Malloy[35] described attention deficit hyperactivity disorder children who were socially insensitive and scored more poorly on arithmetic than on verbal tests. The basis for assigning these deficit patterns to the right hemisphere combines a smattering of neurologic signs with inference from the effects of focal-hemisphere lesions on adults, as follows: (1) Right hemisphere lesions, especially posterior parietal, result in visuospatial and visuomotor impairments. However, LH lesions also do so, but they are of a different type.[36] (2) Right-hemisphere lesions are assumed to induce arithmetic problems because of the presumed reliance of arithmetic on spatial subskills. But LH lesions as often cause acalculia.[37] (3) Right hemisphere lesions leave some patients unable to appreciate socioemotional cues in speech intonation, gestures, and facial expression and oblivious to humor, irony, and sarcasm, though less often than is usually assumed. But social obliviousness is rather widespread in learning disability[38] and not of proven lateralizing value. An appropriately diagnosed person with RH learning disability not only selectively combines these three deficits but also offers independent evidence that the RH, and it only, is at fault.

The term *nonverbal learning disability* describes a range of behavioral phenotypes rather than a single type. Sampling biases have been inadequately considered. Ostensible nonverbal learning disability cases are typically drawn from clinic referrals for school problems. By definition, their problems are not language-based. This leads to an accumulation of classroom misfits with miscellaneous behavioral and attentional concerns. The syndrome status of such a sample and its RH learning disability status are tenuous, based on a facile identification of sundry problems in attention and calculation as well as internalizing psychopathology with RH dysfunction. Objective correlates—electrophysiologic, metabolic, and structural asymmetries—remain to be documented. Alternative interpretations exist for most cases, particularly those diagnosed purely by neuropsychological battery.

DIFFERENTIAL DIAGNOSIS OF NONVERBAL LEARNING DISABILITY

Attention Deficit Hyperactivity Disorder

Neuropsychological test batteries are notoriously insensitive to attentional pathology. Attention deficit hyperactivity disorder is not itself based on right-hemisphere abnormality (see Chap. 65). But some ADHD individuals have difficulty "automatizing"—for instance, arithmetic tables or number facts. Some do appear socially insensitive, largely on account of their lack of impulse control.

Depression

Whereas major depression in childhood is rare in the absence of gross abuse or neglect, many ADHD children are periodically dysthymic or characterologically depressed. Depression is thought to engender impaired visuospatial performance[39] and perhaps even mild left-sided neurologic signs.[40] A dysthymic child may be mistaken for one with nonverbal learning disability.

Overfocused Attention

Often associated with ADHD but orthogonal to it is an attentional style that is perseverative, isolating, and narrowly focused.[41] Overfocused children work slowly, and, like those who are depressed, tend to do poorly on timed tests, which, in turn, cluster in the nonverbal sections of intelligence test batteries. They may also balk at arithmetic problems, more for fear of failure than actual difficulty in learning the computational rules. Their internally directed focus of attention makes them socially oblivious; they give priority to meeting their own idiosyncratic need for predictability over acting prosocially and addressing mainstream concerns, so they can simulate a nonverbal learning disability profile.

Autistic Spectrum Disorder

Individuals with Asperger syndrome or high-functioning autism who do not have the more usual autistic language disorder are conspicuous mostly for their rigid manner and circumscribed interests (see Chap. 67). They may differ from overfocusers in degree rather than in kind.

Overanxious Disorder

Anxiety affects arithmetic more than reading. This is perhaps because arithmetic problems more explicitly challenge the anxious child, evoking fear of failure and consequent avoidance. The repeatedly remarked upon association of poor calculation and interpersonal difficulties[42,43] can reflect a primary anxiety rather than a cognitive deficit. The historically overused special education category "emotionally disturbed" may comprise anxious, neglected, and abused children, and only a few with undiagnosed ADHD.

Social Learning Disability

This pragmatic category designates the many persons with learning disability who experience social difficulties and might benefit from social-skills training (see Chap. 64). Nonverbal learning disability cannot be diagnosed based on social learning disability alone.

REFERENCES

1. Siegel L: IQ is irrelevant to the definition of learning disabilities. *J Learn Disabil* 22:469–478, 1989.
2. Foss JM: Nonverbal learning disabilities and remedial interventions. *Ann Dyslexia* 41:128–140, 1991.
3. Badian NA: Dyscalculia and nonverbal disorders of learning, in Myklebust HR (ed): *Progress in Learning Disabilities.* New York: Grune & Stratton, 1983, pp 235–264.
4. Chandler HN: Confusion confounded: A teacher tries to use research results to teach maths. *J Learn Disabil* 11:361–369, 1987.
5. Hazel JS, Schyumaker JB: Social skills and learning disabilities: Current issues and recommendations for future research, in Kavanaugh JF, Truss TJ (eds): *Learning Disabilities.* Parkton, MD: York Press, 1988, pp 293–345.
6. Bakker D, Licht R: Learning to read: Changing horses in mid-stream, in Pavlidis GT, Fisher DF

(eds): *Dyslexia: Its Neuropsychology and Treatment.* New York: Wiley, 1986, pp 87–96.

7. Kinsbourne M, Rufo DT, Gamzu E, et al: Neuropsychological deficits in adults with dyslexia. *Dev Med Child Neurol* 33:763–775, 1991.

8. Johnson DJ, Blalock JW: *Adults with Learning Disabilities: Clinical Studies.* New York: Grune & Stratton, 1987.

9. Fletcher JM: Memory for verbal and nonverbal stimuli in learning disabled subgroups: Analysis by selective reminding. *J Exp Child Psychol* 40:244–259, 1985.

10. Kosc L: Neuropsychological implications of diagnosis and treatment of mathematical learning disabilities. *Topics Learning Learning Disabil* 9:19–30, 1981.

11. Moses J: Neurological analysis of calculation deficits. *Focus Learn Disabil Math* 6:1–12, 1984.

12. Temple CM: Digit dyslexia: A category-specific disorder in developmental dyscalculia. *Cog Neuropsychol* 6:93–119, 1989.

13. Ackerman P, Anhalt J, Dykman R: Arithmetic automization failure in children with attention and reading disorders: Associations and sequels. *J Learn Disabil* 19:222–232, 1986.

14. Greenstein J, Strain PS: The utility of the Key Math Diagnostic arithmetic test for adolescent learning disabled students. *Psychol Schools* 14:275–282, 1977.

15. Temple CM: Procedural dyscalculia and number fact dyscalculia: Double dissociation in developmental dyscalculia. *Cog Neuropsychol* 8:155–176, 1991.

16. Rosenberger P: Perceptual-motor and attentional correlates of developmental dyscalculia. *Ann Neurol* 26:216–220, 1989.

17. Kinsbourne M, Warrington EK: The developmental Gerstmann syndrome. *Arch Neurol* 8:490–501, 1963.

18. Benson DF, Geschwind N: Developmental Gerstmann syndrome. *Neurology* 20:293, 1970.

19. Siegel I, Heaven RK: Categorization of learning disabilities, in Ceci SJ (ed): *Handbook of Cognitive, Social and Neuropsychological Aspects of Learning Disabilities.* Hillsdale, NJ: Erlbaum, 1986, pp 95–121.

20. Fleischner J, Frank B: Visual-spatial ability and mathematics achievement in learning disabled and normal body. *Focus Learn Prob Math* 1:7–22, 1979.

21. Kiesseling LS, Denckla MB, Carlton M: Evidence for differential hemispheric function in children with hemiplegic cerebral palsy. *Dev Med Child Neurol* 25:727–734, 1983.

22. Shalev RS, Manor O, Amir N, et al: Developmental dyscalculia and brain laterality. In press.

23. Siegel LS, Ryan EB: Development of grammatical sensitivity; phonological, and short-term memory skills in normally achieving and learning disabled children. *Dev Psychol* 24:28–37, 1988.

24. Shafir U, Siegel LS: Subtypes of learning disabilities in adolescents and adults. *J Learn Disabil* 27:123–134, 1994.

25. Shalev RS, Wertman R, Amir N: Developmental dyscalculia. *Cortex* 24:555–561, 1988.

26. Kemper MB, Hagerman RJ, Ahmad RS, Mariner R: Cognitive profiles and the spectrum of clinical manifestations in heterozygous fra x females. *Am J Med Genet* 23:139–156, 1986.

27. Money J: Turner's syndrome and parietal lobe functions. *Cortex* 9:387–393, 1973.

28. Pennington BF: Genetics of learning disabilities. *Semin Neurol* 11:28–34, 1991.

29. Aldenkamp AP, Alpherts WCJ, Dekker MJA, Overweg J: Neurophysiological aspects of learning disabilities in epilepsy. *Epilepsia* 31(suppl 4):S9–S20, 1990.

30. Myklebust HR: Nonverbal learning disabilities: Assessment and intervention, in Myklebust HR (ed): *Progress in Learning Disabilities.* New York: Grune & Stratton, 1975, pp 85–121.

31. Weintraub S, Mesulam M-M: Developmental learning disabilities of the right hemisphere: Emotional, interpersonal, and cognitive components. *Arch Neurol* 40:463–468, 1983.

32. Tranel D, Hall LE, Olson S, Tranel NN: Evidence for a right hemisphere developmental learning disability. *Dev Neuropsychol* 3:113–127, 1987.

33. Rourke B, ed. *Nonverbal Learning Disabilities.* New York: Guilford, 1995.

34. Voeller KKS. Right hemisphere deficit syndrome in children. *Am J Psychiatry* 143:1004–1009, 1986.

35. Grace J, Malloy P: Neuropsychiatric aspects of right hemisphere learning disability. *Neuropsychiatry Neuropsychol Behav Neurol* 5:194–204, 1992.

36. Warrington EK, James M, Kinsbourne M: Drawing disability in relation to laterality of cerebral lesions. *Brain* 89:53–82, 1966.

37. Grafman J, Pasafiume D, Faglioni P, Boller F: Calculation disturbances in adults with focal hemispheric damage. *Cortex* 18:37–50, 1982.

38. Bryan TH, Bryan JH: Social interactions of LD children. *Learn Disabil Q* 1(1):33–38, 1978.

39. Kinsbourne M: Hemisphere interactions in depression, in Kinsbourne M (ed): *Cerebral Hemisphere Function in Depression.* Washington, DC: American Psychiatric Association, 1988, pp 135–162.

40. Brumback RA, Staton RD: A hypothesis regarding the commonality of right hemisphere involvement in learning disability, attentional disorder and childhood major depressive disorder. *Percept Motor Skills* 55:1091–1097, 1982.

41. Kinsbourne M: Overfocusing: An apparent subtype of attention deficit-hyperactivity disorder, in Amir N, Rapin I, Branski D (eds): *Pediatric Neurology: Behavior and Cognition of the Child with Brain Dysfunction.* Basel: Karger, 1991, pp 18–35.

42. Johnson DJ, Myklebust HR: *Learning Disabilities.* New York: Grune & Stratton, 1971.

43. Semrud-Clikeman M, Hynd GW: Right hemisphere dysfunction in nonverbal learning disabilities: Social, academic and adaptive functioning in adults and children. *Psychol Bull* 107:196–209, 1990.

Chapter 64

SOCIAL AND EMOTIONAL LEARNING DISABILITIES

Kytja K. S. Voeller

WHAT IS SOCIAL AND EMOTIONAL LEARNING DISABILITY?

Social and emotional learning disability (SELD) is a subset of disorders characterized by chronic difficulties in social relationships that first appear in childhood. Children with SELD are highly verbal, not at all aggressive, and have the best of social intentions. They wish to make friends and be popular but lack the ability to do so. Other children consider them "weird" and avoid them. The deficits lie in the area of reading social signals, making correct inferences about them (and social situations in general), understanding that other people may have viewpoints and motivations different from one's own, developing internal representations of societal norms and expectations, and effectively using this information to guide one's behavior.

The recognition of a behavioral profile in children characterized by deficits in social relatedness dates back to the late 1960s and early 1970s. Social and emotional learning impairments were noted in association with nonverbal learning disability[1,2] and with neurological signs,[3] especially left-sided signs implicating right hemisphere dysfunction.[4] Neuropsychological research documented associations between social and emotional deficits and a variety of other deficits, including mathematical and perceptual deficits,[5] as well as impairments in processing affect from facial expression and tone of voice, arousal, and attention (compromised in adults after right hemisphere damage).[6–9] The likely role of developmental right hemisphere dysfunction was confirmed by a series of studies starting in the 1980s[10–16] (see Ref. 17 for a review).

There is a marked overlap between SELD and psychiatric pathology. Children and adults with SELD are often first seen by psychiatrists[18] and can be classified as falling into the category of social communication spectrum disorder.[19] Many different psychiatric diagnostic labels are applied to these patients. If they are severely enough impaired, they may be diagnosed as having autistic disorder, pervasive developmental disorder (although this would be unusual), or Asperger syndrome.[20] The major differential diagnostic points favoring Asperger syndrome involve the presence of constricted intellectual interests (such as an encyclopedic knowledge of all the subway cars in New York City) or a remarkable cognitive ability (e.g., calendar calculation) combined with stereotypies (e.g., hand-flapping and unusual posturing). The most common comorbid psychiatric diagnosis is depression, which often emerges in SELD children as they approach adolescence.[21] Another frequently encountered comorbid condition is anxiety disorder (patients with SELD are typically shy, inhibited, and socially anxious). Other psychiatric diagnoses, such as obsessive-compulsive disorder (repetitive worries and special interests), schizoid/schizotypal (emotionally distant), or attention deficit disorder (ADD; particularly without hyperactivity) are often made for patients with SELD.

THE NEUROPSYCHOLOGICAL AND BEHAVIORAL CHARACTERISTICS OF PATIENTS WITH SELD

The neuropsychological profile of many of these patients is characterized by deficits in the area of visuospatial and mathematical ability and thus would also be subsumed under the label of nonverbal learning disability. However, the two diagnoses are not the same: The social deficits seen in SELD can be dissociated from the neuropsychological and academic deficits seen in nonverbal learning disability. A child can have nonverbal learning disability without the array of social deficits and the child with SELD can be quite competent in math and lack the visuoperceptual deficits that characterize nonverbal learning disability.

The fundamental deficit seen in SELD involves the computation of social-emotional information. Deficits involve impaired processing of the facial, gestural, and vocal prosodic signals of others. Thus, these individuals may perform more poorly when tested on instruments designed to assess facial affect recognition. Manoach and co-workers[16] demonstrated that those subjects tested in a formal manner on such instruments also had difficulty on auditory prosody. These patients may also have difficulty with the motor programming of face and limb affective gestures and affective prosody, so that they have an emotional flatness, robotic speech, and an array of atypical social behaviors.[4,10,12,13,17] They may have difficulty in integrating social gaze into other aspects of social interactions. They do not maintain eye contact and do not use gaze in a reciprocal, socially communicative fashion. They often violate societal rules of distance by standing too close and impinging on the social space of the person they are talking to. They may also be inappropriately affectionate and "sticky"—they put forth affectionate displays that are not really proper for the situation. The lack of normal affective expression, gaze disturbance, violation of social space, and "stickiness" all contribute to their oddness.

Finally, individuals with SELD often appear to have difficulty making correct inferences about the meaning of social cues. Here one can only speculate as to what is involved. Possibly they lack the ability to make appropriate representations of expected social behaviors and to judge what they are observing against these internal representations. An area that has not been fully explored in these patients is their ability to process higher-level representations of the "minds" of other individuals. In other words, it is not clear if they can differentiate between "propositional attitudes" (the perception of reality— i.e., "I think the coffee pot is empty") and "propositional contents" (the state of physical reality—"the coffee pot is empty"). This involves an awareness that other persons may have perceptions and motivations that differ from one's own; it is referred to as *theory of mind.*[22,23] Based on observations of their behavior, there is a strong suggestion that they do, in fact, not understand the perspectives of others; as a result, they are apt to make disastrous social faux pas. In addition, they manifest many deficits in the pragmatic use of language. Their choice of topics may be grossly irrelevant to the situation; they may wish to dazzle peers with a list of the numbers of the subway cars in New York City or an enumeration of all the astronauts who flew NASA missions, suggesting that they are unable to adjust their conversational content to their listeners.

Although the description above encompasses the child with full-blown SELD (that is, involving the perceptual, motor, and cognitive aspects of social-emotional behaviors), not all individuals show all of the manifestations. There may be a dissociation between the perception and expression of social-emotional information. Thus, some children have relatively intact signal perception but difficulty generating social-emotional displays, or they may have impairment in perception of such displays with intact motor output. There may also be modality-specific forms of SELD, characterized by the inability to read social signals through the visual modality but not auditory prosodic cues, or vice versa. We also postulate that there is a relatively rare affect-specific form, in which some individuals are relatively blind to cues that map onto certain classes of affect (e.g., they can read the word *happy* but do not effectively discriminate anger from sadness).

ETIOLOGIC FACTORS

Both genetic factors as well as acquired encephalopathic factors (either prenatal strokes or postnatal brain injury) have been implicated in the etiology of SELD. *Genetic* factors play a substantial role, accounting for over half of the subjects in the series reported by Weintraub and Mesulam,[10] Voeller,[12] and Manoach.[16] The genetic contribution may, in fact, be as important as early strokes or trauma or more so. A number of the children that I have examined have relatives (parents or parents' siblings) who are quite odd and socially remote. This is congruent with the report that some family members of autistic individuals and those with Asperger syndrome have been described as being remote and odd, with inadequate social use of language.[20,24] Moreover, atypical social behaviors are seen in association with several specific genetic syndromes—girls with Turner syndrome[25] and fragile X carrier females.[26] This would suggest that neural modules subserving social-emotional processing are affected in some systematic but as yet obscure fashion by genetic factors affecting brain growth.

The impact of early *brain lesions* on social behaviors is also quite complex. Recent animal studies of brain development indicate that the response to brain injury early in development depends on multiple factors, such as the timing, site, and size of the lesion. The sex of the fetus also plays an important role in determining the outcome of early lesions,[27] as does postnatal experience.[28] Thus, although lesions involving the right hemisphere in the adult have a major impact on the processing of facial affective information,[9] the situation in the developing brain may not be as straightforward. For instance, lesions occurring at specific times during embryogenesis may disrupt the normal development of remote areas of the same hemisphere or the contralateral hemisphere.[29]

Moreover, it is possible that the distinction between "acquired" and "genetic" lesions is not as well defined as one would like. It is clear that structural lesions may arise as a result of genetic factors. We do not have enough information at this time to settle this issue, but several intriguing studies point up the complexity of the problem. A recent positron emission tomography study in healthy women volunteers suggests that the brain substrate for processing emotion involves the right anterior cingulate and the inferior frontal gyri *bilaterally*.[30] Berthier and coworkers,[31] studying two young men with Asperger syndrome (of the type overlapping with the SELD diagnosis), reported neuroradiologically identified neuromigrational anomalies involving the left frontal region in one patient and the bilateral frontal opercular region, particularly on the left. The mother of one of the patients also had a left temporal macrogyrus. Of particular interest was the fact that both patients showed *left*-sided neurologic signs (pointing to *right* hemispheric involvement) and cognitive impairments suggesting right hemispheric dysfunction. Another patient with Asperger syndrome, whose symptoms grew more severe with age, was described in association with partial (anterior) agenesis of the corpus callosum.[32] Anterior agenesis of the corpus callosum often affects development of the neighboring cingulate cortex as well as other regions of the frontal lobe and could clearly result in impaired social behavior. Parenthetically, it should be noted that although some patients may have evidence of bilateral involvement on neurologic examination, right hemispheric lesions appear to be a sufficient cause of SELD-like behavior. Whether bilateral lesions increase the deficit is not clear.

Finally, on a theoretical basis, one would predict that SELD might be associated with *left* hemispheric dysfunction in a small subset of patients. There may be several different reasons for this. First, one can suggest that rare cases of *developmental crossed aprosodia,* analogous to the crossed aprosodias described in adults,[33] will be encountered. Another explanation was advanced regarding such a patient, described by Sandson and coworkers.[34] This patient had anomalous dominance, atypical social development and evidence of left hemispheric dysfunction. Manoach and associates[16] have suggested that in some of these patients with left hemispheric damage and the resulting shift of language-processing to the right hemisphere, the phenomenon of *crowding* exists, in which the neural substrates of the right hemisphere do not have the capacity to compute both social-emotional information and propositional language.

WORKUP AND DIAGNOSTIC EVALUATIONS

The diagnosis of SELD requires an approach from a broad neuropsychiatric perspective. A careful psychiatric and neurologic history must be obtained, with attention to the patient's developmental history. (For a more detailed review of approaches to the assessment of social-emotional behaviors in children, including the maturation of social behaviors, the reader is referred to a recent summary by Voeller.[35]) In addition to standard assessments of intelligence and academic achievement, a neuropsychological/neurobehavioral evaluation focusing on executive function, attention, memory, language (particularly the pragmatic/semantic aspects of language), praxis, and visuospatial ability is necessary. In the course of the interview and examination, observation of the patient's social behaviors and ability to engage in reciprocal social interaction should be carefully assessed. Does the patient manifest social anxiety, inability to maintain eye contact, aprosodia, constricted affect? The patient's *internal* social-emotional experiences and social judgment must be explored: what makes him or her happy? Sad? Angry? Frightened? (The examiner must also evaluate the affect generated in the course of this discussion.) Does the patient have an adequate vocabulary of words to describe emotions and internal states? How much insight does the patient have? How well does the patient appear to understand the perceptions and motivations of others? The neurologic examination often supplies important evidence of lateralizing signs suggesting subtle right hemispheric dysfunction (e.g., growth asymmetries of the face and extremities, posturing of the left upper extremity with stress gait, left-sided hyperreflexia, left parietal sensory deficits).[36] Patients should be carefully screened for evidence of a subclinical seizure disorder. Neurophysiologic and neuroimaging examinations may contribute valuable information to the clinical picture.

DIFFERENTIAL DIAGNOSIS

It is important to note that there are many reasons why a child may have difficulty relating to peers (e.g., motor handicap, impaired communication skills, or an impulsive, angry, aggressive, antisocial array of behaviors—e.g., oppositional defiant disorder or conduct disorder). Not all problems with social behaviors can be diagnosed as SELD. Although children with SELD are rarely aggressive, aggression is occasionally seen.[19] It is here that the detailed developmental neuropsychiatric history and behavioral neurologic/neuropsychological assessment provides converging evidence for this diagnosis.

TREATMENT

Approaches to the treatment of SELD have yet to be developed, so that the following suggestions should be considered as possibilities rather than as interventions of demonstrated efficacy.

One exception is the treatment of seizures, which may not be readily apparent. Manoach and coworkers[16] reported that one of their patients improved significantly following treatment with anticonvulsant medication: mood, eye contact, social interaction, and prosody improved markedly, and the episodes (presumably seizure equivalents) of sudden dread, dissociation, and unprecipitated crying, sadness, and confusion) diminished. Treatment of ADD (often a comorbid condition) may be helpful. Some patients may benefit from treatment of depression. If obsessive-compulsive symptoms are particularly striking, clomipramine or a similar drug may be helpful.

Several patient variables should be factored into the treatment plan. The patient must be examined to determine (1) if there is any dissociation between the expression and comprehension of affective signals, (2) whether the deficit is modality-specific, (3) if the patient has the ability to represent mental states of others, (4) if the patient has *metaawareness* of the deficits, (5) if the patient is able to use social-emotional information to guide behavior, and (6) whether the patient can regulate his or her behavior. For example, patients who are aprosodic, with a constricted array of affective expression, may or may not be proportionately impaired in processing incoming social signals. Thus, one should carefully evaluate both the expression and comprehension of social signals. Some of these patients can be trained to generate more appropriate motor behaviors and will benefit from such training. Patients who cannot maintain eye contact can sometimes be trained to stare fixedly at the nasal bridge of the person talking to them, which often minimizes the impression created by the eye-contact problem. Patients who cannot "read" social signals can sometimes be taught to ask for verbal information about the emotional state of others. It is much more difficult to work with patients who have difficulty understanding the mental states of others or who lack any inkling of the severity or nature of their deficits (metaawareness). Also, these techniques will not work with patients who cannot regulate their behaviors and are impulsive or impersistent.

The basic principles to be applied in managing patients with other types with neuropsychological deficits should also be utilized in the management of patients with SELD. This starts out by helping the patient understand the specific areas of deficit. Most SELD patients do not attempt to obfuscate or deny their social deficits but are typically exquisitely sensitive to them. However, since social-emotional behaviors are typically interpreted as "psychiatric," they have learned to interpret them in that light and often view themselves as "weird" or "crazy." Recasting these deficits as a neurologically based disability is often helpful to them. Showing them specifically the impact of aprosodia or inability to maintain gaze is often helpful. One can utilize videotaping with instant replay for this purpose. A supportive "coach" who can steer them in the direction of types of work that demand verbal skills and minimize heavy "on-line" computation of social situations is helpful. Some SELD adults have been able to work successfully in job situations of this type. Others may require considerable counseling in order to find and function in the appropriate vocational niche.

The age of the patient must be factored into this equation, because the management of children with SELD is quite different from that of adults. For instance, youngsters with SELD benefit from external structuring of their social environment and often benefit from modeling of appropriate social behaviors. The goal should be to reduce the "odd" behaviors to the minimum and program appropriate social behaviors that will get these children through some of their social interactions. Although these patients may not be able to spontaneously select the correct social motor program 100 percent of the time, even modest improvements in appropriateness improve their chances of surviving in the community. Although "social skills" programs are often available for children, these may not be helpful to children with SELD. Such training programs are typically conducted in group settings and are directed to children with behavioral problems in the realm of oppositional defiant disorder/conduct disorder and aggression; they focus heavily on self-control issues. Because most children with oppositional defiant/conduct disorder usually do not have deficits in social perception, this issue is not addressed here, but it is the crucial one for the management of SELD.

There is still a great deal to learn about the neurobiology, clinical manifestations, and treatment of disorders in the realm of the social emotional learning disabilities. However, there is increasing awareness among professionals of the existence of disorders of this type, and in the next decade we can look forward to an expansion of our knowledge about this fascinating entity.

RFERENCES

1. Johnson DJ, Myklebust HR: *Learning Disabilities.* New York: Grune & Stratton, 1971.
2. Myklebust HR: Nonverbal learning disabilities: Assessment and intervention, in Myklebust HR (ed): *Progress in Learning Disabilities.* New York: Grune & Stratton, 1975, vol 3, pp 281–301.
3. Rudel RG, Teuber HL, Twitchell TE: Levels of impairment of sensorimotor functions in children with early brain damage. *Neuropsychologia* 12:95–108, 1974.

4. Denckla MB: Minimal brain dysfunction, in Chall J, Mirsky A (eds): *Education and the Brain.* Chicago: National Society for the Study of Education and the University of Chicago Press, 1978, pp 223–268.

5. Rourke BP, Finlayson MAJ: Neuropsychological significance of variations in patterns of academic performance: Verbal and visual-spatial abilities. *J Abnorm Child Psychol* 6:121–133, 1978.

6. Tucker DM, Watson RT, Heilman KM: Discrimination and evocation of affectively intoned speech in patients with right parietal disease. *Neurology* 27:947–950, 1977.

7. Heilman KM, Schwartz HD, Watson RT: Hypoarousal in patients with the neglect syndrome and emotional indifference. *Neurology* 28:229–232, 1978.

8. Heilman KM, Bowers D, Speedie L, Coslett HB: Comprehension of affective and nonaffective prosody. *Neurology* 34:917–921, 1984.

9. Bowers D, Bauer RM, Coslett HB, Heilman KM: Processing of faces by patients with unilateral hemisphere lesions: I. dissociation between judgments of facial affect and facial identity. *Brain Cogn* 4:258–272, 1985.

10. Weintraub S, Mesulam MM: Developmental learning disabilities of the right hemisphere: Emotional, interpersonal and cognitive components. *Arch Neurol* 40:463–468, 1983.

11. Tranel D, Hall LE, Olson S, Tranel NN: Evidence for a right-hemisphere developmental learning disability. *Dev Neuropsychol* 3:113–117, 1987.

12. Voeller KKS: Right hemisphere deficit syndrome in children. *Am J Psychiatry* 143:1004–1009, 1986.

13. Voeller KKS, Hanson JA, Wendt RN: Facial affect recognition in children: Comparison of the performance of children with right and left hemisphere lesions. *Neurology* 38:1744–1748, 1988.

14. Abramson R, Katz DA: A case of developmental right hemisphere dysfunction: Implications for psychiatric diagnosis and management. *J Clin Psychiatry* 50:70–71, 1989.

15. Sandson TA, Manoach DS, Price BH, et al: "Right hemisphere learning disability" associated with left hemisphere dysfunction: Anomalous dominance and development. *J Neurol Neurosurg Psychiatry* 57:1129–1132, 1994.

16. Manoach DS, Sandson TA, Weintraub S: The developmental social-emotional processing disorder is associated with right hemisphere abnormalities. *Neuropsychiatry Neuropsychol Behav Neurol* 8:99–105, 1995.

17. Semrud-Clikeman M, Hynd GW: Right hemispheric dysfunction in nonverbal learning disabilities: Social, academic, and adaptive functioning in adults and children. *Psychol Bull* 107:196–209, 1990.

18. Grace J, Malloy P: Neuropsychiatric aspects of right hemisphere learning disability. *Neuropsychiatry Neuropsychol Behav Neurol* 5:194–204, 1992.

19. Tanguay PE: Infantile autism and social communication spectrum disorder. *J Am Acad Child Adolesc Psychiatry* 29:854, 1990.

20. Szatmari P, Bremner R, Nagy J: Asperger's syndrome: A review of clinical features. *Can J Psychiatry* 34:554–560, 1989.

21. Rourke BP, Young GC, Leenaars AA: A childhood learning disability that predisposes those afflicted to adolescent and adult depression and suicide risk. *J Learn Disabil* 22:169–175, 1989.

22. Frith U, Morton J, Leslie AM: The cognitive basis of a biological disorder: Autism. *TINS* 14:433–438, 1991.

23. Baron-Cohen S, Leslie AM, Frith U: Does the autistic child have a "theory of mind?" *Cognition* 21:37–46, 1985.

24. Landa R, Piven J, Wzorek MM, et al: Social language use in parents of autistic individuals. *Psychol Med* l22:245–254, 1992.

25. McCauley E, Kay T, Ito J, Treder R: The Turner syndrome: Cognitive deficits, affective discrimination, and behavior problems. *Child Dev* 58:464–473, 1987.

26. Reiss AL, Hagerman RJ, Vinogradov S, et al: Psychiatric disability in female carriers of the fragile X chromosome. *Arch Gen Psychiatry* 45:25–30, 1988.

27. Clark AS, Goldman-Rakic PS: Gonadal hormones influence the emergence of cortical function in nonhuman primates. *Behav Neurosci* 103:1287–1295, 1991.

28. Goldman PS, Mendelson MJ: Salutary effects of early experience on deficits caused by lesions of frontal association cortex in developing rhesus monkeys. *Exp Neurol* 57:588–602, 1977.

29. Goldman-Rakic PS, Rakic P: Experimental modification of gyral patterns, in Geschwind N, Galaburda AM (eds): *Cerebral Dominance: The Biological Foundations.* Cambridge, MA: Harvard University Press, 1985, pp 179–192.

30. George MS, Ketter TA, Gill DS, et al: Brain regions involved in recognizing facial emotion or identity: An oxygen-15 PET study. *J Neuropsychiatry Clin Neurosci* 5:384–394, 1993.

31. Berthier ML, Starkstein SE, Leiguarda IR: Devel-

opmental cortical anomalies in Asperger's syndrome: Neuroradiological findings in two patients. *J Neuropsychiatry Clin Neurosci* 2:197–201, 1990.

32. David AS, Wacharasindhu A, Lishman WA: Severe psychiatric disturbance and abnormalities of the corpus callosum: Review and case series. *J Neurol Neurosurg Psychiatry* 56:85–93, 1993.

33. Ross ED, Anderson B, Morgan-Fisher A: Crossed aprosodia in strongly dextral patients. *Arch Neurol* 46:206–209, 1989.

34. Sandson TA, Manoach DS, Price BH, et al: "Right hemisphere learning disability" associated with left hemisphere dysfunction: Anomalous dominance and development. *J Neurol Neurosurg Psychiatry* 57:1129–1132, 1994.

35. Voeller KKS: Techniques for measuring social competence in children, in Lyon GR (ed): *Frames of Reference for the Assessment of Learning Disability: New Views on Measurement Issues.* Baltimore: Brooks, 1994, pp 523–554.

36. Voeller KKS: Clinical neurological aspects of the right hemisphere deficit syndrome. *J Child Neurol* 10:S16–S22, 1995.

Chapter 65

ATTENTION DEFICIT HYPERACTIVITY DISORDER

Bruce F. Pennington

BACKGROUND AND CLINICAL FEATURES

Attention deficit hyperactivity disorder (ADHD) is one of the most common chronic disorders of childhood, with a prevalence of 1 to 7 percent according to recent epidemiologic studies.[1] Of course, prevalence depends on definition and definitions vary in how pervasive they require the ADHD symptoms to be. In a careful epidemiologic study that required pervasiveness across three different reporters—parents, teachers, and a physician—the prevalence was only 1.2 percent.[2] Sex ratios in referred samples have been reported to be as high as 9:1 (males:females), but one epidemiologic study found a sex ratio of 3:1.[3] Thus, as in other disorders, such as reading disability, males are more likely to be referred than females. Because much of the research on ADHD has relied on referred samples, we know much more about ADHD in males than in females.

The cardinal symptoms of ADHD are hyperactivity, impulsivity, and distractibility as reported by parents, teachers, and health-care professionals, usually by means of standardized questionnaires. Although the reliability of such questionnaires has been amply demonstrated and the cutoffs for ADHD are empirically derived, the construct validity of what is measured by such questionnaires is another matter. It seems unlikely that adult perceptions of these troublesome, molar behaviors carve out a "natural kind," and indeed

the net cast by this broad definition captures many other disorders. These comorbid disorders include reading disability,[4–6] conduct disorder,[7] depression,[8–10] Tourette syndrome,[11,12] and possibly others. In fact, more than half of the children with ADHD qualify for a comorbid diagnosis.[13,14] The causal relations between ADHD and these comorbid disorders are largely unknown, but behavior genetic studies are now being conducted to test whether the observed comorbidities are due to a common etiology, an etiologic subtype, or one disorder producing a secondary phenocopy of the other.[4,15,16]

In terms of natural history, the age of onset is usually in toddlerhood, with a peak "age of onset" between ages 3 and 4.[17] Symptoms of ADHD may appear earlier, even in utero. It is becoming clearer that ADHD is a chronic disorder across the life span[18] and that the clinical pattern observed in adults is similar to that observed in school-aged children.

ETIOLOGY

There has been considerable progress in examining the genetics of ADHD in the last few years, and we now have evidence that it is familial, moderately heritable, and may be transmitted in a major locus fashion. In terms of familiality, the rate of ADHD in families of ADHD male probands has been found to be over seven times the rate of the disorder in nonpsychiatric control families;[8] a later study reported a similar increase in risk among relatives of female probands.[19,20] Stevenson[21] found a heritability of 0.76 for ADHD in his twin study, and several other twin studies have found similar results.[22–23] There has been one recent segregation analysis of ADHD,[20] which found autosomal dominant transmission with considerably reduced penetrance of the hypothesized major gene. Taken together, this evidence indicates genetic influence on ADHD, some of which may be due to a locus of sizable effect.

Finally, there are recent reports of linkage between ADHD and specific genetic markers. One report involved a thyroid gene,[24] but this can only be a small genetic subtype, since the frequency of this gene is much lower than the frequency of ADHD.[25] Subsequently, a different group of investigators found a linkage between the dopamine transporter locus (DAT1) and ADHD.[26] That DAT1 locus was chosen as a candidate gene because stimulant medications effective in treating ADHD inhibit the dopamine transporter. A third possible linkage involves the C4B gene on the short arm of chromosome 6.[27] Replication in an independent sample is needed for these linkage results.

BRAIN MECHANISMS

The hypothesis of frontal lobe dysfunction in ADHD has been advanced by several researchers[28–33] based on the observation that frontal lesions in both experimental animals and human patients sometimes produce hyperactivity, distractibility, or impulsivity, alone or in combination.[34–36] Of course, lesions in other parts of the brain can also produce these symptoms.

The best evidence for brain differences in ADHD comes from measures of brain function, including measures of electrophysiology, regional cerebral blood flow, and catecholamines (dopamine and norepinephrine). With regard to brain structure, earlier work[37–38] found no evidence of structural differences in CT scan studies of ADHD children. However, using magnetic resonance imaging (MRI) Hynd and colleagues[39] did find absence of the usual right greater than left frontal asymmetry in ADHD children. They contrasted ADHD subjects with both dyslexics and controls; the frontal finding was present in both clinical groups but did not differentiate between them, even though the dyslexic group was selected to be non-ADHD. There is an association between the right frontal lobe and measures of sustained attention, so this neuroanatomic difference has theoretical relevance to ADHD. Obviously more studies are needed to examine the replicability and specificity of this candidate neuroanatomic difference in ADHD.

In terms of brain function, the electrophysiologic measures have supported the hypothesis of central nervous system (CNS) underarousal in at least a subgroup of hyperactive children.[40] Likewise, Lou and colleagues[41] found decreased blood flow to the frontal lobes in ADHD children, which increased after the children received Ritalin (methylphenidate). Ritalin treatment also decreased blood flow to the motor cortex and primary sensory cortex, "suggesting an inhibition of function of these structures, seen clinically as less distractibility and decreased motor activity during treatment" (p. 829). These investigators have replicated this result in an expanded sample;[42] in this second report they emphasize the basal ganglia as the locus of reduced blood flow in ADHD. Zametkin and colleagues[43] used positron emission tomography (PET) to study the parents of ADHD children who themselves had residual-type ADHD. They found an overall reduction in cerebral glucose utilization, particularly in right frontal areas, but increased utilization in posterior medial orbital areas. A second study by this group[44] investigating teenagers with ADHD replicated some but not all of those findings. This second study found significant reductions in the ADHD group in normalized glucose metabolism in 6 of 60 brain regions, including the left anterior frontal lobe. Metabolism in that region correlated inversely with ADHD symptom severity across the combined sample of patients and controls. Since hyperfrontality of blood flow is characteristic of the normal brain, hypofrontality in ADHD could explain the low central arousal found in the electrophysiologic studies.

In terms of brain biochemistry, Shaywitz and coworkers[45] found lower levels of homovanillic acid (HVA; the main dopamine metabolite) in the cerebrospinal fluid of ADHD children compared to controls. Dopamine has a preponderant distribution in the frontal regions of the cortex. Moreover, a well-validated animal model of ADHD involves dopamine depletion.[38]

In summary, one plausible theory of brain mechanisms in ADHD is as follows: The symptoms of ADHD are caused by functional hypofrontality, which, in turn, is caused by either structural and/or biochemical changes in the prefrontal lobes or closely related structures, such as the basal ganglia, and is detectable as reduced frontal blood flow. Biochemically, the cause would be low dopamine levels, which Ritalin treatment reverses, at least in part.

Unfortunately, the story is not that simple. One study found that dopamine agonists were not effective in treating hyperactive children,[46] whereas certain dopamine antagonists did have unexpected beneficial effects in ADHD children.[33] Both of these results are opposite to what would be predicted by the dopamine depletion hypothesis. Therefore the neurochemical mechanisms may be more complex, although the ubiquitous problem of heterogeneity in ADHD samples is another explanation.

Zametkin and Rapoport[33] argue that no single neurotransmitter is exclusively involved in the pathogenesis of ADHD, both because stimulant medications always affect more than one neurotransmitter and because of the multiple interrelations among specific catecholamines and their precursors and metabolites. They[33] and Oades[47] both argue that the combined action of dopaminergic and noradrenergic systems should be considered in the biology of ADHD.

Obviously, much more research is needed, preferably using familial samples that are as phenotypically homogeneous as possible. If the recent linkage between ADHD and either the DAT1 or C4B loci is replicated, then neurobiological research could focus on a genetic subtype of ADHD.

COGNITIVE PHENOTYPE

There is a fairly extensive literature on cognitive processes in ADHD, which has lately become more explicitly neuropsychological in the hypotheses tested. Virginia Douglas has been a pioneer in this area, establishing that there is a distinctive cognitive phenotype in ADHD that needs to be explained. She and others have found that children with ADHD are impaired on tasks requiring vigilance, systematic search, and motor control and inhibition but unimpaired on basic verbal and nonverbal memory tasks.[48]

Neuropsychological studies of ADHD have mainly focused on the frontal lobe or executive function hypothesis, for reasons discussed earlier. We recently reviewed published studies of executive functions in ADHD.[49]

We found that 15/18 studies reported a significant difference between ADHD subjects and controls on one or more executive function measures. A total of 60 executive function measures were used across studies; for 40 of these (67 percent), there was significantly worse performance in the ADHD group. In contrast, *none* of the 60 measures was significantly better in the ADHD group.

There also appears to be some specificity to the finding of executive function deficits in ADHD; only 19 (35 percent) of the 54 nonexecutive function measures administered across studies found significant group differences. When these nonexecutive function measures are categorized into different domains, it becomes clear that some domains are more likely to be impaired than others. Children with ADHD in these studies were generally unimpaired on measures of verbal memory, other verbal processes, or visuospatial processing. They were fairly consistently impaired on measures of vigilance and perceptual speed, consistent with previous research. Of course, vigilance and perceptual speed tasks may be influenced by executive functions.

In summary, there is evidence for a somewhat specific executive function deficit in ADHD. Future work must elucidate which specific executive functions are impaired (and intact) in ADHD and to relate these to its neurobiological mechanisms and etiologies. Further specifying the neuropsychological phenotype of ADHD will also benefit diagnosis and treatment.

ACKNOWLEDGMENTS

This work was supported by NICHD grants P50 HD27802 and P30 HD04024 and NIMH grants 5 K02 MH00419 (RSA), 5 R37 MH38820 (MERIT), and R01 MH45916.

REFERENCES

1. Hinshaw SP: *Attention Deficits and Hyperactivity in Children.* London: Sage, 1994.
2. Spreen O, Tupper D, Risser A, et al: *Human Developmental Neuropsychology.* New York: Oxford University Press, 1984.
3. Szatmari P, Offord DR, Boyle M: Correlates, associated impairments, and patterns of service utilization of children with attention deficit disorders: Findings from the Ontario Child Health Study. *J Child Psych Psychiatry* 30:205–217, 1989.
4. Gilger JW, Pennington BF, DeFries JC: A twin study of the etiology of comorbidity: Attention-deficit hyperactivity disorder and dyslexia. *J Am Acad Child and Adolesc Psychiatry* 31:343–348, 1992.
5. McGee R, Share DL: Attention deficit disorder-hyperactivity and academic failure: Which comes first and what should be treated? *J Am Acad Child Adolesc Psychiatry* 27:318–325, 1988.
6. Shaywitz SE, Shaywitz BE: Attention deficit disorder: Current perspectives, in Kavanaugh JF, Truss TJ (eds): *Learning Disabilities: Proceedings of the National Conference.* Parkton, MD: York Press, 1988.
7. Moffitt TE, Silva PA: Self-reported delinquency, neuropsychological deficit, and history of attention deficit disorder. *J Abnorm Child Psychol* 16:553–569, 1988.
8. Biederman J, Faraone SV, Keenan K, et al: Family-genetic and psychosocial risk factors in DSM III attention deficit disorder. *J Am Acad Child Adolesc Psychiatry* 29:526–533, 1990.
9. Livingston R, Dykman R, Ackerman P: The frequency and significance of additional self-reported psychiatric diagnoses in children with attention deficit disorder. *J Abnorm Child Psychol* 18:465–478, 1990.
10. Anderson J, Williams S, McGee R, Silva P: DSM-III disorders in pre-adolescent children. *Arch Gen Psychiatry* 44:69–76, 1987.
11. Sverd J, Curley AD, Jandorf L, Volkersz L: Behavior disorder and attention deficits in boys with Tourette syndrome. *J Am Acad Child Adolesc Psychiatry* 27:413–417, 1988.
12. Towbin KE, Riddle MA: Attention deficit hyperactivity disorder, in Kurlan R (ed): *Handbook of Tourette Syndrome and Related Tic and Behavioral Disorders.* New York: Dekker, 1993, pp 89–109.
13. Biederman J, Faraone SV, Keenan K, et al: Further evidence for family-genetic risk factors in attention deficit hyperactivity disorder: Patterns of comorbidity in probands and relatives in psychiatrically and pediatrically referred samples. *Arch Gen Psychiatry* 49:728–738, 1992.
14. Sprich-Buckminster S, Biederman J, Milberger S, et al: Are perinatal complications relevant to the manifestation of ADD? Issues of comorbidity and familiality. *J Am Acad of Child Adolesc Psychiatry* 32:1032–1037, 1993.
15. Faraone SV, Biederman J, Kritcher B, et al: Evidence for the independent familial transmission of attention deficit hyperactivity disorder and learning disabilities: Results from a family genetic study. *Am J Psychiatry* 150:891–895, 1993.
16. Stevenson J, Pennington BF, Gilger JW, et al: Hyperactivity and spelling disability: Testing for shared genetic etiology. *J Child Psychol Psychiatry* 34:1137–1152, 1993.
17. Palfrey JS, Levine MD, Walker DK, Sullivan M, et al: The emergence of attention deficits in early childhood: A prospective study. *J Dev Behav Pediatr* 6:339–348, 1985.
18. Gittleman R, Mannuzza S, Shenker R, Gonagura N: Hyperactive boys almost grown up. *Arch Gen Psychiatry* 42:937–947, 1985.
19. Faraone S, Biederman J, Keenan K, Tsuang MT: A family genetic study of girls with DSM-III attention deficit disorder. *Am J Psychiatry* 148:112–117, 1991.
20. Faraone S, Biederman J, Chen WJ, et al: Segregation analysis of attention deficit hyperactivity disorder: Evidence for single major gene transmission. *Psychiatr Genet* 2:257–275, 1992.
21. Stevenson J: Evidence for a genetic etiology in hy-

peractivity in children. *Behav Genet* 22:337–344, 1992.

22. Eaves L, Silberg J, Hewitt JK, et al: Genes, personality, and psychopathology: A latent class analysis of liability to symptoms of attention-deficit hyperactivity disorder in twins, in Plomin R, McClearn GE (eds): *Nature, Nurture and Psychology.* Washington, DC: APA Books, 1993.

23. Willerman L: Activity level and hyperactivity in twins. *Child Dev* 44:288–293, 1973.

24. Hauser P, Zametkin AJ, Martinez P, et al: Attention deficit-hyperactivity disorder in people with generalized resistance to thyroid hormone. *N Engl J Med* 328:997–1001, 1993.

25. Elia J, Gulotta C, Rose SR, et al: Thyroid function and attention-deficit hyperactivity disorder. *J Am Acad Adolesc Psychiatry* 33:169–172, 1994.

26. Cook EH, Stein MA, Krasowski MD, et al: Association of attention deficit disorder and the dopamine transporter gene. *Am J Hum Genet* 56:993–998, 1995.

27. Warren RP, Odell JD, Warren WL, et al: Reading disability, attention deficit hyperactivity disorder, and the immune system. *Lett Sci* 268:786–787, 1995.

28. Gualtieri CT, Hicks RE: Neuropharmacology of methylphenidate and a neural substrate for childhood hyperactivity. *Psychiatr Clin North Am* 6:875–892, 1985.

29. Mattes JA: The role of frontal lobe dysfunction in childhood hyperkinesis. *Comp Psychiatry* 21:358–369, 1989.

30. Pontius AA: Dysfunctional patterns analogous to frontal lobe system and caudate nucleus syndromes in some groups of minimal brain dysfunction. *J Am Med Women Assoc* 28:285–292, 1973.

31. Rosenthal RH, Allen TW: An examination of attention, arousal and learning dysfunctions of hyperkinetic children. *Psychol Bull* 85:689–715, 1978.

32. Stamm JS, Kreder SV: Minimal brain dysfunction: Psychological and neuropsychological disorders in hyperkinetic children, in Gazzaniga MS (ed): *Handbook of Behavioral Neurology: Neuropsychology.* New York: Plenum Press, 1979, vol 2.

33. Zametkin AJ, Rapoport JL: The pathophysiology of attention deficit disorders, in Lahey BB, Kadzin AE (eds): *Advances in Clinical Child Psychology.* New York: Plenum Press, 1986.

34. Fuster JM: *The prefrontal cortex: Anatomy, Physiology and Neuropsychology of the Frontal Lobe,* 2d ed. New York: Raven Press, 1989.

35. Levin HS, Eisenberg HM, Benton AL: *Frontal Lobe Function and Dysfunction.* New York: Oxford University Press, 1991.

36. Stuss DT, Benson DF: *The Frontal Lobes.* New York: Raven Press, 1986.

37. Harcherick DF, Cohen DJ, Ort S, et al: Computed tomography brain scanning in four neuropsychiatric disorders of childhood. *Am J Psychiatry* 142:731–737, 1985.

38. Shaywitz SE, Shaywitz BA, Cohen DJ, Young JG: Monoaminergic mechanisms in hyperactivity, in Rutter M (ed): *Developmental Neuropsychiatry.* New York: Guilford, 1983.

39. Hynd GW, Semrud-Clikeman M, Lorys AR, et al: Brain morphology in developmental dyslexia and attention deficit disorder/hyperactivity. *Arch Neurol* 47:919–926, 1990.

40. Ferguson HB, Rappaport JL: Nosological issues and biological validation, in Rutter M (ed): *Developmental Neuropsychiatry.* New York: Guilford, 1983.

41. Lou HC, Henriksen L, Bruhn P: Focal cerebral hypoperfusion in children with dysphasia and/or attention deficit disorder. *Arch Neurol* 41:825–829, 1984.

42. Lou HC, Henriksen L, Bruhn P: Strial dysfunction in attention deficit and hyperkinetic disorder. *Arch Neurol* 46:48–52, 1989.

43. Zametkin AJ, Nordahl TE, Gross M, et al: Cerebral glucose metabolism in adults with hyperactivity of childhood onset. *N Engl J Med* 323:1361–1366, 1990.

44. Zametkin AJ, Liebenauer LL, Fitzgerald GA, et al: Brain metabolism in teenagers with attention-deficit hyperactivity disorder. *Arch Gen Psychiatry* 50:333–340, 1993.

45. Shaywitz BA, Cohen DJ, Bowers MB: CSF monoamine metabolites in children with minimal brain dysfunction: Evidence for alteration of brain dopamine. *J Pediatr* 90:67–71, 1977.

46. Mattes JA, Gittelman R: A pilot trial of amantadine in hyperactive children. Paper presented at the NCDEU meeting, Key Biscayne, FL, 1979.

47. Oades RD: Attention deficit disorder with hyperactivity: The contribution of catecholaminergic activity. *Progr Neurobiol* 29:365–391, 1987.

48. Douglas VI: Cognitive deficits in children with attention deficit disorder with hyperactivity, in Bloomindale LM, Sergeant J (eds): *Attention Deficit Disorder: Criteria, Cognition, Intervention.* New York: Pergamon Press, 1988.

49. Pennington BF, Ozonoff S: Annotation: Executive functions and developmental psychopathologies. *J Child Psychol Psychiatry* 37:51–87, 1996.

Chapter 66

MENTAL RETARDATION

Marcel Kinsbourne

Mental retardation is typically conceptualized as a global underdevelopment of mental function. In fact, an across-the-board impairment, which includes both mental operations (processing), and the means for selecting adaptively among them (attention), applies most literally to the most severely affected individuals, who have effectively no cognitive functioning at all. The idea that when mental impairment is less severe it can still be global, that is, comparable in degree of impairment across the cognitive profile, is an application of the notion that a single factor, general intelligence (g), accounts for the bulk of the interindividual variance in intelligence. Studies that compare monozygotic and dizygotic twin pairs separated at birth give solid support to this idea, showing that more than half the variance in intelligence is indeed inherited, that is, genetic.[1] Degradation of g would implicate cognitive function in a domain-general manner.

The construct of a global mental capacity seems to be at odds with the widely favored notion that the brain representation of cognitive function is domain-specific—that is, modular—with much intraindividual variability in the efficiency of different modules. Each person is even said to house "multiple intelligences."[2] The unchallengeable validity of the construct of general intelligence can be reconciled with the equally robust reality of cerebral functional localization if g is taken to represent not some single "basic" mental operation or attribute (problem-solving ability, speed of responding) but the general well-formedness of the brain. Note that regional cerebral surface area has been shown by twin studies to be under tight genetic control.[3] The extent to which the brain is "well formed" may vary within the intact general population, depending on genotype, giving rise to the normal (gaussian) distribution of intelligence test scores. But when brain development is adversely affected by gene malfunction or insult early in gestation, such widespread ill-formedness of brain regions results, compromising so many cognitive functions (modules), that global mental retardation is approximated. To such cases, traditional measures of intelligence, based on which mental retardation is stratified into four levels of functioning, can reasonably be applied.

To the extent that mental retardation is not global but disproportionately implicates some cognitive domains, the opportunity arises for neuropsychological analysis. Instances are Down syndrome, Williams syndrome, congenital hydrocephalus, autistic spectrum disorder, and x chromosome aneuploidies (see section on mild mental retardation). Finer-grained neuropsychological analysis in severe mental retardation is obstructed by a dearth of valid and reliable neuropsychological tests for the severely mentally retarded population.

MENTAL TESTING

Mental tests typically sample a range of cognitive domains in different subtests, and the subject's mental age, intelligence quotient, and/or developmental quotient is a performance average. Averaging is not warranted if there is major "scatter" between scores in different domains; it overestimates the weaker and underestimates the stronger skills and does not capture any aspect of the individual's cognitive profile. Striking dissociations between cognitive domains are surprisingly prevalent in mental retardation (see below).

Those persons with mental retardation whose IQ ranges between 50 and 70 are usually considered "educable"; those with scores below 50 are considered "trainable" only. The latter are further subdivided into those who are moderately (35 to 49), severely (20 to 34), and profoundly (less than 20) retarded.[4] The cutoff points, 70, 50, 35, and 20 roughly correspond to two, three, four, and five standard deviations below the population mean, respectively.

These categories are subject to qualification by additional considerations, which are incorporated into the overall clinical judgment. Maladaptive personality traits, personality disorders, and deviant attention can depress the ability of persons with mental retardation to perform activities of daily living to well below the predicted level. Examples are social withdrawal (autism), impulsive restlessness (hyperactivity), and thought disorder (psychosis). Cerebral palsy and epilepsy often further compromise independent functioning.

The ninth and most recent classification by the American Association for Mental Retardation embodies such qualifications in its definition and forgoes global stratification.[5] Mental retardation is present if there exist "limitations in two or more of the following adaptive skill areas: communication, self-care, home living, functional academics, leisure and work." Each of these domains considered separately may call for one of the following "intensities of support": intermittent, limited, extensive, or pervasive. The Social Security Administration is equally pragmatic, defining mental retardation as "mental incapacity as evidenced by dependence upon others for personal needs" and directs services toward those with "impairment which substantially limits one or more life activity."

Instruments used to evaluate aspects of cognitive function include those shown in Table 66-1. These well-normed instruments lose accuracy below IQ 50. Also, the predictive validity of early childhood intelligence tests is low. The standard tests can be supplemented with the following:

Leiter International Scale (nonverbal)

Denver Developmental Screening Test II, by pediatrician's testing, observation, and history, birth to age 6 years

Vineland Social Maturity Scale (by caregiver)

Criterion-referenced adaptive behavior inventories include the following:

Comprehensive Test of Adaptive Behavior

Scales of Independent Behavior

Vineland Adaptive Behavior Scales

These instruments are applicable to trainable mental retardation, from birth to adult age.

The definition of mental retardation stipulates onset at any age up to 18 years. Therefore,

Table 66-1

Instruments used to evaluate cognitive function

Instrument	Applicable age range		
	Years, months		Years, months
Bailey Scales of Mental Development	2	to	2, 6
McCarthy Scales of Mental Development	2, 6	to	8, 6
Kaufman Assessment Battery (children)	2, 6	to	12, 5
Stanford Binet (4th ed)	2, 0	to	23, 0
Wechsler Preschool and Primary Scale	4, 0	to	6, 6

although development is usually uniformly slow from the start, the term *mental retardation* can also be applied to development that levels off with increasing age or that is initially normal but then declines, either abruptly (static encephalopathy) or gradually (progressive encephalopathy). These trajectories cannot be retrospectively inferred based on the behavioral end state alone.

MILD MENTAL RETARDATION

The prevalence of mild mental retardation overall is about 1.25 percent[6] but only reaches this level well into school age (because of delays in recognition). It varies with setting (urban or rural) and somewhat with gender (3 boys per 2 girls), the latter partly accounted for by X-linked syndromes.[7] Euphemistic labeling classifies some persons with urban mild mental retardation as "learning-disabled." In a nationwide study,[8] the three strongest predictors of mild mental retardation, in descending order, were maternal education, socioeconomic index, and mother's nonverbal intelligence. In all three predictors, polygenic inheritance and substandard environment are confounded; some 75 percent of those with mild mental retardation live in poverty. Early assessment of the home environment yields powerful predictors of cognitive development and school performance.[9]

Suggested additional etiologies for mild mental retardation include:

1. "Suboptimal pregnancy and delivery,"[10] notably prematurity.[11]

2. Diet of the expectant mother and later of the child that is deficient in animal proteins and micronutrients (vitamins and minerals) though not in calories.[12] Iron deficiency is known to cause mild mental retardation.[13] Like mild/moderate malnutrition, it is widespread in developing countries. Malnutrition also affects personality, rendering the child withdrawn, incurious, and lethargic, thereby compounding the adverse effects on cognition by minimizing exposure to learning opportunities. Supplemental feeding allegedly yields long-term benefit, independent of and additive with the effect of concurrent environmental enrichment.[14]

3. Subclinical lead burdens (sampled in blood and teeth) have negligible effects on intelligence once the usually concomitant low parental intelligence and unstimulating home environment are factored out.[15,16]

Dissociations between Cognitive Domains in Mild Mental Retardation

Another (though spurious) way of being included in the mild mental retardation group is by averaging across very impaired function in some domains and normal function in others. Whatever their overall level of functioning is, autistic individuals are typically disproportionately impaired in language (especially pragmatics) and in social cognition. The latter includes face perception and "theory of mind"—inferring the perspective or point of view of another person.[17] Conversely, children with Williams syndrome (infantile hypercalcemia) are relatively strong in language and social cognition (including theory of mind), but weak in spatial and number sense.[18] Efficient phonological and syntactic language skill dissociates from impaired social cognition and face recognition in hydrocephalus-meningomyelocele, taking the form of vapid "cocktail chatter."[19] Conversely, Down syndrome individuals are disproportionately impaired in language (as well as in motor skills).[20] Among x chromosomal aneuploidies, XO (Turner syndrome) is characterized by selectively impaired visuospatial, arithmetic, and memory skills,[21] whereas XXX have a selectively verbal deficit.[22] Individuals with fragile-X, though usually more than mildly mentally retarded, are particularly handicapped in language development.[23]

Dissociations between language and other cognitive skills argue against the view that language enables or organizes thought; if it did, the level of language development would impose a ceiling on cognitive development in general. The dissociations favor the view that language is one of a set of independent cognitive systems, each dedicated to solving a different problem that was adaptively significant to evolving human beings. Within the overall language domain, studies of atypical cognitive development have demonstrated, with striking clarity, independence of semantic from phonological/syntactical skill (Williams syndrome, congenital hydrocephalus) and of pragmatics from the rest (austistic spectrum disorder).

Attentional and temperamental styles also dissociate between subgroups of mental retardation. Some globally mentally retarded people exhibit "splinter skill": hyperlexics' mechanical reading skills far outstrip their spoken and reading comprehension,[24] and calendar savants can fluently relate date to day of the week across several decades.[25] Hyperlexics and savants are credited with an unusually persistent focus of attention on idiosyncratically chosen content areas rather than with specific supernormal cognitive skills. Not only do they engage in repetitive behavior, but they exhibit deficient orienting to novel stimuli. Their stimulus overselectivity is thought to be secondary to the difficulty in disengaging attention.[26] Dissociations in temperament are exemplified by the talkative but also fearful and obsessional child with Williams syndrome,[18] the sociable verbose child with hydrocephalus-meningomyelocele, and the shy, withdrawn child with autistic spectrum disorder,[27] including that caused by fragile-X.[28] The fact that abnormal development can bias temperament toward either an outgoing (externalizing) or a withdrawn (internalizing) extreme cannot be regarded as secondary to the adaptive issues that are involved. It demonstrates that temperament, like cognition, has a neuropsychological basis, perhaps involving opponent mechanisms that drive the individuals' attentional focus in opposite directions.

SEVERE MENTAL RETARDATION

The prevalence of mental retardation below IQ 50 is 3 to 4 per 1000, with half in the moderate range, three in eight severe, and one in eight profound.[29] Children with severe mental retardation are considered to be brain-damaged, and the sub-

stantial positive correlation between proband and mid-parent IQ found in mild mental retardation is not in evidence in severe mental retardation. Absent autopsy, estimates of etiology are largely subjective, unreliable, and widely variable. Judges who undertake record reviews typically underestimate multifactorial causation[30] and favor prenatal causes when in doubt. Prenatal factors are estimated to affect 13 to 50 percent via chromosomal and genetic disorder and 20 to 30 percent via malformation. Perinatal causes are invoked in between 10 and 15 percent, and postnatal causes in 3 to 12 percent. Some 18 to 40 percent of cases are considered unexplained in different studies.[31] Among autopsied mental retardation, a biased sample, major structural abnormality is the rule.[32]

LONG-TERM OUTCOMES

Life expectancy for mental retardation is curtailed only by fatal associated disease or when a profoundly retarded individual who cannot move and has to be tube-fed[33] dies from intercurrent infection, usually respiratory. In Down syndrome, there is additional mortality through early-onset Alzheimer disease.[34] Alzheimer neuropathology (plaques and tangles) is widespread in Down syndrome brains before age 40. Behavioral regression, characterized by social withdrawal and loss of self-help skills, is followed by early demise.

DEVIANT BEHAVIOR

Atypical behavior is often ascribed to the mental insufficiency itself. In fact, the sources of abnormal behavior are as follow:

1. Defense against excessive and overwhelming demands. This elicits avoidance behavior, including stereotypies.[35]

2. Environmental deprivation, including the effects of institutionalization.

3. Cerebral dysfunction, including toxic effects of psychoactive drugs, akathisia (restless shuffling), and dystonia (notably tardive dyskinesias).

4. Psychopathology; some 10 percent of persons with mental retardation have a severe mental illness,[36] including schizophrenia (3 percent; five times the population incidence). If there is associated epilepsy, the risk of psychopathology rises to about 50 percent.[37]

Psychiatric disorders in mental retardation respond to the same psychoactive drug regimens as they do in the general population. However, there is a risk that toxic effects can be overlooked when patients are nonverbal or uncommunicative or may be confused with the disordered behavior being treated. Self-injurious behavior is relatively frequent and characteristic of Lesch-Nyhan syndrome and Prader-Willie syndrome. Treatment with serotonergic agents is recommended.[38] A comprehensive up-to-date review of mental health in mental retardation is available.[39]

MANAGEMENT

Management options subdivide into prevention and cure of the causative disorder, which are beyond the scope of this chapter, and behavioral measures—those that attempt to raise intelligence level and those that offer the requisite external supports to enable the mentally retarded individuals to use their existing capabilities to the fullest extent.

Enrichment programs, such as Head Start, do indeed engender gains in IQ, but these gradually dissipate after the program is concluded.[40] However, some persons with high-level mental retardation benefit from lasting spin-off gains in self-confidence and motivation.

Mainstreaming persons with mental retardation—defined as maintaining them at least half the time in a regular classroom—helps them only when it is combined with individually programmed educational support. The quality of the home environment is a critically important moderator variable.[41] Afforded appropriate home and classroom conditions, most persons with mild mental retardation will become independent and self-sufficient in routine manual occupations.

Facilitated communication, promoted as "unlocking" latent intelligence in the person with mental retardation, has no scientific validity. In experiments, the communicative output is revealed as that of the facilitator rather than that of the person with mental retardation.[42]

Disruptive and maladaptive behaviors that are reactive to the environment rather than manifestations of psychopathology; they are managed by behavior therapy, using positive reinforcement scheduling. Aversive reinforcement is not recommended.

MENTAL RETARDATION AND BEHAVIORAL NEUROSCIENCE

Neuropsychological investigation has paid scant attention to mental retardation, for the same reason that, until recently, it virtually ignored dementia. Global depression of higher mental function seems to offer little promise to its core agenda of discovering double dissociations that reveal how the components of cognitive systems are organized or how that organization develops. But dissociations do occur in mental retardation and are being used to elucidate the genesis and epigenesis of developing cognitive domains.[43]

An overall head circumference (and, by inference, brain size) at birth below the normal range (i.e., microcephaly) is the single most powerful prediction of impaired cognitive development. Excessive brain size (cerebral gigantism) is also associated with mental retardation (e.g., Ref. 44). Systematic differences in brain morphology between mental retardation syndromes are being revealed by magnetic resonance imaging (MRI),[45,46] and the size of a brain part does seem to relate, albeit not straightforwardly, to its efficiency (e.g., Ref. 47). (Overall brain size correlates modestly with IQ even in the normal populations.[48]) Noninvasive measurements of regional cerebral blood flow by functional MRI will evaluate claims for anomalous brain organization in specific mental retardation syndromes, such as Down syndrome[49] and Williams syndrome.[50] Computerized surveys of regional cell populations in autopsied brain further enrich a cross-disciplinary approach to neurobehavioral development.

EARLY IDENTIFICATION OF DEVELOPMENTAL DELAY

Although early identification of delayed development does not usually lead to a specific diagnosis, it has practical benefits for children and their parents. Early intervention services are mandated for all handicapped children and their families (Public Law 99-457). The clinical evaluation of developmentally delayed children has been recently well summarized, with tabulations of biomedical and neurodevelopmental risk factors.[51]

REFERENCES

1. Bouchard TJ, Lykken DT, McGue M, et al: Sources of human psychological differences: The Minnesota study of twins reared apart. *Science* 252:223–228, 1990.
2. Gardner H: *Frames of Mind.* New York: Basic Books, 1983.
3. Tramo MJ, Loftus WC, Thomas CE, et al: Surface area of human cerebral cortex and its gross morphological subdivisions: In vivo measurements in monozygotic twins suggest differential hemisphere effects of genetic factors. *J Cogn Neurosc* 7:293–301, 1995.
4. Grossman HJ (ed): *Classification in Mental Retardation.* Washington, DC: American Association on Mental Deficiency, 1983.
5. Luckasson R, Coulter DL, Pollaway EA, et al: Mental retardation: Definition, classification and systems of support. Washington, DC: American Association of Mental Retardation, 1992.
6. Schalock RL, Stark JA, Snell ME, et al: The changing conception of mental retardation: Implications for the field. *Ment Retard* 32:181–193, 1994.
7. Herbst DS, Baird DA: Nonspecific mental retardation in British Columbia as ascertained through a registry. *Am J Ment Defic* 87:506–517, 1983.
8. Broman SH, Nichols PL, Kennedy WA: *Preschool IQ: Prenatal and Early Developmental Correlates.* Hillsdale, NJ: Erlbaum, 1975.
9. Barnard K: Prevention of parenting alterations for women with low social support. *Psychiatry* 51:248–253, 1988.
10. Gilberg C, Gilberg IC: Note on the relationship between clinical and epidemiological samples: The question of reduced optimality in the pre-, peri-, and neonatal periods. *J Autism Dev Disord* 21:251–253, 1991.
11. McCormich MC, Brooks-Gunn J, Workman-Daniels K, et al: The health and developmental status of very low birthweight children at school age. *JAMA* 267:2204–2208, 1992.
12. Sigman M: Nutrition and child development: More food for thought. *Curr Dir Psychol Sci* 4:52–55, 1995.
13. Lozoff B, Jiminez E, Wolf AW: Long-term effects of iron deficiency anemia in infancy. *N Engl J Med* 325:687–694, 1991.
14. Pollitt E, Gorman K, Engle P, et al: Early supplementary feeding and cognition: Effects over two decades. *Monogr Soc Res Child Dev* 7:1–99, 1993.
15. Pocock SJ, Smith M, Baghurst P: Environmental lead and children's intelligence: A systematic review of the epidemiological evidence. *Br Med J* 309:1189–1197, 1994.
16. Wolf AW, Jiminez E, Lozoff B: No evidence of developmental ill effects of low-level lead exposure in a developing country. *Dev Behav Pediatr* 15:224–231, 1994.
17. Prior M, Dahlstrom B, Squires T: Autistic children's knowledge of thinking and feeling states in other people. *J Child Psychol Psychiatry* 31:587–602, 1990.
18. Udwin O: A survey of adults with Williams syndrome and idiopathic infantile hypercalcemia. *Dev Med Child Neurol* 32:129–136, 1990.
19. Dennis M, Jacennik B, Barnes MA: The content of narrative discourse in children and adolescents after early-onset hydrocephalus and in normally developing age peers. *Brain Lang* 46:129–165, 1994.
20. Dykens EM, Hodapp RM, Evans DW: Profiles and development of adaptive behavior in children with Down syndrome. *Am J Ment Retard* 98:580–587, 1994.
21. Rovet JF: The psychoeducational characteristics of children with Turner syndrome. *J Learn Disabil* 26:333–341, 1993.
22. Pennington B, Puck M, Robinson A: Language and cognitive development in 47 XXX females followed since birth. *Behav Genet* 10:31–41, 1980.
23. Wiesniewski KF, French JH, Fernando S, et al: Fragile-X syndrome: Associated neurological abnormality and developmental disabilities. *Ann Neurol* 18:665–669, 1985.
24. Siegel LS: A longitudinal study of a hyperlexic child: Hyperlexia as a language disorder. *Neuropsychologia* 22:577–585, 1984.

25. Young RL, Nettelbeck E: The "intelligence" of calendrical calculators. *Am J Ment Retard* 99:186–200, 1994.

26. Casey BJ, Gordon CT, Mannheim GB, Rumsey JM: Dysfunctional attention in autistic servants. *J Clin Exp Neuropsychol* 15:933–946, 1993.

27. Pascualvaca DM: Attention capacities in children with pervasive developmental disorders. *Int Pediat* 10:166–170, 1995.

28. Kerby DS, Dawson BL: Autistic features, personality, and adaptive behavior in males with the fragile-X syndrome and no autism. *Am J Ment Retard* 98:455–462, 1994.

29. Hagberg B, Kyllerman M: Epidemiology of mental retardation: A Swedish survey. *Brain Dev* 5:441–449, 1983.

30. McLaren J, Bryson SE: Review of recent epidemiological studies of mental retardation: Prevalence, associated disorders and etiology. *Am J Ment Retard* 92:243–254, 1987.

31. Wellesley D, Hockey A, Stanely F: The aetiology of intellectual disability in Western Australia: A community-based study. *Dev Med Child Neurol* 33:963–973, 1991.

32. Freytag E, Lindenberg R: Neuropathological findings in patients of a hospital for the mentally deficient: A survey of 359 cases. *Johns Hopkins Med J* 121:379–395, 1967.

33. Eyman RK, Borthwick-Duffy SA, Call TL, White JF: Prediction of mortality in institutional and community settings. *J Ment Def Res* 32:203–213, 1988.

34. Rasmussen DE, Sobody D: Age, adaptive behavior, and Alzheimer disease in Down syndrome: Cross-sectional and longitudinal analyses. *Am J Ment Retard* 99:151–165, 1994.

35. Kinsbourne M: Do repetitive movement patterns in children and animals serve a dearousing function? *J Dev Behav Pediatr* 1:39–42, 1980.

36. Parsons JA, May JG, Menolascino FJ: The nature and incidence of mental illness in mentally retarded individuals, in Menolascino FJ, Stark JA (eds): *Handbook of Mental Illness in the Mentally Retarded.* New York: Plenum Press, 1984, pp 3–43.

37. Rutter M, Graham P, Yule W: A neuropsychiatric study in childhood. *Clin Dev Med* 35/36:1–272, 1970.

38. Pies RW, Popli AP: Self-injurious behavior: Pathophysiology and implications for treatment. *J Clin Psychiatry* 56:580–588, 1995.

39. Bouras N: *Mental Health in Mental Retardation.* New York: Cambridge University Press, 1994.

40. Ottenbacher K, Petersen P: The efficacy of early intervention programs for children with organic handicaps. *Eval Progr Plan* 8:135–148, 1985.

41. Helper MM: Follow-up of children with minimal brain dysfunction: Outcomes and predictors, in Rie HE, Rie ED (ed): *Handbook of Minimal Brain Dysfunctions: A Critical Review.* New York: Wiley, 1980.

42. Wheeler DL, Jacobson JW, Paglieri RA, Schwartz AA: An experimental assessment of facilitated communication. *Ment Retard* 31:49–60, 1993.

43. Karmiloff-Smith A: *Beyond Modularity: A Developmental Perspective on Cognitive Science.* Cambridge, MA: MIT Press, 1992.

44. Beemer FA, Veenema H, dePater JM: Cerebral gigantism (Sotos syndrome) in two patients with Fra(x) chromosome. *Am J Med Genet* 23:221–226, 1986.

45. Courchesne E, Yeung-Courchesne R, Press GA, et al: Hypoplasia of cerebellar vermal lobules VI and VII in autism. *N Engl J Med* 318:1349–1354, 1988.

46. Jernigan TL, Bellugi U: Anomalous brain morphology on magnetic resonance imaging in Williams and Down syndromes. *Arch Neurol* 47:529–533, 1990.

47. Yazgan MY, Wechsler BE, Kinsbourne M, et al: Functional significance of individual variations in callosal ara. *Neuropsychologia* 33:769–779, 1995.

48. Andreasson NC, Flauer M, Swayze V, et al: Intelligence and brain structure in normal individuals. *Am J Psychiatry* 150:130–134, 1993.

49. Piccirilli M, D'Alessandro M, Mazzi P, et al: Cerebral organization for language in Down syndrome patients. *Cortex* 27:41–47, 1991.

50. Karmiloff-Smith A, Klima E, Bellugi U, et al: Is there a social module? Language, face processing, and theory of mind in individuals with Williams syndrome. *J Cog Neurosc* 7:196–208, 1995.

51. First LR, Palfrey JS: The infant or young child with developmental delay. *N Engl J Med* 330:478–483, 1994.

Chapter 67

PERVASIVE DEVELOPMENTAL DISORDERS: AUTISM AND SIMILAR DISORDERS

Nancy J. Minshew

The category of pervasive developmental disorder (PDD) was introduced to classification systems in 1980 when it became clear that autism was not a psychotic disorder and could no longer be classified with the childhood psychoses. The term was coined to reflect the full range of IQs in autism, the selective nature of the deficits, and the severity of their impact on adaptive function. The PDD diagnostic category is stipulated for disorders characterized by specific qualitative impairments in social interactions, verbal and nonverbal language and their use for communication, symbolic and imaginative play, and abstract reasoning and related complex behavior. Impairments are selective—i.e., disproportionate to age and IQ expectations—and also have distinctive qualitative characteristics. A variety of other more subtle or nonspecific abnormalities—ranging from delayed motor development and hyperactivity to relative insensitivity to pain, sound sensitivity, and exaggerated fears—are often also present but are considered minor or peripheral features. From the beginning it was clear that there were disorders other than autism in this category, but the capacity for differentiating and defining them was essentially nonexistent. The classification and criteria for these disorders remain in evolution.

The PDD category has been part of three diagnostic classification systems since its introduction. The diagnostic criteria and disorders in this category have varied over time, reflecting existing hypotheses about the importance of particular clinical features in reliably delineating valid syndromes and the results of field trials testing these hypotheses (see Tables 67-1 and 67-2). The first classification of the PDDs in DSM-III[1] reflected the hypothesis that high- and low-functioning autistic individuals had different clinical disorders. When field trials failed to support the validity of this distinction, autism was presented in DSM-III-R[2] as a single disorder of widely varying severity, and the focus of differential diagnosis shifted to the boundaries of autism. Several issues then came under investigation. The first pertained to the differentiation of autism from general mental retardation, Rett syndrome, and fragile-X syndrome, as well as the clinical significance of presentation with regression past the time typical for autism. A second focus of investigation was distinguishing high-functioning autism from Asperger syndrome and the nonverbal learning disability (NLD) syndrome. The third issue was the specificity of diagnostic criteria across the severity spectrum for differentiating autism from "not autism," otherwise known as PDD not otherwise specified. In the majority of cases, this distinction is based on deficits that are less severe than expected for autism at a particular age and IQ rather than the absence of symptoms in one or more areas. Such distinctions require extensive clinical experience with autism across the age and severity spectrum and are unlikely to be amenable to the checklist format of the diagnostic criteria in classification systems. At present, such distinctions are not of primary importance for clinical practice, as interventions are not geared to such subtle distinctions but rather

Table 67-1
Pervasive developmental disorders: 1980–1995

1. DSM-III
Infantile autism
Childhood onset pervasive developmental disorder
Atypical pervasive developmental disorder

2. DSM-III-R
Autistic disorder
Pervasive developmental disorder not otherwise
  specified

3. DSM-IV
Autistic disorder   299.00
Childhood disintegrative disorder   299.10
Asperger's disorder   299.80
Pervasive developmental disorder not other-
  wise specified   299.80
Rett's disorder   299.80

to the quality of the deficits that characterize the PDDs as a group.

The most recent classifications of the PDDs provided in DSM-IV[3] and ICD-10[4] have expanded the number of PDDs, reflecting some but not all of the diagnostic issues under study. These two classifications are quite similar, with ICD-10 providing some additional categories for deviations from autism, which in DSM-IV are subserved under the single heading of PDD not otherwise specified (NOS).

Table 67-2
*DSM-IV and ICD-10 pervasive
developmental disorders*

1. DSM-IV and ICD-10
Autistic disorder   299.00, F84.0
Childhood disintegrative disorder   299.10, F84.3
Asperger's disorder   299.80, F84.6
Pervasive developmental disorder not
  otherwise specified   299.80, F84.9
Rett's disorder   299.80, F84.2

2. ICD-10
Additional diagnosis not included in DSM-IV
Atypical autism   F84.1
Overactive disorder with mental retardation   F84.4
  and stereotyped movements
Other pervasive developmental disorder   F84.8

CLINICAL SYNDROME OF AUTISM

The clinical description of the PDDs is largely that of autism. Current clinical distinctions between the different PDDs are largely defined in terms of deviations from autism. With the exception of Rett syndrome and the nonverbal learning disability syndrome, not enough is known about the other PDDs to make distinctions independent of the definition of autism.

Presentation

Autism has two modes of presentation, the more common being in the form of developmental delays. In the majority of autistic children, the central impairments become apparent as skills fail to appear at the usual time in development and the resulting abnormal behavior is displayed. The language delay often becomes the sole or dominant clinical concern, but developmental delays are also present if assessed in social skills, play skills, range of interests, and fine motor praxis. These delays may be identified, but their significance for diagnosis is often not appreciated. A subset of these autistic children will, in addition, have a modest gross motor delay, with walking achieved by 18 to 22 months. The remaining one-fourth of autistic children present between 12 and 24 months with regression and loss of previously acquired skills in involved areas following a period of largely normal development. Gross motor skills are not lost, which is one important point of departure from Rett syndrome. The manifestations of autism appear the same thereafter, regardless of mode of presentation.

Clinical Features

The signs and symptoms of autism are most severe in early childhood in all autistic children, but the course diverges dramatically thereafter, with a wide range of outcomes. Approximately one-half of autistic children make no developmental progress and their presentation remains unchanged from early childhood. The other one-half make small to substantial developmental gains in the social, language, reasoning, and behavior domains between 3 and 8 years of age; thus the manifestations of autism may be substantially altered with age. Despite the dramatic improvement in abilities and behavior over the early years in these individuals, major difficulties persist throughout life. The natural history of autism and similar disorders is therefore one of substantial improvement by school age in a significant percentage of cases. In these children, the history of deficits and behavior during early childhood provides critical clues to the basis of the difficulties experienced in later life.

Social Impairment

The autistic type of social deficit is characterized by an impairment in the reciprocal quality of interactions. The term *social reciprocity* refers to the dynamic capacity for maintaining appropriate interactions from moment to moment. Social reciprocity is not a single skill but rather the result of a composite of skills, only some of which have been defined. In verbal interactions, the essence of reciprocity is manifest in the capacity for "chit chat," which is conversation that is not structured or guided by another individual, a predetermined topic, or a rote script of questions and responses. Repeated clinical contact may be necessary in some verbal autistic individuals to determine whether their contributions to conversation are dependent on the question-and-answer structure of the evaluation or follow an unvarying preset format of stock questions and answers. In preverbal children, reciprocity is manifest in the dynamic interplay involved in teasing around limits. A typical example is the toddler's attempts to get into a forbidden drawer while a parent is on the phone, all the while watching the parent's reaction and adjusting the provocation to elicit a tease but not an outright limit-setting reaction from the parent. Regardless of language status, both examples of reciprocity require the capacity to accurately judge and predict the other individual's reaction, a clear grasp of the situation and of social cause and effect, and the ability to subtly manipulate both. All of these components underlying reciprocity are seriously impaired in autism.

The social deficit is manifest across a wide range of severity depending on the individual's age and general level of function. In its severest form, the social deficit is manifest by a complete lack of both comprehension of the social behavior of others and the innate capacity for a social response. In moderate forms, the individual has only a rudimentary comprehension of the social behavior of others and has a few simple, stereotyped ways of interacting. In its least severe form, the autistic type of social deficit is manifest by only partial understanding of the social behavior of others and awkward, limited ways of interacting. These individuals are extremely naive, often failing to understand what is automatically obvious to others about social situations. They are prone to being exploited on the one hand and, on the other, to unknowingly committing significant violations of social conventions and infringing on the social rights of other people. Their behavior is often interpreted to be purposefully offensive and rude, when in reality it is the consequence of a skill deficit.

Language Impairment

The autistic type of language deficit is characterized by the involvement of all forms of language, the consequent failure to compensate for verbal language deficits with nonverbal language, a delay in the onset of all language development or loss of these forms of language as a result of a regression, a deviant pattern of language development, abnormalities in the use of all forms of language for social communication, and substantial residual deficits despite developmental progress. Impairments are therefore present in the comprehension and expression of verbal language as well as nonverbal language such as eye contact, facial expression, gestures, and prosody. When language is present, impairments in comprehension are disproportionate to expressive language and thus are easily underestimated.

As with the social deficit, there is a wide range of language outcomes in autism. Approximately 50 percent of autistic children develop no comprehension or expression of language in any of these modalities. Thus, the most severely impaired autistic individual does not develop the capacity to use or understand words, tone of voice, eye contact, facial expression, gesture, or pantomime. Because nonverbal language and prosody are also impaired, nonverbal autistic children, unlike nonautistic language-delayed children, do not use alternate forms of communication to compensate for their verbal language deficit. Of the remaining 50 percent of autistic children, about 25 percent develop only rudimentary and abnormal verbal and nonverbal language, reflecting an arrest of developmental progress in one of the disordered phases of development that characterize autism. The remaining 25 percent develop sentence language, eye contact, and limited nonverbal language between 4 and 8 years of age after following the typical disordered pattern of language development. However, even the best language outcome is associated with substantial residual deficits in the comprehension and expression of higher-order language abilities, such as pragmatics and semantics, satire and innuendo in voice tones, gaze and facial expression for social communication, and longer or more complex units of language.

The abnormal pattern of verbal language development in autism follows a distinctive sequence that includes simple immediate echolalia, complex delayed echolalia, the functional use of echolalia to communicate needs resulting in pronoun reversals, original or nonechoed language with grammatical errors or grammatically correct language that is stereotyped, grammatically correct simple sentences, and complex sentences.

Eye contact follows a similar sequence, with initially no eye contact followed by glancing contact at a distance, watching of others at a distance, glancing eye contact in social situations, prolonged eye contact in social situations, and eye contact that is normal in quantity in social situations. Residual deficits are subtle but functionally substantial and involve the comprehension and use of gaze for social communication. Abnormalities of facial expression consist of the presence of a constant neutral expression during social communication

or frequent unvarying smiling. Similarly, the individual will have difficulty comprehending the meaning of even basic facial expressions but may eventually comprehend obviously displayed emotions in familiar individuals. Other aspects of nonverbal language—such as raising of the arms to signal the desire to be picked up, pointing, and nodding of the head for yes and no—likewise fail to develop or develop far past the usual time.

In addition to these abnormalities in the form of language, the use of language that is present for communication and the content are typically abnormal. Again, there is a wide range of expression of these deficits, but common examples are the failure of the individual to speak other than for needs and the endless perseveration on a single topic of conversation.

Impairment in Symbolic and Pretend Play

Interest in toys and the capacity for playing with them in normal ways are delayed in developing well past the usual time and fail to develop completely in severe autism. These abnormalities appear to be related to the delayed and only partial development of comprehension of the symbolic meaning of toys. Initially, such children are not interested in toys. When and if toy play develops, play is abnormal and involves simple uses that do not reflect the overall symbolic meaning of the toy. Thus, toys are put in lines or taken apart, moving parts are set in motion and observed intently, or they are assembled into precisely arranged collections without being used for play. With further developmental progress, isolated appropriate actions emerge and then sequences of actions. Despite progress, play remains repetitive and never acquires the imaginative quality seen in normal children. The capacity of some high-functioning autistic children for verbatim memorization of television and videotape shows can be considerable, and such imitations should be distinguished from true original, imaginative play.

Pretend play involving others is also similarly impaired, with initially no interest in play with others and failure to imitate common infant games like patty cake or household chores, followed by the emergence of simple forms of play such as tickling and chase or ball rolling and eventually parallel play. Ultimately, the less severely autistic children will play hide and seek and board games with others, but team sports and complex imaginative or cooperative play usually remain beyond their abilities. High-functioning autistic children soon become obsessed with games that capitalize on visuospatial and rote memory skills rather than imagination.

Restricted Range of Interests and Activities

The final symptom category is defined in behavioral terms and refers to several types of abnormal behavior associated with autism. The deficit underlying these peculiar behaviors has not been documented, but they likely reflect the peculiar two-part cognitive deficit in autism consisting of a heightened awareness of detail coupled with impaired abstract reasoning abilities.

Abnormal behavior in this category is of several types: interest in the elementary sensory aspects or the parts of an object, difficulty coping with change, and a narrow range of interests with a focus on details. These odd behaviors appear to reflect the autistic individual's unusual awareness of the more elementary details about objects or topics combined with the failure to organize the world along conceptual lines. Interest in the elementary sensory aspects of objects and object parts and difficulty coping with everyday changes are typical of the younger or more impaired autistic individual, whereas difficulty limited to unusual changes and obsessions and a narrow range of interests are typical of higher-functioning autistic individuals.

Associated Signs and Symptoms

Some signs and symptoms are common in autism but are not considered central features of the disorder. These include hyperactivity, delayed motor development, apraxia, relative insensitivity to pain, sensory sensitivities, and abnormalities in the intensity and focus of attention.

In addition, autism is associated with mental retardation in 70 percent of cases. The cooccurrence of autism and mental retardation cannot, however, be explained by chance. Rather, mental retardation appears to be the more severe expression of the peculiar cognitive deficit in autism. As IQ declines in autism, abstract reasoning falls disproportionately, whereas immediate recall and visuospatial ability are unusually preserved. The predictable outcome with increasing severity of such a profile is mental retardation with an unusual preservation of memory for details and visuospatial ability and unusually poor adaptive behavior relative to IQ.

Neurologic Examination

The neurologic examination in autism is remarkable for the absence of findings other than those described above and for above-average head circumference.[5] Dysmorphic features are absent, as are obvious long-tract signs. Tone is generally but subtly decreased. Reflexes are either generally increased (3+) or absent in the upper extremities and at the knees but brisk at the ankles. Babinski signs are absent.

Pervasive Developmental Disorders Other Than Autism

Two disorders—Asperger syndrome[6] and the syndrome of the developmental learning disabilities of the right hemisphere (DLDRH),[7] also known as the nonverbal learning disability syndrome[8]—are restricted to verbal individuals with IQs above 70. In the past, the term *Asperger syndrome* was commonly used as a synonym for high-functioning autism. In DSM-IV, Asperger syndrome is distinguished from autism by the absence of early developmental language abnormalities. The validity of this criterion in identifying a clinical syndrome distinguishable from autism will be assessed in field trials. The developmental right hemisphere syndrome is not part of the formal classification systems but is readily identified by a constellation of impairments in social abilities, prosody, facial expression and eye contact, facial recognition, arithmetic, visuospatial ability, and attention to left space. The social impairment in these individuals has not been characterized but appears to be less severe than in autism, as evidenced by the ability of such persons to function in the mainstream of society without support. The abnormalities in nonverbal language are not distinguishable from autism, but the localized signs of right parietal dysfunction constitute a clear departure from autism and provide a ready basis for distinguishing the two disorders clinically.

In mentally retarded individuals, additional considerations in the PDD category are Rett syndrome, fragile-X syndrome, and probably also tuberous sclerosis. Of these, only Rett syndrome is presently included in classification systems. Rett syndrome presents with a regression in the first to second years of life, which is the basis for confusion with autism. Beyond this overlap, these are two entirely different disorders. Rett syndrome is limited to females and is distinguished from autism by the presence of decelerating head growth and eventual microcephaly, loss of voluntary hand movements, loss of walking ability if acquired, periodic breathing, and difficulty swallowing. Death typically occurs in the second to third decade of life. Rett syndrome is very rare, even compared to autism, and although it is a differential diagnostic consideration in females presenting with regression, it is much less likely than autism and has a fatal outcome. Fragile-X syndrome, named for its association with the fragile-X chromosomal abnormality, occurs in males, often several in the same family, and is distinguished by testicular enlargement after puberty. Other physical features such as a long, narrow facies, prominent ears, hyperextensible joints, and flat feet are variable and may not be present in affected individuals. If present, they are helpful in identifying prepubescent mentally retarded individuals at high risk for fragile-X syndrome. Fragile-X syndrome may be confused with autism because of the presence of deficits in social and language abilities and stereotypic motor movements. The social and language deficits in fragile-X individuals have different characteristics than in autism but have not been suffi-

ciently described to be of general use in differential diagnosis. In autism research centers, the incidence of fragile-X syndrome in individuals diagnosed as autistic is less than 1 percent. Tuberous sclerosis is accompanied by a high incidence of autistic behavior, but a specific syndrome or PDD has not yet been defined. Such cases are considered cases of autism with a known etiology but clinical differences from the typical case of autism have not been examined. As in Rett and fragile-X syndromes, such differences may become obvious on investigation.

The remaining nonautism PDDs consist of childhood disintegrative disorder, pervasive developmental disorder not otherwise specified, and mental retardation associated with hyperactivity and stereotypic movements. Childhood disintegrative disorder is defined by presentation with regression between 2 and 12 years of age.[9] A significant percentage of children in this category are eventually found to have a degenerative neurologic disorder. Pervasive developmental disorder not otherwise specified is a catch-all for cases that fail to meet the criteria for autism or for one of the other specifically defined PDDs. In most cases, this diagnosis is the result of less severe deficits in one or more areas than expected in autism at that age and general ability level. Such distinctions require a level of experience usually confined to research centers; they are not amenable to the current checklist format of diagnostic criteria. Such distinctions do not have clinical implications in terms of intervention and thus the autism/PDD designation for this entitlement category is a practical one. In ICD-10 but not DSM-IV, an additional category for mental retardation with hyperactivity and stereotypic motor activity is included to represent the constellation known as Wing's triad.[10] In contrast with the mental retardation in Down syndrome, mental retardation is often associated with declining sociability, diminishing language ability, and stereotypies. This additional category was provided to acknowledge Wing's triad and to accommodate these individuals separately from autism and general mental retardation.

Medical Disorders Associated with a Pervasive Developmental Disorder

About 5 percent of cases of autism are associated with an identifiable neurologic, genetic, or infectious disorder, with tuberous sclerosis being the most common. Other causes include fragile-X syndrome, fetal infection with either rubella or cytomegalovirus, and untreated phenylketonuria. A wide variety of metabolic disorders have been identified on a single-case basis. Depending on how broad a definition is used for PDD, a wide variety of etiologies has been associated with a clinical syndrome similar to autism.[11] Again, clinical discrepancies between cases with and without such etiologies have not been examined.

Complications

Seizure disorder and affective disorder are relatively common complications in autism and similar disorders and should be suspected as causes of any sustained deterioration in function and behavior not explained by change or adverse environmental conditions. The cumulative prevalence of generalized seizures by young adulthood was determined to be 25 and 33 percent in two longitudinal studies, which is equivalent to the results of cross-sectional studies. Onset of seizures may occur at any age, but early childhood and adolescence are common. The occurrence of partial complex seizures in autistic individuals and others with similar disorders has also been documented and found to be difficult to recognize clinically except by a significant and unexplained deterioration in function.

Less is known about the occurrence of affective disorder. At present, depressive episodes are thought to be a complication of the second or later decades of life in higher-functioning autistic individuals, but the apparent predilection for older higher-functioning autistic individuals may be only a detection artifact. Manic episodes have also been documented.

Neuropsychology

The neuropsychology of autism was largely limited to conclusions drawn from studies of Weschler IQ profiles until the general acceptance of diagnostic criteria for autism in high-functioning individuals made neuropsychological testing feasible. The IQ-based studies emphasized disparities between verbal and performance IQ scores (VIQ < PIQ), relative weakness on the comprehension subtest, and relative strength on block design. However, studies of autistic individuals who were not mentally retarded have demonstrated that these Wechsler profile characteristics are not universal in autism and should not be used in diagnosis or differential diagnosis.[12,13] Neuropsychological studies in autism have demonstrated predominant deficits in abstract reasoning and problem-solving abilities, higher-order language abilities, and complex memory abilities.[14-16] More subtle deficits have also been documented in complex motor abilities or praxis and higher cortical sensory abilities. Together these findings have provided evidence of a generalized deficit in the processing of complex information that transcends domains and sensory modalities, with deficits present on tasks with a high information-processing load relative to age and IQ and preserved function on simpler tasks in these same functional domains. Academic achievement in high-functioning autistic individuals was similarly characterized by deficits on higher-order language comprehension tasks involving analytic and interpretive abilities, with preserved performance on basic procedural or mechanical tasks such as reading decoding, spelling, and vocabulary.[17,18] The learning disability associated with autism and similar disorders is essentially the converse of the pattern associated with the traditional learning disabilities such as dyslexia and dyscalculia.

Neurophysiology

The neurophysiology of autism is largely a research issue, aside from the clinical usefulness of brainstem auditory evoked potentials in assessing hearing. One recent summary of this literature has emphasized the occurrence of hearing loss in this population and has advocated vigorous evaluation of hearing status.[19] Neurophysiologic functioning in autism has been demonstrated to be characterized by abnormalities in cognitive potentials with preservation of early and middle latency potentials. From a pathophysiologic perspective, this profile implicates complex cognitive processes and higher brain regions. A recent study of eye movement physiology in autism[20] has revealed a similar profile with prominent abnormalities in cortically controlled eye movements subserved by frontal and parietal circuitry and intact basic and reflex eye movements subserved by subcortical and posterior fossa structures.

Neuropathology

The description of the neuropathology of autism[21] has been limited to the examination of a small number of cases and to clinical pathology methods. Quantitative measurements of cell number and structure volume are notably lacking. The neuropathologic abnormalities described in autism are subtle overall and consist of a 100- to 200-g increase in brain weight in most cases and histologic abnormalities in the limbic system and cerebellum. In the small, compact gray matter structures of the limbic system, the neurons were immature in appearance and exhibited a truncation in dendritic tree development. In addition, there was an increase in cell-packing density, which appeared to be the consequence of a decrease in the neuropil. In the cerebellum, there was a decrease in Purkinje and granule cells throughout the hemispheres but greatest in neocerebellar regions. These findings have been of major importance in providing definitive evidence of the neurologic basis of autism and have characterized it as a disorder of neuronal organization.

Neuroradiology

The most common neuroradiologic finding in autism is of normal neuroanatomy when cases associated with disorders such as tuberous sclerosis, fetal rubella, or fetal cytomegalovirus are excluded from consideration. Mild to moderate enlargement of the lateral ventricles occurs in a minority of autistic individuals but is not related to autism severity or hydrocephalus.

Reports of other imaging findings in autism have been based on research protocols and quantitative measurements rather than clinically apparent imaging abnormalities. These studies are in the preliminary phase and the majority have had significant methodologic limitations. Initial reports of selective hypo- or hyperplasia of the neocerebellar vermis[22,23] have not been replicated by studies that controlled for age, gender, and IQ of subjects.[24–26] An increase in the midsagittal area of supratentorial brain and in supratentorial brain volume has been reported in two separate studies.[26,27] The increase in white matter volume observed radiologically may provide the first explanation for the increase in brain weight that has been observed neuropathologically.

Pathophysiology

The pathophysiology of the clinical syndrome of autism is controversial, with multiple different hypotheses as to the central neuropsychologic deficit and central nervous system localization. Regardless of differences, most current theories propose a primary deficit in higher-order cognitive abilities and localization at the neural systems level or at multiple levels of the neuraxis. The predominant theories propose a core deficit in executive functions,[28] control of attention,[23] or complex information processing.[29] Localizations proposed for these deficits include frontal systems, frontal cortex–parietal cortex–neocerebellar vermis, and generalized involvement of neocortical systems, repectively.

Treatment

The treatment of autism and similar disorders involves primarily an environmental and behavioral approach, as there are no medications with demonstrated efficacy against the primary deficits in autism. However, the value of medications directed against secondary or associated signs and symptoms such as anxiety, attention deficit disorder, depression or mania, and seizure disorder should not be underestimated. Academic intervention should employ a model that is the converse of the traditional learning disability approach, with a particular emphasis on interpretative and problem-solving deficits. Social skills training at a basic level usually reserved for mentally retarded individuals and protection from scapegoating by peers is equally essential. The same principles apply to the job setting. Jobs should be selected that make little demand on social abilities, interpretation of oral or written information, and problem solving; more suitable jobs involve a solitary work setting and repetitive tasks that do not require problem solving. Again, monitoring and protection from scapegoating by peers is essential. In both the school and job setting, an explanation to peers of the autistic individual's deficits and examples of appropriate responses from peers improves the chances of success.

In terms of behavior modification, which is the mainstay of treatment, several guidelines are essential to the successful application of such techniques to individuals with pervasive developmental disorders. The underlying principle is the recognition that autism and the pervasive developmental disorders directly involve the very skills that are the basis of adaptive function in society and thus the capacity for adapting to real life. Thus, these individuals should not be expected to adapt to the environment but rather the environment should be adapted to them. Second, staff should be highly familiar with the deficits in autism and their behavioral manifestations, so that these individuals are not expected to do things that involve their deficits and that odd behavior which is not hindering the individual's function is accepted as hard-wired rather than targeted for change because it looks odd to others. Difficulty in coping with the presence of others and with change and ritualistic obsessive compulsive behavior are the sources of most undesirable behavior. Thus, if a behavior problem develops, the social demands and amount of change occurring in the environment at the time need to be assessed to determine if they exceed the individual's usual tolerance limits. Rituals that do not interfere with function should generally be respected as a means of coping with change.

REFERENCES

1. American Psychiatric Association: *Diagnostic and Statistical Manual of Mental Disorders,* 3d ed. Washington, DC: American Psychiatric Association Press, 1980.
2. American Psychiatric Association: *Diagnostic and Statistical Manual of Mental Disorders,* 3d ed rev. Washington, DC: American Psychiatric Association Press, 1987.
3. American Psychiatric Association: *Diagnostic and Statistical Manual of Mental Disorders,* 4th ed. Washington, DC: American Psychiatric Association Press, 1994.
4. World Health Organization: *International Classification of Diseases: 10. Classification of Mental and Behavioural Disorders: Clinical Descriptions and Diagnostic Guidelines.* Geneva: WHO 1992.
5. Bailey A, Luthert P, Bolton P, et al: Autism and megalencephaly. *Lancet* 341:1225–1226, 1993.
6. Wing L: Asperger's syndrome: A clinical account. *Psychol Med* 11:115–129, 1981.
7. Weintraub S, Mesulam MM: Developmental learning disabilities of the right hemisphere: Emotional, interpersonal, and cognitive components. *Arch Neurol* 40:463–468, 1983.
8. Rourke BP: *Nonverbal Learning Disabilities: The Syndrome and the Model.* New York, Guilford Press, 1989.
9. Volkmar FR: Childhood disintegrative disorder. *Child Adolesc Psychiatr Clin North Am* 3:119–129, 1994.
10. Wing L, Gould J: Severe impairments of social interaction and associated abnormalities in children: Epidemiology and classification. *J Autism Dev Disord* 9:11–29, 1979.
11. Gillberg C, Coleman M: *The Biology of the Autistic Syndromes,* 2d ed. London: MacKeith, 1992.
12. Minshew NJ, Goldstein G, Siegel DJ: Speech and language in high functioning autistic individuals. *Neuropsychology* 9:255–261, 1995.
13. Siegel DJ, Minshew NJ, Goldstein G: Wechsler IQ profiles in diagnosis of high-functioning autism. *J Autism Dev Disord,* 1996. In press.
14. Minshew NJ, Goldstein G, Muenz LR, Payton JB: Neuropsychological functioning in non-mentally retarded autistic individuals. *J Clin Exp Neuropsychol* 14:740–761, 1992.
15. Minshew NJ, Goldstein G, Siegel DJ, Nicholson M: Selective pattern of cognitive functioning in autism:

A function of information processing load (abstr). *Biol Psychiatry* 35:632, 1994.

16. Rumsey JM, Hamburger SD: Neuropsychological findings in high-functioning men with infantile autism, residual state. *J Clin Exp Neuropsychol* 10:201–221, 1988.

17. Goldstein G, Minshew NJ, Siegel DJ: Age differences in academic achievement in high-functioning autistic individuals. *J Clin Exp Neuropsychol* 5:671–680, 1994.

18. Minshew NJ, Goldstein G, Taylor HG, Siegel DJ: Academic achievement in high functioning autistic individuals. *J Clin Exp Neuropsychol* 2:261–270, 1994.

19. Klin A: Auditory brainstem responses in autism: brainstem dysfunction or peripheral hearing loss. *J Autism Dev Dis* 23:15–35, 1993.

20. Minshew NJ, Sweeney JA, and Furman JM: Evidence for a primary neocortical systems abnormality in autism. *Soc Neurosci Abstr* 21:735, 1995.

21. Bauman ML, and Kemper TL: Neuroanatomic observations of the brain in autism, in Bauman ML, Kemper TL (eds): *The Neurobiology of Autism.* Baltimore: Johns Hopkins University Press, 1994, pp 86–101.

22. Courchesne E, Yeung-Courchesne R, Press GA, et al: Hypoplasia of cerebellar vermal lobules VI and VII in autism. *N Engl J Med* 318:1349–1354, 1988.

23. Courchesne E, Townsend JP, Akshoomoff NA, et al: A new finding: Impairment in shifting attention in autistic and cerebellar patients, in Broman SH, Grafman J (eds): *Atypical Deficits in Developmental Disorders: Implications for Brain Function.* Hillsdale, NJ: Erlbaum, 1994, pp 101–317.

24. Kleiman MD, Neff S, Rosman NP: The brain in infantile autism: Is the cerebellum really abnormal? *Neurology* 2:753–760, 1992.

25. Holttum JR, Minshew NJ, Sanders RS, Phillips NE: Magnetic resonance imaging of the posterior fossa in autism. *Biol Psychiatry* 32:1091–1101, 1992.

26. Piven J, Nehme E, Simon J, et al: Magnetic resonance imaging in autism: Measurement of the cerebellum, pons and fourth ventricle. *Biol Psychiatry* 31:491–504, 1992.

27. Piven J, Arnt S, Bailey J, et al: An MRI study of brain size in autism. *Am J Psychiatry,* 152:1145–1149, 1995.

28. Ozonoff S, Strayer DL, McMahon WM, et al: Executive function abilities in autism: An information processing approach. *J Child Psychol Psychiatry* 35:659–685, 1994.

29. Minshew NJ, Goldstein G, Siegel DJ: Profile of neuropsychologic functioning in autism: A generalized disorder of complex information processing. *J Int Neuropsychol Soc.* Submitted.

GLOSSARY OF LINGUISTIC TERMS*

Affix A MORPHEME that must be attached to another morpheme. Also known as a bound morpheme. Prefixes attach to the beginning of a morpheme (e.g., *re-* in *redefine*), and suffixes attach to the end of a morpheme (e.g., *-er* in *worker*).

Case A set of affixes or word forms that are used to distinguish the roles of nouns. For example, in English, *I, me,* and *my* have different cases.

Categorical perception The phenomenon whereby a continuous change in a physical characteristic of a speech signal is perceived discontinuously. For example, "ba" and "pa" differ in voice onset time (VOT). If one starts with a "ba" and gradually increases VOT, English speakers find it difficult to detect any change until a categorical boundary is reached. When the categorical boundary is crossed, subjects' perception of the sound suddenly switches from voiced (ba) to unvoiced (pa).

Closed class word See FUNCTION WORD.

Content word A word that has lexical meaning (SEMANTIC content). Examples include nouns, verbs, adjectives, and adverbs. Because new lexical words such as *modem* or *fax* can freely be invented (i.e., the number of possible lexical words is infinite), lexical words are sometimes referred to as OPEN CLASS WORDS.

Discourse The organization of continuous stretches of language larger than a sentence in a conversation or text.

Function word or functor A word or bound morpheme whose role is strictly or mostly to signal grammatical relationships. Examples include INFECTIONS, conjunctions, articles, auxiliary verbs, and pronouns. A given language has a limited and finite number of functors and, hence, function words are sometimes referred to as CLOSED CLASS WORDS or closed class morphemes.

Inflection Refers to affixes that signal grammatical relationships such as plural, past tense, progressive tense, and possession (in English, *-s*, *-ed*, *-ing*, and *'s*, respectively).

Lexical access The process of looking words up in one's lexicon (mental dictionary).

Lexical decision In psycholinguistic experiments, subjects are sometimes asked to decide whether a string of letters (or sounds) is a word in their language. For example, subjects might be presented English words such as "table" and non-words such as "bivel." Because the only way to determine that "table" is a word and "bivel" is not a word is to determine whether they are in one's lexicon, lexical decision tasks are used to study LEXICAL ACCESS.

Morpheme The minimal distinctive unit of meaning that can be combined to form words. Morphemes can be bound (see AFFIX) or free (able to appear by themselves).

Morphology The branch of linguistics that investigates the form or structure of words and

*Prepared by Karin Stromswold.

the processes and rules that govern the ways in which MORPHEMES are combined.

Open class word   See CONTENT WORD.

Orthography   The writing system of a language.

Phoneme   The minimal unit of the sound system of a language that can be used to signal a potential difference in meaning. For example, /b/ and /p/ are phonemes in English because there are minimal pairs of words such as /bat/ and /pat/ and /cab/ and /cap/ that differ only in whether a /b/ or a /p/ is present.

Phonemic awareness   The awareness that words and morphemes are composed of PHONEMES. Specifically, phonemic awareness refers to the ability to break words into their component phonemes (e.g., /bat/ → /b/ + /a/ + /t/), report the number of syllables in a word, report whether a particular phoneme appears in a word, etc.

Phonology   The branch of linguistics that studies the sound systems of languages, including the sounds that are used in a language and the way these sounds may be combined.

Pragmatics   The branch of linguistics that investigates phenomena associated with the use of the language by individuals. Of particular interest is the constraints that people encounter when they use language in social settings and the effect their language has on the people with whom they are talking.

Prosody   The overall sound pattern or contour of a word or sentence, including pitch, loudness, tempo, and rhythm.

Semantics   The branch of linguistics that studies meaning in language.

Syntax   The branch of linguistics that studies the grammar of language, particularly the rules that govern the way words combine to form sentences.

Thematic role   A term used for semantic roles such as agent, patient, location, source, or goal. For example, in the sentence *John eats spaghetti, John* is the agent and *spaghetti* is the patient. In Government Binding Theory, every argument is given a particular thematic role by its predicate. Thematic roles are drawn from a universal set of thematic relations.

INDEX

Page numbers followed by *f* or *t* refer to illustrations or tables, respectively.

ISBN 0-07-020361-X

9 780070 203617

90000>